Ansel's Pharmaceutical Dosage Forms and Drug Delivery Systems

EIGHTH EDITION

Ansel's Pharmaceutical Dosage Forms and Drug Delivery Systems

EIGHTH EDITION

Loyd V. Allen, Jr., PhD
Professor and Chair Emeritus
Department of Medicinal Chemistry and Pharmaceutics
College of Pharmacy
University of Oklahoma
Editor-in-Chief
International Journal of Pharmaceutical Compounding

Nicholas G. Popovich, PhD
Professor and Head
Department of Pharmacy Administration
College of Pharmacy
University of Illinois at Chicago

Howard C. Ansel, PhD
Professor and Dean Emeritus
College of Pharmacy
The University of Georgia

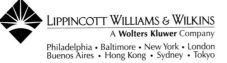

LIPPINCOTT WILLIAMS & WILKINS
A **Wolters Kluwer** Company
Philadelphia • Baltimore • New York • London
Buenos Aires • Hong Kong • Sydney • Tokyo

Senior Acquisitions Editor: David B. Troy
Senior Managing Editor: Matthew J. Hauber
Marketing Manager: Christen DeMarco
Production Editor: Jennifer Ajello
Designer: Doug Smock
Compositor: Peirce Graphic Services, LLC.
Printer: Courier—Kendallville

351 West Camden Street
Baltimore, MD 21201

530 Walnut Street
Philadelphia, PA 19106

Printed in the United States of America

Library of Congress Cataloging-in-Publication Data

Allen, Loyd V.
   Ansel's pharmaceutical dosage forms and drug delivery systems / Loyd V. Allen Jr., Nicholas G. Popovich, Howard C. Ansel.—8th ed.
      p. ; cm.
   Rev. Ed. of: Pharmaceutical dosage forms and drug delivery systems / Howard C. Ansel, Loyd V. Allen, Jr., Nicholas G. Popovich. 7th ed. c1999.
   Includes bibliographical references and index.
   ISBN 13: 978-0-7817-4612-0
   ISBN 10: 0-7817-4612-4
   1. Drugs—Dosage forms. 2. Drug delivery systems. I. Title: Pharmaceutical dosage forms and drug delivery systems. II. Popovich, Nicholas G. III. Ansel, Howard C., 1933– IV. Ansel, Howard C., 1933– Pharmaceutical dosage forms and drug delivery systems. V. Title.
   [DNLM: 1. Dosage Forms. 2. Drug Delivery Systems. QV 785 A427a2004]
   RS200.A57 2004
   615'.1—dc22   2004048276

To purchase additional copies of this book, call our customer service department at **(800) 638-3030** or fax orders to **(301) 824-7390**. International customers should call **(301) 714-2324**.

Visit Lippincott Williams & Wilkins on the Internet: http://www.LWW.com. Lippincott Williams & Wilkins customer service representatives are available from 8:30 am to 6:00 pm, EST.

08 09
7 8 9 10

Preface

The purpose of this text is to introduce pharmacy students to the principles and technologies applied in the preparation of pharmaceutical dosage forms and drug delivery systems. An integrated presentation is used to demonstrate the interrelationships between pharmaceutical and biopharmaceutical principles, product design, formulation, manufacture, and the clinical application of the various dosage forms in patient care. Regulations governing the manufacturing and compounding of pharmaceuticals are also presented.

As has been the hallmark of this textbook since its first edition more than 30 years ago, each chapter is written at a level consistent with the requirements of students being introduced to this area of study. Because this textbook often is used early in the professional curriculum, it contains important introductory topics, such as the historical development of drugs and pharmacy, the role of the pharmacist in contemporary practice, standards of the *United States Pharmacopeia–National Formulary,* systems and techniques of pharmaceutical measurement, pharmaceutical and biopharmaceutical principles applicable to drug product development, current good manufacturing practice and current good compounding practice standards, and the regulatory process by which pharmaceuticals are approved for marketing by the federal Food and Drug Administration.

The Eighth Edition

The eighth edition presents a significant rewrite of some of the sections of the previous edition. We have reorganized the book into eight divisions, containing 20 chapters, based upon traditional pharmaceutic pedagogy. This allows the systematic presentation of dosage forms according to their physical form and characteristics. The Physical Pharmacy Capsules introduced in the sixth edition continue to emphasize important underlying pharmaceutical principles. Also continued in this edition is the Chapter at a Glance at the beginning of each chapter.

Other important changes:

- Enhanced considerations of dosage form design and formulation
- Two case studies (one pharmaceutical and one clinical) in each of the dosage form chapters (see "Introduction to the SOAP Format for Case Studies," next)
- An update of the current good compounding practices
- Expanded clinical considerations in the use of the dosage forms
- Two new glossaries in the appendix, one listing dosage forms and one listing pharmaceutical terms, back as a result of numerous requests of students and faculty.

Introduction to the SOAP Format for Case Studies[a]

The most commonly used documentation format for case studies is referred to by the mnemonic SOAP, which stands for *Subjective* information, *Objective* information, *Assessment*, and *Plan.*

---

[a]Adapted with permission from O'Sullivan TA, Wittkowsky AK. Clinical drug monitoring. In Boh LE, ed. Pharmacy Practice Manual: A Guide to the Clinical Experience, 2nd ed. Baltimore: Lippincott Williams & Wilkins, 2001;594.

The content of a SOAP note written by a pharmacist will be slightly different from that written by another type of health care provider, primarily in the assessment section; a pharmacist's SOAP note will primarily identify problems of diagnosis.

Before a SOAP note is begun, the following must be clearly defined:

- What are the patient's most important problems that must be addressed and/or resolved *now*?
- What is the evidence that each problem exists?
- What are the therapeutic goals and options for each problem?

The answers to each of these questions will form the content of the assessment section of the SOAP note. Therefore, the assessment is written mentally before the actual SOAP note is begun. After the problems are defined, subjective and objective information needed to justify why those problems exist should be written down.

The first paragraph begins with "**S:**" and contains subjective information, which is obtained from the patient interview. Examples of subjective information include patient-provided information about disease symptoms, over-the-counter medications, drug allergy descriptions, and compliance.

The second paragraph begins with "**O:**" and contains objective information obtained by physically examining the patient, reading laboratory data, checking prescription records for doses and refill patterns, locating medication costs from a printed or on-line formulary, and so on. Some information can be either subjective or objective, depending on how it is obtained. The most important thing to remember when composing the subjective and objective portions of notes is that *only information pertaining directly to the assessment should be included.*

The third paragraph begins with "**A:**" and contains the pharmacist's assessment of the patient's medical and pharmacologic problem or problems. If the subjective and objective paragraphs are written well, the problem should be obvious to the reader. Other types of information included in the assessment paragraph are the therapeutic goals and a brief discussion of the therapeutic alternatives.

The fourth paragraph begins with either "**P:**" or "**R:**" and details either a plan (P), or recommendation (R), whichever is more appropriate for the situation. The plan should include individualized instructions (drug by generic name, dose, route, frequency, and when applicable, duration of therapy). The exact dose and frequency should be identified.

Also, the monitoring plan must be detailed, including specifically what (e.g., laboratory test, symptom) should be measured, who should measure it (patient, caregiver, pharmacist), when and how frequently the measuring should occur, and at what point changing therapy will be considered. A backup plan for use in the event of therapeutic failure should also be noted here. Finally, instructions for the proper use of prescribed medication or medications should be included to enhance the therapeutic outcome.

Acknowledgments

I acknowledge with grateful appreciation the major contributions and foresight of Howard C. Ansel, the originator of the textbook, whose guidance and hard work over the years have significantly contributed to the education of tens of thousands of pharmacists worldwide. Deep appreciation to Nicholas G. Popovich for his extensive contribution to this textbook in clinical pharmacy and pharmacy practice and his unique ability to present the integrated approach used in this work. Together, we extend our gratitude to students and academic colleagues who have shared their thoughts with us on this revision; we hope that we have been successful in responding to their thoughtful suggestions. We also acknowledge with appreciation our colleagues in industry who have generously provided scientific and technical information and updated figures and photos for our use.

We gratefully acknowledge the following individuals who contributed to the development of this book through their critiques, review, and suggestions of the individual chapters. Chapter 15 (Parenterals): Jane A. Gottlieb, RPh; David Donley RPh, Manager of the Pharmacy Department at Clarian Health, Indianapolis, Indiana; and Mary Baker, PharmD, MBA, Senior Medical Manager, Global Medical Affairs, Hospira, Inc. Chapter 16 (Biologics): Mary Ann Kliethermes, PharmD, Pharmacotherapist, Clinical Assistant Professor of the Ambulatory Care Pharmacy and Manager of the Refill-10 Program of the Pharmaceutical Care Center; and Leslie Ann Briars, PharmD, Clinical Assistant Professor and Pediatric Clinical Pharmacist of Ambulatory Care Pharmacy Services at the University of Illinois at Chicago, College of Pharmacy. Chapter 18 (Radiopharmaceuticals): Dan Murphy, RPh, Regional Pharmacy Compliance Specialist, West Hartford, Connecticut; Peter Sposato, RPh, Pharmacy Manager at Syncor International Corporation, Glastonbury, Connecticut; and Louis Juliano, RPh, Senior Director of Operations, Northeast at the Cardinal Health Nuclear Pharmacy Services, Kings Park, New York. In addition, we thank the following former doctoral students at the University of Illinois at Chicago College of Pharmacy and Purdue University School of Pharmacy and Pharmacal Sciences for their critiques, review, and suggestions of the individual chapters. They are Raoof R. Abdellatif, PharmD; Nancy J. Costlow, PharmD; Paul S. Djuricich, PharmD; Huzefa H. Master, PharmD; Mary E. Kiersma, PharmD; and Jennifer Thomas, PharmD.

New to this edition are the dosage form chapter case studies. A number of former doctoral students at the University of Illinois at Chicago College of Pharmacy and the Purdue University School of Pharmacy and Pharmacal Sciences prepared the clinical case studies, and we sincerely appreciate their contribution to the text. Those participating and the chapters in which their cases appear are as follows: Chapters 6 and 9, Yamini Shah, PharmD; Chapters 7 and 8, Sumi Patel, PharmD; Chapters 10 and 11, Rebecca L. Roche, PharmD; Chapter 12, Malisa H. Patel, PharmD; Chapter 13, Kristin M. Hurt, PharmD; Chapters 14 and 17, Kristin M. Hurt PharmD and Malisa H. Patel, PharmD; Chapter 15, Natalie Y. Vazzana, PharmD, and Elizabeth Chu, PharmD; and Chapters 16 and 19, James Song, PharmD. Nicki L. Hilliard, PharmD, MSHA, BCNP, FAPhA, Associate Professor of Nuclear Pharmacy at the University of Arkansas College of Pharmacy, created the clinical case for Chapter 18.

We especially thank the staff at Lippincott Williams & Wilkins who have contributed so expertly to the planning, preparation, and production of this new edition: David Troy, Matt Hauber, Samantha Smith, and Jennifer Ajello.

LOYD V. ALLEN, JR.
Edmond, Oklahoma

Contents

x   Contents

Appendices

List of Physical Pharmacy Capsules

Introduction to Drugs and Pharmacy

1

Chapter at a glance

A drug is defined as an agent intended for use in the diagnosis, mitigation, treatment, cure, or prevention of disease in humans or in other animals. One of the most astounding qualities of drugs is the diversity of their actions and effects on the body. This quality enables their selective use in the treatment of a range of common and rare conditions in-volving virtually every body organ, tissue, and cell.

Some drugs selectively stimulate the cardiac muscle, the central nervous system, or the gastrointestinal tract, whereas other drugs have the opposite effect. Mydriatic drugs dilate the pupil of the eye, and miotics constrict or diminish pupillary size. Drugs can render blood more coagulable or less coagulable; they can increase the hemoglobin content of the erythrocytes, reduce serum cholesterol, or expand blood volume.

Drugs termed emetics induce vomiting, whereas antiemetic drugs prevent vomiting. Diuretic drugs increase the flow of urine; expectorant drugs increase respiratory tract fluid; and cathartics or laxatives evacuate the bowel. Other drugs decrease the flow of urine, diminish body secretions, or induce constipation.

Drugs may be used to reduce pain, fever, thyroid activity, rhinitis, insomnia, gastric acidity, motion sickness, blood pressure, and mental depression. Other drugs can elevate mood, blood pressure, or activity of the endocrine glands. Drugs can combat infectious disease, destroy intestinal worms, or act as antidotes against the poisoning effects of other drugs. Drugs can assist in smoking cessation or alcohol withdrawal or can modify obsessive-compulsive disorders.

Drugs are used to treat common infections, AIDS, benign prostatic hyperplasia, cancer, cardiovascular disease, asthma, glaucoma, Alzheimer's disease, and male impotence. They can protect against the rejection of transplanted tissues and organs and reduce the incidence of measles and mumps. Antineoplastic drugs provide one means of attacking the cancerous process; radioactive pharmaceuticals provide another.

Drugs may be used to diagnose diabetes, liver malfunction, tuberculosis, or pregnancy. They can replenish a body deficient in antibodies, vitamins, hormones, electrolytes, protein, enzymes, or blood. Drugs can prevent pregnancy, assist fertility, and sustain life itself.

Certainly the vast array of effective medicinal agents available today is one of our greatest scientific accomplishments. It is difficult to conceive our civilization devoid of these remarkable and beneficial agents. Through their use, many of the diseases that have plagued humans throughout history, such as smallpox and poliomyelitis, are now virtually extinct. Illnesses such as diabetes, hypertension, and mental depression are effectively controlled with modern drugs. Today's surgical procedures would be virtually impossible without the benefit of anes-

thetics, analgesics, antibiotics, blood transfusions, and intravenous fluids.

New drugs may be derived from plant or animal sources, as byproducts of microbial growth, or through chemical synthesis, molecular modification, or biotechnology. Computer libraries and data banks of chemical compounds and sophisticated methods of screening for potential biologic activity assist drug discovery.

The process of drug discovery and development is complex. It entails the collective contributions of many scientific specialists, including organic, physical, and analytical chemists; biochemists; molecular biologists; bacteriologists; physiologists; pharmacologists; toxicologists; hematologists; immunologists; endocrinologists; pathologists; biostatisticians; pharmaceutical scientists; clinical pharmacists; physicians; and many others.

After a potential new drug substance is discovered and undergoes definitive chemical and physical characterization, a great deal of biologic information must be gathered. The basic pharmacology, or the nature and mechanism of action of the drug on the biologic system, must be determined including toxicologic features. The drug's site and rate of absorption, its pattern of distribution and concentration within the body, its duration of action, and the method and rate of its elimination or excretion must be studied. Information on the drug's metabolic degradation and the activity of any of its metabolites must be obtained. A comprehensive study of the short-term and long-term effects of the drug on various body cells, tissues, and organs must be made. Highly specific information, such as the effect of the drug on the fetus of a pregnant animal or its ability to pass to a nursing baby through the breast milk of its mother, may be obtained. Many a promising new drug has been abandoned because of its potential to cause excessive or hazardous adverse effects.

The most effective routes of administration (e.g., oral, rectal, parenteral, topical) must be determined, and guidelines for the dosages recommended for persons of varying ages (e.g., neonates, children, adults, geriatrics), weights, and states of illness have to be established. It has been said that the only difference between a drug and a poison is the dose. To facilitate administration of the drug by the selected routes, appropriate dosage forms, such as tablets, capsules, injections, suppositories, ointments, aerosols, and others, are formulated and prepared. Each of these dosage units is designed to contain a specified quantity of medication for ease and accuracy of dosage administration. These dosage forms are highly sophisticated delivery systems. Their design, development, production, and use are the product of application of the pharmaceutical sciences—the blending of the basic, applied, and clinical sciences with pharmaceutical technology.

Each particular pharmaceutical product is a formulation unique unto itself. In addition to the active therapeutic ingredients, a pharmaceutical formulation contains a number of nontherapeutic or pharmaceutical ingredients. It is through their use that a formulation achieves its unique composition and characteristic physical appearance. Pharmaceutical ingredients include such materials as fillers, thickeners, solvents, suspending agents, tablet coatings and disintegrants, penetration enhancers, stabilizing agents, antimicrobial preservatives, flavors, colorants, and sweeteners.

To ensure the stability of a drug in a formulation and the continued effectiveness of the drug product throughout its usual shelf life, the principles of chemistry, physical pharmacy, microbiology, and pharmaceutical technology must be applied. The formulation must be such that all components are physically and chemically compatible, including the active therapeutic agents, the pharmaceutical ingredients, and the packaging materials. The formulation must be preserved against decomposition due to chemical degradation and protected from microbial contamination and the destructive influences of excessive heat, light, and moisture. The therapeutic ingredients must be released from the dosage form in the proper quantity and in such a manner that the onset and duration of the drug's action is that which is desired. The pharmaceutical product must lend itself to efficient administration and must possess attractive features of flavor, odor, color, and texture that enhance acceptance by the patient. Finally, the product must be effectively packaged and clearly and completely labeled according to legal regulations.

Once prepared, the pharmaceutical product must be properly administered if the patient is to receive maximum benefit. The medication must be taken in sufficient quantity, at specified intervals, and for an indicated duration to achieve the desired therapeutic outcomes. The effectiveness of the medication in achieving the prescriber's objectives should be reevaluated at regular intervals and necessary adjustments made in the dosage, regimen, schedule, or form, or indeed, in the choice of the drug administered. Patients' expressions of disappointment in the rate of progress or complaints of side effects to the prescribed drug should be evaluated and decisions made as to the continuance, adjustment, or major change in drug therapy. Before initially taking a medication, a patient should be advised of any expected side effects and of foods, beverages, and/or other drugs that may interfere with the effectiveness of the medication.

Through professional interaction and communication with other health professionals the pharmacist can contribute greatly to patient care. An intimate knowledge of drug actions, pharmacotherapeutics, formulation and dosage form design, available pharmaceutical products, and drug information sources makes the pharmacist a vital member of the health care team. The pharmacist is entrusted with the legal responsibility for the procurement, storage, control, and distribution of effective pharmaceutical products and for the compounding and filling of prescription orders. Drawing on extensive training and knowledge, the pharmacist serves the patient as an advisor on drugs and encourages their safe and proper use. The pharmacist delivers pharmaceutical services in a variety of community and institutional health care environments and effectively uses medication records, patient monitoring, and assessment techniques in safeguarding the public health.

To appreciate the progress that has been made in drug discovery and development and to provide background for the study of modern drugs and pharmaceutical dosage forms, it is important to examine pharmacy's heritage.

The Heritage of Pharmacy

Drugs, in the form of vegetation and minerals, have existed as long as humans. Human disease and the instinct to survive have led to their discovery through the ages. The use of drugs, crude though they may have been, undoubtedly began long before recorded history, for the instinct of primitive man to relieve the pain of a wound by bathing it in cool water or by soothing it with a fresh leaf or protecting it with mud is within the realm of belief. From experience, early humans would learn that certain therapy was more effective than others, and from these beginnings came the practice of drug therapy.

Among many early races, disease was believed to be caused by the entrance of demons or evil spirits into the body. The treatment naturally involved ridding the body of the supernatural intruders. From the earliest records, the primary methods of removing spirits were through the use of spiritual incantations, the application of noisome materials, and the administration of specific herbs or plant materials.

The First Apothecary

Before the days of the priestcraft, the wise man or woman of the tribe, whose knowledge of the healing qualities of plants had been gathered through experience or handed down by word of mouth, was called upon to attend to the sick or wounded and prepare the remedy. It was in the preparation of the medicinal materials that the art of the apothecary originated.

The art of the apothecary has always been associated with the mysterious, and its practitioners were believed to have connection with the world of spirits and thus performed as intermediaries between the seen and the unseen. The belief that a drug had magical associations meant that its action, for good or for evil, did not depend upon its natural qualities alone. The compassion of a god, the observance of ceremonies, the absence of evil spirits, and the healing intent of the dispenser were individually and collectively needed to make the drug

therapeutically effective. Because of this, the tribal apothecary was one to be feared, respected, trusted, sometimes mistrusted, worshiped, and revered, for it was through his potions that spiritual contact was made, and upon that contact the cures or failures depended.

Throughout history, the knowledge of drugs and their application to disease has always meant power. In the Homeric epics, the term *pharmakon* (Gr.), from which our word pharmacy was derived, connotes a charm or a drug that can be used for good or for evil. Many of the tribal apothecary's failures were doubtless due to impotent or inappropriate medicines, underdosage, overdosage, and even poisoning. Successes may be attributed to experience, mere coincidence of appropriate drug selection, natural healing, inconsequential effect of the drug, or placebo effects, that is, successful treatment due to psychologic rather than therapeutic effects. Even today, placebo therapy with inert or inconsequential chemicals is used successfully to treat individual patients and is a routine practice in the clinical evaluation of new drugs, in which subjects' responses to the effects of the actual drug and the placebo are compared and evaluated.

As time passed, the art of the apothecary combined with priestly functions, and among the early civilizations, the priest–magician or priest–physician became the healer of the body as well as of the soul. Pharmacy and medicine are indistinguishable in their early history because their practice was the combined function of the tribal religious leaders.

Early Drugs

Because of the patience and intellect of the archeologist, the types and specific drugs used in the early history of drug therapy are not as indefinable as one might suspect. Numerous ancient tablets, scrolls, and other relics as early as 3000 BC have been uncovered and deciphered by archaeologic scholars to the delight of historians of both medicine and pharmacy; these ancient documents are specific associations with our common heritage (Fig. 1.1).

Perhaps the most famous of these surviving memorials is the Ebers papyrus, a continuous scroll some 60 feet long and a foot wide dating to the 16th century BC. This document, which is now preserved at the University of Leipzig, is named for the noted German Egyptologist Georg Ebers, who discovered it in the tomb of a mummy and partly translated it during the last half of the 19th century. Since that time many scholars have participated in the translation of the document's challenging hieroglyphics, and although they are not unanimous in their interpretations, there is little doubt that by 1550 BC, the Egyptians were using some drugs and dosage forms that are still used today.

The text of the Ebers papyrus is dominated by drug formulas, with more than 800 formulas or prescriptions being described and more than 700 drugs mentioned. The drugs are chiefly botanical, although mineral and animal drugs are also noted. Such botanical substances as acacia, castor bean (from which we express castor oil), and fennel are mentioned along with apparent references to such minerals as iron oxide, sodium carbonate, sodium chloride, and sulfur. Animal excrements were also used in drug therapy.

The vehicles of the day were beer, wine, milk, and honey. Many of the pharmaceutical formulas employed two dozen or more medicinal agents, a type of preparation later called polypharmacal. The Egyptians commonly used mortars and pestles, hand mills, sieves, and balances in their compounding of suppositories, gargles, pills, inhalations, troches, lotions, ointments, plasters, and enemas.

Introduction of the Scientific Viewpoint

Throughout history, many individuals have contributed to the advancement of the health sciences. Notable among those whose genius and creativeness had a revolutionary influence on the development of pharmacy and medicine were Hippocrates (ca. 460–377 BC), Dioscorides (1st century AD), Galen (ca. 130–200 AD), and Paracelsus (1493–1541 AD).

Hippocrates, a Greek physician, is credited with the introduction of scientific pharmacy and medicine. He rationalized medicine, systematized medical knowledge, and put the practice of medicine on a high ethical plane. His thinking on the ethics and science of medicine dominated the medical writings of his and successive generations, and his concepts and precepts are embodied in the renowned Hippocratic oath of ethical behavior for the healing professions. His works included the descriptions of hundreds of drugs, and it was during this period that the term *pharmakon* came to mean a purifying remedy for good only, transcending the previous connotation of a charm or drug for good or for evil purposes. Because of his pioneering work in medical science and his inspirational teachings and advanced philosophies that have become a part of modern medicine, Hippocrates is honored by being called the Father of Medicine.

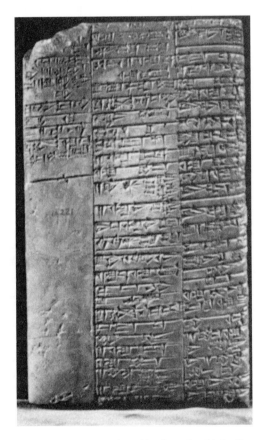

FIGURE 1.1 Sumerian clay tablet from the third millennium BC on which are believed to be the world's oldest written prescriptions. Among them are a preparation of the seed of carpenter plant, gum resin of markhazi, and thyme, all pulverized and dissolved in beer, and a combination of powdered roots of "Moon plant" and white pear tree, also dissolved in beer. (Courtesy of the University Museum, University of Pennsylvania.)

Dioscorides, a Greek physician and botanist, was the first to deal with botany as an applied science of pharmacy. His work, *De Materia Medica*, is considered a milestone in the development of pharmaceutical botany and in the study of naturally occurring medicinal materials. This area of study is today known as pharmacognosy, a term formed from two Greek words, *pharmakon*, drug, and *gnosis*, knowledge. Some of the drugs Dioscorides described, including opium, ergot, and hyoscyamus, continue to have use in medicine. His descriptions of the art of identifying and collecting natural drug products, the methods of their proper storage, and the means of detecting adulterants or contaminants were the standards of the period, established the need for additional work, and set guidelines for future investigators.

Claudius Galen, a Greek pharmacist–physician who attained Roman citizenship, aimed to create a perfect system of physiology, pathology, and treatment. Galen formulated doctrines that were followed for 1500 years. He was one of the most prolific authors of his or any other era, having been credited with 500 treatises on medicine and some 250 others on philosophy, law, and grammar. His medical writings include descriptions of numerous drugs of natural origin with a profusion of drug formulas and methods of compounding. He originated so many preparations of vegetable drugs by mixing or melting the individual ingredients that the field of pharmaceutical preparations was once commonly referred to as "Galenic pharmacy." Perhaps the most famous of his formulas is one for a cold cream, called Galen's Cerate, which has similarities to some in use today.

Pharmacy remained a function of medicine until the increasing variety of drugs and the growing complexity of compounding demanded specialists who could devote full attention to the art. Pharmacy was officially separated from medicine for the first time in 1240 AD, when a decree of Emperor Frederick II of Germany regulated the practice of pharmacy within the part of his kingdom called the Two Sicilies. His edict separating the two professions acknowledged that pharmacy required special knowledge, skill, initiative, and responsibility if adequate care to the medical needs of the people was to be guaranteed. Pharmacists were obligated by oath to prepare reliable drugs of uniform quality according to their art. Any exploitation of the patient through business relations between the pharmacist and the physician was strictly forbidden. Between that time and the evolution of chemistry as an exact science, pharmacy and chemistry became united as pharmacy and medicine had been.

Perhaps no person in history exercised such a revolutionary influence on pharmacy and medicine as did Aureolus Theophrastus Bombastus von Hohenheim (1493–1541), a Swiss physician and chemist who called himself Paracelsus. He influenced the transformation of pharmacy from a profession based primarily on botanical science to one based on chemical science. Some of his chemical observations were astounding for his time and for their anticipation of later discoveries. He believed it was possible to prepare a specific medicinal agent to combat each specific disease and introduced a host of chemical substances to internal therapy.

Early Research

As the knowledge of the basic sciences increased, so did their application to pharmacy. The opportunity was presented for the investigation of medicinal materials on a firm scientific basis, and the challenge was accepted by numerous pharmacists who conducted their research in the back rooms and basements of their pharmacies. Noteworthy among them was the Swede Karl Wilhelm Scheele (1742–1786), perhaps the most famous of all pharmacists because of his scientific genius and dramatic discoveries. Among his discoveries were the chemicals lactic acid, citric acid, oxalic acid, tartaric acid, and arsenic acid. He identified glycerin, invented new methods of preparing calomel and benzoic acid, and discovered oxygen a year before Priestley.

The isolation of morphine from opium by the German pharmacist Friedrich Sertürner (1783–1841) in 1805 prompted a series of isolations of other active materials from medicinal plants by a score of French pharmacists. Joseph Caventou (1795–1877) and Joseph Pelletier

(1788–1842) combined their talents and isolated quinine and cinchonine from cinchona and strychnine and brucine from nux vomica. Pelletier together with Pierre Robiquet (1780–1840) isolated caffeine, and Robiquet independently separated codeine from opium. Methodically one chemical after another was isolated from plant drugs and identified as an agent responsible for the plants' medicinal activity. Today we are still engaged in this fascinating activity as we probe nature for more useful and more specific therapeutic agents. Contemporary examples of drugs isolated from a natural source include paclitaxel (Taxol), an agent with antitumor activity derived from the Pacific yew tree (*Taxus baccata*) and employed in the treatment of metastatic carcinoma of the ovary; vincaleukoblastine, another antineoplastic drug, from *Vinca rosea*; and digoxin, a cardiac glycoside, from *Digitalis lanata*.

Throughout Europe during the late 18th century and the beginning of the 19th century, pharmacists like Pelletier and Sertürner were held in great esteem because of their intellect and technical abilities. They applied the art and the science of pharmacy to the preparation of drug products with the highest standards of purity, uniformity, and efficacy possible at that time. The extraction and isolation of active constituents from crude (unprocessed) botanical drugs led to the development of dosage forms of uniform strength containing singly effective therapeutic agents of natural origin. Many pharmacists of the period began to manufacture quality pharmaceutical products on a small but steadily increasing scale to meet the growing needs of their communities. Some of today's largest pharmaceutical research and manufacturing companies developed from these progressive prescription laboratories of two centuries ago.

Although many of the drugs indigenous to America and first used by the American Indian were adopted by the settlers, most drugs needed in this country before the 19th century were imported from Europe, either as the raw materials or as finished products. With the Revolutionary War, however, it became more difficult to import drugs, and the American pharmacist was stimulated to acquire the scientific and technologic expertise of his European contemporary. From this period until the Civil War, pharmaceutical manufacture was in its infancy in this country. A few of the pharmaceutical firms established during the early 1800s are still in operation. In 1821, the Philadelphia College of Pharmacy was established as the nation's first school of pharmacy.

Drug Standards

As the scientific basis for drugs and drug products developed, so did the need for uniform standards to ensure quality. This need led to the development and publication of monographs and reference books containing such standards to be used by those involved in the production of drugs and pharmaceutical products. Organized sets of monographs or books of these standards are called pharmacopeias or formularies.

The *United States Pharmacopeia* and the *National Formulary*

The term pharmacopeia comes from the Greek *pharmakon*, meaning drug, and *poiein*, meaning make, and the combination indicates any recipe or formula or other standards required to make or prepare a drug. The term was first used in 1580 in connection with a local book of drug standards in Bergamo, Italy. From that time on countless city, state, and national pharmacopeias were published by various European pharmaceutical societies. As time passed, the value of a uniform set of national drug standards became apparent. In Great Britain, for example, three city pharmacopeias—the London, the Edinburgh, and the Dublin—were official until 1864, when they were replaced by the *British Pharmacopoeia* (BP).

In the United States, drug standards were first provided on a national basis in 1820, when the first *United States Pharmacopeia* (USP) was published. However, the need for drug standards was recognized in this country long before the first USP was published. For convenience and because of their familiarity with them, colonial physicians and apothecaries used the pharmacopeias and other references of their various homelands. The first American pharmacopeia was the so-called *Lititz Pharmacopeia*, published in 1778 at Lititz, Pennsylvania, for use by the Military Hospital of the United States Army. It was a 32-page booklet containing information on 84 internal and 16 external drugs and preparations.

During the last decade of the 18th century, several attempts were made by various local medical societies to collate drug information, set appropriate standards, and prepare an extensive American pharmacopeia of the drugs in use at that time. In 1808, the Massachusetts Medical Society published a 272-page pharmacopeia containing information or monographs on 536 drugs and pharmaceutical preparations. Included were monographs on many drugs indigenous to America, which were not described in the European pharmacopeias of the day.

On January 6, 1817, Lyman Spalding, a physician from New York City, submitted a plan to the Medical Society of the County of New York for the creation of a national pharmacopeia. Spalding's efforts were later to result in his being recognized as the Father of the *United States Pharmacopeia*. He proposed dividing the United States as then known into four geographic districts—northern, middle, southern, and western. The plan provided for a convention in each of these districts, to be composed of delegates from all medical societies and medical schools within them. Where there was as yet no incorporated medical society or medical school, voluntary associations of physicians and surgeons were invited to assist in the undertaking. Each district's convention was to draft a pharmacopeia and appoint delegates to a general convention to be held later in Washington, D.C. At the general convention, the four district pharmacopeias were to be compiled into a single national pharmacopeia.

Draft pharmacopeias were submitted to the convention by only the northern and middle districts. These were reviewed, consolidated, and adopted by the first United States Pharmacopeial Convention assembled in Washington, D.C., on January 1, 1820. The first USP was published on December 15, 1820, in English and Latin, then the international language of

medicine, to render the book more intelligible to physicians and pharmacists of any nationality. Within its 272 pages were listed 217 drugs considered worthy of recognition; many of them were taken from the *Massachusetts Pharmacopeia*, which is considered by some to be the precursor to the USP. The objective of the first USP was stated in its preface and remains important. It reads in part:

> It is the object of a Pharmacopeia to select from among substances which possess medicinal power, those, the utility of which is most fully established and best understood; and to form from them preparations and compositions, in which their powers may be exerted to the greatest advantage. It should likewise distinguish those articles by convenient and definite names, such as may prevent trouble or uncertainty in the intercourse of physicians and apothecaries (1).

Before adjourning, the convention adopted a constitution and bylaws, with provisions for subsequent meetings of the convention leading to a revised USP every 10 years. As many new drugs entered use, the need for more frequent issuance of standards became increasingly apparent. In 1900, the Pharmacopeial Convention granted authority to issue supplements to the USP whenever necessary to maintain satisfactory standards. At the 1940 meeting of the convention, it was decided to revise the USP every 5 years while maintaining the use of periodic supplements.

The first United States Pharmacopeial Convention was composed exclusively of physicians. In 1830 and again in 1840, prominent pharmacists were invited to assist in the revision, and in recognition of their contributions pharmacists were awarded full membership in the convention of 1850 and have participated regularly ever since. By 1870, the USP was so nearly in the hands of pharmacists that vigorous efforts were required to revive interest in it among physicians. The present constitution and bylaws of the United States Pharmacopeial Convention provide for accredited delegates representing educational institutions, professional and scientific organizations, divisions of governmental bodies, non–United States international organizations and pharmacopeial bodies, persons who possess special scientific competence or knowledge of emerging technologies, and public members (2). Of the seven elected members of the board of trustees, at least two must be representatives of the medical sciences, two others must be representatives of the pharmaceutical sciences, and at least one must be a public member.

After the appearance of the first USP, the art and science of both pharmacy and medicine changed remarkably. Before 1820, drugs to treat disease had been the same for centuries. The USP of 1820 reflected the fact that the apothecary of that day was competent at collecting and identifying botanical drugs and preparing from them the mixtures and preparations required by the physician. The individual pharmacist seemed fulfilled as he applied his total art to the creation of elegant pharmaceutical preparations from crude botanical materials. It was a time that would never be seen again because of the impending upsurge in technologic capabilities and the steady development of the basic sciences, particularly synthetic organic chemistry.

The second half of the 19th century brought great and far-reaching changes. The industrial revolution was in full swing in the United States. The steam engine, which used water power to turn mills that powdered crude botanical drugs, was replaced by the gas, diesel, or electric motor. New machinery was substituted for the old whenever possible, and often machinery from other industries was adapted to the special needs of pharmaceutical manufacturing. Mixers from the baking industry, centrifugal machines from the laundry industry, and sugarcoating pans from the candy industry were a few examples of improvisations. Production increased rapidly, but the new industry had to wait for the scientific revolution before it could claim newer and better drugs for mankind. A symbiosis between science and the advancing technology was needed.

By 1880, the industrial manufacture of chemicals and pharmaceutical products had become well established in this country, and the pharmacist was relying heavily on commercial sources for drug supply. Synthetic organic chemistry began to have its influence on drug therapy. The isolation of some active constituents of plant drugs led to knowledge of their chemical structure. From this arose methods of synthetically duplicating the same structures, as well as manipulating molecular structure to produce organic chemicals yet undiscovered in nature. In 1872, the synthesis of salicylic acid from phenol inaugurated the synthesis of a group of analgesic compounds including acetylsalicylic acid (aspirin), which was introduced into medicine in 1899. Among other chemicals synthesized for the first time were sleep-producing derivatives of barbituric acid called barbiturates. This new source of drugs—synthetic organic chemistry—welcomed the turn into the 20th century.

Until this time, drugs created through the genius of the synthetic organic chemist relieved a host of maladies, but none had been found to be curative—none, that is, until 1910, when arsphenamine, a specific agent against syphilis, was introduced to medical science. This was the start of an era of chemotherapy, an era in which the diseases of humans became curable through the use of specific chemical agents. The concepts, discoveries, and inspirational work that led mankind to this glorious period are credited to Paul Ehrlich, the German bacteriologist who together with a Japanese colleague, Sahachiro Hata, discovered arsphenamine. Today most of our new drugs, whether they are curative or palliative, originate in the flask of the synthetic organic chemist.

The advancement of science, both basic and applied, led to drugs of a more complex nature and to more of them. The standards advanced by the USP were more than ever needed to protect the public by ensuring the purity and uniformity of drugs.

When the American Pharmaceutical Association (APhA) was organized in 1852, the only authoritative and recognized book of drug standards available was the third revision of the USP. To serve as a therapeutic guide to the medical profession, its scope, then as now, was restricted to drugs of established therapeutic merit. Because of strict selectivity, many drugs and formulas that were accepted and used by the medical profession were not granted admission to early revisions of the USP. As a type of protest, and in keeping with the original objectives of the APhA to standardize drugs and formulas, certain pharmacists, with the sanction of their national organization, prepared a formulary containing many of the popular drugs and formulas denied admission to the USP. The first edition was published in 1888 under the title *National Formulary of Unofficial Preparations* (3). The designation "unofficial preparations" reflected the protest mood of the authors, since the USP had earlier adopted the term "official" as applying to the drugs for which it provided standards. The title was changed to *National Formulary* (NF) on June 30, 1906, when President Theodore Roosevelt signed into law the first federal Pure Food and Drug Act, designating both the USP and NF as establishing legal standards for medicinal and pharmaceutical substances. Thus the two publications became official compendia. Among other things, the law required that whenever the designation USP or NF was used or implied on drug labeling, the products must conform to the physical and chemical standards set forth in the compendium monograph.

The early editions of the NF served mainly as a convenience to practicing pharmacists by providing uniform names of drugs and preparations and working directions for the small-scale manufacture of popular pharmaceutical preparations prescribed by physicians. Before 1940, the NF, like the USP, was revised every 10 years. After that date, new editions appeared every 5 years, with supplements issued periodically as necessary.

In 1975, the United States Pharmacopeial Convention, Inc., purchased the NF, unifying the official compendia and providing the mechanism for a single national compendium.

The first combined compendium, comprising the USP XX and NF XV, became official on July 1, 1980. All monographs on therapeutically active drug substances appeared in the USP section of the volume, whereas all monographs on pharmaceutical agents appeared in the NF section. This format has been continued in subsequent revisions. The USP 23–National Formulary 18, which became official in 1995, was the first edition to drop the use of roman numerals in favor of arabic numerals to indicate the edition. The USP-NF became an annual publica-

tion in 2002 with USP 25–NF 20, and the 2003 edition, USP 26–NF 21, contains approximately 4000 drug monographs and is published both in print and on CD-ROM.

The standards advanced by the USP and the NF are put to active use by all members of the health care industry who share the responsibility and enjoy the public's trust for ensuring the availability of quality drugs and pharmaceutical products. Included in this group are pharmacists, physicians, dentists, veterinarians, nurses, producers, and suppliers of bulk chemicals for use in drug production, large and small manufacturers of pharmaceutical products, drug procurement officers of various private and public health agencies and institutions, drug regulatory and enforcement agencies, and others.

USP and NF Monographs

The USP and NF adopt standards for drug substances, pharmaceutical ingredients, and dosage forms reflecting the best in the current practices of medicine and pharmacy and provide suitable tests and assay procedures for demonstrating compliance with these standards. In fulfilling this function, the compendia become legal documents, every statement of which must be of a high degree of clarity and specificity.

Many pharmaceutical products on the market, especially combinations of therapeutic ingredients, are not described in formulation or dosage form monographs in the official compendia. However, the individual components in these products are described in monographs in the compendia, in supplements to the compendia, or in drug applications for marketing approved by the Food and Drug Administration (FDA).

An example of a typical monograph for a drug substance appearing in the USP is shown in Figure 1.2. This monograph demonstrates the type of information that appears for organic medicinal agents.

The initial part of the monograph consists of the official title (generic or nonproprietary name) of the drug substance. This is followed by its graphic or structural formula, empirical

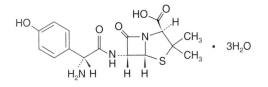

$C_{16}H_{19}N_3O_5S \cdot 3H_2O$ 419.45

4-Thia-1-azabicyclo[3.2.0]hepane-2-carboxylic acid,
  6-[[amino(4-hydroxyphenyl)acetyl]amino-3,
  3-dimethyl-7-oxo-, trihydrate 2S-[2α,[5α,6β(S^*)]]-.
  (2S,5R,6R)-6-[(R)-(−)-2-Amino-2-(p-hydroxyphenyl)
  acetamido]-3,3-dimethyl-7-oxo-4-thia-1-azabicyclo
  [3.2.0]heptane-2-carboxylic acid trihydtate   [61336-
  70-7].
Anhydrous   365.41   [26787-78-0].

Amoxicillin contains not less than 900 μg and not more
than 1050 μg of $C_{16}H_{19}N_3O_5S$ per mg, calculated on the
anhydrous basis.
Packaging and storage—Preserve in tight containers, at
controlled room temperature.
Labeling—Where it is intended for use in preparing injectable dosage forms, the label states that it is intended for
veterinary use only and that it is sterile or must be subjected
to further processing during the preparation of injectable
dosage forms. Label all other Amoxicillin to indicate that it
is to be used in the manufacture of nonparenteral drugs only.
USP Reference standards [11]—*USP Amoxicillin RS. USP
Endotoxin RS.*
Identification, *Infrared Absorption* (197K).
Crystallinity [695]: meets the requirements.
pH [791]: between 3.5 and 6.0, in a solution containing 2
mg per mL.
Water, *Method I* [921]: between 11.5% and 14.5%.
Dimethylaniline [223]: meets the requirement.
Other requirements—Where the label states that Amoxicillin is sterile, it meets the requirements for *Sterility* and
Bacterial endotoxins under *Amoxicillin for Injectable Suspension.* Where the label states that Amoxicillin must be subjected to further processing during the preparation of injectable dosage forms, it meets the requirements for *Bacterial
endotoxins* under *Amoxicillin for Injectable Suspension.*

Assay—
  Diluent—Dissolve 13.6 g of monobasic potassium phosphate in 2000 mL of water, and adjust with a 45% (w/w)
solution of potassium hydroxide to a pH of 5.0±0.1.
  Mobile phase—Prepare a suitable filtered mixture of
Diluent and acetonitrile (96:4). Make adjustments if necessary (see *System Suitability* under *Chromatography* [621]).
Decrease the acetonitrile concentration to increase the retention time of amoxicillin.
  Standard preparation—Dissolve an accurately weighed
quantity of USP Amoxicillin RS quantitatively in *Diluent* to
obtain a solution having a known concentration of about
1.2 mg per mL. Use this solution within 6 hours.
  Assay preparation—Transfer about 240 mg of Amoxicillin, accurately weighed, to a 200-mL volumetric flask,
dissolve in and dilute with *Diluent* to volume, and mix. Use
this solution within 6 hours.
  Chromatographic system (see *Chromatography* [621])—
The liquid chromatograph is equipped with a 230-nm detector and a 4-mm × 25-cm column that contains packing
L1. The flow rate is about 1.5 mL per minute. Chromatograph the *Standard preparation,* and record the peak responses as directed for *Procedure:* the capacity factor, k^r, is
between 1.1 and 2.8, the column efficiency is not less than
1700 theoretical plates, the tailing factor is not more than
2.5, and the relative standard deviation for replicate injections is not more than 2.0%.
  Procedure—Separately inject equal volumes (about 10
μL) of the *Standard preparation* and the *Assay preparation*
into the chromatograph, record the chromatograms, and
measure the responses for the major peaks. Calculate the
quantity, in μg, of $C_{16}H_{19}N_3O_5S$ per mg of the Amoxicillin
taken by the formula:

$$200(CP/W)(r_u/r_s),$$

in which C is the concentration, in mg per mL, of USP
Amoxicillin RS in the *Standard preparation, P* is the stated
amoxicillin content, in μg per mg, of USP Amoxicillin S,
W is the quantity, in mg, of Amoxicillin taken to prepare
the *Assay preparation,* and r_u and r_s are the amoxicillin
peak responses obtained from the *Assay preparation* and
the *Standard preparation,* respectively.

FIGURE 1.2 Amoxicillin.

formula, molecular weight, established chemical names, and the drug's Chemical Abstracts
Service (CAS) registry number. The CAS registry
number identifies each compound uniquely in
the CAS computer information retrieval system. Appearing next in the monograph is a
statement of chemical purity, a cautionary
statement that reflects the toxic nature of the
agent, packaging and storage recommendations, and chemical and physical tests and the
prescribed method of assay to substantiate the
identification and purity of the chemical.

In each monograph, the standards set forth
are specific to the individual therapeutic agent,
pharmaceutical material, or dosage form
preparation to ensure purity, potency, and
quality.

The USP Drug Research and Testing Laboratory provides direct laboratory assistance to
the USP and the NF. The laboratory's main
functions are the evaluation of USP reference
standards and the evaluation and development of analytical methods to be used in the
compendia.

Other Pharmacopeias

In addition to the USP and the NF, other references to drug standards, such as the *Homeopathic Pharmacopeia of the United States* (HPUS) and the *Pharmacopeia Internationalis*, or *International Pharmacopeia* (IP), provide additional guidelines for drug quality required by certain practitioners and agencies. HPUS is used by pharmacists and homeopathists as well as by law enforcement agencies that must ensure the quality of homeopathic drugs. The term homeopathy was coined by Samuel Hahnemann (1755–1843) from the Greek homoios, meaning similar, and pathos, meaning disease. In essence, the basis of homeopathy is the law of similarities, or that like cures like: that is, a drug that produces symptoms of the illness in healthy persons will also be capable of treating those same symptoms and curing the disease. Embodied in the homeopathic approach are (*a*) the testing of a drug on healthy persons to find the drug's effects so that it may be employed against the same symptoms manifesting a disease in an ill person; (*b*) the use of only minute doses of drugs in therapy, employed in dilutions expressed as "1x" (a 1:10 dilution), "2x" (a 1:100 dilution), and so on; (*c*) the administration of not more than one drug at a time; and (*d*) the treatment of the entire symptom complex of the patient, not just one symptom (4–6). The HPUS is essential for pharmacists who prepare drugs to be used in the practice of homeopathy.

The IP is published by the World Health Organization (WHO) of the United Nations with the cooperation of member countries. It is intended as a recommendation to national pharmacopeial revision committees to modify their pharmacopeias according to international standards. It has no legal authority, only the respect and recognition accorded it by the participating countries in their effort to provide acceptable drug standards on an international basis. The first volume of the IP was published in 1951. It has been revised periodically since that time.

Over the years, a number of countries have published their own pharmacopeias, including the United Kingdom, France, Italy, Japan, India, Mexico, Norway, and the former Union of Soviet Socialist Republics. These pharmacopeias and the *European Pharmacopeia* (EP or Ph Eur) are used within their legal jurisdictions and by multinational pharmaceutical companies that develop and market products internationally. Countries not having a national pharmacopeia frequently adopt one of another country for use in setting and regulating drug standards. Selection of the pharmacopeia is usually based on geographic proximity, a common heritage or language, or a similarity of drugs and pharmaceutical products used. For example, Canada, which does not have its own national pharmacopeia, has traditionally used USP–NF standards. The Mexican pharmacopeia (*Farmacopea de los Estados Unidos Mexicanos*) is the only other actively maintained pharmacopeia in this hemisphere (7).

Standards Set Forth in FDA-Approved New-drug applications

In the United States, in addition to the official compendia, some initial drug and drug product standards and assay methods are established as set forth in new drug and antibiotic applications approved by the FDA (see Chapter 2). The manufacturer must rigidly adhere to these initial standards to maintain product quality and continued FDA approval for marketing. Ultimately, these or subsequently developed standards are adopted as new monographs by the USP–NF.

International Organization for Standardization

The International Organization for Standardization (ISO) is an international consortium of representative bodies constituted to develop and promote uniform or harmonized international standards. Representing the United States in the consortium is the American National Standards Institute.

Among the various ISO standards used in the pharmaceutical industry are those in the series ISO 9000 to ISO 9004. Included here are standards pertaining to development, production, quality assurance (QA), quality control (QC), detection of defective products, quality management (QM), and other issues, such as product safety and liability. Industry compliance with the standards is voluntary. However, many firms find it advantageous to their business to comply with ISO standards and to be identified within their industry as having an internationally recognized QM system. Some companies choose to become ISO certified through a rigorous evaluation and accreditation process (8).

Drug Regulation and Control

The first federal law in the United States designed to regulate drug products manufactured domestically was the Food and Drug Act of 1906. The law required drugs marketed interstate to comply with their claimed standards for strength, purity, and quality. Manufacturers' claims of therapeutic benefit were not regulated until 1912, when the passage of the Sherley Amendment specifically prohibited false claims of therapeutic effects, declaring such products misbranded.

The Federal Food, Drug, and Cosmetic Act of 1938

The need for additional drug standards was tragically demonstrated in 1938. The then-new wonder drug sulfanilamide, which was not soluble in most common pharmaceutical solvents of the day, was prepared and distributed by an otherwise reputable manufacturer as an elixir using as the solvent diethylene glycol, a highly toxic agent used in antifreeze solutions. Before the product could be removed from the market, more than 100 persons died of diethylene glycol poisoning. The necessity for proper product formulation and thorough pharmacologic and toxicologic testing of the therapeutic agent, pharmaceutical ingredients, and the completed product was painfully recognized. Congress responded with passage of the Federal Food, Drug, and Cosmetic Act of 1938 and the creation of the FDA to administer and enforce it. The 1938 act prohibits the distribution and use of any new drug or drug product without the prior filing of a new-drug application (NDA) and approval of the FDA. It became the responsibility of the FDA to either grant or deny permission to distribute a new product after reviewing the applicant's filed data on the product's ingredients, methods of assay and quality standards, formulation and manufacturing processes, preclinical (animal, tissue, or cell culture) studies including pharmacology and toxicology, and clinical trials on human subjects. Although the act of 1938 required pharmaceutical products to be safe for human use, it did not require them to be efficacious.

Durham-Humphrey Amendment of 1952

Drugs approved for marketing by the FDA are categorized according to the manner in which they may be legally obtained by the patient. Drugs deemed safe enough for use by the layman in the self-treatment of simple conditions for which competent medical care is not sought are classified as over the counter (OTC) or nonprescription drugs and may be sold without a physician's or other legally authorized prescriber's prescription. The OTC status of a drug may be changed if more stringent control over the drug's distribution and use is warranted later. Other drugs that are considered useful only after expert diagnosis or too dangerous for use in self-medication are made available to the patient only by prescription. These drugs must bear the symbol "Rx Only" or the legend "Caution: Federal Law Prohibits Dispensing Without Prescription." New drug substances are limited to prescription-only dispensing. However, their legal status may be changed to OTC, albeit usually at lower recommended dosage, should they later be considered useful and safe enough for the lay person's discretionary use. Examples of such drugs include ibuprofen, ketoprofen, cimetidine, loratadine, and ranitidine.

According to the Durham-Humphrey Amendment, prescriptions for legend drugs may not be refilled (dispensed again after the initial filling of the prescription) without the express consent of the prescriber. The refill status of prescriptions for certain legend drugs known to be subject to public abuse was further regulated with the passage of the Drug Abuse Control Amendments of 1965 and then by the Comprehensive Drug Abuse Prevention and Control Act of 1970.

Kefauver-Harris Amendments of 1962

A tragedy in 1960 led to the passage of the Kefauver-Harris Amendments to the Federal Food Drug and Cosmetic Act of 1938. A new synthetic drug, thalidomide, recommended as a sedative and tranquilizer, was being sold OTC in Europe. It was a drug of special interest because of its apparent lack of toxicity even at extreme dosage levels. It was hoped that it would replace the barbiturates as a sedative and therefore prevent the frequent deaths caused from accidental and intentional barbiturate overdosage. A pharmaceutical company was awaiting FDA approval for marketing in the United States when reports of a toxic effect of the drug's use in Europe began to appear. Thalidomide given to women during pregnancy produced birth defects, most notably phocomelia, an arrested development of the limbs of the affected newborn. Thousands of children were affected to various extents (9). Some were born without arms or legs; others, with partially formed limbs. The more fortunate were born with only disfigurations of the nose, eyes, and ears. The most severely afflicted died of malformation of the heart or gastrointestinal tract. This drug catastrophe spurred Congress to strengthen the existing laws regarding new drugs. Without dissent, on October 10, 1962, the Kefauver-Harris Drug Amendments to the Food, Drug, and Cosmetic Act of 1938 were passed by both houses of Congress. The purpose of the enactment was to ensure a greater degree of safety for approved drugs, and manufacturers were now required to prove a drug both safe and effective before it would be granted FDA approval for marketing.

Under the Food, Drug, and Cosmetic Act as amended, the sponsor of a new drug is required to file an investigational new-drug application (IND) with the FDA before the drug may be clinically tested on human subjects. Only after carefully designed and structured human clinical trials, in which the drug is evaluated for safety and effectiveness, may the drug's sponsor file a NDA seeking approval for marketing. The requirements for these and other submissions to the FDA are presented in Chapter 2.

Interestingly, WHO now considers thalidomide to be the standard treatment for the fever and painful skin lesions associated with erythema nodosum leprosum (ENL) in patients with leprosy and has been used for this purpose worldwide for many years (10). In 1997, an FDA advisory committee recommended that the agency approve thalidomide for treatment of ENL in the United States under strict distribution controls and with appropriate patient education programs (11). The potential usefulness of thalidomide in other conditions, such as rheumatoid arthritis, multiple sclerosis, AIDS- and cancer-related cachexia, HIV/AIDS progression, and aphthous ulcers, is under investigation (12).

Comprehensive Drug Abuse Prevention and Control Act of 1970

The Comprehensive Drug Abuse Prevention and Control Act of 1970 served to consolidate and codify control authority over drugs of abuse into a single statute. Under its provisions, the Drug Abuse Control Amendments of 1965, the Harrison Narcotic Act of 1914, and other related laws governing stimulants, depressants, narcotics, and hallucinogens were repealed and replaced by regulatory framework now administered by the Drug Enforcement Administration (DEA) in the Department of Justice.

The Comprehensive Drug Abuse Prevention and Control Act of 1970 established five "schedules," for the classification and control of drug substances that are subject to abuse. These schedules provide for decreasing levels of control, from schedule I to schedule V. The drugs in the five schedules may be described as follows:

Schedule I: Drugs with no accepted medical use, or other substances with a high potential for abuse. In this category are agents including heroin, LSD, mescaline, peyote, methaqualone, marijuana, and similar items. Any nonmedical substance that is being abused can be placed in this category.

Schedule II: Drugs with accepted medical uses and a high potential for abuse that if abused may lead to severe psychologic or physical dependence. In this category are morphine, cocaine, methamphetamine, amobarbital, and other such drugs.

Schedule III: Drugs with accepted medical uses and a potential for abuse less than those listed in schedules I and II that if abused may lead to moderate psychologic or physical dependence. In this category are specified quantities of codeine, hydrocodone, and similar agents.

Schedule IV: Drugs with accepted medical uses and low potential for abuse relative to those in Schedule III that if abused may lead to limited physical dependence or psychologic dependence relative to drugs in schedule III. In this category are specified quantities of diphenoxin, diazepam, oxazepam, and similar agents.

Schedule V—Drugs with accepted medical uses and low potential for abuse relative to those in schedule IV that if abused may lead to limited physical dependence or psychologic dependence relative to drugs in schedule IV. Included in this category are specified quantities of dihydrocodeine, diphenoxylate, and similar agents.

In all instances, local and state laws may strengthen the federal drug laws but may not be used to weaken them.

Drug Listing Act of 1972

The Drug Listing Act was enacted to provide the FDA with the legislative authority to compile a list of marketed drugs to assist in the enforcement of federal laws requiring that drugs be safe and effective and not adulterated or misbranded. Under the regulations of the act, each firm that manufactures or repackages drugs for ultimate sale or distribution to patients or consumers must register with the FDA and submit appropriate information for listing. All foreign drug manufacturing and distributing firms whose products are imported into the United States are also included in this regulation. Exempt from the registration and listing requirements are hospitals, clinics, and the various health practitioners who prepare pharmaceutical products for use in their respective institutions and practices. Also exempt are research and teaching institutions in which drug products are prepared for purposes other than sale. Each registrant is assigned a permanent registration number, following the format of the National Drug Code (NDC) numbering system. Under this system, the first 4 numbers, the labeler code of the 10-character code, identify the manufacturer or distributor. The last 6 numbers identify the drug formulation and the trade package size and type. The segment that identifies the drug formulation is the product code, and the segment that identifies the trade package size and type is the package code. The manufacturer or distributor determines the ratio of use of the last 6 digits for the two codes, as a 3:3 digit product code to package code configuration (e.g., 542-112) or a 4:2 digit configuration (e.g., 5421-12). Only one such type of configuration may be selected for use by a manufacturer or distributor, who then assigns a code number to each product to be included in the drug listing. A final code number is presented as the example: NDC 0081-5421-12.

The NDC numbers appear on all manufacturers' drug labeling. In some instances, manufacturers imprint the NDC number directly on the dosage units, such as capsules and tablets, for rapid and positive identification when the number is matched in the NDC Directory or against a decoding list provided by the manufacturer. Once a number is assigned to a drug product, it is a permanent assignment. Even when a drug manufacturer discontinues the manufacture and distribution of a product, the number may not be used again. If a drug product is substantially changed, as through an alteration in the active ingredients, dosage form, or product name, the registrant assigns a new NDC number and advises the FDA accordingly.

The product information received by the FDA from each registrant is processed and stored in computer files to provide easy access to the following types of information:

1. List of all drug products
2. List of all drug products by labeled indications or pharmacologic category

3. List of all drug products by manufacturer
4. List of a drug product's active ingredients
5. List of a drug product's inactive ingredients
6. List of drug products containing a particular ingredient
7. List of drug products newly marketed or remarketed
8. List of drug products discontinued
9. All labeling of drug products
10. All advertising of drug products

The drug listing program enables the FDA to monitor the quality of all drugs on the market in the United States.

In a continuing effort to ensure the standards for drug quality control, the FDA's regulations provide not only for the inspection and certification of pharmaceutical manufacturing procedures and facilities but also for field surveillance and assay of products obtained from the shelves of retail distributors. If a manufacturer is not meeting the established standards for drug product quality, that manufacturer will be denied permission to continue to produce products for distribution until compliance with the standards is attained.

Drug Price Competition and Patent Term Restoration Act of 1984

Changes to speed FDA approval of generic drugs and the extension of patent life for innovative new drugs were the major components of the Drug Price Competition and Patent Restoration Act of 1984.

Under the provisions of the legislation, applications for generic copies of an originally approved new drug can be filed through an abbreviated new-drug application (ANDA) and not require the extensive animal and human studies of an NDA. This reduces considerably the time and expense of bringing a generic version of the drug to market. The FDA evaluates the chemistry, manufacturing, control standards, and the drug's bioavailability in determining that the generic version is equivalent to the originally approved drug.

For holders of patented drugs, the legislation provides an extension of patent life equal to the time required for FDA review of the NDA plus half the time spent in the testing phase, up to a maximum of 5 years and not to exceed the usual 20-year patent term. This extends the effective patent life and exclusive marketing period for innovative new drug products, thereby encouraging pioneering research and development.

Prescription Drug Marketing Act of 1987

The Prescription Drug Marketing Act of 1987 established new safeguards on the integrity of the nation's supply of prescription drugs. Because of its author, Representative John Dingell, and its purpose to prevent drug diversion, the act has often been referred to as the Dingell bill and the Drug Diversion Act. The act is intended to reduce the risks of adulterated, misbranded, repackaged, or mislabeled drugs entering the legitimate marketplace through "secondary sources." The primary sections of the Act are summarized as follows:

1. Reimportation: Prohibits the reimportation of drug products manufactured in the United States except by the manufacturer of the product.
2. Sales restrictions: Prohibits selling, trading, purchasing, or the offer to sell, trade, or purchase a drug sample. It also prohibits resale by health care institutions of pharmaceuticals purchased explicitly for the use of the institution. Charitable institutions that receive drugs at reduced prices or no cost cannot resell the drugs.
3. Distribution of samples: Samples may be distributed only to (a) practitioners licensed to prescribe such drugs and (b) at the written request of the practitioner, to pharmacies of hospitals or other health care institutions. Sample distribution must be made through mail or common carrier and not directly by employees or agents of the manufacturer.
4. Wholesale distributors: Manufacturers are required to maintain a list of their authorized distributors. Wholesalers who desire to distribute a drug for which they are not authorized distributors must inform their wholesale customers, prior to the sale, of the name of the person from whom they obtained the goods and all previous sales.

Dietary Supplement Health and Education Act of 1994

In passing the Dietary Supplement Health and Education Act (DSHEA) of 1994, Congress recognized the growing interest in the use of various herbs and dietary supplements and addressed the need to regulate the labeling claims made for these products. These products, which include vitamins, minerals, amino acids, and botanicals, legally are not considered drugs if they have not been submitted for review on NDAs and thus have not been evaluated for safety and efficacy by the FDA. However, as with drugs, their safe use is a concern to the FDA.

The act forbids manufacturers or distributors of these products to make any advertising or labeling claims that indicate that the use of the product can prevent or cure a specific disease. In fact, a disclaimer must appear on the product: "This product is not intended to diagnose, treat, cure, or prevent any disease." However, the law does permit claims of benefit as they may properly relate to a nutrient deficiency disease or based on scientific evidence, how an ingredient may affect the body's "structure or function" (e.g., increase circulation or lower cholesterol) or how use of the product can affect a person's general well-being. But before any promotional or labeling claims may be made, they first must be submitted to the FDA as being truthful and not misleading (13).

The use of herbs and nutritional supplements are part of today's milieu of "alternative" therapies, and as such are receiving increased attention on the part of the scientific community and the FDA. Many of these agents, including ginseng, ginkgo, saw palmetto, St. John's wort, and Echinacea, are used worldwide and have been the subject of literature reports and research conducted in Europe and Asia. In 1997, a report of the U.S. Presidential Commission on Dietary Supplement Labels called for more research in this country on the health benefits of dietary supplements. In response, academic and National Institutes of Health (NIH) studies are being undertaken to assess the therapeutic usefulness of some of these agents and to determine their safety. The USP–NF is adopting standards for many of these products using marker ingredients that must be present within specified ranges if the product is labeled USP–NF.

The FDA and the Food and Drug Administration Modernization Act of 1997

As noted previously, the FDA was established in 1938 to administer and enforce the Federal Food Drug and Cosmetic Act. Starting with this initial authority, today the FDA is responsible for enforcing many additional pieces of legislation.

The mission of the FDA is to protect the public health against risks associated with the production, distribution, and sale of food and food additives, human drugs and biologicals, radiologic and medical devices, animal drugs and feeds, and cosmetics. In carrying out the intent of legislation it is mandated to enforce, the FDA

- Sets policies, establishes standards, issues guidelines, and promulgates and enforces rules and regulations governing the affected industries and their products
- Monitors for regulatory compliance through reporting requirements, product sampling and testing, and establishment inspections
- Establishes product labeling requirements, disseminates product use and safety information, issues product warnings, and directs product recalls
- Acts as the government's gatekeeper in making safe and effective new drugs, clinical laboratory tests, and medical devices available through a carefully conducted application and review process.

The FDA, an agency of the Department of Health and Human Services, is organized into appropriate units to support its various responsibilities and functions (e.g., new drug evaluation, regulatory compliance). The Center for Drug Evaluation and Research and the Center for Biologics Evaluation and Research are responsible for the drug and biologicals approval process as described in Chapter 2. The FDA is headquartered in Rockville, Maryland, with employees throughout the United States in six regions, each with district offices and resident inspection posts.

The FDA Modernization Act of 1997 was enacted to streamline FDA policies and to codify many of the agency's newer regulations (14). The bill expanded patient access to investigational treatments for AIDS, cancer, Alzheimer's disease, and other serious or life-threatening illnesses. It also provided for faster new drug approvals by using drug sponsor's fees to hire additional internal reviewers, by the authorized use of external reviewers, and by changes in the requirements demonstrating a drug's clinical effectiveness. It also provided incentives for investigations of drugs for children.

The legislation included provisions to track clinical trial data in a joint program with the NIH, established a system to follow and review studies of the safety and efficacy of marketed drug products, established a program for the dissemination of information on off-label uses of marketed drugs and encouraged applications for additional therapeutic indications, and fostered the expansion of the FDA's information management system and the agency's progress toward paperless systems for human drug applications.

To codify, enable, and enforce legislative authority, the FDA develops relevant guidelines and regulations. These are first published in the *Federal Register* for public comment, and when finalized, in the *Code of Federal Regulations*.

Code of Federal Regulations and Federal Register

Title 21 of the *Code of Federal Regulations* (CFR) consists of eight volumes containing all regulations issued under the Federal Food, Drug and Cosmetic Act and other statutes administered by the FDA. A ninth volume contains regulations issued under statutes administered by the DEA. The volumes are updated each year to incorporate all regulations issued during the preceding 12-month period. The *Federal Register* (FR) is issued each workday by the Superintendent of Documents, U.S. Government Printing Office (GPO) and contains proposed and final regulations and legal notices issued by federal agencies, including the FDA and the DEA. These publications provide the most definitive information on federal laws and regulations pertaining to drugs. The FR and the CFR are available in print and online through GPO Access (http://www.access.gpo.gov/nara/cfr).

Drug Product Recall

If the FDA or a manufacturer finds that a marketed product presents a threat or a potential threat to consumer safety, that product may be recalled, or sought for return to the manufacturer from its depth of distribution. The pharmaceutical manufacturer is legally bound to report serious unlabeled adverse reactions to the FDA through the FDA MedWatch Program (800-FDA-1088 or www.FDA.gov). A practitioner also has a responsibility to report a problem with any drug product or medical device using the MedWatch program. Reported problems may include product defects, product adulteration, container leakage, improper labeling, unexpected adverse reactions, and others.

A drug product recall may be initiated by the FDA or by the manufacturer, the latter being termed a voluntary recall. A numerical classification, as follows, indicates the degree of hazard associated with the product being recalled:

Class I: There is a reasonable probability that the use of or exposure to a violative product will cause serious adverse health consequences or death.

Class II: The use of or exposure to a violative product may cause temporary or medically reversible adverse health consequences or the probability of serious adverse health consequences is remote.

Class III: The use of or exposure to a violative product is not likely to cause adverse health consequences.

The depth of recall, or the level of market removal or correction (e.g., wholesaler, retailer, consumer), depends on the nature of the product, the urgency of the situation, and depth to which the product has been distributed. The lot numbers of packaging control numbers on the containers or labels of the products help in identifying the product to be recalled.

The Pharmacist's Contemporary Role

Pharmacy graduates holding the Bachelor of Science in Pharmacy (BS) degree or the Doctor of Pharmacy (PharmD) degree practice in a variety of settings, applying the basic pharmaceutical sciences, the clinical sciences, and professional training and experience. This includes practice in community pharmacies, patient care institutions, managed care, home health care, military and government service, academic settings, professional associations, and the pharmaceutical research and manufacturing industry, as well as in other positions requiring the pharmacist's expertise.

Historically, the abbreviation RPh (registered pharmacist) has been used as the professional designation of a pharmacist licensed by a state board of pharmacy to practice in that state. Doctors of Pharmacy use the PharmD after their name in place of RPh. To minimize any confusion from patients, some states now use the title DPh (Doctor of Pharmacy) to designate licensed pharmacists. This designation is used by pharmacists who have earned a Bachelor of Science in Pharmacy. Under this format, all pharmacists in the states where this has been implemented can be called doctor; one is a professional degree designation and the other a licensure designation.

Most pharmacists practice within an ambulatory care or community pharmacy setting. In this setting the pharmacist plays an active role in the patient's use of prescription and nonprescription medication, diagnostic agents, durable medical equipment and devices, and other health care products. The pharmacist develops individual patient medication profiles, issues patient information leaflets (PILs), counsels patients on their health status, and provides information on the use of drug and nondrug measures. As members of the health care team, pharmacists serve as a source of drug information and participate in the selection, monitoring, and assessment of drug therapy.

A substantial number of pharmacists practice in institutional settings, such as hospitals, clinics, extended care facilities, and health maintenance organizations (HMOs). In these settings, pharmacists manage drug distribution and control systems and provide a variety of clinical services, including drug utilization reviews (DURs), drug use evaluations, therapeutic drug monitoring, intravenous admixture programs, pharmacokinetic consulting services, investigational drug supplies, and poison control and drug information.

The Board of Pharmaceutical Specialties certifies practice specialties in nuclear pharmacy, nutrition support pharmacy, pharmacotherapy, psychiatric pharmacy, and oncology pharmacy.

In recent years, managed health care programs have grown extraordinarily. Managed health care organizations have enrolled a large and rapidly growing base of patients and thus have assumed major responsibilities in the delivery of health care, including the delivery of pharmaceutical services. Many new positions have evolved for pharmacists within the managed care industry, including positions for pharmacy benefits managers, disease management specialists, drug formulary managers, therapeutic outcomes researchers, drug utilization review specialists, and others (15, 16). In these functions, managed care pharmacists apply administrative, epidemiological, clinical, financial, research, information technology, and communication skills to their practice.

A number of pharmacy graduates, particularly those having an interest in institutional practice, participate in postgraduate residency and/or fellowship programs to enhance their practice and/or research skills. A pharmacy residency is an organized, directed postgraduate training program in a defined area of practice. The chief purpose is to train pharmacists in professional practice and management skills. Residency programs are conducted primarily in institutional practice settings. A fellowship to develop skill in research is a directed, highly individualized postgraduate program designed to prepare the participant to become an independent researcher. Both pharmacy residencies and fellowships last 12 months or longer and require the close direction of a qualified preceptor.

Pharmacists working for pharmaceutical research, development, and manufacturing firms can participate in a range of activities, including drug discovery, drug analysis and quality control, product development and production, clinical studies and drug evaluation, labeling and drug literature, marketing and sales, and management. The pharmacist's knowledge of the basic chemical, biological, and pharmaceutical sciences, along with technical knowledge of product formulation, dosage form design, and clinical use meshes well with the requirements of the pharmaceutical industry. Pharmacists with advanced degrees (Master of Science [MS] or Doctor of Philosophy [PhD]) in the basic or pharmaceutical sciences or in health care administration are highly sought in the pharmaceutical industry.

In government service, pharmacists perform professional and administrative functions in the development and implementation of pharmaceutical care delivery programs and in the design and enforcement of regulations involving drug distribution and drug quality standards. Career opportunities for pharmacists in government service at the federal level include positions in the military service, in the public health service, and in such civil service agencies as the FDA, Veterans Administration, Department of Health and Human Services, DEA, NIH, and others. At the state and local levels, many pharmacists find rewarding careers in health departments, family and children's services, drug investigation and regulatory control, clinics and other health care institutions, and with state boards of pharmacy.

Schools of pharmacy hire pharmacists, some with and some without advanced degrees, to serve as preceptors within the practice setting, to teach specific courses and/or laboratories within the academic institution, to participate in extramural research, and to contribute to the service and continuing education mission of the school. Some pharmacists work full time in the academic setting, whereas many others provide part-time professional instruction in community or hospital pharmacies, teaching hospitals and clinics, drug information centers, nursing homes and extended care facilities, health departments, home health

care, managed care, and other areas in which pharmaceutical services are delivered.

A number of pharmacists serve their profession in volunteer or professional positions with local, state, and national pharmaceutical associations.

Pharmacists exercise a vital health education role in their communities through participation in drug and health education community forums, by speaking on drug issues in schools, by conducting in-service education programs in patient care settings, and by providing input on drug and health issues to legislators and other community leaders and officials.

The Mission of Pharmacy

In 1990, the board of trustees of the APhA adopted the following mission statement for pharmacy (17):

> The mission of pharmacy is to serve society as the profession responsible for the appropriate use of medications, devices, and services to achieve optimal therapeutic outcomes.

The elements of the statement were defined as follows:

> Pharmacy is the health profession that concerns itself with the knowledge system that results in the discovery, development, and use of medications and medication information in the care of patients. It encompasses the clinical, scientific, economic, and educational aspects of the profession's knowledge base and its communication to others in the health-care system.
>
> Society encompasses patients, other health-care providers, health-policy decision makers, corporate health benefits managers, the healthy public, and other individuals and groups to whom health care and medication use are important.
>
> Appropriate refers to the pharmacist's responsibility to ensure that a medication regimen is specifically tailored for the individual patient, based on accepted clinical and pharmacological parameters. Further, the pharmacist should evaluate the regimen to assure maximum safety, cost effectiveness, and compliance by the patient.
>
> Medications refers to legend and nonlegend agents used in the diagnosis, treatment, prevention, and/or cure of disease. The term is specifically and purposefully used and is distinguished from the term drug, which has a negative and nontherapeutic public image.
>
> Devices refers to the equipment, process, biotechnological entities, diagnostic agents, or other products that are used to assist in effective management of the medication regimen.

Services refers to patient, health professional and public education services, screening and monitoring programs, medication-regimen management, and related activities that contribute to effective medication use by patients.

Optimal therapeutic outcomes declares the profession's ultimate contribution to public health. Pharmacy asserts it unique rights, privileges, and responsibilities—and accepts the attendant liabilities—associated with medication use. Pharmacy recognizes the need effectively to integrate its healthcare role with the complementary roles of the patient and other health care professionals.

Definition of Pharmaceutical Care

Today, the role of the pharmacist in contemporary practice is the delivery of pharmaceutical care, which was first proposed in 1975 by Mikeal and others as "the care that a given patient requires and receives which assures rational drug usage" (18). Since then, the term has been redefined by many authors, including Strand and others who in 1992 stated (19):

> Pharmaceutical care is that component of pharmacy practice which entails the direct interaction of the pharmacist with the patient for the purpose of caring for that patient's drug-related needs.

The American Society of Health-System Pharmacists (ASHP), a national organization that represents pharmacists who practice in hospitals, HMOs, long-term care facilities, home care agencies, and other components of health care systems, advanced the following statement on pharmaceutical care in 1993 (20):

> The mission of the pharmacist is to provide pharmaceutical care. Pharmaceutical care is the direct, responsible provision of medication-related care for the purpose of achieving definite outcomes that improve a patient's quality of life.

The American Pharmaceutical Association in 1996 issued its Principles of Practice for Pharmaceutical Care, including the following general statement (21):

> Pharmaceutical care is a patient-centered, outcomes-oriented pharmacy practice that requires the pharmacist to work in concert with the patient and the patient's other healthcare providers to promote health, to prevent disease, and to assess, monitor, initiate, and modify medication use to assure that drug therapy regimens are safe and effective.
>
> The goal of pharmaceutical care is to optimize the patient's health-related quality of life and achieve positive clinical outcomes, within realistic economic expenditures.

Implicit in all of these statements is the requirement of pharmacists to participate fully in all aspects of medication distribution and their appropriate clinical use to achieve optimal therapeutic outcomes. The contemporary pharmacy literature is replete with research papers and articles in support of the concept and practice of pharmaceutical care, including: clinical skill development (22), pharmaceutical care databases (23), information technology (24), literature retrieval (25), therapeutic drug monitoring and outcomes assessment (26–29), drug utilization review (30), pharmacotherapy and disease management (31–32), drug treatment protocols (33), adverse drug reaction monitoring (34), pharmacokinetic services (35), and strategies to implement pharmaceutical care (36).

In 1997, the American Association of Colleges of Pharmacy's Janus Commission issued a report, *Approaching the Millennium*, which stated that to provide pharmaceutical care, the successful pharmacy graduate must be (37):

- A problem solver, capable of adapting to changes in health care
- Able to achieve health outcomes through effective medication use that are valued by the health care system
- Able to collaborate with and be a resource to physicians, nurses, and other health care team members
- A committed life-long learner

Pharmacy Practice Standards

The scope and standards of pharmacy practice are established in each state through laws and regulations promulgated by the state's board of pharmacy. Together with applicable federal laws, they constitute the basis for the legal practice of pharmacy.

Over the years, various professional associations in pharmacy have developed documents termed standards of practice. One such document, *Practice Standards of the American Society of Health-System Pharmacists*, is updated and published annually. In 1991, the APhA, the American Association of Colleges of Pharmacy, and the National Association of Boards of Pharmacy studied the scope of pharmacy practice to revalidate the Standards of Practice for the Profession of Pharmacy (which were published in 1979 and updated in 1986 as Competency Statements for Pharmacy Practice (38). They can be summarized as follows:

> General management and administration of the pharmacy: Selects and supervises pharmacists and nonprofessionals for pharmacy staff; establishes a pricing structure for pharmaceutical services and products; administers budgets and negotiates with vendors; develops and maintains a purchasing and inventory system for all drugs and pharmaceutical supplies; initiates a formulary system. In general, establishes and administers pharmacy management, personnel and fiscal policy.
>
> Processing the prescription: Verifies prescription for legality and physical and chemical compatibility; checks patient's record before dispensing prescription; measures quantities needed to dispense prescription; performs final check of finished prescription; dispenses prescription.
>
> Patient care functions: Clarifies patient's understanding of dosage; integrates drug with patient information; advises patient of potential drug-related conditions; refers patient to other health care resources; monitors and evaluates therapeutic response of patient; reviews and/or seeks additional drug-related information.
>
> Education of health care professionals and patients: Organizes, maintains, and provides drug information to other health care professionals; organizes and/or participates in in-pharmacy education programs for other pharmacists; makes recommendations regarding drug therapy to physician or patient; develops and maintains system for drug distributions and quality control.

In 1998, a consortium of 10 pharmacy organizations undertook a pharmacy practice activity classification project to develop uniform language in describing practice activities in such areas as pharmacotherapy, monitoring and therapeutic outcomes, dispensing medications,

health promotion and disease prevention, and health systems management (39). The developed classification is intended to provide the common language to be used and understood within and outside of the profession in describing the practice activities of pharmacists.

The Omnibus Budget Reconciliation Act of 1990

The Omnibus Budget Reconciliation Act of 1990 (OBRA 90), which became effective on January 1, 1993, established a requirement for each state to develop and mandate DUR programs to improve the quality of pharmaceutical care provided to patients covered by the federal medical assistance (Medicaid) program (40, 41). The statute was designed to ensure that prescriptions are appropriate, medically necessary, and not likely to result in adverse medical effects. The statute required that each state's plan provide for a review of drug therapy before each prescription is filled and delivered to an eligible patient.

The regulations required patient medication monitoring for therapeutic appropriateness, therapeutic duplication, overuse, underuse, drug–disease contraindications, drug–drug interactions with other prescribed and OTC medications, drug–allergy interactions, correct drug dosage, duration of treatment, and clinical abuse or misuse. They also required that pharmacists offer therapeutic counseling to each recipient of a prescription or the recipient's caregiver regarding the drug, dosage and duration of use, route of administration, side effects, contraindications, techniques for self-monitoring drug therapy, proper storage, refill information, and action to be taken in the event of a missed dose. Pharmacists are to maintain patient medication profiles and therapeutic counseling records.

In designing the DUR programs, state boards of pharmacy commonly included the federal requirements in the state's pharmacy practice regulations, thereby applying them to each recipient of a prescription, not only to patients receiving benefits under the Medicaid program. Many states used the model regulations for the practice of pharmaceutical care developed by the National Association of Boards of Pharmacy.

Code of Ethics for Pharmacists of the American Pharmaceutical Association

By definition, a profession is founded on an art, built on specialized intellectual training, and has as its primary objective the performing of a service. The principles on which the professional practice of pharmacy is based are embodied in the Code of Ethics of the APhA.

The APhA Code of Ethics has been revised over the years to reflect dynamic changes in the profession. The current version is as follows.

These principles of professional conduct for Pharmacists are established to guide the pharmacist in his relationship with patients, fellow practitioners, other health professionals, and the public.

- A Pharmacist should hold the health and safety of patients to be of first consideration; he should render to each patient the full measure of his ability as an essential health practitioner.
- A Pharmacist should never condone the dispensing, promoting, or distributing of drugs or medical devices, or assist therein, which are not of good quality, which do not meet standards required by law or which lack therapeutic value for the patient.
- A pharmacist should always strive to perfect and enlarge his professional knowledge. He should utilize and make available this knowledge as may be required in accordance with his best professional judgment.
- A Pharmacist has the duty to observe the law, to uphold the dignity and honor of the profession, and to accept its ethical principles. He should not engage in any activity that will bring discredit to the profession and should expose, without fear or favor, illegal or unethical conduct in the profession.
- A Pharmacist should seek at all times only fair and reasonable remuneration for his services. He should never agree to or participate in transactions with practitioners of other health professions or any other person under which fees are divided or which may cause financial or other exploitation in connection with the rendering of his professional services.
- A Pharmacist should respect the confidential and personal nature of his professional records; except where the best interest of the patient requires or the law demands, he should not disclose such information to anyone without proper patient authorization.
- A Pharmacist should not agree to practice under terms or conditions which tend to interfere with or impair the proper exercise of his professional judgment and skill, which tend to cause a deterioration of the quality of his service or which require him to consent to unethical conduct.

- A Pharmacist should strive to provide information to patients regarding professional services truthfully, accurately, and fully, and should avoid misleading patients regarding the nature, cost, or value of the Pharmacist's professional services.
- A Pharmacist should associate with organizations having for their objective the betterment of the profession of pharmacy; he should contribute of his time and funds to carry on the work of these organizations.

Code of Ethics of the American Association of Pharmaceutical Scientists

Like pharmacy practitioners, pharmaceutical scientists recognize their special obligation to society and to the public welfare. Members of the American Association of Pharmaceutical Scientists (AAPS) have adopted the following code of ethics (42).

In their scientific pursuits, they:

Conduct their work in a manner that adheres to the highest principles of scientific research so as to merit the confidence and trust of peers and the public in particular regarding the rights of human subjects and concern for the proper use of animals involved and provision for suitable safeguards against environmental damage.

Avoid scientific misconduct and expose it when encountered. AAPS uses the current federal definition of scientific misconduct, 65 FR 76260-76264: Fabrication, falsification, and plagiarism in proposing, performing, or reviewing research or reporting research results.

Recognize latitude for differences of scientific opinion in the interpretation of scientific data and that such differences of opinion do not constitute unethical conduct.

Disclose sources of external financial support for, or significant financial interests in the content of, research reports/publications and avoid the manipulation of the release of such information for illegal financial gain.

Report results accurately, stating explicitly any known or suspected bias, opposing efforts to improperly modify data or conclusions and offering professional advice only on those subjects concerning which they regard themselves competent through scientific education, training or experience.

Respect the known ownership rights of others in scientific research and seek prior authorization from the owner before disclosure or use of such information including the contents of manuscripts submitted for prepublication review.

Support in their research and among their employers the participation and employment of all qualified persons regardless of race, gender, creed or national origin.

REFERENCES

1. History of the Pharmacopeia of the United States. In: United States Pharmacopeia, 23rd rev. Rockville, MD: United States Pharmacopeial Convention, Inc., 1995;xlii–xlv.
2. Constitution and bylaws. USP 26-NF 21, The United States Pharmacopeial Convention, Rockville, MD, 2003, pp 2865–2875.
3. History of the National Formulary. In: National Formulary, 18th ed. Rockville, MD: United States Pharmacopeial Convention, 1995;2196–2200.
4. Chavez ML. Homeopathy. Hosp Pharm 1998;33: 41–49.
5. Der Marderosian AH. Understanding homeopathy. J Am Pharm Assoc 1996;NS36:317–321.
6. Pray WS. The challenge to professionalism presented by homeopathy. Am J Pharm Ed 1996;60:198–204.
7. The United States Pharmacopeia, 23rd rev. Rockville, MD: United States Pharmacopeial Convention, 1995:liv.
8. Hassler J, Yankowsky, A. An overview of ISO 9001 certification. BioPharm 1995;19:48–50.
9. FDA. The thalidomide tragedy—25 years ago. FDA Consumer 1987;21:14–17.
10. Safety issues raised as thalidomide is considered for approval. Pharm Today 1997;3:1.
11. FDA talk paper. Rockville, MD: Food and Drug Administration 1997;T97–43:1–4.
12. Levien T, Baker DE, Ballasiotes, AA. Reviews of dexrazoxane and thalidomide. Hosp Pharm 1996;31:487–510.
13. Bonnell L. Packaging nutritional supplements. Pharmaceut Med Packaging News 1997;5:42–50.
14. Wechsler J. Congress modernizes FDA. Pharm Tech 1997;21:16–26.
15. Wynn P. New directions in pharmacy careers. Managed Care Pharm Prac 1996;3:14–19.
16. Vogenberg FR. Managed health care: a review. Hosp Pharm 1997;32:975–982.
17. The mission of pharmacy. Washington: American Pharmaceutical Association. http://www.pharmacyandyou.org/about/aboutapha.html; accessed 8/9/2003.
18. Mikeal RL, Brown TP, Lazarus HL, Vinson MC. Quality of pharmaceutical care in hospitals. Am J Hosp Pharm 1975;32:567–574.
19. Strand LM, Cipolle RJ, Morley PC. Pharmaceutical care: an introduction. Current Concepts. Kalamazoo MI: Upjohn, 1992.
20. American Society of Health-System Pharmacists. ASHP Guidelines on a Standardized Method of Pharmaceutical Care. Am J Health-Syst Pharm 1996;53:1713–1716.
21. Principles of practice for pharmaceutical care. Washington: American Pharmaceutical Association. http://www.aphanet.org/pharmcare/prinprac.html; accessed 8/9/2003.

22. Barnette DJ, Murphy CM, Carter BL. Clinical skill development for community pharmacists. JAPhA 1996;NS36:573–579.
23. Rodriquez de Bittner M, Michocki R. Pharmaceutical care databases. JAPhA 1997;NS37:595–596.
24. West DS, Szeinbach S. Information technology and pharmaceutical care. JAPhA 1997;NS37:497–501.
25. Grant KL, Herrier RN, Armstrong EP. Teaching a systematic search strategy improves literature retrieval skills of pharmacy students. Am J Pharm Ed 1996;60:281–286.
26. Madan PL. Therapeutic drug monitoring. US Pharm 1996;21:92–105.
27. McDonough RP. Interventions to improve patient pharmaceutical care outcomes. JAPhA 1996;NS36: 453–459.
28. Grainger-Rousseau TJ, Miralles MA, Hepler CH, et al. Therapeutic outcomes monitoring: application of pharmaceutical care guidelines to community pharmacy. JAPhA 1997;NS37:647–661.
29. Mullins, CD, Baldwin R, Perfetto, EM. What are outcomes? JAPhA 1996;NS36:39–49.
30. Kubacka RT. A primer on drug utilization review. JAPhA 1996;NS36:257–261.
31. Armstrong EP, Langley PC. Disease management programs. Am J Health-Syst Pharm 1996;53:53–58.
32. Rodriques de Bittner M, Haines ST. Pharmacy-based diabetes management: a practical approach. JAPhA 1997;NS37:443–455.
33. APhA Guide to drug treatment protocols. Washington: American Pharmaceutical Association, 1997.
34. ASHP guidelines on adverse drug reaction monitoring and reporting. Bethesda MD: American Society of Health-System Pharmacists, 1995.
35. ASHP statement on the pharmacist's role in clinical pharmacokinetic services. Bethesda MD: American Society of Health-System Pharmacists, 1989.
36. Chrymko MM. Strategies for implementing pharmaceutical care in a community health system. Hosp Pharm 1996;31:1567–1576.
37. Approaching the Millennium: The Report of the AACP Janus Commission. Alexandria VA: American Association of Colleges of Pharmacy, 1997.
38. Pancorbo SA, Campagna KD, Davenport JK, et al. Task force report of competency statements for pharmacy practice. Am J Pharm Ed 1987;51:196–206.
39. Pharmacy Practice Classification. JAPhA 1998;38: 139–148.
40. Medicaid program: drug use review program and electronic claims management system for outpatient drug claims. Washington: Health Care Financing Administration, Department of Health and Human Services, 1992; Federal Register 57:49397–49412.
41. Brushwood DB, Catizone CA, Coster J M. OBRA 90: what it means to your practice. US Pharm 1992;17: 64–73.
42. American Association of Pharmaceutical Scientists, Alexandria, VA.

New Drug Development and Approval Process

2

The federal Food, Drug, and Cosmetic Act, as regulated through Title 21 of the U.S. *Code of Federal Regulations*, requires a new drug to be approved by the Food and Drug Administration (FDA) before it may be legally introduced in interstate commerce (1). The regulations apply to drug products manufactured domestically and those imported into the United States.

To gain approval for marketing, a drug's sponsor (e.g., a pharmaceutical company) must demonstrate, through supporting scientific evidence, that the new drug or drug product is safe and effective for its proposed use. The sponsor must also demonstrate that the various processes and controls used in producing the drug substance and in manufacturing, packaging, and labeling are properly controlled and validated to ensure that the product meets established standards of quality.

The process and time course from drug discovery to approval for marketing can be lengthy and tedious but are well defined and understood in the pharmaceutical industry. A schematic representation of the process for new drug development is shown in Figure 2.1 and the usual time course is depicted in Figure 2.2. After the discovery (e.g., synthesis) of a proposed new drug, the agent is biologically characterized for pharmacologic and toxicologic effects and for potential therapeutic application. Preformulation studies are initiated to define the physical and chemical properties of the agent. Formulation studies follow to develop the initial features of the proposed pharmaceutical product or dosage form. To obtain the required evidence demonstrating the drug's safety and effectiveness for its proposed use, a carefully designed and progressive sequence of preclinical (e.g., cell culture, whole animal) and clinical (human) studies are undertaken.

Only when the preclinical studies demonstrate adequate safety and the new agent shows promise as a useful drug will the drug's sponsor file an investigational new drug application (IND) with the FDA for initial testing in humans. If the drug demonstrates adequate safety in these initial human studies, termed Phase 1, progressive human trials through Phases 2 and 3 are undertaken to assess safety and efficacy. As the clinical trials progress, laboratory work continues toward defining the agent's basic and clinical pharmacology and toxicology, product design and development, manufacturing scale-up and process controls, analytical methods development, proposed labeling and package design, and initial plans for marketing. At the completion of the carefully designed preclinical and clinical studies, the drug's sponsor may file a new drug application (NDA) seeking approval to market the new product.

The FDA's approval of an NDA indicates that the body of scientific evidence submitted sufficiently demonstrates that the drug or drug product is safe and effective for the proposed clinical indications, that there is adequate assurance of its proper manufacture and control, and that the final labeling accurately presents the necessary information for its proper use. Some products, however, have been approved and later removed from the market for safety reasons, including grepafloxacin HCl (Raxar), bromfenac sodium (Duract), cisapride (Propulsid), alosetron HCl (Lotrovec), fenfluramine HCl (Pondimin), dexfenfluramine HCl (Redux), terfenadine (Seldane), cerivastatin (Baycol), mibefradil (Posicor), astemizole (Hismanal), and troglitazone (Rezulin).

The content of a product's approved labeling, represented by the package insert, is a summary of the entire drug development process because it contains the essential chemistry, pharmacology, toxicology, indications and contraindications for use, adverse effects, formulation composition, dosage, and storage requirements, as ascertained during the research and development.

In addition to the general new drug approval process, special regulations apply for the approval of certain new drugs to treat serious or life-threatening illnesses, such as AIDS and cancer. These may be placed on an accelerated or fast-track program for approval. Also, if there are no satisfactory approved drug or treatment alternatives for a serious medical condition, special protocols may be issued permitting use of an investigational drug to treat some patients prior to approval of the NDA. This type of protocol is termed a treatment IND. Treatment INDs often are sought for orphan drugs, which are targeted for small

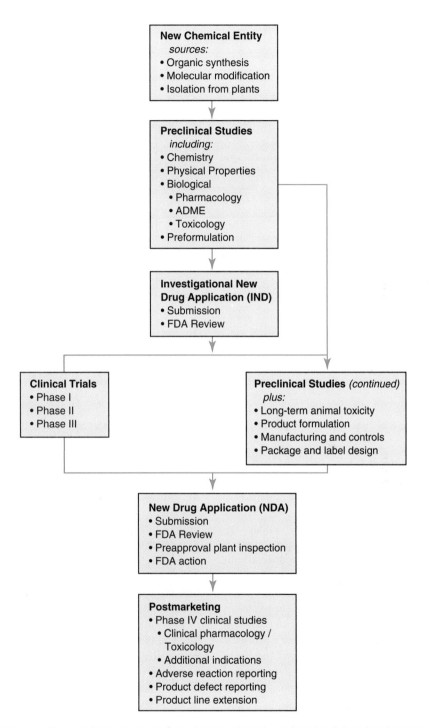

FIGURE 2.1 The new drug development process from discovery through preclinical and clinical studies, FDA review of the new drug application, and postmarketing activities.

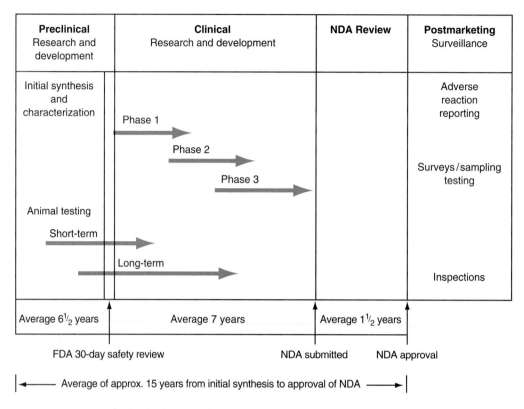

FIGURE 2.2 Time course for the development of a new drug. (Adapted from FDA Consumer, 21:5,1987; New Drug Approvals in 1997, Pharmaceutical Research and Manufacturers Association, Washington, DC, January 1998.)

numbers of patients who have rare conditions or diseases for which there are no satisfactory alternative treatments.

For certain changes in a previously approved NDA, such as a labeling or formulation change, a manufacturer is required to submit for approval a supplemental new drug application (SNDA).

An abbreviated new drug application (ANDA) is used to gain approval to market a duplicate (usually a competing generic product) of a product that is already approved and being marketed by the pioneer, or original sponsor, of the drug. In these instances, the sponsor of the ANDA provides documentation on the chemistry, manufacturing, controls, and bioavailability of the proposed product to demonstrate biologic equivalence to the original product (2). Clinical data on the drug's safety and efficacy are not required because clinical studies were provided by the pioneer sponsor.

Federal regulations are varied and specific for antibiotic drugs (3); for biologics, such as human blood products and vaccines, which require approval of a biologics licensing application (BLA) for distribution (4); for over-the-counter (OTC) drugs (5); and for animal drugs, which may require an investigational new animal drug application (INADA), a new animal drug application (NADA) or a supplemental new animal drug application (SNADA) (6). Medical devices, such as catheters and cardiac pacemakers, follow a separate approval process as defined in the *Code of Federal Regulations* (7).

The following sections are intended to serve as an overview of the new drug development and approval process. More specific and detailed information may be obtained directly from the referenced sections of the *Code of Federal Regulations* (1–7), from relevant entries in the *Federal Register* (8), and from other treatises on the topic (9–13).

Drug Discovery and Drug Design

The discovery of new drugs and their development into commercial products takes place across the broad scope of the pharmaceutical industry. The basic underpinning for this effort is the cumulative body of scientific and biomedical information generated worldwide in research institutes, academic centers, and industry. The combined efforts of chemists, biologists, molecular biologists, pharmacologists, toxicologists, statisticians, physicians, pharmacists and pharmaceutical scientists, engineers, and many others participate in drug discovery and development.

Some pharmaceutical firms focus their research and development (R&D) activities on new prescription drugs for human use, whereas other firms concentrate on the development of OTC medications, generic drugs, biotechnology products, animal health care drugs, diagnostic products, and/or medical devices. Many of the large pharmaceutical companies develop and manufacture products of various types, with some firms having subsidiary companies for specialized functions and products.

The pharmaceutical industry in the United States grew rapidly during World War II and in the years immediately following. The upsurge in the domestic production of drugs and pharmaceutical products stemmed in part from the wartime hazards and consequent undependability of overseas shipping, the unavailability of drugs from previous sources, and the increased need for drugs of all kinds, but especially those with life-saving capabilities. One such drug is penicillin, the antibiotic that became commercially available in 1944, 15 years after its discovery in England by Sir Alexander Fleming and 1 year before the end of the war.

After the war, other antibiotics were developed, and today there is a host of them, with effectiveness against a range of pathogens. The postwar boom in drug discovery continued with the development of many new agents, such as vaccines to protect against poliomyelitis, measles, and influenza, and new pharmacologic categories of drugs including oral hypoglycemic drugs effective against certain types of diabetes mellitus, antineoplastic or anticancer drugs, immunosuppressive agents to assist the body's acceptance of organ transplants, oral contraceptives to prevent pregnancy, and a host of tranquilizers and antidepressant drugs to treat the emotionally distressed.

In recent years, many new and important innovative therapeutic agents have been developed and approved by the FDA, including drugs to treat AIDS (efavirenz [Sustiva], didanosine [Videx EC], tenofovir [Viread]), prostate cancer (leuprolide acetate [Eligard], triptorelin pamoate [Trelstar]), hyperlipidemia (lovastatin [Mevacor]), pulmonary arterial hypertension (treprostinil sodium [Remodulin]); infectious diseases (moxifloxacin hydrochloride [Avelox], voriconazole [Vfend]); chronic asthma (montelukast sodium [Singulair]); irritable bowel syndrome in women (tegaserod maleate [Zelnorm]); cataplexy in patients with narcolepsy (sodium oxybate [Xyrem]), dementia associated with Alzheimer's disease (galantamine hydrochloride [Reminyl]), deep vein thrombosis (fondaparinux sodium [Arixtra]), and other diseases and conditions, with literally hundreds of potential therapeutic agents in various stages of clinical evaluation. Annually, approximately 40 new molecular entities receive FDA approval for marketing. In addition, many new dosage strengths and dosage forms of previously approved drugs, new generic products, and new biologics are approved each year.

Not all drugs are discovered, developed, and first approved in the United States. Many pharmaceutical companies do drug research and development in other countries, and many drugs are first marketed abroad. Many of the world's largest pharmaceutical companies are multinational firms with facilities for research and development, manufacturing, and distribution in countries around the world. Irrespective of country of origin, a drug may be proposed by its sponsor for regulatory approval for marketing in the United States and/or in other countries. These approvals do not occur simultaneously, as they are subject to the laws, regulations, and requirements peculiar to each country's governing authority.

However, the international effort to harmonize regulations through the work of the International Conference on Harmonization (ICH) as described at the end of this chapter fosters multinational drug approvals.

Sources of New Drugs

New drugs may be discovered from a variety of natural sources or synthesized in the laboratory. They may be discovered by accident or as the result of many years of tireless pursuit.

Throughout history, plant materials have served as a reservoir of potential new drugs. Yet only a small portion of the approximately 270,000 known plants thus far have been investigated for medicinal activity. Certain major contributions to modern drug therapy may be attributed to the successful conversion of botanic folklore remedies into modern wonder drugs. The chemical reserpine, a tranquilizer and hypotensive agent, is an example of a medicinal chemical isolated by design from the folklore remedy *Rauwolfia serpentina*. Another plant drug, periwinkle, or *Vinca rosea*, was first scientifically investigated as a result of its reputation in folklore as an agent useful in the treatment of diabetes mellitus. Plant extracts from *Vinca rosea* yield two potent drugs, which when screened for pharmacologic activity, surprisingly exhibited antitumor capabilities. These two materials, vinblastine and vincristine, since have been used successfully in the treatment of certain types of cancer, including acute leukemia, Hodgkin's disease, lymphocytic lymphoma, and other malignancies. Another example, paclitaxel (Taxol), prepared from an extract of the Pacific yew tree, is used in the treatment of ovarian cancer.

After the isolation and structural identification of active plant constituents, organic chemists may recreate them by total synthesis in the laboratory or more important, use the natural chemical as the starting material in the creation of slightly different chemical structures through molecular manipulation. The new structures, termed semisynthetic drugs, may have a slightly or vastly different pharmacologic activity from that of the starting substance, depending on the nature and extent of chemical alteration. Other plant constituents that in themselves may be inactive or rather unimportant therapeutically may be chemically modified to yield important drugs with profound pharmacologic activity. For example, the various species of *Dioscorea*, popularly known as Mexican yams, are rich in the chemical *steroid structure* from which cortisone and estrogens are semisynthetically produced.

Animals have served humans in their search for drugs in a number of ways. They not only have yielded to drug testing and biologic assay but also have provided drugs that are mannered from their tissues or through their biologic processes. Hormonal substances, such as thyroid extract, insulin, and pituitary hormone obtained from the endocrine glands of cattle, sheep, and swine, are lifesaving drugs used daily as replacement therapy in the human body. The urine of pregnant mares is a rich source of estrogens. Knowledge of the structural architecture of the individual hormonal substances has produced a variety of synthetic and semisynthetic compounds with hormone-like activity. The synthetic chemicals used as oral contraceptives are notable examples.

The use of animals in the production of various biologic products, including serums, antitoxins, and vaccines, has had lifesaving significance ever since the pioneering work of Edward Jenner on the smallpox vaccine in England in 1796. Today the poliomyelitis vaccine is prepared in cultures of renal monkey tissue, the mumps and influenza vaccines in fluids of chick embryo, the rubella (German measles) vaccine in duck embryo, and the smallpox vaccine from the skin of bovine calves inoculated with vaccinia virus. New vaccines for diseases as AIDS and cancer are being developed through the use of cell and tissue cultures.

Today we are witnessing a new era in the development of pharmaceutical products as a result of the advent of genetic engineering, the submicroscopic manipulation of the double helix, the spiral DNA chain of life. Through this process will come more abundant and vastly purer antibiotics, vaccines, and yet unknown chemical and biologic products to combat human disease.

The two basic technologies that drive the genetic field of drug development are recombinant DNA and monoclonal antibody production (14–16). Common to each technique is the ability to manipulate and produce proteins, the building blocks of living matter. Proteins are an almost infinite source of drugs. Made up of long chains of amino acids, their sequence and spatial configuration offer a staggering number of possibilities. Both recombinant rDNA and monoclonal antibody production techniques influence cells' ability to produce proteins.

The more fundamental of the two techniques is recombinant DNA. It has the potential to produce almost any protein. Genetic material can be transplanted from higher species, such as humans, into a lowly bacterium. This so-called gene splicing can induce the lower organism to make proteins it would not otherwise have made. Such drug products as human insulin, human growth hormone, hepatitis B vaccine, epoetin-alpha, and interferon are being produced in this manner.

Whereas recombinant DNA techniques involve the manipulation of proteins within the cells of lower animals, monoclonal antibody production is conducted entirely within the cells of higher animals, including the patient. The technique exploits the ability of cells with the potential to produce a desired antibody and stimulates an unending stream of pure antibody production. These antibodies have the capacity to combat the specific target.

Monoclonal antibodies have an enormous potential to change the face of medicine and pharmacy in the next decade, and applications for their use are already in progress. Diagnostically, for example, monoclonal antibodies are used in home pregnancy testing products. Their use ensures that a woman can perform the test easily in a short period with high reproducibility and in an inexpensive manner. In these tests, the monoclonal antibody is highly sensitive to binding on one site on the human chorionic gonadotropin (HCG) molecule, a specific marker to pregnancy because in healthy women, HCG is synthesized exclusively by the placenta. In medicine, monoclonal antibodies are being used to stage and to localize malignant cells of cancer, and it is anticipated that they will be used in the future to combat disease such as lupus erythematosus, juvenile-onset diabetes, and myasthenia gravis.

Human gene therapy, used to prevent, treat, cure, diagnose, or mitigate human disease caused by genetic disorders, is another promising new technology. The human body contains up to 100,000 genes. Genes that are aligned on a double strand of DNA in the nucleus of every cell control all of the body's functions. Base pairs of adenine and thymine (A and T, respectively) and cytosine and guanine (C and G, respectively) constitute the instructions on a gene. Only genes necessary for a specific cell's function are active or expressed. When a gene is expressed, a specific type of protein is produced. In genetic diseases, gene expression may be altered and/or gene sequences may be mismatched, partly missing, or repeated too many times, causing cellular malfunction and disease.

Gene therapy is a medical intervention based on the modification of the genetic material of living cells. Cells may be modified outside the body (ex vivo) for subsequent administration, or they may be modified within the body (in vivo) by gene therapy products given directly to the patient. In either case, gene therapy entails the transfer of new genetic material to the cells of a patient with a genetic disease. The genetic material, usually cloned DNA, may be transferred into the patient's cells physically, as through microinjection, through chemically mediated transfer procedures, or through disabled retroviral gene transfer systems that integrate genetic material directly into the host cell chromosomes (17–19).

The first human gene therapy used was to treat adenosine deaminase (ADA) deficiency, a condition that results in abnormal functioning of the immune system. Therapy consisted of the administration of genetically modified cells capable of producing ADA (18). Many emerging biopharmaceutical companies are exploring the application of gene therapy to treat sickle cell anemia, malignant melanoma, renal cell cancer, heart disease, familial hypercholesterolemia, cystic fibrosis, lung and colorectal cancer, and AIDS (20).

Although there is justified excitement and great expectation for the potential of the new biotechnologies in the development of advanced therapies, the work of the synthetic organic chemist remains today's most usual source of new drugs. The modern chemist's work is enhanced by computer-based molecular modeling, access to huge chemical libraries, and the use of high-throughput screening to discover compounds having an affinity for specific biologic target sites (21–22).

A Goal Drug

In theory, a goal drug would produce the specifically desired effect, be administered by the most desired route (generally orally) at minimal dosage and dosing frequency, have optimal onset and duration of activity, exhibit no side effects, and following its desired effect would be eliminated from the body efficiently, completely, and without residual effect. It would also be easily produced at low cost, pharmaceutically elegant, and physically and chemically stable in various conditions of use and storage. Although not completely attainable in practice, these qualities and features are sought in drug and dosage form design.

Methods of Drug Discovery

Although some drugs may be the result of fortuitous discovery, most drugs are the result of carefully designed research programs of screening, molecular modification, and mechanism-based drug design (23).

Random or untargeted screening involves the testing of large numbers of synthetic organic compounds or substances of natural origin for biologic activity. Random screens may be used initially to detect an unknown activity of the test compound or substance or to identify the most promising compounds to be studied by more sophisticated *nonrandom* or targeted screens to determine a specific activity.

Although random and nonrandom screening programs can examine a host of new compounds for activity, sometimes promising compounds may be overlooked if the screening models are not sensitive enough to reflect ac-

curately the specific disease against which the agent or its metabolites may be useful (24).

To detect and evaluate biologic activity, *bioassays* are used to differentiate the effect and potency (strength of effect) of the test agent from those of controls of known action and effect. The initial bioassays may be performed in vitro using cell cultures to test the new agent's effect against enzyme systems or tumor cells, whereas subsequent bioassays may be performed in vivo and use more expensive and disease-specific animal models.

Newer methods, such as high-throughput screening, are capable of examining 15,000 chemical compounds a week using 10 to 20 biologic assays (22). To be effective, this requires a sizable and chemically diverse collection of compounds to examine, which many pharmaceutical and chemical companies have in chemical libraries. Frequently these libraries, which may contain hundreds of thousands of compounds, are purchased or licensed from academic or commercial sources. With the advent of techniques like combinatorial chemistry, it has become feasible to increase substantially the size and diversity of a chemical library (22).

Molecular modification is chemical alteration of a known and previously characterized organic compound (frequently a *lead compound*; see next section) for the purpose of enhancing its usefulness as a drug. This could mean enhancing its specificity for a particular body target site, increasing its potency, improving its rate and extent of absorption, modifying to advantage its time course in the body, reducing its toxicity, or changing its physical or chemical properties (e.g., solubility) to provide desired features (23). The molecular modifications may be slight or substantial, involving changes in functional groups, ring structures, or configuration. Knowledge of chemical structure–pharmacologic activity relationships plays an important role in designing new drug molecules. Molecular modification produces new chemical entities and improved therapeutic agents. Figure 2.3, *A* and *B* shows the molecular modifications that led to the discoveries of the first commercial beta blocker, propranolol, and the first commercial histamine H_2-receptor blocking agent, cimetidine.

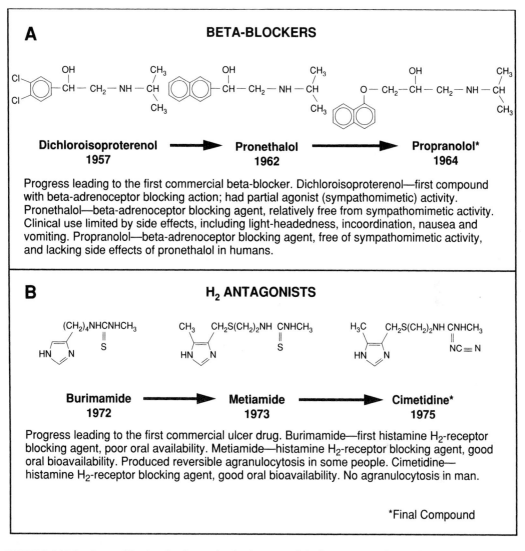

FIGURE 2.3 Molecular modifications leading to the development of the first commercial beta blocker, propranolol, and the first commercial histamine H_2-receptor blocking agent, cimetidine. (Reprinted with permission from Maxwell RA. The state of the art of the science of drug discovery. Drug Development Research 1984;4:375–389; through Pharmaceutical Research: Therapeutic and Economic Value of Incremental Improvements, 1990;12. Courtesy of National Pharmaceutical Council, Reston, VA).

Mechanism-based drug design is molecular modification to design a drug that interferes specifically with the known or suspected biochemical pathway or mechanism of a disease process. The intention is the interaction of the drug with specific cell receptors, enzyme systems, or the metabolic processes of pathogens or tumor cells, resulting in a blocking, disruption, or reversal of the disease process. For this it is essential to understand the biochemical pathway of the disease process and the manner in which it is regulated. *Molecular graphics*, the use of computer graphics to represent and manipulate the structure of the drug molecule to fit the simulated molecular structure of the receptor site, is a useful complementary tool in drug molecule design.

An example of mechanism-based drug design is the compound enalaprilat (Vasotec), which inhibits the angiotensin-converting enzyme (ACE) that catalyzes the conversion of angiotensin I to the vasoconstrictor substance angiotensin II. Inhibition of the enzyme results in decreased plasma angiotensin II, leading to decreased vasopressor effects and lower blood pressure. Another example is ranitidine (Zantac), an inhibitor of histamine at the histamine H_2-receptors, including receptors on the gastric cells. This inhibits gastric acid secretion, making the drug effective in the treatment of gastric ulcers and other gastrointestinal conditions related to the production of gastric acid. A third example is sertraline (Zoloft), which inhibits the central nervous system's neuronal uptake of serotonin, making the drug useful in the treatment of depression.

A Lead Compound

A lead compound is a prototype chemical compound that has a fundamental desired biologic or pharmacologic activity. Although active, the lead compound may not possess all of the features desired, such as potency, absorbability, solubility, low toxicity, and so forth. Thus, the medicinal chemist may seek to modify the lead compound's chemical structure to achieve the desired features while reducing the undesired ones. The chemical modifications produce analogs with additional or different functional chemical groups, altered ring structures, or different chemical configurations. The results are modified chemical compounds capable of having different interactions with the body's receptors, thereby eliciting different actions and intensities of action.

The synthesis of derivatives of the prototype chemical may ultimately lead to successive generations of new compounds of the same pharmacologic type. This may be exemplified by the development of new generations of cephalosporin antibiotics; additional H_2-antagonists from the pioneer drug cimetidine; and the large series of antianxiety drugs derived from the benzodiazepine structure and the innovator drug chlordiazepoxide (Librium).

Most drugs exhibit activities secondary to their primary pharmacologic action. It is fairly common to take advantage of a secondary activity by using molecular modification to develop new compounds that amplify the second-

ary use of the drug or by gaining approval to market the drug for a secondary indication. For example, the drug finasteride (Proscar) was originally developed and approved to treat benign prostatic hyperplasia. Later, the same drug (as Propecia) was approved at a lower recommended dosage to treat male pattern baldness.

Prodrugs

Prodrug is a term used to describe a compound that requires metabolic biotransformation after administration to produce the desired pharmacologically active compound. The conversion of an inactive prodrug to an active compound occurs primarily through enzymatic biochemical cleavage. Depending on the specific prodrug–enzyme interaction, the biotransformation may occur anywhere along the course of drug transit or at the body site where the requisite enzymes are sufficiently present. An example of a prodrug is enalapril maleate (Vasotec) which, after oral administration, is bioactivated by hydrolysis to enalaprilat, an ACE inhibitor used in the treatment of hypertension. Prodrugs may be designed preferentially for solubility, absorption, biostability, and prolonged release (23).

Solubility

A prodrug may be designed to possess solubility advantages over the active drug, enabling the use of specifically desired dosage forms and routes of administration. For example, if an active drug is insufficiently soluble in water to prepare a desired intravenous injection, a water-soluble prodrug could be prepared through the addition of a functional group that later would be detached by the metabolic process to yield, once again, the active drug molecule.

Absorption

A drug may be made more water or lipid soluble, as desired, to facilitate absorption via the intended route of administration.

Biostability

If an active drug is prematurely destroyed by biochemical or enzymatic processes, the design of a prodrug may protect the drug during its transport in the body. In addition, the use of a prodrug could result in site-specific action of greater potency.

Prolonged Release

Depending on a prodrug's rate of metabolic conversion to active drug, it may provide prolonged drug release and extended therapeutic activity.

FDA's Definition of a New Drug

According to the FDA, a new drug is any that is not recognized as being safe and effective in the conditions recommended for its use among experts who are qualified by scientific training and experience (1).

A drug need not be a new chemical entity to be considered new. A change in a previously approved drug product's formulation or method of manufacture constitutes newness under the law, since such changes can alter the therapeutic efficacy and/or safety of a product.

A combination of two or more old drugs or a change in the usual proportions of drugs in an established combination product is considered new if the change introduces a question of safety or efficacy.

A proposed new use for an established drug, a new dosage schedule or regimen, a new route of administration, or a new dosage form all cause a drug or drug product's status to new and triggers reconsideration for safety and efficacy.

Drug Nomenclature

When first synthesized or identified from a natural source, an organic compound is represented by an *empirical formula*, for example $C_{16}H_{19}N_3O_5S.3H_2O$ for amoxicillin, which indicates the number and relationship of the atoms in the molecule. As knowledge of the relative locations of these atoms increases, the compound receives a *systematic chemical name*, such as 4-Thia-1-azabicylco[3.2.0]heptane-2-carboxylic acid, 6-[[amino(4-hydroxyphenyl) acetyl]amino-3, 3-dimethyl-7-oxo, trihydrate 2S-[2α, [5α,6β(S*)]]-. To be adequate and fully specific, the name must reveal every part of the compound's molecular structure, so that it describes only that compound and no other. The systematic name is generally so formidable that it soon is replaced in scientific communication by a shortened name, which, although less descriptive chemically, is understood to refer only to that chemical compound. This shortened name is the chemical's *nonproprietary* (or generic) name (e.g., amoxicillin; see Fig. 1.2).

Today many companies give their new compounds *code numbers* before assigning a nonproprietary name. These code numbers take the form of an identifying prefix letter or letters that identify the drug's sponsor, followed by a number that further identifies the test compound (for example, SQ 14,225, the investigational code number for the drug captopril, initially developed by Squibb). The code number frequently stays with a compound from its initial preclinical laboratory investigation through human clinical trials.

When the results of testing indicate that a compound shows sufficient promise of becoming a drug, the sponsor may formally propose a nonproprietary name and may also apply to the U.S. Patent Office (and foreign agencies as well) for a proprietary or trademark name. Should the drug receive recognition in an official compendium, the nonproprietary name established during the drug's early usage is adopted. Nonproprietary names are issued only for single agents, whereas proprietary or trademark names may be associated with a single chemical entity or with a mixture of chemicals constituting a specific proprietary product.

The task of designating appropriate nonproprietary names for chemical agents rests primarily with the United States Adopted Names (USAN) Council. This organized effort at coining nonproprietary names for drugs was inaugurated in 1961 as a joint project of the American Medical Association and the United States Pharmacopeial Convention. They were joined in 1964 by the American Pharmacists Association (formerly the American Pharmaceutical Association) to form the USAN Council; in 1967, the FDA was invited to take part in the work of the council.

The United States Pharmacopeial Convention publishes the USAN and the *USP Dictionary of Drug Names*. In addition to listing the US-ANs, the reference also includes brand names of research-oriented firms, investigational drug code designations, official names of United States Pharmacopeia (USP) and National Formulary (NF) articles with their chemical names and graphic formulas, and international nonproprietary names published by the World Health Organization. This reference of drug names now includes more than 9500 nonproprietary drug name entries. It also includes formerly used brand names of commercially available drugs; these names are sometimes changed, but practitioners may need to know what the previous names have been.

A proposal for a USAN usually originates from a firm or individual who has developed a substance of potential therapeutic usefulness to the point that there is a distinct possibility of its being marketed in the United States. Occasionally, the initiative is taken by the USAN Council in the form of a request to parties interested in a substance for which a nonproprietary name appears to be lacking. Proposals are expected to conform to the council's guidelines for coining nonproprietary names. The name should (*a*) be short and distinctive in sound and spelling and not be such that it is easily confused with existing names, (*b*) indicate the general pharmacologic or therapeutic class into which the substance falls or the general chemical nature of the substance if the latter is associated with the specific pharmacologic activity, and (*c*) embody the syllable or syllables characteristic of a related group of compounds.

When general agreement on a name has been reached between the council and the drug's sponsor, it is announced as a proposed USAN. This indicates the council's intention to adopt the name and serves notice to those who wish to protest the selection. The tentatively adopted USAN is then submitted for consideration by various American and foreign drug regulatory agencies, including the World Health Organization, the British Pharmacopoeia Commission, the French Codex, the Nordic Pharmacopeia, the USP–NF, and the FDA. Under the 1962 Drug Amendments, the Secretary of the Department of Health and Human Services has authority to designate the nonproprietary name for any drug in the interest of usefulness or simplicity. The authority is delegated to the commissioner of the FDA. If no objections are raised, adoption is considered final, and the USAN is published in the literature of the medical and pharmaceutical professions. On rare occasions a USAN-adopted name is changed to foster clarity or uniformity. With the creation of the USAN Council and the cooperation of the interested parties on a worldwide basis, nonproprietary drug nomenclature has become standardized. The USP Expert Committee on Nomenclature and Labeling has been developing a standardized pronunciation for the drugs within each class; this will be important for voice recognition computer software.

Biologic Characterization

Prospective drug substances must undergo preclinical testing for biologic activity to assess their potential as useful therapeutic agents. These studies, which fall into the general areas of pharmacology, drug metabolism, and toxicology, involve many types of scientists, including general biologists, microbiologists, molecular biologists, biochemists, geneticists, pharmacologists, physiologists, pharmacokineticists, pathologists, toxicologists, statisticians, and others. Their work leads to the determination of whether a chemical agent possesses adequate features of safety and sufficient promise of usefulness to pursue as a prospective new drug.

To judge whether a drug is safe and effective, information must be gained on how it is absorbed, distributed throughout the body, stored, metabolized, and excreted and how it affects the action of the body's cells, tissues, and organs. Scientists have developed studies that may be conducted outside the living body by using cell and tissue culture and computer programs that simulate human and animal systems. Cell cultures are being used increasingly to screen for toxicity before progressing to whole-animal testing. Computer models help to predict the properties of substances and their probable actions in living systems. Although these systems have reduced dependence on the use of animals in drug studies, they have not completely replaced the need to study drugs in whole animals as a safeguard before their administration to humans.

Pharmacology

Within its broad definition, pharmacology (pharmaco, drugs; logos, study of) is the science concerned with drugs, their sources, appearance, chemistry, actions, and uses.(25) The term in general can be expanded to include properties, biochemical and physiologic effects, mechanisms of action, absorption, distribution, biotransformation, and excretion. From this basic field of study come such subareas as *pharmacodynamics*, the study of the biochemical and physiologic effects of drugs and their mechanisms of action; *pharmacokinetics*, which deals with the absorption, distribution, metabolism or biotransformation, and excretion (ADME) of drugs; and *clinical pharmacology*, which applies pharmacologic principles to the study of the effects and actions of drugs in humans.

Today's emphasis in the development of new drugs is on identifying the cause and process of a disease and then designing molecules capable of interfering with that process. Although the precise cause of each disease is not yet known, what is known is that most diseases arise from a biochemical imbalance, an abnormal proliferation of cells, an endogenous deficiency, or an exogenous chemical toxin or invasive pathogen.

The biochemical processes in the body's cells involve intricate enzymatic reactions. An understanding of the role of a particular enzyme system in the body's healthy state and disease state can lead to the design of drugs that affect the enzyme system with positive results, as exemplified earlier in this chapter for the drug enalaprilat.

Different drug substances produce different effects on the biologic system because of the specific interactions between a drug's chemical structure and specific cells or cellular components of a particular tissue or organ, termed receptor sites (Fig. 2.4). The action of most drugs takes place at the molecular level, with the drug molecules interacting with the molecules of the cell structure or its contents. The selectivity and specificity of drugs for a certain body tissue—for example, drugs that act primarily on the nerves, heart, or kidney—are related to specific sites on or within the cells, receptive only to chemicals of a particular chemical structure and configuration. This is the basis for *structure–activity relationships* established for drugs and for families of drugs within ther-

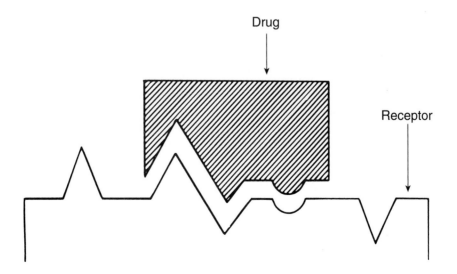

FIGURE 2.4 Receptor site and substrate (drug). (Reprinted with permission from Clark FH, ed. How modern medicines are discovered. Courtesy of Futura Publishing.)

apeutic categories. Studies of the pharmacologic activities of a series of analogs with varied functional groups and side chains can reveal the most specific structure for a given drug–cell or drug–enzyme interaction.

Although receptors for many drugs have yet to be identified, they, like the active centers of enzymes, are considered to be carboxyl, amino, sulfhydryl, phosphate, and similar reactive groups oriented on or in the cell in a pattern complementary to that of the drugs with which they react. The binding of a drug to the receptor is thought to be accomplished mainly by ionic, covalent, and other relatively weak reversible bonds. Occasionally firm covalent bonding is involved, and the drug effect is then slowly reversible.

There is a relationship between the *quantity* of drug molecules available for interaction and the capacity of the specific receptor site. For instance, after a dose of drug and its transit to the site of action, the cell's receptors may or may not become fully saturated with interacting drug. When the receptors *are* saturated, the effects of the specific interaction are maximized. Any additional drug present (as in the circulation) and not participating in the interaction may serve as a reservoir to replace drug molecules released from the complex. Two drugs in a biologic system may compete for the same binding sites, with the drug having the stronger bonding attraction for the site generally prevailing. Already bound molecules of the more weakly bound drug may be displaced from the binding site and left free in the circulation.

Certain cells within the body are capable of binding drugs without eliciting a drug effect. These cells act as carriers and may be important to a drug's transport to active sites or to sites of the drug's biotransformation and elimination.

The process of evaluating chemical compounds for biologic activity and the determination of their mechanisms of action is the responsibility of the pharmacologist. In vitro cultures of cells and enzymes systems and in vivo animal models are used to define a chemical's *pharmacologic profile*.

To define a pharmacologic profile, pharmacologists progress stepwise through increasingly sophisticated levels of evaluation, based on the test compound's success in prior studies. Whole-animal studies are reserved for test compounds that have demonstrated reasonable potential as a drug candidate.

Among the early studies are the determination of a compound's selectivity for various receptors and its activity against select enzyme systems. Studies of the compound's effects on cell function are then performed to detect evidence of efficacy and to determine whether the compound is an agonist or antagonist. These are followed by studies with isolated animal tissues to define further the compound's activity and selectivity. Then whole-animal studies are used to evaluate the pharmacologic effects of the agent on specific organ systems. Finally, studies are undertaken using animal models of human disease for which the compound is considered a drug candidate.

Most animal testing is done on small animals, usually rodents (mouse, rat) for a number of reasons including cost, availability, the small amount of drug required for a study, the ease of administration by various routes (oral, inhalation, intravenous), and experience with drug testing in these species. However, in final pharmacologic and toxicologic studies, two or more animal species are used as required by the FDA, including a rodent and an animal from another order. Drugs are studied at various dose levels to determine effect, potency, and toxicity.

The primary objective of the animal studies is to obtain basic information on the drug's effects that may be used to predict safe and effective use in humans. This is a difficult task because of species variation and the fact that animals are not absolute predictors of human response. However, a number of animal models have been developed to mimic certain human diseases, and these are used effectively. For instance, there are animal models for type I diabetes and hypertension, using genetically diabetic and hypertensive animals, respectively, and for tumor growth, using tumor transplants into various species. Certain animal species have been determined to be best for certain studies of organ systems, or as human disease models, including the dog and rat for hypertension, the dog and guinea pig for respiratory effects, the dog for diuretic activity, the rabbit for blood coagulation, and the mouse and rat for central nervous system studies (26–27). Unfortunately, useful animal models are not available for every human disease. As a drug candidate progresses in its preclinical pharmacologic evaluation, drug metabolism and toxicity tests are initiated.

Drug Metabolism

A series of animal studies of a proposed drug's ADME are undertaken to determine (*a*) the *extent* and *rate* of drug absorption from various routes of administration, including the one intended for human use; (*b*) the rate of distribution of the drug through the body and the site or sites and duration of the drug's residence; (*c*) the rate, primary and secondary sites, and mechanism of the drug's metabolism in the body and the chemistry and pharmacology of any metabolites; and (*d*) the proportion of administered dose eliminated from the body and its rate and route of elimination. In these studies, a minimum of two animal species are employed (generally the same as used in the pharmacologic and toxicologic studies), a rodent and one other, usually a dog.

The biochemical transformation or metabolism of drug substances is the body's means of transforming nonpolar drug molecules into polar compounds, which are more readily eliminated. Specific and nonspecific enzymes participate in drug metabolism, primarily in the liver but also in the kidneys, lung, and gastrointestinal tract. Drugs that enter the hepatic circulation after absorption from the gut, as after oral administration, are particularly exposed to rapid drug metabolism. This transit through the liver and exposure to the hepatic enzyme system is termed the *first-pass effect*. If the first-pass effect is to be avoided, other routes of administration (buccal, rectal) may be used that allow the drug to be absorbed into the systemic circulation through blood vessels other than hepatic.

Drug metabolism or biotransformation frequently results in the production of one or more metabolites of the administered drug, some of which may be pharmacologically active compounds, others not. As noted previously, drug metabolism may be essential to convert prodrugs to active compounds. For reasons of safety, it is important to determine whether a drug's metabolic products are toxic or nontoxic to the animal and later to the human. When metabolites are found, they are chemically and biologically characterized for activity and toxicity. Some new drugs have been discovered as metabolic byproducts, or metabolites, of parent compounds.

ADME studies are performed through the timely collection and analysis of urine, blood, and feces samples and through a careful examination of animal tissues and organs upon autopsy. In addition, special studies are undertaken to determine the presence, if any, of a test drug or its metabolites in the milk of lactating animals; the ability of the drug to cross the placental barrier and enter the fetal blood supply; and the long-term retention of drug or metabolites in the body. In studying the formation and disposition of metabolites, a radioactive label is commonly incorporated into the administered compound and traced in the animal's waste products and tissues.

The relationship between ADME and drug product development is discussed in Chapter 5.

Toxicology

Toxicology deals with the adverse or undesired effects of drugs (25). Although the ability to predict the safe use of a new drug in humans based on preclinical animal studies is desirable, it is not entirely achievable. The direct extrapolation of preclinical animal safety data to humans is difficult because of species variation, different dose–response relationships, immunologic differences, subjective reactions that are not deducible in animals (such as headache), and for other reasons (27). Although many adverse reactions in humans cannot be predicted in advance through animal studies, the greater the number of animal species tested that demonstrate a toxic effect, the greater the likelihood the effect will also be seen in humans.

In drug development programs, preclinical drug safety evaluation or toxicity studies are undertaken to determine (*a*) the substance's potential for toxicity with short-term (acute effects) or long-term use (chronic effects); (*b*) the substance's potential for specific organ toxicity; (*c*) the mode, site, and degree of toxicity; (*d*) dose–response relationships for low, high, and intermediate doses over a specified time; (*e*) gender, reproductive, or teratogenic toxicities; and (*f*) the substance's carcinogenic and genotoxic potential.

Initial toxicology studies are conducted on rodents. After successful initial testing, another animal, usually a dog, is added to the testing program to develop the FDA-required two-order toxicology profile. The toxicology profile includes acute or short-term toxicity; subacute or subchronic toxicity; chronic toxicity; carcinogenicity testing; reproduction studies; and mutagenicity screening (9, 28–29). Figure 2.1 shows that short-term and long-term toxicity studies span the entire program of drug development, from preclinical studies through clinical trials and into postmarketing surveillance.

Acute or Short-Term Toxicity Studies

These studies are designed to determine the toxic effects of a test compound when administered in a single dose and/or in multiple doses over a short period, usually a single day. Although various routes of administration may be used (such as lavage dosing via gastric tube), the studies should be conducted to represent the intended route for human use.

The test compound is administered at various dose levels, with toxic signs observed for onset, progression or reversal, severity, mortality, and rates of incidence. Doses are ranged, to find the largest single dose of the test compound that will not produce a toxic effect; the dose level at which severe toxicity occurs; and intermediate toxicity levels. The animals are observed and compared with controls for eating and drinking habits, weight change, toxic effects, psychomotor changes, and any other signs of untoward effects, usually over a 30-day postdose period. Feces and urine specimens are collected and clinical laboratory tests performed to detect changes in clinical chemistry

and other changes that could indicate toxicity. When they occur, animal deaths are recorded, studied by histology and pathology, and statistically evaluated on the basis of dose–response, gender, age, intraspecies and interspecies findings, and against laboratory controls.

Subacute or Subchronic Studies

In designing an animal toxicology program, relationships to projected human clinical studies for safety must be considered. For example, animal toxicity studies of a minimum of 2 weeks of daily drug administration at three or more dosage levels to two animal species are required to support the initial administration of a single dose in human clinical testing (8). These studies are termed *subacute* or *subchronic*. The initial human dose is usually one-tenth of the highest nontoxic dose (in milligrams per kilogram of subject's weight) shown during the animal studies. For drugs intended to be given to humans for a week or more, animal studies of 90 to 180 days must demonstrate safety. These are termed *chronic toxicity* studies. And if the drug is to be used for a chronic human illness, animal studies 1 year or longer must be undertaken to support human use. Some animal toxicity studies last 2 years or longer and may be used to corroborate findings obtained during the course of human clinical trials.

Included in the subchronic and chronic studies are comparative data of test and control animal species, strain, sex, age, dose levels and ranges, routes of administration, duration of treatment, observed effects, mortality, body weight changes, food and water consumption, physical examinations (e.g., electrocardiography, ophthalmic examination), hematology, clinical chemistry, organ weights, gross pathology, neoplastic pathology, histopathology, urinalysis, ADME data, and other factors (28). Figure 2.5 shows a toxicologist examining research data of body weight changes during preclinical rodent studies.

Carcinogenicity Studies

Carcinogenicity testing is usually a component of chronic testing and is undertaken when the

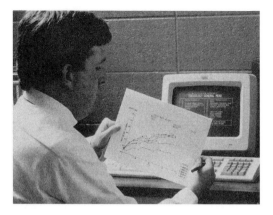

FIGURE 2.5 A toxicologist examining research data of body weight changes during preclinical studies in mice. (Courtesy of Toxicology Research Laboratories, Lilly Research Laboratories, Division of Eli Lilly and Company.)

compound has shown sufficient promise as a drug to enter human clinical trials. Carcinogenicity studies are usually carried out in a limited number of rat and mouse strains for which there is reasonable information on spontaneous tumor incidence.

Dose-ranging studies are done with female and male animals using high, intermediate, and low doses over a 90-day period. For carcinogenicity studies, the high dose should be only high enough (the maximum tolerated dose) to elicit signs of minimal toxicity without significantly altering the animal's normal lifespan by effects other than carcinogenicity (30).

Carcinogenicity studies are long term (18–24 months), with surviving animals killed and studied at defined weeks during the test period. Data on the causes of animal death (other than killing), tumor incidence, type and site, and necropsy findings are collected and evaluated. Any preneoplastic lesions and/or tissue-specific proliferative effects are important findings.

Reproduction Studies

Reproduction studies are undertaken to reveal *any* effect of an active ingredient on mammalian reproduction. Included in these studies are fertility and mating behavior; early embryonic, prenatal, and postnatal development; multigenerational effects; and teratology. The combination of studies allows exposure from conception to sexual maturity and allows immediate and latent effects to be detected through complete life cycles and through successive generations.

In these studies, the maternal parent, fetus, neonates, and weaning offspring are evaluated for anatomic abnormalities, growth, and development. The same species of animal used in other toxicity studies are used in reproductive studies, usually the rat. In *embryotoxicity* studies only, a second mammalian species traditionally has been required. The rabbit is the preferred choice for practicality and the extensive background knowledge accumulated on this species.

In reproductive studies, as is the case for other toxicity studies, the doses selected and the routes of administration used are critical. A high dose, based on previous acute and chronic toxicity and pharmacokinetic studies, is selected, with lower dosages chosen in descending sequence. Setting close dosage intervals is useful to reveal trends in dose-related toxicity. Although once daily dosing is usual, the drug's pharmacokinetics may influence the frequency of dosing (31). The route or routes of administration used should be similar to those intended for human use. A single route of administration may be acceptable if it can be shown that a similar drug distribution (kinetic profile) results from different routes of administration.

Genotoxicity or Mutagenicity Studies

Genotoxicity studies are performed to determine whether the test compound can affect gene mutation or cause chromosome or DNA damage. Strains of *Salmonella typhimurium* are routinely used in assays to detect mutations (9, 32).

Early Formulation Studies

As a promising compound is characterized for biologic activity, it is also evaluated with regard to chemical and physical properties that have a bearing on its ultimate and successful formulation into a stable and effective pharmaceutical product. This is the area of responsibility of pharmaceutical scientists and formulation pharmacists trained in *pharmaceutics*.

When sufficient information is gleaned on the compound's physical and chemical properties, initial formulations of the dosage form are developed for use in human clinical trials. During the course of the clinical trials, the proposed product is developed further, from initial formulation to final formulation and from pilot plant (or small-scale production) to scale-up, in preparation for large-scale manufacturing.

To provide sufficient quantities of the bulk chemical (drug) compound for the sequence of preclinical studies, clinical trials, and small-scale and large-scale dosage form production, the careful planning, scheduling, and implementation of the bulk chemical's production must be undertaken by chemical engineers. Quality control and validation must be built into each step of the process.

Full documentation of the chemistry, manufacturing, and controls is an essential part of all drug applications filed with the FDA (1, 33).

Preformulation Studies

Each drug substance has intrinsic chemical and physical characteristics that must be considered before the development of a pharmaceutical formulation. Among these are the drug's solubility, partition coefficient, dissolution rate, physical form, and stability. These and other factors, considered more fully in Chapter 4 and throughout the text, are briefly noted here as an introduction to their importance in the preparation of dosage forms for drug evaluation in human clinical trials and in the development of a final product submitted to the FDA for marketing approval. The relatively new Biopharmaceutic Drug Classification System is discussed in more detail in Chapter 5 and is designed to correlate in vitro drug product dissolution and in vivo bioavailability, since drug dissolution and gastrointestinal permeability are the fundamental parameters controlling the rate and extent of drug absorption (34).

Drug Solubility

A drug substance administered by any route must possess some aqueous solubility for systemic absorption and therapeutic response.

Poorly soluble compounds (e.g., less than 10 mg/mL aqueous solubility) may exhibit incomplete, erratic, and/or slow absorption and thus produce a minimal response at desired dosage. Enhanced aqueous solubility may be achieved by preparing more soluble derivatives of the parent compound, such as salts or esters; by chemical complexation; or by reducing the drug's particle size.

Partition Coefficient

To produce a pharmacologic response, a drug molecule must first cross a biologic membrane of protein and lipid, which acts as a lipophilic barrier to many drugs. The ability of a drug molecule to penetrate this barrier is based in part on its preference for lipids (lipophilic) versus its preference for an aqueous phase (hydrophilic). A drug's partition coefficient is a measure of its distribution in a lipophilic–hydrophilic phase system and indicates its ability to penetrate biologic multiphase systems.

Dissolution Rate

The speed at which a drug substance dissolves in a medium is called its *dissolution rate*. Dissolution rate data, when considered along with data on a drug's solubility, dissolution constant, and partition coefficient, can provide an indication of the drug's absorption potential. For a chemical entity, its acid, base, or salt forms, as well as its physical form (e.g., particle size), may result in substantial differences in the dissolution rate.

Physical Form

The crystal or amorphous forms and/or the particle size of a powdered drug can affect the dissolution rate, thus the rate and extent of absorption, for a number of drugs. For example, by reducing particle size and increasing powder fineness and therefore the surface area of a poorly soluble drug, its dissolution rate in the gut is enhanced (through greater exposure of the drug to gastrointestinal fluid) and its biologic absorption increased. Small and controlled particle size is also critical for drugs administered to the lung by inhalation. The smaller the particle, the deeper is the penetration into the alveoli. Thus, by selective control of the physical parameters of a drug, biologic response may be optimized.

Stability

The chemical and physical stability of a drug substance alone, and when combined with formulation components, is critical to preparing a successful pharmaceutical product. For a given drug, one type of crystal structure may provide greater stability than other structures and may therefore be preferred. For drugs susceptible to oxidative decomposition, the addition of antioxidant stabilizing agents to the formulation may be required to protect potency. For drugs destroyed by hydrolysis, protection against moisture in formulation, processing, and packaging may be required to prevent decomposition. In every case, drug stability testing at various temperatures, conditions of relative humidity (RH)—as 40°C 75% RH/30°C 60% RH—durations, and environments of light, air, and packaging is essential in assessing drug and drug product stability. Such information is vital in developing label instructions for use and storage, assigning product expiration dating, and packaging and shipping.

Initial Product Formulation and Clinical Trial Materials

An initial product is formulated using the information gained during the preformulation studies and with consideration of the dose or doses, dosage form, and route of administration desired for the clinical studies and for the proposed marketed product. Thus, depending upon the design of the clinical protocol and desired final product, formulation pharmacists are called upon to develop a specific dosage form (e.g., capsule, suppository, solution) of one or more dosage strengths for administration by the intended route of administration (e.g., oral, rectal, intravenous). Additional dosage forms for other than the initial route of administration may later be developed, depending on patients' requirements, therapeutic utility, and marketing assessments. This is es-

pecially important if the drug may be administered to children.

The initial formulations prepared for Phase 1 and Phase 2 of the clinical trials, although not as sophisticated and elegant as the final formulation, should be of high pharmaceutical quality, meet analytical specifications for composition, manufacturing, and control, and be sufficiently stable for the period of use.

Often during Phase 1 studies, for orally administered drugs, capsules are employed containing the active ingredient alone, without pharmaceutical excipients. Excipients are included in the formulation for Phase 2 trials. During human trials, studies of the drug's ADME are undertaken to obtain a profile of the drug's human pharmacokinetics and biologic availability from the formulation administered. Different formulations may be prepared and examined to develop the one having the desired characteristics (see Chapter 5). During Phase 2, the final dosage form is selected and developed for Phase 3 trials; this is the formulation that is submitted to the FDA for marketing approval.

Clinical supplies or *clinical trial materials* comprise all dosage formulations used in the clinical evaluation of a new drug. This includes the proposed new drug, *placebos* (inert substances for controlled studies) and drug products against which the new drug is to be compared (*comparator* drugs or drug products). They all must be prepared in indistinguishable dosage forms (look alike, taste alike, and so on) and packaged with coded labels to reduce possible bias when *blinded* studies are called for in the clinical protocol. Blinded studies are controlled studies in which at least one of the parties (e.g., patient, physician) does not know which product is being administered. At the conclusion of the clinical study, the codes for the products administered are broken and the clinical results statistically evaluated. Some studies are *open label*, in which case all parties may know what products are administered.

Some pharmaceutical companies have special units for the preparation, analytical control, coding, packaging, labeling, shipping, and record maintenance of clinical supplies. Other companies integrate this activity within their existing drug product development and production operations. Still other companies employ contract firms specializing in this field to prepare and manage their clinical trial materials program.

In all clinical study programs, the package label of the investigational drug must bear the statement "Caution: new drug—limited by federal [or United States] law to investigational use." Once received by the investigator, the clinical supplies may be administered only to subjects in the study. Blister packaging is commonly used in clinical studies, with immediate labels containing the clinical study or protocol number, patient identification number, sponsor number, directions for use, code number to distinguish between investigational drug, placebo, and/or comparator product, and other relevant information. Records of the disposition of the drug must be maintained by patient number, dates, and quantities administered. When there is a department of pharmacy at the site of the clinical study (e.g., university teaching hospital) pharmacists frequently assist in the control and management of clinical supplies. When an investigation is terminated, suspended, discontinued, or complete, all unused clinical supplies must be returned to the sponsor and an accounting made of used and unused product.

All formulations, from those developed initially through the final marketed version, must be prepared under the conditions and procedures set out by the FDA in its Current Good Manufacturing Practice guidelines (35), as outlined in Chapter 3.

The Investigational New Drug Application

Under the Food, Drug, and Cosmetic Act as amended, the sponsor of a new drug is required to file with the FDA an *IND* before the drug may be given to human subjects (1). This is to protect the rights and safety of the subjects and to ensure that the investigational plan is sound and is designed to achieve the stated objectives. The *sponsor* of an IND takes responsibility for and initiates a clinical investigation. The sponsor may be an individual (a sponsor–investigator),

a pharmaceutical company, governmental agency, academic institution, or other private or public organization. The sponsor may actually conduct the study or employ, designate, or contract other qualified persons to do so. Nowadays many *contract research organizations* conduct all or designated portions of clinical studies or clinical drug trials for others through contractual arrangements.

After submission of the IND, the sponsor must delay use of the drug in human subjects for not less than 30 days from the date the FDA acknowledges receipt of the application. An IND automatically goes into effect following this period unless the FDA notifies the sponsor that as a result of its review of the submission, it is waiving the period and the sponsor may initiate the study early or the investigation is being placed on a *clinical hold*.

A *clinical hold* is an order issued by the FDA to delay the start of a clinical investigation or to suspend an ongoing study. During a clinical hold, the investigational drug may not be administered to human subjects (unless specifically permitted by the FDA for individual patients in an ongoing study). A clinical hold is issued when there is concern that human subjects will be exposed to unreasonable and significant risk of illness or injury; when there is a question of the qualifying credentials of the clinical investigators; or when the IND is considered incomplete, inaccurate, or misleading. If the concerns raised are addressed to the FDA's satisfaction, a clinical hold may be lifted and clinical investigations resumed; if not, an IND may be maintained in a clinical hold, declared inactive, withdrawn by the sponsor, or terminated by the FDA.

Content of the IND

The content of an IND is prescribed in the *Code of Federal Regulations* and is submitted under a cover sheet (*Form FDA-1571*) (1).

Among the items required:

- Name, address, and telephone number of the sponsor of the drug
- Name and title of the person responsible for monitoring the conduct and progress of the investigation

- Names and titles of the persons responsible for the review and evaluation of information relevant to the safety of the drug
- Name and address of any contract research organization involved in the study
- Identification of the phase or phases of the clinical investigation to be conducted
- Introductory statement and general investigational plan: the name of the drug and all active ingredients, the drug's structural formula and pharmacologic class, the formulation of the dosage form and route of administration, and the broad objectives and planned duration of the study
- Description of the investigational plan: the rationale for the drug or research study, the indication or indications to be studied, the approach to evaluating the drug, the types of studies to be conducted, the estimated number of subjects to be given the drug, and any serious risks anticipated based on animal studies or other human experiences with the drug
- Brief summary of previous human experience with the drug (domestic or foreign), including the reasons if the drug has been withdrawn from any other investigation and/or marketing
- Chemistry, manufacturing, and control information: a complete description of the drug substance, including its physical, chemical, and biologic characteristics; its method of preparation and analytical methods to ensure its identity, strength, quality, purity, and stability; a quantitative list of the active and inactive components of the dosage form to be administered; the methods, facilities, and controls employed in the manufacture, processing, packaging and labeling of the new drug to ensure appropriate qualitative and quantitative standards and product stability during the clinical investigation
- Pharmacology and toxicology information: the drug's mechanism of action if known; information on the drug's absorption, distribution, metabolism, and excretion; and acute, subacute, chronic, and reproductive and developmental toxicity studies

- If the new drug is a combination of previously investigated components, a complete preclinical and clinical summary of these components when administered singly and any data or expectations relating to the effect when combined
- *Clinical protocol* for each planned study (discussed in the next section)
- Commitment that an *Institutional Review Board* (IRB) has approved the clinical study and will continue to review and monitor the investigation (discussed in the next section)
- *Investigator brochure* (discussed in the next section)
- Commitment not to begin clinical investigations until the IND is in effect, the signature of the sponsor or authorized representative, and the date of the signed application

The Clinical Protocol

As a part of the IND application, a *clinical protocol* must be submitted to ensure the appropriate design and conduct of the investigation. Clinical protocols include

- Statement of the purpose and objectives of the study
- Outline of the investigational plan and study design, including the kind of control group and methods to minimize bias on the part of the subjects, investigators, and analysts
- Estimate of the number of patients to be involved
- Basis for subject selection, with inclusion and exclusion criteria
- Description of the dosing plan, including dose levels, route of administration, and duration of patient exposure
- Description of the patient observations, measurements, and tests to be used
- Clinical procedures, laboratory tests, and monitoring to be used in minimizing patient risk
- Names, addresses, and credentials of the principal investigators and coinvestigators
- Locations and descriptions of the clinical research facilities to be used
- Approval of the authorized IRB

Once an IND is in effect, a sponsor must submit an amendment for approval of any proposed changes. This may involve changes of dosing levels, testing procedures, the addition of new investigators, additional sites for the study, and so on.

For many years, women and the elderly were included only rarely in clinical drug investigations. Women of childbearing age were excluded from early drug tests out of fear that the subject would become pregnant during the investigation with possible harm to the fetus. Exceptions were made only in cases of potentially lifesaving drugs. However, in recognition that the general exclusion of women from drug investigations results in inadequate data on any gender-based differences in a drug's effects, the FDA now calls for the inclusion of women in numbers adequate to allow detection of clinically significant differences in drug response.

The FDA *Guideline for the Study and Evaluation of Gender Differences in the Clinical Evaluation of Drugs* issued in 1993 states the agency's gender inclusion policy (36). Although the guideline does not require participation of women in any particular trial, it sets forth FDA's general expectations regarding the inclusion of both women and men in drug development, analysis of clinical data by gender, and assessment of potential pharmacokinetic differences between genders. In 1994, the National Institutes of Health (NIH) similarly issued its policy that women and minorities be included in all NIH-supported biomedical and behavioral research projects involving human subjects "unless there is a clear and compelling rationale and justification that their inclusion is inappropriate with respect to the health of the subjects or the purpose of the research" (37).

Pregnancy is a concern in drug investigations because drugs are readily transported from the maternal to the fetal circulation (38). Because of undeveloped drug detoxication and excretion mechanisms in the fetus, concentrations of drugs may actually reach a higher level in the fetus than in the maternal circulation, with toxic levels resulting. To reduce the risk of fetal exposure to investigational drugs in women of childbearing age, the FDA guideline calls for pregnancy testing, use of contraception, and full information disclosure of potential fetal risks to prospective study subjects. The FDA has made a special effort to ensure that women who have a life-threatening disease (e.g., AIDS-related) are not *automatically* excluded from investigational trials of drug products for that disease because of a perceived risk of reproductive or developmental toxicity from use of the investigational drug (39). There are other instances in which drug studies or use during pregnancy are justified, for example, agents intended to prevent Rh immunization and hemolytic disease of the newborn (40).

When a proposed drug is likely to have significant use in the elderly, elderly patients are required to be included in clinical studies to yield age-related data of a drug's effectiveness and any adverse effects. Older people handle a drug differently because of altered body functions such as diminished liver and kidney function, reduced circulation, and changes in drug ADME. Furthermore, the elderly have a greater incidence of chronic illness and multiple disease states than younger adults, and as a result, take multiple medications daily, increasing the potential for drug–drug interactions. This potential is studied and defined.

Recognition of the need to examine in children new drugs intended for the pediatric patient has a similar requirement to ensure a drug's safe and effective use in this population. Also, differentiation in a drug's activity in minority groups and their subpopulations is important in the full assessment of a drug's potential. It is well known that there are interethnic variations both in disease incidence and in biologic response to some medications, and these factors must be considered in the clinical evaluation of drug substances.(41)

Each IND submission must have the prior approval of the IRB with jurisdiction over the site of the proposed clinical investigation. An IRB is a body of professional and public members that has the responsibility for reviewing and approving any study involving human subjects in the institution they serve. The purpose of the IRB is to protect the safety of human subjects by assessing a proposed clinical protocol, evaluating the benefits against risks, and ensuring that the plan includes all needed measures for subject protection. By law, the IRB shall be constituted to include persons competent to review clinical research proposals and be diverse in membership, with consideration of race, gender, cultural background, and sensitivity to issues affecting the subjects and the community (42). Any substantive change or amendment to an originally approved clinical protocol must be submitted, reviewed, and approved by the IRB and the FDA before implementation.

Each clinical investigator must receive from the sponsor an *investigator's brochure,* which contains all of the pertinent information developed during the preclinical studies, including summary information on the drug's chemistry, pharmacology, toxicology, pharmacokinetics; formulation of the clinical trial materials; any known information related to the drug's safety and effectiveness; a description of possible risks and side effects that may be anticipated and special monitoring required; the clinical protocol and study design; criteria for patient inclusion and exclusion; laboratory and clinical tests to be performed; and drug control and record keeping information.

Each study has defined criteria for *subject inclusion or exclusion.* These criteria may relate to age, sex (as qualified earlier), smoking, health status, and other factors deemed necessary in a given phase of investigation. Each subject in a clinical investigation must participate willingly and with full knowledge of the benefits and risks associated with the investigation.

The sponsor of the study must certify that each person who will receive the investigational drug has given *informed consent*—that is, has been informed of the following: participation in the study is voluntary; the purpose and nature of the study; the procedures involved; a description of any foreseeable risks or discomforts; the potential benefits for patients; disclosure of alternative procedures or courses of treatments, if any; the extent of confidentiality of records; conditions under which the subject's participation in the study may be terminated; consequences of a patient's decision to withdraw from the study; the approximate number of subjects to be enrolled; and whom to contact for answers to pertinent questions

and/or in case of research-related illness or injury. These elements of informed consent, and additional protections that apply to prisoners in clinical investigations, must be in conformance with the *Code of Federal Regulations* (43). Individuals who agree to be subjects in an investigation indicate their consent by signing the form or document containing this information.

Investigators selected by the sponsor to conduct a clinical investigation must be qualified as experts by training and experience to investigate a particular drug. Each investigator's qualifications are submitted to the FDA as a part of the IND application. To participate in an investigation, each investigator signs a form agreeing to comply with and to be responsible for ensuring that the study is conducted according to the IND's investigational plan and clinical protocol; protecting the rights, safety, and welfare of the human subjects; control of the investigational drug; written records of case histories and clinical observations; and the timely submission of progress reports, safety reports, and a final report. It is the responsibility of the sponsor to monitor the progress of all clinical investigations under its IND. If a sponsor discovers that an investigator is not in compliance with the investigational plan, it is the sponsor's responsibility to gain compliance or to terminate the investigator's participation in the study.

Any serious, unexpected, life-threatening, or fatal adverse experience that may be associated with the use of the drug during a clinical investigation must be reported promptly to the sponsor and subsequently to the FDA for investigation. Depending on the severity and assessment of the adverse experience, an alert notice may be sent to other investigators, a clinical hold may be placed on the study for further evaluation and assessment, or the IND may be withdrawn by the sponsor, placed on inactive status, or terminated by the FDA.

Pre-IND Meetings

On request, the FDA will advise a sponsor on scientific, technical, or formatting concerns relating to the preparation and submission of an IND. This may include advice on the adequacy of data to support an investigational plan, the design of a clinical trial, or whether the proposed investigation is likely to produce the data needed to meet the requirements of the next step, the filing of a NDA to gain approval for marketing.

FDA Review of an IND Application

The FDA's objectives in reviewing an IND are to protect the safety and rights of the human subjects and to help ensure that the study allows the evaluation of the drug's safety and effectiveness. These objectives are best met by the accuracy and completeness of the IND submission, the design and conduct of the investigational plan, and the expertise and diligence of the investigators.

When received by the FDA, the IND submission is stamped with the date of receipt, assigned an application number, and forwarded to either the Center for Drug Evaluation and Research (CDER) or the Center for Biologics Evaluation and Research (CBER) for review. Applications for chemical agents are sent to CDER and applications for biologics to CBER.

Within CDER, applications are forwarded to the appropriate office of drug evaluation and then to one of its divisions for review as follows:

Office of Drug Evaluation I
Division of Neuropharmacological Drug
  Products
Division of Oncology Drug Products
Division of Cardio-Renal Drug Products

Office of Drug Evaluation II
Division of Metabolic and Endocrine Drug
  Products
Division of Pulmonary Drug Products
Division of Reproductive and Urologic
  Drug Products

Office of Drug Evaluation III
Division of Gastro-Intestinal and Coagula-
  tion Drug Products
Division of Anesthetic, Critical Care, and
  Addiction Drug Products
Division of Medical Imaging and Radio-
  pharmaceutical Drug Products

Office of Drug Evaluation IV
Division of Anti-Viral Drug Products
Division of Anti-Infective Drug Products
Division of Special Pathogen and Immuno-
  logic Drug Products

Office of Drug Evaluation V
Division of Anti-Inflammatory, Analgesic,
  and Ophthalmologic Drug Products
Division of Dermatologic and Dental Drug
  Products
Division of Over-The-Counter Drug
  Products

After assignment to one of the divisions, the content of the application is thoroughly reviewed to determine whether the preclinical data indicate that the drug is sufficiently safe for administration to human subjects and that the proposed clinical studies are designed to provide the desired data on drug safety and efficacy while not exposing the human subjects to unnecessary risks.

Although the discussion in this chapter is based principally on the evaluation and approval of new chemical entities and products, for biologic products there is a similar but necessarily distinct procedure of application review and product licensing for biologics through CBER and its divisions (4):

Division of Allergenic Products and
  Parasitology
Division of Bacterial Products
Division of Viral products
Division of Vaccines and Related
  Products
Division of Hematologic Products
Division of Blood Establishment and
  Products
Division of Cellular and Gene Therapy
Division of Monoclonal Antibodies Appli-
  cations.

FDA Drug Classification System

Upon receipt and examination of an IND or NDA, the FDA classifies the drug by chemical type and therapeutic potential, as shown in Table 2.1. The classification system allows the FDA to base review priorities on the level of therapeutic advance or need (44).

TABLE 2.1 FDA DRUG CLASSIFICATION SYSTEM

By chemical type

Type 1	New molecular entity; not marketed in United States
Type 2	New ester, new salt, or other derivative of an approved active moiety
Type 3	New formulation of a drug marketed in United States
Type 4	New combination of two or more compounds
Type 5	New manufacturer of a drug marketed in United States
Type 6	New therapeutic indication for an approved drug

Note: a drug may receive a single or multiple classification, as 3 and 4.

By therapeutic classification

Type P	Priority review; a therapeutic gain
Type S	Standard review; similar to other approved drugs

Additional classifications

Type AA	For treatment of AIDS or HIV-related disease
Type E	For life-threatening or severely debilitating disease
Type F	Review deferred pending data validation
Type G	Data validated; removal of F rating
Type N	Nonprescription drug
Type V	Drug having orphan drug status

Note: a drug may receive a single or multiple classification, as P, AA, and V.

Adapted from Mathieu M. New drug development: a regulatory overview, 3rd ed. Cambridge, MA: PAREXEL International, 1994; and Hunter JR, Rosen DL, DeChristoforo R. How FDA expedites evaluation of drugs for AIDS and other life-threatening illnesses. Wellcome Programs in Hospital Pharmacy, No. 67930093009, 1993.

Phases of a Clinical Investigation

An IND may be submitted for one or more *phases* of a clinical investigation, namely Phase 1, Phase 2, or Phase 3 (Fig. 2.2, Table 2.2). Although the phases are conducted sequentially, certain studies may overlap.

Phase 1 includes the initial introduction of an investigational drug into humans and is primarily for the purpose of assessing safety. The studies are closely monitored by clinicians expert in such investigations. The human subjects are usually healthy volunteers, although in certain protocols they may be patients. The total number of subjects included in Phase 1 studies varies with the drug but is usually in the range of 20 to 100. The initial dose of the drug is usually low, usually one-tenth of the highest no-effect dose observed during the animal studies. If the first dose is well tolerated, the investigation continues with the administration of progressively greater doses (to new subjects) until some evidence of the drug's effects are observed.

Phase 1 studies are designed to determine the human pharmacology of the drug, structure–activity relationships, side effects associated with increasing doses, and if possible, early evidence of effectiveness. Among the basic data collected are the rate of absorption; the concentration of drug in the blood over time; the rate and mechanism of drug metabolism and elimination; toxic effects, if any, in body tissues and major organs; and changes in physiologic processes from baseline. The subjects' ability to tolerate the drug and any unpleasant effects of the drug are observed and recorded. Phase 1 studies are often useful in selecting from among different chemical analogs of a lead compound. As noted previously, capsules without excipients are used for orally administered drugs in Phase 1 studies. If the studies demonstrate sufficient merit and if the order of drug toxicity is low, *Phase 2* begins, studying up to several hundred patients.

Phase 2 trials are controlled clinical studies to evaluate the effectiveness of a drug in patients with the condition for which the drug is intended and to assess side effects and risks that may be revealed. Because this phase uses patients as subjects, side effects or toxicity symptoms that were not shown in the preclinical animal studies or in Phase 1 studies with healthy volunteers may be revealed for the first time. Only clinicians expert in the disease being treated are used as investigators during Phase 2 studies (Fig. 2.6). During this phase, additional data are collected on the drug's pharmacokinetics and studies undertaken to

TABLE 2.2 PHASES OF CLINICAL TESTING

	NUMBER OF PATIENTS	LENGTH	PURPOSE	PERCENT SUCCESSFULLY COMPLETING*
Phase 1	20–100	Several months	Mainly safety	67
Phase 2	Up to several hundred	Several months to 2 years	Some short-term safety but mainly effectiveness	45
Phase 3	Several hundred to several thousand	1–4 years	Safety, effectiveness, dosage	5–10

*For example, of 20 drugs entering clinical testing, 13 or 14 successfully complete Phase 1 trials and go on to Phase 2; about 9 will complete Phase 2 and go to Phase 3; only 1 or 2 will clear Phase 3, and on average about 1 of the original 20 will ultimately be approved for marketing. (Source: FDA Consumer, 1987;21:12.)

determine dose–response and dose ranging (often called *Phase 2a studies*). Each patient is monitored for the appearance of the drug's effects while the dose is carefully increased to determine the minimal effective dose. Then the dose is extended beyond the minimally effective dose to the level at which a patient reveals extremely undesirable or intolerable toxic or adverse effects. The greater the range between the dose of drug determined to be minimally effective and that which causes severe side effects, the greater is the drug's safety margin. These dose determination studies (often called *Phase 2b studies*) result in the specific doses and

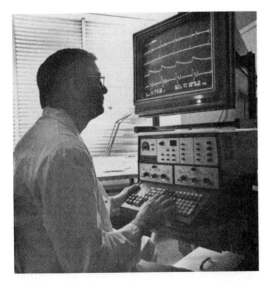

FIGURE 2.6 Monitoring the effects for cardiac function of an un investigational drug as a part of its clinical evaluation. (Courtesy of Eli Lilly and Company.)

the dose range to be used in *Phase 3* studies. During Phase 2 trials, the drug product is refined, with the final formulation developed for use during late Phase 2 and Phase 3 trials.

If the clinical results of Phase 2 trials indicate continued promise for the new drug and if the margin of safety appears to be good, *end-of-Phase 2* meetings between the drug's sponsor and the FDA's review division are held to analyze the data from Phases 1 and 2, to resolve any questions and issues, and to establish investigational plans for Phase 3 studies.

Phase 3 studies may include several hundred to several thousand patients in controlled and uncontrolled trials. The objective is to determine the usefulness of the drug in an expanded patient base. Many additional clinicians having patients with the condition for drug's intended use are recruited to participate in this trial. Several dosage strengths of the proposed drug may be evaluated during this phase, using formulations intended to be proposed in the NDA and for marketing. Sufficient information on the drug's effectiveness and safety is expected to be gathered during Phase 3 to evaluate the overall benefit–risk relationship of the drug and to file a complete NDA.

It is fairly common for certain Phase 3 studies to be continued after an NDA is filed but *prior to* approval. In these instances, the completed studies (*Phase 3a studies*) are considered sufficient for the NDA. The additional studies (*Phase 3b studies*) are used to gather supplemental information that may support certain labeling requests, provide information on patients' quality of life issues, reveal product advantages over already marketed competing drugs, provide evidence in support of possible additional drug indications, or provide other clues for prospective postmarketing studies (*Phase 4*).

Clinical Study Controls and Designs

As indicated, Phase 2 and some Phase 3 studies are *controlled*, that is, the effects of the investigational drug are compared with another agent. The second agent may be a placebo (*placebo control*) or an active drug (*positive control*), a standard or comparator drug product. Both a placebo and an active drug may be used as controls in the same study. For studies that are *blinded*, the identities of the investigational drug and the control or controls are not revealed to certain participants to decrease bias. In *single blind* studies, the patient is unaware of the agent administered. In *double blind* studies, neither the patient nor the clinician is aware of the agent administered. In preparing dosage forms for blinded studies, all of the agents administered, investigational drug, placebo, and/or comparator drug, must be indistinguishable to the blinded individuals. This requires the preparation of clinical trial materials of the same dosage form, having the same size, shape, color, flavor, texture, and so forth. Indistinguishable clinical trial materials are not necessary for *open label* studies, in which all parties are aware of the identities of the agents administered.

In designing a clinical trial, many additional factors are considered, including the scheme of the study design and the duration of the treatment period. Before treatment, *baseline data* are obtained on each subject through physical examination and appropriate laboratory tests and procedures. Subjects are randomly assigned to different treatment groups to allow treatment comparisons. Some common parallel and crossover study designs are depicted in Figure 2.7 (45). These studies may be blinded or not, using placebo and/or active drug controls. The parallel designs are applicable to most clinical trials. Crossover designs are useful in comparing different treatments within individuals, since following one treatment a

patient is crossed over to a different treatment. Between treatment periods, subjects may be given no drugs as a *washout* period to allow return to baseline.

Drug Dosage and Terminology

A major part of any clinical drug study is the determination of a drug's safe and effective dose. As noted earlier, dose and dose ranging studies are conducted during Phase 2 and concluded during Phase 3 clinical trials.

The safe and effective dose of a drug depends on a number of factors, including characteristics of the drug substance, the dosage form and its route of administration, and a variety of patient factors including age, body weight, general health status, any pathologic conditions, and concomitant drug therapy. All of these factors and others are integral to clinical drug trials.

For convenience of dosage administration, most products are formulated to contain a drug's usual dose within a single unit (e.g., capsule), or within a specified volume (e.g., 5 mL or a teaspoonful) of a liquid dosage form. To serve varying dosage requirements, manufacturers often formulate a drug into more than one dosage form and in more than a single strength.

The dose of a drug may be described as an amount that is enough but not too much; the idea is to achieve the drug's optimum therapeutic effect with safety but at the lowest possible dose. The effective dose of a drug may be different for different patients. The familiar bell curve presented in Figure 2.8 shows that in a normal distribution sample, a drug's dose will provide what might be called an average effect in most individuals. However, in a portion of the population the drug will produce little effect, and in another portion the drug will produce an effect greater than average. The amount of drug that will produce the desired effect in most adult patients is considered the drug's *usual adult dose* and the likely starting dose for a patient. From this initial dose the physician may, if necessary, increase or decrease subsequent doses to meet the particular requirements of the patient. Certain drugs may

SOME CLINICAL TRIAL PARALLEL STUDY DESIGNS

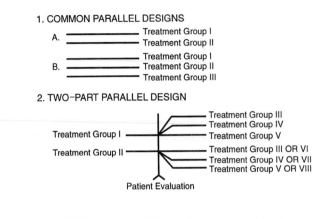

1. COMMON PARALLEL DESIGNS

A. ——————— Treatment Group I
   ——————— Treatment Group II

B. ——————— Treatment Group I
   ——————— Treatment Group II
   ——————— Treatment Group III

2. TWO-PART PARALLEL DESIGN

Treatment Group I ———— Treatment Group III
                       Treatment Group IV
                       Treatment Group V

Treatment Group II ——— Treatment Group III OR VI
                       Treatment Group IV OR VII
                       Treatment Group V OR VIII

Patient Evaluation

3. INTRODUCTION OF PLACEBO DURING TREATMENT

Treatment Group I	Placebo	Treatment Group I
Treatment Group II	Placebo	Treatment Group II
Treatment Group III	Placebo	Treatment Group III

4. MULTIPLE DOSES WITHIN EACH TREATMENT GROUP

| Treatment Group I | Dose A | Dose B | Dose C | Dose D |
| Treatment Group II | Dose E | Dose F | Dose G | Dose H |

SOME CLINICAL TRIAL CROSSOVER STUDY DESIGNS

1. SINGLE CROSSOVER WITH NO INTERVENING BASELINE

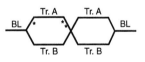

2. SINGLE CROSSOVER WITH INTERVENING BASELINE

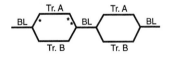

3. EXTRA PERIOD CROSSOVER

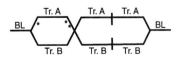

FIGURE 2.7 Some common clinical study designs. (Reprinted with permission from Spilker B. Guide to Clinical Trials, New York: Raven, 1991).

produce more than one effect, depending on the dose. For example, a low dose of a barbiturate produces sedation, whereas a larger dose produces hypnotic effects. The *usual dosage range* indicates the quantitative range or amounts of the drug that may be prescribed safely within the framework of usual medical practice. Doses falling outside of the usual range may result in underdosage or overdosage or may reflect a patient's special requirements. For drugs administered to children, a *usual pediatric dose* may be determined, as discussed later in this section.

The schedule of dosage, or the *dosage regimen*, is determined during the clinical investigation and is based largely on a drug's inherent duration of action, its pharmacokinetics, and the characteristics of the dosage form (e.g., immediate release or modified release). Because of these factors, some drugs are recommended for once-a-day dosage and others more frequently.

For certain drugs, an *initial*, *priming*, or *loading* dose may be required to attain the desired concentration of the drug in the blood or tissues, after which the blood level may be maintained through subsequent administration of regularly scheduled *maintenance doses*.

Certain biologic products, such as tetanus immune globulin, may have two usual doses, a *prophylactic dose*, or the amount administered to protect the patient from contracting the illness, and the *therapeutic dose*, which is administered to a patient after exposure or contraction of the illness. The doses of vaccines and other biologic products, like insulin, sometimes are expressed in *units of activity* rather than in specific quantitative amounts of the drug. This is because the unavailability of suitable chemical assay methods for the active biologic component necessitates the use of biologic assays to determine a product's potency.

To provide systemic effects, a drug must be absorbed from its route of administration at a suitable rate, be distributed in adequate concentration to the receptor sites, and remain there for a sufficient period. One measure of a drug's absorption characteristics is its blood serum concentration at various intervals after administration. Certain drugs have a correlation between blood serum concentration and the presentation of drug effects. For these drugs, an average blood serum concentration represents the minimum concentration that can be expected to produce the drug's desired effects in a patient. This concentration is the *minimum effective concentration (MEC)*. As shown in Figure 2.9, the serum concentration of a hypothetical drug reaches the MEC 2 hours after its administration, achieves a peak concentration in 4 hours, and decreases below

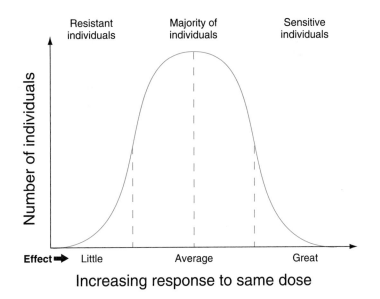

FIGURE 2.8 Drug effect in a population sample.

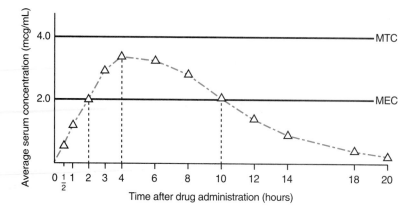

FIGURE 2.9 Example of a blood level curve for a hypothetical drug as a function of time following oral administration. MEC, minimum effective concentration; MTC, minimum toxic concentration.

the MEC in 10 hours. If it were desired to maintain the drug serum concentration above the MEC for a longer period, a second dose of the drug would be required at approximately 8 hours. The time–blood level curve presented in Figure 2.9 is hypothetical. In practice, the curve would vary, depending on the nature of the drug substance, its chemical and physical characteristics, the dosage form administered, and individual patient factors. The second level of serum concentration of drug refers to the *minimum toxic concentration* (MTC). Drug serum concentrations above this level would be expected to produce dose-related toxic effects in the average individual. Ideally, the serum drug concentration in a well-dosed patient would be maintained between the MEC and the MTC (the therapeutic window for the drug) for the period that drug effects are desired. Table 2.3 presents examples of therapeutic, toxic, and considered lethal concentrations for some drug substances.

The *median effective dose* of a drug is the amount that will produce the desired intensity of effect in 50% of the individuals tested. The *median toxic dose* is the amount that will produce a defined toxic effect in 50% of the individuals tested. The relationship between the desired and undesired effects of a drug is commonly expressed as the *therapeutic index* and is defined as the ratio between a drug's median toxic dose and its median effective dose, TD50/ED50. Thus, a drug with a therapeutic index of 15 would be expected to have a greater margin of safety in its use than a drug with a

therapeutic index of 5. For certain drugs, the therapeutic index may be as low as 2, and extreme caution must be exercised in their administration. Examples of therapeutic indices for some drugs are shown in Table 2.4.

Some factors of patients considered in determining a drug's dose in clinical investigations and in medical practice include the following.

Age

The age of the patient may be a consideration in the determination of drug dosage. Age is particularly important in the treatment of neonatal, pediatric, and geriatric patients. Infants, especially newborns and those born prematurely, have immature hepatic and renal function, the means by which drugs are normally inactivated and eliminated from the body. A reduced capacity to detoxify and eliminate drugs can result in drug accumulation in the tissues to toxic levels. Often drug blood levels are determined in these patients and are carefully monitored.

Before there was sufficient understanding of the capacity of the young to detoxify and eliminate drugs, infants and children were dosed by fractions of the adult dose determined by an age-based formula. Age alone is no longer considered to be a particularly valid criterion in the determination of pediatric dosage. Today, doses for many drugs are determined through pediatric clinical trials under special protocols and subject safeguards (46). Many pediatric doses are based on body weight or body surface area, as noted later in this section.

TABLE 2.3 THERAPEUTIC AND TOXIC BLOOD LEVEL CONCENTRATIONS OF SOME DRUG SUBSTANCES

DRUG SUBSTANCE	DRUG SUBSTANCE CONCENTRATION, MILLIGRAMS/LITER		
	THERAPEUTIC	TOXIC	LETHAL
Acetaminophen	10–20	400	1500
Amitriptyline	0.5–0.20	0.4	10–20
Barbiturates			
Short acting	1	7	10
Intermediate acting	1–5	10–30	30
Long acting	~10	40–60	80–150
Dextropropoxyphene	0.05–0.2	5–10	57
Diazepam	0.5–2.5	5–20	:50
Digoxin	0.0006–0.0013	0.002–0.009	—
Imipramine	0.05–0.16	0.7	2
Lidocaine	1.2–5.0	6	—
Lithium	4.2–8.3	13.9	13.9–34.7
Meperidine	0.6–0.65	5	30
Morphine	0.1	—	0.05–4
Phenytoin	5–22	50	100
Quinidine	3–6	10	30–50
Theophylline	20–100	—	—

Adapted from Winek CL. Clin Chem 1976;22:832; and Goth A. Medical Pharmacology, 11th ed. St. Louis: Mosby, 1984;757–759.

Elderly persons also present unique therapeutic and dosing problems that require special attention. Most physiologic functions begin to diminish in adults after the third decade of life. For example, cardiac output declines approximately 1% per year from age 20 to age 80. Glomerular filtration rate falls progressively until age 80, at which time it is only about half of what it was at age 20. Vital capacity, immune capacity, and liver microsomal enzyme function also decrease (47). The decline in renal and hepatic function in the elderly slows the drug clearance rate and increases the possibility of drug accumulation and toxicity. Elderly persons may also respond differently to drugs than younger patients because of changes in drug receptor sensitivity or because of age-related alterations in target tissues or organs (48).

TABLE 2.4 THERAPEUTIC INDICES FOR VARIOUS DRUG SUBSTANCES

LESS THAN 5	BETWEEN 5 AND 10	GREATER THAN 10
Amitriptyline	Barbiturates	Acetaminophen
Chlordiazepoxide	Diazepam	Bromide
Diphenhydramine	Digoxin	Chloral hydrate
Ethchlorvynol	Imipramine	Glutethimide
Lidocaine	Meperidine	Meprobamate
Methadone	Paraldehyde	Nortriptyline
Procainamide	Primidone	Pentazocine
Quinidine	Thioridazine	Propoxyphene

Reprinted with permission from Niazi S. Textbook of Biopharmaceutics and Clinical Pharmacokinetics. New York: Appleton-Century-Crofts, 1979;254.

Furthermore, the chronic disorders in most geriatric patients requires concomitant drug therapy, increasing the possibility of drug–drug interactions and adverse drug effects. In the clinical evaluation of a new drug, consideration is given to other drugs most likely to be taken concomitantly by the intended patient, with studies directed toward determining potential drug–drug effects or interactions.

To assist the pharmacist in pediatric and geriatric patient dosing, the American Pharmacists Association offers the *Pediatric Dosage Handbook* and the *Geriatric Dosage Handbook* (49).

Body Weight

The usual doses for drugs are considered generally suitable for 70-kg (150 pound) individuals. The ratio between the amount of drug administered and the size of the body influences drug concentration in body fluids. Therefore, drug dosage may require adjustment from the usual adult dose for abnormally lean or heavy patients. The doses for certain drugs are based on body weight and are expressed on a *milligram* (drug) *per kilogram* (body weight) basis (e.g., 1 mg/kg).

As noted earlier, body weight is considered more dependable than age as determinant of drug dosage for youngsters, and for many drugs the dose is based on milligrams per kilogram. In some instances, a pediatric dose may be based on a combination of age and weight (e.g., 6 months to 2 years of age: 3 mg/kg/day).

Body Surface Area

Because of the correlation between a number of physiologic processes and body surface area (BSA), some drug doses are based on this relationship (e.g., 1 mg/M^2 BSA). The BSA for a child or adult may be determined using a nomogram (Fig. 2.10). The BSA is determined at the intersect of a straight line drawn to connect an individual's height and weight. For example, an adult measuring 67 inches in height and weighing 132 pounds would have a BSA of approximately 1.7 square meters.

Sex

Because biochemical and physiologic factors produce different responses to certain drugs and drug dosages in men and women due to, biochemical and physiological factors, both sexes should be included in clinical drug trials. Pharmacokinetic differences between women and men may be particularly important for drugs having a narrow therapeutic index, in which the smaller average size of women may necessitate modified dosing. Drugs with narrow therapeutic indices carry the inherent risk that drug blood levels may increase to toxic levels or decrease to ineffective levels with minimal dosing changes. Other important studies on women include the effects of the menstrual cycle and menopausal status on a drug's pharmacokinetics and the drug interaction potential of concomitant estrogen or oral contraceptive use (50).

Because virtually no clinical investigations have included pregnant women in their study protocols and thus drug effects are undetermined in these circumstances, great caution is advised for use of most drugs during pregnancy and in women of childbearing age. Similar caution is applicable to drug use in nursing mothers because transfer from mother's milk to an infant is well documented for a variety of drugs (51, 52).

Pathologic State

The effects of certain drugs may be modified by the pathologic condition of the patient. For example, if certain drugs are used in the presence of renal impairment, excessive systemic accumulation of the drug may occur, risking toxicity. In such conditions, lower than usual doses are indicated, and if therapy is prolonged, blood serum levels of the drug should be assessed and the patient monitored at regular intervals to ensure the maintenance of nontoxic levels of the drug. In these instances, pharmacokinetic dosing is an integral part of the clinical study protocol and of approved product labeling.

Tolerance

The ability to endure the influence of a drug, particularly during continued use, is referred to as *drug tolerance*. It is usually developed to a specific drug and to its chemical congeners; in the latter instance, it is referred to as *cross-tolerance*. The result is that drug dosage must be

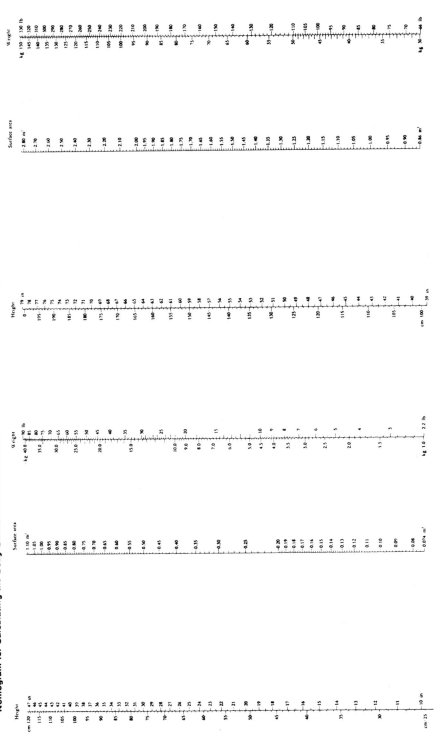

FIGURE 2.10 Nomograms for calculating body surface area. **A.** For children. **B.** For adults. (From the formula of Du Bots and Du Bots, Arch Intern Med 1916;17:863: $S = W^{0.425} \times H^{0.725} \times 71.84$, or log S = log $W \times 0.425$ + log $H \times 0.725$ + 1.8564, where S = body surface in square centimeters, W = weight in kilograms, H = height in centimeters. Reprinted with permission from R.J. Geigy S.A. Documenta Geigy Scientific Tables, 7th ed. Basel: Ciba-Geigy, 537–538.)

increased over time to maintain a desired therapeutic response. Tolerance is common with the use of antihistamines and narcotic analgesics. After the development of tolerance, normal response may be regained by suspending the drug's administration for a while.

Concomitant Drug Therapy

The effects of a drug may be modified by the prior or concurrent administration of another drug. Such interference, a *drug–drug interaction*, may be due to a chemical or physical interaction between the drugs or to an alteration of the absorption, distribution, metabolism, or excretion patterns of one of the drugs. Certain clinical protocols include the evaluation of a new drug in the presence of other drugs most likely to be included in the target patient's therapeutic regimen.

Important drug–drug interactions that are identified during a drug's clinical trials are included in approved product labeling. Additional drug interactions that become known after the drug is marketed are added in labeling revisions. Drug–drug interactions may include "social" agents such as tobacco and alcohol, which affect the pharmacokinetics of a number of drugs and require an alteration in a drug's usual dose.

Time and Conditions of Administration

The time at which a drug is administered may influence dosage. This is true especially for oral therapy in relation to meals. Absorption proceeds more rapidly if the stomach and upper portions of the intestinal tract are empty of food. A dose of a drug that is effective when taken before a meal may be less effective if administered during or after eating. Drug–food interactions can affect a drug's usual absorption pattern. When such interactions are determined, appropriate guidance is provided in the product literature.

Dosage Form and Route of Administration

The effective dose of a drug may vary with the dosage form and the route of administration.

Drugs administered intravenously enter the blood stream directly and completely. In contrast, drugs administered orally are rarely if ever fully absorbed into the blood stream because of the various physical, chemical, and biologic barriers to their absorption. Thus, in many instances a lower parenteral (injectable) dose of a drug is required than the oral dose to achieve the same blood levels or clinical effects. Varying rates and degrees of absorption can occur from drug administration in the rectum, in the gastrointestinal tract, under the tongue, via the skin, and to other sites. Therefore, for a given drug, different dosage forms and routes of administration are considered new by the FDA and must be evaluated individually through clinical studies to determine the effective doses.

Treatment IND

A *Treatment IND* or a *treatment protocol* permits the use of an investigational drug in the treatment of patients *not enrolled* in the clinical study but who have a serious or immediately life-threatening disease for which there is no satisfactory alternative therapy. The objective is to make promising new drugs available to desperately ill patients as early as possible in the drug development process. By FDA definition, "*immediately life-threatening*" means "a stage of a disease in which there is a reasonable likelihood that death will occur within a matter of months or in which premature death is likely without early treatment" (1). This includes such conditions as advanced cases of AIDS, herpes simplex encephalitis, advanced metastatic refractory cancers, bacterial endocarditis, Alzheimer's disease, advanced multiple sclerosis, advanced Parkinson's disease, and others.

For products to be considered for a treatment IND, the drug must be under active investigation in a controlled clinical trial with sufficient evidence of its safety and efficacy demonstrated to support its use in the intended patients. Depending on the sponsor's clinical safety and efficacy data, a drug may be approved for treatment use during Phase 2 or Phase 3 of the clinical trials. In applying for a drug's treatment use, a sponsor must submit a *treatment protocol* in addition to the information normally included in an IND application. In making its decision, the FDA renders a risk–benefit judgment after considering the severity of the disease, any alternative therapy, and the potential benefits of the drug against the known and possible risks. In addition to the treatment IND, the law provides for the *emergency use* of an investigational drug in rare situations before a sponsor's submission of an IND application (1).

IND for an Orphan Drug

Under the Orphan Drug Act of 1983 as amended, an *orphan disease* is defined as a rare disease or condition that affects fewer than 200,000 people in the United States and for which there is no reasonable expectation that costs of research and development for the indication can be recovered by sales of the product in the United States. Examples of such illnesses are chronic lymphocytic leukemia, Gaucher's disease, cystic fibrosis, and conditions related to AIDS.

The FDA Office of Orphan Products Development was established to identify and facilitate the development of orphan products, including drugs, biologics, and medical devices. To foster the necessary research and development, the FDA provides support grants to conduct clinical trials on safety and effectiveness. Applicants first request orphan status designation for the disease and file an IND or an investigational device exemption with their grant application. In most cases, grants are awarded for Phase 2 and Phase 3 clinical studies based on preliminary clinical research. Regular and treatment IND protocols may be included in orphan drug clinical trials. An incentive to orphan product development is a provision for a 7-year period of exclusive marketing rights after regulatory approval of a product.

Withdrawal or Termination of an IND

A sponsor may withdraw an IND at any time, ending all clinical investigations. All stock of clinical supplies must be returned to the sponsor or otherwise destroyed. If an IND is withdrawn for safety reasons, the FDA, IRB, and all investigators must be so advised.

If no subjects are entered in an IND for 2 years or more or if investigations remain on a clinical hold for 1 year or more, the FDA may place the IND on inactive status upon proper notification of the sponsor. An IND may also be placed on inactive status on the initiative of the sponsor.

The FDA may terminate an IND and end related clinical investigations for reasons of safety, efficacy, or regulatory compliance.

The New Drug Application

If the three phases of clinical testing during the IND period demonstrate sufficient drug safety and therapeutic effectiveness, the sponsor may file a NDA with the FDA. This filing may be preceded by a pre-NDA meeting between the sponsor and the FDA to discuss the content and format of the new drug application. The purpose of the NDA is to gain permission to market the drug product in the United States.

General Content of the NDA Submission

A NDA contains a complete presentation of all of the preclinical and clinical results that the sponsor has obtained during investigation of the drug. It is a highly organized document that may contain several hundred volumes of information. In recent years, a computer-assisted new drug application process has been implemented whereby the sponsor may interact by computer with the FDA reviewers to facilitate the application review.

The applicant submits three copies of the NDA: an *archival copy*, maintained by the FDA as the reference document; a *review copy*, used by the FDA review division, and a *field copy*, used by the FDA district office and field inspectors in an on-site *preapproval inspection* (1). The preapproval inspection is conducted in the facilities in which the approved product is to be produced. The inspectors assess the sponsor's capability to comply with all control and quality standards contained in the application, including the FDA's Current Good Manufacturing Practice standards (discussed in Chapter 3). Final approval of an NDA can be contingent upon this inspection.

In part, an application for a new chemical entity contains the following components:

- Application form (form FDA 356h) with the name, address, date, and signature of the applicant or the applicant's authorized representative
- Chemical, nonproprietary, code, and proprietary names of the drug, the dosage form, its strength, and route of administration
- Statement regarding the applicant's proposal to market the drug product as prescription only or as an OTC product
- Detailed summary of all aspects of the application, including the proposed text of the product's intended labeling, chemistry, manufacturing and controls, nonclinical and clinical pharmacology and toxicology, human pharmacokinetics and bioavailability, statistical analysis, clinical trial data, benefit and risk considerations, and proposed additional or planned postmarketing studies
- Detailed technical sections on the chemistry, manufacturing, and controls for the drug substance, including its physical and chemical characteristics, methods of identification, assay, and controls, and the drug product, including its composition, specifications, methods of manufacture and equipment used, in-process controls, batch and master production records, container and closure systems, stability, and expiration dating
- Detailed technical sections for nonclinical pharmacology and toxicology in relation to the proposed therapeutic indication, including acute, subacute, and chronic toxicology, carcinogenicity, reproductive toxicology, and animal studies of absorption, distribution, metabolism, and excretion
- Detailed technical sections for human pharmacokinetics and bioavailability along with microbiology for antibiotic applications
- Detailed technical sections for clinical data for each controlled and uncontrolled study

relating to the proposed indication, a copy of the study protocol, effectiveness and safety data including any updates on safety information, comparison of human and animal pharmacology and toxicology data, support for the dosage and dose intervals and modifications for specific subgroups, such as pediatric, geriatric, and renally impaired subjects
- Statement regarding compliance to IRB and informed consent requirements
- Statistical methods and analysis of the clinical data
- Samples of the drug substance, drug product proposed for marketing, reference standards, and finished market package, as requested
- Clinical case report forms for the archival copy of the application

The FDA accepts foreign clinical data if they are applicable to the United States population and domestic medical practice; if the studies were conducted by clinical investigators of recognized competence; and if the FDA considers the data to be valid without the need for an on-site inspection. The FDA has entered into bilateral agreements with some countries whereby inspections performed by regulatory personnel of those countries are acceptable to the FDA.

Drug Product Labeling

The labeling of all drug products distributed in the United States must meet the specific labeling requirements set forth in the *Code of Federal Regulations* and approved for each product by the FDA (53). Specific labeling requirements differ for prescription drugs, nonprescription drugs, and animal drugs. In each instance, however, the objective is the same—to ensure the appropriate and safe use of the approved product.

According to federal regulations, *drug labeling* includes not only the labels placed on an immediate container but also the information on the packaging, in package inserts, and in company literature, advertising, and promotional materials.

For prescription drugs, labeling is a summary of all of the preclinical and clinical studies conducted over the period from drug discovery through product development to FDA approval. The essential prescribing information for a human prescription drug is provided in the package insert, which by law contains a balanced presentation of the usefulness and the risks associated with the product to enable safe and effective use. The package insert is required to contain the following summary information in the order listed.

1. *Description* of the product, including the proprietary and nonproprietary names, dosage form and route of administration, quantitative product composition, pharmacologic or therapeutic class of the drug, chemical name and structural formula of the drug compound, and important chemical and physical information (e.g., pH, sterility).
2. *Clinical pharmacology*, including a summary of actions of the drug in humans, relevant in vitro and animal studies essential to the biochemical and/or physiologic basis for action, pharmacokinetic information on rate and degree of absorption, biotransformation and metabolite formation, degree of drug binding to plasma proteins, rate or half-time of elimination, uptake by a particular organ or fetus, and any toxic effects.
3. *Indications and usage*, including the FDA-approved indications in the treatment, prevention, or diagnosis of a disease or condition, evidence of effectiveness demonstrated by results of controlled clinical trials, and special conditions to the drug's use for short-term or long-term use.
4. *Contraindications*, situations in which the drug should not be used because the risk of use clearly outweighs any possible beneficial effect. Contraindications may be associated with drug hypersensitivity, concomitant therapy, disease state, pregnancy, and/or factors of age or gender.
5. *Warnings*, including descriptions of serious adverse reactions and potential safety hazards, limitations to use imposed by them, and steps to be taken if they occur. Especially serious warnings are called black box warnings, as they are set off in the product's labeling within a black box.
6. *Precautions*, including special care to be exercised by prescriber and patient in the use of the drug; these include drug–drug, drug–food, drug–laboratory test interactions, effects on fertility, use in pregnancy, and use in nursing mothers and children.
7. *Adverse reactions*, including predictable and potential unpredictable undesired (side) effects, categorized by organ system or severity of reaction and frequency of occurrence.
8. *Drug abuse and dependence*, including legal schedule if a controlled substance, types of abuse and resultant adverse reactions, psychologic and physical dependence potential, and treatment of withdrawal.
9. *Overdosage*, including signs, symptoms, and laboratory findings of acute overdosage, along with specifics or principles of treatment.
10. *Dosage and administration*, stating the recommended usual dose, the usual dosage range, the safe upper limit of dosage, duration of treatment, modification of dosage in special patient populations (children, elders, patients with kidney and/or liver dysfunction), and special rates of administration (as with parenteral medications).
11. *How supplied*, including information on available dosage forms, strengths, and means of dosage form identification, as color, coating, scoring, and National Drug Code.

FDA Review and Action Letters

The completed NDA is carefully reviewed by the FDA, which decides whether to allow the sponsor to market the drug, to disallow marketing, or to require additional data before rendering a judgment. By regulation, the FDA must respond within 180 days of receipt of an application. This 180-day period is called the *review clock* and is often extended by agreement between the applicant and the FDA, as additional information, studies, or clarifications are sought.

The NDA is reviewed by the same FDA division that reviewed the sponsor's original IND. However, for the NDA review, the FDA also obtains the recommendation of an outside advisory review committee composed of persons of recognized competence and stature in the clinical area of the proposed drug's use. Although not binding, this committee's recommendation has influence in the FDA's decision to issue one of the following action letters after the entire review of the application is completed.

> *Approvable letter:* The agency will approve the application if specific additional data or other requested material is submitted or if specified conditions are met. This frequently pertains to development or wording of the final product labeling.
> *Approval letter:* Approval of the application permitting marketing.
> *Not approvable letter:* The application is not considered approvable because of one or more deficiencies.

After an NDA is approved and the product marketed, the FDA requires periodic safety and other reports, schedules plant inspections, and requires continued compliance with control and quality standards and current good manufacturing practices.

Phase 4 Studies and Postmarketing Surveillance

The receipt of marketing status for a new drug product does not necessarily end a sponsor's investigation of the drug. Continued clinical investigations, often called Phase 4 studies, may contribute to the understanding of the drug's mechanism or scope of action, may indicate possible new therapeutic uses for the drug, and/or may demonstrate the need for additional dosage strengths, dosage forms, or routes of administration. Postmarketing studies may also reveal additional side effects, serious and unexpected adverse effects, and/or drug interactions.

In applying for a new use, strength, dosage form, or route of administration for a previously approved drug, the sponsor must file a new IND, conduct all necessary additional nonclinical and clinical studies, and file a new NDA for FDA review.

Postmarketing Reporting of Adverse Drug Experiences

A drug's sponsor is required to report to the FDA each adverse drug experience that is both serious (life-threatening or fatal) and unexpected (not contained in the approved drug product labeling), regardless of the source of the information, within 15 working days of receipt of the information. These 15-day alert reports must then be investigated by the sponsor with a follow-up report submitted to the FDA, again within 15 working days. Other adverse events, not considered serious and unexpected, are reported quarterly for 3 years following the date of approval of the NDA and annually thereafter. Practicing pharmacists and other health care professionals participate in adverse drug experience reporting through the FDA's MedWatch program, using forms provided for this purpose (54).

Depending on the nature, causal relationship, and seriousness of an adverse drug reaction report, the FDA may require revised product labeling to reflect the new findings, ask the sponsor to issue special warning notices to health care professionals, undertake or require the sponsor to undertake a review of all available clinical data, restrict the marketing of the product during a review period, issue a product recall notice, or withdraw product approval for marketing.

In the event of information on or a confirmed incident of a mislabeled, contaminated, or deteriorated product in distribution, the sponsor is required to file an NDA field alert report to the FDA district office by telephone or other rapid communication within 3 working days of receipt of the information. The FDA follows up with appropriate action.

Annual Reports

Each year the sponsor of an approved drug must file with the FDA division responsible for the NDA review a report containing the following information:

- An annual summary of significant new information that might affect the safety, effectiveness, or labeling of the drug product

- Data on the quantity of dosage units of the drug product distributed domestically and abroad
- A sample of professional labeling, patient brochures, or package inserts, and a summary of any changes since the previous report
- Reports of experiences, investigations, studies, or tests involving chemical or physical properties of the drug that may affect its safety or effectiveness
- A full description of any manufacturing and controls changes not requiring a supplemental new drug application
- Copies of unpublished reports and summaries of published reports of new toxicologic findings in vitro and animal studies conducted or obtained by the sponsor
- Full or abstract reports on published clinical trials of the drug, including studies on safety and effectiveness; new uses; biopharmaceutical, pharmacokinetic, clinical pharmacologic, and epidemiologic reports; pharmacotherapeutic and lay press articles on the drug; summaries of unpublished clinical trials or prepublication manuscripts, as available, conducted or obtained by the sponsor
- A statement on the current status of any postmarketing studies performed by or on behalf of the sponsor
- Specimens of mailing pieces or other forms of promotion of the drug product

Failure to make required reports may lead to FDA withdrawal of approval for marketing.

Supplemental, Abbreviated, and Other Applications

In addition to the IND and NDA, the following types of applications are filed with the FDA for the purposes described.

Supplemental New Drug Application

A sponsor of an approved NDA may make changes in that application through the filing of a supplemental new drug application (SNDA). Depending on the changes proposed, some re-quire FDA approval before implementing; others do not. Among the changes requiring prior approval:

- A change in the method of synthesis of the drug substance
- Use of a different facility to manufacture the drug substance where the facility has not been approved through inspection for Current Good Manufacturing Practice standards within the previous 2 years
- Change in the formulation, analytical standards, method of manufacture, or in-process controls of the drug product
- Use of a different facility or contractor to manufacture, process, or package the drug product
- Change in the container and closure system for a drug product
- Extension of the expiration date for a drug product based on new stability data
- Any labeling change that does not add to or strengthen a previously approved label statement

Examples of changes that may be made without prior approval are minor editorial or other changes in the labeling that add to or strengthen an approved label section; any analytical changes made to comply with the USP–NF; an extension of the product's expiration date based on full shelf-life data obtained from a protocol in the approved application; and a change in the size (not the type of system) of the container for a solid dosage form.

Abbreviated New Drug Application

An abbreviated new drug application (ANDA) is one in which nonclinical laboratory studies and clinical investigations may be omitted, except those pertaining to the drug's bioavailability. These applications are usually filed for duplicates (generic copies) of drug products previously approved under a full NDA and for which the FDA has determined that information on the exempted nonclinical and clinical studies is already available at the agency. ANDAs commonly are filed by competing companies following the expiration of patent term protection of the innovator drug or drug product.

Bioavailability and product bioequivalency are discussed in Chapter 5.

Biologics License Application

Biologics License Applications (BLAs) are submitted to the FDA's CBER for the manufacture of biologics, such as blood products, vaccines, and toxins. The applications for biologics approvals follow the regulatory requirements as stated specifically for these products in the relevant parts of the *Code of Federal Regulations* (4).

Animal Drug Applications

The Federal Food, Drug, and Cosmetic Act, as amended, contains specific regulations pertaining to approval for the marketing and labeling of drugs intended for animal use (6). Regulations apply to investigational new animal drug applications, new animal drug applications (NADA), supplemental new animal drug applications, and abbreviated new animal drug applications.

On October 22, 1994, the Animal Medicinal Drug Use Clarification Act of 1994 was signed into law. It allows veterinarians to prescribe extralabel uses of approved animal drugs and approved human drugs for animals.

Medical Devices

The FDA has regulatory authority over the manufacture and licensing of all medical devices, from surgical gloves and catheters to cardiac pacemakers and cardiopulmonary bypass blood gas monitors (7). Included in the regulations are standards and procedures for manufacturer registration, investigational studies, good manufacturing practices, and premarket approval.

International Conference on Harmonization of Technical Requirements for Registration of Pharmaceuticals for Human Use

In recognition of the international marketplace for pharmaceuticals and in an effort to achieve global efficiencies for both regulatory agencies and the pharmaceutical industry, the FDA, counterpart agencies of the European Union and Japan, and geographic representatives of the pharmaceutical industry formed a tripartite organization in 1991 to discuss, identify, and address relevant regulatory issues. This organization, named the International Conference on Harmonization of Technical Requirements for Registration of Pharmaceuticals for Human Use (ICH) has worked toward harmonizing, or bringing together, regulatory requirements with the long-range goal of establishing a uniform set of standards for drug registration within these geographic areas.

With ICH success, duplicative technical requirements for registering pharmaceuticals would be eliminated; new drug approvals would occur more rapidly; patients' access to new medicines would be enhanced worldwide; the quality, safety, and efficacy of imported products would be improved; and there would be an increase in information transfer between participating countries (55–56).

The ICH's work toward uniform standards is focused on three general areas, quality, safety, and efficacy.

The quality topics include stability, light stability, analytical validation, impurities, and biotechnology. The safety topics include carcinogenicity, genotoxicity, toxicokinetics, reproduction toxicity, and single- and repeat-dose toxicity. The efficacy topics include population exposure, managing clinical trials, clinical study reports, dose response, ethnic factors, good clinical practices, and geriatrics. For each topic, relevant regulations are identified, addressed, and consensus guidelines developed. The intention is that these guidelines will be incorporated into domestic regulations. In the United States, the resulting guidelines are published in the *Federal Register* as notices, with accompanying statements indicating that the guideline should be "useful" or "considered" by applicants conducting required studies or submitting registration applications. Examples of specific ICH-developed guidelines:

Stability testing of new drug substances and products

Validation of analytical procedures for
pharmaceuticals

Impurities in new drug substances

Impurities in new drug products

Nonclinical safety studies for the conduct of
human clinical trials for pharmaceuticals

Preclinical testing of biotechnology-
derived pharmaceuticals

General considerations for clinical trials

Studies in support of special populations:
geriatrics

Ethnic factors in the acceptability of foreign data

Repeated dose tissue distribution studies

Dose selection for carcinogenicity studies
of pharmaceuticals

Dose response information to support drug
registration

REFERENCES

1. Code of Federal Regulations, Title 21, Parts 300–314.
2. Code of Federal Regulations, Title 21, Part 320.
3. Code of Federal Regulations, Title 21, Part 430.
4. Code of Federal Regulations, Title 21, Parts 600–680.
5. Code of Federal Regulations, Title 21, Part 330.
6. Code of Federal Regulations, Title 21, Parts 510–555.
7. Code of Federal Regulations, Title 21, Parts 800–895.
8. Federal Register, U.S. Washington: Government Printing Office, Superintendent of Documents.
9. Mathieu M. New Drug Development: A Regulatory Overview. 3rd ed. Cambridge, MA: PAREXEL International, 1994.
10. Guarino RA, ed. New Drug Approval Process. New York: Marcel Dekker, 1987.
11. Smith CG. The Process of New Drug Discovery and Development. Boca Raton, FL: CRC, 1992.
12. Sneader W. Drug Development: From Laboratory to Clinic. New York: John Wiley & Sons, 1986.
13. Spilker B. Multinational Pharmaceutical Companies Principles and Practices. 2nd ed. New York: Raven Press, 1994.
14. Wordell CJ. Biotechnology update. Hosp Pharm 1991;26:897–900.
15. Tami JA, Parr MD, Brown SA, Thompson, JS. Monoclonal antibody technology. Am J Hosp Pharm 1986;43:2816–2826.
16. Brodsky FM. Monoclonal antibodies as magic bullets. Pharm Res 1988;5:1–9.
17. Parasrampuria DA, Hunt CA. Therapeutic delivery issues in gene therapy, part 2: targeting approaches. Pharm Tech 1998;22:34–43.
18. Chew NJ. Cellular and gene therapies, part 1: regulatory health. BioPharmacy 1995;8:22–23.
19. Smith TJ. Gene therapy: opportunities for pharmacy in the 21st century. Am J Pharm Ed 1996;60:213–215.
20. Milestones in gene therapy. BioPharmacy 1997;10:17.
21. Kauvar, LM. Affinity fingerprinting: implications for drug discovery. Pharm News 1996;3:12–15.
22. Harris, AL. High throughput screening and molecular diversity. Pharm News 1995;2:26–30.
23. Silverman RB. Drug discovery, design, and development. In: The Organic Chemistry of Drug Design and Drug Action. New York: Academic Press, 1992;4–51.
24. Perun TJ, Propst CL, eds. Computer-aided Drug Design: Methods and Applications. New York: Marcel Dekker, 1989.
25. Spraycar M (Ed.). Stedman's Medical Dictionary, 26th ed. Baltimore: Williams & Wilkins, 1995;1340.
26. Katzung BG. Basic and Clinical Pharmacology. Norwalk, CT: Appleton & Lange, 1987;44–51.
27. Spilker B. Extrapolation of preclinical safety data to humans. Drug News Perspect 1991;4:214–216.
28. Guideline for the Format and Content of the Nonclinical/Pharmacology/Toxicology Section of an Application. Rockville, MD: Food and Drug Administration, 1987.
29. 60 Federal Register 11263–11268. International conference on harmonization; guideline on the assessment of systemic exposure in toxicity studies, 1995.
30. 60 Federal Register 11277–11281. International conference on harmonization; guidance on dose selection for carcinogenicity study of pharmaceuticals, 1995.
31. 58 Federal Register 21073–21080. International conference on harmonization; draft guideline on detection of toxicity to reproduction for medicinal products, 1993.
32. 59 Federal Register 48734–48737. International conference on harmonization, draft guideline on specific aspects of regulatory genotoxicity tests, 1994.
33. Guideline for the Format and Content of the Chemistry, Manufacturing, and Controls Section of an Application. Rockville, MD: Food and Drug Administration, 1987.
34. Amidon GL, Lennarnas H, Shah VP, Crison JR. A theoretical basis for a biopharmaceutic drug classification: the correlation of in vitro drug product dissolution and in vivo bioavailability. Pharm Res 12(3):1995;413–420.
35. Code of Federal Regulations, Title 21, Parts 210–211.
36. 58 Federal Register 39405–39416. Guideline for the study and evaluation of gender differences in the clinical evaluation of drugs, 1993.
37. 59 Federal Register 11145–11151. NIH guidelines on the inclusion of women and minorities as subjects in clinical research, 1994.
38. Richardson ER. Drugs and pregnancy. Wellcome Trends in Pharmacy 1983;7:4.
39. 62 Federal Register 49946–49954. Investigational new drug applications; proposed amendment to clinical hold regulations for products intended for life-threatening diseases, 1997.
40. Wright DT, Chew NJ. Women as subjects in clinical research. Appl Clin Trials 1996;5:44–52.
41. Wick JY. Culture, ethnicity, and medications. JAPhA 1996;NS36:555–563.

42. Code of Federal Regulations, Title 21, Part 56.

43. Code of Federal Regulations, Title 21, Part 50.

44. Hunter JR, Rosen DL, DeChristoforo R. How FDA expedites evaluation of drugs for AIDS and other life-threatening illnesses. Wellcome Programs in Hosp Pharm 1993 (January).

45. Spilker B. Guide to Clinical Trials. New York: Raven, 1991.

46. Bush C. When your subject is a child. Appl Clin Trials 1997;6:54–56.

47. Cohen HJ. The elderly patient: a challenge to the art and science of medicine. Drug Ther 1983; 13:41.

48. Futerman SS. The geriatric patient: pharmacy care can make a difference. Apothecary 1982;94:34.

49. Lexi-Comp's Drug Information Series; Pediatric Dosage Handbook and Geriatric Dosage Handbook; Lexi-Comp, Hudson, Ohio; American Pharmacists Association, Washington, DC.

50. Food and Drug Administration. FDA Med Bull 1993:23:2–4.

51. Logsdon BA. Drug use during lactation. JAPhA 1997;NS37:407–418.

52. The transfer of drugs and other chemicals into human breast milk. Washington: American Pharmacists Association, 1983.

53. Code of Federal Regulations, Title 21, Part 201.

54. MedWatch. Rockville, MD: Food and Drug Administration.

55. Heydorn WE. ICH: background and current status. Pharm News 1994;1:22–24.

56. Report of the FDA task force on international harmonization. Rockville, MD: Food and Drug Administration, 1992.

Current Good Manufacturing Practices and Current Good Compounding Practices

3

Chapter at a glance

Standards for Current Good Manufacturing Practice

Current Good Manufacturing Practice (cGMP or GMP) regulations are established by the Food and Drug Administration (FDA) to ensure that minimum standards are met for drug product quality in the United States. The first GMP regulations were promulgated in 1963 under the provisions of the Kefauver-Harris Drug Amendments and since then they have been periodically revised and updated.

The cGMP regulations establish requirements for all aspects of pharmaceutical manufacture. They apply to domestic and to foreign suppliers and manufacturers whose bulk components and finished pharmaceutical products are imported, distributed or sold in this country. To ensure compliance, the FDA inspects the facilities and production records of all firms covered by these regulations.

The Code of Federal Regulations contains requirements for the "Current Good Manufacturing Practice for Finished Pharmaceuticals,"

(1) and additional cGMP requirements for biologic products (2), medicated articles (3), and medical devices (4). Currency and compliance with cGMP regulations is supported through notices in the Federal Register and through the FDA's Compliance Policy Guide and various other Guidances issued by the FDA.

A topical outline of the cGMP regulations for finished pharmaceuticals is presented in Table 3.1 and summarized in the sections that follow.

TABLE 3.1 TOPICAL OUTLINE OF CURRENT GOOD MANUFACTURING PRACTICE REGULATIONS

General Provisions
Scope
Definitions

Organization and Personnel
  Responsibilities of quality control unit
  Personnel qualifications
  Personnel responsibilities
  Consultants

Buildings and Facilities
  Design and construction features
  Lighting
  Ventilation, air filtration, air heating and
    cooling
  Plumbing
  Sewage and refuse
  Washing and toilet facilities
  Sanitation
  Maintenance

Equipment
  Equipment design, size, and location
  Equipment construction
  Equipment cleaning and maintenance
  Automatic, mechanical, and electronic
    equipment
  Filters

Control of Components and Drug Product Containers and Closures
  General requirements
  Receipt and storage of untested components,
    drug product containers, and closures
  Testing and approval or rejection of components,
    drug product containers, and closures
  Use of approved components, drug product
    containers, and closures
  Retesting of approved components, drug product
    containers, and closures
  Rejected components, drug product containers,
    and closures
  Drug product containers and closures

Production and Process Controls
  Written procedures; deviations
  Charge-in of components
  Calculation of yield
  Equipment identification
  Sampling and testing of in-process materials and
    drug products
  Time limitations on production
  Control of microbiological contamination
  Reprocessing

Packaging and Labeling Control
  Materials examination and usage criteria
  Labeling issuance
  Packaging and labeling operations
  Tamper-resistant packaging requirements for
    over-the-counter human drug products
  Drug product inspection
  Expiration dating

Holding and Distribution
  Warehousing procedures
  Distribution procedures

Laboratory Controls
  General requirements
  Testing and release for distribution
  Stability testing
  Special testing requirements
  Reserve samples
  Laboratory animals
  Penicillin contamination

Records and Reports
  General requirements
  Equipment cleaning and use log
  Component, drug product container, closure, and
    labeling records
  Master production and control records
  Batch production and control records
  Production record review
  Laboratory records
  Distribution records
  Complaint files

Returned and Salvaged Drug Products
  Returned drug products
  Drug product salvaging

Code of Federal Regulations 21, part 211, revised April 1, 1996.

cGMP for Finished Pharmaceuticals

General Provisions: Scope and Definitions

The regulations in 21 CFR, Part 211 contain the minimum good manufacturing practice requirements for the preparation of finished pharmaceutical products for administration to humans or animals.

Common terms used in these regulations are defined as follows:

Active ingredient or active pharmaceutical ingredient: Any component that is intended to furnish pharmacologic activity or other direct effect in the diagnosis, cure, mitigation, treatment or prevention of disease or to affect the structure or function of the body of man or other animals.

Batch: A specific quantity of a drug of uniform specified quality produced according to a single manufacturing order during the same cycle of manufacture.

Batchwise control: The use of validated in-process sampling and testing methods in such a way that results prove the process has done what it purports to do for the specific batch concerned.

Certification: Documented testimony by qualified authorities that a system qualification, calibration, validation, or revalidation has been performed appropriately and that the results are acceptable.

Compliance: Determination through inspection of the extent to which a manufacturer is acting in accordance with prescribed regulations, standards, and practices.

Component: Any ingredient used in the manufacture of a drug product, including those that may not be present in the finished product.

Drug product: A finished form that contains an active drug and inactive ingredients. The term may also include a form that does not contain an active ingredient, such as a placebo.

Inactive ingredient: Any component other than the active ingredients in a drug product.

Lot: A batch or any portion of a batch having uniform specified quality and a distinctive identifying lot number.

Lot number, control number, or batch number: Any distinctive combination of letters, numbers, or symbols from which the complete history of the manufacture, processing, packaging, holding, and distribution of a batch or lot of a drug product may be determined.

Master record: Record containing the formulation, specifications, manufacturing procedures, quality assurance requirements, and labeling of a finished product.

Quality assurance: Provision to all concerned the evidence needed to establish confidence that the activities relating to quality are being performed adequately.

Quality audit: A documented activity performed in accordance with established procedures on a planned and periodic basis to verify compliance with the procedures to ensure quality.

Quality control: The regulatory process through which industry measures actual quality performance, compares it with standards, and acts on the difference.

Quality control unit: An organizational element designated by a firm to be responsible for the duties relating to quality control.

Quarantine: An area that is marked, designated, or set aside for the holding of incoming components prior to acceptance testing and qualification for use.

Representative sample: A sample that accurately portrays the whole.

Reprocessing: The activity whereby the finished product or any of its components is recycled through all or part of the manufacturing process.

Strength: The concentration of the drug substance per unit dose or volume.

Verified: Signed by a second individual or recorded by automated equipment.

Validation: Documented evidence that a system (e.g., equipment, software, controls) does what it purports to do.

Process validation: Documented evidence that a process (e.g., sterilization) does what it purports to do.

Validation protocol: A prospective experimental plan to produce documented evidence that the system has been validated.

Organization and Personnel

The organization and personnel section of the regulations deals with the responsibilities of the quality control unit, employees, and consultants. The regulations require that a quality control unit have the authority and responsibility for all functions that may affect product quality. This includes accepting or rejecting product components, product specifications, finished products, packaging, and labeling. Adequate laboratory facilities shall be provided, written procedures followed, and all records maintained.

All personnel engaged in the manufacture, processing, packing, or holding of a drug product, including those in supervisory positions, are required to have the education, training, and/or experience needed to fulfill the assigned responsibility. Appropriate programs of skill development, continuing education and training, and performance evaluations are essential for maintaining quality assurance. Any consultants advising on scientific and technical matters should possess requisite qualifications for the tasks.

Buildings and Facilities

As outlined in Table 3.1, the regulations in this section include the design, structural features, and functional aspects of buildings and facilities. Each building's structure, space, design, and placement of equipment must be such to enable thorough cleaning, inspection, and safe and effective use for the designated operations. Proper considerations must be given to such factors as water quality standards; security; materials used for floors, walls, and ceilings; lighting; segregated quarantine areas for raw materials and product components subject to quality control ap-

proval; holding areas for rejected components; storage areas for released components; weighing and measuring rooms; sterile areas for ophthalmic and parenteral products; flammable materials storage areas; finished products storage; control of heat, humidity, temperature, and ventilation; waste handling; employee facilities and safety procedures in compliance with the Occupational Safety and Health Administration regulations; and procedures and practices of personal sanitation.

All work in the manufacture, processing, packing, or holding of a pharmaceutical product must be logged in, inspected by a supervisor, and signed off. Similarly, a log of building maintenance must be kept to document this component of the regulations.

Equipment

Each piece of equipment must be of appropriate design and size and suitably located to facilitate operations for its intended use, cleaning, and maintenance. The equipment's surfaces and parts must not interact with the processes or product's components so as to alter the purity, strength, or quality.

Standard operating procedures must be written and followed for the proper use, maintenance, and cleaning of each piece of equipment, and appropriate logs and records must be kept. Automated equipment and computers used in the processes must be routinely calibrated, maintained, and validated for accuracy.

Filters used in the manufacture or processing of injectable drug products shall not release fibers into such products. If fiber-releasing filters must be used, non–fiber-releasing filters also must be used to reduce any fiber content.

Control of Components, Containers, and Closures

Written procedures describing the receipt, identification, storage, handling, sampling, testing, and approval or rejection of all drug product components, product containers, and closures must be maintained and followed. Bulk pharmaceutical chemicals, containers, and closures must meet the exact physical and chemical specifications established with the supplier at the time of ordering.

When product components are received from a supplier, each lot must be logged in with the purchase order number, date of receipt, bill of lading, name and vital information of the supplier, supplier's stock or control number, and quantity received. The component is assigned a control number that identifies both the component and the intended product. Raw materials are quarantined until they are verified through representative sampling and careful qualitative and quantitative analysis. The quality control unit approves and releases for use in manufacture only those that meet the specifications. The assigned control number follows the component throughout production so it can be traced if necessary.

Rejected components, drug product containers, and closures are identified and controlled under a quarantine system to prevent their use in manufacturing and processing operations.

Production and Process Controls

Written procedures are required for production and process controls to ensure that the drug products have the correct identity, strength, quality, and purity. These procedures, which include the charge-in of all components, use of in-process controls, sample testing, and process and equipment validation, must be followed for quality assurance. Any deviation from the written procedures must be recorded and justified. In most instances, the operator records time and date of each key operation and the supervisor signs off on it. When operations are controlled by automated equipment, such equipment must be validated regularly for precision.

All product ingredients, equipment, and drums or other containers of bulk finished product must be distinctively identified by labeling as to content and/or status.

In-process samples are taken from production batches periodically for product control. In-process controls are of two general types: (*a*) those performed by production personnel at the time of operation to ensure that the machinery is producing output within preestab-lished control limits (e.g., tablet size, hardness), and (*b*) those performed by the quality control laboratory personnel to ensure compliance with all product specifications (e.g., tablet content, dissolution) and batch-to-batch consistency. Product found out of standard sometimes may be reprocessed for subsequent use. However, in this, as in all instances, procedures must be performed according to established protocol, all materials must be accounted for, all specifications met, and all records meticulously maintained.

Packaging and Labeling Control

Written procedures are required for the receipt, identification, storage, handling, sampling, and testing of drug product and issuance of labeling and packaging materials. Labeling for each variation in drug product—strength, dosage form, or quantity of contents—must be stored separately with suitable identification. Obsolete and outdated labels and other packaging materials must be destroyed. Access to the storage area must be limited to authorized personnel.

All materials must be withheld for use in the packaging and labeling of product until approved and released by the quality control unit. Control procedures must be followed and records maintained for the issuance and use of product labeling. Quantities issued, used, and returned must be reconciled and discrepancies investigated. Before labeling operations commence, the labeling facilities must be inspected to ensure that all drug products and labels have been removed from the previous operations. During and at the conclusion of an operation, the products are visually or electronically inspected for correct labeling and packaging. All of these procedures are essential to avoid label mixups and the mislabeling of products. All records of inspections and controls must be documented in the batch production records.

Labels must meet the legal requirements for content as outlined in Chapter 2 and later in this chapter. Each label must contain expiration dating and the production batch or lot number to facilitate product identification. Special packaging requirements may apply in certain instances, as with tamper-evident packaging for over-the-counter (OTC) products.

Expiration Dating

To ensure that a drug product meets applicable standards of identity, strength, quality, and purity at the time of use, it must bear an expiration date determined by appropriate stability testing. Exempt from this requirement are homeopathic drug products, allergenic extracts, and investigational drugs that meet the standards established during preclinical and clinical studies.

Tamper-Evident Packaging

On November 5, 1982, the FDA published initial regulations on tamper-resistant packaging in the *Federal Register*. These regulations were promulgated after criminal tampering with OTC drug products earlier in that year resulted in illness and deaths. In the primary incident, cyanide was surreptitiously placed in acetaminophen capsules in commercial packages.

Today, the cGMP regulations require tamper-evident packaging for OTC drug products to improve their security and to ensure their safety and effectiveness. All OTC drug products offered for retail sale are required to have tamper-evident packaging except for some categories, such as dentifrices, skin care products, insulin, and throat lozenges. For other product categories, a manufacturer may file with the FDA a Request for Exemption From Tamper Evident Rule. The petition is required to contain specific information on the drug product, the reasons the requirement is unnecessary or cannot be achieved, and alternative steps the petitioner has taken or may take to reduce the likelihood of malicious adulteration of the product. Generally exempt from these regulations are products not packaged for retail sale but rather distributed to hospitals, nursing homes, and health care clinics for institutional use.

A tamper-evident package is defined as "one having one or more indicators or barriers to entry which, if breached or missing, can reasonably be expected to provide visible evidence to consumers that tampering has occurred" (1). The indicators or barriers may involve the immediate drug product container and/or an outer container or carton. For two-piece hard gelatin capsule products, a minimum of two tamper-evident packaging features is required unless the capsules are sealed with tamper-resistant technology.

Even with these safeguards in effect, the possibility of drug product tampering requires the pharmacist and consumer to remain constantly vigilant for signs of product entry. Pharmaceutical manufacturers have the option of determining the type of tamper-resistant packaging to use. Table 3.2 presents some examples of tamper-evident packaging.

Holding and Distribution

Written procedures must be established and followed for the holding and distribution of product. Finished pharmaceuticals must be quarantined in storage until released by the quality control unit. Products must be stored and shipped under conditions that do not affect product quality. Ordinarily, the oldest approved stock is distributed first. The distribution control system must allow the distribution point of each lot of drug product to be readily determined to facilitate its recall if necessary.

Laboratory Controls

Laboratory controls are requirements for the establishment of and conformance to written specifications, standards, sampling plans, test procedures, and other such mechanisms. The specifications, which apply to each batch of drug product, include provisions for sample size, test intervals, sample storage, stability testing, and special testing requirements for certain dosage forms, including parenterals, ophthalmics, controlled-release products, and radioactive pharmaceuticals. Reserve samples must be retained for distributed products for specified periods depending on their category. Reserve samples must be maintained for 1 to 3 years after the expiration date of the last lot of the drug product.

Records and Reports

Production, control, and distribution records must be maintained for at least a year follow-

TABLE 3.2 EXAMPLES OF TAMPER-EVIDENT PACKAGING

PACKAGE TYPE	TAMPER PROTECTION
Film wrapper	Sealed around product and/or product container; film must be cut or torn to remove product.
Blister/strip pack	Individually sealed dose units; removal requires tearing or breaking individual compartment.
Bubble pack	Product and container sealed in plastic, usually mounted on display card; plastic must be cut or broken open to remove product.
Shrink seal, band	Band or wrapper shrunk by heat or drying to conform to cap; must be torn to open package.
Foil, paper, plastic pouch	Sealed individual packet; must be torn to reach product.
Bottle seal	Paper or foil sealed to mouth of container under cap; must be torn or broken to reach product.
Tape seal	Paper or foil sealed over carton flap or bottle cap; must be torn or broken to reach product.
Breakable cap	Plastic or metal tearaway cap over container; must be broken to remove.
Sealed tube	Seal over mouth of tube; must be punctured to reach product.
Sealed carton	Carton flaps sealed; carton cannot be opened without damage.
Aerosol container	Tamper-resistant by design.

ing the expiration date of a product batch. This includes equipment cleaning and maintenance logs; specifications and lot numbers of product components, including raw materials and product containers and closures; and label records. Complete master production and control records for each batch must be kept and must include the following:

Name and strength of the product
Dosage form
Quantitative amounts of components and dosage units
Complete manufacturing and control procedures
Specifications
Special notations
Equipment used
In-process controls
Sampling and laboratory methods and assay results
Calibration of instruments
Distribution records
Dated and employee-identified records

These master records must document that each step in the production, control, packaging, labeling, and distribution of the product was ac-complished and approved by the quality control unit. Depending on the operation, the operator's and/or supervisor's full signatures, initials, or other written or electronic identification codes are required.

Records of written and oral complaints regarding a drug product (e.g., product failure, adverse drug experience) must also be maintained, along with information regarding the internal disposition of each complaint. All records must be made available at the time of inspection by FDA officials.

Returned and Salvaged Drug Products

Returned drug products (e.g., from wholesalers) must be identified by lot number and product quality determined through appropriate testing. Drug products that meet specifications may be salvaged or reprocessed. Those that do not, along with those that have been subjected to improper storage (e.g., extremes in temperature), shall not be returned to the marketplace. Records for all returned products must be maintained and must include the date and reasons for the return; quantity and lot number of product returned; procedures employed for holding, testing, and reprocessing the product; and the product's disposition.

Information Technology and Automation

Although not part of the cGMP requirements, the effective deployment of information technologies and automated systems can enhance pharmaceutical process development, production efficiencies, product quality, and regulatory compliance (5).

Computers are used extensively in plant operations such as production scheduling, in-process manufacturing, quality control, and packaging and labeling. The networking of computers in the production and quality control areas fully integrates laboratory information and manufacturing operations into sophisticated management systems. These integrated systems support cGMP compliance, process validation, resource management, and cost control. Figure 3.1 presents an example of computer use in the pharmaceutical industry for the management of plant operations.

Robotic devices increasingly are being employed to replace manual operations in production lines, analytical sampling, and packaging. Figure 3.2 presents an example of robot use in the laboratory. Laboratory robotics provides automation in areas such as sample preparation and handling, wet chemistry procedures, laboratory process control, and instrumental analysis (6). Pharmaceutical applications of robotics include automated product handling in production lines and in procedures such as sampling and analysis, tablet content uniformity, and dissolution testing.

Additional cGMP Regulatory Requirements

Active Pharmaceutical Ingredients and Pharmaceutical Excipients

The manufacture of active pharmaceutical ingredients (APIs) comes under the aegis of cGMP regulations and requirements. The FDA publication *Guide to the Inspection of Bulk Pharmaceutical Chemicals* (7) identifies the inspection program for manufacture of chemical components of pharmaceutical products to ensure that all required standards for quality are met. Because the quality of any finished pharmaceutical product depends on the quality of the various components, including the active ingredients, compliance with cGMPs is a critical part of the FDA's preapproval inspection program for new drug applications (NDAs) and abbreviated new drug applications (ANDAs).

The broad cGMP areas described previously for finished pharmaceuticals (e.g., facilities, personnel, production and process controls, process validation) apply but are directed toward the process-specific aspects of bulk pharmaceutical chemicals. The application of the regulations is focused on all of the defining elements of chemical purity and quality, including the following (8, 9):

Specifications and analytical methods for all reactive and nonreactive components used in synthesis
Critical chemical reaction steps

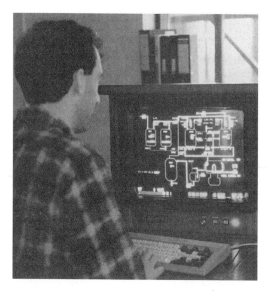

FIGURE 3.1 Example of computer use in the pharmaceutical industry. The machine shown is an Allen Bradley Advisor 21 operator interface. This allows the plant operator to communicate with the main programmable logical controller. The Advisor 21 gives a constant real-time update of the process on a series of screens and allows an operator to perform programmed operations at the push of a button. (Courtesy of Elan Corporation, plc.)

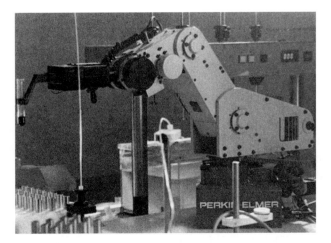

FIGURE 3.2 Robotics in laboratory use. Perkin-Elmer Robotic Arm and Perkin-Elmer Lambda 1a UV/VIS Spectropho-tometer. (Courtesy of Elan Corporation, plc.)

Handling of chemical intermediates

Effect of scale-up of chemical batches on the yield

Quality of the water systems

Solvent handling and recovery systems

Analytical methods to detect impurities or chemical residues and the limits set

Stability studies of the bulk pharmaceutical chemical

Pharmaceutical excipients, as they too are components of finished pharmaceutical products, must be produced in accordance with cGMP standards as certified on the application by each sponsor of an NDA or ANDA. Although there is no FDA approval system specific for pharmaceutical excipients, a comprehensive good manufacturing practices guide has been established by the U.S. affiliate of the International Pharmaceutical Excipients Council and is harmonized with the European counterpart organization (10).

Clinical Trial Materials

Clinical trial materials (CTM) must be produced in conformance with cGMP regulations. This applies to both the production of the active pharmaceutical ingredients (API) and investigational drug products.

The API used in a clinical investigation is subject to all of the requirements for the production of bulk pharmaceutical chemicals.

However, the batch size is different from the commercial scale used in the production of an FDA-approved product. In some cases, technology transfer in the production of an API from one production site or laboratory to another may require validation to ensure purity and quality standards.

The CTMs used in clinical investigations must be produced in compliance with the cGMP regulatory requirements and standardized as to identity, purity, strength, and quality (11). However, during preclinical testing and the early phases of clinical evaluation, a product's formulation and many of the production processes and analytical controls are under development. Thus, during this period, the regulatory requirements are applied with flexibility. As the clinical trials progress from Phase 1 to Phase 2, the processes are being characterized and refined, and during Phase 3 they are expected to meet all regulatory requirements. It is during Phase 3 that process optimization is demonstrated to the FDA by the production of at least one-tenth of a commercial-size batch (e.g., 100,000 capsules) of the proposed product. Prior to that, adequate supplies of dosing units from a few hundred to a few thousand may be prepared by hand or in pilot plant–scale operations as is necessary for the clinical trials.

In addition to the active drug product, matching placebo and/or comparator products must be prepared. Specific labeling, coding, packaging design, assembly, and distribution protocols are in effect for CTMs to accommodate the clinical trial design and the requirements for investigational drugs as discussed in Chapter 2.

Biologics

As noted previously, current good manufacturing practice standards are defined for biologic products in the *Code of Federal Regulations* (2). While the basic regulations for finished pharmaceuticals apply to biologic products as well, the nature of blood, bacterial, and viral products requires specific additional mandates. A full discussion of the cGMP requirements and standards for biologics are beyond the scope of this text; however, these example areas of activity demonstrate the scope of the additional regulatory content: blood collection procedures; environmental controls; segregation of activities; containment; cell bank and cell line characterization and testing; cell propagation and fermentation; inactivation of infectious agents; aseptic processing validation; use of bioassays; live vaccine work areas; work with spore-bearing organisms; and evaluation, quantification, and validation of risk factors.

Medical Devices

Medical devices follow a path for FDA approval that resembles that for pharmaceuticals. For instance, clinical investigations of devices are conducted on approval of an investigational device exemption and approved for marketing when shown to be safe and effective through a premarket approval application, similar to an investigational new drug (IND) and NDA, respectively. Medical devices also are subject to the reporting of adverse events, to recall, and to termination of approval.

The regulations for "good manufacturing practice for medical devices" are similar in organizational structure to those for finished pharmaceuticals. They include sections on personnel; buildings; equipment; control of components; production and process controls; packaging and labeling; holding, distri-

bution, and installation; device evaluation; and records (4).

Literally thousands of medical devices are regulated by the provisions of the *Code of Federal Regulations*. Each device has a specific design with individual performance features and utility. For many devices, specific standards are stated in the regulations. Devices covered by cGMP regulations include intraocular lenses, hearing aids, intrauterine devices, cardiac pacemakers, clinical chemistry analyzers, catheters, cardiopulmonary bypass heart-lung machine console, dental x-ray equipment, surgical gloves, condoms, prosthetic hip joints, traction equipment, computed tomography equipment, and powered wheelchairs.

Noncompliance with cGMP Regulations

Noncompliance with cGMP regulations can lead to a number of regulatory actions by the FDA. Noncompliance determined during a premarket approval inspection of facilities as part of an NDA or ANDA application likely would result in a delay of approval of an otherwise approvable application. Noncompliance with cGMP regulations during a regularly scheduled FDA inspection can lead to various actions, depending on the severity of the offenses. In most instances time for corrective action is given, with the firm required to institute and document corrective measures and undergo another inspection. In a worst-case scenario, the FDA is empowered to remove violative products from the market, withdraw product approvals, and restrict further applications. All FDA actions are subject to appeal.

cGMP Requirements for Manufacturing in Pharmacies

The FDA's cGMP regulations apply to community or institutional pharmacies engaged in the manufacture, repackaging, or relabeling of drugs and drug products in a supplier function and beyond the usual conduct of professional dispensing. Pharmacies that engage in such activities must register with the FDA as a manufacturer or distributor and be subject to FDA inspection at regular intervals. Included are hospital pharmacies that repackage drug products for their own use and for the use of other hospitals; chain pharmacy operations that repackage and relabel bulk quantities of products for distribution in the chain; and similar repackaging and relabeling by individual pharmacists or pharmacies for distribution to other pharmacies or retailers.

Recently, professional and legislative attention has been directed toward differentiating between pharmaceutical manufacturing and compounding as practiced by community pharmacists (12). Pharmaceutical manufacturing is large-scale production of drugs or drug products for distribution and sale, whereas compounding is professional preparation of prescriptions for specific patients as a part of the traditional practice of pharmacy.

Current Good Compounding Practices

In recent years pharmacists have increased the practice of compounding patient-specific medications. An increase in the incidence of pharmaceutical compounding was noted in the 1970s and continued into the 1980s. By the early to mid 1990s, compounding was making a dramatic comeback in pharmacy practice. A number of reasons have been presented for the increase in preparing patient-specific medications, including the following:

1. Many patients need drug dosages or strengths that are not commercially available.
2. Many patients need dosage forms, such as suppositories, oral liquids, or topicals, that are not commercially available.
3. Many patients are allergic to excipients in commercially available products.
4. Children's medications must be prepared as liquids, flavored to enhance compliance, and prepared in alternative dosage forms, such as lozenges, gumdrops, and lollipops.
5. Some medications are not very stable and require preparation and dispensing every few days; they are not suitable to be manufactured products.

6. Many products are reported in the literature but are not manufactured yet, so pharmacists can compound them for their physicians' and patients' use.
7. Many physicians desire to try products in innovative ways, and pharmacists can work with them to solve medication problems.
8. Most products are not available for veterinary patients and must be compounded.
9. Home health care and the treatment of an increasing number of patients at home has resulted in many community pharmacies and home health care pharmacies preparing sterile products for home use; formerly, most sterile products were compounded in hospital pharmacies.
10. Hospice care has resulted in new approaches to pain management and higher concentrations and combinations of drugs that are now used.

As the extent of compounding increased, many standard-setting agencies and regulatory bodies wanted to ensure quality compounded products; consequently, there was a lot of activity during the mid 1990s to establish guidelines for pharmaceutical compounding.

U.S. Pharmacopeia–National Formulary

In 1990 the U.S. Pharmacopeial Convention approved the appointment of an expert panel on pharmacy compounding practices. The activities of the panel initially were to prepare a chapter for the United States Pharmacopeia (USP) and to begin preparing monographs of compounded products for inclusion in the National Formulary (NF). The prepared chapter, "Pharmacy Compounding Practices," was published and became official in 1996 (13). The first of the compounding monographs became official in 1998, and some monographs that were previously published in the USP–NF are being reintroduced.

Chapter <795>, "Pharmacy Compounding," includes the following discussions: (*a*) compounding environment; (*b*) stability of compounded preparations; (*c*) ingredient selection and calculations; (*d*) checklist for acceptable strength, quality and purity; (*e*) compounded preparations; (*f*) compounding process; (*g*) compounding records and documents; (*h*) quality control; and (*i*) patient counseling.

The introduction to the chapter discusses the difference between manufacturing and compounding. Generally speaking, compounding differs from manufacturing in the specific practitioner–patient–pharmacist relationships, the quantity of medication prepared in anticipation of receiving a prescription or a prescription order, and the conditions of sale, which are limited to specific prescription orders.

The compounding environment section discusses the design and maintenance of the facilities to be used and the equipment selected for compounding. It refers to other specific chapters in the USP, namely "Weights and Balances and the Prescription Balances" and "Volumetric Apparatus." Any equipment used for compounding must be of appropriate design and size for compounding and suitable for the intended use.

The discussion of stability includes packaging, sterility, and stability criteria and guidelines for assigning beyond-use dates for compounded preparations; the latter are detailed as follows:

"In the absence of stability information that is applicable to a specific drug and preparation, the following maximum beyond-use dates are recommended for nonsterile compounded drug preparations that are packaged in tight, light-resistant containers and stored at controlled room temperature unless otherwise indicated" (15).

For nonaqueous liquids and solid formulations, (*a*) where the manufactured drug product is the source of active ingredient, the beyond-use date is not later than 25% of the time remaining until the product's expiration date or 6 months, whichever is earlier; (*b*) where a USP or NF substance is the source of active ingredient, the beyond-use date is not later than 6 months.

For water-containing formulations prepared from ingredients in solid form, the beyond-use date is not later than 14 days when stored at cold temperatures.

For all other formulations, the beyond-use date is not later than the intended duration of therapy or 30 days, whichever is earlier.

The chapter goes on to detail that these beyond-use date limits can be exceeded if there is supporting valid scientific stability information that is directly applicable to the product being compounded. The product must be the same drug in a similar concentration, pH, excipients, vehicle, water content, and so on.

The section on ingredient selection describes sources for drugs and excipients as follows:

1. A USP- or NF-grade substance is the preferred source for compounding.
2. A drug of the highest quality, reasonably available, may be used, preferably one listed as ACS (American Chemical Society) or FCC (Food and Chemicals Codex) grade. Material safety data sheets should be maintained on all materials used for compounding in the pharmacy.
3. A manufactured drug product can be used as a source of a drug, excipient, or vehicle. If manufactured drugs are used as the source for the active drugs, then the presence of all excipients must be considered in the overall acceptability of the final product.

Calculations are discussed as they relate to the amount of concentration of drug substances in each unit or dosage portion of a compounded preparation. Special emphasis is placed on calculations involving the purity and potency of drugs, their salt forms, and equivalent potencies.

The chapter also details a checklist that can be used to consider the advisability of preparing a compounded dosage form. It then details many dosage forms and some quality control characteristics that can be checked in the final compounded products. Following is a discussion of the steps in a compounding process that can be used as a template for compounding prescriptions. Record-keeping requirements of various states generally include a formulation record and a compounding record.

Quality control and the responsibility of the pharmacist in reviewing each procedure and observing the finished preparation are discussed. The chapter ends with the importance of patient counseling in the proper use, storage, and observation for instability of the dispensed product. The overall emphasis of the chapter is to support the pharmacist in the compounding of products of acceptable strength, quality, and purity.

During the early to mid 1990s, the FDA district offices began investigating a number of pharmacies that were compounding very large quantities of drug products and shipping them throughout the United States. It was the opinion of the FDA that these pharmacies were actually involved in manufacturing, not compounding.

At the American Pharmaceutical Association meeting in 1993, FDA Commissioner Kesler stated that it was not the purpose of the FDA to stop the compounding activities of pharmacists but to stop the practice of manufacturing under the guise of compounding. However, over the next few years, the activities of the FDA inspectors and district personnel increased, and some pharmacists were threatened with arrest and legal proceedings. The FDA was determined to require that all compounded medications meet the requirements set forth as a new drug, or else they could not be dispensed to patients. Obviously, this was impossible and seriously threatened pharmaceutical compounding.

The national pharmacy organizations united to protect the rights of pharmacists to compound. The National Association of Boards of Pharmacy promulgated the Good Compounding Practices, which have been either adopted or modified and adopted by many states. The U.S. Pharmacopeial Convention renewed its commitment to compounding by the preparation of chapters for the USP–NF and in establishing monographs for the compendia. In 1997, the efforts of many organizations, politicians, and pharmacists resulted in a section of the Food and Drug Administration Modernization Act of 1997 (12) being aimed at supporting pharmacists' right to compound, with some guidelines.

Food and Drug Modernization Act of 1997

The purpose of Section 127 of Public Law 105–115 was to ensure patients' access to individualized drug therapy and prevent unnecessary FDA regulation of health professional practice. This legislation exempted pharmacy compounding from several regulatory requirements but did not exempt drug manufacturing. The legislation also set forth conditions that must be met to qualify for exemption from the act's requirements.

The act states that a compounded product is exempt if the drug product is compounded for an individual patient based on the unsolicited receipt of a valid prescription order or a notation, approved by the prescribing practitioner, on the prescription order that a compounded product is necessary for the identified patient, if the product meets certain requirements outlined in the act. In April 2002, however, the U.S. Supreme Court found unconstitutional one of the provisions of the act related to the advertising restrictions on compounding. This section was ruled not to be separable from the rest of the pharmacy compounding provisions, so the entire section was thrown out. New legislation may be forthcoming.

The Food and Drug Modernization Act of 1997 removed any doubt that compounding is legal under the FDC Act, and Congress has clearly recognized the importance of compounding.

National Association of Boards of Pharmacy

"The Good Compounding Practices Applicable to State-Licensed Pharmacies" (14), developed by the National Association of Boards of Pharmacy, discusses eight recommendations. The subparts include (A), general provisions; (B), organization and personnel; (C), drug compounding facilities; (D), equipment; (E), control of components and drug product containers and closures; (F), drug compounding controls; and (G), labeling control of excess products and records and reports.

Subpart (A), General Provisions, provides two important definitions:

Compounding: The preparation, mixing, assembling, packaging, or labeling of a drug or device (i) as the result of a practitioner's prescription drug order or initiative based on the practitioner–patient–pharmacist relationship in the course of professional practice, or (ii) for the purpose of or as an incident to research, teaching, or chemical analysis and not for sale or dispensation. Compounding also includes preparation of drugs or devices in anticipation of prescription drug orders based on routine regularly observed prescribing patterns.

Manufacturing: the production, preparation, propagation, conversion, or processing of a drug or device, either directly or indirectly, by extraction from substances of natural origin or independently by means of chemical or biological synthesis; it includes any packaging or repackaging of the substance or substances or labeling or relabeling of its container and promotion and marketing of such drugs or devices. Manufacturing also includes preparation and promotion of commercially available products from bulk compounds for resale by pharmacies, practitioners, or other persons.

Subpart (B), Organization and Personnel, discusses the responsibilities of pharmacists and other personnel engaged in compounding. It also stresses that only personnel authorized by the responsible pharmacist shall be in the immediate vicinity of the drug compounding operation.

Subpart (C), Drug Compounding Facilities, describes the areas that should be set aside for compounding, either sterile or not. Special attention is required for radiopharmaceuticals and for products requiring special precautions to minimize contamination, such as penicillin.

Subpart (D), Equipment, states that equipment used must be of appropriate design, adequate size, and suitably located to facilitate operation for its intended use and for its cleaning and maintenance. If mechanical or electronic equipment is used, controls must be in place to ensure proper performance.

Subpart (E), Control of Components and Drug Product Containers and Closures, describes the packaging requirements for compounded products.

Subpart (F), Drug Compounding Controls, discusses the written procedures to ensure that the finished products are of the proper identity, strength, quality and purity, as labeled.

Subpart (G), Labeling Control of Excess Products and Records and Reports, describes the various records and reports that are required under these guidelines.

Many individual states have used this model and implemented their own version. All pharmacists and pharmacy students should become familiar with the individual state requirements in the state in which they practice.

It will be important as compounding pharmacy increases to ensure reasonable agreement between the national and state agencies so pharmacists will have a set of guidelines within which they can work to provide their patients the needed individualized medications.

Packaging, Labeling, and Storage of Pharmaceuticals

The proper packaging, labeling, and storage of pharmaceutical products are all essential for product stability and efficacious use.

Containers

Standards for the packaging of pharmaceuticals by manufacturers are contained in the "Current Good Manufacturing Practice" section of the *Code of Federal Regulations* (1), in the USP–NF (15), and in the FDA's *Guideline for Submitting Documentation for Packaging for Human Drugs and Biologics* (16). When submitting a new drug application, the manufacturer must include all relevant specifications for packaging the product. During the initial stages of clinical investigations, the packaging must be shown to provide adequate drug stability for the duration of the clinical trials. As the clinical trials advance to their final stage, information on the chemical and physical characteristics of the container, closure, and other component parts of the package system for the proposed product must be developed to ensure drug stability for its anticipated shelf life.

Different specifications are required for parenteral, nonparenteral, pressurized, and bulk containers and for those made of glass, plastic, and metal. In each instance, the package and closure system must be shown to be effective for the particular product for which it is intended. Depending on the intended use and type of container, among the qualities tested are the following:

Physicochemical properties
Light-transmission for glass or plastic
Drug compatibility
Leaching and/or migration
Vapor transmission for plastics
Moisture barrier
Toxicity for plastics
Valve, actuator, metered dose, particle size, spray characteristics, and leaks for aerosols
Sterility and permeation for parenteral containers
Drug stability for all packaging

Compendium terms applying to types of containers and conditions of storage have defined meanings (15). According to the USP, a container is "that which holds the article and is or may be in direct contact with the article." The immediate container is "that which is in direct contact with the article at all times." The closure is part of the container. The container, including the closure, should be clean and dry before it is filled with the drug. The container must not interact physically or chemically with the drug so as to alter its strength, quality, or purity beyond the official requirements.

The USP classifies containers according to their ability to protect their contents from external conditions (15). The minimally acceptable container is termed a well-closed container. It "protects the contents from extraneous solids and from loss of the article under ordinary conditions of handling, shipment, storage, and distribution." A tight container "protects the contents from contamination by extraneous liquids, solids, or vapors, from loss of the article, and from efflorescence, deliquescence, or evaporation under the ordinary or customary conditions of handling, shipment, storage, and distribution and is capable of tight re-closure." A hermetic container "is impervious to air or any other gas under the ordinary or customary

conditions of handling, shipment, storage, and distribution." Sterile hermetic containers are generally used to hold preparations intended for injection or parenteral administration. A single-dose container is one that holds a quantity of drug intended as a single dose and when opened cannot be resealed with assurance that sterility has been maintained. These containers include fusion-sealed ampuls and prefilled syringes and cartridges. A multiple-dose container is a hermetic container that permits withdrawal of successive portions of the contents without changing the strength or endangering the quality or purity of the remaining portion. These containers are commonly called vials. Examples of single-dose and multiple-dose products are shown in Figure 3.3.

Dosage forms, such as tablets, capsules, and oral liquids, may be packaged in single-unit or multiple-unit containers. A single-unit container is designed to hold a quantity of drug intended for administration as a single dose promptly after the container is opened. Multiple-unit containers contain more than a single unit or dose of the medication. Examples of single-unit and multiple-unit packages are shown in Figure 3.4. A single-unit package is termed a unit dose package. The single-unit packaging of drugs may be performed on a large scale by a manufacturer or distributor or

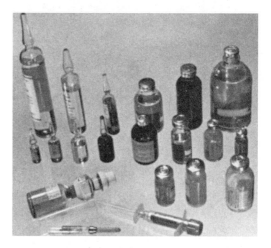

FIGURE 3.3 Injectable products packaged in single-dose (ampul) and multiple-dose (vial) containers and in unit dose syringes.

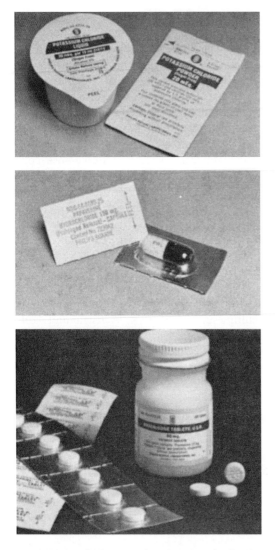

FIGURE 3.4 Multiple-unit and single-unit packaging, including patient cup, unit dose of powder, blister packaging of single capsule, and strip packaging of tablets. (Courtesy of Roxane Laboratories.)

unit packages a convenient and sanitary means of maintaining and using their medication. Among the advantages cited for single-unit packaging and unit dose dispensing are positive identification of each dosage unit and reduction of medication errors, reduced contamination of the drug because of its protective wrapping, reduced dispensing time, greater ease of inventory control in the pharmacy or nursing station, and elimination of waste through better medication management with less discarded medication.

Many hospitals with unit dose systems strip-package oral solids (Fig. 3.5). Such equipment seals solid dosage forms into four-sided pouches and imprints dose identification on each package at the same time. The equipment can be adjusted to produce individual single-cut packages or perforated strips or rolls of doses. The packaging materials may be combinations of paper, foil, plastic, or cellophane. Some drugs must be packaged in foil-to-foil wrappings to prevent the deteriorating effects of light or permeation of moisture. The packaging of solid

on a smaller scale by the pharmacy dispensing the medication. In either instance, the single-unit package must be appropriately labeled with the product identity, quality and/or strength, name of manufacturer, and lot number to ensure positive identification of the medication.

Although single-unit packaging has particular usefulness in institutional settings such as hospitals and extended care facilities, it is not limited to them. Many outpatients find single-

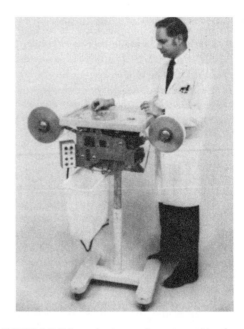

FIGURE 3.5 Strip packaging equipment capable of producing 50 packages per minute. Seals solid dosage units in a variety of wrapping materials and labels each package simultaneously. (Courtesy of Packaging Machinery Associates.)

dosage forms in clear plastic or aluminum blister wells is perhaps the most popular method of single-unit packaging (Fig. 3.6).

Oral liquids may be dispensed in single units in paper, plastic, or foil cups or prepackaged and dispensed in glass containers having threaded caps or crimped aluminum caps. A number of hospital pharmacies package oral liquids for children's use in disposable plastic oral syringes with rubber or plastic tips on the orifice for closure. In these instances, the nursing staff must be fully aware of the novel packaging and special labeling used to indicate that they are not for injection. These oral syringes are designed so they will not accept a needle. Other dosage forms, such as suppositories, powders, ointments, creams, and ophthalmic solutions, are also commonly found in single-unit packages provided by their manufacturers. However, the relatively infrequent use of these dosage forms in a given hospital, extended care facility, or community pharmacy does not generally justify the expense of pur-

chasing the specialized packaging machinery necessary for the small-scale packaging of these forms.

Some pharmaceutical manufacturers use unit-of-use packaging; that is, the quantity of drug product prescribed is packaged in a container. For example, if certain antibiotic capsules are usually prescribed to be taken 4 times a day for 10 days, unit-of-use packaging would contain 40 capsules. Other products may be packaged to contain a month's supply.

Many pharmaceutical products require light-resistant containers. In most instances a container made of a good quality of amber glass or a light-resistant opaque plastic will reduce light transmission sufficiently to protect a light-sensitive pharmaceutical. Agents termed ultraviolet absorbers may be added to plastic to decrease the transmission of short ultraviolet rays. The USP provides tests and standards for glass and plastic containers with respect to their ability to prevent the transmission of light (15). Containers intended to provide protec-

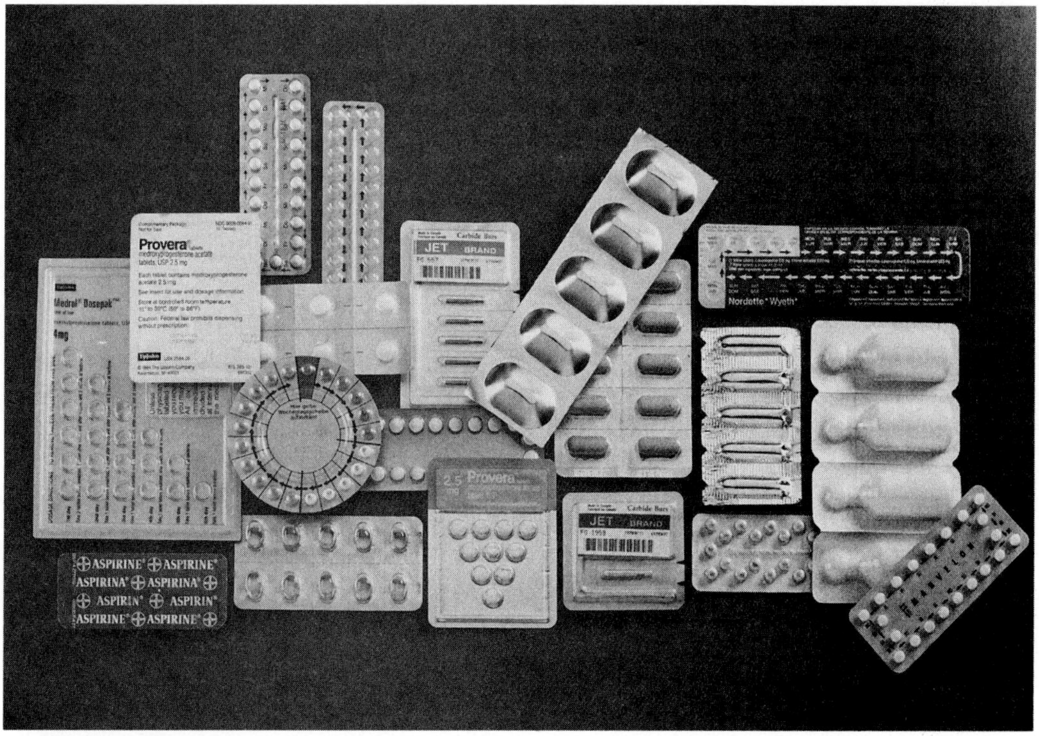

FIGURE 3.6 Commercial blister packaging of pharmaceuticals. (Courtesy of Hueck Foils L.L.C.)

tion from light or those offered as light-resistant containers must meet the USP standards that define the acceptable limits of light transmission at any wavelength between 290 and 450 nm. A recent innovation in plastic packaging is the coextruded two-layer high-density polyethylene bottle, which has an inner layer of black polyethylene coextruded with an outer layer of white polyethylene. The container provides both light resistance (exceeding amber glass) and moisture protection. It is increasingly being used in the packaging of tablets and capsules.

The glass used in packaging pharmaceuticals falls into four categories, depending on the chemical constitution of the glass and its ability to resist deterioration. Table 3.3 presents the chemical makeup of the various glasses; types I, II, and III are intended for parenteral products, and type NP is intended for other products. Each type is tested according to its resistance to water attack. The degree of attack is determined by the amount of alkali released from the glass in the specified test conditions. Obviously, leaching of alkali from the glass into a pharmaceutical solution or preparation could alter the pH and thus the stability of the product. Pharmaceutical manufacturers must use containers that do not adversely affect the composition or stability of their products. Type I is the most resistant glass of the four categories.

Today most pharmaceutical products are packaged in plastic. The modern compact-type container used for oral contraceptives, which contains sufficient tablets for a monthly cycle of administration and permits the scheduled removal of one tablet at a time, is a prime example of contemporary plastic packaging (Fig. 3.6). Plastic bags for intravenous fluids, plastic

ointment tubes, plastic film–protected suppositories, and plastic tablet and capsule vials are other examples of plastics used in pharmaceutical packaging.

The widespread use of plastic containers arose from a number of factors, including the following:

Its advantage over glass in lightness of weight and resistance to impact, which reduces transportation costs and losses due to container damage

The versatility in container design and consumer acceptance

Consumer preference for plastic squeeze bottles in administration of ophthalmics, nasal sprays, and lotions

The popularity of blister packaging and unit-dose dispensing, particularly in health care institutions

The term *plastic* does not apply to a single type of material but rather to a vast number of materials, each developed to have desired features. For example, the addition of methyl groups to every other carbon atom in the polymer chains of polyethylene will give polypropylene, a material that can be autoclaved, whereas polyethylene cannot. If a chlorine atom is added to every other carbon in the polyethylene polymer, polyvinyl chloride (PVC) is produced. This material is rigid and has good clarity, making it particularly useful in the blister packaging of tablets and capsules. However, it has a significant drawback for packaging medical devices (e.g., syringes): it is unsuitable for gamma sterilization, a method that is being used increasingly. The placement of other functional groups on the main chain of polyethylene or added to other types of polymers can give a variety of alterations to the final plastic material. Among the newer plastics are polyethylene terephthalate (PET), amorphous polyethylene terephthalate glycol (APET), and polyethylene terephthalate glycol (PETG). Both APET and PETG have excellent transparency and luster and can be sterilized with gamma radiation (17).

Among the problems encountered in the use of plastics in packaging are (*a*) permeability of the containers to atmospheric oxygen and to

TABLE 3.3 CONSTITUTION OF OFFICIAL GLASS TYPES

TYPE	GENERAL DESCRIPTION
I	Highly resistant borosilicate glass
II	Treated soda lime glass
III	Soda lime glass
NP	General purpose soda lime glass

moisture vapor (*b*) leaching of the constituents of the container to the internal contents (*c*) absorption of drugs from the contents to the container (*d*) transmission of light through the container, and (*e*) alteration of the container upon storage. Agents frequently added to alter the properties of plastic include plasticizers, stabilizers, antioxidants, antistatic agents, antifungal agents, colorants, and others.

Permeability is considered a process of solution and diffusion, with the penetrant dissolving in the plastic on one side and diffusing through to the other side. Permeability should not be confused with porosity, in which minute holes or cracks in the plastic allow gas or moisture vapor to move through directly. The permeability of a plastic is a function of several factors, including the nature of the polymer itself; the amounts and types of plasticizers, fillers, lubricants, pigments and other additives; pressure; and temperature. Generally, increases in temperature, pressure, and the use of additives tend to increase the permeability of the plastic. Glass containers are less permeable than plastic containers.

The movement of moisture vapor or gas, especially oxygen, through a pharmaceutical container can pose a threat to the stability of the product. In the presence of moisture, solid dosage forms may lose their color or physical integrity. A host of pharmaceutical adjuncts, especially those used in tablet formulations, as diluents, binders, and disintegrating agents, are affected by moisture. Most of these adjuncts are carbohydrates, starches, and natural or synthetic gums, and because of their hygroscopicity, they hold moisture and may even serve as nutrient media for the growth of microorganisms. Many of the tablet-disintegrating agents act by swelling, and if they are exposed to high moisture vapor during storage, they can cause tablet deterioration. Many medicinal agents, including aspirin and nitroglycerin, are adversely affected by moisture and require special protection. Sublingual nitroglycerin tablets must be dispensed in their original glass container.

Specially developed high-barrier packaging can provide added protection to pharmaceutical products against the effects of humidity. Such packaging meets the drug stability requirements adopted by the International Committee on Harmonization, which call for testing of packaged products for a minimum for 12 months at 25°C (77°F) at 60% relative humidity (18). Many capsule and other products are liable to deteriorate in humidity unless protected by high-barrier packaging. Desiccant protectants, such as silica gel in small packets, are commonly included in solid-form packaging as added protection against the effects of moisture vapor.

Drug substances that are subject to oxidative degradation may undergo a greater degree of degradation when packaged in plastic than in glass. In glass, the container's void space is confined and presents only a limited amount of oxygen to the drug contents, whereas a drug packaged in a gas-permeable plastic container may be constantly exposed to oxygen because of the replenished air supply entering through the container. Liquid pharmaceuticals packaged in permeable plastic may lose drug molecules or solvent to the container, altering the concentration of the drug in the product and affecting its potency.

Leaching is a term used to describe the movement of components of a container into the contents. Compounds leached from plastic containers are generally the polymer additives, such as the plasticizers, stabilizers, or antioxidants. The leaching of these additives occurs predominantly when liquids or semisolids are packaged in plastic. Little leaching occurs when tablets or capsules are packaged in plastic.

Leaching may be influenced by temperature, excessive agitation of the filled container, and the solubilizing effect of liquid contents on one or more of the polymer additives. The leaching of polymer additives from plastic containers of fluids intended for intravenous administration is a special concern that requires careful selection of the plastic used. Leached material, whether dissolved in an intravenous fluid or in minute particles, poses a health hazard to the patient. Thus, studies of the leaching characteristics of each plastic considered for use are undertaken as a part of the drug development process. Soft-walled plastic containers of PVC are used to package intravenous solutions and blood for transfusion.

Sorption, a term used to indicate the binding of molecules to polymer materials, includes both adsorption and absorption. Sorption occurs through chemical or physical means due to the chemical structure of the solute molecules and the physical and chemical properties of the polymer. Generally, the un-ionized species of a solute has a greater tendency to be bound than the ionized species. Because the degree of ionization of a solute may be affected by the pH of a solution, the pH may influence the sorption tendency of a particular solute. Furthermore, the pH of a solution may affect the chemical nature of a plastic container so as to increase or decrease the active bonding sites available to the solute molecules. Plastic materials with polar groups are particularly prone to sorption. Because sorption depends on the penetration or diffusion of a solute into the plastic, the pharmaceutical vehicle or solvent used can also play a role by altering the integrity of the plastic.

Sorption may occur with active pharmacologic agents or with pharmaceutical excipients. Thus, each ingredient must be examined in the proposed plastic packaging to determine its tendency. Sorption may be initiated by the adsorption of a solute to the inner surface of a plastic container. After saturation of the surface, the solute may diffuse into the container and be bound within the plastic. The sorption of an active pharmacologic agent from a pharmaceutical solution would reduce its effective concentration and render the product's potency unreliable. The sorption of pharmaceutical excipients such as colorants, preservatives, or stabilizers would likewise alter the quality of the product.

Deformations, softening, hardening, and other physical changes in plastic containers can be caused by the action of the container's contents or external factors, including changes in temperature and the physical stress placed upon the container in handling and shipping.

It is always good practice to dispense medication to patients in the same type and quality of container as that used by the manufacturer. In some instances the original container may be used to dispense the medication.

Child-Resistant and Adult–Senior Use Packaging

To reduce accidental poisonings through the ingestion of drugs and other household chemicals, the Poison Prevention Packaging Act was passed into law in 1970. Responsibility for administration and enforcement, originally with the FDA, was transferred to the Consumer Product Safety Commission in 1973, when this agency was created by passage of the Consumer Product Safety Act. The initial regulations called for the use of childproof closures for aspirin products and certain household chemical products shown to have a significant potential for causing accidental poisoning in youngsters.

As the technical capability to produce effective closures was developed, the regulations were extended to include the use of safety closures in the packaging of both legend and OTC medications. At present all legend drugs intended for oral use must be dispensed by the pharmacist to the patient in a container having a child-resistant closure unless the prescriber or the patient specifically requests otherwise or unless the product is specifically exempt from the requirement.

The Consumer Product Safety Commission may propose exemption of certain drugs and drug products from the regulations based on toxicologic data or on practical considerations. For instance, certain cardiac drugs, such as sublingual tablets of nitroglycerin, are exempt from the regulations because of the importance of a patient's immediate access to the medication. Exemptions are also permitted in the case of OTC products for one package size or specially marked package to be available to consumers for whom safety closures are unnecessary or too difficult to manipulate. These consumers include childless persons, arthritic patients, and the debilitated. These packages must be labeled "This package for households without young children" or "Package not child-resistant."

A child-resistant container is defined as one that is significantly difficult for children under 5 years of age to open or to obtain a harmful amount of its contents within a reasonable time and that is not difficult for "normal adults" to use properly (19, 20). The Consumer Product Safety Commission evaluates the effectiveness of such containers using children aged 42 to 51 months. The four basic designs commonly used are align the arrows, press down and turn, squeeze and turn, and latch top. A child-resistant prescription container is shown in Figure 3.7.

In recognition that many adults, particularly the elderly and those with arthritis or weakened hand strength, have difficulty opening child-resistant packages, the regulations were amended (effective in 1998) to require that child-resistant containers be readily opened by senior adults. The previous requirement, which used adults 18 to 45 years of age in the testing evaluation, was replaced by protocols using adults in three age groups: 50 to 54, 55 to 59, and 60 to 70 (20). A specially designed child-resistant and adult-friendly closure for packaging and dispensing medication is shown in Figure 3.8.

Drugs that are used or dispensed in patient care institutions, including hospitals, nursing homes, and extended care facilities, need not be dispensed with safety closures unless they are intended for patients who are leaving institution.

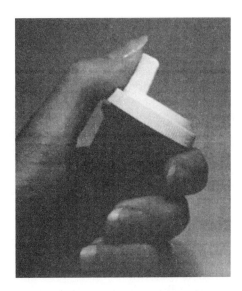

FIGURE 3.8 A senior-friendly child-resistant prescription container. When the arrows on the cap and vial are lined up, leverage on the large tab enables the senior adult patient to push off the cap using a thumb or the side of a hand. The snap cap may also be reversed, with the tab facing in the container, for non–child-resistant use. (Courtesy of Lermer Packaging Corporation.)

Tamper-Evident Packaging

The discussion of tamper-evident packaging born out of incidents in which the contents of OTC products were adulterated with toxic substances was presented earlier in this chapter in the cGMP section "Packaging and Label Control."

Compliance Packaging

Many patients are not compliant with the prescribed schedule for taking their medications. The many factors associated with noncompliance include misunderstanding the dosing schedule, confusion because the patient is taking multiple medications, forgetfulness, and a feeling of well-being leading to premature discontinuance of medication.

To assist patients in taking their medications on schedule, manufacturers and pharmacists have devised numerous educational techniques, reminder aids, compliance packages, and devices. The oral contraceptive compact was among the earliest packages developed to assist adherence to a prescribed dosing schedule.

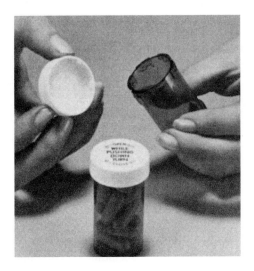

FIGURE 3.7 Child-resistant safety closure on a prescription container. (Courtesy of Owens-Brockway Prescription Products.)

Many subsequent packaging innovations include blister packaging in a calendar pack. For prescriptions dispensed in traditional containers (e.g., capsule vials), pharmacists often provide calendar medication schedules or commercial pillboxes with daily or weekly compartments. These medication compliance techniques and devices are particularly useful for patients taking multiple medications.

Labeling

All drug products distributed in the United States must meet the labeling requirements in the *Code of Federal Regulations* (1–4, 21, 22). Different labeling requirements apply to investigational drugs, manufacturer's prescription drugs, controlled substances, dispensed prescription medication, OTC products, products for animals, medical devices, and other specific categories and specific products. In every instance, federal labeling requirements may be strengthened by state law.

According to federal regulations, manufacturers' drug product labeling includes not only the labels on the immediate container and packaging but also inserts; company literature; advertising and promotional material, including brochures, booklets, mailing pieces, file cards, bulletins, price lists, catalogs, sound recordings, film strips, motion picture films, slides, exhibits, displays, literature reprints, and computer-accessed information; and other materials related to the product.

Important information for a prescription-only drug is provided to health professionals through the manufacturer's product package insert. As discussed in Chapter 2, the package insert must provide full disclosure, that is, a full and balanced presentation of the drug product to enable the prescriber to use the drug with sufficient knowledge of important benefit to risk factors.

Manufacturer's Label

Included in the information usually appearing on the manufacturer's or distributor's immediate label affixed to the container of legend drugs is the following:

1. The established or nonproprietary name of the drug or drugs and the proprietary name of the product if one is used
2. The name of the manufacturer, packer, or distributor of the product
3. A quantitative statement of the amount of each drug per unit of weight, volume, or dosage unit, whichever is most appropriate
4. The pharmaceutical type of dosage form constituting the product
5. The net amount of drug product contained in the package, in units of weight, volume, or number of dosage units, as appropriate
6. The logo "Rx only" or the federal legend "Caution—Federal law prohibits dispensing without prescription" or a similar statement.
7. A label reference to see the accompanying package insert or other product literature for dosage and other information
8. Special storage instructions when applicable
9. The National Drug Code identification number for the product (and often a bar code)
10. An identifying lot or control number
11. An expiration date
12. For controlled drug substances, the DEA symbol "C" together with the schedule assigned (e.g., III). The statement "Warning—May be habit forming" may appear also.

Prescription Label

When filling a prescription, by federal law the pharmacist must include the following information on the label of the dispensed medication:

The name and address of the pharmacy
The serial number of the prescription
The date of the prescription or the date of its filling or refilling (state law often determines which date is to be used)
The name of the prescriber
The name of the patient
Directions for use, including any precautions, as indicated on the prescription

In addition, state laws may require additional information:

The address of the patient

The initials or name of the dispensing pharmacist

The telephone number of the pharmacy

The drug name, strength, and manufacturer's lot or control number

The expiration date of the drug

The name of the manufacturer or distributor

OTC Labeling

In 1997 the FDA undertook an initiative to develop a standard format for OTC drug product labeling. This initiative was the result of findings that the design and format of labeling information varied considerably among OTC products, making it difficult for consumers to read and understand the information (23). The FDA called for standardized headings and subheadings, a standard order of presentation, standard type style, and labeling language revised to be simpler to read and more easily understood by the consumer.

The label on the container of OTC products includes the following:

Product name.

Name and address of the manufacturer, packer or distributor.

Statement of the net quantity of the contents.

Established names and quantities of all active ingredients per dosage unit. Inactive ingredients are also listed.

The name of any habit-forming substance or substances in the preparation.

Statement of pharmacologic category or principal intended action (e.g., antacid) and adequate directions for safe and effective use, for example, dose, frequency of dose, dose and age considerations, route of administration, and preparation for use, such as shaking or dilution.

Cautions and warnings to protect the consumer, for example, maximum duration of administration prior to consulting a physician, anticipated side effects, appropriate instructions in the event of accidental overdose, conditions against which the drug is contraindicated or to be used only with professional supervision, drug interaction precautions, pregnancy and nursing warning if the drug is intended for systemic absorption (unless specifically exempted from this requirement): "Warning: As with any drug, if you are pregnant or nursing a baby, seek the advice of a health professional before using this product."

Sodium content for certain oral products intended for ingestion, when the product contains 5 mg of sodium or more per single dose or 140 mg or more in the maximum daily dose.

Storage conditions, including storage in a safe place out of the reach of children.

Description of tamper-evident feature

Lot number and expiration date

As noted, OTC package labeling must include appropriate warning statements whenever indiscriminate use of the medication may lead to serious medical complications or mask a condition more serious than that for which the medication was intended. For example, the use of laxatives is dangerous when symptoms of appendicitis are present because they can intensify the problem and even bring on rupture of the appendix. For this reason the following statement is required by law to appear on laxative preparations:

Warning: Do not use when abdominal pain, nausea, or vomiting is present. Frequent or prolonged use of this preparation may result in dependence on laxatives.

A patient may underestimate the seriousness of a cough if a proprietary cough syrup temporarily relieves it; however, coughing is a symptom of many serious conditions requiring specific treatment. OTC cough remedies must therefore bear the following warning statement:

Warning: A persistent cough may be a sign of a serious condition. If cough persists for more than 1 week, tends to recur, or is accompanied by a fever, rash, or persistent headache, consult a doctor.

These are but two examples of the warning statements required on various types of proprietary products. Serious conditions cannot be diagnosed or successfully treated by the lay person with OTC medications.

Storage

To ensure the stability of a pharmaceutical preparation for the period of its intended shelf life, the product must be stored in proper conditions. The labeling of each product includes the desired conditions of storage. The terms generally employed in such labeling have meanings defined by the USP (15):

Cold: Any temperature not exceeding 8°C (46°F). A refrigerator is a cold place in which the temperature is maintained thermostatically between 2° and 8°C (36° and 46°F). A freezer is a cold place in which the temperature is maintained thermostatically between –25° and –10°C (–13° and 14°F).

Cool: Any temperature between 8° and 15°C (46° and 59°F). An article for which storage in a cool place is directed may alternatively be stored in a refrigerator unless otherwise specified in the individual monograph.

Room temperature: The temperature prevailing in a working area. A controlled room temperature encompasses the usual working environment of 20° to 25°C (68° to 77°F) but also allows for temperature variations between 15°C and 30°C (59° and 86°F) that may be found in pharmacies, hospitals, and drug warehouses.

Warm: Any temperature between 30° and 40°C (86° and 104°F).

Excessive heat: Above 40°C (104°F).

Protection from freezing: Where in addition to the risk of breakage of the container, freezing subjects a product to loss of strength or potency or to destructive alteration of the dosage form, the container label bears an appropriate instruction to protect the product from freezing.

Transportation

The stability protection of a pharmaceutical product during transportation is an important consideration. However, maintenance of satisfactory conditions of temperature and humidity during shipment is not always practiced (24). Temperature and humidity variations may occur during shipment from a manufacturer to a wholesaler or to a pharmacy, from a pharmacy to a patient, during mail order shipment of prescriptions and their time in the mailbox, and in emergency care vehicles. Transportation to and within geographic areas of extreme temperatures and humidity requires special consideration.

REFERENCES

1. Code of Federal Regulations, Title 21, Parts 210–211.
2. Code of Federal Regulations, Title 21, Part 606.
3. Code of Federal Regulations, Title 21, Part 226.
4. Code of Federal Regulations, Title 21, Part 820.
5. A strategic view of information technology in the pharmaceutical industry. Philadelphia: Deloitte & Touche, 1994.
6. Laboratory robotics handbook. Hopkinton, MA: Zymark, 1988.
7. Guide to inspection of bulk pharmaceutical chemicals. Rockville, MD: Food & Drug Administration, 1991.
8. Moore RE. FDA's guideline for bulk pharmaceutical chemicals: a consultant's interpretation. Pharm Tech 1992;16:88–100.
9. Avallone HL. GMP inspections of drug-substance manufacturers. Pharm Tech 1992;16:46–55.
10. Mercill A. A good manufacturing practices guide for bulk pharmaceutical excipients. Pharm Tech 1995;19: 34–40.
11. Bernstein DF. Investigational clinical trial material supply operations in new product development. Appl Clin Trials 1993;2:59–69.
12. FDA Modernization Act. Washington: Congress of the United States, 1997.
13. Selections from USP 23-NF 18: Pharmacy compounding practices and sterile drug products for home use. Rockville, MD: United States Pharmacopeial Convention, 1996.
14. Model State Pharmacy Act and Model Rules of the National Association of Boards of Pharmacy. Park Ridge, IL: National Association of Boards of Pharmacy, 1993.
15. United States Pharmacopeia 27–National Formulary 22. Rockville, MD: United States Pharmacopeial Convention, 1995.
16. Guideline for submitting documentation for packaging of human drugs and biologics. Rockville MD: Food & Drug Administration, 1987.
17. Hacker D. Extruder sees future of medical market: rigid PET. Pharmaceut Med Packaging News 1994; 2:22.
18. Wagner J. Pending ICH guidelines and sophisticated drugs add up to the need for higher moisture protec-

tion. Pharmaceut Med Packaging News 1996;4:
20–24.

19. 60 Federal Register 38671–38674.

20. 60 Federal Register 37709–37744.

21. Code of Federal Regulations, Title 21, Parts 500–599.

22. Code of Federal Regulations, Title 21, Part 1300.

23. 62 Federal Register 9023–9061.

24. Okeke CC, Bailey LC, Medwick T, Grady LT. Temperature fluctuations during mail order shipment of pharmaceutical articles using mean kinetic temperature approach. Pharmaceut Forum 1997;23:4155–4182.

Dosage Form Design: Pharmaceutical and Formulation Considerations

4

Chapter at a glance

Drug substances are seldom administered alone; rather they are given as part of a formulation in combination with one or more nonmedicinal agents that serve varied and specialized pharmaceutical functions. Selective use of these nonmedicinal agents, referred to as *pharmaceutical ingredients* or *excipients*, produces dosage forms of various types. The pharmaceutical ingredients solubilize, suspend, thicken, dilute, emulsify, stabilize, preserve, color, fla-

vor, and fashion medicinal agents into efficacious and appealing dosage forms. Each type of dosage form is unique in its physical and pharmaceutical characteristics. These varied preparations provide the manufacturing and compounding pharmacist with the challenges of formulation and the physician with the choice of drug and delivery system to prescribe. The general area of study concerned with the formulation, manufacture, stability, and effectiveness of pharmaceutical dosage forms is termed *pharmaceutics.*

The proper design and formulation of a dosage form requires consideration of the physical, chemical, and biologic characteristics of all of the drug substances and pharmaceutical ingredients to be used in fabricating the product. The drug and pharmaceutical materials must be compatible with one another to produce a drug product that is stable, efficacious, attractive, easy to administer, and safe. The product should be manufactured with appropriate measures of quality control and packaged in containers that keep the product stable. The product should be labeled to promote correct use and be stored under conditions that contribute to maximum shelf life.

Methods for the preparation of specific types of dosage forms and drug delivery systems are described in subsequent chapters. This chapter presents some general considerations regarding physical pharmacy, drug product formulation, and pharmaceutical ingredients.

The Need for Dosage Forms

The potent nature and low dosage of most of the drugs in use today precludes any expectation that the general public could safely obtain the appropriate dose of a drug from the bulk material. Most drug substances are administered in milligram quantities, much too small to be weighed on anything but a sensitive prescription or electronic analytical balance. For instance, how could the lay person accurately obtain from a bulk supply the 325 mg of aspirin found in the common tablet? Not possible. Yet compared with many other drugs, the dose of aspirin is formidable (Table 4.1). For example, the dose of ethinyl estradiol, 0.05 mg, is 1/6500 the amount of aspirin in an aspirin tablet. To put it another way, 6500 ethinyl estradiol tablets, each containing 0.05 mg of drug, could be made from an amount of ethinyl estradiol equal to the amount of aspirin in just one standard tablet. When the dose of the drug is minute, as with ethinyl estradiol, solid dosage forms such as tablets and capsules must be prepared with fillers or diluents so that the dosage unit is large enough to pick up with the fingertips.

Besides providing the mechanism for the safe and convenient delivery of accurate dosage, dosage forms are needed for additional reasons:

1. To protect the drug substance from the destructive influences of atmospheric oxygen or humidity (coated tablets, sealed ampuls)
2. To protect the drug substance from the destructive influence of gastric acid after oral administration (enteric-coated tablets)
3. To conceal the bitter, salty, or offensive taste or odor of a drug substance (capsules, coated tablets, flavored syrups)
4. To provide liquid preparations of substances that are either insoluble or unstable in the desired vehicle (suspensions)
5. To provide clear liquid dosage forms of substances (syrups, solutions)
6. To provide rate-controlled drug action (various controlled-release tablets, capsules, and suspensions)
7. To provide optimal drug action from topical administration sites (ointments, creams, transdermal patches, and ophthalmic, ear, and nasal preparations)
8. To provide for insertion of a drug into one of the body's orifices (rectal or vaginal suppositories)
9. To provide for placement of drugs directly in the bloodstream or body tissues (injections)
10. To provide for optimal drug action through inhalation therapy (inhalants and inhalation aerosols)

General Considerations in Dosage Form Design

Before formulating a drug substance into a dosage form, the desired product type must be determined insofar as possible to establish the framework for product development. Then, various initial formulations of the product are developed and examined for desired features (e.g., drug release profile, bioavailability, clinical effectiveness) and for pilot plant studies and production scale-up. The formulation that best meets the goals for the product is selected to be its *master formula.* Each batch of product subsequently prepared must meet the specifications established in the master formula.

TABLE 4.1 SOME DRUGS WITH RELATIVELY LOW USUAL DOSES

DRUG	USUAL DOSE (MG)	CATEGORY
Betaxolol HCl	10.00	Antianginal
Clotrimazole	10.00	Antifungal
Methylphenidate HCl	10.00	CNS stimulant
Medroxyprogesterone acetate	10.00	Progestin
Mesoridazine besylate	10.00	Antipsychotic
Morphine sulfate	10.00	Narcotic analgesic
Nifedipine	10.00	Coronary vasodilator
Omeprazole	10.00	Antiulcerative
Quinapril HCl	10.00	Antihypertensive
Chlorazepate dipotassium	7.50	Tranquilizer
Buspirone HCl	5.00	Antianxiety
Enalapril maleate	5.00	Antihypertensive
Hydrocodone	5.00	Narcotic analgesic
Prednisolone	5.00	Adrenocortical steroid
Albuterol sulfate	4.00	Bronchodilator
Chlorpheniramine maleate	4.00	Antihistaminic
Felodipine	2.50	Vasodilator
Glyburide	2.50	Antidiabetic
Doxazosin mesylate	2.00	Antihypertensive
Levorphanol tartrate	2.00	Narcotic analgesic
Prazosin HCl	2.00	Antihypertensive
Risperidone	2.00	Antipsychotic
Estropipate	1.25	Estrogen
Bumetanide	1.00	Diuretic
Clonazepam	1.00	Anticonvulsant
Ergoloid mesylates	1.00	Cognitive adjuvant
Alprazolam	0.50	Antianxiety
Colchicine	0.50	Gout suppressant
Nitroglycerin	0.40	Antianginal
Digoxin	0.25	Cardiotonic (maintenance)
Levothyroxine	0.10	Thyroid
Misoprostol	0.10	Antiulcerative
Ethinyl estradiol	0.05	Estrogen

There are many different forms into which a medicinal agent may be placed for the convenient and efficacious treatment of disease. Most commonly, a manufacturer prepares a drug substance in several dosage forms and strengths for the efficacious and convenient treatment of disease (Fig. 4.1). Before a medicinal agent is formulated into one or more dosage forms, among the factors considered are such therapeutic matters as the nature of the illness, the manner in which it is treated (locally or through systemic action), and the age and anticipated condition of the patient.

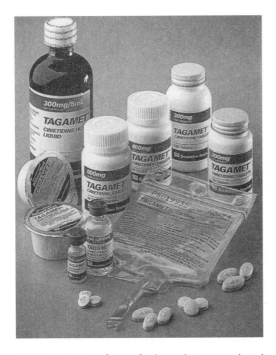

FIGURE 4.1 Various forms of a drug substance marketed by a pharmaceutical manufacturer to meet the special requirements of the patient. (Courtesy of SmithKline Beecham.)

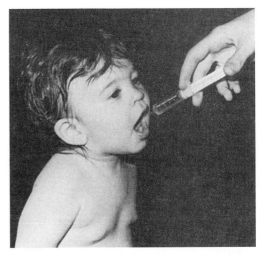

FIGURE 4.2 Pee Dee Dose brand of dispense used to administer measured volumes of liquid oral medication to youngsters. (Courtesy of Baxa Corporation.)

If the medication is intended for systemic use and oral administration is desired, tablets and/or capsules are usually prepared because they are easily handled by the patient and are most convenient in the self-administration of medication. If a drug substance has application in an emergency in which the patient may be comatose or unable to take oral medication, an injectable form of the medication may also be prepared. Many other examples of therapeutic situations affecting dosage form design could be cited, including motion sickness, nausea, and vomiting, for which tablets and skin patches are used for prevention and suppositories and injections for treatment.

The age of the intended patient also plays a role in dosage form design. For infants and children younger than 5 years of age, pharmaceutical liquids rather than solid forms are preferred for oral administration. These liquids, which are flavored aqueous solutions, syrups, or suspensions, are usually administered directly into the infant's or child's mouth by drop, spoon, or oral dispenser (Fig. 4.2) or incorporated into the child's food. A single liquid pediatric preparation may be used for infants and children of all ages, with the dose of the drug varied by the volume administered. When a young patient has a productive cough or is vomiting, gagging, or simply rebellious, there may be some question as to how much of the medicine administered is actually swallowed and how much is expectorated. In such instances, injections may be required. Infant-size rectal suppositories may also be employed, although drug absorption from the rectum is often erratic.

During childhood and even adulthood, a person may have difficulty swallowing solid dosage forms, especially uncoated tablets. For this reason, some medications are formulated as chewable tablets. Many of these tablets are comparable in texture to an after-dinner mint and break down into a pleasant-tasting creamy material. Newly available tablets dissolve in the mouth in about 10 to 15 seconds; this allows the patient to take a tablet but actually swallow a liquid. Capsules have been found by many to be more easily swallowed than whole tablets. If a capsule is moistened in the mouth before it is swallowed, it becomes slippery and readily slides down the throat with water. Also, a teaspoonful of gelatin dessert, liquid candy, or syrup placed in the mouth and partially swallowed before placing the solid dosage form in the mouth aids in swallowing them. Also, if a person has difficulty swallowing a capsule, the contents may be emptied into a spoon, mixed with jam, honey, or other similar food to mask the taste of the medication, and swallowed. Medications intended for the elderly are commonly formulated into oral liquids or may be extemporaneously prepared into an oral liquid by the pharmacist. However, certain tablets and capsules that are designed for controlled release should not be crushed or chewed, because that would interfere with their integrity and intended performance.

Many patients, particularly the elderly, take multiple medications daily. The more distinctive the size, shape, and color of solid dosage forms, the easier is proper identification of the medications. Errors in taking medications among the elderly occur frequently because of their multiple drug therapy and impaired eyesight. Dosage forms that allow reduced frequency of administration without sacrifice of efficiency are particularly advantageous.

In dealing with the problem of formulating a drug substance into a proper dosage form, research pharmacists employ knowledge gained through experience with other chemically similar drugs and through the proper use of the physical, chemical, biologic, and pharmaceutical sciences. The early stages of any new formulation include studies to collect basic information on the physical and chemical characteristics of the drug substance. These basic studies are the *preformulation* work needed before actual product formulation begins.

Preformulation Studies

Before the formulation of a drug substance into a dosage form, it is essential that it be chemically and physically characterized. The following *preformulation studies* (1) and others provide the type of information needed to define the nature of the drug substance. This information provides the framework for the drug's combination with pharmaceutical ingredients in the fabrication of a dosage form.

Physical Description

It is important to understand the physical description of a drug substance prior to dosage form development. Most drug substances in use today are solid materials, pure chemical compounds of either crystalline or amorphous constitution. The purity of the chemical substance is essential for its identification and for evaluation of its chemical, physical, and biologic properties. Chemical properties include structure, form, and reactivity. Physical properties include such characteristics as its physical description, particle size, crystalline structure, melting point, and solubility. Biologic properties relate to its ability to get to a site of action and elicit a biologic response.

Drugs can be used therapeutically as solids, liquids, and gases. Liquid drugs are used to a much lesser extent than solid drugs; gases, even less frequently.

Liquid drugs pose an interesting problem in the design of dosage forms and delivery systems. Many liquids are volatile and must be physically sealed from the atmosphere to prevent evaporation loss. Amyl nitrite, for example, is a clear yellowish liquid that is volatile even at low temperatures and is also highly flammable. It is kept for medicinal purposes in small sealed glass cylinders wrapped with gauze or another suitable material. When amyl nitrite is administered, the glass is broken between the fingertips, and the liquid wets the gauze covering, producing vapors that are inhaled by the patient requiring vasodilation. Propylhexedrine is another volatile liquid that must be contained in a closed system. This drug is used as a nasal inhalant for its vasoconstrictor action. A cylindrical roll of fibrous material is impregnated with propylhexedrine, and the saturated cylinder is placed in a suitable, usually plastic, sealed nasal inhaler. The inhaler's cap must be securely tightened each time it is used. Even then, the inhaler maintains its effectiveness for only a limited time because of the volatility of the drug.

Another problem associated with liquid drugs is that those intended for oral administration cannot generally be formulated into tablet form, the most popular form of oral medication, without chemical modification. An exception to this is the liquid drug nitroglycerin, which is formulated into sublingual tablets that disintegrate within seconds after placement under the tongue. However, because the drug is volatile, it has a tendency to escape from the tablets during storage, and it is critical that the tablets be stored in a tightly sealed glass container. For the most part, when a liquid drug is to be administered orally and a solid dosage form is desired, one of two approaches is used. First, the liquid substance may be sealed in a soft gelatin capsule. Vitamins A, D, and E, cyclosporin (Neoral, Sandimmune), and ergoloid mesylates (Hydergine LC) are liquids commercially available in capsule form. Second, the liquid drug may be developed into a solid ester or salt form that will be suitable for tablets or drug capsules. For instance, scopolamine hydrobromide is a solid salt of the liquid drug scopolamine and is easily pressed into tablets. Another approach to formulate liquids into solids is by mixing the drug with a solid or melted semisolid material, such as a high-molecular-weight polyethylene glycol. The melted mixture is poured into hard gelatin capsules to harden and the capsules sealed.

For certain liquid drugs, especially those taken orally in large doses or applied topically, their liquid nature may have some advantage in therapy. For example, 15-mL doses of mineral oil may be administered conveniently as such. Also, the liquid nature of undecylenic acid certainly does not hinder but rather enhances its use topically in the treatment of fungus infections of the skin. However, for the most part, pharmacists prefer solid materials in formulation work because they can easily form them into tablets and capsules.

Formulation and stability difficulties arise less frequently with solid dosage forms than with liquid preparations, and for this reason many new drugs first reach the market as tablets or dry-filled capsules. Later, when the pharmaceutical problems are resolved, a liquid form of the same drug may be marketed. This procedure is doubly advantageous, because for the most part physicians and patients alike prefer small, generally tasteless, accurately dosed tablets or capsules to the analogous liquid forms. Therefore, marketing a drug in solid form first is more practical for the manufacturer and suits most patients. It is estimated that tablets and capsules constitute the dosage form dispensed 70% of the time by community pharmacists, with tablets dispensed twice as frequently as capsules.

Microscopic Examination

Microscopic examination of the raw drug substance is an important step in preformulation work. It gives an indication of particle size and size range of the raw material along with the crystal structure. Photomicrographs of the initial and subsequent batch lots of the drug substance can provide important information in case of problems in formulation processing attributable to changes in particle or crystal characteristics of the drug. During some processing procedures, the solid drug powders must flow freely and not become entangled. Spherical and oval powders flow more easily than needle-shaped powders and make processing easier.

Melting Point Depression

A characteristic of a pure substance is a defined melting point or melting range. If not pure, the substance will exhibit a change in melting point. This phenomenon is commonly used to determine the purity of a drug substance and in some cases the compatibility of various substances before inclusion in the same dosage form. This characteristic is further described in Physical Pharmacy Capsule 4.1, Melting Point Depression.

The Phase Rule

Phase diagrams are often constructed to provide a visual picture of the existence and extent of the presence of solid and liquid phases in binary, ternary, and other mixtures. Phase diagrams are normally two-component (binary) representations, as shown in Physical Pharmacy Capsule 4.2, The Phase Rule, but multicomponent phase diagrams can also be constructed.

Particle Size

Certain physical and chemical properties of drug substances, including dissolution rate, bioavailability, content uniformity, taste, texture, color, and stability, are affected by the particle size distribution. In addition, flow characteristics and sedimentation rates, among other properties, are important factors related

PHYSICAL PHARMACY CAPSULE 4.1

Melting Point Depression

The *melting point*, or *freezing point*, of a pure crystalline solid is defined as the temperature at which the pure liquid and solid exist in equilibrium. Drugs with a low melting point may soften during a processing step in which heat is generated, such as particle size reduction, compression, sintering, and so on. Also, the melting point or range of a drug can be used as an indicator of purity of chemical substances (a pure substance is ordinarily characterized by a very sharp melting peak). An altered peak or a peak at a different temperature may indicate an adulterated or impure drug. This is explained as follows.

The *latent heat of fusion* is the quantity of heat absorbed when 1 g of a solid melts; the molar heat of fusion (ΔH_f) is the quantity of heat absorbed when 1 mole of a solid melts. High-melting-point substances have high heat of fusion, and low-melting-point substances have low heat of fusion. These characteristics are related to the types of bonding in the specific substance. For example, ionic materials have high heats of fusion (NaCl melts at 801°C with a heat of fusion of 124 cal/G), and those with weaker van der Waals forces have low heats of fusion (paraffin melts at 52°C with a heat of fusion of 35.1 cal/g). Ice, with weaker hydrogen bonding, has a melting point of 0°C and a heat of fusion of 80 cal/g.

The addition of a second component to a pure compound (A), resulting in a mixture, will result in a melting point that is lower than that of the pure compound. The degree to which the melting point is lowered is proportional to the mole fraction (N_A) of the second component that is added. This can be expressed thus:

$$\Delta T = \frac{2.303\ RTT_0}{\Delta H_f} \log N_A$$

where

ΔH_F is the molar heat of fusion,
T is the absolute equilibrium temperature,
T_0 is the melting point of pure A, and
R is the gas constant.

Two noteworthy things contribute to the extent of lowering of the melting point:

1. Evident from this relationship is the inverse proportion between the melting point and the heat of fusion. When a second ingredient is added to a compound with a low molar heat of fusion, a large lowering of the melting point is observed; substances with a high molar heat of fusion will show little change in melting point with the addition of a second component.
2. The extent of lowering of the melting point is also related to the melting point itself. Compounds with low melting points are affected to a greater extent than compounds with high melting points upon the addition of a second component (i.e., low-melting-point compounds will result in a greater lowering of the melting point than those with high melting points).

to particle size. It is essential to establish as early as possible how the particle size of the drug substance may affect formulation and efficacy. Of special interest is the effect of particle size on absorption. Particle size significantly influences the oral absorption profiles of certain drugs, including griseofulvin, nitrofurantoin, spironolactone, and procaine penicillin. Also, satisfactory content uniformity in solid dosage forms depends to a large degree on

PHYSICAL PHARMACY CAPSULE 4.2

The Phase Rule

A phase diagram, or temperature-composition dia-gram, represents the melting point as a function of composition of two or three component systems. The figure is an example of such a representation for a two-component mixture. This phase diagram depicts a two-component mixture in which the components are completely miscible in the molten state and no solid so-lution or addition compound is formed in the solid state. As is evident, starting from the extremes of either pure component A or pure component B, as the sec-ond component is added, the melting point of the pure component decreases. There is a point on this phase diagram at which a minimum melting point occurs (i.e., the eutectic point). As is evident, four regions, or phases, in this diagram, represent the following:

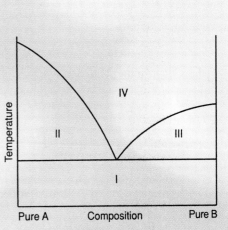

I.   Solid A + solid B
II. Solid A + melt
III. Solid B + melt
IV. Melt

Each phase is a homogenous part of the system, physically separated by distinct boundaries.

A description of the conditions under which these phases can exist is called the *Phase Rule*, which can be presented thus:

$$F = C - P + X$$

where

    F is the number of degrees of freedom,
    C is the number of components,
    P is the number of phases, and
    X is a variable dependent upon selected considerations of the phase diagram (1, 2 or 3).

C describes the minimum number of chemical components to be specified to define the phases. The F is the number of independent variables that must be specified to define the complete system (e.g., temperature, pressure, concentration).

EXAMPLE 1

In a mixture of menthol and thymol, a phase diagram similar to that illustrated can be obtained. To describe the number of degrees of freedom in the part of the graph moving from the curved line starting at pure A, progressing downward to the eutectic point, and then following an increasing melting point to pure B, it is evident from this presentation that either temperature or composition will describe this system, since it is assumed in this instance that pressure is constant. Therefore, the number of degrees of freedom to describe this portion of the phase diagram is given thus:

$$F = 2 - 2 + 1 = 1$$

In other words, along this line either temperature or composition will describe the system.

Physical Pharmacy Capsule 4.2 cont.

EXAMPLE 2

When in the area of a single phase of the diagram, such as the melt (IV), the system can be described thus:

$$F = 2 - 1 + 1 = 2$$

In this portion of the phase diagram, two factors, temperature and composition, can be varied without a change in the number of phases in the system.

EXAMPLE 3

At the eutectic point,

$$F = 2 - 3 + 1 = 0$$

and any change in the concentration or temperature may cause disappearance of one of the two solid phases or the liquid phase.

Phase diagrams are valuable for interpreting interactions between two or more components, relating not only to melting point depression and possible liquefaction at room temperature but also the formation of solid solutions, coprecipitates, and other solid-state interactions.

---

particle size and the equal distribution of the active ingredient throughout the formulation. Particle size is discussed further in Chapter 6.

Polymorphism

An important factor on formulation is the crystal or amorphous form of the drug substance. Polymorphic forms usually exhibit different physicochemical properties, including melting point and solubility. Polymorphic forms in drugs are relatively common: it has been estimated that at least one-third of all organic compounds exhibit polymorphism.

In addition to polymorphic forms, compounds may occur in noncrystalline or amorphous forms. The energy required for a molecule of drug to escape from a crystal is much greater than is required to escape from an amorphous powder. Therefore, the amorphous form of a compound is always more soluble than a corresponding crystal form.

Evaluation of crystal structure, polymorphism, and solvate form is an important preformulation activity. The changes in crystal characteristics can influence bioavailability and chemical and physical stability and can have important implications in dosage form process functions. For example, it can be a significant factor relating to tablet formation because of flow and compaction behaviors, among others. Various techniques are used to determine crystal properties. The most widely used methods are hot stage microscopy, thermal analysis, infrared spectroscopy, and x-ray diffraction.

Solubility

An important physicochemical property of a drug substance is solubility, especially aqueous system solubility. A drug must possess some aqueous solubility for therapeutic efficacy. For a drug to enter the systemic circulation and exert a therapeutic effect, it must first be in solution. Relatively insoluble compounds often exhibit incomplete or erratic absorption. If the solubility of the drug substance is less than desirable, consideration must be given to improve its solubility. The methods to accomplish this depend on the chemical nature of the drug and the type of drug product under consideration. Chemical modification of the drug into salt or ester forms is frequently used to increase solubility.

A drug's solubility is usually determined by

the equilibrium solubility method, by which an excess of the drug is placed in a solvent and shaken at a constant temperature over a long period until equilibrium is obtained. Chemical analysis of the drug content in solution is performed to determine degree of solubility.

Solubility and Particle Size

Although solubility is normally considered a physicochemical constant, small increases in solubility can be accomplished by particle size reduction as described in the Physical Pharmacy Capsule 4.3, Solubility and Particle Size.

Solubility and pH

Another technique, if the drug is to be formulated into a liquid product, is adjustment of the pH of the solvent to enhance solubility. However, for many drug substances pH adjustment is not an effective means of improving solubility. Weak acidic or basic drugs may require extremes in pH that are outside accepted physiologic limits or that may cause stability problems with formulation ingredients. Adjustment of pH usually has little effect on the solubility of substances other than electrolytes. In many cases, it is desirable to use cosolvents or other techniques such as complexation, micronization, or solid dispersion to improve aqueous solubility. A review of pH is provided in Physical Pharmacy Capsule 4.4, Principles of pH. The effect of pH on solubility is illustrated in Physical Pharmacy Capsule 4.5, Solubility and pH.

In recent years, more and more physicochemical information on drugs is being made

PHYSICAL PHARMACY CAPSULE 4.3

Solubility and Particle Size

The particle size and surface area of a drug exposed to a medium can affect actual solubility within reason, for example, in the following relationship:

$$\log \frac{S}{S_0} = \frac{2\gamma V}{2.303\ RTr}$$

where

S is the solubility of the small particles,
S_0 is the solubility of the large particles,
γ is the surface tension,
V is the molar volume,
R is the gas constant,
T is the absolute temperature, and
r is the radius of the small particles.

The equation can be used to estimate the decrease in particle size required to increase solubility. For example, a desired increase in solubility of 5% would require an increase in the S/So ratio to 1.05; that is, the left term in the equation would become log 1.05. If a powder has a surface tension of 125 dynes per centimeter, molar volume of 45 cm³, and temperature of 27°C, what is the particle size required to obtain the 5% increase in solubility?

$$\log 1.05 = \frac{(2)(125)(45)}{(2.303)(8.314 \times 10^7)(300)r}$$

$$r = 9.238 \times 10^{-6}\ cm\ or\ 0.09238\mu$$

A number of factors are involved in actual solubility enhancement, and this is only an introduction to the general effects of particle size reduction.

Principles of pH

pH is a critical variable in pharmaceutics, and a basic understanding of its principles and measurement are important. Let's begin with a definition of the term pH. The p comes from the word power. The H, of course, is the symbol for hydrogen. Together, the term pH means the hydrogen ion exponent.

The pH of a substance is a measure of its acidity, just as a degree is a measure of temperature. A specific pH value tells the exact acidity. Rather than stating general ideas, such as cherry syrup is acidic or the water is hot, a specific pH value gives the same relative point of reference, thus providing more exact communication. "The cherry juice has a pH of 3.5" or "the water is at 80°C" provides an exact common language.

pH is defined in terms of the hydrogen ion activity:

$$pH = -\log_{10} a_{H+} \text{ or } 10^{-pH} = a_{H+}$$

pH equals the negative logarithm of the hydrogen ion activity, or the activity of the hydrogen ion is 10 raised to the exponent –pH. The latter expression renders the use of the p exponent more obvious. The activity is the effective concentration of the hydrogen ion in solution. The difference between effective and actual concentration decreases as one moves toward more dilute solutions, in which ionic interaction becomes progressively less important.

Normally reference is made to the hydrogen ion when reference should be made to the hydronium ion (H_3O^+). It is a matter of convenience and brevity that only the hydrogen ion is mentioned, even though it is normally in its solvated form:

$$H^+ + H_2O = H_3O^+$$

The complexing of the hydrogen ion by water affects activity and applies to other ions, which partially complex or establish an equilibrium with the hydrogen ion. In other words, equilibrium such as

$$H_2CO_3 = H^+ + HCO_3^-$$

$$HC_2H_3O_2 = H^+ + C_2H_3O_2^-$$

complexes the hydrogen ion so that it is not sensed by the pH measuring system. This is why an acid-base titration is performed if the total concentration of acid (H^+) is needed. These effects on hydrogen ion activity are obvious, but other more subtle effects are involved in the correlation of activity and concentration.

The activity of the hydrogen ion can be defined by its relation to concentration (C_{H}^+, molality) and the activity coefficient f_H+:

$$aH^+ = f_H+ \, C_H+$$

If the activity coefficient is unity, activity is equal to concentration. This is nearly the case in dilute solutions, whose ionic strength is low. Since the objective of most pH measurements is to find a stable and reproducible reading that can be correlated to the results of some process, it is important to know what influences the activity coefficient and therefore the pH measurement.

Physical Pharmacy Capsule 4.4 cont.

The factors that affect the activity coefficient are the temperature (T), the ionic strength (μ), the dielectric constant (ϵ), the ion charge (Zi), the size of the ion in angstroms (Å), and the density of the solvent (d). All of these factors are characteristics of the solution that relate the activity to the concentration by two main effects, the salt effect and the medium effect; the latter relates the influence that the solvent can have on the hydrogen ion activity. Thus, hydrogen activity is related to concentration through a salt effect and a solvent effect. Because of these influences, a sample pH value cannot be extrapolated to another temperature or dilution. If the pH value of a particular solution is known at 40°C, it is not automatically known at 25°C.

THE pH SCALE

In pure water, hydrogen and hydroxyl ion concentrations are equal at 10^{-7} M at 25°C. This is a neutral solution. Since most samples encountered have less than 1 M H^+ or OH^-, the extremes of pH 0 for acids and pH 14 for bases are established. Of course, with strong acids or bases, pH values below 0 and above 14 are possible but infrequently measured.

MEASUREMENT OF pH

The activity of the hydrogen ion in solution is measured with a glass electrode, a reference electrode, and a pH meter.

COMBINATION ELECTRODES

A combination electrode is a combination of the glass and reference electrodes into a single probe. The main advantage in using a combination electrode is with the measurement of small volume samples or samples in limited-access containers.

available to pharmacists in routinely used reference books. This type of information is important for pharmacists in different types of practice, especially those involved in compounding and pharmacokinetic monitoring.

Dissolution

Variations in the biologic activity of a drug substance may be brought about by the rate at which it becomes available to the organism. In many instances, dissolution rate, or the time it takes for the drug to dissolve in the fluids at the absorption site, is the rate-limiting step in absorption. This is true for drugs administered orally in solid forms such as tablets, capsules, or suspensions, and for those administered intramuscularly. When the dissolution rate is the rate-limiting step, anything that affects it will also affect absorption. Consequently, dissolu-

tion rate can affect the onset, intensity, and duration of response and control the overall bioavailability of the drug from the dosage form, as discussed in the previous chapter.

The dissolution rate of drugs may be increased by decreasing the drug's particle size. It may also be increased by increasing its solubility in the diffusion layer. The most effective means of obtaining higher dissolution rates is to use a highly water soluble salt of the parent substance. Although a soluble salt of a weak acid will precipitate as the free acid in the bulk phase of an acidic solution, such as gastric fluid, it will do so in the form of fine particles with a large surface area.

The dissolution rates of chemical compounds are determined by two methods: the constant-surface method, which provides the intrinsic dissolution rate of the agent, and particulate dissolution, in which a suspension of

PHYSICAL PHARMACY CAPSULE 4.5

Solubility and pH

pH is one of the most important factors in the formulation process. Two areas of critical importance are the effects of pH on solubility and stability. The effect of pH on solubility is critical in the formulation of liquid dosage forms, from oral and topical solutions to intravenous solutions and admixtures.

The solubility of a weak acid or base is often pH dependent. The total quantity of a monoprotic weak acid (HA) in solution at a specific pH is the sum of the concentrations of both the free acid and salt (A^-) forms. If excess drug is present, the quantity of free acid in solution is maximized and constant because of its saturation solubility. As the pH of the solution increases, the quantity of drug in solution increases because the water-soluble ionizable salt is formed. The expression is

$$HA \xrightarrow{\quad K_a \quad} H^+ + A^-$$

where K_a is the dissociation constant.

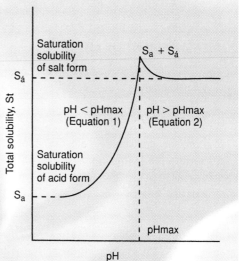

There may be a certain pH level reached where the total solubility (S_T) of the drug solution is saturated with respect to both the salt and acid forms of the drug, that is, the pH_{max}. The solution can be saturated with respect to the salt at pH values higher than this, but not with respect to the acid. Also, at pH values less than this, the solution can be saturated with respect to the acid but not to the salt. This is illustrated in the accompanying figure.

To calculate the total quantity of drug that can be maintained in solution at a selected pH, either of two equations can be used, depending on whether the product is to be in a pH region above or below the pH_{max}. The following equation is used when below the pH_{max}:

$$S_T = S_a \left(1 + \frac{K_a}{[H^+]} \right) \quad \textit{(Equation 1)}$$

The next equation is used when above the pH_{max}:

$$S_T = S'_a \left(1 + \frac{K_a}{[H^+]} \right) \quad \textit{(Equation 2)}$$

where

S_a is the saturation solubility of the free acid and
S'_a is the saturation solubility of the salt form.

EXAMPLE

A pharmacist prepares a 3.0% solution of an antibiotic as an ophthalmic solution and dispenses it to a patient. A few days later the patient returns the eye drops to the pharmacist because the product contains a precipitate. The pharmacist, checking the pH of the solution and finding it to be 6.0, reasons that the problem may be pH related. The physicochemical information of interest on the antibiotic includes the following:

Molecular weight	285 (salt) 263 (free acid)
3.0% solution of the drug	0.1053 molar solution
Acid form solubility (S_a)	3.1 mg/mL (0.0118 molar)
K_a	5.86×10^{-6}

Using Equation 1, the pharmacist calculates the quantity of the antibiotic in solution at a pH of 6.0 (*Note*: pH of 6.0 = [H$^+$] of 1×10^{-6})

$$S_T = 0.0118\,[1 + \,] = 0.0809 \text{ molar}$$

From this the pharmacist knows that at a pH of 6.0, a 0.0809-molar solution can be prepared. However, the concentration that was to be prepared was a 0.1053 molar solution; consequently, the drug will not be in solution at that pH. The pH may have been all right initially but shifted to a lower pH over time, resulting in precipitation of the drug. The question is at what pH (hydrogen ion concentration) the drug will remain in solution. This can be calculated using the same equation and information. The S_T value is 0.1053 molar.

$$0.1053 = 0.0118 \left[1 + \frac{5.86 \times 10^{-6}}{[\text{H}^+]} \right]$$

$$[\text{H}^+] = 7.333 \times 10^{-7}, \text{ or a pH of } 6.135$$

The pharmacist prepares a solution of the antibiotic, adjusting the pH to above about 6.2, using a suitable buffer system, and dispenses the solution to the patient—with positive results.

An interesting phenomenon concerns the close relationship of pH to solubility. At a pH of 6.0, only a 0.0809 molar solution could be prepared, but at a pH of 6.13 a 0.1053 molar solution could be prepared. In other words, a difference of 0.13 pH units resulted in

$$\frac{0.1053 - 0.0809}{0.0809} = 30.1\%$$

more drug going into solution at the higher pH than at the lower pH. In other words, a very small change in pH resulted in about 30% more drug going into solution. According to the figure, the slope of the curve would be very steep for this example drug, and a small change in pH (x-axis) results in a large change in solubility (y-axis). From this, it can be reasoned that if one observes the pH–solubility profile of a drug, it is possible to predict the magnitude of the pH change on its solubility.

In recent years more and more physicochemical information on drugs is being made available to pharmacists in routinely used reference books. This type of information is important for pharmacists in different types of practice, especially those who compound and do pharmacokinetic monitoring.

the agent is added to a fixed amount of solvent without exact control of surface area.

The constant-surface method uses a compressed disc of known area. This method eliminates surface area and surface electrical charges as dissolution variables. The dissolution rate obtained by this method, the *intrinsic* *dissolution rate*, is characteristic of each solid compound and a given solvent in the fixed experimental conditions. The value is expressed as milligrams dissolved per minute per centimeters squared. It has been suggested that this value is useful in predicting probable absorption problems due to dissolution rate. In particulate dissolution, a weighed amount of powdered sample is added to the dissolution medium in a constant agitation system. This method is frequently used to study the influence of particle size, surface area, and excipients upon the active agent. Occasionally, the surface properties of the drug produce an inverse relationship of particle size to dissolution. In these instances, surface charge and/or agglomeration results in the reduced particle size form of the drug presenting a lower effective surface area to the solvent due to incomplete wetting or agglomeration. Fick's laws describe the relationship of diffusion and dissolution of the active drug in the dosage form and when administered in the body, as shown in Physical Pharmacy Capsule 4.6, Fick's Laws of Diffusion and the Noyes-Whitney Equation.

Early formulation studies should include the effects of pharmaceutical ingredients on the dissolution characteristics of the drug substance.

Membrane Permeability

Modern preformulation studies include an early assessment of passage of drug molecules across biologic membranes. To produce a biologic response, the drug molecule must first cross a biologic membrane. The biologic membrane acts as a lipid barrier to most drugs and permits the absorption of lipid-soluble substances by passive diffusion, while lipid insoluble substances can diffuse across the barrier only with considerable difficulty if at all. The interrelationship of the dissociation constant, lipid solubility, and pH at the absorption site with the absorption characteristics of various drugs are the basis of the pH partition theory.

Data obtained from the basic physicochemical studies, specifically, pKa, solubility, and dissolution rate, provide an indication of absorption. To enhance these data, a technique using the everted intestinal sac may be used to evaluate absorption characteristics of drug substances. In this method, a piece of intestine is removed from an intact animal, everted, filled with a solution of the drug substance, and the degree and rate of passage of the drug through the membrane sac is determined. This method allows evaluation of both passive and active transport.

In the latter stages of preformulation testing or early formulation studies, animals and man must be studied to assess the absorption efficiency and pharmacokinetic parameters and to establish possible in vitro and in vivo correlation for dissolution and bioavailability.

Partition Coefficient

The use of the partition coefficient is described in some detail in Physical Pharmacy Capsule 4.7, Partition Coefficient. Inherent in this procedure is the selection of appropriate extraction solvents, drug stability, use of salting-out additives, and environmental concerns. The octanol–water partition coefficient is commonly used in formulation development. Following the illustrations provided earlier, it is defined as

$$P = \frac{(\text{Conc. of drug in octanol})}{(\text{Conc. of drug in water})}$$

P depends on the drug concentration only if the drug molecules have a tendency to associate in solution. For an ionizable drug, the following equation is applicable:

$$P = \frac{(\text{Conc. of drug in octanol})}{[1 - \alpha](\text{Conc. of drug in water})}$$

where α equals the degree of ionization.

pKa/Dissociation Constants

Among the physicochemical characteristics of interest is the extent of dissociation or ionization of drug substances. This is important because the extent of ionization has an important effect on the formulation and pharmacokinetic parameters of the drug. The extent of dissociation or ionization in many cases is highly dependent on the pH of the medium containing the drug. In formulation, often the vehicle is adjusted to a certain pH to obtain a certain level of ionization of the drug for solubility and stability. In the pharmacokinetic area, the extent of ionization of a drug has a strong effect on its extent of absorption, distribution, and elimination. Dissociation constant, or pKa, is usually determined by potentiometric titration. For the practicing

PHYSICAL PHARMACY CAPSULE 4.6

Fick's Laws of Diffusion and the Noyes-Whitney Equation

All drugs must diffuse through various barriers when administered to the body. For example, some drugs must diffuse through the skin, gastric mucosa, or some other barrier to gain access to the interior of the body. Parenteral drugs must diffuse through muscle, connective tissue, and so on to get to the site of action; even intravenous drugs must diffuse from the blood to the site of action. Drugs must also diffuse through various barriers for metabolism and excretion.

Considering all the diffusion processes that occur in the body (passive, active, and facilitated), it is not surprising that the laws governing diffusion are important to drug delivery systems. In fact, diffusion is important not only in the body but also in some quality control procedures used to determine batch-to-batch uniformity of products (dissolution test for tablets based on the Noyes-Whitney equation, which can be derived from Fick's law).

When individual molecules move within a substance, diffusion is said to occur. This may occur as the result of a concentration gradient or by random molecular motion.

Probably the most widely used laws of diffusion are known as Fick's first and second laws. Fick's first law involving steady-state diffusion (where dc/dx does not change) is derived from the following expression for the quantity of material (M) flowing through a cross-section of a barrier (S) in unit time (t) expressed as the flux (J):

$$J = dM/(S\ dt)$$

Under a concentration gradient (dc/dx), Fick's first law can be expressed thus:

$$J = D[(C_1 - C_2)/h]\ \text{or}\ J = -D\ (dC/dx)$$

where

  J is the flux of a component across a plane of unit area,
  C_1 and C_2 are the concentrations in the donor and receptor compartments,
  h is the membrane thickness, and
  D is the diffusion coefficient (or diffusivity).

The sign is negative, denoting that the flux is in the direction of decreasing concentration. The units of J are grams per square centimeter; C, grams per cubic centimeter; M, grams or moles; S, square centimeters; x, centimeters; and D, square centimeters per second.

D is appropriately called a diffusion coefficient, not a diffusion constant, as it is subject to change. D may change in value with increased concentrations. Also, D can be affected by temperature, pressure, solvent properties, and the chemical nature of the drug itself. To study the rate of change of the drug in the system, one needs an expression that relates the change in concentration with time at a definite location in place of the mass of drug diffusing across a unit area of barrier in unit time; this expression is known as Fick's second law. This law can be summarized as stating that the change in concentration in a particular place with time is proportional to the change in concentration gradient at that particular place in the system.

In summary, Fick's first law relates to a steady-state flow, whereas Fick's second law relates to a change in concentration of drug with time, at any distance, or an unsteady state of flow.

The diffusion coefficients ($D \times 10^{-6}$) of various compounds in water (25°C) and other media have been determined as follows: ethanol, 12.5 cm^2/second; glycine, 10.6 cm^2/second; sodium lauryl sulfate, 6.2 cm^2/second; glucose, 6.8 cm^2/second.

Physical Pharmacy Capsule 4.6 cont.

The concentration of drug in the membrane can be calculated using the partition coefficient (K) and the concentration in the donor and receptor compartments.

$$K = C_1/C_d = C_2/C_r$$

where

C_1 and C_d are the concentrations in the donor compartment (g/cm³)
and C_2 and C_r are the concentrations in the receptor compartment (g/cm³).

K is the partition coefficient of the drug between the solution and the membrane. It can be estimated using the oil solubility of the drug versus the water solubility of the drug. Usually the higher the partition coefficient, the more the drug will be soluble in a lipophilic substance. We can now write the expression:

$$dM/dt = [DSK(C_d - C_r)]/h$$

or in sink conditions,

$$dM/dt = DSKC_d/h = PSC_d$$

The permeability coefficient (centimeters per second) can be obtained by rearranging to:

$$P = DK/h$$

EXAMPLE 1

A drug passing through a 1-mm-thick membrane has a diffusion coefficient of 4.23×10^{-7} cm²/second and an oil–water partition coefficient of 2.03. The radius of the area exposed to the solution is 2 cm, and the concentration of the drug in the donor compartment is 0.5 mg/mL. Calculate the permeability and the diffusion rate of the drug.

h = 1 mm = 0.1 cm
D = 4.23×10^{-7} cm²/second
K = 2.03
r = 2 cm, S = $\pi(2cm)^2$ = 12.57 cm²
Cd = 0.5 mg/mL
P = $[(4.23 \times 10^{-7}$ cm²/second) $(2.03)]/0.1$ cm = 8.59×10^{-6} cm/second
dM/dt = $(8.59 \times 10^{-6}$ cm/second) (12.57 cm²)(0.5 mg/mL) = 5.40×10^{-5} mg/second
$(5.40 \times 10^{-5}$ mg/second)(3600 second/hour) = 0.19 mg/hour

In the dissolution of particles of drug, the dissolved molecules diffuse away from the individual particle body. An expression to describe this, derived from Fick's equations, is known as the Noyes and Whitney expression, proposed in 1897. It can be written as follows:

$$dC/dt = (DS/Vh)(Cs - C)$$

where

C is the concentration of drug dissolved at time t,
D is the diffusion coefficient of the solute in solution,
S is the surface area of the exposed solid,
V is the volume of solution,
h is the thickness of the diffusion layer,
Cs is the saturation solubility of the drug, and
C is the concentration of solute in the bulk phase at a specific time, t.

Physical Pharmacy Capsule 4.6 cont.

It is common practice to use sink conditions in which C does not exceed about 20% of the solubility of the drug being investigated. Under these conditions, the expression simplifies to

$$dC/dt = DSC_s/Vh$$

and incorporating the volume of solution (V), the thickness of the diffusion layer (h), and the diffusivity coefficient (D) into a coefficient k (to take into account the various factors in the system), the expression becomes

$$dC/dt = kSC_s$$

As the factors are held constant, it becomes apparent that the dissolution rate of a drug can be proportional to the surface area exposed to the dissolution medium. A number of other expressions have been derived for specific application to various situations and conditions.

These relationships expressed as Fick's first and second laws and the Noyes-Whitney equation have great importance and relevance in pharmaceutical systems.

EXAMPLE 2

The following information was obtained using the USP 26–NF 21 dissolution apparatus I. The drug is soluble 1 g in 3 mL of water, so sink conditions were maintained; the surface area of the tablet exposed was 1.5 cm^2 (obtained by placing the tablet in a special holder exposing only one side to the dissolution medium); and the dosage form studied was a 16-mg sustained-release tablet; the release pattern should be zero order. What is the rate of release of drug?

TIME (HOURS)	DRUG CONCENTRATION (MG/900 ML OF SOLUTION)	GRAPH OF RELEASE PROFILE
0.0	0.0	
0.5	1.0	
1.0	1.9	
2.0	4.1	
4.0	8. 0	
6 0	11.8	
8.0	15.9	

In this problem, since the surface area (S) was maintained constant at 1.5 cm^2 and the solubility (Cs) of the drug is constant at 1 g in 3 mL of water, the plot of concentration (C) versus time (t) yields a slope with a value of kSCs, or k$_2$, expressing the rate of release of the drug.

$$dC/dt = kSC_s$$

The slope of the line $= \Delta y/\Delta x = (y_2 - y_1)/(x_2 - x_1)$
$= (15.9 \text{ mg} - 0 \text{ mg})/(8.0 \text{ h} - 0 \text{ h})$
$= 15.9/8 = 1.99 \text{ mg/h}$

Therefore, the rate of release of the sustained-release preparation is 1.99, or approximately 2 mg per hour. From this, the quantity of drug released at any time (t) can be calculated.

PHYSICAL PHARMACY CAPSULE 4.7

Partition Coefficient

The oil–water partition coefficient is a measure of a molecule's lipophilic character; that is, its preference for the hydrophilic or lipophilic phase. If a solute is added to a mixture of two immiscible liquids, it will distribute between the two phases and reach an equilibrium at a constant temperature. The distribution of the solute (unaggregated and undissociated) between the two immiscible layers can be described thus:

$$K = C_U/C_L$$

where

K is the distribution constant or partition constant,
C_U is the concentration of the drug in the upper phase, and
C_L is the concentration of the drug in the lower phase.

This information can be effectively used in the

1. Extraction of crude drugs
2. Recovery of antibiotics from fermentation broth
3. Recovery of biotechnology-derived drugs from bacterial cultures
4. Extraction of drugs from biologic fluids for therapeutic drug monitoring
5. Absorption of drugs from dosage forms (ointments, suppositories, transdermal patches)
6. Study of the distribution of flavoring oil between oil and water phases of emulsions
7. In other applications

This basic relationship can be used to calculate the quantity of drug extracted from or remaining behind in a given layer and to calculate the number of extractions required to remove a drug from a mixture.

The concentration of drug found in the upper layer (U) of two immiscible layers is given thus:

$$U = Kr/(Kr + 1)$$

where

K is the distribution partition constant and
r is V_u/V_l, or the ratio of the volume of upper and lower phases.

The concentration of drug remaining in the lower layer (L) is given thus:

$$L = 1/(Kr + 1)$$

If the lower phase is successively extracted again with n equal volumes of the upper layer, each upper (U_n) contains the following fraction of the drug:

$$U_n = Kr/(Kr + 1)^n$$

where

U_n is the fraction contained in the nth extraction and
n is the nth successive volume.

The fraction of solute remaining in the lower layer (L_n) is given thus:

$$L_n = 1/(kr + 1)^n$$

Physical Pharmacy Capsule 4.7 cont.

More efficient extractions are obtained using successive small volumes of the extraction solvent than single larger volumes. This can be calculated as follows when the same volume of extracting solvent is used in divided portions. For example, the fraction L_n remaining after the nth extraction:

$$L_n = \frac{1}{\left(\dfrac{Kr}{n}+1\right)^n}$$

EXAMPLE 1

At 25°C and pH 6.8, the K for a second generation cephalosporin is 0.7 between equal volumes of butanol and the fermentation broth. Calculate the U, L, and L_n (using the same volume divided into fourths).

$$U = 0.7/(0.7 + 1) = 0.41 \text{ The fraction of drug extracted into the upper layer}$$

$$L = 1/(0.7 + 1) = 0.59 \text{ The fraction of drug remaining in the lower layer}$$

The total of the fractions in the U and L = 0.41 + 0.59 = 1.

If the fermentation broth is extracted with four successive extractions accomplished by dividing the quantity of butanol used into fourths, the quantity of drug remaining after the fourth extraction is

$$L_{4th} = \frac{1}{\left(\dfrac{0.7 \times 1}{4}+1\right)^4} = 0.525$$

From this, the quantity remaining after a single volume, single extraction is 0.59, but when the single volume is divided into fourths and four successive extractions are done, the quantity remaining is 0.525; therefore, more was extracted using divided portions of the extracting solvent. Inherent in this procedure is the selection of appropriate extraction solvents, drug stability, use of salting-out additives, and environmental concerns.

pharmacist, it is important in predicting precipitation in admixtures and in calculating the solubility of drugs at certain pH values. Physical Pharmacy Capsule 4.8, pKa/Dissociation Constants, presents a brief summary of dissociation and ionization concepts.

Drug and Drug Product Stability

One of the most important activities of preformulation work is evaluation of the physical and chemical stability of the pure drug substance. It is essential that these initial studies be conducted using drug samples of known purity. The presence of impurities can lead to erroneous conclusions in such evaluations. Stability studies conducted in the preformulation phase include solid-state stability of the

drug alone, solution phase stability, and stability in the presence of expected excipients. Initial investigation begins with knowledge of the drug's chemical structure, which allows the preformulation scientist to anticipate the possible degradation reactions.

Drug Stability: Mechanisms of Degradation

Chemical instability of medicinal agents may take many forms, because the drugs in use today are of such diverse chemical constitution. Chemically, drug substances are alcohols, phenols, aldehydes, ketones, esters, ethers, acids, salts, alkaloids, glycosides, and others, each with reactive chemical groups having different susceptibilities to chemical instability. Chemi-

pKa/Dissociation Constants

The dissociation of a weak acid in water is given by this expression:

$$HA \leftrightarrow H^+ + A^-$$
$$K_1[HA] \leftrightarrow K_2[H^+][A^-]$$

At equilibrium, the reaction rate constants K_1 and K_2 are equal. This can be rearranged, and the dissociation constant defined as

$$K_a = \frac{K_1}{K_2} = \frac{[H^+][A^-]}{[HA]}$$

where K_a is the acid dissociation constant.

For the dissociation of a weak base that does not contain a hydroxyl group, the following relationship can be used:

$$BH^+ \leftrightarrow H^+ + B$$

The dissociation constant is described by

$$K_a = \frac{[H^+][B]}{[BH^+]}$$

The dissociation of a hydroxyl-containing weak base,

$$B + H_2O \leftrightarrow OH^- + BH^+$$

The dissociation constant is described by

$$K_b = \frac{[OH^-][BH^+]}{[B]}$$

The hydrogen ion concentrations can be calculated for the solution of a weak acid using

$$[H^+] = \sqrt{K_a c}$$

Similarly, the hydroxyl ion concentration for a solution of a weak base is approximated by

$$[OH^-] = \sqrt{K_b c}$$

Some practical applications of these equations are as follows.

EXAMPLE 1

The K_a of lactic acid is 1.387×10^{-4} at 25°C. What is the hydrogen ion concentration of a 0.02 M solution?

$$[H^+] = \sqrt{1.387 \times 10^{-4} \times 0.02} = 1.665 \times 10^{-3} \text{ G-ion/L.}$$

EXAMPLE 2

The K_b of morphine is 7.4×10^{-7}. What is the hydroxyl ion concentration of a 0.02 M solution?

$$[OH] = \sqrt{7.4 \times 10^{-7} \times 0.02} = 1.216 \times 10^{-4} \text{ G-ion/L.}$$

cally, the most frequently encountered destructive processes are hydrolysis and oxidation.

Hydrolysis is a solvolysis process in which (drug) molecules interact with water molecules to yield breakdown products. For example, aspirin, or acetylsalicylic acid, combines with a water molecule and hydrolyzes into one molecule of salicylic acid and one molecule of acetic acid.

Hydrolysis is probably the most important single cause of drug decomposition, mainly because a great number of medicinal agents are esters or contain such other groupings as substituted amides, lactones, and lactams, which are susceptible to the hydrolytic process (2).

Another destructive process is oxidation, which destroys many drug types, including aldehydes, alcohols, phenols, sugars, alkaloids, and unsaturated fats and oils. Chemically, oxidation is loss of electrons from an atom or a molecule. Each electron lost is accepted by some other atom or molecule, reducing the recipient. In inorganic chemistry, oxidation is accompanied by an increase in the positive valence of an element, for example, ferrous ($+2$) oxidizing to ferric ($+3$). In organic chemistry, oxidation is frequently considered synonymous with the loss of hydrogen (dehydrogenation) from a molecule. Oxidation frequently involves free chemical radicals, which are molecules or atoms containing one or more unpaired electrons, such as molecular (atmospheric) oxygen ($\bullet O$—$O\bullet$) and free hydroxyl ($\bullet OH$). These radicals tend to take electrons from other chemicals, thereby oxidizing the donor.

Many of the oxidative changes in pharmaceutical preparations have the character of autoxidations. Autoxidations occur spontaneously under the initial influence of atmospheric oxygen and proceed slowly at first and then more rapidly. The process has been described as a type of chain reaction commencing with the union of oxygen with the drug molecule and continuing with a free radical of this oxidized molecule participating in the destruction of other drug molecules and so forth.

In drug product formulation work, steps are taken to reduce or prevent deterioration due to hydrolysis, oxidation, and other processes. These techniques are discussed later.

Drug and Drug Product Stability: Kinetics and Shelf Life

Stability is the extent to which a product retains within specified limits and throughout its period of storage and use (i.e., its shelf life) the same properties and characteristics that it possessed at the time of its manufacture.

Five types of stability concern pharmacists:

1. *Chemical*: Each active ingredient retains its chemical integrity and labeled potency within the specified limits.
2. *Physical*: The original physical properties, including appearance, palatability, uniformity, dissolution, and suspendability are retained.
3. *Microbiologic*: Sterility or resistance to microbial growth is retained according to the specified requirements. Antimicrobial agents retain effectiveness within specified limits.
4. *Therapeutic*: The therapeutic effect remains unchanged.
5. *Toxicologic*: No significant increase in toxicity occurs.

Chemical stability is important for selecting storage conditions (temperature, light, humidity), selecting the proper container for dispensing (glass vs. plastic, clear vs. amber or opaque, cap liners), and anticipating interactions when mixing drugs and dosage forms. Stability and expiration dating are based on reaction kinetics, that is, the study of the rate of chemical change and the way this rate is influenced by concentration of reactants, products, and other chemical species and by factors such as solvent, pressure, and temperature.

In considering chemical stability of a pharmaceutical, one must know the reaction order and reaction rate. The reaction order may be the overall order (the sum of the exponents of the concentration terms of the rate expression), or the order with respect to each reactant (the exponent of the individual concentration term in the rate expression).

Rate Reactions

The reaction rate is a description of the drug concentration with respect to time. Most commonly, zero-order and first-order reactions are encountered in pharmacy. These are presented in Physical Pharmacy Capsule 4.9, Rate Reactions, along with some appropriate examples.

Q_{10} Method of Shelf Life Estimation

The Q_{10} method of shelf life estimation lets the pharmacist estimate shelf life for a product that has been stored or is going to be stored under a different set of conditions. It is explained in Physical Pharmacy Capsule 4.10, Q_{10} Method of Shelf Life Estimation.

Enhancing Stability of Drug Products

Many pharmaceutical ingredients may be used to prepare the desired dosage form of a drug substance. Some of these agents may be used to achieve the desired physical and chemical characteristics of the product or to enhance its appearance, odor, and taste. Other substances may be used to increase the stability of the drug substance, particularly against hydrolysis and oxidation. In each instance, the added pharmaceutical ingredient must be compatible with and must not detract from the stability of the drug substance.

There are several approaches to the stabilization of pharmaceutical preparations containing drugs subject to hydrolysis. Perhaps the most obvious is the reduction or elimination of water from the pharmaceutical system. Even solid dosage forms containing water-labile drugs must be protected from humidity in the atmosphere. This may be accomplished by applying a waterproof protective coating over tablets or by keeping the drug in a tightly closed container. It is fairly common to detect hydrolyzed aspirin by noticing an odor of acetic acid upon opening a bottle of aspirin tablets. In liquid preparations, water can frequently be replaced or reduced in the formulation through the use of substitute liquids such as glycerin, propylene glycol, and alcohol. In certain injectable products, anhydrous vegetable oils may be used as the drug's solvent to reduce the chance of hydrolytic decomposition.

Decomposition by hydrolysis may be prevented in other liquid drugs by suspending them in a nonaqueous vehicle rather than dissolving them in an aqueous solvent. In still other instances, particularly for certain unstable antibiotic drugs, when an aqueous preparation is desired, the drug may be supplied to the pharmacist in a dry form for *reconstitution* by adding a specified volume of purified water just before dispensing. The dry powder is actually a mixture of the antibiotic, suspending agents, flavorants, and colorants; when reconstituted by the pharmacist, it remains stable for the period over which the preparation is normally consumed. Refrigeration is advisable for most preparations considered subject to hydrolysis. Together with temperature, pH is a major determinant of the stability of a drug prone to hydrolytic decomposition. Hydrolysis of most drugs depends on the relative concentrations of the hydroxyl and hydronium ions, and a pH at which each drug is optimally stable can be easily determined. For most hydrolyzable drugs optimum stability is on the acid side, somewhere between pH 5 and 6. Therefore, through judicious use of buffering agents, the stability of otherwise unstable compounds can be increased. Buffers are used to maintain a certain pH, as described in Physical Pharmacy Capsule 4.11, Buffer Capacity.

Pharmaceutically, oxidation of a susceptible drug substance is most likely to occur when it is not kept dry in the presence of oxygen or when it is exposed to light or combined with other chemical agents without proper regard to their influence on oxidation. Oxidation of a chemical in a pharmaceutical preparation is usually accompanied by an alteration in the color of that preparation. It may also result in precipitation or a change in odor.

The oxidative process is diverted and the stability of the drug is preserved by agents called *antioxidants*, which react with one or more compounds in the drug to prevent progress of the chain reaction. In general, antioxidants act by providing electrons and easily available hydrogen atoms that are accepted more readily by the free radicals than are those of the drug being protected. Various antioxidants are employed in pharmacy. Among those most frequently used in aqueous preparations are sodium sulfite (Na_2SO_3, at high pH values), sodium bisulfite ($NaHSO_3$, at intermediate pH values), sodium metabisulfite ($Na_2S_2O_5$ at low

PHYSICAL PHARMACY CAPSULE 4.9

Rate Reactions

ZERO-ORDER RATE REACTIONS

If the loss of drug is independent of the concentration of the reactants and constant with respect to time (i.e., 1 mg/mL/hour), the rate is called zero order. The mathematical expression is

$$\frac{-dC}{dt} = k_0$$

where k_0 is the zero-order rate constant [concentration(C)/time(t)].

The integrated and more useful form of the equation:

$$C = -k_0 t + C_0$$

where C_0 is the initial concentration of the drug.

The units for a zero rate constant k_o are concentration per unit time, such as moles per liter-second or milligrams per milliliter per minute.

It is meaningless to attempt to describe the time required for *all* material in a reaction to decompose, that is, infinity. Therefore, reaction rates are commonly described by k or by their half-life, $t_{1/2}$.

The half-life equation for a zero order reaction:

$$t_{1/2} = 1/2 \, (C_0/k_0)$$

If the C_o changes, the $t_{1/2}$ changes. There is an inverse relationship between the $t_{1/2}$ and k.

EXAMPLE 1

A drug suspension (125 mg/mL) decays by zero-order kinetics with a reaction rate constant of 0.5 mg/mL/hour. What is the concentration of intact drug remaining after 3 days (72 hours), and what is its $t_{1/2}$?

$$C = -(0.5 \text{ mg/mL/hour}) \, (72 \text{ hour}) + 125 \text{ mg/mL}$$
$$C = 89 \text{ mg/mL after 3 days}$$
$$t_{1/2} = 1/2 \, (125 \text{ mg/mL})/(0.5 \text{ mg/mL/hour})$$
$$t_{1/2} = 125 \text{ hours}$$

EXAMPLE 2

How long will it take for the suspension to reach 90% of its original concentration?

$$90\% \times 125 \text{ mg/mL} = 112.5 \text{ mg/mL}$$

$$t = \frac{C - C_0}{-k_0} - \frac{112.5 \text{ mg/mL} - 125 \text{ mg/mL}}{-0.5 \text{ mg/mL/hour}} = 25 \text{ hours}$$

Drug suspensions are examples of pharmaceuticals that ordinarily follow zero-order kinetics for degradation.

Physical Pharmacy Capsule 4.9 cont.

FIRST-ORDER RATE REACTIONS

If the loss of drug is directly proportional to the concentration remaining with respect to time, it is called a first-order reaction and has the units of reciprocal time, that is, time^{-1}. The mathematical expression is

$$\frac{-dC}{dt} = kC$$

where

C is the concentration of intact drug remaining,
t is time,
(dC/dt) is the rate at which the intact drug degrades, and
k is the specific reaction rate constant.

The integrated and more useful form of the equation:

$$\log C = \frac{-kt}{2.303} + \log C_0$$

where C_0 is the initial concentration of the drug.
In natural log form, the equation is

$$\ln C = -kt + \ln C_0$$

The units of k for a first-order reaction are per unit of time, such as per second.
    The half-life equation for a first-order reaction is

$$t_{1/2} = 0.693/k$$

and can be easily derived from the first-order equation by substituting values of C = 50% and C_o = 100%, representing a decrease in concentration by 50%.

EXAMPLE 3

An ophthalmic solution of a mydriatic drug at 5 mg/mL exhibits first-order degradation with a rate of 0.0005/day. How much drug will remain after 120 days, and what is its half-life?

$$\ln C = -(0.0005/day)\,(120) + \ln (5 \text{ mg/mL})$$
$$\ln C = -0.06 + 1.609$$
$$\ln C = 1.549$$
$$C = 4.71 \text{ mg/mL}$$
$$t_{1/2} = 0.693/0.0005/day$$
$$t_{1/2} = 1{,}386 \text{ days}$$

EXAMPLE 4

In Example 3, how long will it take for the drug to degrade to 90% of its original concentration?

$$90\% \text{ of } 5 \text{ mg/mL} = 4.5 \text{ mg/mL}$$
$$\ln 4.5 \text{ mg/mL} = -(0.0005/day)t + \ln (5 \text{ mg/mL})$$
$$t = \frac{\ln 4.5 \text{ mg/mL} - \ln 5 \text{ mg/mL}}{-0.0005/day}$$
$$t = 210 \text{ days}$$

Physical Pharmacy Capsule 4.9 cont.

ENERGY OF ACTIVATION: ARRHENIUS EQUATION

Stability projections for shelf life (t_{90}, or the time required for 10% of the drug to degrade with 90% of the intact drug remaining) are commonly based on the Arrhenius equation:

$$\log = \frac{k_2}{k_1} = \frac{Ea\,(t_2 - T_1)}{2.3\,RT_1T_2}$$

which relates the reaction rate constants (k) to temperatures (T) with the gas constant (R) and the energy of activation (Ea).

The relationship of the reaction rate constants at two different temperatures provides the energy of activation for the degradation. By performing the reactions at elevated temperatures instead of allowing the process to proceed slowly at room temperature, the Ea can be calculated and a k value for room temperature determined with the Arrhenius equation.

EXAMPLE 5

The degradation of a new cancer drug follows first-order kinetics and has first-order degradation rate constants of 0.0001/hour at 60°C and 0.0009 at 80°C. What is its Ea?

$$\log = \frac{(0.0009)}{(0.0001)} = \frac{EA\,(353 - 333)}{(2.3)\,(1.987)\,(353)\,(333)}$$

$$Ea = 25{,}651\ \text{kcal/mol}$$

pH values), hypophosphorous acid (H_3PO_2), and ascorbic acid. In oleaginous (oily or unctuous) preparations, alpha-tocopherol, butyl hydroxy anisole, and ascorbyl palmitate find application.

In June 1987, U.S. Food and Drug Administration (FDA) labeling regulations went into effect requiring a warning about possible allergic-type reactions, including anaphylaxis, in the package insert for prescription drugs to whose final dosage form sulfites have been added. Sulfites are used as preservatives in many injectable drugs, such as antibiotics and local anesthetics. Some inhalants and ophthalmic preparations also contain sulfites, but relatively few oral drugs contain these chemicals. The purpose of the regulation is to protect the estimated 0.2% of the population who are subject to allergic reactions to the chemicals. Many sulfite-sensitive persons have asthma or other allergic conditions. Previous to the regulations dealing with prescription medication, the FDA issued regulations for the use of sulfites in food. Asthmatics and other patients who may be sulfite sensitive

should be reminded to read the labels of packaged foods and medications to check for the presence of these agents. Sulfite agents covered by the regulations are potassium bisulfite, potassium metabisulfite, sodium bisulfite, sodium metabisulfite, sodium sulfite, and sulfur dioxide. The FDA permits the use of sulfites in prescription products, with the proper labeling, because there are no generally suitable substitutes for sulfites to maintain potency in certain medications. Some but not all epinephrine injections contain sulfites.

The proper use of antioxidants permits their specific application only after appropriate biomedical and pharmaceutical studies. In certain instances other pharmaceutical additives can inactivate a given antioxidant. In other cases certain antioxidants can react chemically with the drugs they were intended to stabilize without a noticeable change in the appearance of the preparation.

Because oxygen may adversely affect their stability, certain pharmaceuticals require an oxygen-free atmosphere during preparation and

PHYSICAL PHARMACY CAPSULE 4.10

Q_{10} Method of Shelf Life Estimation

The Q_{10} approach, based on Ea, which is independent of reaction order, is described as

$$Q_{10} = e^{\{(Ea/R)[(1/T + 10) - (1/T)]\}}$$

where

Ea is the energy of activation,
R is the gas constant, and
T is the absolute temperature.

In usable terms, Q_{10}, the ratio of two different reaction rate constants, is defined thus:

$$Q_{10} = \frac{K_{(T + 10)}}{K_T}$$

The commonly used Q values of 2, 3, and 4 relate to the energies of activations of the reactions for temperatures around room temperature (25°C). For example, a Q value of 2 corresponds to an Ea (kcal/mol) of 12.2, a Q value of 3 corresponds to an Ea of 19.4, and a Q value of 4 corresponds to an Ea of 24.5. Reasonable estimates can often be made using the value of 3.

The equation for Q_{10} shelf life estimates is

$$t_{90}(T_2) = \frac{t_{90}(T_1)}{Q_{10}^{(\Delta T/10)}}$$

where

$t_{90}T_2$ is the estimated shelf life,
$t_{90}T_1$ is the given shelf life at a given temperature, and
ΔT is the difference in the temperatures T_1 and T_2.

As is evident from this relationship, an increase in ΔT will decrease the shelf life and a decrease in ΔT will increase shelf life. This is the same as saying that storing at a warmer temperature will shorten the life of the drug and storing at a cooler temperature will increase the life of the drug.

EXAMPLE 1

An antibiotic solution has a shelf life of 48 hours in the refrigerator (5°C). What is its estimated shelf life at room temperature (25°C)?
Using a Q value of 3, we set up the relationship as follows:

$$t_{90}(T_2) = \frac{t_{90}(T_1)}{Q_{10}^{(\Delta T/10)}} = \frac{48}{3^{[(25 - 5)/10]}} = \frac{48}{3^2} = 5.33 \text{ hours}$$

EXAMPLE 2

An ophthalmic solution has a shelf life of 6 hours at room temperature (25°C). What is the estimated shelf life in a refrigerator at 5°C? (*Note:* Since the temperature is decreasing, ΔT will be negative.)

$$t_{90}(T_2) = \frac{6}{3^{[(5 - 25)/10]}} = \frac{6}{3^{-2}} = 6 \times 3^2 = 54 \text{ hours}$$

These are estimates, and actual energies of activation can be often be obtained from the literature for more exact calculations.

PHYSICAL PHARMACY CAPSULE 4.11

Buffer Capacity

pH, buffers, and buffer capacity are especially important in drug product formulation, since they affect the drug's solubility, activity, absorption, and stability and the patient's comfort.

A buffer is a system, usually an aqueous solution, that can resist changes in pH upon addition of an acid or base. Buffers are composed of a weak acid and its conjugate base or a weak base and its conjugate acid. Buffers are prepared by one of these processes:

1. Mixing a weak acid and its conjugate base or a weak base and its conjugate acid
2. Mixing a weak acid and a strong base to form the conjugate base or a weak base and a strong acid to form the conjugate acid

Using the Henderson-Hasselbach equation:

$$pH = pKa + \log (base/acid)$$

Remember that the acid is the proton donor and the base is the proton acceptor.

EXAMPLE 1

A buffer is prepared by mixing 100 mL of 0.2 M phosphoric acid with 200 mL of 0.08 M sodium phosphate monobasic. What is the pH of this buffer? (K_a of phosphoric acid = 7.5×10^{-3})

Moles acid = (0.2 mol/1000 mL)(100 mL) = 0.02 mol; (0.02 mol)/(0.3 L) = 0.067 M

Moles base = (0.08 mol/1000 mL)(200 mL) = 0.016 mol; (0.016 mol/(0.3 L) = 0.053 M

$$pKa = -\log 7.5 \times 10^{-3} = 2.125$$

$$pH = 2.125 + \log (0.016\ mol/0.02\ mol) = 2.028$$

EXAMPLE 2

Determine the pH of the buffer prepared as shown:

Sodium acetate 50 g
Conc. HCl 10 mL
Water q.s. 2 L
Helpful numbers:
  pK_a acetic acid = 4.76
  m.w. sodium acetate = 82.08
  m.w. acetic acid = 60.05
  m.w. HCl = 36.45
  Conc. HCl ~ 44% HCl w/v

NaAc	+	HCl	→	NaCl	+	HAc	+	NaAc
(0.609 mol)		(0.121 mol)		(0.121 mol)		((0.121 mol)		(0.488 mol)

HCl: {(10 mL) [(44g)/(100 mL)] (l mol)/(36.45g)} = 0.121 mol
NaAc: {(50 g)[(1 mol)/(82.08g)]} = 0.609 mol
    (0.609 mol) − (0.121 mol) = 0.488 mol
pH = 4.76 + log (0.488 mol)/(0.121 mol) = 5.367

Physical Pharmacy Capsule 4.11 cont.

The ability of a buffer solution to resist changes in pH upon the addition of an acid or a base is called buffer capacity (β) and is defined thus:

$$\beta = \Delta B/\Delta pH$$

where

  ΔB is molar concentration of acid or base added,
  ΔpH is change in pH due to addition of acid or base, and
  ΔpH can be determined experimentally or calculated using the Henderson-Hasselbach equation.

EXAMPLE 3

If 0.2 mole of HCl is added to a 0.015 M solution of ammonium hydroxide and the pH falls from 9.5 to 8.9, what is the buffer capacity?

$$\Delta pH = 9.5 - 8.9 = 0.6$$
$$\Delta B = 0.2 \text{ mol/L} = 0.2 \text{ M}$$
$$\beta = 0.2 \text{ M}/0.6 = 0.33 \text{ M}$$

EXAMPLE 4

If 0.002 mole of HCl is added to the buffer in Example 1, what is its buffer capacity? After adding 0.002 mole HCl:

H_3PO_4: 0.02 mol + 0.002 mol = 0.022 mol
NaH_2PO_4: 0.016 mol − 0.002 mL = 0.014 mol
pH = 2.125 + log (0.014 mol/0.022 mol) = 1.929
ΔpH = 2.028 − 1.929 = 0.099
ΔAB = 0.002 mol/0.3 L = 0.0067 M
β = 0.0067 M/0.099 = 0.067 M

Another approach to calculating buffer capacity involves the use of Van Slyke's equation:

$$\beta = 2.3C \{Ka[H^+]/(Ka[H^+])2\}$$

where

  C is the sum of the molar concentrations of the acid and base, and $[H^+] = 10^{-pH}$.

EXAMPLE 5

What is the Van Slyke buffer capacity of the buffer prepared in Example 1?

$$C = 0.0067 \text{ M} + 0.0053 \text{ M} = 0.12 \text{ M}$$
$$Ka = 7.5 + 10^{-3}$$
$$[H^+] = 10^{-2.028} = 9.38 \times 10^{-3} \text{ M}$$
$$\beta = 2.3(0.12M)\{[(7.5 \times 10^{-3}M)(9.38 \times 10^{-3}M)/[(7.5 \times 10^{-3}M)/(9.38 \times 10^{-3}M)^2]\} = 0.68 \text{ M}$$

storage. Oxygen may be present in pharmaceutical liquids in the airspace within the container or may be dissolved in the liquid vehicle. To avoid these exposures, oxygen-sensitive drugs may be prepared in the dry state and packaged in sealed containers with the air replaced by an inert gas such as nitrogen, as may liquid preparations. This is common practice in commercial production of vials and ampuls of easily oxidizable preparations intended for parenteral use.

Trace metals originating in the drug, solvent, container, or stopper are a constant source of difficulty in preparing stable solutions of oxidizable drugs. The rate of formation of color in epinephrine solutions, for instance, is greatly increased by the presence of ferric, ferrous, cupric, and chromic ions. Great care must be taken to eliminate these trace metals from labile preparations by thorough purification of the source of the contaminant or by chemically complexing or binding the metal through the use of specialized agents that make it chemically unavailable for participation in the oxidative process. These chelating agents are exemplified by calcium disodium edetate and ethylenediamine tetra-acetic acid (EDTA).

Light can also act as a catalyst to oxidation reactions, transferring its energy (photons) to drug molecules, making the latter more reactive through increased energy capability. As a precaution against acceleration of oxidation, sensitive preparations are packaged in light-resistant or opaque containers.

Because most drug degradations proceed more rapidly as temperature increases, it is also advisable to maintain oxidizable drugs in a cool place. Another factor that can affect the stability of an oxidizable drug in solution is the pH of the preparation. Each drug must be maintained in solution at the pH most favorable to its stability. This varies from preparation to preparation and must be determined on an individual basis for the drug in question.

Statements in the USP, as with those in Table 4.2, warn of the oxidative decomposition of drugs and preparations. In some instances the specific agent to employ as a stabilizer is mentioned in the monograph, and in others the term "suitable stabilizer" is used. An example in which a particular agent is designated for use is in the monograph for potassium iodide oral solution, USP. Potassium iodide in solution is prone to photocatalyzed oxidation and the release of free iodine, with a resultant yellow to brown discoloration of the solution. The use of light-resistant containers is essential to its stability. As a further precaution against decomposition if the solution is not to be used within a short time, the USP recommends the addition of 0.5 mg of sodium thiosulfate for each gram of potassium iodide. In the event free iodine is released during storage, the sodium thiosulfate converts it to colorless and soluble sodium iodide:

$$I_2 + 2Na_2S_2O_3 \rightarrow 2\,NaI + Na_2S_4O_6$$

In summary, for easily oxidizable drugs, the formulation pharmacist may stabilize the preparation by the selective exclusion from the system of oxygen, oxidizing agents, trace metals, light, heat, and other chemical catalysts to the oxidation process. Antioxidants, chelating agents, and buffering agents may be added to create and maintain a favorable pH.

In addition to oxidation and hydrolysis, destructive processes include polymerization,

TABLE 4.2 SOME USP DRUGS AND PREPARATIONS ESPECIALLY SUBJECT TO CHEMICAL OR PHYSICAL DETERIORATION

PREPARATION	CATEGORY	MONOGRAPH OR LABEL WARNING
Epinephrine bitartrate ophthalmic solution Epinephrine inhalation solution Epinephrine injection Epinephrine nasal solution Epinephrine ophthalmic solution	Adrenergic	Do not use inhalation, injection, nasal, or ophthalmic solution if it is brown or contains a precipitate.
Isoproterenol sulfate inhalation, solution Isoproterenol inhalation solution	Adrenergic (bronchodilator)	Do not use inhalation or injection if it is pink to brown or contains a precipitate.
Nitroglycerin tablets	Antianginal	To prevent loss of potency, keep in original container or supplemental container specifically labeled suitable for nitroglycerin tablets.
Paraldehyde	Hypnotic	Subject to oxidation to form acetic acid.

chemical decarboxylation, and deamination. However, these processes occur less frequently and are peculiar to only small groups of chemical substances. Polymerization is a reaction between two or more identical molecules that forms a new and generally larger molecule. Formaldehyde is an example of a drug capable of polymerization. In solution it may polymerize to paraformaldehyde $(CH_2O)_n$, a slowly soluble white crystalline substance that may cloud the solution. The formation of paraformaldehyde is enhanced by cool storage, especially in solutions with high concentrations of formaldehyde. The official formaldehyde solution contains approximately 37% formaldehyde and according to the USP should be stored at temperatures not below 15°C (59°F). If the solution becomes cloudy upon standing in a cool place, it usually may be cleared by gentle warming. Formaldehyde is prepared by the limited oxidation of methanol (methyl alcohol), and the USP permits a residual amount of this material to remain in the final product, since it can retard the formation of paraformaldehyde. Formaldehyde solution must be maintained in a tight container because oxidation of the formaldehyde yields formic acid.

$$CH_3OH \xrightarrow{(O)} HCHO \xrightarrow{(O)} HCOOH$$
$$\text{methanol} \qquad \text{formaldehyde} \qquad \text{formic acid}$$

Other organic drug molecules may be degraded through processes in which one or more of their active chemical groups are removed. These processes may involve various catalysts, including light and enzymes. Decarboxylation and deamination are examples of such processes; the former is decomposition of an organic acid (R•COOH) and release of carbon dioxide gas, and the latter is removal of the nitrogen-containing group from an organic amine. For example, insulin, a protein, deteriorates rapidly in acid solutions as a result of extensive deamination (3). Thus, most preparations of insulin are neutralized to reduce the rate of decomposition.

Stability Testing

FDA's Current Good Manufacturing Practice regulations include sections on stability and stability testing of pharmaceutical components and finished pharmaceutical products. In addition, FDA and International Conference on Harmonization (ICH) guidelines and guidances provide working recommendations to support the regulatory requirements. Among these are the following (4):

> "Stability Testing of New Drug Substances and Products"
> "Quality of Biotechnological Products: Stability Testing of Biotechnology/Biological Drug Products"
> "Photostability Testing of New Drug Substances and Products"
> "Stability Testing of New Dosage Forms"

Drug and drug product stability testing during every stage of development is critical to the quality of the product. Drug stability is important during preclinical testing and in clinical (human) trials to obtain a true and accurate assessment of the product being evaluated. For a marketed drug product, assurance of stability is vital to its safety and effectiveness during the course of its shelf life and use.

The FDA-required demonstration of drug stability is necessarily different for each stage of drug development, such as for a 2-week preclinical study, an early Phase I study, a limited Phase II trial, a pivotal Phase III clinical study, or for a new drug application. As a drug development program progresses, so do the requisite data to demonstrate and document the product's stability profile. Before approval for marketing, a product's stability must be assessed with regard to its formulation; the influence of its pharmaceutical ingredients; the influence of the container and closure; the manufacturing and processing conditions (e.g., heat); packaging components; conditions of storage; anticipated conditions of shipping, temperature, light, and humidity; and anticipated duration and conditions of pharmacy shelf life and patient use. Holding intermediate product components (such as drug granulations for tablets) for long periods before processing into finished pharmaceutical products can affect the stability of both the intermediate component and the finished product. Therefore, in-process stability testing, including retesting of intermediate components, is important.

Product containers, closures, and other packaging features must be considered in stability testing. For instance, tablets or capsules packaged in glass or plastic bottles require different stability test protocols from those for blister packs or strip packaging. Drugs particularly subject to hydrolysis or oxidative decomposition must be evaluated accordingly. And sterile products must meet sterility test standards to ensure protection against microbial contamination. Any preservatives must be tested for effectiveness in the finished product.

As noted elsewhere in this section, drug products must meet stability standards for long-term storage at room temperature and relative humidity. Products are also subjected to accelerated stability studies as an indication of shelf life stability. It is an FDA requirement that if the data are not submitted in the approved application, the first three postapproval production batches of a drug substance be subjected to long-term stability studies and the first three postapproval production batches of drug product be subjected to both long-term and accelerated stability studies (5, 6).

Drug instability in pharmaceutical formulations may be detected in some instances by a change in the physical appearance, color, odor, taste, or texture of the formulation, whereas in other instances chemical changes may not be self-evident and may be ascertained only through chemical analysis. Scientific data pertaining to the stability of a formulation can lead to prediction of the expected shelf life of the proposed product, and when necessary to redesign of the drug (e.g., into more stable salt or ester form) and to reformulation of the dosage form. Obviously, the rate at which a drug product degrades is of prime importance. The study of the rate of chemical change and the way it is influenced by such factors as the concentration of the drug or reactant, the solvent, temperature and pressure, and other chemical agents in the formulation is reaction kinetics.

In general a kinetic study begins by measuring the concentration of the drug at given intervals under a specific set of conditions including temperature, pH, ionic strength, light intensity, and drug concentration. The measurement of the drug's concentration at the various times reveals the stability or instability of the drug under the specified conditions with the passage of time. From this starting point, each of the original conditions may be varied to determine the influence of such changes on the drug's stability. For example, the pH of the solution may be changed while the temperature, light intensity, and original drug concentration are held constant.

The findings may be presented graphically, by plotting the drug concentration as a function of time. From the experimental data, the reaction rate may be determined and a rate constant and half-life calculated.

The use of exaggerated conditions of temperature, humidity, light, and others to test the stability of drug formulations is termed accelerated stability testing. Accelerated temperature stability studies, for example, may be conducted for 6 months at 40°C with 75% relative humidity. If a significant change in the product occurs under these conditions, lesser temperature and humidity may be used, such as 30°C and 60% relative humidity. Short-term accelerated studies are used to determine the most stable of the proposed formulations for a drug product. In stress testing, temperature elevations, in 10°C increments higher than used in accelerated studies, are employed until chemical or physical degradation. Once the most stable formulation is ascertained, its long-term stability is predicted from the data generated from continuing stability studies. Depending on the types and severity of conditions employed, it is fairly common to maintain samples under exaggerated conditions of both temperature and varying humidity for 6 to 12 months. Such studies lead to the prediction of shelf life for a drug product.

In addition to the accelerated stability studies, drug products are subjected to long-term stability studies under the usual conditions of transport and storage expected during product distribution. In conducting these studies, the different national and international climate zones to which the product may be subjected must be borne in mind and expected variances in conditions of temperature and humidity included in the study design. Geographic regions are defined by zones: zone I, temperate; zone II, subtropical; zone III, hot and dry; and zone IV, hot and humid. A given drug product may encounter more than a single zone of temperature and humidity variations during its production and shelf life. Furthermore, it may be warehoused, transported, placed on a pharmacy's shelf, and subsequently in the patient's medicine cabinet, over a varying time course and at a wide range of temperature and humidity. In general, however, the long-term (12 months minimum) testing of new drug entities is conducted at 25°C ± 2°C and at a relative humidity of 60% ± 5%. Samples maintained under these conditions may be retained for 5 years or longer, during which time they are observed for physical signs of deterioration and chemically assayed. These studies, considered with the accelerated stability studies previously performed, lead to a more precise determination of drug product stability, actual shelf life, and the possible extension of expiration dating.

When chemical degradation products are detected, the FDA requires the manufacturer to report their chemical identity, including structure, mechanism of formation, physical and chemical properties, procedures for isolation and purification, specifications and directions for determination at levels expected to be present in the pharmaceutical product, and their pharmacologic action and biologic significance, if any.

In addition, signs of degradation of the specific dosage forms must be observed and reported. For the various dosage forms, this includes the following (1):

Tablets: Appearance (cracking, chipping, mottling), friability, hardness, color, odor, moisture content, clumping, disintegration, and dissolution.

Capsules: Moisture tackiness, color, appearance, shape, brittleness, and dissolution.

Oral solutions and suspensions: Appearance, precipitation, pH, color, odor, redispersibility (suspensions), and clarity (solutions).

Oral powders: Appearance, color, odor, moisture.

Metered-dose inhalation aerosols: Delivered dose per actuation, number of metered doses, color, particle size distribution, loss of propellant, pressure, valve corrosion, spray pattern, absence of pathogenic microorganisms.

Topical nonmetered aerosols: Appearance, odor, pressure, weight loss, net weight dispensed, delivery rate, and spray pattern.

Topical creams, ointments, lotions, solutions, and gels: Appearance, color, homogeneity, odor, pH, resuspendibility (lotions), consistency, particle-size distribution, strength, weight loss.

Ophthalmic and nasal and oral inhalation preparations: Appearance, color, consistency, pH, clarity (solutions), particle size and resuspendibility (suspensions, ointments), strength, and sterility.

Small-volume parenterals: Appearance, color, particulate matter, dispersibility (suspensions), pH, sterility, pyrogenicity, and closure integrity.

Large-volume parenterals: Appearance, color, clarity, particulate matter, pH, volume and extractables (when plastic containers are used), sterility, pyrogenicity, and closure integrity.

Suppositories: Softening range, appearance, and melting.

Emulsions: Appearance (such as phase separation), color, odor, pH, and viscosity.

Controlled-release membrane drug delivery systems: Seal strength of the drug reservoir, decomposition products, membrane integrity, drug strength, and drug release rate.

Under usual circumstances, most manufactured products must have a shelf life of 2 or more years to ensure stability at the time of consumption. Commercial products must bear an appropriate expiration date that sets out the time during which the product may be expected to maintain its potency and remain stable under the designated storage conditions. The expiration date limits the time during which the product may be dispensed by the pharmacist or used by the patient.

Prescriptions requiring extemporaneous compounding by the pharmacist do not require the extended shelf life that commercially manufactured and distributed products do because they are intended to be used immediately on receipt by the patient and used only during the immediate course of the prescribed treatment. However, these compounded prescriptions must remain stable and efficacious during the course of use, and the compounding pharmacist must employ formulative components and techniques that will result in a stable product (7).

In years past pharmacists were confronted primarily with innocuous topical prescriptions that required extemporaneous formulation. However, in recent years there has been a need to compound other drug delivery systems, for example progesterone vaginal suppositories and oral suspensions, from tablets or capsules. When presented with a prescription that requires extemporaneous compounding, the pharmacist is confronted with a difficult situation, because the potency and stability of these prescriptions is a serious matter. Occasionally, the results of compatibility and stability studies on such prescriptions are published in scientific and professional journals. These are very useful; however, for some prescriptions stability and compatibility information is not readily available. In these instances, it behooves the pharmacist to contact the manufacturer of the active ingredient or ingredients to solicit stability information. Also, a compilation of published stability information is included in *Trissel's Stability of Compounded Formulations* (8). The published stability data are applicable only to products that are prepared identically to the products that are reported.

USP guidelines on stability of extemporaneous compounded formulations state that in the absence of stability information applicable to a specific drug and preparation, the following guidelines can be used: nonaqueous liquids and solid formulations in which the manufactured drug is the source of the active ingredient, not later than 25% of the time remaining until the product's expiration date or 6 months, whichever is earlier; nonaqueous liq-

uids and solid formulations in which a USP or NF substance is the source of active ingredient, a beyond-use date of 6 months; for water-containing formulations prepared from ingredients in solid form, a beyond-use date not later than 14 days in storage at cold temperatures; for all other formulations, a beyond-use date of the intended duration of therapy or 30 days, whichever is earlier (9). Thus, if an oral aqueous liquid preparation is made from a tablet or capsule formulation, the pharmacist should make up only at most 14 days' supply, and it must be stored in a refrigerator. Furthermore, the pharmacist must dispense the medication in a container conducive to stability and use and must advise the patient of the proper method of use and conditions of storage of the medication.

Finally, when compounding on the basis of extrapolated or less than concrete information, the pharmacist is well advised to keep the formulation simple and not to shortcut but use the necessary pharmaceutical adjuvants to prepare the prescription.

Pharmaceutical Ingredients and Excipients

Definitions and Types

To produce a drug substance in a final dosage form requires pharmaceutical ingredients. For example, in the preparation of solutions, one or more *solvents* are used to dissolve the drug substance, *flavors* and *sweeteners* are used to make the product more palatable, *colorants* are added to enhance appeal, *preservatives* may be added to prevent microbial growth, and *stabilizers*, such as antioxidants and chelating agents, may be used to prevent decomposition, as previously discussed. In the preparation of tablets, *diluents* or *fillers* are commonly added to increase the bulk of the formulation, *binders* to cause adhesion of the powdered drug and pharmaceutical substances, *antiadherents* or *lubricants* to assist smooth tablet formation, *disintegrating agents* to promote tablet breakup after administration, and coatings to improve stability, control disintegration, or enhance appearance. Ointments, creams, and suppositories acquire their characteristic features from their pharmaceutical bases. Thus, for each dosage form, the pharmaceutical ingredients establish the primary features of the product and contribute to the physical form, texture, stability, taste, and overall appearance.

Table 4.3 presents the principal categories of pharmaceutical ingredients, listing some of the official and commercial agents in use. Additional discussion of many ingredients may be found in the chapters where they are most relevant; for example, pharmaceutical materials used in tablet and capsule formulations are discussed in Chapters 7 and 8 and those used in modified-release solid oral dosage forms and drug delivery systems in Chapter 9.

Handbook of Pharmaceutical Excipients

The *Handbook of Pharmaceutical Excipients* (10) presents monographs on more than 250 excipients used in dosage form preparation. Each monograph includes such information as nonproprietary, chemical, and commercial names; empirical and chemical formulas and molecular weight; pharmaceutical specifications and chemical and physical properties; incompatibilities and interactions with other excipients and drug substances; regulatory status; and applications in pharmaceutical formulation or technology.

Harmonization of Standards

There is great interest in the international harmonization of standards applicable to pharmaceutical excipients. This is because the pharmaceutical industry is multinational, with major companies having facilities in more than a single country, with products sold in markets worldwide, and with regulatory approval for these products required in each country. Standards for each drug substance and excipient used in pharmaceuticals are contained in pharmacopeias—or for new agents, in an application for regulatory approval by the relevant governing authority. The four pharmacopeias with the largest international use are the *United States Pharmacopeia–National Formulary* (USP–NF), *British Pharmacopeia* (BP), *European Pharma-*

copeia (EP), and *Japanese Pharmacopeia* (JP). Uniform standards for excipients in these and other pharmacopeias would facilitate production efficiency, enable the marketing of a single formulation of a product internationally, and enhance regulatory approval of pharmaceutical products worldwide. The goal of harmonization is an ongoing effort by corporate representatives and international regulatory authorities.

A few of the more common and widely used pharmaceutical excipients, including sweeteners, flavors, colors, and preservatives, are discussed here.

Appearance and Palatability

Although most drug substances in use today are unpalatable and unattractive in their natural state, their preparations present them to the patient as colorful, flavorful formulations attractive to the sight, smell, and taste. These qualities, which are the rule rather than the exception, have virtually eliminated the natural reluctance of many patients to take medications because of disagreeable odor or taste. In fact, the inherent attractiveness of today's pharmaceuticals has caused them to acquire the dubious distinction of being a source of accidental poisonings in the home, particularly among children who are lured by their organoleptic appeal.

There is some psychologic basis to drug therapy, and the odor, taste, and color of a pharmaceutical preparation can play a part. An appropriate drug has its most beneficial effect when it is accepted and taken properly by the patient. The proper combination of flavor, fragrance, and color in a pharmaceutical product contributes to its acceptance.

Flavoring Pharmaceuticals

The flavoring of pharmaceuticals applies primarily to liquids intended for oral administration. The 10,000 taste buds on the tongue, roof of the mouth, cheeks, and throat have 60 to 100 receptor cells each (11). These receptor cells interact with molecules dissolved in the saliva and produce a positive or negative taste sensation. Medication in liquid form comes into immediate and direct contact with these

TABLE 4.3 EXAMPLES OF PHARMACEUTICAL INGREDIENTS

INGREDIENT TYPE	DEFINITION	EXAMPLES
Acidifying agent	Used in liquid preparations to provide acidic medium for product stability.	Citric acid Acetic acid Fumaric acid Hydrochloric acid Nitric acid
Alkalinizing agent	Used in liquid preparations to provide alkaline medium for product stability.	Ammonia solution Ammonium carbonate Diethanolamine Monoethanolamine Potassium hydroxide Sodium bicarbonate Sodium borate Sodium carbonate Sodium hydroxide Trolamine
Adsorbent	An agent capable of holding other molecules onto its surface by physical or chemical (chemisorption) means.	Powdered cellulose Activated charcoal
Aerosol propellant	Agent responsible for developing the pressure within an aerosol container and expelling the product when the valve is opened.	Carbon dioxide Dichlorodifluoromethane Dichlorotetrafluoroethane Trichloromonofluoromethane
Air displacement	Agent employed to displace air in a hermetically sealed container to enhance product stability.	Nitrogen Carbon dioxide
Antifungal preservative	Used in liquid and semisolid preparations to prevent growth of fungi. Effectiveness of parabens is usually enhanced by use in combination.	Butylparaben Ethylparaben Methylparaben Benzoic acid Propylparaben Sodium benzoate Sodium propionate
Antimicrobial preservative	Used in liquid and semisolid preparations to prevent growth of microorganisms.	Benzalkonium chloride Benzethonium chloride Benzyl alcohol Cetylpyridinium chloride Chlorobutanol Phenol Phenylethyl alcohol Phenylmercuric nitrate Thimerosal
Antioxidant	Used to prevent deterioration of preparations by oxidation.	Ascorbic acid Ascorbyl palmitate Butylated hydroxyanisole Butylated hydroxytoluene Hypophosphorous acid Monothioglycerol Propyl gallate Sodium ascorbate Sodium bisulfite Sodium formaldehyde Sulfoxylate Sodium metabisulfite

(continued)

TABLE 4.3 EXAMPLES OF PHARMACEUTICAL INGREDIENTS

INGREDIENT TYPE	DEFINITION	EXAMPLES
Buffering agent	Used to resist change in pH upon dilution or addition of acid or alkali.	Potassium metaphosphate Potassium phosphate, monobasic Sodium acetate Sodium citrate, anhydrous and dihydrate
Chelating agent	Substance that forms stable water-soluble complexes (chelates) with metals; used in some liquid pharmaceuticals as stabilizers to complex heavy metals that might promote instability. In such use they are also called *sequestering* agents.	Edetic acid Edetate disodium
Colorant	Used to impart color to liquid and solid (e.g., tablets and capsules) preparations.	FD&C Red No. 3 FD&C Red No. 20 FD&C Yellow No. 6 FD&C Blue No. 2 D&C Green No. 5 D&C Orange No. 5 D&C Red No. 8 Caramel Ferric oxide, red
Clarifying agent	Used as a filtering aid for its adsorbent qualities.	Bentonite
Emulsifying agent	Used to promote and maintain dispersion of finely subdivided particles of liquid in a vehicle in which it is immiscible. End product may be a liquid emulsion or semisolid emulsion (e.g., a cream).	Acacia Cetomacrogol Cetyl alcohol Glyceryl monostearate Sorbitan monooleate Polyoxyethylene 50 stearate
Encapsulating agent	Used to form thin shells to enclose a drug for ease of administration.	Gelatin Cellulose acetate phthalate
Flavorant	Used to impart a pleasant flavor and often odor to a preparation. In addition to the natural flavorants listed, many synthetic ones are used.	Anise oil Cinnamon oil Cocoa Menthol Orange oil Peppermint oil Vanillin
Humectant	Used to prevent drying of preparations, particularly ointments and creams.	Glycerin Propylene glycol Sorbitol
Levigating agent	Liquid used as an intervening agent to reduce the particle size of a powder by grinding, usually in a mortar.	Mineral oil Glycerin Propylene glycol
Ointment base	Semisolid vehicle for medicated ointments.	Lanolin Hydrophilic ointment Polyethylene glycol ointment Petrolatum Hydrophilic petrolatum White ointment Yellow ointment Rose water ointment

(continued)

TABLE 4.3 EXAMPLES OF PHARMACEUTICAL INGREDIENTS

INGREDIENT TYPE	DEFINITION	EXAMPLES
Plasticizer	Component of film-coating solutions to make film more pliable, enhance spread of coat over tablets, beads, and granules.	Diethyl phthalate Glycerin
Solvent	Used to dissolve another substance in preparation of a solution; may be aqueous or not (e.g., oleaginous). Cosolvents, such as water and alcohol (hydroalcoholic) and water and glycerin, may be used when needed. Sterile solvents are used in certain preparations (e.g., injections).	Alcohol Corn oil Cottonseed oil Glycerin Isopropyl alcohol Mineral oil Oleic acid Peanut oil Purified water Water for injection Sterile water for injection Sterile water for irrigation
Stiffening agent	Used to increase thickness or hardness of a preparation, usually an ointment.	Cetyl alcohol Cetyl esters wax Microcrystalline wax Paraffin Stearyl alcohol White wax Yellow wax
Suppository base	Vehicle for suppositories.	Cocoa butter Polyethylene glycols (mixtures)
Surfactant (surface active agent)	Substances that absorb to surfaces or interfaces to reduce surface or interfacial tension. May be used as wetting agents, detergents, or emulsifying agents.	Benzalkonium chloride Nonoxynol 10 Octoxynol 9 Polysorbate 80 Sodium lauryl sulfate Sorbitan monopalmitate
Suspending agent	Viscosity-increasing agent used to reduce sedimentation rate of particles in a vehicle in which they are not soluble; suspension may be formulated for oral, parenteral, ophthalmic, topical, or other route.	Agar Bentonite Carbomer (e.g., Carbopol) Carboxymethylcellulose sodium Hydroxyethyl cellulose Hydroxypropyl cellulose Hydroxypropyl methylcellulose Kaolin Methylcellulose Tragacanth Veegum
Sweetening agent	Used to impart sweetness to a preparation.	Aspartame Dextrose Glycerin Mannitol Saccharin sodium Sorbitol Sucrose
Tablet antiadherents	Prevent tablet ingredients from sticking to punches and dies during production.	Magnesium stearate Talc

(continued)

TABLE 4.3 EXAMPLES OF PHARMACEUTICAL INGREDIENTS

INGREDIENT TYPE	DEFINITION	EXAMPLES
Tablet binders	Substances used to cause adhesion of powder particles in tablet granulations.	Acacia Alginic acid Carboxymethylcellulose sodium Compressible sugar (e.g., Nu-Tab) Ethylcellulose Gelatin Liquid glucose Methylcellulose Povidone Pregelatinized starch
Tablet and capsule diluent	Inert filler to create desired bulk, flow properties, and compression characteristics of tablets and capsules.	Dibasic calcium phosphate Kaolin Lactose Mannitol Microcrystalline cellulose Powdered cellulose Precipitated calcium carbonate Sorbitol Starch
Tablet coating agent	Used to coat a tablet to protect against decomposition by atmospheric oxygen or humidity, to provide a desired release pattern, to mask taste or odor, or for aesthetic purposes. Coating may be sugar, film, or enteric. Sugar coating is water-based; forms a thick covering around a tablet. Sugar-coated tablets generally start to break up in the stomach. Film forms a thin cover around a formed tablet or bead. Unless it is enteric, film dissolves in the stomach. Enteric coating passes through the stomach to break up in the intestines. Some water-insoluble coatings (e.g., ethylcellulose) are used to slow the release of drug in the gastrointestinal tract.	
Sugar coating		Liquid glucose Sucrose
Film coating		Hydroxyethyl cellulose Hydroxypropyl cellulose Hydroxypropyl methylcellulose Methylcellulose (e.g., Methocel) Ethylcellulose (e.g., Ethocel)
Enteric coating		Cellulose acetate phthalate Shellac (35% in alcohol, pharmaceutical glaze)
Tablet direct compression excipient	Used in direct compression tablet formulations.	Dibasic calcium phosphate (e.g., Ditab)
Tablet disintegrant	Used in solid forms to promote disruption of the mass into smaller particles more readily dispersed or dissolved.	Alginic acid Carboxymethylcellulose calcium Microcrystalline cellulose (e.g., Avicel) Polacrilin potassium (e.g., Amberlite)

(continued)

TABLE 4.3 EXAMPLES OF PHARMACEUTICAL INGREDIENTS

INGREDIENT TYPE	DEFINITION	EXAMPLES
		Sodium alginate
		Sodium starch glycolate
		Starch
Tablet glidant	Used in tablet and capsule formulations to improve flow properties of the powder mixture.	Colloidal silica
		Cornstarch
		Talc
Tablet lubricant	Used in tablet formulations to reduce friction during tablet compression.	Calcium stearate
		Magnesium stearate
		Mineral oil
		Stearic acid
		Zinc stearate
Tablet or capsule opaquant	Used to render a coating opaque. May be used alone or with a colorant.	Titanium dioxide
Tablet polishing agent	Used to impart an attractive sheen to coated tablets.	Carnauba wax
		White wax
Tonicity agent	Used to render solution similar in osmotic dextrose characteristics to physiologic fluids, e.g., in ophthalmic, parenteral, and irrigation fluids.	Sodium chloride
Vehicle	Carrying agent used in formulating a variety of liquids for oral and parenteral administration. Generally, oral liquids are aqueous (e.g., syrups) or hydroalcoholic (e.g., elixirs). Solutions for intravenous use are aqueous, whereas intramuscular injections may be aqueous or oleaginous.	
Flavored, sweetened		Acacia syrup
		Aromatic syrup
		Aromatic elixir
		Cherry syrup
		Cocoa syrup
		Orange syrup
		Syrup
Oleaginous		Corn oil
		Mineral oil
		Peanut oil
		Sesame oil
Sterile		Bacteriostatic sodium chloride injection
		Bacteriostatic water for injection
Viscosity-increasing agent	Used to render preparations more resistant to flow. Used in suspensions to deter sedimentation, in ophthalmic solutions to enhance contact time (e.g., methylcellulose), to thicken topical creams, etc.	Alginic acid
		Bentonite
		Carbomer
		Carboxymethylcellulose
		Sodium
		Methylcellulose
		Povidone
		Sodium alginate
		Tragacanth

taste buds. The addition of flavoring agents to liquid medication can mask the disagreeable taste. Drugs placed in capsules or prepared as coated tablets may be easily swallowed with no contact between the drug and the taste buds. Tablets containing drugs that are not especially distasteful may remain uncoated and unflavored. Swallowing them with water usually is sufficient to avoid undesirable taste sensations. However, chewable tablets, such as certain antacid and vitamin products, usually are sweetened and flavored to improve acceptance.

The flavor sensation of a food or pharmaceutical is actually a complex blend of taste and smell, with lesser influences of texture, temperature, and even sight. In flavor-formulating a pharmaceutical product, the pharmacist must give consideration to the color, odor, texture, and taste of the preparation. It would be incongruous, for example, to color a liquid pharmaceutical red and give it a banana taste and a mint odor. The color of a pharmaceutical must have a psychogenic balance with the taste, and the odor must also enhance that taste. Odor greatly affects the flavor of a preparation or foodstuff. If one's sense of smell is impaired, as during a head cold, the usual flavor sensation of food is similarly diminished.

The medicinal chemist and the formulation pharmacist are well acquainted with the taste characteristics of certain chemical types of drugs and strive to mask the unwanted taste through the appropriate use of flavoring agents. Although there are no rules for unerringly predicting the taste sensation of a drug based on its chemical constitution, experience permits the presentation of several observations. For instance, although we recognize and assume the salty taste of sodium chloride, the formulation pharmacist knows that not all salts are salty but that their taste is a function of both cation and anion. Whereas salty tastes are evoked by chlorides of sodium, potassium, and ammonium and by sodium bromide, bromides of potassium and ammonium elicit bitter and salty sensations, and potassium iodide and magnesium sulfate (epsom salt) are predominantly bitter. In general, low-molecular-weight salts are salty, and high-molecular-weight salts are bitter.

With organic compounds, an increase in the number of hydroxyl groups (—OH) seems to increase the sweetness of the compound. Sucrose, which has eight hydroxyl groups, is sweeter than glycerin, another pharmaceutical sweetener, which has but three hydroxyl groups. In general, the organic esters, alcohols, and aldehydes are pleasant to the taste, and since many of them are volatile, they also contribute to the odor and thus the flavor of preparations in which they are used. Many nitrogen-containing compounds, especially the plant alkaloids (e.g., quinine) are extremely bitter, but certain other nitrogen-containing compounds (e.g., aspartame) are extremely sweet. The medicinal chemist recognizes that even the most simple structural change in an organic compound can alter its taste. D-Glucose is sweet, but L-glucose has a slightly salty taste; saccharin is very sweet, but N-methyl-saccharin is tasteless (12).

Thus, prediction of the taste characteristics of a new drug is only speculative. However, it is soon learned, and the formulation pharmacist is then put to the task of increasing the drug's palatability in the environment of other formulative agents. The selection of an appropriate flavoring agent depends on several factors, primarily the taste of the drug substance itself. Certain flavoring materials are more effective than others in masking or disguising the particular bitter, salty, sour, or otherwise undesirable taste of medicinal agents. Although individuals' tastes and flavor preferences differ, cocoa-flavored vehicles are considered effective for masking the taste of bitter drugs. Fruit or citrus flavors are frequently used to combat sour or acid-tasting drugs, and cinnamon, orange, raspberry, and other flavors have been successfully used to make preparations of salty drugs more palatable.

The age of the intended patient should also be considered in the selection of the flavoring agent, because certain age groups seem to prefer certain flavors. Children prefer sweet candylike preparations with fruity flavors, but adults seem to prefer less sweet preparations with a tart rather than a fruit flavor.

Flavors can consist of oil- or water-soluble liquids and dry powders; most are diluted in carriers. Oil-soluble carriers include soybean and other edible oils; water-soluble carriers include water, ethanol, propylene glycol, glycerin, and emulsifiers. Dry carriers include maltodextrins, corn syrup solids, modified starches, gum arabic, salt, sugars, and whey protein. Flavors can degrade as a result of exposure to light, temperature, head space oxygen, water, enzymes, contaminants and other product components, so they must be carefully selected and checked for stability.

The different types of flavors include natural, artificial, and spice:

Natural flavor: Essential oil, oleoresin, essence or extractive, protein hydrolysate, distillate, or any product of roasting, heating or enzymolysis, which contains the flavoring constituents derived from a spice, fruit or fruit juice, vegetable or vegetable juice, edible yeast, herb, bark, bud, root, leaf or similar plant material, meat, seafood, poultry, eggs, dairy products, or fermentation products thereof whose significant function in food is flavoring rather than nutritional. [CFR 101.22(a)(3)] In "all natural" flavors, one doesn't necessarily know the exact chemical composition.

Artificial flavor: Any substance used to impart flavor that is not derived from a spice, fruit or fruit juice, vegetable or vegetable juice, edible yeast, herb, bark, bud, root, leaf or similar plant material, meat, fish, poultry, eggs, dairy products, or fermentation products thereof. [CFR 101.22(a)(1)]

Spice: Any aromatic vegetable substance in whole, broken, or ground form, except substances traditionally regarded as foods, such as onions, garlic, and celery; whose significant function in food is seasoning rather than nutritional; that is true to name; and from which no portion of any volatile oil or other flavoring principle has been removed. [CFR 101.22(a)(2)]

In addition to the types of flavors, you should be aware of commercial flavor designa-tions, including the following (*Note*: ABCD would be the flavor name, e.g., cherry):

Natural ABCD flavor	All components derived from ABCD.
ABCD flavor, natural and artificial	At least one component derived from ABCD. No definition of natural to artificial ratio.
ABCD flavor, WONF[a]	All components natural. At least one component derived from ABCD.
Natural flavor, ABCD type	All components natural. No components derived from ABCD.
ABCD flavor, artificial	All components are artificial.
Conceptual flavors	May contain artificial flavors. No reference point. May only have to declare in ingredient declaration.

[a]WONF, with other natural flavors.

A general guide to using flavors is to start as follows (keep in mind it is usually possible to add more flavor, but once it is added, it's too late to remove it).

Water-soluble flavors	Generally start at 0.2% for artificial and 1–2% for natural flavors.
Oil-soluble flavors	Generally start at 0.1% in finished product for artificial flavors and 0.2% for natural flavors.
Powdered flavors	Generally start at 0.1% in finished product for artificial flavors and 0.75% for natural flavors.

Sweetening Pharmaceuticals

In addition to sucrose, a number of artificial sweetening agents have been used in foods and pharmaceuticals over the years. Some of these, including aspartame, saccharin, and cyclamate, have faced challenges over their safety by the FDA and restrictions to their use and sale; in fact, in 1969 FDA banned the cyclamates from use in the United States.

The introduction of diet soft drinks in the 1950s provided the spark for the widespread use of artificial sweeteners today. Besides dieters, diabetics are regular users of artificial sweeteners. Over the years, each of the artificial sweeteners has undergone long periods of review and debate. Critical to the evaluation of food additives are issues of metabolism and toxicity. For example, almost none of the saccharin a person consumes is metabolized; it is excreted by the kidneys virtually unchanged. Cyclamate, on the other hand, is metabolized, or processed, in the digestive tract, and its byproducts are excreted by the kidneys. Aspartame breaks down in the body into three basic components: the amino acids phenylalanine and aspartic acid, and methanol. These three components, which also occur naturally in various foods, are in turn metabolized through regular pathways in the body. Because of its metabolism to phenylalanine, the use of aspartame by persons with phenylketonuria (PKU) is discouraged, and diet foods and drinks must bear an appropriate label warning indicating that the particular foodstuff not be consumed by such individuals. They cannot metabolize phenylalanine adequately, so they undergo an increase in the serum levels of the amino acid (hyperphenylalaninemia). This can result in mental retardation and can affect the fetus of a pregnant woman who has PKU.

Passage in 1958 of the Food Additives Amendment to the Food, Drug, and Cosmetic Act produced a major change in how the federal government regulates food additives. For one thing, no new food additive may be used if animal feeding studies or other appropriate tests showed that it caused cancer. This is the famous Delaney Clause. The *amount* of the substance one would have to consume to induce cancer is not significant under the Delaney Clause.

Another critical feature of the 1958 amendment was that it did not apply to additives that were generally recognized by experts as safe for their intended uses. Saccharin, cyclamate, and a long list of other substances were being used in foods before the amendment's passage and were "generally recognized as safe"—or what is known today as GRAS. Aspartame, on the other hand, was the first artificial sweetener to fall under the 1958 amendment's requirement for premarketing proof of safety, because the first petition to FDA for its approval was filed in 1973. In 1968, the Committee on Food Protection of the National Academy of Sciences issued an interim report on the safety of nonnutritive sweeteners, including saccharin. In the early 1970s, FDA began a major review of hundreds of food additives on the GRAS list to determine whether current studies justified their safe status. In 1972, with new studies under way, FDA decided to take saccharin off the GRAS and establish interim limits that would permit its continued use until additional studies were completed. (Previous studies indicated that male and female rats fed doses of saccharin developed a significant incidence of bladder tumors.) In November 1977, Congress passed the Saccharin Study and Labeling Act, which permitted saccharin's continued availability while mandating that warning labels be used to advise consumers that saccharin caused cancer in animals. The law also directed FDA to arrange further studies of carcinogens and toxic substances in foods.

Cyclamate was introduced into beverages and foods in the 1950s and dominated the artificial sweetener market in the 1960s. After much controversy regarding its safety, the FDA issued a final ruling in 1980 stating that safety has not been demonstrated. Since that date, scientific studies have continued the search for conclusive support or rejection of the FDA decision. At question is cyclamate's possible carcinogenicity and its possible causation of genetic damage and testicular atrophy. See the indicated references for a review of the recent history of sweeteners, including saccharin, cyclamate, fructose, polyalcohols, sucrose, and aspartame (13–16).

Acesulfame potassium, a nonnutritive sweetener discovered in 1967, was approved in 1992 by the FDA. It previously was used in a number of other countries. Structurally similar to saccharin, it is 130 times as sweet as sucrose and is excreted unchanged in the urine. Acesulfame is more stable than aspartame at elevated temperatures and FDA initially approved it for use in candy, chewing gum, confectionery, and instant coffees and teas.

A relatively new sweetening agent in U.S. commerce is Stevia powder, the extract from the leaves of the plant *Stevia rebaudiana bertoni*. It is natural, nontoxic, safe, and about 30 times as sweet as cane sugar, or sucrose. It can be used in both hot and cold preparations. Table 4.4 compares three of the most commonly used sweeteners in the food and drug industry.

Most large pharmaceutical manufacturers have special laboratories for taste-testing proposed formulations of their products. Panels of employees or interested community participants participate in evaluating the various formulations, and their assessments become the basis for the firm's flavoring decisions.

The flavoring agent in liquid pharmaceutical products is added to the solvent or vehicle component of the formulation in which it is most soluble or miscible. That is, water-soluble flavorants are added to the aqueous component of a formulation and poorly water-soluble flavorants are added to the alcoholic or other nonaqueous solvent component of the formulation. In a hydroalcoholic or other multisolvent system, care must be exercised to maintain the flavorant in solution. This is accomplished by maintaining a sufficient level of the flavorant's solvent.

Coloring Pharmaceuticals

Coloring agents are used in pharmaceutical preparations for esthetics. A distinction should be made between agents that have inherent color and those that are employed as colorants. Certain agents—sulfur (yellow), riboflavin (yellow), cupric sulfate (blue), ferrous sulfate (bluish green), cyanocobalamin (red), and red mercuric iodide (vivid red)—have inherent color and are not thought of as pharmaceutical colorants in the usual sense of the term.

Although most pharmaceutical colorants in use today are synthetic, a few are obtained from natural mineral and plant sources. For example, red ferric oxide is mixed in small proportions with zinc oxide powder to give calamine its characteristic pink color, which is intended to match the skin tone upon application.

The synthetic coloring agents used in pharmaceutical products were first prepared in the middle of the 19th century from principles of coal tar. Coal tar (*pix carbonis*), a thick, black viscid liquid, is a byproduct of the destructive distillation of coal. Its composition is extremely complex, and many of its constituents may be separated by fractional distillation. Among its products are anthracene, benzene, naphtha, creosote, phenol, and pitch. About 90% of the dyes used in the products FDA regulates are synthesized from a single colorless derivative of benzene called aniline. These aniline dyes are also known as synthetic organic dyes or as coal tar dyes, since aniline was originally obtained from bituminous coal. Aniline dyes today come mainly from petroleum.

Many coal tar dyes were originally used indiscriminately in foods and beverages to en-

TABLE 4.4 COMPARISON OF SWEETENERS

	SUCROSE	SACCHARIN	ASPARTAME
Source	Sugar cane; sugar beet	Chemical synthesis; phthalic anhydride, a petroleum product	Chemical synthesis; methyl ester dipeptide of phenylalanine and aspartic acid
Relative sweetness	1	300	180–200
Bitterness	None	Moderate to strong	None
Aftertaste	None	Moderate to strong; sometimes metallic or bitter	None
Calories	4/g	0	4/g
Acid stability	Good	Excellent	Fair
Heat stability	Good	Excellent	Poor

hance their appeal without regard to their toxic potential. It was only after careful scrutiny that some dyes were found to be hazardous to health because of either their own chemical nature or the impurities they carried. As more dyestuffs became available, some expert guidance and regulation were needed to ensure the safety of the public. After passage of the Food and Drug Act in 1906, the U.S. Department of Agriculture established regulations by which a few colorants were *permitted* or *certified* for use in certain products. Today, the FDA regulates the use of color additives in foods, drugs, and cosmetics through the provisions of the Federal Food, Drug, and Cosmetic Act of 1938, as amended in 1960 with the Color Additive Amendments. Lists of color additives *exempt* from certification and those *subject* to certification are codified into law and regulated by the FDA (17). Certified color additives are classified according to their approved use: (*a*) FD&C color additives, which may be used in foods, drugs, and cosmetics; (*b*) D&C color additives, some of which are approved for use in drugs, some in cosmetics, and some in medical devices; and (*c*) external D&C color additives, the use of which is restricted to external parts of the body, not including the lips or any other body surface covered by mucous membrane. Each certification category has a variety of basic colors and shades for coloring pharmaceuticals. One may select from a variety of FD&C, D&C, and external D&C reds, yellows, oranges, greens, blues, and violets. By selective combinations of the colorants one can create distinctive colors (Table 4.5).

As a part of the National Toxicology Program of the U.S. Department of Health and Human Services, various substances, including color additives, are studied for toxicity and carcinogenesis. For color additives, the study protocols usually call for a 2-year study in which groups of male and female mice and rats are fed diets containing various quantities of the colorant. The killed and surviving animals are examined for evidence of long-term toxicity and carcinogenesis. Five categories of evidence of carcinogenic activity are used in reporting observations: (*a*) "clear evidence" of carcinogenic activity; (*b*) "some evidence"; (*c*) "equivocal

TABLE 4.5 EXAMPLES OF COLOR FORMULATIONS

SHADE OR COLOR	FD&C DYE	% OF BLEND
Orange	Yellow #6	100
	or	
	Yellow #5	95
	Red #40	5
Cherry	Red #40	100
	or	
	Red #40	99
	Blue #1	1
Strawberry	Red #40	100
	Or	
	Red #40	95
	Red #3	5
Lemon	Yellow #5	100
Lime	Yellow #5	95
	Blue #1	5
Grape	Red #40	80
	Blue #1	20
Raspberry	Red #3	75
	Yellow #6	20
	Blue #1	5
Butterscotch	Yellow #5	74
	Red #40	24
	Blue #1	2
Chocolate	Red #40	52
	Yellow #5	40
	Blue #1	8
Caramel	Yellow #5	64
	Red #3	21
	Yellow #6	9
	Blue #1	6
Cinnamon	Yellow #5	60
	Red #40	35
	Blue #1	5

From literature of Warner-Jenkinson Co., St. Louis, Mo.

evidence," indicating uncertainty; (*d*) "no evidence," indicating no observable effect; and (*e*) "inadequate study," for studies that cannot be evaluated because of major flaws.

The certification status of the colorants is continually reviewed, and changes are made in the list of certified colors in accordance with toxicology findings. These changes may be (*a*) the withdrawal of certification, (*b*) the transfer of a colorant from one certification category to another, or (*c*) the addition of new colors to the list. Before gaining certification, a color additive must be demonstrated to be safe. In the case of pharmaceutical preparations, color additives, as with all additives, must not interfere with therapeutic efficacy, nor may they interfere with the prescribed assay procedure for the preparation.

In the 1970s, concern and scientific questioning of the safety of some color additives heightened. A color that drew particular attention was FD&C Red No. 2, because of its extensive use in foods, drugs, and cosmetics. Researchers in Russia reported that this color, also known as amaranth, caused cancer in rats. Although the FDA was never able to determine the purity of the amaranth tested in Russia, these reports led to FDA investigations and a series of tests that eventually resulted in withdrawal of FD&C Red No. 2 from the FDA certified list in 1976 because its sponsors were unable to prove safety. That year, FDA also terminated approval for use of FD&C Red No. 4 in maraschino cherries and ingested drugs because of unresolved safety questions. FD&C Red No. 4 is now permitted only in externally applied drugs and cosmetics.

FD&C Yellow No. 5 (also known as tartrazine) causes allergic-type reactions in many people. People who are allergic to aspirin are also likely to be allergic to this dye. As a result, the FDA requires listing of this dye by name on the labels of foods (e.g., butter, cheese, ice cream) and ingested drugs containing it.

A colorant becomes an integral part of a pharmaceutical formulation, and its exact quantitative amount must be reproducible each time the formulation is prepared, or else the preparation would have a different appearance from batch to batch. This requires a high degree of skill, for the amount of colorant generally added to liquid preparations ranges from 0.0005 to 0.001% depending upon the colorant and the depth of color desired. Because of their color potency, dyes generally are added to pharmaceutical preparations in the form of diluted solutions rather than as concentrated dry powders. This permits greater accuracy in measurement and more consistent color production.

In addition to liquid dyes in the coloring of pharmaceuticals, lake pigments may also be used. Whereas a chemical material exhibits coloring power or tinctorial strength when dissolved, pigment is an insoluble material that colors by dispersion. An FD&C lake is a pigment consisting of a substratum of alumina hydrate on which the dye is adsorbed or precipitated. Having aluminum hydroxide as the substrate, the lakes are insoluble in nearly all solvents. FD&C lakes are subject to certification and must be made from certified dyes. Lakes do not have a specified dye content; they range from 10 to 40% pure dye. By their nature, lakes are suitable for coloring products in which the moisture levels are low.

Lakes in pharmaceuticals are commonly used in the form of fine dispersions or suspensions. The pigment particles may range in size from less than 1 μm up to 30 μm. The finer the particle, the less chance for color speckling in the finished product. Blends of various lake pigments may be used to achieve a variety of colors, and various vehicles, such as glycerin, propylene glycol, and sucrose-based syrup, may be employed to disperse the colorants.

Colored empty gelatin capsule shells may be used to hold a powdered drug mixture. Many commercial capsules are prepared with a capsule body of one color and a cap of a different color, resulting in a two-colored capsule. This makes certain commercial products more readily identifiable than solid-colored capsules. For powdered drugs dispensed as such or compressed into tablets, a generally larger proportion of dye is required (about 0.1%) to achieve the desired hue than with liquid preparations.

Both dyes and lakes are used to color sugar-coated tablets, film-coated tablets, direct-compression tablets, pharmaceutical suspensions, and other dosage forms (18). Traditionally, sugar-coated tablets have been colored with syrup solutions containing varying amounts of the water-soluble dyes, starting with very dilute solutions, working up to concentrated color syrup solutions. As many as 30 to 60 coats are common. With the lakes, fewer color coats are used. Appealing tablets have been made with as few as 8 to 12 coats using lakes dispersed in syrup. Water-soluble dyes in aqueous vehicles or lakes dispersed in organic solvents may be effectively sprayed on tablets to produce attractive film coatings. There is continued interest today in chewable tablets, because of the availability of many direct-compression materials such as dextrose, sucrose, mannitol, sorbitol, and spray-dried lactose. The direct-compression colored chewable tablets may be prepared with 1 pound of lake per 1000 pounds of tablet mix. For aqueous suspensions, FD&C water-soluble colors or lakes may be satisfactory. In other suspensions, FD&C lakes are necessary. The lakes, added to either the aqueous or nonaqueous phase, generally at a level of 1 pound of color per 1000 pounds of suspension, require homogenization or mechanical blending to achieve uniform coloring.

For the most part, ointments, suppositories, and ophthalmic and parenteral products assume the color of their ingredients and do not contain color additives. Should a dye lose the certification status it held when a product was first formulated, manufactured, and marketed, the manufacturer must reformulate within a reasonable length of time, using only color additives certified at the new date of manufacture.

In addition to esthetics and the certification status of a dye, a formulation pharmacist must select the dyes to be used in a particular formula on the basis of their physical and chemical properties. Of prime importance is the solubility of a prospective dye in the vehicle to be used for a liquid formulation or in a solvent to be employed during a pharmaceutical process, as when the dye is sprayed on a batch of tablets. In general, most dyes are broadly grouped into those that are water soluble and those that are oil soluble; few if any dyes are both. Usually a water-soluble dye is also adequately soluble in commonly used pharmaceutical liquids like glycerin, alcohol, and glycol ethers. Oil-soluble dyes may also be soluble to some extent in these solvents and in liquid petrolatum (mineral oil), fatty acids, fixed oils, and waxes. No great deal of solubility is required, since the concentration of dye in a given preparation is minimal.

Another important consideration when selecting a dye for use in a liquid pharmaceutical is the pH and pH stability of the preparation to be colored. Dyes can change color with a change in pH, and the dye must be selected so

that no anticipated pH change will alter the color during the usual shelf life. The dye also must be chemically stable in the presence of the other formulative ingredients and must not interfere with the stability of the other agents. To maintain their original colors, FD&C dyes must be protected from oxidizing agents, reducing agents (especially metals, including iron, aluminum, zinc, and tin), strong acids and alkalis, and excessive heating. Dyes must also be reasonably photostable; that is, they must not change color when exposed to light of anticipated intensities and wavelengths under the usual conditions of shelf storage. Certain medicinal agents, particularly those prepared in liquid form, must be protected from light to maintain their chemical stability and their therapeutic effectiveness. These preparations are generally kept in dark amber or opaque containers. For solid dosage forms of photolabile drugs, a colored or opaque capsule shell may enhance the drug's stability by shielding out light rays.

Preservatives

In addition to the stabilization of pharmaceutical preparations against chemical and physical degradation due to changed environmental conditions within a formulation, certain liquid and semisolid preparations must be preserved against microbial contamination.

Sterilization and Preservation

Although some types of pharmaceutical products, for example ophthalmic and injectable preparations, are sterilized by physical methods (autoclaving for 20 minutes at 15 pounds pressure and 121°C, dry heat at 180°C for 1 hour, or bacterial filtration) during manufacture, many of them also require an antimicrobial preservative to maintain their aseptic condition throughout storage and use. Other types of preparations that are not sterilized during their preparation but are particularly susceptible to microbial growth because of the nature of their ingredients are protected by the addition of an antimicrobial preservative. Preparations that provide excellent growth media for microbes are most aqueous preparations, especially syrups, emulsions, suspensions, and some semisolid preparations, particularly creams. Certain hydroalcoholic and most alcoholic preparations may not require the addition of a chemical preservative when the alcoholic content is sufficient to prevent microbial growth. Generally, 15% alcohol will prevent microbial growth in acid media and 18% in alkaline media. Most alcohol-containing pharmaceuticals, such as elixirs, spirits, and tinctures, are self-sterilizing and do not require additional preservation. The same applies to other individual pharmaceuticals that by virtue of their vehicle or other formulative agents may not permit the growth of microorganisms.

Preservative Selection

When experience or shelf storage experiments indicate that a preservative is required in a pharmaceutical preparation, its selection is based on many considerations, including some of the following:

1. The preservative prevents the growth of the type of microorganisms considered the most likely contaminants of the preparation.
2. The preservative is soluble enough in water to achieve adequate concentrations in the aqueous phase of a system with two or more phases.
3. The proportion of preservative remaining undissociated at the pH of the preparation makes it capable of penetrating the microorganism and destroying its integrity.
4. The required concentration of the preservative does not affect the safety or comfort of the patient when the pharmaceutical preparation is administered by the usual or intended route; that is, it is nonirritating, nonsensitizing, and nontoxic.
5. The preservative has adequate stability and will not be reduced in concentration by chemical decomposition or volatilization during the desired shelf life of the preparation.
6. The preservative is completely compatible with all other formulative ingredients and does not interfere with them, nor do they interfere with the effectiveness of the preservative agent.

7. The preservative does not adversely affect the preparation's container or closure.

General Preservative Considerations

Microorganisms include molds, yeasts, and bacteria, with bacteria generally favoring a slightly alkaline medium and the others an acid medium. Although few microorganisms can grow below pH 3 or above pH 9, most aqueous pharmaceutical preparations are within the favorable pH range and therefore must be protected against microbial growth. To be effective, a preservative agent must be dissolved in sufficient concentration in the aqueous phase of a preparation. Furthermore, only the undissociated fraction or molecular form of a preservative possesses preservative capability, because the ionized portion is incapable of penetrating the microorganism. Thus the preservative selected must be largely undissociated at the pH of the formulation being prepared. Acidic preservatives like benzoic, boric, and sorbic acids are more undissociated and thus more effective as the medium is made more acid. Conversely, alkaline preservatives are less effective in acid or neutral media and more effective in alkaline media. Thus, it is meaningless to suggest preservative effectiveness at specific concentrations unless the pH of the system is mentioned and the undissociated concentration of the agent is calculated or otherwise determined. Also, if formulative materials interfere with the solubility or availability of the preservative agent, its chemical concentration may be misleading, because it may not be a true measure of the effective concentration. Many incompatible combinations of preservative agents and other pharmaceutical adjuncts have been discovered in recent years, and undoubtedly many more will be uncovered in the future as new preservatives, pharmaceutical adjuncts, and therapeutic agents are combined for the first time. Many of the recognized incompatible combinations that inactivate the preservative contain macromolecules, including various cellulose derivatives, polyethylene glycols, and natural gums. These include tragacanth, which can attract and hold preservative agents, such as the parabens and phenolic compounds, rendering them unavailable for their preservative function. It is essential for the research pharmacist to examine all formulative ingredients as one affects the other to ensure that each agent is free to do its job. In addition, the preservative must not interact with a container, such as a metal ointment tube or a plastic medication bottle, or with an enclosure, such as a rubber or plastic cap or liner. Such an interaction could result in decomposition of the preservative or the container closure or both, causing decomposition and contamination. Appropriate tests should be devised and conducted to prevent this type of preservative interaction.

Mode of Action

Preservatives interfere with microbial growth, multiplication, and metabolism through one or more of the following mechanisms:

1. Modification of cell membrane permeability and leakage of cell constituents (partial lysis)
2. Lysis and cytoplasmic leakage
3. Irreversible coagulation of cytoplasmic constituents (e.g., protein precipitation)
4. Inhibition of cellular metabolism, such as by interfering with enzyme systems or inhibition of cell wall synthesis
5. Oxidation of cellular constituents
6. Hydrolysis

A few of the commonly used pharmaceutical preservatives and their probable modes of action are presented in Table 4.6.

Preservative Utilization

Suitable substances may be added to a pharmaceutical preparation to enhance its permanency or usefulness. Such additives are suitable only if they are nontoxic and harmless in the amounts administered and do not interfere with the therapeutic efficacy or tests or assays of the preparation. Certain intravenous preparations given in large volumes as blood replenishers or as nutrients are not permitted to contain bacteriostatic additives, because the amounts required to preserve such large volumes would constitute a health hazard when administered to the patient. Thus preparations like dextrose injection, USP, and others commonly given as fluid and nutrient replenishers by intravenous injections in amounts of 500 to 1000 mL may not contain antibacterial preservatives. On the other hand, injectable preparations given in small volumes—for example, morphine sulfate injection, USP, which provides a therapeutic amount of morphine sulfate in approximately a 1-mL volume—can be preserved with a suitable preservative without the danger of the patient receiving an excessive amount of the preservative.

Examples of the preservatives and their concentrations commonly employed in pharmaceutical preparations are benzoic acid (0.1–0.2%), sodium benzoate (0.1–0.2%), alcohol (15–20%), phenylmercuric nitrate and acetate (0.002–0.01%), phenol (0.1–0.5%), cresol (0.1–0.5%), chlorobutanol (0.5%), benzalkonium chloride (0.002–0.01%), and com-

TABLE 4.6 PROBABLE MODES OF ACTION OF SOME PRESERVATIVES

PRESERVATIVE	PROBABLE MODES OF ACTION
Benzoic acid, boric acid, p-hydroxybenzoates	Denaturation of proteins
Phenols and chlorinated phenolic compounds	Lytic and denaturation action on cytoplasmic membranes and for chlorinated preservatives, also by oxidation of enzymes
Alcohols	Lytic and denaturation action on membranes
Quaternary compounds	Lytic action on membranes
Mercurials	Denaturation of enzymes by combining with thiol (-SH) groups

binations of methylparaben and propylparaben (0.1–0.2%), the latter being especially good against fungus. The required proportion varies with the pH, dissociation, and other factors already indicated as well with the presence of other formulative ingredients with inherent preservative capabilities.

For each type of preparation to be preserved, the research pharmacist must consider the influence of the preservative on the comfort of the patient. For instance, a preservative in an ophthalmic preparation must have an extremely low degree of irritant qualities, which is characteristic of chlorobutanol, benzalkonium chloride, and phenylmercuric nitrate, frequently used in ophthalmic preparations. In all instances, the preserved preparation must be biologically tested to determine its safety and efficacy and shelf-tested to determine its stability for the intended shelf life of the product.

REFERENCES

 1. Poole JW. Preformulation. FMC Corporation, 1982.
 2. Brange J, Langkjaer L, Havelund S, Vølund A. Chemical stability of insulin: hydrolytic degradation during storage of pharmaceutical preparations. Pharm Res 1991;9:715–726.
 3. Guideline for submitting documentation for the stability of human drugs and biologics. Rockville, MD: Food & Drug Administration, 1987.
 4. FDA/ICH Regulatory Guidance on Stability. In: Federal Register. Washington: Food & Drug Administration, 1998; 63:9795–9843.
 5. Sheinin EB. ICH guidelines: History, present status, intent. Athens, GA: International Good Manufacturing Practices Conference, 1998.
 6. Rothman B. Stability is the issue. Athens, GA: International Good Manufacturing Practices Conference, 1998.
 7. Guidelines on compounding of nonsterile products in pharmacies. Bethesda MD: Am Society Hospital Pharm, 1996.
 8. Trissel L. Trissel's Stability of Compounded Formulations, 11th ed. Washington: American Pharmaceutical Association, 2002.
 9. U.S. Pharmacopeia 26–National Formulary 21. Rockville, MD: U.S. Pharmacopeial Convention, 2003.
10. Handbook of Pharmaceutical Excipients, 4th ed. Washington: American Pharmaceutical Association, 2003.
11. Lewis R. When smell and taste go awry. FDA Consumer 1991;25:29–33.
12. Hornstein I, Teranishi R. The chemistry of flavor. Chem Eng News 1967;45:92–108.
13. Murphy DH. A practical compendium on sweetening agents. Am Pharm 1983; NS23:32–37.
14. Jacknowitz AI. Artificial sweeteners: How safe are they? U.S. Pharmacist 1988;13:28–31.
15. Krueger RJ, Topolewski M, Havican S. In search of the ideal sweetener. Pharmacy Times 1991;July:72–77.
16. Lecos CW. Sweetness minus calories = controversy. FDA Consumer 1985;19:18–23.
17. Code of federal regulations, Title 21, Parts 70–82.
18. Colorants for drug tablets and capsules. Drug and Cosmetic Industry 1983;133(2):44.

Chapter at a glance

As discussed in Chapter 4, the biologic response to a drug is the result of an interaction between the drug substance and functionally important cell receptors or enzyme systems. The response is due to an alteration in the biologic processes that were present prior to the drug's administration. The magnitude of the response is related to the concentration of the drug achieved at the site of its action. This drug concentration depends on the dosage of the drug administered, the extent of its absorption and distribution to the site, and the rate and extent of its elimination from the body. The physical and chemical constitution of the drug substance—particularly its lipid solubility, degree of ionization, and molecular size—determines to a great extent its ability to carry out its biologic activity. The area of study embracing this relationship between the physical, chemical, and biologic sciences as they apply to drugs, dosage forms, and drug action has been given the descriptive term *biopharmaceutics*.

In general, for a drug to exert its biologic effect, it must be transported by the body fluids, traverse the required biologic membrane barriers, escape widespread distribution to unwanted areas, endure metabolic attack, penetrate in adequate concentration to the sites of action, and interact in a specific fashion, causing an alteration of cellular function. A simplified diagram of this complex series of events between a drug's administration and its elimination is presented in Figure 5.1.

The absorption, distribution, biotransformation (metabolism), and elimination of a drug from the body are dynamic processes that continue from the time a drug is taken until all of the drug has been removed from the body. The *rates* at which these processes occur affect the onset, intensity, and duration of the drug's activity within the body. The area of study that elucidates the time course of drug concentration in the blood and tissues is termed *pharmacokinetics*. It is the study of the kinetics of absorption, distribution, metabolism, and excretion (ADME) of drugs and their corresponding pharmacologic, therapeutic, or toxic effects in animals and man. Furthermore, since one drug may alter the ADME of another drug, pharmacokinetics may be applied in the study of interactions between drugs.

Once a drug is administered and absorption begins, the drug does not remain in a single body location but rather is distributed throughout the body until its ultimate elimination. For instance, following the oral administration of a drug and its entry into the gastrointestinal tract, a portion of the drug is absorbed into the circulatory system, from which it is distributed to the various other body fluids, tissues, and organs. From these sites the drug may return to the circulatory system and be excreted through the kidney as such or metabolized by the liver or other cellular site and be excreted as one or more metabolites. As shown in Figure 5.1, drugs administered by intravenous injection are introduced directly into the circulatory system, avoiding absorption, which is required for systemic effects from all other routes of administration.

The various body locations to which a drug travels may be viewed as separate compartments, each containing some fraction of the administered dose of drug. The transfer of drug from the blood to other body locations is generally a rapid and reversible process; that is, the drug may diffuse back into the circulation. The drug in the blood therefore exists in equilibrium with the drug in the other compartments. However, in this equilibrium state, the concentration of the drug in the blood may be quite different (greater or lesser) than the concentration of the drug in the other compartments. This is due largely to the physicochemical properties of the drug and its resultant

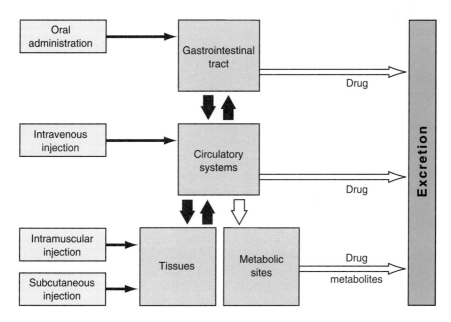

FIGURE 5.1 Events of absorption, metabolism, and excretion of drugs after their administration by various routes.

ability to leave the blood and traverse the biologic membranes. Certain drugs leave the circulatory system rapidly and completely, whereas other drugs do so slowly and with difficulty. A number of drugs become bound to blood proteins, particularly the albumins, and only a small fraction of the drug administered may actually be found outside of the circulatory system at a given time. The transfer of drug from one compartment to another is mathematically associated with a specific rate constant describing that particular transfer. Generally, the rate of transfer of a drug from one compartment to another is proportional to the concentration of the drug in the compartment from which it exits; the greater the concentration, the greater is the amount of drug transfer.

Metabolism is the major process by which foreign substances, including drugs, are eliminated from the body. During metabolism a drug substance may be biotransformed into pharmacologically active or inactive metabolites. Often, both the drug substance and its metabolite or metabolites are active and exert pharmacologic effects. For example, the anticonvulsant drug carbamazepine is metabolized in the liver to an active epoxide metabolite. In some instances a pharmacologically inactive drug (termed a *prodrug*) may be administered for the known effects of its active metabolites. Dipivefrin, for example, is a prodrug of epinephrine formed by the esterification of epinephrine and pivalic acid. This enhances the lipophilic character of the drug, and as a consequence its penetration into the anterior chamber of the eye is 17 times that of epinephrine. Within the eye, dipivefrin HCl is converted by enzymatic hydrolysis to epinephrine.

The metabolism of a drug to inactive products is usually an irreversible process that culminates in the excretion of the drug from the body, usually via the urine. The pharmacokineticist may calculate an elimination rate constant (k_{el}) for a drug to describe its rate of elimination from the body. The term *elimination* refers to both metabolism and excretion. For drugs that are administered intravenously and therefore are not absorbed, the task is much less complex than for drugs administered by other routes. Except with intravenous administration absorption and elimination occur simultaneously but at different rates.

Principles of Drug Absorption

Before an administered drug can arrive at its site of action in effective concentrations, it must surmount a number of barriers. These barriers are chiefly a succession of biologic membranes such as those of the gastrointestinal epithelium, lungs, blood, and brain. Body membranes are generally classified as three main types: (*a*) those composed of several layers of cells, like the skin; (*b*) those composed of a single layer of cells, like the intestinal epithelium; and (*c*) those less than one cell thick, like the membrane of a single cell. In most instances a drug substance must pass more than one of these membrane types before it reaches its site of action. For instance, a drug taken orally must first traverse the gastrointestinal membranes (stomach and intestines), gain entrance to the general circulation, pass to the organ or tissue with which it has affinity, gain entrance to that tissue, and then enter its individual cells.

Although the chemistry of body membranes differs one from another, the membranes may be viewed in general as a bimolecular lipoid (fat containing) layer attached on both sides to a protein layer. Drugs are thought to penetrate these biologic membranes in two general ways: (*a*) by passive diffusion and (*b*) through specialized transport mechanisms. Within each of these main categories, more clearly defined processes have been ascribed to drug transfer.

Passive Diffusion

The term *passive diffusion* is used to describe the passage of (drug) molecules through a membrane that does not actively participate in the process. Drugs absorbed according to this method are said to be *passively absorbed*. The absorption process is driven by the concentration gradient (that is, the differences in concentration) across the membrane, with the passage of drug molecules occurring primarily from the side of high concentration. Most drugs pass through biologic membranes by diffusion.

Passive diffusion is described by *Fick's first law*, which states that the rate of diffusion or transport across a membrane (dc/dt) is proportional to the difference in drug concentration on both sides of the membrane:

$$-\frac{dc}{dt} = P(C_1 - C_2)$$

where

C₁ and C₂ are the drug concentrations on each side of the membrane and
P is a permeability coefficient or constant.

The term C_1 is customarily used to represent the compartment with the greater concentration of drug, and thus the transport of drug proceeds from compartment 1 (e.g., absorption site) to compartment 2 (e.g., blood).

The concentration of drug at the site of absorption (C_1) is usually much greater than on the other side of the membrane because of the rapid dilution of the drug in the blood and its subsequent distribution to the tissues, so for practical purposes the value of $C_1 - C_2$ may be taken simply as that of C_1 and the equation written in the standard form for a first-order rate equation:

$$-\frac{dc}{dt} = PC_1$$

The gastrointestinal absorption of most drugs from solution occurs in this manner in accordance with *first-order kinetics*, in which the rate depends on drug concentration; that is, doubling the dose doubles the transfer rate. The magnitude of the permeability constant depends on the diffusion coefficient of the drug, the thickness and area of the absorbing membrane, and the permeability of the membrane to the particular drug.

Because of the lipoid nature of the cell membrane, it is highly permeable to lipid-soluble substances. The rate of diffusion of a drug across the membrane depends not only on its concentration but also on the relative extent of its affinity for lipid and rejection of water (a high lipid partition coefficient). The greater its affinity for lipid and the more hydrophobic it is, the faster will be its rate of penetration into the lipid-rich membrane. Erythromycin base, for example, possesses a higher partition coefficient than other erythromycin compounds,

for example, estolate and gluceptate. Consequently, the base is the preferred agent for the topical treatment of acne where penetration into the skin is desired.

Because biologic cells are also permeated by water and lipid-insoluble substances, it is thought that the membrane also contains water-filled pores or channels that permit the passage of these types of substances. As water passes in bulk across a porous membrane, any dissolved solute with small enough molecules to traverse the pores passes in by *filtration*. Aqueous pores vary in size from membrane to membrane and thus in their individual permeability characteristics for certain drugs and other substances.

Most drugs today are weak organic acids or bases. Knowledge of their individual ionization or dissociation characteristics is important, because their absorption is governed to a large extent by their degrees of ionization as they are presented to the membrane barriers. Cell membranes are more permeable to the un-ionized forms of drugs than to their ionized forms, mainly because of the greater lipid solubility of the un-ionized forms and the highly charged nature of the cell membrane, which results in binding or repelling of the ionized drug and thereby decreases cell penetration. Also, ions become hydrated through association with water molecules, resulting in larger particles than the undissociated molecule and again decreased penetrating capability.

The degree of a drug's ionization depends both on the pH of the solution in which it is presented to the biologic membrane and on the pK_a, or dissociation constant, of the drug (whether an acid or base). The concept of pK_a is derived from the Henderson-Hasselbalch equation.

For an acid:

$$pH = pK_a + \log \frac{\text{ionized conc. (salt)}}{\text{un-ionized conc. (acid)}}$$

For a base:

$$pH = pK_a + \log \frac{\text{un-ionized conc. (base)}}{\text{ionized conc. (salt)}}$$

Since the pH of body fluids varies (stomach, pH 1; lumen of the intestine, pH 6.6; blood plasma, pH 7.4), the absorption of a drug from various body fluids will differ and may dictate to some extent the type of dosage form and the route of administration preferred for a given drug.

Rearranging the equation for an acid yields

$$pK_a - pH = \log \frac{\text{un-ionized concentration (acid)}}{\text{ionized concentration (salt)}}$$

and one can theoretically determine the relative extent to which a drug remains un-ionized under various conditions of pH. This is particularly useful when applied to body fluids. For instance, if a weak acid having a pK_a of 4 is assumed to be in an environment of gastric juice with a pH of 1, the left side of the equation yields the number 3, which means that the ratio of un-ionized to ionized drug particles is about 1000:1, and gastric absorption is excellent. At the pH of plasma the reverse is true, and in the blood the drug is largely in the ionized form. Table 5.1 presents the effect of pH on the ionization of weak electrolytes, and Table 5.2 offers some representative pK_a values of common drug substances.

The equation and Table 5.1 show that a drug substance is half ionized at a pH value equal to

TABLE 5.1 THE EFFECT OF PH ON THE IONIZATION OF WEAK ELECTROLYTES PK_A-PH % UN-IONIZED

	IF WEAK ACID	IF WEAK BASE
−3.0	0.10	99.90
−2.0	0.99	99.00
−1.0	9.09	90.90
−0.7	16.60	83.40
−0.5	24.00	76.00
−0.2	38.70	61.30
0.0	50.00	50.00
+0.2	61.30	38.70
+0.5	76.00	24.00
+0.7	83.40	16.60
+1.0	90.90	9.09
+2.0	99.00	0.99
+3.0	99.90	0.10

Reprinted with permission from Doluisio JT, Swintosky JV. Factors influencing drug distribution in the body. Am J Pharm 1965;137:149.

TABLE 5.2. PK_A VALUES FOR SOME ACIDIC AND BASIC DRUGS

	PK_A
Acids	
Acetylsalicylic acid	3.5
Barbital	7.9
Benzylpenicillin	2.8
Boric acid	9.2
Dicoumarol	5.7
Phenobarbital	7.4
Phenytoin	8.3
Sulfanilamide	10.4
Theophylline	9.0
Thiopental	7.6
Tolbutamide	5.5
Warfarin	4.8
Bases	
Amphetamine	9.8
Apomorphine	7.0
Atropine	9.7
Caffeine	0.8
Chlordiazepoxide	4.6
Cocaine	8.5
Codeine	7.9
Guanethidine	11.8
Morphine	7.9
Procaine	9.0
Quinine	8.4
Reserpine	6.6

its pK_a. Thus pK_a may be defined as the pH at which a drug is 50% ionized. For example, phenobarbital has a pK_a value of about 7.4, and in plasma (pH 7.4) it is present as ionized and un-ionized forms in equal amounts. However, a drug substance cannot reach the blood plasma unless it is placed there directly through intravenous injection or is favorably absorbed from a site along its route of entry, such as the gastrointestinal tract, and allowed to pass into the general circulation. As shown in Table 5.2, phenobarbital, a weak acid with a pK_a of 7.4, would be largely undissociated in the gastric environment of pH 1 and would likely be well absorbed. A drug may enter the circulation rapidly and at high concentrations if membrane penetration is easily accomplished or at a low rate and low level if the drug is not readily absorbed from its route of entry. The pH of the drug's current environment influences the rate and degree of its further distribution because under one condition of pH it becomes more or less un-ionized and therefore more or less lipid penetrating than under another. If an un-ionized molecule is able to diffuse through the lipid barrier and remain un-ionized in the new environment, it may return to its former location or go on to a new one. However, if in the new environment it is greatly ionized because of the influence of the pH of the second fluid, it likely will be unable to cross the membrane with its former ability. Thus a concentration gradient of a drug usually is reached at equilibrium on each side of a membrane because different degrees of ionization occur on each side. A summary of the concepts of dissociation and ionization is found in Physical Pharmacy Capsule 4.8.

It is often desirable for pharmaceutical scientists to make structural modifications in organic drugs and thereby favorably alter their lipid solubility, partition coefficients, and dissociation constants while maintaining the same basic pharmacologic activity. These efforts frequently result in increased absorption, better therapeutic response, and lower dosage.

Specialized Transport Mechanisms

In contrast to the passive transfer of drugs and other substances across a biologic membrane, certain substances, including some drugs and biologic metabolites, are conducted across a membrane through one of several postulated *specialized transport* mechanisms. This type of transfer seems to account for substances, many naturally occurring as amino acids and glucose, that are too lipid insoluble to dissolve in the boundary and too large to flow or filter through the pores. This type of transport is thought to involve membrane components that may be enzymes or some other type of agent capable of forming a complex with the drug (or other agent) at the surface membrane. The complex moves across the membrane, where the drug is released, with the carrier returning to the original surface. Figure 5.2 presents the simplified scheme of this process. Specialized transport may be differentiated from passive transfer in that the former process may become saturated as the amount of carrier for a given substance becomes completely bound with that sub-

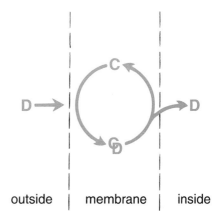

FIGURE 5.2 Active transport mechanism. D, drug molecule; C, the carrier in the membrane. (Modified with permission from O'Reilly W. Aust J Pharm 1966;47:568.)

stance, resulting in a delay in transport. Other features of specialized transport include the specificity by a carrier for a particular type of chemical structure, so that if two substances are transported by the same mechanism or carrier, one will competitively inhibit the transport of the other. Furthermore, the transport mechanism is inhibited in general by substances that interfere with cell metabolism. The term *active transport* as a subclassification of specialized transport denotes a process with the additional feature of the solute or drug being moved across the membrane against a concentration gradient, that is, from a solution of lower concentration to one of a higher concentration, or if the solute is an ion, against an electrochemical potential gradient. In contrast to active transport, *facilitated diffusion* is a specialized transport mechanism having all of the described characteristics except that the solute is not transferred against a concentration gradient and may attain the same concentration inside the cell as on the outside.

Many body nutrients, such as sugars and amino acids, are transported across the membranes of the gastrointestinal tract by carrier processes. Certain vitamins, such as thiamine, niacin, riboflavin, and pyridoxine, and drug substances, such as methyldopa and 5-fluorouracil, require active transport mechanisms for their absorption.

Investigations of intestinal transport have often used in situ (at the site) or in vivo (in the body) animal models or ex vivo (outside the body) transport models; however, recently cell culture models of human small intestine absorptive cells have become available to investigate transport across intestinal epithelium (1). Both passive and transport-mediated studies have been conducted to investigate mechanisms and rates of transport.

Dissolution and Drug Absorption

For a drug to be absorbed, it must first be dissolved in the fluid at the absorption site. For instance, a drug administered orally in tablet or capsule form cannot be absorbed until the drug particles are dissolved by the fluids in the gastrointestinal tract. When the solubility of a drug depends on either an acidic or basic medium, the drug dissolves in the stomach or intestines respectively (Fig. 5.3). The process by which a drug particle dissolves is termed *dissolution*.

As a drug particle undergoes dissolution, the drug molecules on the surface are the first to enter into solution, creating a saturated layer of drug solution that envelops the surface of the solid drug particle. This layer of solution is the *diffusion layer*. From this diffusion layer the drug molecules pass throughout the dissolving fluid and make contact with the biologic membranes, and absorption ensues. As the molecules of drug continue to leave the diffusion layer, the layer is replenished with dissolved drug from the surface of the drug particle, and the process of absorption continues.

If the dissolution of a given drug particle is rapid or if the drug is administered as a solution and remains present in the body as such, the rate at which the drug becomes absorbed depends mainly on its ability to traverse the membrane barrier. However, if the rate of dissolution for a drug particle is slow because of the physicochemical characteristics of the drug substance or the dosage form, dissolution itself is a rate-limiting step in absorption. Slowly soluble drugs such as digoxin may not only be absorbed at a slow rate; they may be incompletely

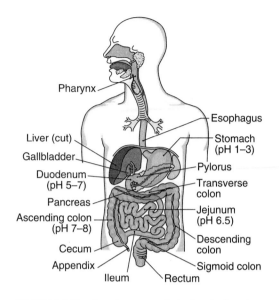

FIGURE 5.3 The digestive system, including the locations of drug absorption and their respective pH values. (Adapted with permission from Cohen BJ, Wood DL. Memmler's the human body in health and disease, 9th ed. Philadelphia: Lippincott Williams & Wilkins, 2000.)

absorbed or in some cases largely unabsorbed following oral administration because of the natural limitation of time that they may remain within the stomach or the intestinal tract. Thus, poorly soluble drugs or poorly formulated drug products may be incompletely absorbed and pass unchanged out of the system via the feces.

Under normal circumstances a drug may be expected to remain in the stomach for 2 to 4 hours (*gastric emptying time*) and in the small intestine for 4 to 10 hours, although there is substantial variation between people and even in the same person on different occasions. Various techniques have been used to determine gastric emptying time and the gastrointestinal passage of drug from various oral dosage forms, including tracking dosage forms labeled with gamma-emitting radionuclides through gamma scintigraphy (2, 3). The gastric emptying time for a drug is most rapid with a fasting stomach, becoming slower as the food content is increased. Changes in gastric emptying time and/or in intestinal motility can affect drug transit time and thus the opportunity for drug dissolution and absorption.

These changes can be affected by drugs. Certain drugs with anticholinergic properties, for example dicyclomine HCl and amitriptyline HCl, can slow gastric emptying. This can enhance the rate of absorption of drugs normally absorbed from the stomach and reduce the rate of absorption of drugs that are primarily absorbed from the small intestine. Alternatively, drugs that enhance gastric motility, for example laxatives, may cause some drugs to move through the gastrointestinal system and past their absorptive site at such a rate as to reduce the amount of drug absorbed. This effect has been demonstrated with digoxin, whose absorption is significantly decreased by accelerating gastrointestinal motility.

Aging may also influence gastrointestinal absorption. In the elderly, gastric acidity, the number of absorptive cells, intestinal blood flow, the rate of gastric emptying, and intestinal motility are all decreased. However, drugs in which absorption depends on passive processes are not affected by these factors as much as those that depend on active transport mechanisms, such as calcium, iron, thiamine, and sugars. A decrease in gastric emptying time is advantageous for drugs that are absorbed from the stomach but disadvantageous for those that are prone to acid degradation, such as penicillins and erythromycin, or inactivated by stomach enzymes, such as L-dopa.

The dissolution of a substance may be described by the modified Noyes-Whitney equation:

$$\frac{dc}{dt} = kS(c_s - c_t)$$

where

c d c/dt is the rate of dissolution,
k is the dissolution rate constant,
S is the surface area of the dissolving solid,
c_s is the saturation concentration of drug in the diffusion layer (which may be approximated by the maximum solubility of the drug in the solvent, since the diffusion layer is considered saturated), and
c_t is the concentration of the drug in the

dissolution medium at time t ($c_s - c_t$ is the concentration gradient).

The rate of dissolution is governed by the rate of diffusion of solute molecules through the diffusion layer into the body of the solution. The equation reveals that the dissolution rate of a drug may be increased by increasing the surface area (reducing the particle size) of the drug, by increasing the solubility of the drug in the diffusion layer, and by factors embodied in the dissolution rate constant, k, including the intensity of agitation of the solvent and the diffusion coefficient of the dissolving drug. For a given drug, the diffusion coefficient and usually the concentration of the drug in the diffusion layer will increase with increasing temperature. Also, increasing the rate of agitation of the dissolving medium will increase the rate of dissolution. A reduction in the viscosity of the solvent employed is another means to enhance the dissolution rate of a drug. Changes in the pH or the nature of the solvent that influence the solubility of the drug may be used to advantage in increasing dissolution rate. Effervescent buffered aspirin tablet formulations use some of these principles to their advantage. The alkaline adjuvants in the tablet enhance the solubility of the aspirin within the diffusional layer, and the evolution of carbon dioxide agitates the solvent system, that is, gastric juices. Consequently, the rate of absorption of aspirin into the blood stream is faster than from a conventional aspirin tablet formulation. If this dosage form is acceptable to the patient, it provides a quicker means for the patient to gain relief from a troublesome headache. Many manufacturers use a particular amorphous, crystalline, salt, or ester form of a drug that will exhibit the solubility characteristics needed to achieve the desired dissolution characteristics. Some of these factors that affect drug dissolution briefly are discussed in the following paragraphs, whereas others will be discussed in succeeding chapters in which they are relevant.

The chemical and physical characteristics of a drug substance that can affect safety, efficacy, and stability must be carefully defined by appropriate standards in an application for U.S. Food and Drug Administration (FDA) approval and then sustained and controlled throughout product manufacture.

Surface Area

When a drug particle is broken up, the total surface area is increased. For drug substances that are poorly or slowly soluble, this generally results in an increase in the *rate* of dissolution. This is explained in Physical Pharmacy Capsule 5.1, Particle Size, Surface Area, and Dissolution Rate.

Increased therapeutic response to orally administered drugs due to smaller particle size has been reported for a number of drugs, among them theophylline, a xanthine derivative used to

treat bronchial asthma; griseofulvin, an antibiotic with antifungal activity; sulfisoxazole, an anti-infective sulfonamide, and nitrofurantoin, a urinary anti-infective drug. To increase surface area, pharmaceutical manufacturers frequently use *micronized* powders in their solid products. Micronized powders consist of drug particles reduced in size to about 5 microns and smaller. A slight variation on this is accomplished by blending and melting poorly water-soluble powders with a water-soluble polymer, such as polyethylene glycol (PEG). In the molten state and if the drug dissolves in the carrier, a molecular dispersion of the drug in the carrier results. Solidification produces a solid dispersion that

PHYSICAL PHARMACY CAPSULE 5.1

Particle Size, Surface Area, and Dissolution Rate

Particle size has an effect on dissolution rate and solubility. As shown in the Noyes-Whitney equation,

$$\frac{dC}{dT} = kS(C_s - C_t)$$

where

dC/dT is the rate of dissolution (concentration with respect to time),
K is the dissolution rate constant
S is the surface area of the particles,
C_s is the concentration of the drug in the immediate proximity of the dissolving particle, that is, the solubility of the drug, and
C_t is the concentration of the drug in the bulk fluid.

It is evident that C_s cannot be significantly changed, C_t is often under sink conditions (an amount of the drug is used that is less than 20% of its solubility) and k comprises many factors, such as agitation and temperature. This leaves the S, surface area, as a factor that can affect the rate of dissolution.

An increase in the surface area of a drug will, within reason, increase the dissolution rate. Circumstances in which it may decrease the rate include a decrease in the effective surface area, that is, a condition in which the dissolving fluid cannot wet the particles. Wetting is the first step in dissolution. This can be demonstrated by visualizing a tablet of diameter 0.75 inch by thickness 0.25 inch. The surface area of the tablet can be increased by drilling a series of 0.0625-inch holes in the tablet. However, even though the surface area has been increased, the dissolution fluid—water—because of surface tension and so on cannot necessarily penetrate the new holes and displace the air. Adsorbed air and other factors can decrease the effective surface area of a dosage form, including powders. This is the reason that particle size reduction does not always raise the dissolution rate. One can also visualize a powder that has been comminuted to a very fine state of subdivision; when it is placed in a beaker of water, the powder floats because of the entrapped and adsorbed air. The effective surface area is not the same as the actual surface area of the powder.

can be pulverized and formed into tablets or capsules. When this powder is placed in water, the water-soluble carrier rapidly dissolves, leaving the poorly soluble drug molecules enveloped in water, thus forming a solution.

The use of micronized drugs is not confined to oral preparations. For example, ophthalmic and topical ointments use micronized drugs for their preferred release characteristics and nonirritating quality after application.

Because of the different rates and degrees of absorption obtainable from drugs of various particle size, products of the same drug substance prepared by two or more reliable pharmaceutical manufacturers may result in different degrees of therapeutic response in the same individual. A classic example of this occurs with phenytoin sodium capsules, which have two distinct forms. The first is the rapid-release type, that is, Prompt Phenytoin Sodium Capsules, USP, and the second is the slow-dissolution type, that is, Extended Phenytoin Sodium Capsules, USP. The former has a dissolution rate of not less than 85% in 30 minutes and is recommended for use 3 to 4 times per day. The latter has a slower dissolution rate, for example, 15 to 35% in 30 minutes, which lends itself to use in patients who can be dosed less frequently. Because of such differences in formulation for a number of drugs and drug products, it is generally advisable for a person to continue taking the same brand of medication, provided it produces the desired therapeutic effect. Patients who are stabilized on one brand of drug should not be switched to another unless necessary. However, when a change is necessary, appropriate blood or plasma concentrations of the drug should be monitored until the patient is stabilized on the new product.

Occasionally, a rapid rate of drug absorption is not desired in a pharmaceutical preparation. Research pharmacists who wish to provide sustained rather than rapid action may employ agents of varying particle size to provide controlled dissolution and absorption. Summaries of the physicochemical principles of particle size reduction and the relation of particle size to surface area, dissolution, and solubility may be found in the Physical Pharmacy Capsules in Chapter 4.

Crystal or Amorphous Drug Form

Solid drug materials may occur as pure crystalline substances of definite identifiable shape or as amorphous particles without definite structure. The amorphous or crystalline character of a drug substance may be of considerable importance to its ease of formulation and handling, its chemical stability, and as has been recently shown, even its biologic activity. Certain medicinal agents may be produced to exist in either a crystalline or an amorphous state. Since the amorphous form of a chemical is usually more soluble than the crystalline form, different extents of drug absorption may result with consequent differences in the degree of pharmacologic activity obtained from each. Two antibiotic substances, novobiocin and chloramphenicol palmitate, are essentially inactive when administered in crystalline form, but when they are administered in the amorphous form, absorption from the gastrointestinal tract proceeds rapidly, with good therapeutic response. In other instances, crystalline forms of drugs may be used because of greater stability than the corresponding amorphous forms. For example, the crystalline forms of penicillin G as the potassium salt or sodium salt are considerably more stable than the analogous amorphous forms. Thus, in formulation work on penicillin G, the crystalline forms are preferred and result in excellent therapeutic response.

The hormone insulin presents another striking example of the different degree of activity that may result from the use of different physical forms of the same medicinal agent. Insulin is the active principle of the pancreas and is vital to the body's metabolism of glucose. It is produced by two means. The first is by extraction from pork pancreas. The second is a biosynthetic process with strains of *Escherichia coli*, that is, recombinant DNA. Insulin is used by humans as replacement therapy, by injection, when the body's production of the hormone is insufficient. Insulin is a protein that forms an extremely insoluble zinc–insulin complex when combined with zinc in the presence of acetate buffer. Depending on the pH of the acetate buffer solution, the complex may be an amorphous precipitate or a crystalline material. Each type is produced commercially to take advantage of unique absorption characteristics.

The amorphous form, or Prompt Insulin Zinc Suspension, USP, is rapidly absorbed upon intramuscular or subcutaneous (under the skin) injection. The larger crystalline material, called *ultralente insulin* or Extended Insulin Zinc Suspension, USP, is more slowly absorbed and has a resultant longer duration of action. By combining the two types in various proportions, a physician can provide patients with intermediate-acting insulin of varying degrees of onset and duration of action. A physical mixture of 70% of the crystalline form and 30% of the amorphous form, called *lente insulin* or Insulin Zinc Suspension, USP, is intermediate acting and meets the requirements of many diabetics. Also available is a physical mixture of 50% of the crystalline form and 50% of the amorphous form.

Some crystalline medicinal chemicals are capable of forming different types of crystals, depending on the conditions (temperature, solvent, time) under which crystallization is induced. This property, whereby a single chemical substance may exist in more than one crystalline form, is polymorphism. Only one form of a pure drug substance is stable at a given temperature and pressure, with the other higher-energy forms, called metastable forms, converting in time to the stable crystalline form. It is therefore fairly common for a metastable form of a medicinal agent to change form even in a completed pharmaceutical preparation, although the time required for a complete change may exceed the normal shelf-life of the product. However, from a pharmaceutical point of view, any change in the crystal structure of a medicinal agent may critically affect the stability and even the therapeutic efficacy of the product in which the conversion takes place.

The various polymorphic forms of the same chemical generally differ in many physical properties, including solubility and dissolution, which are of prime importance to the rate and extent of absorption. These differences are manifest so long as the drug is in the solid state. Once solution is effected, the different forms become indistinguishable one from another. Therefore, differences in drug action, pharmaceutically and therapeutically, can be expected from polymorphs contained in solid dosage forms as well as in liquid suspension. The use of metastable forms generally results in higher solubility and dissolution rates than the respective stable crystal forms of the same drug. If all other factors remain constant, more rapid and complete drug absorption will likely result from the metastable forms than from the stable form of the same drug. On the other hand, the stable polymorph is more resistant to chemical degradation and because of its lower solubility is frequently preferred in pharmaceutical suspensions of insoluble drugs. If metastable forms are employed in the preparation of suspensions, their gradual conversion to the stable form may be accompanied by an alteration in the consistency of the suspension itself, which affects its permanency. In all instances, the advantages of the metastable crystalline forms in terms of increased physiologic availability of the drug must be balanced against the increased product stability when stable polymorphs are employed. Sulfur and cortisone acetate exist in more than one crystalline form and are frequently prepared in pharmaceutical suspensions. In fact, cortisone acetate is reported to exist in at least five crystalline forms. It is possible for the commercial products of two manufacturers to differ in stability and therapeutic effect, depending on the crystalline form of the drug used in the formulation.

Salt Forms

The dissolution rate of a salt form of a drug is generally quite different from that of the parent compound. Sodium and potassium salts of weak organic acids and hydrochloride salts of weak organic bases dissolve much more readily than do the respective free acids or bases. The result is a more rapid saturation of the diffusion layer surrounding the dissolving particle and the consequent more rapid diffusion of the drug to the absorption sites.

Numerous examples could be cited to demonstrate the increased rate of drug dissolution due to the use of the salt form of the drug rather than the free acid or base, but the following will suffice: the addition of the ethylenediamine moiety to theophylline increases the water solubility of theophylline fivefold. The use of the ethylenediamine salt of theophylline has allowed the development of oral aqueous solutions of theophylline and diminished the need to use hydroalcoholic mixtures such as elixirs.

Other Factors

The *state of hydration* of a drug molecule can affect its solubility and pattern of absorption. Usually the anhydrous form of an organic molecule is more readily soluble than the hydrated form. This characteristic was demonstrated with the drug ampicillin, when the anhydrous form was shown to have a greater rate of solubility than the trihydrate form (4). The rate of absorption for the anhydrous form was greater than that for the trihydrate form of the drug.

A drug's solubility in the gastrointestinal tract can be affected not only by the pH of the environment but by the normal components of the tract and any foodstuffs. A drug may interact with one of the other agents present to form a chemical complex that may result in reduced drug solubility and decreased drug absorption. The classic example of this complexation is the one between tetracycline analogues and certain cations, for example calcium, magnesium, and aluminum, resulting in decreased absorption of the tetracycline derivative. Also, if the drug

becomes *ad*sorbed onto insoluble material in the tract, its availability for absorption may be correspondingly reduced.

Bioavailability and Bioequivalence

The term *bioavailability* describes the *rate* and *extent* to which an active drug ingredient or therapeutic moiety is absorbed from a drug product and becomes available at the site of action. The term *bioequivalence* refers to the *comparison* of bioavailabilities of different formulations, drug products, or batches of the same drug product.

The availability to the biologic system of a pharmaceutical product is integral to the goals of dosage form design and paramount to the effectiveness of the medication. The study of a drug's bioavailability depends on the drug's absorption or entry into the systemic circulation, and it is necessary to study the pharmacokinetic profile of the drug or its metabolite or metabolites over time in the appropriate biologic system, for example, blood, plasma, urine. Graphically, bioavailability of a drug is portrayed by a concentration time curve of the administered drug in an appropriate tissue system, for example plasma (Fig. 5.4). Bioavailability data are

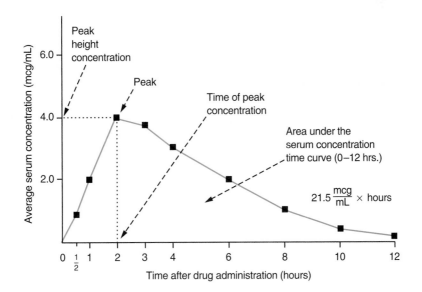

FIGURE 5.4 Serum concentration–time curve showing peak height concentration, time of peak concentration, and AUC. (Courtesy of D. J. Chodos and A. R. DiSanto, Upjohn.)

used to determine (*a*) the amount or proportion of drug absorbed from a formulation or dosage form, (*b*) the rate at which the drug was absorbed, (*c*) the duration of the drug's presence in the biologic fluid or tissue correlated with the patient's response, and (*d*) the relationship between drug blood levels and clinical efficacy and toxicity.

During the product development stages of a proposed drug product, pharmaceutical manufacturers employ bioavailability studies to compare different formulations of the drug substance to ascertain which one allows the most desirable absorption pattern. Later bioavailability studies may be used to compare the availability of the drug substance in different production batches. They may also be used to compare the availability of the drug substance in different dosage forms (e.g., tablets, capsules, elixirs), or in the same dosage form produced by different (competing) manufacturers.

FDA Bioavailability Submission Requirements

The FDA requires bioavailability data submissions in the following instances (5).

1. *New drug applications (NDAs)*: A section of each NDA is required to describe the human pharmacokinetic data and human bioavailability data, or information supporting a waiver of the bioavailability data requirement (see waiver provisions following).
2. *Abbreviated new drug applications (ANDAs)*: In vivo bioavailability data are required unless information is provided and accepted supporting a waiver of this requirement (see waiver provisions following).
3. *Supplemental applications*: In vivo bioavailability data are required if there is a change in the following:
   a. Manufacturing process, product formulation, or dosage strength beyond the variations provided for in the approved NDA.
   b. Labeling to provide for a new indication for use of the drug product and if clinical studies are required, to support the new indication.
   c. Labeling to provide for a new or additional dosage regimen for a special patient population (for example, infants) if clinical studies are required to support the new or additional dosage regimen.

Conditions under which the FDA *may* waive the in vivo bioavailability requirement:

1. The product is a solution intended solely for intravenous administration and contains the same active agent in the same concentration and solvent as a product previously approved through a full NDA.
2. The drug product is administered by inhalation as a gas or vapor and contains the same active agent in the same dosage form as a product previously approved through a full NDA.
3. The drug product is an oral solution, elixir, syrup, tincture, or similar other solubilized form and contains the same active agent in the same concentration as a previously approved drug product through a full NDA and contains no inactive ingredient known to significantly affect absorption of the active drug ingredient.
4. The drug product is a topically applied preparation (for example, ointment) intended for local therapeutic effect.
5. The drug product is an oral form that is not intended to be absorbed (for example, antacid or radiopaque medium).
6. The drug product is a solid oral form that has been demonstrated to be identical or sufficiently similar to a drug product that has met the in vivo bioavailability requirement.

Most bioavailability studies have been applied to drugs in solid forms intended to be administered orally for systemic effects. The emphasis in this direction has been primarily due to the proliferation of competing products in recent years, particularly the nonproprietary (generic) capsules and tablets, and the knowledge that certain drug entities when formulated and manufactured differently into solid dosage forms are particularly prone to variations in biologic availability. Thus, these present discussions will focus on solid dosage forms. However, this is not to imply that systemic drug absorption is not intended from other routes of administration or other dosage forms or that these products may have no bioavailability problems. Indeed, drug absorption from other routes is affected by the physicochemical properties of the drug and the formulative and manufacturing aspects of the dosage form design.

Blood, Serum, or Plasma Concentration Time Curve

Following oral administration of a medication, if blood samples are drawn from the patient at specific time intervals and analyzed for drug content, the resulting data may be plotted on ordinary graph paper to yield the type of drug blood level curve presented in Figure 5.4. The vertical axis of this type of plot characteristically presents the concentration of drug in the blood (or serum or plasma), and the horizontal axis presents the time the samples were obtained following the administration of the drug. When the drug is first administered (time zero), the blood concentration of the drug should also be zero. As the drug passes into the stomach and/or intestine, it is released from the dosage form, eventually dissolves, and is absorbed. As the sampling and analysis continue, the blood samples reveal increasing concentrations of drug (positive slope of the curve) until the maximum (peak) concentration (C_{max}) is reached. Then the blood level of the drug decreases (negative slope of the curve), and if no additional dose is given, it eventually falls to zero. The diminished blood level of drug after the peak height is reached indicates that the rate of elimination from the blood stream is greater than the rate of absorption into the circulatory system. Absorption does not terminate after the peak blood level is reached; it may continue for some time. Similarly, the process of drug elimination is continuous. It begins as soon as the drug first appears in the blood stream and continues until all of the drug has been eliminated. The positive or negative slope of the curve indicates which process is faster. When the drug leaves the blood, it may be found in various body tissues and cells for which it has an affinity until ultimately it is excreted as such or as drug metabolites in the urine or via some other route (Fig. 5.5). A urinalysis for the drug or its metabolites may be used to indicate the extent of absorption and/or the rate of elimination.

Parameters for Assessment and Comparison of Bioavailability

In discussing the important parameters to be considered in the comparative evaluation of the blood level curves following the oral administration of single doses of two formulations of the same drug entity, Chodos and DiSanto (6) list the following:

1. The peak height concentration (C_{max})
2. The time of the peak concentration (T_{max})
3. The area under the blood (or serum or plasma) concentration time curve (AUC)

Using Figure 5.4 as an example, the height of the peak concentration is equivalent to 4.0 µg/mL of drug in the serum; the time of the peak concentration is 2 hours after administration; and the AUC from 0 to 12 hours is calculated as 21.5 µg/mL × hours. The meaning and use of these parameters are further explained as follows.

Peak Height

Peak height concentration is the C_{max} observed in the blood plasma or serum following a dose of the drug, indicating a slope of zero, meaning the rates of absorption and elimination are equal. For conventional dosage forms, such as tablets and capsules, the C_{max} will usually occur at only a single time, T_{max}. The amount of drug is usually expressed in terms of its concentration in relation to a specific volume of blood, serum, or plasma. For example, the concentration may be expressed as grams per 100 mL, micrograms per milliliter, or milligrams per 100 mL. Figure 5.6 depicts concentration time curves showing different peak height concentrations for *equal* amounts of drug from two different formulations following oral administration. The horizontal line drawn across the figure indicates that the minimum effective concentration (MEC) for the drug substance is

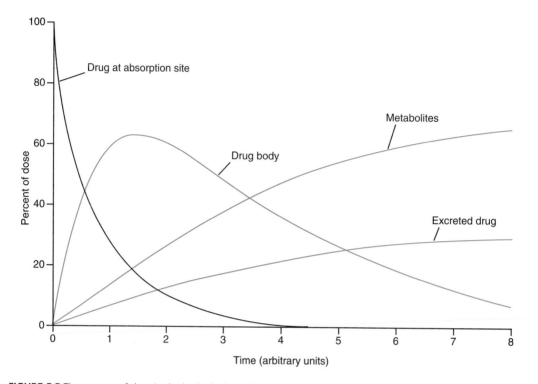

FIGURE 5.5 Time course of drug in the body. (Adapted with permission from Rowland M, Tozer TN. Clinical pharmacokinetics, 2nd ed. Philadelphia: Lea & Febiger, 1989.)

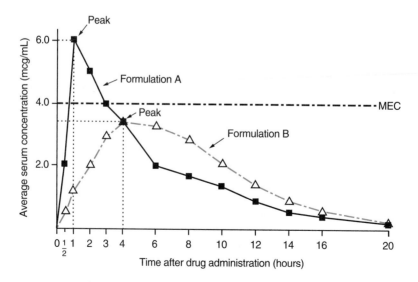

FIGURE 5.6 Serum concentration–time curve showing different peak height concentrations for equal amounts of drug from two different formulations following oral administration. (Courtesy of D. J. Chodos and A. R. DiSanto, Upjohn.)

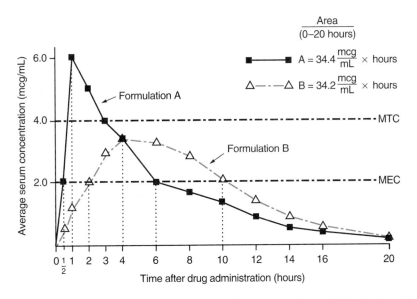

FIGURE 5.7 Serum concentration–time curve showing peak height concentrations, peak height times, times to reach MEC and areas under the curves for equal amounts of drug from two different formulations following oral administration. (Courtesy of D. I. Chodos and A. R. DiSanto, Upjohn.)

4.0 μg/mL. This means that for the patient to exhibit an adequate response to the drug, this concentration in the blood must be achieved. Comparing the blood levels of drug achieved after oral administration of equal doses of formulations A and B in Figure 5.6, formulation A will achieve the required blood levels of drug to produce the desired pharmacologic effect, whereas formulation B will not. On the other hand, if the MEC for the drug is 2.0 μg/mL and the minimum toxic concentration (MTC) is 4.0 μg/mL, as depicted in Figure 5.7, equal doses of the two formulations result in toxic effects produced by formulation A but only desired effects by formulation B. The objective in the individual dosing of a patient is to achieve the MEC but not the MTC.

The *size* of the dose influences the blood level concentration and C_{max} for that substance. Figure 5.8 depicts the influence of dose on the blood level–time curve for a hypothetical drug administered by the same route and in the same dosage form. In this example, it is assumed that all doses are completely absorbed and eliminated at the same rates. As the dose increases, the C_{max} is proportionally higher and the AUC proportionally greater. T_{max}, is the same for each dose.

Time of Peak

The second important parameter in assessing the comparative bioavailability of two formulations is T_{max}. In Figure 5.6, T_{max} is 1 hour for formulation A and 4 hours for formulation B.

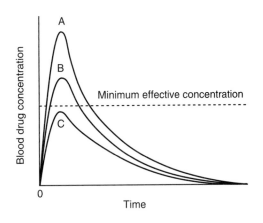

FIGURE 5.8 The influence of dose size on the blood drug concentration–time curves when three different doses of the same drug are administered and the rates of drug absorption and elimination are equal after the three doses. A, 100 mg; B, 80 mg; C, 50 mg. (Adapted with permission from Ueda CT. Concepts in clinical pharmacology: essentials of bioavailability and bioequivalence. Upjohn, 1979).

This parameter reflects the *rate* of absorption from a formulation, which determines the time needed for the MEC to be reached and thus for initiation of the desired effect. The rate of absorption also influences the period over which the drug enters the blood stream and therefore affects the duration that the drug is maintained in the blood. In Figure 5.7, formulation A allows the drug to reach the MEC within 30 minutes following administration and a peak concentration in 1 hour. Formulation B has a slower rate of release. Drug from this formulation reached the MEC 2 hours after administration and its peak concentration 4 hours after administration. Thus formulation A permits the greater rate of drug absorption; it allows drug to reach both the MEC and its peak height sooner than formulation B. On the other hand, formulation B provides more time for drug concentrations maintained above the MEC, 8 hours (2 to 10 hours following administration) compared to 5.5 hours (30 minutes to 6 hours following administration) for formulation A. Thus, if a rapid onset of action is desired, a formulation similar to A is preferred, but if a long duration rather than a rapid onset of action is desired, a formulation similar to B is preferred.

In summary, changes in the *rate* of drug absorption change the values of both C_{max} and T_{max}. Each product has its own characteristic rate of absorption. When the *rate* of absorption is decreased, the C_{max} is lowered and T_{max} occurs at a later time. If the doses of the drugs are the same and presumed completely absorbed, as in Figure 5.7, the AUC for each is essentially the same.

Area Under the Serum Concentration Time Curve

The AUC of a concentration–time plot (Fig. 5.4) is considered representative of the total amount of drug absorbed into the circulation following the administration of a single dose of that drug. Equivalent doses of a drug, when fully absorbed, produce the same AUC. Thus, two curves dissimilar in terms of peak height and time of peak, like those in Figure 5.7, may be similar in terms of AUC and thus in the amount of drug absorbed. As indicated in Figure 5.7, the AUC for formulation A is 34.4 µg/mL × hours and for formulation B is 34.2 µg/mL × hours, essentially the same. If equivalent doses of drug in different formulations produce *different* AUC values, differences exist in the *extent* of absorption between the formulations. Figure 5.9 depicts concentration–time curves for three different formulations of equal amounts of drug with greatly different AUC. In this example, formulation A delivers a much greater amount of drug

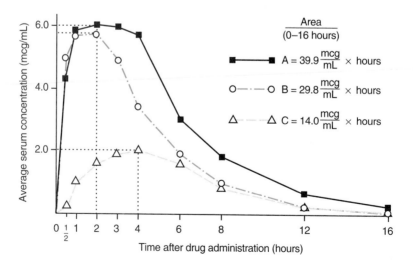

FIGURE 5.9 Serum concentration–time curve showing peak height concentrations, peak height times, and areas under the curves for equal amounts of drugs from three different formulations following oral administration. (Courtesy of D. I. Chodos and A. R. DiSanto, Upjohn.)

to the circulatory system than do the other two formulations. In general, the smaller the AUC, the less drug absorbed.

The fraction (F) (or bioavailability) of an orally administered drug may be calculated by comparison of the AUC after oral administration with that obtained after intravenous administration:

$$F = (AUC)_{oral}/(AUC)_{intravenous}$$

In practice, it is rare for a drug to be completely absorbed into the circulation following oral administration. As noted earlier, many drugs undergo a first-pass effect resulting in some degree of metabolic degradation before entering the general circulation. In addition, factors of product formulation, dissolution, chemical and physical interactions with the gastrointestinal contents, gastric emptying time, intestinal motility, and others limit the absorption of an administered dose of a drug. The oral dosage strengths of many commercial products are based on considerations of the proportion of the dose administered that is expected to be absorbed and available to its site of action to produce the desired drug blood level and/or therapeutic response. The absolute bioavailability following oral dosing is generally compared to intravenous dosing. As examples, the mean oral absorption of a dose of verapamil (Calan) is reported to be 90%; enalapril (Vasotec), 60%; diltiazem (Cardizem), about 40%, lisinopril (Zestril), about 25%; and alendronate sodium about 0.64%. However, there is large intersubject variability, and the absorbed doses may vary from patient to patient.

Bioequivalence of Drug Products

A great deal of discussion and scientific investigation have been devoted recently to the problem of determining the equivalence between drug products of competing manufacturers.

The rate and extent to which a drug in a dosage form becomes available for biologic absorption or use depends in great measure on the materials in the formulation and on the method of manufacture. Thus, the same drug when formulated in *different* dosage forms may be found to possess different bioavailability

characteristics and hence exhibit different clinical effectiveness. Furthermore, two seemingly identical or equivalent products of the same drug in the same dosage strength and in the *same* dosage form but differing in formulative materials or method of manufacture may vary widely in bioavailability and thus in clinical effectiveness.

Dissolution requirements for capsules and tablets are included in the USP and are integral to bioavailability. Experience has shown that where bioinequivalence has been found between two supposedly equivalent products, dissolution testing can help to define the product differences. According to the USP, significant bioavailability and bioinequivalence problems that may be revealed through dissolution testing are generally the result of one or more of the following factors: the drug's particle size; excessive amounts of a lubricant such as magnesium stearate in the formulation; coating materials; and inadequate amounts of tablet or capsule disintegrants.

The FDA uses the following terms to define the type or level of equivalency between drug products (5).

Pharmaceutical equivalents are drug products that contain identical amounts of the identical active drug ingredient, that is, the same salt or ester of the same therapeutic moiety, in identical dosage forms but not necessarily containing the same inactive ingredients; and that meet the identical compendial or other applicable standard of identity, strength, quality, and purity, including potency and where applicable content uniformity, disintegration times, and/or dissolution rates.

Pharmaceutical alternatives are drug products that contain the identical therapeutic moiety or its precursor but not necessarily in the same amount or dosage form or as the same salt or ester. Each such drug product individually meets either the identical or its own compendial or other applicable standard of identity, strength, quality, and purity, including potency and where applicable content uniformity, disintegration times, and/or dissolution rates.

Bioequivalent drug products are pharmaceutical equivalents or pharmaceutical alternatives whose rate and extent of absorption do not show a significant difference when administered at the same molar dose of the therapeutic moiety under similar experimental conditions, either single dose or multiple dose. Some pharmaceutical equivalents or pharmaceutical alternatives may be equivalent in the extent of their absorption but not in their rate of absorption and yet may be considered bioequivalent because such differences in the rate of absorption are intentional and are reflected in the labeling, are not essential to the attainment of effective body drug concentrations on chronic use, or are considered medically insignificant for the particular drug product studied.

In addition, the term *therapeutic equivalents* has been used to indicate pharmaceutical equivalents that provide essentially the same therapeutic effect when administered to the same individuals in the same dosage regimens.

Differences in bioavailability have been demonstrated for a number of products involving the following and other drugs: tetracycline, chloramphenicol, digoxin, warfarin, diazepam, L-dopa, and oxytetracycline. Not only has bioinequivalence been shown to exist in products of different manufacturers; there have also been variations in the bioavailability of different batches of drug products from the same manufacturer. Variations in the bioavailability of certain drug products have resulted in some therapeutic failures in patients who took two inequivalent drug products in the course of their therapy.

The most common experimental plan to compare the bioavailability of two drug products is the simple *crossover design study*. In this method, each of the 12 to 24 individuals in the group of carefully matched subjects (usually healthy men aged 18 to 40 years and having similar height and weight) is administered both products under fasting conditions and essentially serves as his own control. To avoid bias of the test results, each test subject is randomly assigned one of the two products for the first phase of the study. Once the first assigned product is administered, samples of blood or plasma are drawn from the subjects at predetermined times and analyzed for the active drug moiety and its metabolites as a function of time. The same procedure is then repeated (*crossover*) with the second product after an appropriate interval, that is, a washout period to ensure that there is no residual drug from the first administered product that would artificially inflate the test results of the second product. Afterward, the patient population data are tabulated and the parameters used to assess and compare bioavailability; that is, C_{max}, T_{max}, and AUC are analyzed with statistical procedures. Statistical differences in bioavailability parameters may not always be clinically significant in therapeutic outcomes.

Inherent differences in individuals result in different patterns of drug absorption, metabolism, and excretion. These differences must be statistically analyzed to separate them from the factors of bioavailability related to the products themselves. The value in the crossover experiment is that each individual serves as his own control by taking each of the products. Thus, inherent differences between individuals are minimized.

Absolute bioequivalency between drug products rarely if ever occurs. Such absolute equivalency would yield serum concentration–time curves for the products that would be exactly superimposable. This simply is not expected of products that are made at different times, in different batches, or indeed by different manufacturers. However, some expectations of bioequivalency are expected of products considered to have equivalent merit for therapy.

In most studies of bioavailability, the originally marketed product (often called the prototype, pioneer, innovator, or brand name drug product) is recognized as the established product of the drug and is used as the standard for the bioavailability comparative studies.

As a result of the implementation of the Drug Price Competition and Patent Term Restoration Act of 1984, many additional drugs became available in generic form. Prior to the 1984 act, only drugs marketed before 1962 could be processed by an abbreviated new drug application (ANDA). The ANDA process does not require the sponsor to repeat costly clinical research on active ingredients already found to be safe and effective. The 1984 act extended the eligibility for ANDA processing to drugs first marketed after 1962, making generic versions immediately available for many off-patent drugs previously available only as brand name (pioneer) products.

According to the FDA, a generic drug is considered bioequivalent if the rate and extent of absorption do not show a significant difference from that of the pioneer drug when administered at the same molar dose of the therapeutic ingredient under the same experimental conditions (7). Because in the case of a systemically absorbed drug blood levels even if from an identical product may vary in different subjects, in bioequivalence studies each subject receives both the pioneer and the test drug and thus serves as his own control.

Under the 1984 act, to gain FDA approval a generic drug product must have these characteristics:

- The same active ingredients as the pioneer drug (inert ingredients may vary)
- Identical strength, dosage form, and route of administration
- The same indications and precautions for use and other labeling instructions
- Bioequivalency
- The same batch-to-batch requirements for identity, strength, purity, and quality
- Manufacture under the same strict standards of FDA's Current Good Manufacturing Practice regulations as required for pioneer products

In the design and evaluation of bioequivalence, the FDA employs the 80/20 rule, which requires that a study be large enough to provide an 80% probability to detect a 20% difference in average bioavailability. The allowance of a statistical variability of $\pm 20\%$ in bioequivalence applies to both reformulated pioneer drugs and generics. If a pioneer manufacturer reformulates an FDA-approved product, the subsequent formulation must meet the same bioequivalency standards that are required of generic manufacturers of that product (i.e., the approved bioavailability standard for that product).

The FDA recommends generic substitution only among products that it has evaluated to be therapeutically equivalent. Since 1980, the FDA has prepared an annual *Approved Drug Products with Therapeutic Equivalence Evaluations* (known as the Orange Book), which is published in the USP–DI, Volume III, *Approved Drug Products and Legal Requirements*. This regularly updated publication contains information on about 10,000 approved prescription drug products. About 7,500 of these are available from more than a single manufacturer, with only about 10% considered therapeutically *inequivalent* to the pioneer products. For example, the FDA rates all conjugated estrogens and esterified estrogen products as not therapeutically equivalent because no manufacturer to date has submitted an acceptable in vivo bioequivalence study. Therefore, the FDA does not recommend that these products be substituted for each other.

The variables that can contribute to the differences between products are many (Table 5.3). For instance in the manufacture of a tablet, different materials or amounts of such formulative components as fillers, disintegrating agents, binders, lubricants, colorants, flavorants, and coatings may be used. The particle size or crystalline form of a therapeutic or pharmaceutical component may vary between formulations. The tablet may vary in shape, size, and hardness, depending on the punches, dies, and compression forces used in the process. During packaging, shipping, and storage the integrity of the tablets may be altered by physical impact, changes in humidity and temperature, or through interactions with the components of the container. Each of these factors may affect the rates of tablet disintegration, drug dissolution, and consequently the rate and extent of drug absorption. Although the bioequivalency problems are perhaps greater among tablets than for other dosage forms because of the multiplicity of variables, the same types of problems exist for the other dosage forms and must be considered in assessing bioequivalence.

Sometimes even therapeutically equivalent drugs are not equally suitable for a particular patient. For example, a patient may be hypersensitive to an inert ingredient in one product (brand name or generic) that another product does not contain. Or a patient may become

TABLE 5.3 SOME FACTORS THAT INFLUENCE BIOAVAILABILITY OF ORAL DRUGS

Drug substance physiochemical properties
Particle size
Crystalline or amorphous form
Salt form
Hydration
Lipid or water solubility
pH and pK$_a$

Pharmaceutical ingredients
Fillers
Binders
Coatings
Disintegrating agents
Lubricants
Suspending agents
Surface active agents
Flavoring agents
Coloring agents
Preservative agents
Stabilizing agents

Dosage form characteristics
Disintegration rate (tablets)
Dissolution time of drug in dosage form
Product age and storage conditions

Physiologic factors and patient characteristics
Gastric emptying time
Intestinal Transit Time
Gastrointestinal abnormality or pathologic condition
Gastric contents
Other drugs
Food
Fluids
Gastrointestinal pH
Drug metabolism (gut and during first passage through liver).

confused or upset if dispensed an alternative product that differs in color, flavor, shape, or packaging from that to which he or she is accustomed. Switching between products can generate concern, and thus pharmacists need to be prudent in both initial selection and interchange of products.

Routes of Drug Administration

Drugs may be administered using a variety of dosage forms and routes of administration, as presented in Tables 5.4 and 5.5. One of the fundamental considerations in dosage form design is whether the drug is intended for local or systemic effects. *Local* effects are achieved by direct application of the drug to the desired site of action, such as the eye, nose, or skin. *Systemic* effects result from the entrance of the drug into the circulatory system and transport to the cellular site of its action. For systemic effects, a drug may be placed directly in the blood stream via intravenous injection or absorbed into the venous circulation following oral or other route of administration.

An individual drug substance may be formulated into multiple dosage forms that result in different drug absorption rates and times of onset, peak, and duration of action. Figure

TABLE 5.4 ROUTES OF DRUG ADMINISTRATION

TERM	SITE
Oral	Mouth
Peroral (per os[a])	Gastrointestinal tract via mouth
Sublingual	Under the tongue
Parenteral	Other than the gastrointestinal tract (by injection)
Intravenous	Vein
Intraarterial	Artery
Intracardiac	Heart
Intraspinal or intrathecal	Spine
Intraosseous	Bone
Intraarticular	Joint
Intrasynovial	Joint fluid area
Intracutaneous, intradermal	Skin
Subcutaneous	Beneath the skin
Intramuscular	Muscle
Epicutaneous (topical)	Skin surface
Transdermal	Skin surface
Conjunctival	Conjunctiva
Intraocular	Eye
Intranasal	Nose
Aural	Ear
Intrarespiratory	Lung
Rectal	Rectum
Vaginal	Vagina

[a]The abbreviation *po* is commonly used on prescriptions to indicate oral administration.

TABLE 5.5 ROUTE OF ADMINISTRATION AND DELIVERY SYSTEM OF PRIMARY DOSAGE FORMS

Oral	Tablets
	Capsules
	Solutions
	Syrups
	Elixirs
	Suspensions
	Magmas
	Gels
	Powders
Sublingual	Tablets
	Troches, lozenges
	Drops (solutions)
Parenteral	Solutions
	Suspensions
Epicutaneous, transdermal	Ointments
	Creams
	Infusion pumps
	Pastes
	Plasters
	Powders
	Aerosols
	Lotions
	Transdermal patches, discs, solutions
Conjunctival	Contact lens inserts
	Ointments
Intraocular, intra-aural	Solutions
	Suspensions
Intranasal	Solutions
	Sprays
	Inhalants
	Ointments
Intrarespiratory	Aerosols
Rectal	Solutions
	Ointments
	Suppositories
Vaginal	Solutions
	Ointments
	Emulsion foams
	Gels
	Tablets
	Inserts, suppositories, sponge
Urethral	Solutions
	Suppositories

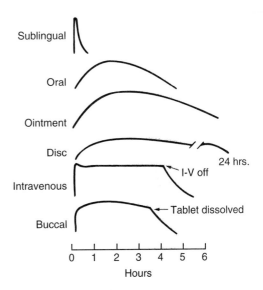

FIGURE 5.10 Blood level curves of nitroglycerin following administration of dosage forms by various routes. (Adapted with permission from Abrams J. Nitroglycerin and long-acting nitrates in clinical practice. Am J Med: Proceedings of the First North American Conference on Nitroglycerin Therapy, June 27, 1983).

5.10 and Table 5.6 demonstrate this for the drug nitroglycerin in various dosage forms. The sublingual, intravenous, and buccal forms present extremely rapid onsets of action, whereas the oral (swallowed), topical ointment, and topical patch present slower onsets of action but greater durations of action. The patch provides the longest duration of action, up to 24 hours following application of a single patch to the skin. The transdermal nitroglycerin patch allows a single daily dose, whereas the other forms require multiple dosing to maintain drug levels within the therapeutic window.

The difference in absorption between dosage forms is a function of the formulation and the route of administration. For example, a problem associated with the oral administration of a drug is that once absorbed through the lumen of the gastrointestinal tract into the portal vein, the drug may pass directly to the liver and undergo the *first-pass effect*. In essence some or all of the drug may be metabolized by the liver. Consequently, its bioavailability is decreased. Thus, the bioavailable fraction is determined by the fraction of drug that is absorbed from the gastrointestinal tract and the fraction that escapes metabolism during its first pass through the liver. The bioavailable

TABLE 5.6 DOSAGE AND KINETICS OF NITROGLYCERIN IN VARIOUS DOSAGE FORMS

NITROGLYCERIN, DOSAGE FORM	USUAL DOSE (MG)	ONSET OF ACTION (MIN)	PEAK ACTION (MIN)	DURATION
Sublingual	0.3–0.8	2–5	4–8	10–30 min
Buccal	1–3	2–5	4–10	30–300 min[a]
Oral	6.5–19.5	20–45	45–120	2–6 hours[b]
Ointment (2%)	0.5–2 inches	15–60	30–120	3–8 hours
Discs	5–10	30–60	60–180	Up to 24 hours

[a]Effect persists so long as tablet is intact.

[b]Some short-term dosing studies have demonstrated effects to 8 hours.

Reprinted with permission from Abrams J. Nitroglycerin and long-acting nitrates in clinical practice. Am J Med. Proceedings of First North American Conference of Nitroglycerin Therapy, June 27, 1983:88.

fraction (f) is the product of these two fractions as follows:

$$f = \text{fraction of drug absorbed} \times \text{fraction escaping first-pass metabolism}$$

The bioavailability is lowest, then, for drugs that undergo a significant first-pass effect. For these drugs, a hepatic extraction ratio, or the fraction of drug metabolized, E, is calculated. The fraction of drug that enters the system circulation and is ultimately available to exert its effect then is equal to the quantity $(1 - E)$. Table 5.7 lists some drugs according to their pharmacologic class that undergo a significant first-pass effect when administered by the oral route.

To compensate for this marked effect, the manufacturer may consider other routes of administration, for example intravenous, intramuscular, or sublingual, that avoid the first-pass effect. Use of these routes must be accompanied by a corresponding adjustment in the dosage.

Another consideration centers on the metabolites themselves and whether they are pharmacologically active or inactive. If they are inactive, a larger oral dose is required to attain the desired therapeutic effect than with a lower dosage in a route with no first-pass effect. The classic example of drug that exhibits this effect is propranolol. However, if the metabolites are the active species, the oral dosage must be carefully tailored to the desired therapeutic effect. First-pass metabolism in this case will result

in a quicker therapeutic response than that achieved by a route with no first-pass effect

Also, the flow of blood through the liver can be decreased under certain conditions. Consequently, the bioavailability of drugs that undergo a first-pass effect can be expected to increase. For example, during cirrhosis the blood flow to the kidney is dramatically decreased, and efficient hepatic extraction by enzymes responsible for a drug's metabolism also falls off. Consequently, in cirrhotic patients the dosage of drug that un-

TABLE 5.7 SOME DRUGS THAT UNDERGO SIGNIFICANT LIVER METABOLISM AND EXHIBIT LOW BIOAVAILABILITY WHEN ADMINISTERED BY FIRST-PASS ROUTES

DRUG CLASS	EXAMPLES
Analgesic	Aspirin, meperidine, pentazocine, propoxyphene
Antianginal	Nitroglycerin
Antiarrhythmic	Lidocaine
Beta-adrenergic blocker	Labetolol, metoprolol, propranolol
Calcium channel blocker	Verapamil
Sympathomimetic amine	Isoproterenol
Tricyclic antidepressant	Desipramine, imipramine, nortriptyline

dergoes a first-pass effect from oral administration will have to be reduced to avoid toxicity.

Oral Route

Drugs are most frequently taken by oral administration. Although a few drugs taken orally are intended to be dissolved in the mouth, nearly all drugs taken orally are swallowed. Of these, most are taken for the *systemic* drug effects that result after absorption from the various surfaces along the gastrointestinal tract. A few drugs, such as antacids, are swallowed for their local action in the gastrointestinal tract.

Compared with alternative routes, the oral route is considered the most natural, uncomplicated, convenient, and safe means of administering drugs. Disadvantages of the oral route include slow drug response (compared with parenterally administered drugs); chance of irregular absorption of drugs, depending upon such factors as constitutional makeup and the amount or type of food in the gastrointestinal tract; and the destruction of certain drugs by the acid reaction of the stomach or by gastrointestinal enzymes.

Dosage Forms Applicable

Drugs are administered by the oral route in a variety of pharmaceutical forms. The most popular are tablets, capsules, suspensions, and various pharmaceutical solutions. Briefly, *tablets* are solid dosage forms prepared by compression or molding that contain medicinal substances with or without suitable diluents, disintegrants, coatings, colorants, and other pharmaceutical adjuncts. Diluents are fillers used to prepare tablets of the proper size and consistency. Disintegrants are used for the breakup or separation of the tablet's compressed ingredients. This ensures prompt exposure of drug particles to the dissolution process, enhancing drug absorption, as shown in Figure 5.11. Tablet coatings are of several types and for several purposes. Some, called *enteric coatings*, are employed to permit safe passage of a tablet through the acid environment of the stomach, where certain drugs may be destroyed, to the more suitable juices of the intestines, where tablet dissolution safely takes

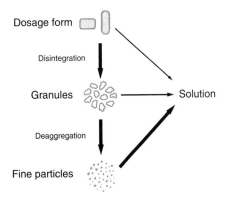

FIGURE 5.11 Disintegration of a tablet dosage form and direct availability of the contents in a capsule dosage form for dissolution and drug absorption after oral administration. (Adapted with permission from Rowland M, Tozer TN. Clinical pharmacokinetics, 2nd ed. Philadelphia: Lea & Febiger, 1989).

place. Other coatings protect the drug substance from the destructive influences of moisture, light, and air during storage or to conceal a bad or bitter taste from the taste buds of a patient. Commercial tablets, because of their distinctive shapes, colors, and frequently employed monograms of company symbols and code numbers, facilitate identification by persons trained in their use and serve as an added protection to public health.

Capsules are solid dosage forms in which the drug substance and appropriate pharmaceutical adjuncts, such as fillers, are enclosed in either a hard or a soft shell, generally composed of a form of gelatin. Capsules vary in size, depending on the amount of drug to be administered, and have distinctive shapes and colors when produced commercially. Drug materials are released from capsules faster than from tablets. Capsules of gelatin, a protein, are rapidly disfigured within the gastrointestinal tract, permitting the gastric juices to permeate and reach the contents. Because unsealed capsules have been subject to tampering by unscrupulous individuals, many capsules nowadays are sealed by fusion of the two capsule shells. Also, capsule-shaped and coated tablets, called caplets, are increasingly used. These are easily swallowed, but their contents are sealed and protected from tampering like tablets.

Suspensions are preparations of finely divided drugs in a suitable fluid vehicle. Suspensions taken orally generally employ an aqueous vehicle, whereas those employed for other purposes may use a different vehicle. Suspensions of certain drugs to be used for intramuscular injection, for instance, may be maintained in a suitable oil. To be suspended, the drug particles must be insoluble in the vehicle. Nearly all suspensions must be shaken before use because they tend to settle. This ensures both uniformity of the preparation and more important, the administration of the proper dosage. Suspensions are a useful means to administer large amounts of solid drugs that would be inconvenient to take in tablet or capsule form. In addition, suspensions have the advantage over solid dosage forms in that they are presented to the body in fine particle size, ready for dissolution immediately upon administration. However, not all oral suspensions are intended to be dissolved and absorbed by the body. For instance, kaolin mixture with pectin, an antidiarrheal preparation, contains suspended kaolin, which acts in the intestinal tract by adsorbing excessive intestinal fluid on the large surface area of its particles.

Drugs administered in aqueous *solution* are absorbed much more rapidly than those administered in solid form, because disintegration and dissolution are not required. Pharmaceutical solutions may differ in the type of solvent employed and therefore in their fluidity characteristics. Among the solutions frequently administered orally are *elixirs*, which are solutions in a sweetened hydroalcoholic vehicle and are more mobile than water; *syrups*, which generally use a sucrose solution as the sweet vehicle, resulting in a viscous preparation; and *solutions* themselves, which officially are preparations in which the drug substance is dissolved predominantly in an aqueous vehicle and do not for reasons of their method of preparation (e.g., injections, which must be sterilized) fall into another category of pharmaceutical preparations.

Absorption

Absorption of drugs after oral administration may occur at the various body sites between the mouth and rectum. In general, the higher up a drug is absorbed along the alimentary tract, the more rapid will be its action, a desirable feature in most instances. Because of the differences in chemical and physical nature among drug substances, a given drug may be better absorbed from one site than from another in the alimentary tract.

Sometimes the oral cavity is the absorption site. Physically, oral absorption of drugs is managed by allowing the drug substance to dissolve within the oral cavity with little or no swallowing until the taste of the drug has dissipated. This process is accommodated by providing the drug as extremely soluble and rapidly dissolving uncoated tablets. Drugs capable of being absorbed in the mouth present themselves to the absorbing surface in a much more concentrated form than when swallowed, since drugs become progressively more diluted with gastrointestinal secretions and contents as they pass along the alimentary tract.

The oral or *sublingual* (beneath the tongue) administration of drugs is regularly used for only a few drugs, with nitroglycerin and certain steroid sex hormones being the best examples. Nitroglycerin, a coronary vasodilator used in the prophylaxis and treatment of angina pectoris, is available in the form of tiny tablets that are allowed to dissolve under the tongue, producing therapeutic effects a few minutes after administration. The dose of nitroglycerin is so small (usually 400 μg) that if it were swallowed, the resulting dilute gastrointestinal concentration might not result in reliable and sufficient drug absorption. Even more important, however, is the fact that nitroglycerin is rapidly destroyed by the liver through the *first-pass effect*. Many sex hormones have been shown to be absorbed materially better from sublingual administration than when swallowed. Although the sublingual route is probably an effective absorption route for many other drugs, it has not been extensively used, primarily because other routes have proven satisfactory and more convenient for the patient. Retaining drug substances in the mouth is unattractive because of the bitter taste of most drugs.

Drugs may be altered within the gastrointestinal tract to render them less available for absorption. This may result from the drug's interaction with or binding to some normal constituent of the gastrointestinal tract or a foodstuff or even another drug. For instance, the absorption of the tetracycline group of antibiotics is greatly interfered with by the simultaneous presence of calcium. Because of this, tetracycline drugs must not be taken with milk or other calcium-containing foods or drugs.

Sometimes the pharmacist intends to prepare a formulation that releases the drug slowly over an extended time. There are many methods by which slow release is accomplished, including the complexation of the drug with another material, the combination of which is only slowly released from the dosage form. An example of this is slow-release waxy-matrix potassium chloride tablets. These are designed to release their contents gradually as they are shunted through the gastrointestinal tract. Because their contents are leached out gradually, there is little incidence of gastric irritation. The intermingling of food and drug generally results in delayed drug absorption. Since most drugs are absorbed more effectively from the intestines than from the stomach, when rapid absorption is intended, it is generally desirable to have the drug pass from the stomach into the intestines as rapidly as possible. Therefore, gastric emptying time is an important factor in drug action dependent on intestinal absorption. Gastric emptying time may be increased by a number of factors, including the presence of fatty foods (more effect than proteins, which in turn have more effect than carbohydrates) or lying on the back when bedridden (lying on the right side facilitates passage in many instances), or decreased, as by the presence of drugs (e.g., morphine) that have a quieting effect on the movements of the gastrointestinal tract. If a drug is administered in the form of a solution, it may be expected to pass into the intestines more rapidly than drugs administered in solid form. As a rule, large volumes of water taken with medication facilitate gastric emptying and passage into the intestines.

The pH of the gastrointestinal tract increases progressively along its length from about pH 1 in the stomach to approximately pH 8 at the far end of the intestines. pH has a definite bearing on the degree of ionization of most drugs, and this in turn affects lipid solubility, membrane permeability, and absorption. Because most drugs are absorbed by passive diffusion through the lipoid barrier, the lipid–water partition coefficient and the pK_a of the drugs are of prime importance to both the degree and the site of absorption within the gastrointestinal tract. As a general rule, weak acids are largely *un-ionized* in the stomach and are absorbed fairly well from this site, whereas weak bases are highly ionized in the stomach and are not significantly absorbed from the gastric surface. Alkalinization of the gastric environment by artificial means (simultaneous administration of alkaline or antacid drugs) would be expected to decrease the gastric absorption of weak acids and to increase that of weak bases. Strong acids and bases are generally poorly absorbed because of their high degree of ionization.

The small intestine serves as the major absorption pathway for drugs because of its suitable pH and the great surface area available for drug absorption along its approximately 20-foot length from the pylorus at the base of the stomach to the large intestine at the cecum. The pH of the lumen of the intestine is about 6.5 (Fig. 5.3), and both weakly acidic and weakly basic drugs are well absorbed from the intestinal surface, which behaves in the ionization and distribution of drugs between it and the plasma on the other side of the membrane as though its pH were about 5.3.

Rectal Route

Some drugs are administered rectally for their local effects and others for their systemic effects. Drugs given rectally may be administered as solutions, suppositories, or ointments. *Suppositories* are solid bodies of various weights and shapes intended for introduction into a body orifice (usually rectal, vaginal, or urethral) where they soften, melt, or dissolve, release their medication, and exert their drug effects. These effects simply may be the promotion of laxation (as with glycerin suppositories), the soothing of inflamed tissues (as with various commercial suppositories used to relieve the discomfort of hemorrhoids), or the promotion of systemic effects (as antinausea or anti motion sickness). The composition of the suppository base, or carrier, can greatly influence the degree and rate of drug release and should be selected on an individual basis for each drug. The use of rectal ointments is generally limited to the treatment of local conditions. Rectal solutions are usually employed as enemas or cleansing solutions.

The rectum and the colon can absorb many soluble drugs. Rectal administration for systemic action may be preferred for drugs destroyed or inactivated by the environments of the stomach and intestines. The administration of drugs by the rectal route may also be indicated when the oral route is precluded because of vomiting or when the patient is unconscious or incapable of swallowing drugs safely without choking. Approximately 50% of a dose of drug absorbed from rectal administration is likely to bypass the liver, an important factor when considering orally administered drugs that are rapidly destroyed in the liver by the first-pass effect. On the negative side, compared with oral administration, rectal administration of drugs is inconvenient, and the absorption of drugs from the rectum is frequently irregular and difficult to predict.

Parenteral Route

The term *parenteral* is derived from the Greek words *para*, meaning beside, and *enteron*, meaning intestine, which together indicate something done outside of the intestine and not by way of the alimentary tract. A drug administered parenterally is one injected through the hollow of a fine needle into the body at various sites and to various depths. The three primary routes of parenteral administration are subcutaneous, intramuscular, and intravenous, although there are others, such as intracardiac and intraspinal.

Drugs destroyed or inactivated in the gastrointestinal tract or too poorly absorbed to provide satisfactory response may be parenterally administered. The parenteral route is also preferred when rapid absorption is essential, as

in emergencies. Absorption by the parenteral route is not only faster than after oral administration, but the blood levels of drug that result are far more predictable, because little is lost after subcutaneous or intramuscular injection and virtually none by intravenous injection; this also generally permits the administration of smaller doses. The parenteral route of administration is especially useful in treating patients who are uncooperative, unconscious, or otherwise unable to accept oral medication.

One disadvantage of parenteral administration is that once the drug is injected, there is no retreat. That is, once the substance is in the tissues or blood stream, removal of the drug warranted by an untoward or toxic effect or an inadvertent overdose is most difficult. By other means of administration, there is more time between drug administration and drug absorption, which becomes a safety factor by allowing for the extraction of unabsorbed drug (as by the induction of vomiting after an orally administered drug). Also, because of the strict sterility requirements for all injections, they are more expensive than other dosage forms and require competent trained personnel for proper administration.

Dosage Forms Applicable

Pharmaceutically, most injectable preparations are either a sterile suspension or solution of a drug substance in water or in a suitable vegetable oil. Drugs in solution act more rapidly than drugs in suspension, with an aqueous vehicle providing faster action in each instance than an oleaginous vehicle. As in other instances of drug absorption, a drug must be in solution to be absorbed, and a suspended drug must first submit to dissolution. Also, because body fluids are aqueous, they are more receptive to drugs in an aqueous vehicle than those in an oily one. For these reasons, the rate of drug absorption can be varied in parenteral products by selective combinations of drug state and supporting vehicle. For instance, a suspension of a drug in a vegetable oil is likely to be much more slowly absorbed than an aqueous solution of the same drug. Slow absorption means prolonged drug action, and when this is achieved through pharmaceutical means, the resulting preparation is referred to as a *depot* or *repository* injection, because it provides a storage reservoir of the drug substance within the body from which it is slowly removed into the systemic circulation. In this regard, even more sustained drug action may be achieved through the use of subcutaneous implantation of compressed tablets, termed pellets, that are only slowly dissolved from their site of implantation, releasing their medication at a fairly constant rate over several weeks to many months. The repository type of injection is mainly limited to the subcutaneous or intramuscular route. It is obvious that drugs injected intravenously do not encounter absorption barriers and thus produce only rapid drug effects. Preparations for intravenous injection must not interfere with the blood components or with circulation and therefore, with few exceptions, are aqueous solutions.

Subcutaneous Injections

The subcutaneous (hypodermic) administration of drugs entails injection through the skin into the loose subcutaneous tissue. Subcutaneous injections are prepared as aqueous solutions or as suspensions and are administered in relatively small volumes, 2 mL or less. Insulin is an example of a drug administered by the subcutaneous route. Subcutaneous injections are generally given in the forearm, upper arm, thigh, or buttocks. If the patient is to receive frequent injections, it is best to alternate injection sites to reduce tissue irritation. After injection, the drug comes into the immediate vicinity of blood capillaries and permeates them by diffusion or filtration. The capillary wall is an example of a membrane that behaves as a lipid pore barrier, with lipid-soluble substances penetrating the membrane at rates varying with their oil–water partition coefficients. Lipid-insoluble (generally more water soluble) drugs penetrate the capillary membrane at rates that appear to be inversely related to their molecular size, with smaller molecules penetrating much more rapidly than larger ones. All substances, whether lipid soluble or not, cross the capillary membrane much

more rapidly than other body membranes. The blood supply to the site of injection is an important factor in considering the rate of drug absorption; consequently, the closer capillaries are to the site of injection, the more prompt is the drug's entrance into the circulation. Also, the more capillaries, the more surface area for absorption and the faster the rate of absorption. Some substances modify the rate of drug absorption from a subcutaneous site of injection. The addition of a vasoconstrictor to the injection formulation (or its prior injection) will generally diminish the rate of drug absorption by causing constriction of the blood vessels in the area of injection and thereby reducing blood flow and the capacity for absorption. This principle is used in the administration of local anesthetics by use of the vasoconstrictor epinephrine. Conversely, vasodilators may be used to enhance subcutaneous absorption by increasing blood flow to the area. Physical exercise can also influence the absorption of drug from an injection site. Diabetic patients who rotate subcutaneous injection sites and then do physical exercise such as jogging must realize that the onset of insulin activity may be influenced by the selected site of administration. Because of the movement of the leg and blood circulation to it during running, the absorption of insulin from a thigh injection site can be expected to be faster than from an abdominal injection site.

Intramuscular Injections

Intramuscular injections are performed deep into the skeletal muscles, generally the gluteal or lumbar muscles. The selected site is where the danger of hitting a nerve or blood vessel is minimal. Aqueous or oleaginous solutions or suspensions may be used intramuscularly. Certain drugs, because of their inherent low solubility, provide sustained drug action after an intramuscular injection. For instance, one deep intramuscular injection of a suspension of penicillin G benzathine results in effective blood levels of the drug for 7 to 10 days.

Drugs that are irritating to subcutaneous tissue are often administered intramuscularly. Also, greater volumes (2–5 mL) may be administered intramuscularly than subcutaneously. When a volume greater than 5 mL is to be injected, it is frequently administered in divided doses to two injection sites. Injection sites are best rotated when a patient is receiving repeated injections over time.

Intravenous Injections

In the intravenous administration of drugs, an aqueous solution is injected directly into the vein at a rate commensurate with efficiency, safety, comfort to the patient, and the desired duration of drug response. Drugs may be administered intravenously as a single, small-volume injection or as a large-volume slow intravenous drip infusion (as is common following surgery). Intravenous injection allows the desired blood level of drug to be achieved in an optimal and quantitative manner. Intravenous injections are usually made into the veins of the forearm and are especially useful in emergencies when immediate drug response is desired. It is essential that the drug be maintained in solution after injection and not be precipitated within the circulatory system, an event that might produce emboli. Because of a fear of the development of pulmonary embolism, oleaginous vehicles are not usually intravenously administered. However, an intravenous fat emulsion is used for patients receiving parenteral nutrition whose caloric requirements cannot be met by glucose. It may be administered either through a peripheral vein or a central venous catheter at a distinct rate to help prevent untoward reactions.

Intradermal Injections

Intradermal injections are administered into the corium of the skin, usually in volumes of about 0.1 mL. Common sites for the injection are the arm and the back. The injections are frequently performed as diagnostic measures, as in tuberculin and allergy testing.

Epicutaneous Route

Drugs are administered topically, or applied to the skin, for their action at the site of application or for systemic drug effects.

Drug absorption via the skin is enhanced if the drug substance is in solution, if it has a favorable lipid–water partition coefficient, and if it is not an electrolyte. Drugs that are absorbed enter the skin by way of the pores, sweat glands, hair follicles, sebaceous glands, and other anatomic structures of the skin's surface. Because blood capillaries lie just below the epidermal cells, a drug that penetrates the skin and is able to traverse the capillary wall finds ready access to the general circulation.

Among the few drugs applied to the skin surface for percutaneous absorption and systemic action are nitroglycerin (antianginal), nicotine (smoking cessation), estradiol (estrogenic hormone), clonidine (antihypertensive), and scopolamine (antinausea, anti–motion sickness). Each of these drugs is available for use in a transdermal delivery system fabricated as an adhesive disc or patch that slowly releases the medication for percutaneous absorption. Additionally, nitroglycerin is available in an ointment for application to the skin for systemic absorption. Nitroglycerin is used therapeutically for ischemic heart disease, with the transdermal dosage forms becoming increasingly popular because of the benefit in patient compliance through their long-acting (24 hours) characteristics. The nitroglycerin patch is generally applied to the arm or chest, preferably in a hair-free or shaven area. The transdermal scopolamine system is also in the form of a patch to be applied to the skin, in this case behind the ear, for the prevention of nausea and vomiting associated with motion sickness. The commercial product is applied several hours before need (as prior to an air or sea trip), where it releases its medication over 3 days. The concepts of transdermal therapeutic systems are discussed further in Chapter 11.

For the most part, pharmaceutical preparations applied to the skin are intended to serve some local action and as such are formulated to provide prolonged local contact with minimal absorption. Drugs applied to the skin for their local action include antiseptics, antifungal agents, anti-inflammatory agents, local anesthetic agents, skin emollients, and protectants against environmental conditions, such as the effects of the sun, wind, pests, and chemical irritants. For these purposes, drugs are most commonly administered in the form of ointments and related semisolid preparations such as creams and pastes, as solid dry powders or aerosol sprays or as liquid preparations such as solutions and lotions.

Pharmaceutically, ointments, creams, and pastes are semisolid preparations in which the drug is contained in a suitable base (ointment base), which is itself semisolid and either hydrophilic or hydrophobic. These bases play an important role in the proper formulation of semisolid preparations, and there is no single base universally suitable as a carrier of all drug substances or for all therapeutic indications. The proper base for a drug must be determined individually to provide the desired drug release rate, staying qualities after application, and texture. Briefly, *ointments* are simple mixtures of drug substances in an ointment base, whereas *creams* are semisolid emulsions less viscid and lighter than ointments. Creams are considered to have greater esthetic appeal for their nongreasy character, ability to vanish into the skin upon rubbing, and ability to absorb serous discharges from skin lesions. *Pastes* contain more solid materials than do ointments and are therefore stiffer and less penetrating. Pastes are usually employed for their protective action. Thus, when protective rather than therapeutic action is desired, the formulation pharmacist will favor a paste, but when therapeutic action is required, he will prefer ointments and creams. Commercially, many therapeutic agents are prepared in both ointment and cream form and are dispensed and used according to the particular preference of the patient and the prescribing practitioner.

Medicinal powders are intimate mixtures of medicinal substances usually in an inert base such as talcum powder or starch. Depending on the particle size of the resulting blend, the powder will have varying dusting and covering capabilities. In any case, the particle should be small enough to ensure against grittiness and consequent skin irritation. Powders are most frequently applied topically to relieve such conditions as diaper rash, chafing, and athlete's foot.

When topical application is desired in liquid form other than solution, lotions are most fre-quently employed. *Lotions* are emulsions or suspensions generally in an aqueous vehicle, although certain solutions have been designated as lotions because of either their appearance or application. Lotions may be preferred over semisolid preparations because of their nongreasy character and their increased spreadability over large areas of skin.

Ocular, Oral, and Nasal Routes

Drugs are frequently applied topically to the eye, ear, and mucous membranes of the nose, usually as ointments, suspensions, and solutions. Ophthalmic solutions and suspensions are sterile aqueous preparations with other ingredients essential to the safety and comfort of the patient. Ophthalmic ointments must be sterile and free of grit. Innovative new delivery systems for ophthalmic drugs continue to be investigated. One dosage form, the Ocusert, is an elliptical unit designed for continuous release of pilocarpine following placement in the cul-de-sac of the eye. Also, case reports of the ability of soft contact lenses to absorb drug from the eye have spawned research on soft contact lenses impregnated with drug. Most nasal preparations are solutions or suspensions administered by drops or as a fine mist. Research is directed toward the feasibility of nasal administration of insulin for diabetes mellitus. Ear preparations are usually viscid so that they have prolonged contact with the affected area. They may be employed simply to soften ear wax, to relieve an earache, or to combat an ear infection. Eye, ear, and nose preparations usually are not used for systemic effects, and although ophthalmic and otic preparations are not usually absorbed to any great extent, nasal preparations *may* be absorbed, and systemic effects after the intranasal application of solution are fairly common.

Other Routes

The lungs provide an excellent absorbing surface for the administration of gases and for aerosol mists of very minute particles of liquids or solids. The gas is usually oxygen, and the drugs are the common general anesthetics administered to patients entering surgery. The rich capillary area of the alveoli of the lungs, which in man covers nearly a thousand square feet, provides rapid absorption and drug effects comparable in speed with those following an intravenous injection. In the case of drug particles, their size largely determines the depth to which they penetrate the alveolar regions; their solubility, the extent to which they are absorbed. After contact with the inner surface of the lungs, an insoluble drug particle is caught in the mucus and is moved up the pulmonary tree by ciliary action. Soluble drug particles that are approximately 0.5 to 1.0 μ in size reach the minute alveolar sacs and are most prompt and efficient in providing systemic effects. Particles smaller than 0.5 μ are expired to some extent, and thus their absorption is not total but variable. Particles 1 to 10 μ effectively reach the terminal bronchioles and to some extent the alveolar ducts and are favored for local therapy. Therefore, in the pharmaceutical manufacture of aerosol sprays for inhalation therapy, the manufacturers not only must attain the proper drug particle size but also must ensure their uniformity for consistent penetration of the pulmonary tree and uniform effects.

In certain instances and for local effects, drugs are inserted into the vagina or the urethra. Drugs are usually presented to the vagina in tablet or other form, such as a suppository, ointment, emulsion foam, gel or solution, and to the urethra as a suppository or solution. Systemic drug effects may result after vaginal or urethral application of drugs following absorption of the drug from the mucous membranes of these sites.

Fate of Drug After Absorption

After absorption into the general circulation from any route of administration, a drug may become bound to blood proteins and delayed in its passage into the surrounding tissues. Many drug substances are highly bound to blood protein and others minimally bound. For instance, in the blood stream naproxen is 99% bound to plasma proteins, penicillin G is 60% bound, amoxicillin only 20% bound, and minoxidil is unbound.

The degree of drug binding to plasma proteins is usually expressed as a percentage or as a fraction (termed *alpha*, or α) of the bound concentration (C_b) to the total concentration (C_t), bound plus unbound (C_u) drug:

$$\alpha = \frac{C_b}{C_u + C_b} = \frac{C_b}{C_t}$$

Thus, if one knows two of the three terms in the equation, the third may be calculated. Drugs having an alpha value above 0.9 are considered highly bound (90%); drugs with an alpha value below 0.2 are considered to be minimally (20% or less) protein bound. Table 5.8 presents approximate serum protein binding characteristics for representative drugs in the blood under conditions associated with usual therapy. The drug–protein complex, which is reversible, involves albumin, although globulins also participate in the binding of drugs, particularly some of the hormones. The binding of drugs to biologic materials entails the formation of relatively weak bonds (e.g., van der Waals, hydrogen, and ionic bonds). The binding capacity of blood proteins is limited, and once they are saturated, additional drug absorbed into the blood stream remains unbound unless bound drug is released, creating a vacant site for another drug molecule to attach. Any unbound drug is free to leave the blood stream for tissues or cellular sites within the body.

Bound drug is neither exposed to the body's detoxication (metabolism) processes nor is it filtered through the renal glomeruli. Bound drug is therefore referred to as the *inactive* portion in the blood, and unbound drug, with its ability to penetrate cells, is termed the *active* blood portion. The bound portion of drug serves as a reservoir or depot from which the drug is released as the free form when the level of free drug in the blood no longer is adequate to ensure protein saturation. The free drug may be only slowly released, which prolongs the drug's stay in the body. For this reason a drug that is highly protein bound may remain in the body longer and require less frequent dosage than another drug that is only slightly protein bound and remains in the body for only a short period. Evidence suggests that the concentra-

TABLE 5.8 EXAMPLES OF DRUG BINDING TO PLASMA PROTEINS

DRUG	PERCENT BOUND
Naproxen (Naprosyn)	>99
Chlorambucil (Leukeran)	>99
Etodolac (Lodine)	>99
Warfarin (Coumadin)	>97
Fluoxetine (Prozac)	>95
Cloxacillin (Tegopen)	>95
Ceftriaxone (Rocephin)	85–95
Cefoperazone (Cefobid)	82–93
Cefonicid (Monocid)	>90
Indomethacin (Indocin)	>90
Spironolactone (Aldactone)	>90
Digitoxin (Crystodigin)	>90
Cyclosporine (Sandimmune)	>90
Sulfisoxazole (Gantrisin)	>85
Diltiazem (Cardizem)	70–80
Penicillin V (Veetids)	>75
Nitroglycerin (Nitro-Bid)	>60
Penicillin G potassium	>60
Methotrexate	>50
Methicillin (Staphcillin)	>40
Ceftizoxime (Cefizox)	>30
Captopril (Capozide)	25–30
Ciprofloxacin (Cipro)	20–40
Digoxin (Lanoxin)	20–25
Ampicillin (Omnipen)	>20
Amoxicillin (Amoxil)	>20
Metronidazole (Flagyl)	<20
Mercaptopurine (Purinethol)	>19
Cephradine (Velosef)	8–17
Ranitidine (Zantac)	>15
Ceftazidime (Tazicef)	<10
Nicotine (ProStep)	<5
Minoxidil (Loniten)	> 0

Average literature values based on conditions usually associated with drug therapy.

tion of serum albumin decreases about 20% in the elderly. This may be clinically significant for drugs that bind strongly to albumin, for example phenytoin, because if there is less albumin available to bind the drug, there will be a corresponding increase of the free drug in the body. Without a downward dosage adjustment in an elderly patient, there could be an increased incidence of adverse effects.

A drug's binding to blood proteins may be affected by the simultaneous presence of another drug or drugs. The additional drug or drugs may produce effects or duration of action quite dissimilar to that found when each is administered alone. Salicylates, for instance, decrease the binding capacity of thyroxin, the thyroid hormone, to proteins. Through this action, the displaced drugs become less protein bound and their activity (and toxicity) may be increased. The intensity of a drug's pharmacologic response is related to the ratio of the bound drug to free active drug and to the therapeutic index of the drug. Warfarin, an anticoagulant, is 97% bound to plasma protein, leaving 3% in free form to exert its effect. If a second drug, such as naproxen, which is strongly bound to plasma proteins, is administered and results in only 90% of the warfarin being bound, 10% of warfarin will be in the free form. Thus, the blood level of the free warfarin (3 to 10%) will triple and possibly result in serious toxicity. The displacement of drugs from plasma protein sites is typical in the elderly, who normally take numerous medicines. Coupled with the aforementioned decrease in serum protein through the aging process, the addition of a highly protein-bound drug to an elderly patient's treatment regimen may pose significant problems if the patient is not monitored carefully for signs of toxicity.

In the same manner as they are bound to blood proteins, drugs may become bound to specific components of certain cells. Thus drugs are not distributed uniformly among all cells of the body, but rather tend to pass from the blood into the fluid bathing the tissues and may accumulate in certain cells according to their permeability and chemical and physical affinities. This affinity for certain body sites influences their action, for they may be brought into contact with reactive tissues (their *receptor sites*) or deposited in places where they are inactive. Many drugs, because of their affinity for and solubility in lipids, are deposited in fatty body tissue, creating a reservoir from which they are slowly released to other tissues.

Drug Metabolism, or Biotransformation

Although some drugs are excreted from the body in their original form, many drugs undergo biotransformation prior to excretion. Biotransformation indicates the chemical changes to drugs within the body as they are metabolized and altered by various biochemical mechanisms. The biotransformation of a drug results in its conversion to one or more compounds that are more water soluble, more ionized, less capable of binding to proteins of the plasma and tissues, less capable of being stored in fat tissue, and less able to penetrate cell membranes, and thereby less active pharmacologically. Because of its new characteristics, a drug so transformed is rendered less toxic and is more readily excreted. It is for this reason that biotransformation is also commonly called detoxification or inactivation. (However, sometimes the metabolites are more active than the parent compound; see *prodrugs*, following.)

The exact metabolic processes (pathways) by which drugs are transformed are an active area of biomedical research. Much work has been done with the processes of animal degradation of drugs, and in many instances the biotransformation in the animal is thought to parallel that in man. Four principal chemical reactions are involved in the metabolism of drugs: oxidation, reduction, hydrolysis, and conjugation. Most oxidation reactions are catalyzed by enzymes (oxidases) bound to the endoplasmic reticulum, a tubular system in liver cells. Only a small fraction of drugs are metabolized by reduction, through the action of reductases in the gut and liver. Esterases in the liver participate in the hydrolytic breakdown of drugs containing ester groups and amides. Glucuronide conjugation is the most common pathway for drug metabolism, through combination of the drug with glucuronic acid, forming ionized compounds that are easily eliminated via the urine (8). Other metabolic processes, including methylation and acylation conjugation reactions, occur with certain drugs to foster elimination.

In recent years, much interest has been shown in the metabolites of drug biotransformation. Certain metabolites may be as active as or even more active pharmacologically than the original compound. Occasionally an active drug is converted into an active metabolite, which must be excreted as such or undergo further biotransformation to an inactive metabolite, for example amitriptyline to nortriptyline. In other instances of drug therapy, an inactive parent compound, referred to as a *prodrug*, may be converted to an active therapeutic agent by chemical transformation in the body. An example is the prodrug enalapril (Vasotec), which after oral administration is hydrolyzed to enalaprilat, an active angiotensin-converting enzyme inhibitor used in the treatment of hypertension. Enalaprilat itself is poorly absorbed when taken orally (and thus the prodrug) but may be administered intravenously in aqueous solution. The use of these active metabolites as original drugs is a new area of investigation and a vast reservoir of potential therapeutic agents.

Several examples of biotransformations occurring within the body are as follows:

(1) Acetaminophen $\xrightarrow{\text{conjugation}}$ Acetaminophen glucuronide
    (active)   (inactive)

(2) Amoxapine $\xrightarrow{\text{oxidation}}$ 8-hydroxy-amoxapine
    (active)   (inactive)

(3) Procainamide $\xrightarrow{\text{hydrolysis}}$ p-Aminobenzoic acid
    (active)   (inactive)

(4) Nitroglycerin $\xrightarrow{\text{reduction}}$ 1–2 and 1–3 dinitroglycerol
    (active)   (inactive)

Some parent compounds undergo full, partial, or no biotransformation following administration. Lisinopril (Zestril), for example, does not undergo metabolism and is excreted unchanged in the urine. On the other hand, verapamil (Calan) metabolizes to at least 12 metabolites, the most prevalent of which is norverapamil. Norverapamil has 20% of the cardiovascular activity of the parent compound. Diltiazem (Cardizem) is partially metabolized (about 20%) to desacetyl diltiazem, which has 10 to 20% of the coronary vasodilator activity of the parent compound. Indomethacin (Indocin) is metabolized in part to desmethyl, desbenzoyl, and desmethyl desbenzoyl metabolites. Propoxyphene napsylate (Darvon N) is metabolized to norpropoxyphene, which has less central nervous system depressant action than the parent compound but greater local anesthetic effects. Most metabolic transformations takes place in the liver, with some drugs, including diltiazem and verapamil, undergoing extensive first-pass effects. Other drugs, such as terazosin (Hytrin), undergo minimal first-pass metabolism. The excretion of both drug and metabolites takes place primarily but to varying degrees via the urine and feces. For example, indomethacin and its metabolites are excreted primarily (60%) in the urine, with the remainder in the feces, whereas terazosin and its metabolites are excreted largely (60%) through the feces and the remainder in the urine.

Several factors influence drug metabolism. For example, there are marked differences between *species* in pathways of hepatic metabolism of a given drug. Species differences make it extremely difficult to extrapolate from one species to another, as with laboratory animals to humans. Furthermore, there are many examples of *interindividual variations* in hepatic metabolism of drugs within one species. Genetic factors affect the basal activity of the drug-metabolizing enzyme systems. Thus, there can be marked intersubject variation in rates of metabolism. Because of this variation, a physician must individualize therapy to maximize the chances for a constructive therapeutic outcome with minimal toxicity. Studies in humans have demonstrated that these differences have occurred within the cytochrome P-450 genetic codes for a family of isoenzymes responsible for drug metabolism.

Age of the patient is another significant factor in drug metabolism. Although pharmacokinetic calculations have not been able to develop a specific correlative relationship with age, it is known that the ability to metabolize drugs is low at the extremes of the age scale, that is, among the elderly and neonates. Liver blood flow is reduced by aging at about 1% per year beginning around age 30 (9). This decreased blood flow to the liver reduces the capacity for hepatic drug metabolism and elimination. For example, the half-life of chlordiazepoxide increases from about 6 hours at age 20 to about 36 hours at age 80. Furthermore, an immature hepatic system disallows the effective metabolism of drugs by the newborn or premature infant. As mentioned earlier, the half-life of theophylline ranges from 14 to 58 hours in the premature infant to 2.5 to 5 hours in young children aged 1 to 4 whose liver enzyme systems are mature.

Diet has also been demonstrated to modify the metabolism of some drugs. For example, the conversion of an asthmatic patient from a high- to a low-protein diet will increase the half-life of theophylline. It has also been demonstrated that the production of polycyclic hydrocarbons by the charcoal broiling of beef enhances the hepatic metabolism and shortens the plasma half-life of theophylline. It is conceivable that this effect also occurs with drugs that are metabolized in similar fashion to theophylline. Diet type, including starvation and intake of certain vegetables (brussels sprouts, cabbage, broccoli), has been shown to influence the metabolism of certain drugs. Finally, exposure to other drugs or chemicals, such as pesticides, alcohol, and nicotine, and the presence of disease states, such as hepatitis, have all demonstrated an influence on drug metabolism and consequently the pharmacokinetic profile of certain drugs.

Excretion of Drugs

The excretion of drugs and their metabolites terminates their activity and presence in the body. They may be eliminated by various routes, with the kidney playing the dominant role by eliminating drugs via the urine. Drug excretion in the feces is also important, especially for drugs that are poorly absorbed and remain in the gastrointestinal tract after oral administration. Exit through the bile is significant only when reabsorption from the gastrointestinal tract is minimal. The lungs provide the exit for many volatile drugs through the expired breath. The sweat glands, saliva, and milk play only minor roles in drug elimination. However, if a drug gains access to the milk of a mother during lactation, it can easily exert its effects in the nursing infant. Drugs that do enter breast milk and may be passed on to nursing infants include theophylline, penicillin, reserpine, codeine, meperidine, barbiturates, diltiazem, and thiazide diuretics. It is generally good practice for the mother to abstain from taking medication until the infant is weaned. If she must take medication, she should abide by a dosage regimen and nursing schedule that permit her own therapy yet ensure the safety of her child. Not all drugs gain entrance into the milk; nevertheless, caution is advisable. Manufacturers' package inserts contain product-specific information (usually in the section on precautions) on drug migration into breast milk.

The unnecessary use of medications during the early stages of pregnancy is likewise restricted by physicians, because certain drugs are known to cross the placental barrier and gain entrance to the tissues and blood of the fetus. Among the many drugs known to do so are all of the anesthetic gases, many barbiturates, sulfonamides, salicylates, and a number of other potent agents like quinine, meperidine, and morphine, the latter two being narcotic analgesics with great potential for addiction. In fact, it is fairly common for an infant to be born addicted because of the addiction of its mother and the passage of the drugs across the placental barrier.

The kidney, as the main organ for the elimination of drugs from the body, must be functioning adequately if drugs are to be efficiently eliminated. For instance, elimination of digoxin occurs largely through the kidney by first-order kinetics; that is, the quantity of digoxin eliminated at any time is proportional to the total body content. Renal excretion of digoxin is proportional to the glomerular filtration rate, which when normal results in a digoxin half-life that may range from 1.5 to 2 days. When the glomerular filtration rate is impaired or disrupted, however, as in an anuric patient, the elimination rate decreases. Consequently, the half-life of digoxin may be 4 to 6 days. Because of this prolongation of digoxin's half-life, the dosage of the drug must be decreased or the dosage interval prolonged. Otherwise, digoxin toxicity will occur. The degree

of impairment can be estimated by measurements of glomerular filtration rates, most often by creatinine clearance. Usually, however, this is not feasible, and the patient's serum creatinine value is used within appropriate pharmacokinetic equations to help determine a drug's dosage regimen.

Some drugs may be reabsorbed from the renal tubule even having been sent there for excretion. Because the rate of reabsorption is proportional to the concentration of drug in un-ionized form, it is possible to modify this rate by adjusting the pH of the urine. By acidifying the urine, as with the oral administration of ammonium chloride, or by alkalinizing it, as with the administration of sodium bicarbonate, one can increase or decrease the ionization of the drug and thereby alter its prospect of being reabsorbed. Alkalinization of the urine has been shown to enhance the urinary excretion of weak acids such as salicylates, sulfonamides, and phenobarbital. The opposite effect can be achieved by acidifying the urine. Thus, the duration of a drug's stay within the body may be markedly altered by changing the pH of the urine. Some foods, such as cranberry juice, can also acidify the urine and may alter drug excretion rates.

The urinary excretion of drugs may also be retarded by the concurrent administration of agents capable of inhibiting their tubular secretion. A well-known example is the use of probenecid to inhibit the tubular secretion of various types of penicillin, thereby reducing the frequency of dosage administrations usually necessary to maintain adequate therapeutic blood levels of the antibiotic drug. In this particular instance, the elevation of penicillin blood levels, by whatever route the antibiotic is administered, to twofold and even fourfold levels has been demonstrated by adjuvant therapy with probenecid. The effects are completely reversible upon withdrawal of the probenecid from concomitant therapy.

The fecal excretion of drugs appears to lag behind the rate of urinary excretion, partly because a day or so elapses before the feces reach the rectum. Drugs administered orally for local activity within the gastrointestinal tract and not absorbed will be eliminated completely via the feces. Unless a drug is particularly irritating to the gastrointestinal tract, there is generally no urgency about removing unabsorbable drugs from the system by means other than normal defecation. Some drugs that are only partially absorbed after oral administration will naturally be partly eliminated through the rectum.

Pharmacokinetic Principles

This section introduces the concept of pharmacokinetics and how it interrelates the various processes that take place when one administers a drug to a patient, that is, absorption, distribution, metabolism, and excretion. It is not intended to be comprehensive, and thus for further information about the subject the reader is referred to other appropriate literature.

A problem encountered when one needs to determine a more accurate dosage of a drug or a more meaningful interpretation of a biologic response to a dose is the inability to determine the drug concentration at the active site in the body. Consequently, the concept of compartmental analysis is used to determine what has become of the drug as a function of time from the moment it is administered until it is no longer in the body. Pharmacokinetic analysis uses mathematical models to simplify or simulate the disposition of the drug in the body. The idea is to begin with a simple model and then modify as necessary. The principal assumption is that the human body may be represented by one or more *compartments* or pools in which a drug resides in a dynamic state for a short time. A compartment is a hypothetical space bound by an unspecified membrane across which drugs are transferred (Fig. 5.12). The transfer of drugs into and out of this compartment is indicated by arrows that point in the direction of drug movement into or out of the compartment. The rate at which a drug is transferred throughout the system is designated by a symbol that usually represents an exponential rate constant. Typically, the letter K or k with numeric or alphanumeric subscripts is used.

Several assumptions are associated with modeling of drug behavior in the body. It is assumed that the volume of each compartment remains constant. Thus, an equation that de-

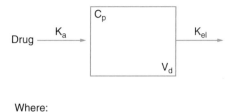

Where:
C_p is the drug concentration in plasma
V_d is the volume of the compartment or volume of distribution

FIGURE 5.12 A one-compartment system.

scribes the time course of the amount of drug in the compartment can be converted to an equation that depicts the time course of the drug concentration in the compartment by dividing both sides of the equation by the volume of the compartment. Second, it is assumed that once a drug enters the compartment, it is instantaneously and uniformly distributed throughout the entire compartment. Thus, it is assumed that a sampling of any one portion of the compartment will yield the drug concentration of the entire compartment.

In compartment models it is assumed that drug passes freely into and out of compartments. Thus, these compartmental systems are known as open systems. Typically, drug transport between compartments follows first-order kinetics, wherein a constant fraction of drug is eliminated per unit of time and can be described by ordinary differential equations. In these linear systems the time constants that describe the rate at which the plasma or blood concentration curve of a drug decays are independent of the dose, the volume of distribution, and the route of administration.

The simplest pharmacokinetic model is the single-compartment *open-model system* (Figure 5.12). This model depicts the body as one compartment characterized by a certain volume of distribution (V_d) that remains constant. Each drug has its own distinct volume of distribution, and this can be influenced by factors including age and disease status. In this scheme a drug can be instantaneously introduced into the compartment, that is, via rapid intravenous administration, or gradually, as with oral administration. In the former case it is assumed that the drug distributes immediately to tissues and instantly attains equilibrium. In the latter case the drug is absorbed at a certain rate and is characterized by the absorption rate constant K_a. Finally, the drug is eliminated from the compartment at a certain rate that is characterized by an elimination rate constant, K_{el}.

It is relevant at this point to consider the *volume of distribution*, V_d, a proportionality constant that refers to the volume into which the total amount of drug in the body must be uniformly distributed to provide the concentration of drug actually measured in plasma or blood. This term can be misleading because it does not represent a specific body fluid or volume. It is influenced by the plasma protein binding and tissue binding of a drug. These then influence the distribution of the drug between plasma water, extracellular fluid, intracellular fluid, and total body water. Furthermore, because a drug can partition between fat and water according to its unique partition coefficient, this can also influence the volume of distribution. Because of these phenomena, pharmacokineticists find it convenient to describe drug distribution in terms of compartmental models.

To determine the rate of drug transfer into and out of the compartment, plasma, serum, or blood samples are drawn at predetermined times after the drug is administered and analyzed for drug concentration. Once a sufficient number of experimental data points is determined, these are plotted on semilogarithmic paper and an attempt is made to fit the experimental points with a smooth curve. Figure 5.13 depicts the plasma concentration–time profile for a hypothetical drug following rapid intravenous injection of a bolus dose of the drug with instantaneous distribution. For drugs whose distribution follows first-order one-compartment pharmacokinetics, a plot of the logarithm of the concentration of drug in the plasma (or blood) versus time will yield a straight line. The equation that describes the plasma decay curve is

$$C_p = C^0_p\, e^{-K_{el}t} \qquad \text{(Equation 5.1)}$$

where

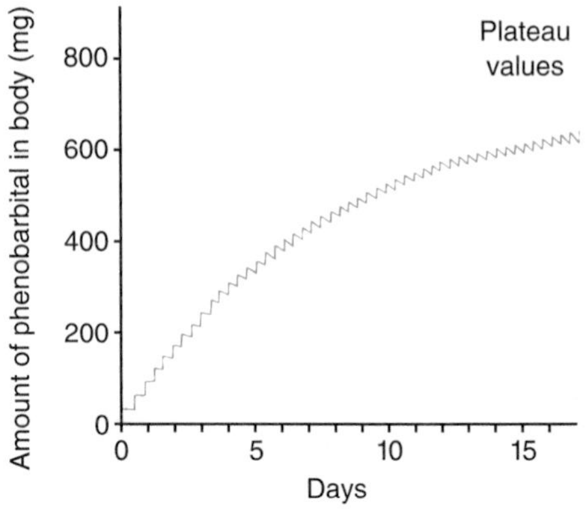

FIGURE 5.13 Plot of the plasma concentration–time data. (Adapted with permission from Rowland M, Tozer TN. Clinical pharmacokinetics, 2nd ed. Philadelphia: Lea & Febiger, 1989.)

K_{el} is the first-order rate of elimination of the drug from the body,

C_p is the concentration of the drug at a time equal to t, and

C^0_p is the concentration of drug at time equal to zero, when all the drug administered has been absorbed but none has been removed from the body through elimination mechanisms, for example, metabolism, renal excretion.

The apparent first-order rate of elimination, K_{el}, is usually the sum of the rate constants of a number of individual processes, for example, metabolic transformation, renal excretion.

For the purpose of pharmacokinetic calculation it is simpler to convert Equation 5.1 to natural logs:

$$\text{Ln } C_p = \text{Ln } C^0_p - K_{el}\,(t) \qquad \text{(Equation 5.2)}$$

and then to log base$_{10}$:

$$\text{Log } C_p = \text{Log } C^0_p - K_{el}\,(t)/2.303 \qquad \text{(Equation 5.3)}$$

Equation 5.3 is then thought of in terms of the Y-intercept form:

$$Y = b + m \times$$
$$\text{Log } C_p = \text{Log } C^0_p - K_{el}/2.303\,(t)$$

and interpreted as such in the semilogarithmic plot illustrated in Figure 5.14. Most drugs administered orally can be adequately described using a one-compartment model, whereas drugs administered by rapid intravenous infusion are usually best described by a two-compartment or three-compartment model system.

Assuming that a drug's volume of distribution is constant within this system, the total amount of drug in the body (Q_b) can be calculated from the following equation:

$$Q_b = [C^0_p] [V_d] \qquad \text{(Equation 5.4)}$$

Usually, C^0_p is determined by extrapolating the drug concentration–time plot to time zero.

In this simple one-compartment system it is assumed that the administered drug is confined to the plasma (or blood) and then excreted. Drugs that exhibit this behavior have small volumes of distribution. For example, a drug such as warfarin, which is extensively bound to plasma albumin, will have a volume of distribution equivalent to that of plasma water, about 2.8 L in an average 70-kg adult. Some drugs, however, are initially distributed at somewhat different rates in various fluids and tissues. Consequently, these drugs' kinetic behavior can best be illustrated by considering an expansion of the one-compartment system to the *two-compartment model* (Fig. 5.15).

In the two-compartment system, a drug enters into and is instantaneously distributed

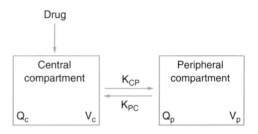

Where:
Q_c = Quantity of drug in central compartment
V_c = Volume of the central compartment
Q_p = Quantity of drug in peripheral compartment
V_p = Volume of the peripheral compartment

FIGURE 5.15 A two-compartment system.

throughout the central compartment. Its subsequent distribution into the second or peripheral compartment is slower. For simplicity, on the basis of blood perfusion and tissue–plasma partition coefficients for a given drug, various tissues and organs are considered together and designated either central compartment or peripheral compartment. The central compartment is usually considered to include the blood, the extracellular space, and organs with good blood perfusion, such as lungs, liver, kidneys, and heart. The peripheral compartment usually comprises tissues and organs that are poorly perfused by blood, such as skin, bone, and fat.

Figure 5.16 depicts the plasma drug concentration–time plot for a rapidly administered intravenous dose of a hypothetical drug that exhibits kinetic behavior exemplifying a two-compartment system. Note the initial steep decline of the plasma drug concentration curve. This typifies the distribution of the drug from the central compartment to the peripheral compartment. During this phase the drug concentration in the plasma will decrease more rapidly than in the postdistributive or elimination phase. Whether this distributive phase is apparent depends on the timing of the plasma samples, particularly in the time immediately following administration. A distributive phase can be very short, a few minutes, or last for hours and even days.

A semilogarithmic plot of the plasma concentration versus time after rapid intravenous

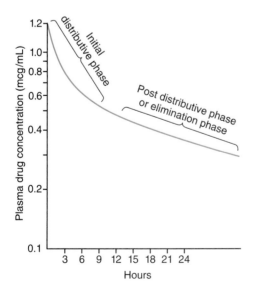

FIGURE 5.14 A semilogarithmic plot of plasma concentration versus time of an intravenous drug that follows first-order two-compartment pharmacokinetics.

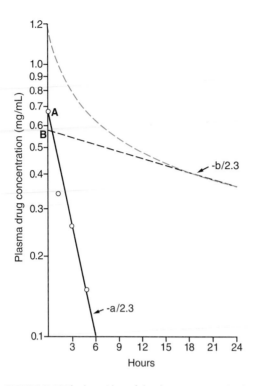

FIGURE 5.16 The logarithm of the drug concentration in plasma plotted versus time (*solid line*) after intravenous administration of a drug whose disposition can be described by a two-compartment model.

injection of a drug best described by a two-compartment model system can often be resolved into two linear components. This procedure can be performed by the method of residuals (or feathering), shown in Figure 5.16. In this procedure, a straight line is fitted through the tail of the original curve and extrapolated to the Y-axis (the value obtained is B). A plot is then made of the absolute difference values of the original curve and the resultant extrapolated straight line. The slope of the feathered line ($-a/2.303$) and the extrapolated line ($-b/2.303$) and the intercepts, A and B, are determined. The following equation describes a two-compartment system:

$$C_p = Ae^{-at} + Be^{-bt} \qquad \text{(Equation 5.5)}$$

This is a two-exponential equation that describes the two-compartment system. In this scheme, the slope of the line, $-a/2.303$, obtained from feathering yields the distributive rate of the drug. The slope of the terminal lin-

ear phase or elimination phase, $-b/2.303$, describes the rate of loss of the drug from the body and usually is considered to be a reflection of the metabolic processes and renal elimination from the body. Appropriate pharmacokinetic formulas allow the clinician to calculate the various volumes of distribution and rates of distribution and elimination for drugs whose pharmacokinetic behavior is exemplified by the two-compartment system.

Half-Life

The half-life ($T_{1/2}$) of a drug describes the time required for a drug's blood or plasma concentration to decrease by half. This fall in drug concentration is a reflection of metabolic processes and/or excretion. The biologic half-life of a drug in the blood may be determined graphically from a pharmacokinetic plot of a drug's blood concentration–time plot, typically after intravenous administration to a sample population. The amount of time required for the concentration of the drug to decrease by half is considered its half-life. The half-life can also be mathematically determined. Recall Equation 5.3 and rearrange the equation as follows:

$$\frac{K_{el}\, t}{2.303} = \text{Log } C^0_p - \text{Log } C_p = \text{Log } \frac{C^0_p}{C_p}$$

$$\text{(Equation 5.6)}$$

Then, if it assumed that C_p is equal to half of C^0_p:

$$\frac{K_{el}\, t}{2.303} = \text{Log } \frac{C^0_p}{0.5\, C^0_p} = \text{Log } 2 \qquad \text{(Equation 5.7)}$$

Thus,

$$t_{1/2} = \frac{2.303 \text{ Log } 2}{K_{el}} = \frac{0.693}{K_{el}} \qquad \text{(Equation 5.8)}$$

If this equation is rearranged, the half-life finds utility in the determination of drug elimination from the body, provided of course that the drug follows first-order kinetics. Rearranging the prior equation:

$$K_{el} = \frac{0.693}{t_{1/2}} \qquad \text{(Equation 5.9)}$$

First-order elimination rate constants are reported in time^{-1}, for example, minutes^{-1} or hours^{-1}. Thus, an elimination constant of a drug of 0.3 hour^{-1} indicates that 30% of the drug is eliminated per hour.

The half-life varies widely between drugs; for some it may be a few minutes, whereas for others it may be hours or even days (Table 5.9). Data on a drug's biologic half-life are useful in determining the most appropriate dosage regimen to achieve and maintain the desired blood level. These determinations usually result in recommended dosage schedules for a drug, such as every 4, 6, or 8 hours. Although these types of recommendations generally suit the requirements of most patients, they do not suit all patients. The most exceptional patients are those with reduced or impaired ability to metabolize or excrete drugs. These patients, most

TABLE 5.9 SOME ELIMINATION HALF-LIFE VALUES

DRUG PRODUCT	ELIMINATION HALF-LIFE[a]
Acetaminophen (Tylenol)	1–4 hours
Amoxicillin (Amoxil)	1 hour
Butabarbital sodium (Butisol sodium)	100 hours
Cimetidine (Tagamet)	2 hours
Digoxin (Lanoxin	1.5–2 days
Diltiazem (Cardizem)	2.5 hours
Ibuprofen (Motrin)	1.8–2 hours
Indomethacin (Indocin)	4.5 hours
Lithium carbonate (Eskalith)	24 hours
Nitroglycerin	3 minutes[b]
Phenytoin sodium (Dilantin)	7–29 hours
Propoxyphene (Darvon)	6–12 hours
Propranolol HCl (Inderal)	4 hours
Ranitidine (Zantac)	2.5–3 hours
Theophylline (Theo-Dur)	3–15 hours
Tobramycin sulfate (Nebcin)	2 hours

[a]Mean, average, or value ranges taken from product information found in *Physicians' Desk Reference*, 57th ed. Montvale, NJ: Thompson PDR, 2003. Half-life values may vary with patient characteristics (e.g., age, liver or renal function, smoking habits), dose levels, and routes of administration.

[b]After intravenous infusion, nitroglycerin is rapidly metabolized to dinitrates and mononitrates.

of whom have liver dysfunction or kidney disease, retain the administered drug in the blood or tissues for extended periods because of their decreased ability to eliminate the drug. The resulting extended biologic half-life of the drug generally necessitates an individualized dosage regimen calling for either less frequent administration than usual or the usual dosage schedule but a decrease in the amount of drug administered.

The drug digoxin presents a good example of a drug having a half-life that is affected by the patient's pathologic condition. Digoxin is eliminated in the urine. Renal excretion of digoxin is proportional to glomerular filtration rate. In subjects with normal renal function, digoxin has a half-life of 1.5 to 2.0 days. In anuric patients (absence of urine formation), the half-life may be prolonged to 4 to 6 days. Theophylline's half-life also varies from population to population. In premature infants with immature liver enzyme systems in the cytochrome P-450 family, the half-life of theophylline ranges from 14 to 58 hours, whereas in children aged 1 to 4 whose liver enzyme systems are more mature, the theophylline half-life ranges from 2 to 5.5 hours. In adult nonsmokers, the half-life ranges from 6.1 to 12.8 hours, whereas in adult smokers the average half-life of theophylline is 4.3 hours. The increase in theophylline clearance from the body among smokers is believed to be due to an induction of the hepatic metabolism of theophylline. The half-life of theophylline is decreased and total body clearance is enhanced to such a degree in smokers that these individuals may actually require a 50 to 100% increase in theophylline dosage to produce effective therapeutic results. The time required to normalize the effect of smoking on theophylline metabolism in the body once the patient stops smoking may range from 3 months to 2 years. Because theophylline is metabolized in the liver, the half-life of theophylline will be extended in liver disease. For example, in one study of 9 patients with decompensated cirrhosis, the average theophylline half-life was 32 hours.

The half-life of a drug in the blood stream may also be affected by a change in the extent to which it is bound to blood protein or cellular components. Such a change in a drug's binding pattern may be brought about by the administration of a second drug having a greater affinity than the first drug for the same binding sites. The result is displacement of the first drug from these sites by the second drug and the sudden availability of free (unbound) drug, which may pass from the blood stream to other body sites, including those concerned with its elimination. Displacement of one drug from its binding sites by another is generally viewed as an undesired event, since the amount of free drug resulting is greater than the level normally achieved during single-drug therapy and may result in untoward drug effects.

Concept of Clearance

The three main mechanisms by which a drug is removed or cleared from the body include (*a*) hepatic metabolism, that is, hepatic clearance, Cl_h, of a drug to either an active or inactive metabolite; (*b*) renal excretion, that is, renal clearance, Cl_r, of a drug unchanged in the urine, and (*c*) elimination of the drug into the bile and subsequently into the intestines for excretion in feces. An alternative way to express this removal or elimination from the body is to use total body clearance (Cl_B), which is defined as the fraction of the total volume of distribution that can be cleared per unit of time. Because most drugs undergo one or more of these processes, the total body clearance, Cl_B, of a drug is the sum of these clearances, usually hepatic, Cl_h, and renal, Cl_r. Clearance via the bile and feces is usually not significant for most drugs.

These processes of elimination work together, so a drug that is eliminated by renal excretion and hepatic biotransformation will have an overall rate of elimination. K_{el} is the sum of the renal excretion, k_u, and hepatic biotransformation, k_m. In the one-compartment model described earlier, total body clearance is the product of the volume of distribution, V_d, and the overall rate of elimination, k_{el}:

$$Cl_B = V_d \times k_{el} \qquad \text{(Equation 5.10)}$$

But recall that k_{el} equals $0.693/t_{1/2}$. If this is substituted in Equation 5.10 and the half-

life, $t_{1/2}$, solved for, the following equation is obtained:

$$t_{1/2} = \frac{0.693V_d}{Cl_b} \qquad \text{(Equation 5.11)}$$

Total body clearance is a function of one or more processes, so if a drug is eliminated from the body through hepatic biotransformation and renal clearance, Equation 5.11 becomes:

$$t_{1/2} = \frac{0.693V_d}{(Cl_h + Cl_r)} \qquad \text{(Equation 5.12)}$$

Thus, a drug's half-life is directly proportional to the volume of distribution and inversely proportional to the total body clearance, which consists of hepatic and renal clearance. In infants and children, who exhibit larger volumes of distribution and have lower clearance values, most drugs have a longer half-life than in adults.

A decrease in the hepatic or renal clearance will prolong the half-life of a drug. This typically occurs in renal failure, and consequently, if one can estimate the percentage decrease in excretion due to renal failure, one can use Equation 5.12 to calculate the new half-life of the drug in the patient. Thus, an adjusted dosage regimen can be calculated to decrease the chance of drug toxicity.

Dosage Regimen Considerations

The previous chapter mentions factors that can influence the dosage of a drug. It is not easy to determine how much drug and how often to administer it for a desired therapeutic effect. There are two basic approaches to the development of dosage regimens. The first is the *empirical approach*, which entails administration of a drug in a certain quantity, noting the therapeutic response, and modifying the amount and interval of dosage accordingly. Unfortunately, experience with administration of a drug usually starts with the first patient, and eventually a sufficient number of patients receive the drug so that a fairly accurate prediction can be made. Besides the desired therapeutic effect, it is necessary to consider the occurrence and severity of side effects. Empirical therapy is usually employed when the drug concentration in serum or plasma does not reflect the concentration of drug at the receptor site in the body or the pharmacodynamic effect of the drug is not related (or correlated) with drug concentration at the receptor site. Empirical therapy is used for many anticancer drugs that demonstrate effects long after they have been excreted from the body. It is difficult to relate the serum level of these drugs with the desired therapeutic effect.

The second approach to the development of a dosage regimen is through the use of pharmacokinetics, or the *kinetic approach*. This approach is based on the assumption that the therapeutic and toxic effects of a drug are related to the amount of drug in the body or to the plasma (or serum) concentration of drug at the receptor site. Through careful pharmacokinetic evaluation of a drug's absorption, distribution, metabolism, and excretion after a single dose, the levels of drug attained from multiple dosing can be estimated. One can then determine the appropriateness of a dosage regimen to achieve a desired therapeutic concentration of drug in the body and evaluate the regimen according to therapeutic response.

Pharmacokinetics is but one of a number of factors that should be considered in the development of a dosage regimen. Table 5.10 illustrates a number of these. Certainly an important factor is the inherent activity, that is,

pharmacodynamics and toxicity. A second consideration is the pharmacokinetics of the drug, which are influenced by the dosage form. The third factor focuses upon the patient to whom the drug will be given and encompasses the clinical state of the patient and how the patient will be managed. Finally, atypical factors may influence the dosage regimen. Collectively, all of these factors influence the dosage regimen.

The regimen of a drug may simply involve a single dose, as with pinworm medication, or may call for multiple doses. In the latter instance, the objective of pharmacokinetic dosing is to design a regimen that will continually maintain a drug's therapeutic serum or plasma concentration within the therapeutic index, that is, above the MEC but below the MTC.

Frequently drugs are administered 1 to 4 times per day, most often in a fixed dose, for example, 75 mg 3 times daily after meals. As mentioned earlier, after a drug is administered, its level within the body varies because of the influence of all of the processes, absorption, distribution, metabolism, and excretion. A drug will accumulate in the body when the dosing interval is less than the time needed for the body to eliminate a single dose. Figure 5.17 illustrates the plasma concentration for a drug given by intravenous administration and oral administration. The 50-mg dose of this drug

TABLE 5.10 FACTORS THAT DETERMINE A DOSAGE REGIMEN

ACTIVITY, TOXICITY		PHARMACOKINETICS
Minimum therapeutic dose		Absorption
Toxic dose	Dosage Regimen	Distribution
Therapeutic index		Metabolism
Side effects		Excretion
Dose-response relationships		

CLINICAL FACTORS		OTHER FACTORS
CLINICAL STATE OF PATIENT	MANAGEMENT OF THERAPY	
Age, weight, urine pH	Multiple drug therapy	Tolerance-dependence
Condition being treated	Convenience of regimen	Pharmacogenetics-idiosyncrasy
Existence of other disease states	Compliance of patient	Drug interactions

Reprinted with permission from Rowland M, Tozer TN. Clinical Pharmacokinetics, 2nd ed. Philadelphia: Lea & Febiger, 1989.

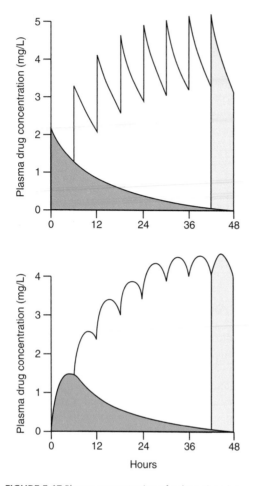

FIGURE 5.17 Plasma concentration of a drug given intravenously (*top*) and orally (*bottom*) on a fixed dose of 50 mg and fixed dosing interval of 8 hours. The half-life is 12 hours. The area under the plasma concentration–time curve during a dosing interval at steady state is equal to the total AUC for a single dose. The fluctuation of the concentration is diminished for oral administration (half-life of absorption is 1.4 hours), but the average steady-state concentration is the same as after intravenous administration, since F = 1. (Adapted with permission from Rowland M, Tozer TN. Clinical pharmacokinetics, 2nd ed. Philadelphia: Lea & Febiger, 1989).

was given at a dosing interval of 8 hours. The drug has an elimination half-life of 12 hours. As one can see, with continued dosing the drug concentration reaches a *steady state* or *plateau* concentration. At this limit the amount of drug lost per interval is replenished when the drug is dosed again. Consequently the concentration of drug in the plasma or serum fluctuates.

Thus, for certain patient types it is optimal to target dosing so that the plateau concentration resides within the therapeutic index of a drug to maintain a MEC. For example, the asthmatic patient maintained on theophylline must have a serum concentration between 10 and 20 µg/mL. Otherwise the patient may be susceptible to an asthma attack. Thus, when dosing the asthmatic patient it is preferable to give theophylline around the clock 4 times daily to sustain levels at least above the minimum effective concentration. If this medicine is administered only every 4 hours during the waking hours, it is possible that the minimum concentration will fall below effective levels between the bedtime dose and the morning dose. Consequently, the patient may awaken in the middle of the night and have an asthma attack.

Patients can be monitored pharmacokinetically through appropriate plasma, serum, or blood samples, and some hospital pharmacies have implemented pharmacokinetic dosing services. The intent is to maximize drug efficacy, minimize toxicity, and keep health care costs at a minimum. Thus complications associated with overdose are controlled and known drug interactions, such as between smoking and theophylline, can be accommodated. In these services once the physician prescribes a certain amount of drug and monitors the clinical response, it is the pharmacist who coordinates the appropriate sample time to determine drug concentration in the appropriate body fluid. After the level of drug is attained, it is the pharmacist who interprets the result and consults with the physician regarding subsequent dosages.

Pharmacokinetic research has demonstrated that the determination of a patient's dosage regimen depends on numerous factors, and daily dose formulas exist for a number of drugs that must be administered on a routine maintenance schedule, for example digoxin, procainamide, and theophylline. For certain drugs such as digoxin, which are not highly lipid soluble, it is preferable to use a patient's lean body weight (LBW) rather than total body weight (TBW) to provide a better estimate of the patient's volume of distribution. Alternatively, even though pharmacokinetic dosing formulas

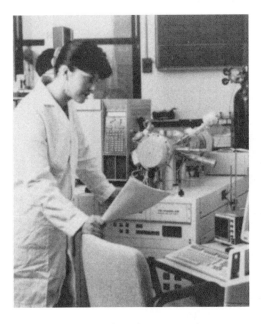

FIGURE 5.18 Computed gas chromatography mass spectrometry used in bioanalytical studies. Consists of Hewlett Packard Gas Chromatograph (Model 5890 A) and VG Mass Spectrometer (Model UG 12–250). (Courtesy of Elan Corporation, plc.)

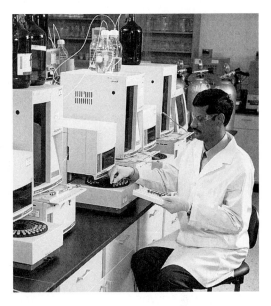

FIGURE 5.19 Assay of product samples using high performance liquid chromatography. (Courtesy of Paddock Laboratories.)

may exist, one must be cognizant that patient factors may be more relevant. For example, with the geriatric patient it is advisable to begin drug therapy with the lowest possible dose and increase the dosage as necessary in small increments to optimize the patient's clinical response. Then the patient should be monitored for drug efficacy and reevaluated periodically. Examples of bioanalytical research laboratories are shown in Figures 5.18 and 5.19.

REFERENCES

1. Cogburn JN, Donovan MG, Schasteen CS. A model of human small intestinal absorptive cells 1: Transport barrier. Pharm Res 1991;8:210–216.

2. Christensen FN et al. The use of gamma scintigraphy to follow the gastrointestinal transit of pharmaceutical formulations. J Pharm Pharmacol 1985; 37:91–95.

3. Coupe AJ, Davis SS, Wilding IR. Variation in gastrointestinal transit of pharmaceutical dosage forms in healthy subjects. Pharm Res 1991;8:360–364.

4. Poole J. Curr Ther Res 1968;10:292–303.

5. Code of Federal Regulations, Title 21, Part 320. Bioavailability and Bioequivalence Requirements.

6. Chodos DJ, DiSanto AR. Basics of Bioavailability. Kalamazoo, MI: Upjohn, 1973.

7. FDA Drug Bulletin, 1986;16, 2:1986, 14–15.

8. Smith HJ. Process of drug handling by the body. Introduction to the Principles of Drug Design, 2nd ed. London: Butterworth, 1988.

9. Cooper JW. Monitoring of drugs and hepatic status. Clinical Consult 1991;10 (6), 1991.

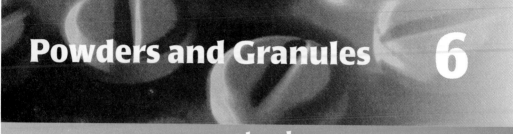

Powders and Granules 6

Chapter at a glance

Most active and inactive pharmaceutical ingredients occur in the solid state as amorphous powders or as *crystals* of various morphologic structure. The term *powder* has more than one connotation in pharmacy. It may be used to describe the physical form of a material, that is, a dry substance composed of finely divided particles. Or it may be used to describe a type of pharmaceutical preparation, that is, a medicated powder intended for internal (i.e., oral powder) or external (i.e., topical powder) use. Powders are intimate mixtures of dry, finely divided drugs and/or chemicals that may be intended for internal or external use.

Although the use of *medicated powders* per se in therapeutics is limited, the use of powdered substances in the preparation of other dosage forms is extensive. For example, powdered drugs may be blended with powdered fillers and other pharmaceutical ingredients to fabricate solid dosage forms as tablets and capsule; they may be dissolved or suspended in solvents or liquid vehicles to make various liquid dosage forms; or they may be incorporated into semisolid bases in the preparation of medicated ointments and creams.

Granules, which are prepared agglomerates of powdered materials, may be used per se for the medicinal value of their content or they may be used for pharmaceutical purposes, as in making tablets, as described later in this and in the next two chapters.

Powders

Before their use in the preparation of pharmaceutical products, solid materials first are characterized to determine their chemical and physical features, including morphology, purity, solubility, stability, particle size, uniformity, and compatibility with any other formulation components (1). Drug and other materials commonly require chemical or pharmaceutical processing to imbue the features desired to enable both the efficient production of a finished dosage form and optimum therapeutic efficacy. This usually includes the adjustment and control of a powder's particle size.

Particle Size and Analysis

The particles of pharmaceutical powders may range from extremely coarse, about 10 mm (1 cm) in diameter, to extremely fine, approaching colloidal dimensions of 1 micron or less. In order to characterize the particle size of a given powder, the *United States Pharmacopeia* (USP) uses these descriptive terms: very coarse, coarse, moderately coarse, fine, and very fine, which are related to the proportion of powder that is capable of passing through the openings of standard sieves of varying fineness in a specified period while being shaken, generally in a mechanical sieve shaker (2). Table 6.1 presents the standard sieve numbers and the openings in each, expressed in millimeters and in microns. Sieves for such pharmaceutical testing and measurement are generally made of wire cloth woven from brass, bronze, or other suitable wire. They are not coated or plated.

TABLE 6.1 OPENING OF STANDARD SIEVES

SIEVE NUMBER	SIEVE OPENING
2.0	9.50 mm
3.5	5.60 mm
4.0	4.75 mm
8.0	2.36 mm
10.0	2.00 mm
20.0	850.00 μm
30.0	600.00 μm
40.0	425.00 μm
50.0	300.00 μm
60.0	250.00 μm
70.0	212.00 μm
80.0	180.00 μm
100.0	150.00 μm
120.0	125.00 μm
200.0	75.00 μm
230.0	63.00 μm
270.0	53.00 μm
325.0	45.00 μm
400.0	38.00 μm

Adapted from USP 26–NF 21.

Powders of vegetable and animal drugs are officially defined as follows (2):

Very coarse (No. 8): All particles pass through a No. 8 sieve and not more than 20% through a No. 60 sieve.

Coarse (No. 20): All particles pass through a No. 20 sieve and not more than 40% through a No. 60 sieve.

Moderately coarse (No. 40): All particles pass through a No. 40 sieve and not more than 40% through a No. 80 sieve.

Fine (No. 60): All particles pass through a No. 60 sieve and not more than 40% through a No. 100 sieve.

Very fine (or a No. 80): All particles pass through a No. 80 sieve. There is no limit to greater fineness.

Granules typically fall within the range of 4- to 12-sieve size, although granulations of powders prepared in the 12- to 20-sieve range are sometimes used in tablet making.

The purpose of particle size analysis in pharmacy is to obtain quantitative data on the size, distribution, and shapes of drug and other components to be used in pharmaceutical formulations. There may be substantial differences in particle size, crystal morphology, and amorphous character within and between substances. Particle size can influence a variety of important factors, including the following:

- Dissolution rate of particles intended to dissolve; drug micronization can increase the rate of drug dissolution and its bioavailability
- Suspendability of particles intended to remain undissolved but uniformly dispersed in a liquid vehicle (e.g., fine dispersions have particles approximately 0.5–10 μm)
- Uniform distribution of a drug substance in a powder mixture or solid dosage form to ensure dose-to-dose content uniformity (3)
- Penetrability of particles intended to be inhaled for deposition deep in the respiratory tract (e.g., 1–5 μm) (4)
- Lack of grittiness of solid particles in dermal ointments, creams, and ophthalmic preparations (e.g., fine powders may be 50–100 μm in size)

A number of methods exist for the determination of particle size, including the following (Physical Pharmacy Capsule 6.1):

- Sieving, in which particles are passed by mechanical shaking through a series of sieves of known and successively smaller size and the determination of the proportion of powder passing through or being withheld on each sieve (range about 40–9500 μm, depending upon sieve sizes) (2, 5)
- Microscopy, in which the particles are sized through the use of a calibrated grid background or other measuring device (range 0.2–100 μm) (6, 7)
- Sedimentation rate, in which particle size is determined by measuring the terminal settling velocity of particles through a liquid medium in a gravitational or centrifugal environment (range 0.8–300 μm) (5). Sedimentation rate may be calculated from Stokes' law.
- Light energy diffraction or light scattering, in which particle size is determined by the reduction in light reaching the sensor as the particle, dispersed in a liquid or gas, passes through the sensing zone (range 0.2–500 μm) (4). Laser scattering, utilizes a He-Ne laser, silicon photo diode detectors and an ultrasonic probe for particle dispersion (range 0.02–2,000 μm) (8).
- Laser holography, in which a pulsed laser is fired through an aerosolized particle spray and photographed in three dimensions with a holographic camera, allowing the particles to be individually imaged and sized (range 1.4–100 μm) (9).
- Cascade impaction is based on the principle that a particle driven by an airstream will hit a surface in its path, provided that its inertia is sufficient to overcome the drag force that tends to keep it in the airstream (10). Particles are separated into various size ranges by successively increasing the velocity of the airstream in which they are carried.

These methods and others may be used for the analysis of particle size and shape. For some materials, a single method may be sufficient; however, a combination of methods is frequently preferred to provide greater certainty of size and shape parameters (7). Most com-

mercial particle size analyzers are automated and linked with computers for data processing, distribution analysis, and printout.

The science of small particles is discussed further in Physical Pharmacy Capsule 6.1, Micromeritics. Physical Pharmacy Capsule 6.2, Particle Size Reduction, points out that a reduction in particle size increases the number of particles and total surface area.

Comminution of Drugs

On a small scale, as in the community pharmacy, the pharmacist reduces the size of chemical substances by grinding with a mortar and pestle. A finer grinding action is accomplished by using a mortar with a rough surface (as a porcelain mortar) than one with a smooth surface (as a glass mortar). Grinding a drug in a mortar to reduce its particle size is termed *trituration*. On a large scale, various types of mills and pulverizers may be used to reduce particle size. Figure 6.1 shows one

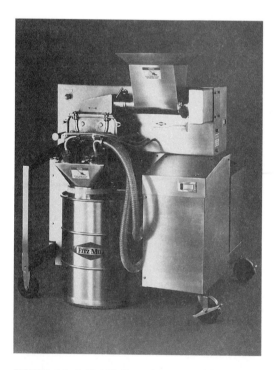

FIGURE 6.1 A FitzMill Comminutor, model VFS-D6A-PCS, used for particle reduction, with attached containment system for protection of environment and prevention of product contamination. (Courtesy of The Fitzpatrick Company.)

Micromeritics

Micromeritics is the science of small particles; a particle is any unit of matter having defined physical dimensions. It is important to study particles because most drug dosage forms are solids, solids are not static systems, the physical state of particles can be altered by physical manipulation, and particle characteristics can alter therapeutic effectiveness.

Micromeritics is the study of a number of characteristics, including particle size and size distribution, shape, angle of repose, porosity, true volume, bulk volume, apparent density, and bulkiness.

PARTICLE SIZE

A number of techniques can be used to determine particle size and size distributions. Particle size determinations are complicated by the fact that particles are not uniform in shape. Only two relatively simple examples are provided for a detailed calculation of the average particle size of a powder mixture. Other methods are generally discussed. The techniques used include the microscopic method and the sieving method.

The microscopic method can include counting not fewer than 200 particles in a single plane using a calibrated ocular on a microscope. Given the following data, what is the average diameter of the particles?

SIZE OF COUNTED PARTICLES (μM)	MIDDLE VALUE μM "D"	NO. PARTICLES PER GROUP "N"	"ND"
40–60	50	15	750
60–80	70	25	1750
80–100	90	95	8550
100–120	110	140	15400
120–140	130	80	10400
		$\Sigma n = 355$	$\Sigma nd = 36850$

$$d_{av} = \frac{\Sigma \, nd}{\Sigma n} = \frac{36{,}850}{355} = 103.8 \; \mu m$$

The sieving method entails using a set of U.S. standard sieves in the size range desired. A stack of sieves is arranged in order, the powder placed in the top sieve, the stack shaken, the quantity of powder resting on each sieve weighed, and this calculation performed:

SIEVE	ARITHMETIC MEAN OPENING (MM)	WEIGHT RETAINED (G)	% RETAINED	% RETAINED × MEAN OPENING (MM)
20/40	0.630	15.5	14.3	9.009
40/60	0.335	25.8	23.7	7.939
60/80	0.214	48.3	44.4	9.502
80/100	0.163	15.6	14.3	2.330
100/120	0.137	3.5	3.3	0.452
		108.7	100.0	29.232

$$d_{av} = \frac{\Sigma \, (\% \text{ retained}) \times (\text{ave. size})}{100} = \frac{29.232}{100} = 0.2923 \text{ mm}$$

Physical Pharmacy Capsule 6.1 cont.

Another method of particle size determination entails sedimentation using the Andreasen pipet, a special cylindrical container from which a sample can be removed from the lower portion at selected intervals. The powder is dispersed in a nonsolvent in the pipet, agitated, and 20-mL samples removed over time. Each 20-mL sample is dried and weighed. The particle diameters can be calculated from this equation:

$$d = \frac{18\, h\eta}{(\rho_i - \rho_e)\, gt}$$

where

d is the diameter of the particles,
h is the height of the liquid above the sampling tube orifice,
η is the viscosity of the suspending liquid,
$\rho_i - \rho_e$ is the density difference between the suspending liquid and the particles,
g is the gravitational constant, and
t is the time in seconds.

Other methods of particle size determinations include elutriation, centrifugation, permeation, adsorption, electronic sensing zone (the Coulter Counter), and light obstruction. The last includes both standard light and laser methods. In general, the resulting average particle sizes by these techniques can provide average particle size by weight (sieve method, light scattering, sedimentation method), and average particle size by volume (light scattering, electronic sensing zone, light obstruction, air permeation, and even the optical microscope).

ANGLE OF REPOSE

The angle of repose is a relatively simple technique for estimating the flow properties of a powder. It can easily be determined by allowing a powder to flow through a funnel and fall freely onto a surface. The height and diameter of the resulting cone are measured and the angle of repose calculated from this equation:

$$\tan \theta = h/r$$

where

h is the height of the powder cone and
r is the radius of the powder cone.

EXAMPLE 1

A powder was poured through the funnel and formed a cone 3.3 cm high and 9 cm in diameter. What is the angle of repose?

$$\tan \theta = h/r = 3.3/4.5 = 0.73$$
$$\text{arc tan } 0.73 = 36.25°$$

Powders with a low angle of repose flow freely, and powders with a high angle of repose flow poorly. A number of factors, including shape and size, determine the flow properties of powders. Spherical particles flow better than needles. Very fine particles do not flow as freely as large particles. In general, particles in the size range of 250 to 2000 μm flow freely if the shape is amenable. Particles in the size range of 75 to 250 μm may flow freely or cause problems, depending on shape and other factors. With most particles smaller than 100 μm, flow is a problem.

Physical Pharmacy Capsule 6.1 cont.

POROSITY, VOID, AND BULK VOLUME

If spheres and the different ways they pack together are used as an example, two possibilities arise. First, the closest packing may be rhombus–triangle, in which angles of 60° and 120° are common. The space between the particles, the void, is about 0.26, resulting in porosity, as described later, of about 26%. Another packing, cubical, with the cubes packed at 90° angles to each other, may be considered. This results in a void of about 0.47, or a porosity of about 47%. This is the most open type of packing. If particles are not uniform, the smaller particles will slip into the void spaces between the larger particles and decrease the void areas.

Packing and flow are important, as they affect the size of container required for packaging, the flow of granulations, the efficiency of the filling apparatus for making tablets and capsules, and the ease of working with the powders.

The characteristics used to describe powders include porosity, true volume, bulk volume, apparent density, true density, and bulkiness. The photo is a tapped density tester.

Porosity is

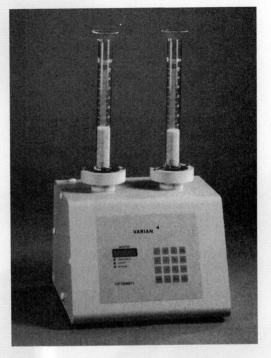

Tapped density tester. (Courtesy of Varian Inc.)

$$\text{Void} \times 100$$

This value should be determined experimentally by measuring the volume occupied by a selected weight of a powder, V_{bulk}. The true volume, V, of a powder is the space occupied by the powder exclusive of spaces greater than the intramolecular space.

Void can be defined as

$$\frac{V_{bulk} - V}{V_{bulk}}$$

therefore, porosity is

$$\frac{V_{bulk} - V}{V_{bulk}} \times 100$$

and the bulk volume is

$$\text{True volume} + \text{porosity}$$

APPARENT DENSITY, TRUE DENSITY, AND BULKINESS

The apparent density, ρ_a, is

$$\frac{\text{Weight of the sample}}{V_{bulk}}$$

Physical Pharmacy Capsule 6.1 cont.

The true density, ρ, is

$$\frac{\text{Weight of the sample}}{V}$$

The bulkiness, B, is the reciprocal of the apparent density,

$$B = 1/\rho_a$$

EXAMPLE 2

A selected powder has a true density (ρ) of 3.5 g/cc. Experimentally, 2.5 g of the powder measures 40 mL in a cylindrical graduate. Calculate the true volume, void, porosity, apparent density, and bulkiness.
True volume:

$$\text{Density} = \text{mass (weight)/volume}$$

$$\text{Volume} = \text{mass (weight)/density}$$

$$= 2.5 \text{ g}/(3.5 \text{ g/cc}) = 0.715 \text{ cc}$$

Void:

$$\frac{V_{bulk} - V}{V_{bulk}} = \frac{40 \text{ mL} - 0.715 \text{ mL}}{40 \text{mL}} = 0.982$$

Porosity:

$$\text{Void} \times 100 = 0.982 \times 100 = 98.2\%$$

Apparent density:

$$(Pa) = \frac{2.5 \text{ g}}{40 \text{ mL}} = 0.0625 \text{ g/mL}$$

Bulkiness:

$$1/Pa = \frac{1}{0.06265 \text{ (g/mL)}} = 16 \text{ mL/g}$$

Powders with a low apparent density and a large bulk volume are considered light, and those with a high apparent density and a small bulk volume are heavy.

such piece of equipment, a FitzMill comminuting machine with a product containment system. Through the grinding action of rapidly moving blades in the comminuting chamber, particles are reduced in size and passed through a screen of desired dimension to the collection container. The collection and containment system protects the environment from chemical dust, reduces product loss, and prevents product contamination.

Levigation is commonly used in small-scale preparation of ointments to reduce the particle size and grittiness of added powders. A mortar and pestle or an ointment tile may be used. A paste is formed by combining the powder and a small amount of liquid (the *levigating agent*) in which the powder is insoluble. The paste is then triturated, reducing particle size. The levigated paste may then be added to the ointment base and the mixture made uniform and smooth by

PHYSICAL PHARMACY CAPSULE 6.2

Particle Size Reduction

Comminution, reduction of the particle size of a solid substance to a finer state, is used to facilitate crude drug extraction, increase the dissolution rates of a drug, aid in the formulation of pharmaceutically acceptable dosage forms, and enhance the absorption of drugs. The reduction in the particle size of a solid is accompanied by a great increase in the specific surface area of that substance. An example of the increase in the number of particles formed and the resulting surface area is as follows.

EXAMPLE

INCREASE IN NUMBER OF PARTICLES

If a powder consists of cubes 1 mm on edge and it is reduced to particles 10 μm on edge, what is the number of particles produced?

1. 1 mm equals 1000 μm.
2. 1000 μm/10 μm = 100 pieces produced on each edge; that is, if the cube is sliced into 100 pieces on the x-axis, each 10 μm long, 100 pieces result.
3. If this is repeated on the y- and z-axes, the result is 100 × 100 × 100 = 1 million particles produced, each 10 μm on edge, for each original particle 1 mm on edge. This can also be written $[(10^2)^3 = 10^6]$.

INCREASE IN SURFACE AREA

What increase in the surface area of the powder is produced by decreasing the particle size from 1 mm to 10 μm?

1. The 1-mm cube has 6 surfaces, each 1 mm on edge. Each face has a surface area of 1 mm^2. Because there are 6 faces, this is 6 mm^2 surface area per particle.
2. Each 10-μm cube has 6 surfaces, each 10 μm on edge. Each face has a surface area of 10 × 10 = 100 μm^2. Because there are 6 faces, this is 6 × 100 μm^2, or 600 μm^2 surface area per particle. Since 10^6 particles resulted from comminuting the 1-mm cube, each 10 μm on edge, the surface are are now is 600 μm^2 × 10^6, or 6 × 10^8 μm^2.
3. To get everything in the same units for ease of comparison, convert the 6 × 10^8 μm^2 into square millimeters as follows.
4. Since there are 1000 μm/mm, there must be 1000^2, or 1 million μm^2/mm^2. This is more appropriately expressed as 10^6 μm^2/mm^2,

$$\frac{6 \times 10^8 \ \mu m^2}{10^6 \ \mu m^2/mm^2} = 6 \times 10^2 \ mm^2$$

The surface areas have been increased from 6 mm^2 to 600 mm^2 by the reduction in particle size of cubes 1 mm on edge to cubes 10 μm on edge, a hundredfold increase in surface area. This can have a significant increase in the rate of dissolution of a drug product.

rubbing them together with a spatula on the ointment tile. A figure-8 track is commonly used to incorporate the materials. Mineral oil and glycerin are commonly used levigating agents.

Blending Powders

When two or more powdered substances are to be combined to form a uniform mixture, it is best to reduce the particle size of each powder individually before weighing and blending. Depending on the nature of the ingredients, amount of powder, and equipment, powders may be blended by spatulation, trituration, sifting, and tumbling.

Spatulation is blending small amounts of powders by movement of a spatula through them on a sheet of paper or an ointment tile. It is not suitable for large quantities of powders or for powders containing potent substances, because homogeneous blending is not as certain as other methods. Very little compression or compacting of the powder results from spatulation, which is especially suited to mixing solid substances that form *eutectic mixtures* (or liquify) when in close and prolonged contact with one another. Substances that form eutectic mixtures when combined include phenol, camphor, menthol, thymol, aspirin, phenyl salicylate, and other similar chemicals. To diminish contact, a powder prepared from such substances is commonly mixed in the presence of an inert diluent, such as light magnesium oxide or magnesium carbonate, to separate physically the troublesome agents.

Trituration may be employed both to comminute and to mix powders. If simple admixture is desired without special need for comminution, the glass mortar is usually preferred. When a small amount of a potent substance is to be mixed with a large amount of diluent, the *geometric dilution* method is used to ensure the uniform distribution of the potent drug. This method is especially indicated when the potent and other ingredients are the same color and a visible sign of mixing is lacking. By this method, the potent drug is placed on an approximately equal volume of the diluent in a mortar and mixed thoroughly by trituration. Then a second portion of diluent equal in volume to the mixture is added, and the trituration repeated. This process is continued by adding equal volumes of diluent to the powder mixture and repeating until all of the diluent is incorporated. Some pharmacists add an inert colored powder to the diluent before mixing to permit visual inspection of the mixing process.

Powders may also be mixed by passing them through sifters like those used in the kitchen to sift flour. Sifting results in a light, fluffy product. This process is not acceptable for the incorporation of potent drugs into a diluent powder.

Another method of mixing powders is tumbling the powder in a rotating chamber. Special small-scale and large-scale motorized powder blenders mix powders by tumbling them (Figs. 6.2 and 6.3). Mixing by this process is thorough but time consuming. Such blenders are widely employed in industry, as are mixers that use motorized blades to blend powder in a large vessel.

Medicated Powders

Some medicated powders are intended to be used internally; others, externally. Most powders for internal use are taken orally after mixing with water. Some powders are intended to be inhaled for local and systemic effects. Other dry powders are commercially packaged for constitution with a liquid solvent or vehicle, some for administration orally, others for use as an injection, and still others for use as a vaginal douche.

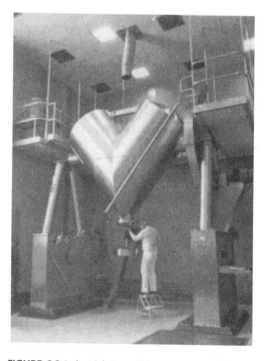

FIGURE 6.2 Industrial-size solid-state processor or twin shell blender used to mix solid particles. (Courtesy of Abbott Laboratories.)

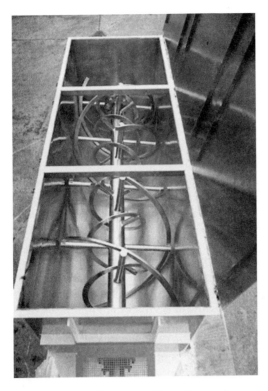

FIGURE 6.3 Ribbon blender used for mixing powders and preparing granulations. (Courtesy of Littleford Day).

Medicated powders for external use are dusted on the affected area from a sifter-type container or applied from a powder aerosol. Powders intended for external use should bear a label marked EXTERNAL USE ONLY or a similar label.

Medicated powders for oral use may be intended for local effects (e.g., laxatives) or systemic effects (e.g., analgesics) and may be preferred to counterpart tablets and capsules by patients who have difficulty swallowing solid dosage forms. The doses of some drugs are too bulky to be formed into tablets or capsules of convenient size, so they may be administered as powders. For administration, they can be mixed with a liquid or soft food. Powders taken orally for systemic use may be expected to result in faster rates of dissolution and absorption than solid dosage forms, since there is immediate contact with the gastric fluids; however, the actual advantage in terms of therapeutic response may be negligible or only minimal, depending on the drug release characteristics of the counterpart products. A primary disadvantage to the use of oral powders is the undesirable taste of the drug.

Some medications, notably antibiotics for children, are intended for oral administration as liquids but are relatively unstable in liquid form. They are provided to the pharmacist by the manufacturer as a dry powder or granule for constitution with a specified quantity of purified water at the time of dispensing. Under labeled conditions of storage, the resultant product remains stable for the prescribed period of use, generally up to 2 weeks. Sterile dry powders intended to be constituted with water for injection or another suitable solvent prior to administration by injection are discussed in Chapter 15.

Aerosol Powders

Some medicated powders are administered by inhalation with the aid of dry-powder inhalers, which deliver micronized particles of medication in metered quantities (Fig. 6.4). Most of

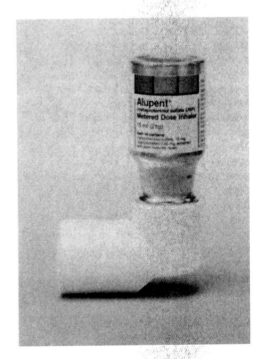

FIGURE 6.4 Metered inhalation aerosol containing a micronized medicated powder and inert propellants. Each dose is delivered through the mouthpiece upon activation of the aerosol unit's valve. (Courtesy of Boehringer Ingelheim Pharmaceuticals.)

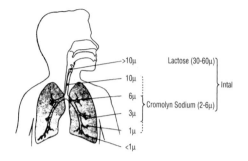

FIGURE 6.5 Relation of particle size to airway penetration (Courtesy of Fisons Corporation.)

these products are used in the treatment of asthma and other bronchial disorders that require distribution of medication deep in the lungs (Fig. 6.5). To accomplish this, the particle size of the micronized medication is prepared in the range of 1 to 6 μm in diameter. In addition to the therapeutic agent, these products contain inert propellants and pharmaceutical diluents, such as crystalline alpha-lactose monohydrate, to aid the formulation's flow properties and metering uniformity and to protect the powder from humidity (11). Powder blowers or insufflators (Fig. 6.6) may be used to deliver dry powders to various parts of the body. Depression of the device's rubber bulb causes turbulence of the powder in the vessel, forcing it out through the orifice in the tip.

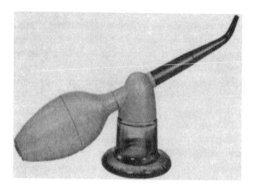

FIGURE 6.6 A general-purpose powder blower or insufflator. The powder is placed in the vessel. When the rubber bulb is depressed, internal turbulence disperses the powder and forces it from the orifice. Powders may be delivered to various body locations, such as the nose, throat, tooth sockets, or skin. (Courtesy of DeVilbiss Company.)

Bulk and Divided Powders

Medicated powders may be provided to the patient in bulk or divided. Some powders are packaged by manufacturers, whereas others are prepared and packaged by the pharmacist.

Bulk Powders

Among the bulk powders available in prepackaged amounts are (a) antacids (e.g., sodium bicarbonate) and laxatives (e.g., psyllium [Metamucil]), which the patient takes by mixing with water or other beverage before swallowing; (b) douche powders (e.g., Massengill Powder), dissolved in warm water by the patient for vaginal use; (c) medicated powders for external application to the skin, usually topical anti-infectives (e.g., bacitracin zinc and polymyxin B sulfate) or antifungals (e.g., tolnaftate); and (d) brewer's yeast powder containing B-complex vitamins and other nutritional supplements. In some cases, a small measuring scoop, spoon, or other device is dispensed with the powder for measuring the dose of the drug.

Dispensing powder medication in bulk quantities is limited to nonpotent substances. Powders containing substances that should be administered in controlled dosage are supplied to the patient in divided amounts in folded papers or packets.

Divided Powders

After a powder has been properly blended (using the geometric dilution method for potent substances), it may be divided into individual dosing units based on the amount to be taken or used at a single time. Each divided portion of powder may be placed on a small piece of paper (Latin chartula; abbrev. chart.; powder paper)that is folded to enclose the medication. A number of commercially prepared premeasured products are available in folded papers or packets, including headache powders (e.g., BC Powders), powdered laxatives (e.g., Perdiem Packets), and douche powders (e.g., Massengill Powder Packettes).

Divided powders may be prepared as follows by the pharmacist. Depending on the potency of the drug substance, the pharmacist decides whether to weigh each portion of powder separately before enfolding in a paper or to approximate each portion by using the block-and-divide method. By the latter method, used only for nonpotent drugs, the pharmacist places the entire amount of prepared powder on a flat surface such as a porcelain or glass plate, pill tile, or large sheet of paper, and with a large spatula forms a rectangular or square block of powder having a uniform depth. Then, using the spatula, the pharmacist cuts into the powder lengthwise and crosswise to delineate the appropriate number of smaller, uniform blocks, each representing a dose or unit of medication. Each of the smaller blocks is separated from the main block with the spatula, transferred to a powder paper, and wrapped.

The powder papers may be of any convenient size to hold the amount of powder required, but the most popular commercially available sizes are 2.75 × 3.75 inches, 3 × 4.5 inches, 3.75 × 5 inches, and 4.5 × 6 inches. The papers may be (a) simple bond paper; (b) vegetable parchment, a thin, semiopaque paper with limited moisture

resistance; (c) glassine, a glazed, transparent paper, also with limited moisture resistance; and (d) waxed paper, a transparent waterproof paper. The selection of the type of paper is based primarily on the nature of the powder. If the powder contains hygroscopic or deliquescent materials, waterproof or waxed paper should be used. In practice, such powders are double-wrapped in waxed paper, and then for aesthetic appeal they are wrapped in bond paper. Glassine and vegetable parchment papers may be used when only a limited barrier against moisture is necessary. Powders containing volatile components should be wrapped in waxed or in glassine papers. Powders containing neither volatile components nor ingredients adversely affected by air or moisture are usually wrapped in white bond paper.

A certain degree of expertise is required in the folding of a powder paper, and practice is required for proficiency. The steps are shown in Figure 6.7 and described as follows:

1. Place the paper flat on a hard surface and fold toward you a uniform flap of about 0.5

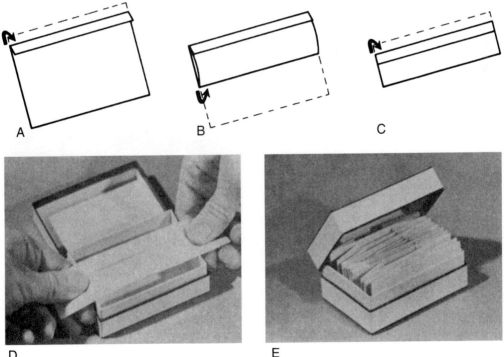

FIGURE 6.7 Steps in folding powder papers.

inch of the long side of the paper. To ensure uniformity of all of the papers, this step should be performed on all the required papers concurrently, using the first folded paper as the guide (Fig. 6.7A).

2. With the flap of each paper away and on top, place the weighed or divided powder in the center of each paper.

3. Being careful not to disturb the powder excessively, bring the lower edge of the paper upward and tuck it into the crease of the flap (Fig. 6.7B).

4. Grasp the flap, press it down upon the tucked-in bottom edge of the paper, and fold again with an amount of paper equal to the size of the original flap (0.5 inch) (Fig. 6.7C).

5. Pick up the paper with the flap on top, being careful not to disturb the position of the powder, and place the partially folded paper over the open powder box (to serve as the container) so that the ends of the paper extend equally beyond the sides (lengthwise) of the open container. Then, press the sides of the box slightly inward and the ends of the paper gently down along the sides of the box to form a crease on each end of the paper. Lift the paper from the box and fold the ends of the paper along each crease sharply so that the powder cannot escape (Fig. 6.7D).

6. Place the folded paper in the box so that the double-folded flaps are at the top, facing you, and the ends are folded away from you (Fig. 6.7E).

Papers folded properly should fit snugly in the box, have uniform folds, and be uniform in length and height. There should be no powder in the folds, and none should escape with moderate agitation. Powder boxes, which are generally pasteboard and hinged, should close easily without touching the tops of the papers. The label for the powders may be placed on the container, but some pharmacists affix a label of directions to each paper.

For convenience and uniformity of appearance, pharmacists may use commercially available small cellophane or plastic envelopes to enclose individual doses or units of use rather than folding individual powder papers. These envelopes are usually moisture resistant, and their use results in uniform packaging.

Granules

As indicated previously, *granules* are prepared agglomerates of smaller particles of powder. They are irregularly shaped but may be prepared to be spherical. They are usually in the 4- to 12-sieve size range, although granules of various mesh sizes may be prepared depending upon their application.

Granules are prepared by wet methods and dry methods. One basic wet method is to moisten the powder or powder mixture and then pass the resulting paste through a screen of the mesh size to produce the desired size of granules. The granules are placed on drying trays and dried by air or under heat. The granules are periodically moved about on the drying trays to prevent adhesion into a large mass. Another type of wet method is fluid bed processing, in which particles are placed in a conical piece of equipment and vigorously dispersed and suspended while a liquid excipient is sprayed on them and the product dried, forming granules or pellets of defined particle size (Fig. 6.8).

The dry granulation method may be performed in a couple of ways. By one method, the dry powder is passed through a roll compactor and then through a granulating machine (Fig.

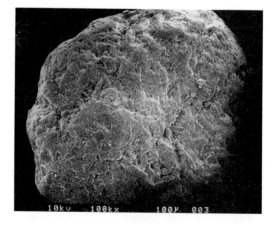

FIGURE 6.8 Granule prepared with fluid bed technology. (Courtesy of Glatt Air Techniques.)

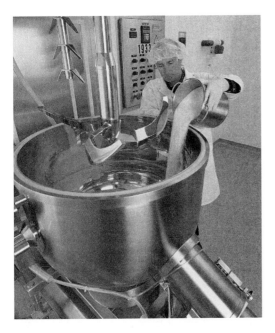

FIGURE 6.9 High speed granulator–mixer. (Courtesy of Paddock Laboratories)

6.9). A roll compactor, also called a roll press or roller compactor, processes a fine powder into dense sheets or forms by forcing it through two mechanically rotating metal rolls running counter to each other (12). The surface of the compacting rolls may be smooth or may have pocket indentations or corrugations that allow compaction of different forms and textures. The compacted powder is granulated to uniform particle size in a mechanical granulator. Powder compactors are generally combined in sequence in integrated compactor–granulation systems.

An alternative dry method, termed slugging, is compression of a powder or powder mixture into large tablets or slugs on a compressing machine under 8,000 to 12,000 pounds of pressure, depending on the physical characteristics of the powder. The slugs are generally flat-faced and about 2.5 cm (1 inch) in diameter (12). The slugs are granulated into the desired particle size, generally for use in the production of tablets. The dry process often results in the production of fines, that is, powder that has not agglomerated into granules. These fines are separated, collected, and reprocessed. The wet and dry granulation methods as they pertain to tablet making are discussed in greater detail in the next chapter.

Granules flow well compared to powders. For comparison, consider the pouring and flowing characteristics of granulated sugar and powdered sugar. Because of their flow properties, granulations are commonly used in tablet making to facilitate the free flow of material from the feeding container (or hopper) into the tablet presses.

Granules have other important characteristics. Because their surface area is less than that of a comparable volume of powder, granules are usually more stable to the effects of atmospheric humidity and are less likely to cake or harden upon standing. Granules also are more easily wetted by liquids than are certain light and fluffy powders (which tend to float on the surface) and are often preferred for dry products intended to be constituted into solutions or suspensions.

A number of commercial products containing antibiotic drugs that are unstable in aqueous solution are prepared as small granules for constitution by the pharmacist with purified water just prior to dispensing. The granules are prepared to contain not only the medicinal agent, but colorants, flavorants, and other pharmaceutical ingredients. Upon constitution, the resultant liquid has all of the desired medicinal and pharmaceutical features of a liquid pharmaceutical.

Other types of granulated commercial products include Lactinex Granules, a mixed culture of *Lactobacillus acidophilus* and *Lactobacillus bulgaricus* in 1-g packets used in the treatment of uncomplicated diarrhea, including that due to antibiotic therapy. The granules are measured and mixed with water or other beverage, sprinkled on food, or eaten plain. Granulations of effervescent products may be compressed into tablet form, as Zantac EFFERdose Tablets (Glaxo Wellcome). Effervescent granules and tablets are dissolved in water before use. The preparation of effervescent granulated salts is as follows.

Effervescent Granulated Salts

Effervescent salts are granules or coarse to very coarse powders containing a medicinal agent in a dry mixture usually composed of sodium bicarbonate, citric acid, and tartaric acid. When added to water, the acids and base react to liberate carbon dioxide, resulting in effervescence. The resulting carbonated solution masks undesirable taste of any medicinal agent. Using granules or coarse particles of the mixed powders rather than small powder particles decreases the rate of solution and prevents violent and uncontrollable effervescence. Sudden and rapid effervescence could overflow the glass and leave little residual carbonation in the solution.

Using a combination of citric and tartaric acids rather than either acid alone avoids certain difficulties. When tartaric acid is used as the sole acid, the resulting granules readily lose their firmness and crumble. Citric acid alone results in a sticky mixture difficult to granulate.

A summary of the chemistry of effervescent granules may be found in Physical Pharmacy Capsule 6.3, Effervescent Granules.

Effervescent granules are prepared by two general methods: (*a*) the dry or fusion method and (*b*) the wet method.

Fusion Method

In the fusion method, the one molecule of water present in each molecule of citric acid acts as the binding agent for the powder mixture. Before mixing the powders, the citric acid crystals are powdered and then mixed with the other powders of the same sieve size to ensure uniformity of the mixture. The sieves and the mixing equipment should be made of stainless steel or other material resistant to the effect of the acids. The mixing of the powders is performed as rapidly as is practical, preferably in an environment of low humidity to avoid absorption of moisture and a premature chemical reaction. After mixing, the powder is placed on a suitable dish in an oven (Fig. 6.10 at 34°C to 40°C. During the heating process, an acid-resistant spatula is used to turn the powder. The heat releases the water of crystallization from the citric acid, which in turn dissolves a portion of the powder mixture, setting the chemical reaction and consequently re-

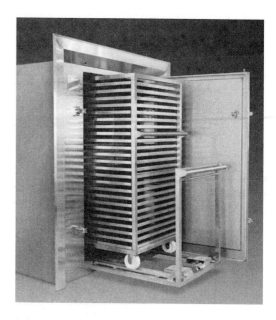

FIGURE 6.10 Large oven for drying granulations. (Courtesy of O'Hara Technologies.)

leasing some carbon dioxide. This causes the softened mass of powder to become somewhat spongy, and when it has reached the proper consistency (as bread dough), it is removed from the oven and rubbed through a sieve to produce granules of the desired size. A No. 4 sieve produces large granules, a No. 8 sieve prepares medium size granules, and a No. 10 sieve prepares small granules. The granules are dried at a temperature not exceeding 54°C and immediately placed in containers and tightly sealed.

Wet Method

The wet method differs from the fusion method in that the source of binding agent is not the water of crystallization from the citric acid but water added to alcohol as the moistening agent, forming the pliable mass for granulation. In this method, all of the powders may be anhydrous as long as water is added to the moistening liquid. Just enough liquid is added (in portions) to prepare a mass of proper consistency; then the granules are prepared and dried in the same manner as described.

PHYSICAL PHARMACY CAPSULE 6.3

Effervescent Granules

Granules are dosage forms that consist of particles ranging from about 4 to 10 mesh in size (4.76–2.00 mm), formed by moistening blended powders and passing through a screen or a special granulator. These moist granules are either air or oven dried. A special form of granules can be used to provide a pleasant vehicle for selected drug products, especially those with a bitter or salty taste. This special formulation, an effervescent granule, may consist of mixtures of citric acid and/or tartaric acid and/or sodium biphosphate combined with sodium bicarbonate.

EXAMPLE

Rx
Active drug   500 mg/5 g tsp
in effervescent granule qs   120 g
Sig: Dissolve 1 teaspoonful in one-half glass of cool water and drink. Repeat every 8 hours.

It is desired to dispense this as a granule, so that the patient will measure out a teaspoonful (5 g) dose, mix, and administer. Since each dose weighs 5 g and the prescription consists of 120 g, there are 24 doses. Each dose contains 0.5 g of active drug, which comes to 12 g of active drug for the entire prescription. This requires 120 g − 12 g = 108 g of effervescent vehicle. A good effervescent blend consists of both citric acid and tartaric acid (1:2 ratio), since the former is rather sticky and the latter produces a chalky, friable granule. It is necessary to calculate the amount of each ingredient required to prepare 108 g of the granulation.

CITRIC ACID

$$3\,NaHCO_3 + C_6H_8O_7.H_2O \rightarrow 4\,H_2O + 3CO_2 + Na_3C_6H_5O_7$$
$$3 \times 84 \qquad 210$$

Citric acid 1 g (MW = 210) reacts with sodium bicarbonate 1.2 g (MW = 84) as obtained from the following:

$$\frac{1}{210} = \frac{x}{3 \times 84}$$

$$x = 1.2\ g$$

TARTARIC ACID

$$2\,NaHCO_3 + C_4H_6O_6 \rightarrow 2\,H_2O + 2CO_2 + Na_2C_4H_4O_6$$
$$2 \times 84 \qquad 150$$

Since it is desired to use a 1:2 ratio of citric acid to tartaric acid, tartaric acid 2 g (MW = 150) reacts with sodium bicarbonate 2.24 g according to the following calculation:

$$\frac{2}{150} = \frac{x}{2} \times 84$$

$$x = 2.24\ g$$

Therefore, sodium bicarbonate 1.2 g and 2.24 g is required to react with 1 + 2 g of the combination of citric acid and tartaric acid. Since it is desired to leave a small amount of the acids unreacted

Physical Pharmacy Capsule 6.3 cont.

to enhance palatability and taste, 2.24 g + 1.2 g = 3.44 g, only 3.4 g of sodium bicarbonate will be used. Therefore, the ratio of the effervescent ingredients is 1:2:3.4 for the citric acid:tartaric acid:sodium bicarbonate. Since the prescription requires 108 g of the effervescent mix, the quantity of each ingredient can be calculated as follows:

$$1 + 2 + 3.4 = 6.4$$
$$1/6.4 \times 108 \text{ g} = 16.875 \text{ g Citric acid}$$
$$2/6.4 \times 108 \text{ g} = 33.750 \text{ g Tartaric acid}$$
$$3.4/6.4 \times 108 \text{ g} = 57.375 \text{ g Sodium bicarbonate}$$
$$\text{Total} = 108 \text{ g}$$

The prescription will require 12 g of the active drug and 108 g of this effervescent vehicle.

CLINICAL CASE STUDY

Subjective

CC: E. M. is an 86-y/o adult ambulatory male (AAM) who resides in a nursing home with complaints of pain in his right heel.

PMH: HTN
Hyperlipidemia
Type II diabetes

Meds: Hydrochlorothiazide 50 mg po q am
Enalapril 5 mg po bid
Atorvastatin 10 mg po qhs
Metformin 1000 mg po bid
Glyburide 5 mg po qd
ASA 81 mg po qd
Centrum 1 tablet po qd

PSH: Tonsillectomy at age 10

FH: Mother HTN, breast cancer, metastatic bone cancer
Father hyperlipidemia, Type II diabetes

SH: (per KF)
(−) Tobacco
(−) EtOH
(−) Illicit drugs
(−) Caffeine

ALL: NKDA

Objective

BP: 125/78
HR: 72
Ht: 5'7"

Wt: 230 lb

Wound with a high volume of yellow slough and exudate on right heel area

Assessment

Decubitus ulcer

Plan

Recommend Debrisan (dextranomer) Beads twice a day. Sprinkle the beads into the ulcer to 3mm (~0.1 inch) thickness. To prevent maceration, apply a nonocclusive dressing and seal on all four sides. Remove the beads before they become fully saturated by irrigating the wound with sterile water or normal saline using a syringe. Apply a new layer of beads while the area is still moist to prevent pain. Change the dressing before the beads become fully saturated. The number of changes per day will depend on the amount of exudate produced and will vary from one to three times a day. Also, it is suggested that for easier removal the dressing be changed before it is completely dry. Avoid contact with the eyes. Contact the physician if the condition worsens or persists beyond 14 to 21 days. The patient's position should be frequently changed to prevent continuous pressure on any single part of the body. Avoid positioning the patient on the right heel.

PHARMACEUTICS CASE STUDY

Subjective Information

A pharmaceutical manufacturer is planning to market a topical powder consisting of an antifungal agent in an inert powder vehicle. However, in the pilot plant scale-up, assay of the containers revealed that they did not have a uniform potency of the antifungal active ingredient. The USP 26–NF 21 monograph for a typical antifungal topical powder states that it is to contain not less than 90.0% and not more than 110.0% of the labeled amount of the active drug. This problem must be corrected before the product can proceed to full-scale manufacturing.

Objective Information

The antifungal occurs as a white or nearly white crystalline powder with not more than a slight odor. It is only very slightly soluble in water and in ether and slightly soluble in alcohol. It has a true density in the range of 4.5 to 5.0 and an apparent density of 0.12 g/mL. It was sifted through a 40-mesh screen prior to blending.

The inert vehicle is talc that occurs as a very fine white or grayish-white crystalline powder. It is unctuous, adheres readily to the skin, and is free of grittiness. It is practically insoluble in dilute acids and alkalis, organic solvents, and water. It has a true density in the range of 2.7 to 2.8 and an apparent density of 0.05 g/mL. It has a specific surface area of 2.41 to 2.42 m^2/g.

The powders are weighed and blended in a large V-blender. The powder is then moved to the hopper of a large packaging device. The machine vibrates significantly during packaging.

Assessment

It appears that the difference in the size and density of the two ingredients is sufficient to suggest a separation in the hopper of the packaging machine. The density of the antifungal is greater than that of the vehicle, and the particle size of the antifungal (40 mesh) is larger than that of the talc (very fine, approximately an 80-mesh powder). One would normally expect the finer powder to settle to the bottom, but since there is a difference in the density of these two powders, the antifungal appears to be settling. This would result in containers that would have varying amounts of active drug.

Plan

One approach to solving this problem is to reduce the particle size of the antifungal agent to be closer to that of the talc so their apparent densities are closer. Another possibility is to use a different packaging device with minimal vibration. Can you think of other reasonable approaches to solving this problem?

REFERENCES

1. Brittain HG. On the physical characterization of pharmaceutical solids. Pharm Tech 1997;21:100–108.
2. The United States Pharmacopeia 26–National Formulary 21. Rockville, MD: U.S. Pharmacopeial Convention, 2003.
3. Yalkowsky SH, Bolton S. Particle size and content uniformity. Pharm Res 1990;7:962–966.
4. Jager PD, DeStefano GA, McNamara DP. Particle-size measurement using right-angle light scattering. Pharm Tech 1993;17:102–110.
5. Carver LD. Particle size analysis. Industrial Res 1971:(August) 39–43.
6. Evans R. Determination of drug particle size and morphology using optical microscopy. Pharm Tech 1993;17:146–152.
7. Houghton ME, Amidon GE. Microscopic characterization of particle size and shape: an inexpensive and versatile method. Pharm Res 1992;9:856–863.
8. Horiba Instruments, Irvine, CA, 1998.
9. Gorman WG, Carroll FA. Aerosol particle-size determination using laser holography. Pharm Tech 1993; 17:34–37.
10. Milosovich SM. Particle-size determination via cascade impaction. Pharm Tech 1992;16:82–86.
11. Hindle M, Byron PR. Size distribution control of raw materials for dry-powder inhalers using aerosizer with aero-dispenser. Pharm Tech 1995:19:64–78.
12. Miller RW. Roller compaction technology. In Parikh DM, ed. Handbook of pharmaceutical granulation technology. New York: Marcel Dekker, 1997;100–150.

Capsules

7

When medications are to be administered orally to adults, capsules and tablets usually are preferred because they are conveniently carried, readily identified, and easily taken.

Consider the convenience of a patient carrying a day's, week's, or month's supply of capsules or tablets compared with equivalent doses of a liquid medication. With capsules and tablets, there is no need for spoons or other measuring devices, which may be inconvenient and may result in less than accurate dosing. Also, most capsules and tablets are tasteless when swallowed, which is not the case with oral liquid medication.

The characteristic shapes and colors of capsules and tablets and the manufacturer's name and product code number commonly embossed or imprinted on their surface make them readily identified. This enhances communication between the patient and health care providers, assists patient compliance, and fosters safe and effective medication use.

Capsules and tablets are available for many medications in a variety of dosage strengths, providing flexibility to the prescriber and accurate individualized dosage for the patient.

From a pharmaceutical standpoint, solid dosage forms are efficiently and productively manufactured; they are packaged and shipped by manufacturers at lower cost and with less breakage than comparable liquid forms; and are more stable and have a longer shelf life than their liquid counterparts.

As discussed later in this chapter, the pharmacist often uses empty hard gelatin capsules for extemporaneous compounding of prescriptions. On occasion, a pharmacist may use commercially available capsules and tablets as the *source* of a medicinal agent when it is not otherwise available. In these instances, the pharmacist must consider any excipients in the commercial product to ensure compatibility with the other ingredients in the compounded prescription. Capsules and tablets designed to provide modified drug release are discussed in Chapter 9.

Overview of Capsules

Capsules are solid dosage forms in which medicinal agents and/or inert substances are enclosed in a small shell of gelatin. Gelatin capsule shells may be *hard* or *soft*, depending on their composition.

Most filled capsules are intended to be swallowed whole. However, it is fairly common in hospitals and extended care facilities for a caregiver to open capsules or crush tablets to mix with food or drink, especially for children or other patients unable to swallow solid dosage forms. This should be done only with the concurrence of the pharmacist, since the drug release characteristics of certain dosage forms can be altered and adversely affect the patient's welfare.

Dosage forms that must be left intact include enteric coated tablets, designed to pass through the stomach for drug release and absorption in the intestine; extended-release dosage forms, designed to provide prolonged release of the medication; and sublingual or buccal tablets, formulated to dissolve under the tongue or in the mouth (1). If the patient cannot swallow an intact solid dosage form, an alternative product, such as a chewable tablet, instant dissolving tablet, oral liquid, oral or nasal inhalation solution, suppository, or injection may be employed.

Hard Gelatin Capsules

Hard gelatin capsule shells are used in most commercial medicated capsules. They are also commonly employed in clinical drug trials, to compare the effects of an investigational drug with those of another drug product or placebo. The community pharmacist also uses hard gelatin capsules in the extemporaneous compounding of prescriptions. The empty capsule shells are made of gelatin, sugar, and water

(Fig. 7.1). As such, they can be clear, colorless, and essentially tasteless; or they may be colored with various FD&C and D&C dyes and made opaque by adding agents such as titanium dioxide. Most commercially available medicated capsules contain combinations of colorants and opaquants to make them distinctive, many with caps and bodies of different colors.

Gelatin is obtained by the partial hydrolysis of collagen obtained from the skin, white connective tissue, and bones of animals. In commerce, it is available in the form of a fine powder, a coarse powder, shreds, flakes, or sheets.

Gelatin is stable in air when dry but is subject to microbial decomposition when it becomes moist. Normally, hard gelatin capsules contain 13 to 16% of moisture (2). However, if stored in an environment of high humidity, additional moisture is absorbed by the capsules, and they may become distorted and lose their rigid shape. In an environment of extreme dryness, some of the moisture normally present in the gelatin capsules is lost, and the capsules may become brittle and crumble when handled. Therefore, it is desirable to maintain hard gelatin capsules in an environment free from excessive humidity or dryness.

Because moisture may be absorbed by gelatin capsules and affect hygroscopic agents within,

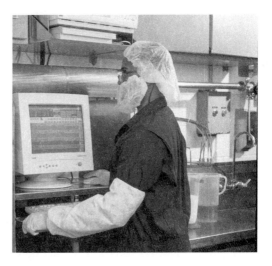

FIGURE 7.1 Preparation of a gelatin mixture for making empty capsules. (Courtesy of Shinogi Qualicaps.)

many capsules are packaged along with a small packet of a desiccant material to protect against the absorption of atmospheric moisture. The desiccant materials most used are dried silica gel, clay, and activated charcoal.

Prolonged exposure to high humidity can affect in vitro capsule dissolution. Such changes have been observed in capsules containing tetracycline, chloramphenicol, and nitrofurantoin (3). Because such changes could forewarn of possible changes in bioavailability, capsules subjected to such stress conditions must be evaluated case by case (3).

Although gelatin is insoluble in cold water, it does soften through the absorption of up to 10 times its weight of water. Some patients prefer to swallow a capsule wetted with water or saliva, because a wetted capsule slides down the throat more readily than a dry capsule. Gelatin is soluble in hot water and in warm gastric fluid; a gelatin capsule rapidly dissolves and exposes its contents. Gelatin, being a protein, is digested by proteolytic enzymes and absorbed.

A number of methods have been developed to track the passage of capsules and tablets through the gastrointestinal tract to map their transit time and drug release patterns. Among these is gamma *scintigraphy*, a noninvasive procedure that entails use of a gamma ray–emitting radiotracer incorporated into the formulation with a gamma camera coupled to a data recording system (4,5). The quantity of material added to allow gamma scintigraphy is small and does not compromise the usual in vivo characteristics of the dosage form being studied. When scintigraphy is combined with pharmacokinetic studies, the resultant *pharmacoscintographic* evaluation provides information about the transit and drug release patterns of the dosage form as well as the rate of drug absorption from the various regions of the gastrointestinal tract (4). This method is particularly useful in (*a*) determining whether a correlation exists between in vitro and in vivo bioavailability for immediate-release products; (*b*) assessing the integrity and transit time of enteric coated tablets through the stomach en route to the intestines; and (*c*) drug and dosage form evaluation in new product development (4, 5). A separate technique using a pH-sensitive

nondigestible radiotelemetric device termed the Heidelberg capsule, the approximate size of a No. 0 gelatin capsule, has been used as a *nonradioactive* means to measure gastric pH, gastric residence time, and gastric emptying time of solid dosage forms in fasting and nonfasting human subjects (6).

As discussed in Chapter 5, drug absorption from the gastrointestinal tract depends on a number of factors, including the solubility of the drug substance, the type of product formulation (i.e., immediate release, modified release, enteric coated), the gastrointestinal contents, and intersubject differences in physiologic character and response.

The Manufacture of Hard Gelatin Capsule Shells

Hard gelatin capsule shells are manufactured in two sections, the capsule body and a shorter cap. The two parts overlap when joined, with the cap fitting snugly over the open end of the capsule body. The shells are produced industrially by the mechanical dipping of pins or pegs of the desired shape and diameter into a temperature-controlled reservoir of melted gelatin mixture (Figs. 7.2 and 7.3). The pegs, made of manganese bronze, are affixed to plates, each capable of holding up to about 500 pegs. Each plate is mechanically lowered to the gelatin bath, the pegs submerged to the desired

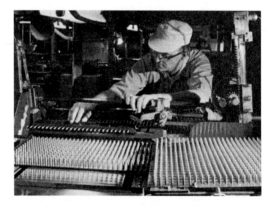

FIGURE 7.2 Body of capsules and their caps are shown as they move through automated capsule-making machine. Each machine is capable of producing 30,000 capsules per hour. It takes a 40-minute cycle to produce a capsule. (Courtesy of SmithKline Beecham.)

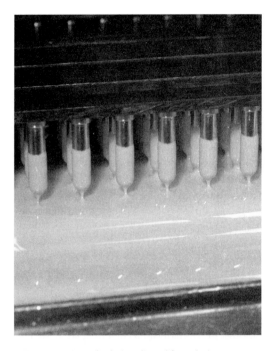

FIGURE 7.3 Capsules being dipped for coloring on automated capsule-making equipment. (Courtesy of Shinogi Qualicaps.)

By tapering the end of the body-producing peg while leaving the cap-making peg rounded, one manufacturer prepares capsules differentiated from those of other manufacturers (Pulvules, Eli Lilly). Another manufacturer uses capsules with the ends of both the bodies and caps highly tapered (Spansule Capsules, SmithKline Beecham). Yet another innovation in capsule shell design is the Snap-fit, Coni-snap, and Coni-snap Supro hard gelatin capsules depicted in Figures 7.4 and 7.5. The original Snap-fit construction enables the two halves of the capsule shells to be positively joined through locking grooves in the shell walls. The two grooves fit into each other and thus ensure reliable closing of the filled capsule. During the closing process, the capsule body is inserted into the cap. With the high-capacity filling rates of the modern capsule filling machines (more than 180,000 capsules per

depth and maintained for the desired period to achieve the proper length and thickness of coating. Then the plate and the pegs are slowly lifted from the bath and the gelatin dried by a gentle flow of temperature- and humidity-controlled air. When dried, each capsule part is trimmed mechanically to the proper length and removed from the pegs, and the capsule bodies and caps are joined together. It is important that the thickness of the gelatin walls be strictly controlled so that the capsule's body and cap fit snugly to prevent disengagement. The pegs on which the caps are formed are slightly larger in diameter than the pegs on which the bodies are formed, allowing the telescoping of the caps over the bodies. In capsule shell production, there is a continuous dipping, drying, removing, and joining of capsules as the peg-containing plates rotate in and out of the gelatin bath. As noted earlier, capsule shells may be made distinctive by adding colorants and/or opaquants to the gelatin bath.

A manufacturer also may prepare distinctive-looking capsules by altering the usual rounded shape of the capsule-making pegs.

CONI-SNAP™

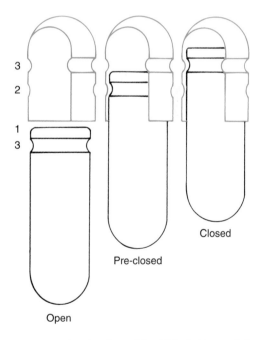

FIGURE 7.4 Line drawings of the CONI-SNAP capsule in open, preclosed, and closed positions. The tapered rims (*1*) avoid telescoping; the indentations (*2*) prevent premature opening; and the grooves (*3*) lock the two capsule parts together after the capsule is filled. (Courtesy of Capsugel Division, Warner-Lambert.)

CONI-SNAP™

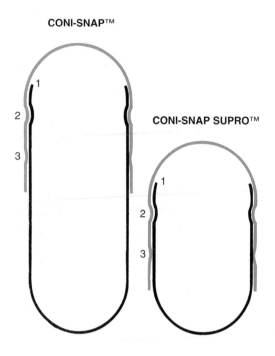

CONI-SNAP SUPRO™

1. Tapered rim to avoid telescoping (CONI-SNAP™)

2. Grooves which lock the two halves together once the capsule has been filled (SNAP-FIT™ principle)

3. Indentations to prevent premature opening

FIGURE 7.5 Line drawings of the CONI-SNAP and CONI-SNAP SUPRO (*right*) capsules. The latter is designed to be smaller and to have the lower portion of the capsule shell concealed except for the rounded end. This makes separation of the two parts more difficult and contributes to capsule integrity. (Courtesy of Capsugel Division, Warner-Lambert.)

latter is visible (Fig. 7.5). Opening of such a filled capsule is difficult because the lower surface offers less gripping surface to pull the two halves apart. This increases the security of the contents and the integrity of the capsule.

After filling, some manufacturers render their capsules tamper evident through various sealing techniques. These methods are discussed later in this section. Capsules and tablets also may be imprinted with the names or monograms of the manufacturer, the assigned national drug code number and other markings making the product identifiable and distinguishable from other products.

Capsule Sizes

Empty gelatin capsules are manufactured in various lengths, diameters, and capacities. The size selected for use is determined by the amount of fill material to be encapsulated. The density and compressibility of the fill will largely determine to what extent it may be packed into a capsule shell (7) (Fig. 7.6). For estimation, a comparison may be made with powders of well-known features (Table 7.1) and an initial judgment made as to the approximate capsule size needed to hold a specific amount of material. However, the final determination may be largely the result of trial and

hour), splitting (telescoping) and/or denting of the capsule shell occurs with the slightest contact between the two rims when they are joined. This problem, which exists primarily with straight-walled capsule shells, led to the development of the Coni-snap capsule, in which the rim of the capsule body is not straight but tapered slightly (Fig. 7.5). This reduces the risk of the capsule rims touching on joining and essentially eliminates the problem of splitting during large-scale filling operations. In the Coni-snap Supro capsules, the upper capsule part extends so far over the lower part that only the rounded edge of the

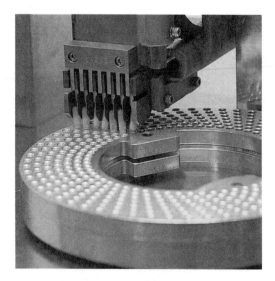

FIGURE 7.6 Capsule ring containing capsule halves being filled with powder. (Courtesy of Shinogi Qualicaps.)

TABLE 7.1 APPROXIMATE CAPACITY OF EMPTY GELATIN CAPSULES

	CAPSULE SIZE							
	000	00	0	1	2	3	4	5
VOLUME (ML)	1.40	0.95	0.68	0.50	0.37	0.30	0.21	0.13
Drug Substance (mg)[a]								
Quinine sulfate	650	390	325	227	195	130	97	65
Sodium bicarbonate	1430	975	715	510	390	325	260	130
Aspirin	1040	650	520	325	260	195	162	97

[a]Amount may vary with the degree of pressure used in filling the capsules.

error. For human use, empty capsules ranging in size from 000 (the largest) to 5 (the smallest) are commercially available (Fig. 7.7). Larger capsules are available for veterinary use.

For prescriptions requiring extemporaneous compounding, hard gelatin capsules permit a wide prescribing latitude by the physician. The pharmacist may compound capsules of a single medicinal agent or combination of agents at the precise dosage prescribed for the individual patient.

Preparation of Filled Hard Gelatin Capsules

The large-scale or small-scale preparation of filled hard gelatin capsules is divided into the following general steps.

1. Developing and preparing the formulation and selecting the size capsule
2. Filling the capsule shells
3. Capsule sealing (optional)
4. Cleaning and polishing the filled capsules

Developing the Formulation and Selection of Capsule Size

In developing a capsule formulation, the goal is to prepare a capsule with accurate dosage, good bioavailability, ease of filling and production, stability, and elegance.

In dry formulations, the active and inactive components must be blended thoroughly to ensure a uniform powder mix for the fill. Care in blending is especially important for low-dose drugs, since lack of homogeneity may result in significant therapeutic consequences. Preformulation studies are performed to determine whether all of the formulation's bulk powders may be effectively blended together as such or require reduction of particle size or other processing to achieve homogeneity.

A diluent or filler may be added to the formulation to produce the proper capsule fill volume. Lactose, microcrystalline cellulose, and starch are commonly used for this purpose. In addition to providing bulk, these materials often provide cohesion to the powders, which is

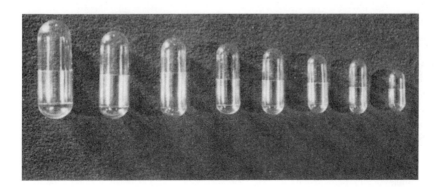

FIGURE 7.7 Actual sizes of hard gelatin capsules. From left to right, sizes 000, 00, 0, 1, 2, 3, 4, and 5.

beneficial in the transfer of the powder blend into capsule shells (2). Disintegrants are frequently included in a capsule formulation to assist the breakup and distribution of the capsule's contents in the stomach. Among the disintegrants used are pregelatinized starch, croscarmellose, and sodium starch glycolate.

To achieve uniform drug distribution, it is advantageous if the density and particle size of the drug and nondrug components are similar. This is particularly important when a drug of low dosage is blended with other drugs or nondrug fill (8). When necessary, particle size may be reduced by *milling* to produce particles ranging from about 50 to 1000 μm. Milled powders may be blended effectively for uniform distribution throughout a powder mix when the drug's dosage is 10 mg or greater (8). For drugs of lower dose or when smaller particles are required, *micronization* is employed. Depending on the materials and equipment used, micronization produces particles ranging from about 1 to 20 μm.

In preparing capsules on an industrial scale using high-speed automated equipment, the powder mix or granules must be free-flowing to allow steady passage of the capsule fill from the hopper through the encapsulating equipment and into the capsule shells. The addition of a *lubricant* or *glidant* such as fumed silicon dioxide, magnesium stearate, calcium stearate, stearic acid, or talc (about 0.25–1%) to the powder mix enhances flow properties (2).

When magnesium stearate is used as the lubricant, the waterproofing characteristics of this water-insoluble material can retard penetration by the gastrointestinal fluids and delay drug dissolution and absorption. A surface-active agent, such as sodium lauryl sulfate, is used to facilitate wetting by the gastrointestinal fluids to overcome the problem (9). Even if a water-insoluble lubricant is used, after the gelatin capsule shell dissolves, gastrointestinal fluids must displace the air that surrounds the dry powder and penetrate the drug before it can be dispersed and dissolved. Powders of poorly soluble drugs have a tendency to resist such penetration. Disintegration agents in a capsule formulation facilitate the breakup and distribution of the capsule's contents.

Whether it be a lubricant, surfactant, disintegrating agent, or some other pharmaceutical excipient, formulation can influence the bioavailability of a drug substance and can account for differences in drug effects between two capsule products of the same medicinal substance. Pharmacists must be aware of this possibility when product interchange is considered.

Inserting tablets or small capsules into capsules is sometimes useful in the commercial production of capsules and in a pharmacist's extemporaneous preparation of capsules (Fig. 7.8). This may be done to separate chemically incompatible agents or to add premeasured amounts of potent drug substances. Rather than weighing a potent drug, a pharmacist may choose to insert a prefabricated tablet of the desired strength in each capsule. Other less potent agents and diluents may then be weighed and added. On an industrial scale, coated pellets designed for modified-release drug delivery are also commonly placed in capsule shells.

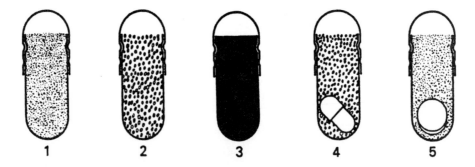

FIGURE 7.8 Examples of fill in hard gelatin capsules. *1*, powder or granulate; *2*, pellet mixture; *3*, paste; *4*, capsule; and *5*, tablet. (Courtesy of Capsugel Division, Warner-Lambert.)

Gelatin capsules are unsuitable for aqueous liquids because water softens gelatin and distorts the capsules, resulting in leakage of the contents. However, some liquids, such as fixed or volatile oils, that do not interfere with the stability of the gelatin shells may be placed in locking gelatin capsules (or the capsules may be sealed with a solution of gelatin thinly coating the interface of the cap and body) to ensure retention of the liquid. Rather than placing a liquid as such in a capsule, the liquid may be mixed with an inert powder to make a wet mass or paste, which may then be placed in capsules in the usual manner (Fig. 7.8). *Eutectic mixtures* of drugs, or mixtures of agents that have a propensity to liquefy when admixed, may be mixed with a diluent or absorbent such as magnesium carbonate, kaolin, or light magnesium oxide to separate the interacting agents and to absorb any liquefied material that may form.

In large-scale capsule production, liquids are placed in *soft gelatin* capsules that are sealed during filling and manufacturing. Soft capsules are discussed later in this chapter.

In most instances the amount of drug in a capsule is a single dose. When the usual dose of the drug is too large for a single capsule, two or more capsules may be required. The total amount of formula prepared is the amount necessary to fill the desired number of capsules. On an industrial scale this means hundreds of thousands of capsules. In community practice, an individual prescription may call for preparation of a few to several hundred capsules. Any slight loss in fill material during preparation and capsule filling will not materially affect an industrial size batch, but in the community pharmacy, a slight loss of powder could result in an inadequate quantity to fill the last capsule. To ensure enough fill in the compounding of small numbers of capsules, the community pharmacist may calculate for the preparation of one or two more capsules than required to fill the prescription. However, this procedure must not be followed for capsules containing a controlled substance, since the amount of drug used and that called for in the prescription must strictly coincide.

The selection of the capsule size for a commercial product is done during product development. The choice is determined by requirements of the formulation, including the dose of the active ingredient and the density and compaction characteristics of the drug and other components. If the dose of the drug is inadequate to fill the volume of the capsule body, a diluent is added. Information on the density and compaction characteristics of a capsule's active and inactive components and comparison to other similar materials and prior experiences can serve as a guide in selecting capsule size (7).

Hard gelatin capsules are used to encapsulate about 65 mg to 1 g of powdered material. As shown in Table 7.1, the smallest capsule (No. 5), may be expected to hold 65 mg of powder or more, depending on the characteristics of the powder. Oftentimes, in the extemporaneous compounding of prescriptions, the best capsule size to use is determined by trial. Use of the smallest size capsule, properly filled, is preferred. A properly filled capsule should have its body filled with the drug mixture, not the cap. The cap is intended to fit snugly over the body to retain the contents.

The following examples demonstrate the drug and nondrug contents of a few commercially available capsules.

Tetracycline Capsules

Active ingredient	Tetracycline hydrochloride 250 mg
Filler	Lactose
Lubricant/glidant	Magnesium stearate
Capsule colorants	FD&C Yellow No. 6, D&C Yellow No. 10, D&C Red No. 28, FD&C Blue No. 1
Capsule opaquant	Titanium dioxide

Acetaminophen With Codeine Capsules

Active ingredients	Acetaminophen 325 mg Codeine phosphate 30 mg
Disintegrant	Sodium starch glycolate
Lubricant/glidants	Magnesium stearate, stearic acid
Capsule colorants	D&C Yellow No. 10, Edible Ink, FD&C Blue No. 1 (FD&C Green No. 3 and FD&C Red No. 40)

Diphenhydramine Hydrochloride Capsules

Active ingredient	Diphenhydramine HCl 25 mg
Filler	Confectioner's sugar
Lubricants/ glidants	Talc, colloidal silicon dioxide
Wetting agent	Sodium lauryl sulfate
Capsule colorants	FD&C Blue No. 1, FD&C Red No. 3
Capsule opaquant	Titanium dioxide

Filling Hard Capsule Shells

When filling a small number of capsules in the pharmacy, the pharmacist may use the punch method. The pharmacist takes the precise number of empty capsules to be filled from the stock container. By counting the capsules as the initial step rather than taking a capsule from stock as each one is filled, the pharmacist guards against filling the wrong number of cap-

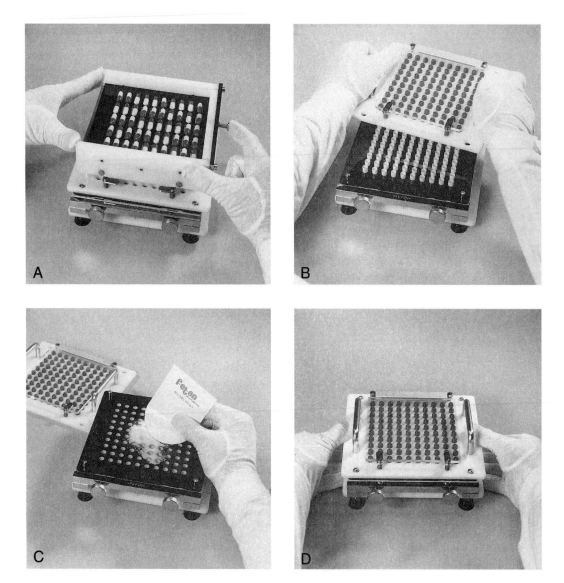

FIGURE 7.9 The Feton capsule-filling machine. **A.** With empty capsules in the loader tray, the tray placed on top of the filler unit. **B.** The loader inserts the capsules into the filling unit and is removed, and the top plate is lifted to separate the caps from the bodies. **C.** The powder is placed on the unit and the capsule bodies filled. **D.** The top plate is returned to the unit and the caps placed on filled capsule bodies. (Courtesy of Chemical and Pharmaceutical Industry Company.)

sules and avoids contaminating the stock container with drug powder. The powder to be encapsulated is placed on a sheet of clean paper or on a glass or porcelain plate. Using the spatula, the powder mix is formed into a cake having a depth of approximately one-fourth to one-third the length of the capsule body. Then an empty capsule body is held between the thumb and forefinger and punched vertically into the powder cake repeatedly until filled. Some pharmacists wear surgical gloves or latex finger cots to avoid handling the capsules with bare fingers. Because the amount of powder packed into a capsule depends on the degree of compression, the pharmacist should punch each capsule in the same manner and after capping weigh the product. When nonpotent materials are placed in capsules, the first filled capsule should be weighed (using an empty capsule of the same size on the opposite balance pan to counter the weight of the shell) to determine the capsule size to use and the degree of compaction to be used. After this determination, the other capsules should be prepared and weighed periodically to check the uniformity of the process. When potent drugs are being used, *each capsule* should be weighed after filling to ensure accuracy. Such weighings protect against uneven filling of capsules and premature exhaustion or underuse of the powder. After the body of a capsule has been filled and the cap placed on the body, the body may be squeezed or tapped gently to distribute some powder to the cap end to give the capsule a full appearance.

Granular material that does not lend itself to the punch method of filling capsules may be poured into each capsule from the powder paper on which it is weighed.

Pharmacists who prepare capsules on a regular or extensive basis may use a hand-operated filling machine (Fig. 7.9). The various types of machines have capacities ranging from 24 to 300 capsules and when efficiently operated are capable of producing about 200 to 2000 capsules per hour.

Machines developed for industrial use automatically separate the caps from empty capsules, fill the bodies, scrape off the excess powder, replace the caps, seal the capsules as

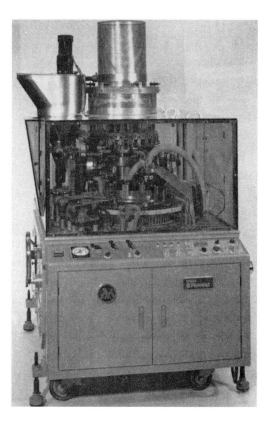

FIGURE 7.10 Osaka Automatic Capsule Filler model R-180, capable of filling up to 165,000 capsules per hour. (Courtesy of Sharples-Stokes Division, Stokes-Merrill, Pennwalt Corporation.)

desired, and clean the outside of the filled capsules at up to 165,000 capsules per hour (Figs. 7.10 and 7.11). The formulation must be such that the filled body contains the accurate drug dosage. This is verified through the use of automated in-process sampling and analysis (Figs. 7.12 and 7.13).

As described later, the USP requires adherence to standards for *content uniformity* and *weight variation* for capsules to assure the accuracy of dosage units.

Capsule Sealing

As mentioned previously, some manufacturers make tamper-evident capsules by sealing the joint between the two capsule parts. One manufacturer makes distinctive-looking capsules by sealing them with a colored band of gelatin (Kapseals, Parke-Davis). If removed, the band

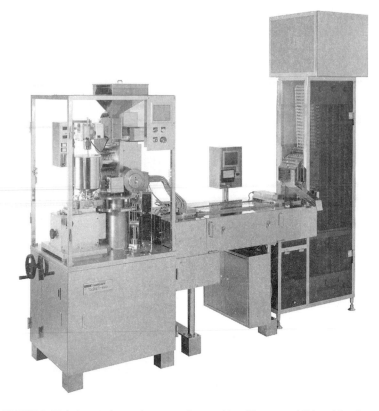

FIGURE 7.11 Automated capsule preparation machine (Courtesy of Shinogi Qualicaps.)

cannot be restored without expert resealing with gelatin. Capsules may also be sealed through a heat welding process that fuses the capsule cap to the body through the double wall thickness at their juncture (10). The process results in a distinctive ring around the capsule where heat welded. Still another process uses a liquid wetting agent that lowers the melting point in the contact areas of the capsule's cap and body and then thermally bonds the two parts using low temperatures (40–45°C) (11). Industrial capsule sealing machines are capable of producing 60,000 to 150,000 gelatin banded, heat welded, or thermally coupled capsules per hour (12). Figure 7.14 depicts a sealed hard gelatin capsule. Although it is difficult and tedious, extemporaneously prepared capsules may be sealed by lightly coating the inner surface of the cap with a warm gelatin solution immediately prior to placement on the filled capsule body.

Cleaning and Polishing Capsules

Small amounts of powder may adhere to the outside of capsules after filling. The powder may be bitter or otherwise unpalatable and should be removed before packaging or dispensing. On a small scale, capsules may be cleaned individually or in small numbers by rubbing them with a clean gauze or cloth. On a large scale, many capsule-filling machines are affixed with a cleaning vacuum that removes any extraneous material from the capsules as they exit the equipment. Figure 7.15 shows industrial cleaning and polishing of filled hard capsules using the Accela-Cota apparatus.

Soft Gelatin Capsules

Soft gelatin capsules are made of gelatin to which glycerin or a polyhydric alcohol such as sorbitol has been added. Soft gelatin capsules,

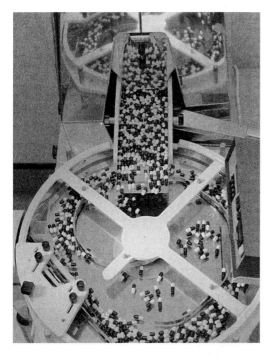

FIGURE 7.12 Automatic capsule weighing apparatus: Vericap 1800A Checkweigher, which rejects capsules not having the precise weight. (Courtesy of Elan Corporation.)

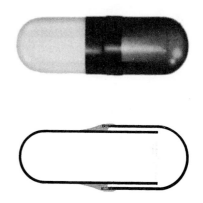

FIGURE 7.14 Z-Weld's gelatin seal fuses the two capsule halves to create a one-piece capsule that is tamper-evident. (Courtesy of Raymond Automation.)

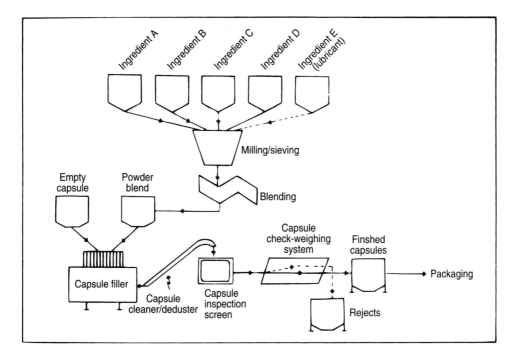

FIGURE 7.13 Process flow diagram for automated capsule filling. (Reprinted with permission from Yelvig M. Principles of process automation for liquid and solid dosage forms. Pharm Technol, 8:47, 1984.)

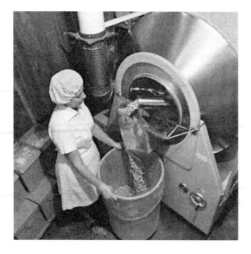

FIGURE 7.15 Cleaning and polishing hard filled capsules using the Accela-Cota apparatus. (Courtesy of Eli Lilly and Company.)

which contain more moisture than hard capsules, may have a preservative, such as methylparaben and/or propylparaben, to retard microbial growth. Soft gelatin capsules may be oblong, oval, or round. They may be a single color or two-tone and may be imprinted with identifying markings. As with hard gelatin capsules, they may be prepared with opaquants to reduce transparency and render characteristic features to the capsule shell.

Soft gelatin capsules are used to encapsulate and hermetically seal liquids, suspensions, pasty materials, dry powders, and even preformed tablets. Soft gelatin capsules are pharmaceutically elegant and are easily swallowed.

Preparation of Soft Gelatin Capsules (13)

Soft gelatin capsules may be prepared by the plate process, using a set of molds to form the capsules, or by the more efficient and productive rotary or reciprocating die processes by which they are produced, filled, and sealed in a continuous operation (Fig. 7.16).

By the plate process, a warm sheet of plain or colored gelatin is placed on the bottom plate of the mold and the liquid-containing medication is evenly poured on it. Then a second sheet of gelatin is carefully placed on top of the med-

ication and the top plate of the mold is put into place. Pressure is then applied to the mold to form, fill, and seal the capsules simultaneously. The capsules are removed and washed with a solvent harmless to the capsules.

Most soft gelatin capsules are prepared by the rotary die process, a method developed in 1933 by Robert P. Scherer. By this method, liquid gelatin flowing from an overhead tank is formed into two continuous ribbons by the rotary die machine and brought together between twin rotating dies (Fig. 7.17). At the same time, metered fill material is injected between the ribbons precisely at the moment that the dies form pockets of the gelatin ribbons. These pockets of fill-containing gelatin are sealed by pressure and heat and then severed from the ribbon. Use of ribbons of two different colors results in bicolored capsules.

The reciprocating die process is similar to the rotary process in that ribbons of gelatin are formed and used to encapsulate the fill, but it differs in the actual encapsulating process. The gelatin ribbons are fed between a set of vertical dies that continually open and close to form rows of pockets in the gelatin ribbons. These pockets are filled with the medication and are sealed, shaped, and cut out of the film as they progress through the machinery. As the capsules are cut from the ribbons, they fall into refrigerated tanks that prevent the capsules from adhering to one another.

Use of Soft Gelatin Capsules

Soft gelatin capsules are prepared to contain a variety of liquid, paste, and dry fills. Liquids that may be encapsulated into soft gelatin capsules include the following (13):

1. Water-immiscible volatile and nonvolatile liquids such as vegetable and aromatic oils, aromatic and aliphatic hydrocarbons, chlorinated hydrocarbons, ethers, esters, alcohols, and organic acids.
2. Water-miscible nonvolatile liquids, such as polyethylene glycols, and nonionic surface active agents, such as polysorbate 80.
3. Water-miscible and relatively nonvolatile compounds, such as propylene glycol and

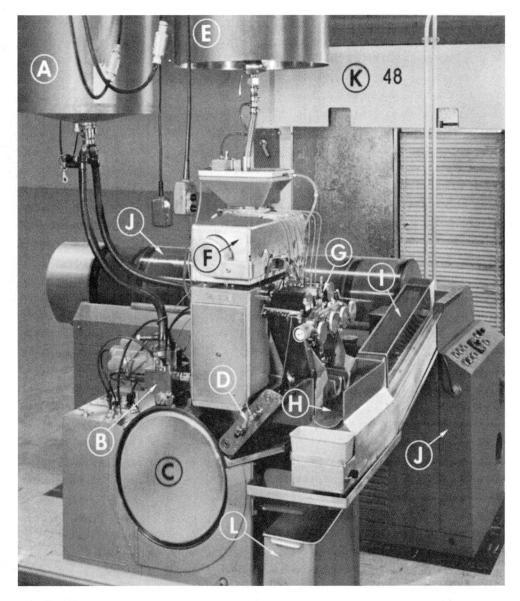

FIGURE 7.16 Rotary die process equipment. *A*, Gelatin tank; *B*, spreader box; *C*, gelatin ribbon casting drum; *D*, mineral oil lubricant bath; *E*, medicine tank; *F*, filling pump; *G*, encapsulating mechanism; *H*, capsule conveyor; *I*, capsule washer; *J*, infrared dryer; *K*, capsule drying tunnel; *L*, gelatin net receiver. (Courtesy of R. P. Scherer Corporation.)

isopropyl alcohol, depending on factors such as concentration used and packaging conditions.

Liquids that can easily migrate through the capsule shell are not suitable for soft gelatin capsules. These materials include water above 5% and low-molecular-weight water-soluble and volatile organic compounds such as alcohols, ketones, acids, amines, and esters.

Solids may be encapsulated into soft gelatin capsules as solutions in a suitable liquid solvent, suspensions, dry powders, granules, pellets, or small tablets.

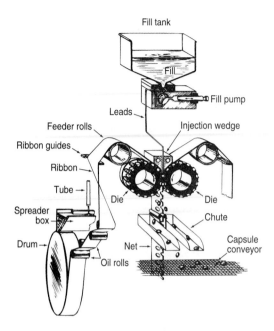

FIGURE 7.17 Rotary die process. (Courtesy of R. P. Scherer Corporation.)

Compendial Requirements for Capsules

Added Substances

Substances added to official preparations, including capsules, to enhance their stability, usefulness, or elegance or to facilitate their manufacture may be used only if they (14)

1. Are harmless in the quantities used
2. Do not exceed the minimum amounts required to provide their intended effect
3. Do not impair the product's bioavailability, therapeutic efficacy or safety
4. Do not interfere with requisite compendial assays and tests

Containers for Dispensing Capsules

The USP lists specifications prescribing the type of container suitable for the repackaging or dispensing of each official capsule and tablet. Depending on the item, the container may be required to be *tight*, *well-closed*, and *light resistant*.

Disintegration Test for Capsules

The disintegration test for hard and soft gelatin capsules follows the same procedure and uses the same apparatus described in the next chapter for uncoated tablets. The capsules are placed in the basket rack assembly, which is immersed 30 times per minute into a thermostatically controlled fluid at 37°C and observed over the time described in the individual monograph. To satisfy the test, the capsules disintegrate completely into a soft mass having no palpably firm core and only some fragments of the gelatin shell.

Dissolution Test for Capsules

The dissolution test for capsules uses the same apparatus, dissolution medium, and test as that for uncoated and plain coated tablets described in Chapter 8. However, if the capsule shells interfere with the analysis, the contents of a specified number of capsules can be removed and the empty capsule shells dissolved in the dissolution medium before proceeding with the sampling and chemical analysis.

Weight Variation

The uniformity of dosage units may be demonstrated by determining *weight variation* and/or *content uniformity*. The weight variation method is as follows.

Hard Capsules

Ten capsules are individually weighed and the contents removed. The emptied shells are individually weighed and the net weight of the contents calculated by subtraction. From the results of an assay performed as directed in the individual monograph, the content of active ingredient in each of the capsules is determined.

Soft Capsules

The gross weight of 10 intact capsules is determined individually. Then each capsule is cut open and the contents removed by washing with a suitable solvent. The solvent is allowed to evaporate at room temperature over about

30 minutes, with precautions to avoid uptake or loss of moisture. The individual shells are weighed and the net contents calculated. From the results of the assay directed in the individual monograph, the content of active ingredient in each of the capsules is determined.

Content Uniformity

Unless otherwise stated in the monograph for an individual capsule, the amount of active ingredient, determined by assay, is within the range of 85% to 115% of the label claim for 9 of 10 dosage units assayed, with no unit outside the range of 70% to 125% of label claim. Additional tests are prescribed when two or three dosage units are outside of the desired range but within the stated extremes.

Content Labeling Requirement

All official capsules must be labeled to express the quantity of each active ingredient in each dosage unit.

Stability Testing

Stability testing of capsules is performed as described in Chapter 4 to determine the intrinsic stability of the active drug molecule and the influence of environmental factors such as temperature, humidity, light, formulative components, and the container and closure system. The battery of stress testing, long-term stability, and accelerated stability tests help determine the appropriate conditions for storage and the product's anticipated shelf life.

Moisture Permeation Test

The USP requires determination of the moisture permeation characteristics of single-unit and unit-dose containers to ensure their suitability for packaging capsules. The degree and rate of moisture penetration is determined by packaging the dosage unit together with a color-revealing desiccant pellet, exposing the packaged unit to known relative humidity over a specified time, observing the desiccant pellet for color change (indicating absorption of moisture) and comparing the pretest and posttest weight of the packaged unit.

Official and Commercially Available Capsules

Approximately 200 officially recognized medications in capsule form are listed in the USP. However, many times this number of capsule products are available from various manufacturers for various drugs and in various dosage strengths.

Examples of official and commercially available medications in hard and soft gelatin capsules are presented in Tables 7.2 and 7.3.

Inspecting, Counting, Packaging, and Storing Capsules

Capsules produced on a small or large scale should be uniform in appearance. Visual or electronic inspection should be undertaken to detect any flaws in the integrity and appearance of the capsules. Defective capsules should be rejected. In commercial manufacture, Current Good Manufacturing Practice regulations require that if the number of production flaws is excessive, the cause must be investigated and documented and steps undertaken to correct the problem.

In the pharmacy, capsules may be counted manually or by automated equipment. Specially designed trays, such as the type depicted in Figure 7.18, are used for counting small numbers of solid dosage units. In using this tray, the pharmacist pours a supply of capsules or tablets from the bulk source onto the clean tray, and using the spatula, counts and sweeps the dosage units into the trough until the desired number is reached. Then the pharmacist closes the trough cover, picks up the tray, returns the uncounted dosage units to the bulk container by means of the lip at the back of the tray, places the prescription container at the opening of the trough, and carefully transfers the capsules or tablets into the container.

TABLE 7.2 EXAMPLES OF SOME OFFICIAL CAPSULES

OFFICIAL CAPSULE	REPRESENTATIVE COMMERCIAL CAPSULES	STRENGTH	CATEGORY
Amoxicillin	Wymox (Wyeth-Ayerst)	250, 500 mg	Antibacterial
Ampicillin	Omnipen (Wyeth-Ayerst)	250, 500 mg	Antibacterial
Cephalexin	Keflex (Dista)	250, 500 mg	Antibacterial
Diphenhydramine HCl	Benadryl HCl (Parke-Davis)	25 mg	Antihistaminic
Doxycycline Hyclate	Vibramycin (Pfizer)	50, 100 mg	Antibacterial
Erythromycin Estolate	Ilosone (Dista)	125, 250 mg	Antibacterial
Fluoxetine HCl	Prozac (Dista)	10, 20 mg	Antidepressant
Flurazepam HCl	Dalmane (Roche)	15, 30 mg	Hypnotic
Gemfibrozil	Lopid (Parke-Davis)	300 mg	Antihyperlipidemic
Griseofulvin	Grisactin (Wyeth-Ayerst)	125, 250 mg	Antifungal
Indomethacin	Indocin (Merck)	25, 50 mg	Anti-inflammatory, antipyretic, analgesic
Levodopa	Larodopa (Roche)	100, 250, 500 mg	Antiparkinsonian
Loperamide HCl	Imodium (Janssen)	2 mg	Antidiarrheal
Oxazepam	Serax (Wyeth-Ayerst)	10, 15, 30 mg	Antianxiety
Propoxyphene HCl	Darvon (Lilly)	32, 65 mg	Analgesic
Tetracycline HCl	Achromycin V (Lederle)	250, 500 mg	Antimicrobial

TABLE 7.3 SOME MEDICATIONS COMMERCIALLY PREPARED INTO SOFT GELATIN CAPSULES

DRUG	TRADE NAME (MANUFACTURER)	CONTENTS AND COMMENTS[a]
Acetazolamide	Diamox Sequels (Lederle)	Carbonic anhydrase inhibitor, slightly water-soluble powder. Contains coated pellets of sustained-release drug.
Cyclosporine	Sandimmune (Novartis)	Immunosuppressive, slightly water-soluble crystalline powder. Contains corn oil, polyoxyethylated glycolyzed glycerides.
Cyclosporine	Neoral (Novartis)	Contains dehydrated alcohol, corn oil mono-, di-, triglycerides, polyoxyl 40 hydrogenated castor oil; forms microemulsion in contact with aqueous fluids for enhanced bioavailability.
Digoxin	Lanoxicaps (Glaxo Wellcome)	Cardiac glycoside, practically water-insoluble powder. Dissolved in polyethylene glycol 400, ethyl alcohol, propylene glycol, water.
Ethosuximide	Zarontin (Parke-Davis)	Anticonvulsant, water-soluble powder. Contains polyethylene glycol 400.
Ranitidine HCl	Zantac GELdose (Glaxo Wellcome)	Histamine H_2-receptor inhibitor, water-soluble granular powder in nonaqueous matrix of synthetic coconut oil, triglycerides.

[a]Only a partial listing of the capsule contents is given. The soft capsule shells may also contain colorants, opaquants, preservatives, and other agents.

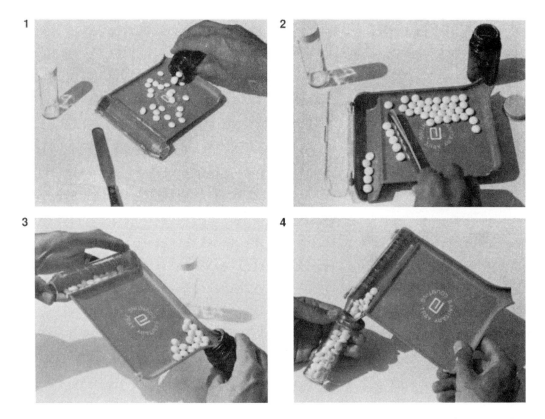

FIGURE 7.18 Steps in counting solid dosage units with the Abbott Sanitary Counting Tray. **1**. Transferring units from stock package to tray. **2**. Counting and transferring units to trough. **3**. Returning excess units to stock container. **4**. Placing counted units in prescription container.

With this method, the dosage units remain untouched by the pharmacist. To prevent batch-to-batch contamination, the tray must be wiped clean after each use, because powder, particularly from uncoated tablets, may remain. In some community and hospital pharmacies, small automated counting and filling machines may be used as shown in Figure 7.19. Computer-based automated dispensing systems are also available that will fill, label, and check the drug using bar code or video systems.

On the industrial scale, solid dosage forms are counted by large automated pieces of equipment that count and transfer the desired number of dosage units into bulk containers. The containers are then mechanically capped, inspected visually or electronically, labeled, and inspected once more. Some filled containers are then placed in outer packaging cartons.

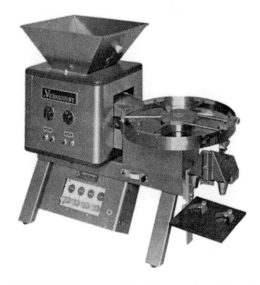

FIGURE 7.19 Versacount Model automatic tablet and capsule counting and filling apparatus. (Courtesy of Production Equipment Co.)

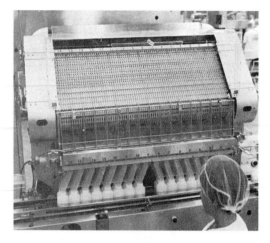

FIGURE 7.20 Large Merrill filling machine that fills 16 bottles with 200 tablets each at one time. A flipper gate in the upper manifold directs the tablets into one row of bottles while the other filled row is evacuated and a new row of bottles

An industrial counting and filling machine is shown in Figure 7.20. Capsules are packaged in glass or in plastic containers, some containing packets of a desiccant to prevent absorption of excessive moisture.

The unit dose and strip packaging of solid dosage forms, particularly by pharmacies that

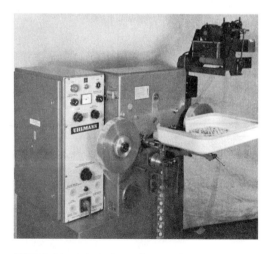

FIGURE 7.21 Strip packager for unit dose dispensing of solid dosage forms. Drug information is imprinted on each package unit. This model has a fully automatic cutoff for 1 to 24 dosage units and is especially suited to unit dose packaging and dispensing in hospitals, dispensaries, nursing homes, and clinics. (Courtesy of Lakso Company.)

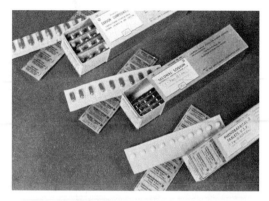

FIGURE 7.22 Unit dose packaging of tablets and capsules. The drug name and other information are imprinted on the backing portion of each unit. (Courtesy of Eli Lilly and Company.)

service nursing homes and hospitals, provides sanitary handling of the medications, ease of identification, and security in accountability for medications. Typical small-scale strip packaging equipment and commercial unit dose packages of capsules and tablets are presented in Figures 7.21 and 7.22, respectively. Capsules should be stored in tightly capped containers in a cool, dry place.

Oral Administration of Solid Dosage Forms

Solid dosage forms (capsules and tablets) for oral administration are best taken by placing the dose upon the tongue and swallowing it with a glassful of water or beverage. Taking solid dosage forms with adequate amounts of water is important. Some patients attempt to swallow a tablet or capsule without water, but this can be dangerous because of the possibility that it will lodge in the esophagus. Esophageal ulceration can occur with dry ingestion of tablets and capsules, particularly taken just before bedtime. Among the drugs of greatest concern in this regard are alendronate sodium, aspirin, ferrous sulfate, any nonsteroidal antiinflammatory drug (NSAID), potassium chloride, and tetracycline antibiotics.

The proper administration of alendronate sodium tablets (Fosamax, Merck), for example, calls for the tablets to be taken with a full

6- or 8-ounce glass of plain water upon rising in the morning and at least half an hour before taking any food, beverage, or other medication to prevent local irritation of the esophagus and other upper gastrointestinal mucosa. The patient is also instructed not to recline for at least 30 minutes and until after the first food of the day is eaten because of the possibility that the drug will reflux into the esophagus.

In general, patients with gastroesophageal reflux disease must take their medications with adequate amounts of water and avoid reclining for at least an hour to avoid reflux.

The administration of oral medication in relation to meals is very important, since the bioavailability and efficacy of certain drugs may be severely affected by food and certain drink. The pharmacist should know about such instances and advise patients accordingly.

As mentioned earlier in this chapter, oral dosage forms with special coatings (e.g., enteric) or are designed to provide controlled drug release, to preserve their drug release features, must not be chewed, broken, or crushed.

When an ordinary tablet is crushed or a capsule opened to facilitate ease of administration, any unpleasant drug taste may be partially masked by mixing with custard, yogurt, rice pudding, other soft food, or fruit juice. The patient should be advised to consume the entire drug–food mixture to obtain the full dose, and to maintain stability the drug should not be premixed and allowed to set.

If a patient cannot swallow a solid dosage form, the pharmacist can suggest a chewable or liquid form of the drug. If these are not available, an extemporaneously compounded liquid form may be prepared.

PHARMACEUTICS CASE STUDY

Subjective Information

You have received the following prescription:
Rx

> Diphenhydramine hydrochloride 25 mg
> Phenyltoloxamine citrate 30 mg
> Acetaminophen 325 mg
> Make #30
> Sig: Caps i–ii po HS PRN sleep

You need to determine the amounts of the ingredients and of lactose to use to make 30 capsules each of sizes 3, 1, or 0.

Objective Information

Volume capacity of capsules

> 3: 0.3 mL
> 1: 0.5 mL
> 0: 0.67 mL

Tapped density of ingredients, excipients

> Lactose: 950 mg/mL
> Diphenhydramine hydrochloride: 800 mg/mL

Phenyltoloxamine citrate: 750 mg/mL
Acetaminophen: 850 mg/mL

Assessment

For each active ingredient, the amount required to make 30 capsules is

> Diphenhydramine HCl 750 mg
> Phenyltoloxamine citrate 900 mg
> Acetaminophen 9.75 g

Determining Amount of lactose required: Method 1 Using #1 capsules

> Weight of five empty #1 capsules: 400 mg
> Weight of five #1 capsules full of lactose: 2.775 g
> Weight of five #1 capsules full of diphenhydramine HCl: 2.4 g
> Weight of five #1 capsules full of phenyltoloxamine citrate: 2.275 g
> Weight of five #1 capsules full of acetaminophen: 2.525 g

Pharmaceutics Case Study cont.

Now average

Lactose: (2775 − 400) / 5 = 475 mg per capsule
Diphenhydramine HCl: (2400 − 400) / 5 = 400 mg per capsule
Phenyltoloxamine citrate: (2275 − 400) / 5 = 375 mg per capsule
Acetaminophen: (2525 − 400) / 5 = 425 mg per capsule

Percent of capsule filled by the required amounts of active ingredient

Diphenhydramine HCl: 25 / 400 × 100 = 6.25%
Phenyltoloxamine citrate: 30 / 375 × 100 = 8%
Acetaminophen: 325 / 425 × 100 = 76.47%

Total = 90.72%, so the remaining 9.28% of each capsule will be lactose. Therefore we require a total of 0.0928 × 475 × 30 = 1.3 g approximately of lactose to make 30 #1 capsules. This calculation can be done in the same way for the #0 capsules, resulting in 6.15 g approximately of lactose required to make 30 #0 capsules. We cannot use #3 capsules for this prescription, as only 255 mg of acetaminophen (and nothing else) will fit into a #3 capsule.

Determining amount of lactose required: Method 2

Calculate the percentage of the volume of a #1 capsule each active ingredient will occupy:

Diphenhydramine HCl: 25 mg / (800 mg/mL) / 0.5 mL × 100 = 6.25%
Phenyltoloxamine citrate: 30 mg / (750 mg/mL) / 0.5 mL × 100 = 8%
Acetaminophen: 325 mg / (850 mg/mL) / 0.5 mL × 100 = 76.47%

Total = 90.72%, so the remaining 9.28% of each capsule will be lactose. The total amount of lactose required:

Lactose: 9.28 / 100 × 0.5 mL × (950 mg/mL) = 1.3 g approx.

Plan

To make 30 #1 capsules, we will require

Diphenhydramine HCl: 750 mg
Phenyltoloxamine citrate: 900 mg
Acetaminophen: 9.75 g
Lactose: 1.3 g

To make 30 #0 capsules, we will require

Diphenhydramine HCl: 750 mg
Phenyltoloxamine citrate: 900 mg
Acetaminophen: 9.75 g
Lactose: 6.15 g

We cannot use #3 capsules for this prescription.

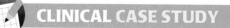

CLINICAL CASE STUDY

Subjective

HPI: K. P. is a 12 y/o WF who is brought to the emergency department by her mother, who states "she went unconscious for about a minute." Mother was teaching her to bake cookies when K. P. asked if there was some-

thing burning in the oven. She described the smell as being that of "gasoline." Mother did not pay much attention to her strange smell, at which time the patient started to "wiggle" both her hands and "smack her lips together." Mother also stated that she started to chew really hard without any food in her

Clinical Case Study cont.

mouth. The episode of strange chewing and lip smacking lasted about a minute, after which K. P. appeared confused and disoriented for several minutes. Her mother recalls asking if something was wrong during the episode, but the patient was unable to respond. Immediately after the episode, mother anxiously drove her to the emergency department. Upon arrival, the patient was oriented to time, place, and people. She denies any nausea, vomiting, dizziness, or confusion. When asked about the episode, patient states she does not recall what her mother described. Patient is otherwise well.

PMH: No hospitalizations since birth

Birth history: Mother was diagnosed with preeclampsia at 8.5 months. Mother denies any use of drugs and alcohol during pregnancy. K. P. was born at 39 weeks gestational age. She was bottle fed as an infant.

Developmental history: Not significant. Patient developed well according to age. Currently developmentally intact.

Immunizations: Up to date

SH: (−) EtOh
    (−) Tobacco
    (−) Caffeine
    (−) Illicit drugs

No siblings, lives with parents in Bloomingdale

FH: Mother with gestational diabetes × 12 years

    Father with HTN × 2 years

Diet: Eats about 5 times a day, mostly snacks (i.e., fruit, granola bars). Does not like to eat breakfast or dinner. Lunch is her biggest meal of the day. Meals consist mostly of cooked vegetables and pasta. Does not like junk food. Does not follow any specific diet.

All: NKDA

PTA: No meds

Objective

Ht: 4'4"
Wt: 102 lb

T: 100.1
Na: 135 mmol/L
K: 4.5 mmol/L
Cl: 102 mmol/L
CO_2: 18 mmol/L
BUN: 3.0 mmol/L
SrCr: 65 mmol/L

Abnormal EEG findings consistent with complex partial seizures: pattern of spikes and slow waves with a frequency of 2 cycles/second.

Assessment

K. P. is a 12 y/o white girl diagnosed with complex partial seizure per EEG and description of episode.

Plan

1. Recommend extended-release carbamazepine (Carbatrol) 200 mg capsule by mouth twice daily. However, mother states that K. P. is unable to swallow capsules or tablets. Counsel mother on gently opening capsule at the seal, being careful not to break the capsule. Tell mother to sprinkle the contents of the capsule into a small amount of food (e.g., a tablespoon of yogurt or applesauce) to ensure that all of the food with the drug is consumed. If contents are sprinkled in a large amount of food, the patient may not finish it all, hence not receive full dose of medication. This may lead to the medication not managing her seizures properly.

2. Teach patient and mother about common side effects of carbamazepine (e.g., dizziness, fatigue, worsening of seizures, nausea, vomiting) that affect a small fraction of patients. Advise patient and mother to report any unusual side effects (e.g., unusual bleeding, bruising, jaundice, dark urine, sore throat, abdominal pain).

Clinical Case Study cont.

3. Teach patient and mother about signs and symptoms of seizures. Inform them that most complex seizures are followed by an aura, which may consist of a strange smell, taste, sound, or visual disturbance. For example, K. P. smelled something burning before she had the seizure. Other signs may include a feeling of fear or anxiety. Inform patient and mother of the tonic-clonic movements that usually follow the aura. Explain to the mother that loss of consciousness is common with this seizure type. Also explain that the patient may appear confused for several minutes after the seizure.

4. Monitoring parameters: carbamazepine plasma levels, signs and symptoms of seizures, frequency of episodes, side effects of the medication. Goals: Increased patient knowledge about condition, no medication side effects, no second episode, therapeutic carbamazepine levels (4–$12\mu g/mL$). Make sure the patient and the mother understand the importance of follow-up physician visits and to exercise caution when purchasing nonprescription and herbal products (i.e., consult a pharmacist).

REFERENCES

1. Mitchell JF. Oral solid dosage forms that should not be crushed: 1996 revision. Hosp Pharm 1996; 31:27–37.
2. Jones BE. Hard gelatin capsules and the pharmaceutical formulator. Pharm Tech 1985;9:106–112.
3. Digenis A, Gold TB, Shah VP. Crosslinking of gelatin capsules and its relevance to their in vitro/in vivo performance. Dissolut Tech 1995;2:1.
4. Gardner D, Casper R, Leith F, Wilding, I. Noninvasive methodology for assessing regional drug absorption from the gastrointestinal tract. Pharm Tech 1997; 21:82–89.
5. Wilding IR. Pharmacoscintigraphic evaluation of oral delivery systems, part I. Pharm Tech 1995; 54–60.
6. Mojaverian P, Reynolds JC, Ouyang A, Wirth F, Kellner PE, Vlasses PH. Mechanism of gastric emptying of a nondisintegrating radiotelemetry capsule in man. Pharm Res 1991;8:97–100.
7. Nash RA. The "rule of sixes" for filling hard-shell gelatin capsules. Int Pharm Compounding 1997;1:40–41.
8. Yalkowsky SH, Bolton S. Particle size and content uniformity. Pharm Res 1990;7:962–966.
9. Caldwell HC. Dissolution of lithium and magnesium from lithium carbonate capsules containing magnesium stearate. J Pharm Sci 1974;63:770–773.
10. Etaseal. Windsor, Ontario: Capsule Technology International.
11. Licaps. Greenwood, SC: Capsugel Division of Warner-Lambert.
12. Quali-seal. Indianapolis: Elanco Qualicaps, Ely Lilly.
13. Stanley JP. Soft gelatin capsules. In: Lachman L, Lieberman HA, Kanig JL eds. The theory and practice of industrial pharmacy, 3rd ed. Philadelphia: Lea & Febiger, 1986, 398–429.
14. The United States Pharmacopeia 26–National Formulary 21. Rockville, MD: U.S. Pharmacopeial Convention, 2003.

Tablets

Chapter at a glance

Tablets are solid dosage forms usually prepared with the aid of suitable pharmaceutical excipients. They may vary in size, shape, weight, hardness, thickness, disintegration, and dissolution characteristics and in other aspects, depending on their intended use and method of manufacture. Most tablets are used in the oral administration of drugs. Many of these are prepared with colorants and coatings of various types. Other tablets, such as those administered sublingually, buccally, or vaginally, are prepared to have features most applicable to their particular route of administration. Advantages of tablets for oral administration are presented in an earlier chapter.

Tablets are prepared primarily by compression, with a limited number prepared by molding. Compressed tablets are manufactured with tablet machines capable of exerting great pressure in compacting the powdered or granulated material (Fig. 8.1). Their shape and di-

mensions are determined by use of various shaped punches and dies (Fig. 8.2). Molded tablets are prepared on a large-scale by tablet machinery or on a small-scale by manually forcing dampened powder material into a mold from which the formed tablet is then ejected and allowed to dry.

Some tablets are *scored*, or grooved, which allows them to be easily broken into two or more parts. This enables the patient to swallow smaller portions as may be desired, or when prescribed, it allows the tablet to be taken in reduced or divided dosage. Some tablets that are not scored are not intended to be broken or cut by the patient, since they may have special coatings and/or drug-release features that would be compromised by altering the tablet's physical integrity.

Types of Tablets

The various types of tablets are described as follows, with their common abbreviations in parentheses.

Compressed Tablets

In addition to the medicinal agent or agents, compressed tablets usually contain a number of pharmaceutical adjuncts, including the following:

Diluents or fillers, which add the necessary bulk to a formulation to prepare tablets of the desired size

Binders or adhesives, which promote adhesion of the particles of the formulation, allowing a granulation to be prepared and maintaining the integrity of the final tablet

Disintegrants or disintegrating agents, which promote breakup of the tablets after administration to smaller particles for ready drug availability

Antiadherents, glidants, lubricants, or lubricating agents, which enhance the flow of the material into the tablet dies, minimize wear of the punches and dies, prevent fill material from sticking to the punches and dies, and produce tablets with a sheen

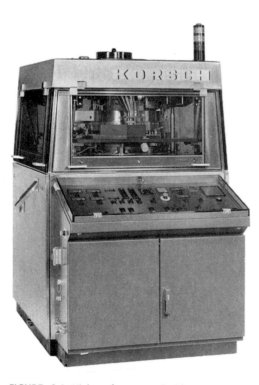

FIGURE 8.1 High-performance double rotary tablet press. The Korsch PharmapressR has a maximum output of 1 million tablets per hour, but for continuous operation it is generally run to produce 600,000 to 800,000 tablets per hour. (Courtesy of Korsch Tableting.)

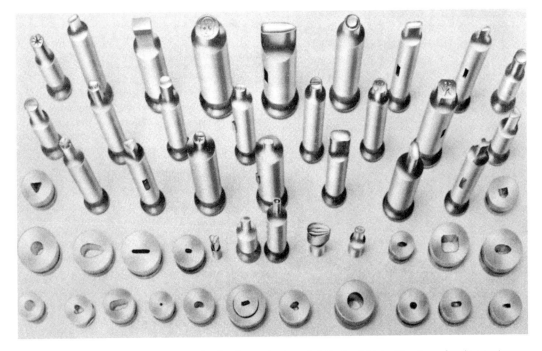

FIGURE 8.2 Various Stokes punches and dies for the production of distinctive tablets. (Courtesy of Stokes Equipment Division, Pennwalt Chemicals.)

Miscellaneous adjuncts such as colorants and flavorants

After compression, tablets may be coated with various materials as described later. Tablets for oral, buccal, sublingual, or vaginal administration may be prepared by compression.

Multiply Compressed Tablets

Multiply compressed tablets are prepared by subjecting the fill material to more than a single compression. The result may be a multiple-layer tablet or a tablet within a tablet, the inner tablet being the *core* and the outer portion being the *shell* (Fig. 8.3). Layered tablets are prepared by initial compaction of a portion of fill material in a die followed by additional fill material and compression to form two- or three-layered tablets, depending on the number of separate fills. Each layer may contain a different medicinal agent, separated for reasons of chemical or physical incompatibility, staged drug release, or simply for the unique appearance of the layered tablet. Usually, each portion of fill is a different color to produce a distinctive-looking tablet. In preparation of tablets within tablets, special machines are required to place the preformed core tablet precisely within the die for application of surrounding fill material.

Sugarcoated Tablets

Compressed tablets may be coated with a colored or an uncolored sugar layer. The coating is water soluble and quickly dissolves after

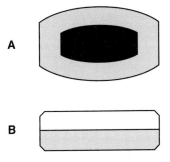

FIGURE 8.3 Multiply compressed tablets. **A.** A core of one drug and a shell of another. **B.** A layered tablet of two drugs.

swallowing. The sugarcoat protects the enclosed drug from the environment and provides a barrier to objectionable taste or odor. The sugarcoat also enhances the appearance of the compressed tablet and permits imprinting of identifying manufacturer's information. Among the disadvantages to sugarcoating tablets are the time and expertise required in the coating process and the increase in size, weight, and shipping costs. Sugarcoating may add 50% to the weight and bulk of the uncoated tablet.

Film-Coated Tablets

Film-coated tablets are compressed tablets coated with a thin layer of a polymer capable of forming a skinlike film. The film is usually colored and has the advantage over sugarcoatings in that it is more durable, less bulky, and less time consuming to apply. By its composition, the coating is designed to rupture and expose the core tablet at the desired location in the gastrointestinal tract.

Gelatin-Coated Tablets

A recent innovation is the gelatin-coated tablet. The innovator product, the gelcap, is a capsule-shaped compressed tablet (Fig. 8.4) that allows the coated product to be about one-third smaller than a capsule filled with an equivalent amount of powder. The gelatin coating facilitates swallowing, and gelatin-coated tablets are more tamper evident than unsealed capsules.

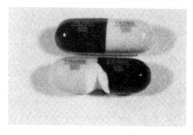

FIGURE 8.4 Cutaway view of Gelcaps dosage form, a gelatin-coated capsule-shaped tablet. Dosage form is more easily swallowed than a comparable tablet, smaller than an equivalent capsule, and tamper evident. (Courtesy of McNeil Consumer Products.)

Enteric-Coated Tablets

Enteric-coated tablets have delayed-release features. They are designed to pass unchanged through the stomach to the intestines, where the tablets disintegrate and allow drug dissolution and absorption and/or effect. Enteric coatings are employed when the drug substance is destroyed by gastric acid or is particularly irritating to the gastric mucosa or when bypass of the stomach substantially enhances drug absorption.

Buccal and Sublingual Tablets

Buccal and sublingual tablets are flat oval tablets intended to be dissolved in the buccal pouch (*buccal tablets*) or beneath the tongue (*sublingual tablets*) for absorption through the oral mucosa. They enable oral absorption of drugs that are destroyed by the gastric juice and/or are poorly absorbed from the gastrointestinal tract. Buccal tablets are designed to erode slowly, whereas those for sublingual use (such as nitroglycerin) dissolve promptly and provide rapid drug effects. *Lozenges* or *troches* are disc-shaped solid dosage forms containing a medicinal agent and generally a flavoring substance in a hard candy or sugar base. They are intended to be slowly dissolved in the oral cavity, usually for local effects, although some are formulated for systemic absorption.

Chewable Tablets

Chewable tablets, which have a smooth, rapid disintegration when chewed or allowed to dissolve in the mouth, have a creamy base, usually of specially flavored and colored mannitol. Chewable tablets are especially useful for administration of large tablets to children and adults who have difficulty swallowing solid dosage forms.

Effervescent Tablets

Effervescent tablets are prepared by compressing granular effervescent salts that release gas when in contact with water. These tablets generally contain medicinal substances that dissolve rapidly when added to water.

Molded Tablets

Certain tablets, such as tablet triturates, may be prepared by molding rather than by compression. The resultant tablets are very soft and soluble and are designed for rapid dissolution.

Tablet Triturates

Tablet triturates are small, usually cylindrical, molded or compressed tablets containing small amounts of usually potent drugs. Today only a few tablet triturate products are available commercially, with most of these produced by tablet compression. Since tablet triturates must be readily and completely soluble in water, only a minimal amount of pressure is applied during their manufacture. A combination of sucrose and lactose is usually the diluent. The few tablet triturates that remain are used sublingually, such as nitroglycerin tablets.

Pharmacists also employ tablet triturates in compounding. For example, triturates are inserted into capsules or dissolved in liquid to provide accurate amounts of potent drug substances.

Hypodermic Tablets

Hypodermic tablets are no longer available in the United States. They were originally used by physicians in extemporaneous preparation of parenteral solutions. The required number of tablets was dissolved in a suitable vehicle, sterility attained, and the injection performed. The tablets were a convenience, since they could be easily carried in the physician's medicine bag and injections prepared to meet the needs of the individual patients. However, the difficulty in achieving sterility, and the availability of prefabricated injectable products, some in disposable syringes, have eliminated the need for hypodermic tablets.

Dispensing Tablets

Dispensing tablets are no longer in use. They might better have been termed *compounding tablets* because the pharmacist used them to compound prescriptions; they were *not* dispensed as such to the patient. The tablets contained large amounts of highly potent drug substances, so that the pharmacist could rapidly obtain premeasured amounts for compounding multiple dosage units. These tablets had the dangerous potential of being inadvertently dispensed as such to patients.

Immediate-Release Tablets

Immediate-release tablets are designed to disintegrate and release their medication with no special rate-controlling features, such as special coatings and other techniques.

Instantly Disintegrating or Dissolving Tablets

Instant-release tablets (rapidly dissolving tablets, or RDTs) are characterized by disintegrating or dissolving in the mouth within 1 minute, some within 10 seconds (e.g., Claritin Reditabs [loratadine], Schering). Tablets of this type are designed for children and the elderly or for any patient who has difficulty in swallowing tablets. They liquefy on the tongue, and the patient swallows the liquid. A number of techniques are used to prepare these tablets, including lyophilization (e.g., Zydis, R. P. Scherer), soft direct compression (e.g., Wow-Tab, Yamanouchi-Shaklee Pharma), and other methods (e.g., Quicksolv, Janssen). These tablets are prepared using very water-soluble excipients designed to wick water into the tablet for rapid disintegration or dissolution. They have the stability characteristics of other solid dosage forms.

The original fast-dissolving tablets were molded tablets for sublingual use. They generally consisted of active drug and lactose moistened with an alcohol–water mixture to form a paste. The tablets were then molded, dried, and packaged. For use, they were simply placed under the tongue to provide a rapid onset of action for drugs such as nitroglycerin. Also, they have been used for drugs that are destroyed in the gastrointestinal tract, such as testosterone, administered sublingually for absorption to minimize the first-pass effect.

The new RDTs are designed for oral use by patients who have difficulty swallowing standard tablets and capsules, such as children and the elderly. These RDTs are more convenient to carry and administer than an oral liquid. There are no standards that define a RDT, but one possibility is dissolution in the mouth within approximately 15 to 30 seconds; anything slower would not be categorized as rapidly dissolving.

Notwithstanding these advantages, there are a number of disadvantages and difficulties associated with formulating RDTs, including drug loading, taste masking, friability, manufacturing costs, and stability of the product.

Drug loading is incorporation of the drug into the dosage form. Some RDTs are made as blanks to which a drug is post loaded, or added after the blank is made. Generally the drug is in solution and is added to the tablet, after which the solvent evaporates. It is also possible for the drug to be added as a dry powder electrostatically at this stage. Most drugs, however, are incorporated into the tablets during manufacturing.

Taste masking poses numerous challenges for RDTs. Since the drug product dissolves in the mouth, any taste of the drug must be covered, either by a flavoring technique or by microencapsulation or nanoencapsulation. The product also should not be gritty, which necessitates very small particle sizes if microencapsulation is used.

Friability is an inherent problem in RDTs. For a product to dissolve instantly, it may be quite friable. Making it more firm and less friable may increase dissolution time. A balance generally must be achieved between friability and speed of dissolution.

Lyophilized Foam

The first entry into the RDT field was the Zydis delivery system. The tablets are prepared by foaming a mixture of gelatin, sugar or sugars, drug, and any other components and pouring the foam into a mold. The mold also serves as the unit dose dispensing package. The foam is lyophilized (Fig. 8.5), and the tablets in the mold are packaged. This system is the fastest disintegrating on the market, as the tablets will dissolve on the tongue in a matter of a few seconds. One disadvantage of this method is that taste masking can be a problem, since the drug is incorporated during the formation of the tablet itself. Another difficulty is that these tablets are sometimes difficult to remove from

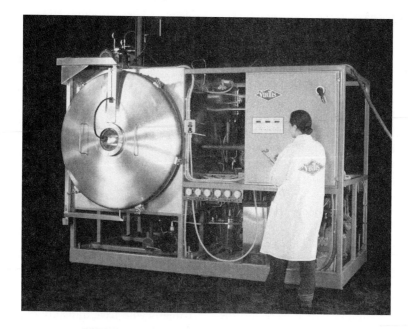

FIGURE 8.5 A large-scale lyophilizer.(Courtesy of Virtis.)

the packaging, since they are soft and one should not press on the dosage unit to remove it but should peel off the material, exposing the tablet in its mold.

Claritin (loratadine) rapidly disintegrating tablets (Reditabs, Schering Corporation) contain 10 mg of micronized loratadine in a base containing citric acid, gelatin, mannitol, and mint flavor formed with the Zydis technology. It disintegrates within seconds after being placed on the tongue, with or without water. Claritin Reditabs have been shown to provide at least equivalent pharmacokinetic parameters to those of traditional tablets in some cases the Reditabs provided greater maximum concentration (C_{max}) and area under the curve (AUC) values. Claritin Reditabs are blister packaged tablets that should be stored in a dry place at 2° to 25°C. They should be used within 6 months of opening the protective laminated foil pouch containing the blister cards; each foil pouch contains one blister card containing 10 individually sealed tablets (1). Other commercial products using this technology include the Maxalt-MLT (Merck), Zofran ODT (GlaxoSmithKline), and Zyprexa Zydis (Eli Lilly) tablets.

Compression

Another method of preparation is using standard tableting technology with a composition that will enhance fluid uptake and tablet disintegration and dissolution. For example, superdisintegrants incorporated with a small quantity of effervescent material will lead to intermediately fast disintegration. The tablets are compressed a little thinner than standard tablets to allow for a larger surface area exposed to the saliva in the mouth. Upon placement in the mouth, the disintegrant starts wicking water into the tablet. The effervescent materials start dissolving and aid in the breakup. This continues until the tablet has disintegrated.

An example product is the Dimetapp ND Orally Disintegrating Tablet (Non-Drowsy Allergy Tablets). These tablets contain loratadine 10 mg in a vehicle of artificial and natural flavor, aspartame, citric acid, colloidal silicon dioxide, corn syrup solids, crospovidone, magnesium stearate, mannitol, microcrystalline cellulose, modified food starch, and sodium bicarbonate. (2)

One product using the DuraSolv and Ora-Solv technologies by Cima Labs is Tempra Quicklets containing acetaminophen 80 mg. These tablets also contain aspartame, citric acid, D&C Red No. 27 Lake, FD&C Blue No. 1 Lake, flavor, magnesium stearate, mannitol, potassium carbonate, silicon dioxide, and sodium bicarbonate. They are somewhat slower than the Zydis tablet, taking about 30 to 45 seconds, unless some tongue pressure is used. These tablets come in a firm molded plastic package to prevent breakage (3). Other commercial products using the same technology include the Alavert (Wyeth Consumer Healthcare), NuLev (Schwarz Pharma), Remeron SolTabs (Organon Teknika), Triaminic Softchews (Novartis Pharmaceutical), and the Zomig Rapidmelt (Zeneca Pharmaceuticals).

The Flashtab technology by Ethypharm is used in Excedrin QuickTabs and an example of the Wowtab® technology by Yamanouchi Pharma is the Benadryl Fastmelt.

Extended-Release Tablets

Extended-release tablets (sometimes called controlled release [CR] tablets) are designed to release their medication in a predetermined manner over an extended period. They are discussed in Chapter 9.

Vaginal Tablets

Vaginal tablets, also called *vaginal inserts*, are uncoated bullet-shaped or ovoid tablets inserted into the vagina for local effects. They are prepared by compression and shaped to fit snugly on plastic inserter devices that accompany the product. They contain antibacterials for the treatment of vaginitis caused by *Haemophilus vaginalis* or antifungals for the treatment of vulvovaginitis candidiasis caused by *Candida albicans* and related species.

Compressed Tablets

The physical features of compressed tablets are well known: round, oblong, or unique in shape; thick or thin; large or small in diameter;

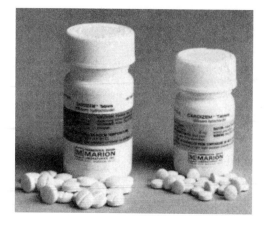

FIGURE 8.6 Packages of a drug product of different tablet strengths, with one scored for ease of breaking in half. (Courtesy of Marion Laboratories.)

flat or convex; unscored or *scored* (Fig. 8.6) in halves, thirds, or quadrants; engraved or imprinted with an identifying symbol and/or code number; coated or uncoated; colored or uncolored; one, two, or three layered.

Tablet diameters and shapes are determined by the die and punches used in compression. The less concave the punches, the flatter the tablets; conversely, the more concave the punches, the more convex the resulting tablets (Fig. 8.7). Punches with raised impressions produce recessed impressions on the tablets; punches with recessed etchings produce tablets with raised impressions or monograms. Monograms may be placed on one or on both sides of a tablet, depending on the punches.

Quality Standards and Compendial Requirements

In addition to the apparent features of tablets, tablets must meet other physical specifications and quality standards. These include criteria for weight, weight variation, content uniformity, thickness, hardness, disintegration, and dissolution. These factors must be controlled during production (in-process controls) and verified after the production of each batch to ensure that established product quality standards are met (Fig. 8.8).

Tablet Weight and USP Weight Variation Test

The quantity of fill in the die of a tablet press determines the weight of the tablet. The volume of fill is adjusted with the first few tablets to yield the *desired weight and content*. For example, if a tablet is to contain 20 mg of a drug substance and if 100,000 tablets are to be produced, 2000 g of drug is included in the formula. After the addition of the pharmaceutical additives, such

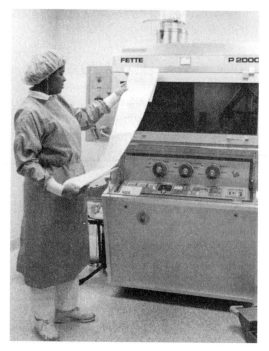

FIGURE 8.8 Quality control in the manufacturing of tablets. (Courtesy of Eli Lilly and Company.)

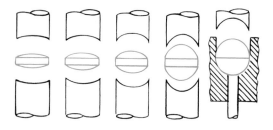

FIGURE 8.7 Contours of the punches determine the shape of the tablets. From left to right, flat face, shallow cup, standard cup, deep cup, and modified ball. (Courtesy of Cherry-Burrell Corporation.)

as the diluent, disintegrant, lubricant, and binder, the formulation may weigh 20 kg, which means that each tablet must weigh 200 mg for 20 mg of drug to be present. Thus, the depth of fill in the tablet die must be adjusted to hold a volume of granulation weighing 200 mg. During production, sample tablets are periodically removed for visual inspection and automated physical measurement (Fig. 8.9).

The USP contains a test for determination of dosage form uniformity by *weight variation* for uncoated tablets (4). In the test, 10 tablets are weighed individually and the average weight calculated. The tablets are assayed and the content of active ingredient in each of the 10 tablets is calculated assuming homogeneous drug distribution.

Content Uniformity

By the USP method 10 dosage units are individually assayed for their content according to the method described in the individual monograph. Unless otherwise stated in the monograph, the requirements for content uniformity are met if the amount of active ingredient in each dosage unit lies within the range of 85% to 115% of the label claim and the standard deviation is less than 6%. If one or more dosage units do not meet these criteria, additional tests as prescribed in the USP are required (4).

Tablet Thickness

The thickness of a tablet is determined by the diameter of the die, the amount of fill permitted to enter the die, the compaction characteristics of the fill material, and the force or pressure applied during compression.

To produce tablets of uniform thickness during and between batch productions for the same formulation, care must be exercised to employ the same factors of fill, die, and pressure. The degree of pressure affects not only thickness but also hardness of the tablet; hardness is perhaps the more important criterion, since it can affect disintegration and dissolution. Thus, for tablets of uniform thickness and hardness, it is doubly important to control pressure. Tablet thickness may be measured by hand gauge during production or by automated equipment (Figs. 8.10, 8.11, and 8.12).

Tablet Hardness and Friability

It is fairly common for a tablet press to exert as little as 3000 and as much as 40,000 lb of force

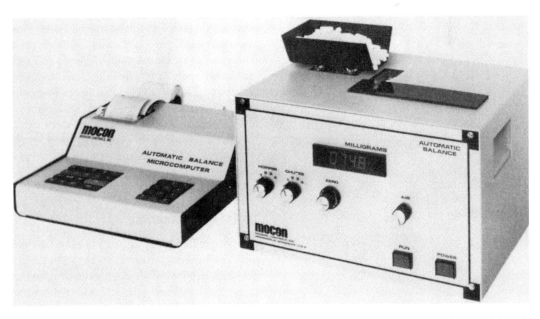

FIGURE 8.9 Automatic balance that weighs product and prints statistics to determine compliance with USP weight variation requirements for tablets. (Courtesy of Mocon Modern Controls.)

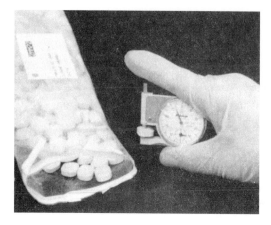

FIGURE 8.10 Tablet thickness gauge. (Courtesy of Eli Lilly and Company.)

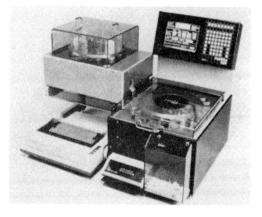

FIGURE 8.12 Automatic weight, hardness, thickness, and tablet diameter test instrument for quality control. Using a microprocessor and monitor for visualization, the instrument can test up to 20 samples at a time. (Courtesy of Scientific Instruments & Technology.)

in production of tablets. Generally, the greater the pressure applied, the harder the tablets, although the characteristics of the granulation also have a bearing on hardness. Certain tablets, such as lozenges and buccal tablets, that are intended to dissolve slowly, intentionally are made hard; other tablets, such as those for immediate drug release, are made soft. In general, tablets should be sufficiently hard to resist breaking during normal handling and yet soft enough to disintegrate properly after swallowing.

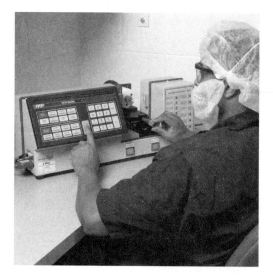

FIGURE 8.11 Tablet diameter testing instrument. (Courtesy of Shinogi Qualicaps.)

Special dedicated hardness testers (Fig. 8.13) or multifunctional systems (Fig. 8.12) are used to measure the degree of force (in kilograms, pounds, or in arbitrary units) required to break a tablet. A force of about 4 kg is considered the minimum requirement for a satisfactory tablet. Multifunctional automated equipment can determine weight, hardness, thickness, and diameter of the tablet.

A tablet's durability may be determined through the use of a *friabilator* (Fig. 8.14). This apparatus determines the tablet's *friability*, or tendency to crumble, by allowing it to roll and fall within the drum. The tablets are weighed before and after a specified number of rotations and any weight loss determined. Resistance to loss of weight indicates the tablet's ability to withstand abrasion in handling, packaging, and shipment. A maximum weight loss of not more than 1% generally is considered acceptable for most products.

Tablet Disintegration

For the medicinal agent in a tablet to become fully available for absorption, the tablet must first disintegrate and discharge the drug to the body fluids for dissolution. Tablet disintegration also is important for tablets containing medicinal agents (such as antacids and antidiarrheals) that are not intended to be ab-

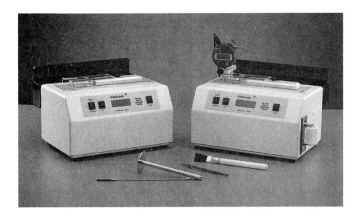

FIGURE 8.13 Tablet hardness tester (Courtesy of Varian Inc.)

sorbed but rather to act locally within the gastrointestinal tract. In these instances, tablet disintegration provides drug particles with an increased surface area for activity within the gastrointestinal tract.

All USP tablets must pass a test for disintegration, which is conducted in vitro using a testing apparatus such as the one shown in Figure 8.15. The apparatus consists of a basket and rack assembly containing six open-ended transparent tubes of USP-specified dimensions, held vertically upon a 10-mesh stainless steel wire screen. During testing, a tablet is placed in each of the six tubes of the basket, and through the use of a mechanical device, the basket is raised and lowered in the immersion fluid at 29

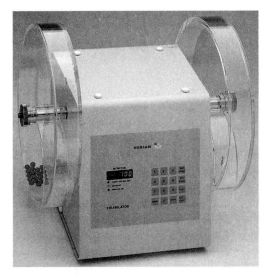

FIGURE 8.14 Varian Friabilator testing apparatus for rolling and impact durability. Tablets are weighed and placed in the acrylic drums, in which a curved baffle is mounted. When the motor is activated by setting the timer, the tablets roll and drop. If the free fall within the drum results in breakage or excessive abrasion of the tablets, they are considered not suited to withstand shipment. The motor makes 20 rpm. When the tablets have been tested, they are removed and weighed again. The difference in weight within a given time indicates the rate of abrasion. (Courtesy of Varian Inc.)

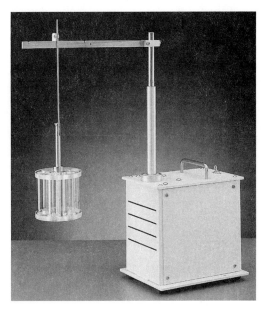

FIGURE 8.15 Tablet disintegration testing apparatus. (Courtesy of Varian Inc.)

to 32 cycles per minute, the wire screen always below the level of the fluid. For uncoated tablets, buccal tablets, and sublingual tablets, water at about 37°C serves as the immersion fluid unless another fluid is specified in the individual monograph. For these tests, complete disintegration is defined as "that state in which any residue of the unit, except fragments of insoluble coating or capsule shell, remaining on the screen of the test apparatus is a soft mass having no palpably firm core" (4).Tablets must disintegrate within the times set forth in the individual monograph, usually 30 minutes, but varying from about 2 minutes for nitroglycerin tablets to up to 4 hours for buccal tablets. If one or more tablets fail to disintegrate, additional tests prescribed by the USP must be performed.

Enteric-coated tablets are similarly tested, except that the tablets are tested in simulated gastric fluid for 1 hour, after which no sign of disintegration, cracking, or softening must be seen. They are then actively immersed in the simulated intestinal fluid for the time stated in the individual monograph, during which time the tablets disintegrate completely for a positive test.

Tablet Dissolution

In vitro dissolution testing of solid dosage forms is important for a number of reasons (5):

1. It guides formulation and product development toward product optimization. Dissolution studies in the early stages of a product's development allow differentiation between formulations and correlations identified with in vivo bioavailability data.
2. Manufacturing may be monitored by dissolution testing as a component of the overall quality assurance program. The conduct of such testing from early product development through approval and commercial production ensures control of any variables of materials and processes that could affect dissolution and quality standards.
3. Consistent in vitro dissolution testing ensures bioequivalence from batch to batch. In assessing such bioequivalence, the U.S. Food and Drug Administration (FDA) allows manufacturers to examine scale-up

batches of 10% of the proposed size of the actual production batch, or 100,000 dosage units, whichever is greater.
4. It is a requirement for regulatory approval of marketing for products registered with the FDA and regulatory agencies of other countries. New drug applications (NDAs) submitted to the FDA contain in vitro dissolution data generally obtained from batches used in pivotal clinical and/or bioavailability studies and from human studies conducted during product development (6). Once the specifications are established in an approved NDA, they become official (USP) specifications for all subsequent batches and bioequivalent products.

The goal of in vitro dissolution testing is to provide insofar as is possible a reasonable prediction of or correlation with the product's in vivo bioavailability. The system relates combinations of a drug's solubility (high or low) and its intestinal permeability (high or low) as a possible basis for predicting the likelihood of achieving a successful in vivo–in vitro correlation (IVIVC) (6, 7). Considered are drugs determined to have

High solubility and high permeability
Low solubility and high permeability
High solubility and low permeability
Low solubility and low permeability

For a high-solubility and high-permeability drug, an IVIVC may be expected if the dissolution rate is slower than the rate of gastric emptying (the rate limiting factor) (8). In the case of a low-solubility and high-permeability drug, dissolution may be the rate-limiting step for absorption, and an IVIVC may be expected. In the case of high solubility and low permeability, permeability is the rate-controlling step, and only a limited IVIVC may be possible. In the case of a drug with low solubility and low permeability, significant problems are likely for oral drug delivery (6).

As noted previously, tablet disintegration is the important first step to the dissolution of the drug in a tablet. A number of formulation and manufacturing factors can affect the disintegration and dissolution of a tablet, including particle size of the drug substance; solubility and hygroscopicity of the formulation; type and concentration of the disintegrant, binder, and lubricant; manufacturing method, particularly the compactness of the granulation and compression force used in tableting; and any in-process variables (9). Together, these factors present a set of complex interrelated conditions that have a bearing on a product's dissolution characteristics. Therefore, batch-to-batch consistency is vitally important to establish dissolution test standards and controls for both materials and processes and to implement them during production and in final testing.

In addition to formulation and manufacturing controls, the method of dissolution testing must be controlled to minimize important variables, such as paddle rotational speed, vibration, and disturbances by sampling probes. Dissolution testing for oral dosage forms has been a component of evaluating product quality in the USP since 1970, when only 12 monographs contained such a requirement. Today the requirement is standard for tablets and capsules.

The USP includes seven apparatus designs for drug release and dissolution testing of immediate-release oral dosage forms, extended-release products, enteric-coated products, and transdermal drug delivery devices. Of primary interest here are USP Apparatus 1 and USP Apparatus 2, used principally for immediate-release solid oral dosage forms.

The equipment consists of (*a*) a variable-speed stirrer motor; (*b*) a cylindrical stainless steel basket on a stirrer shaft (USP Apparatus 1) or a paddle as the stirring element (USP Apparatus 2); (*c*) a 1000-mL vessel of glass or other inert transparent material fitted with a cover having a center port for the shaft of the stirrer and three additional ports, two for removal of samples, and one for a thermometer; and (*d*) a water bath to maintain the temperature of the dissolution medium in the vessel. For use of USP Apparatus 1, the dosage unit is placed inside the basket. For use of USP Apparatus 2, the dosage unit is placed in the vessel.

In each test, a volume of the dissolution medium (as stated in the individual monograph) is placed in the vessel and allowed to come to 37°C ± 0.5°C. Then the stirrer is rotated at the speed specified, and at stated intervals samples of the medium are withdrawn for chemical analysis of the proportion of drug dissolved. The tablet or capsule must meet the stated monograph requirement for rate of dissolution, for example, "not less than 85% of the labeled amount is dissolved in 30 minutes."

There is growing recognition that where inconsistencies in dissolution occur, they occur not between dosage units from the *same* production batch but rather *between batches* or between products from different manufacturers, most likely because of the many factors of formulation, materials, and manufacturing pointed out earlier. However, since dosage units within a batch are generally not the problem, pooled dissolution testing has emerged. This process recognizes batch characteristics and allows pooled specimens to be tested. The pooled specimens may be sampled from the individual dissolution vessels in the apparatus or from multiple dosage units dissolved in a single vessel (10).

Sophisticated and highly automated equipment is continually being developed to provide high levels of quality assurance and control to dissolution testing (Figs. 8.16 and 8.17).

Compressed Tablet Manufacture

Compressed tablets may be made by three basic methods: *wet granulation*, *dry granulation*,

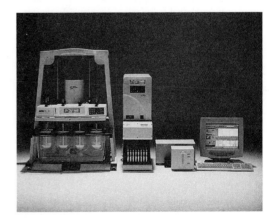

FIGURE 8.16 Hanson Automated Dissolution Test System. Features microprocessor and templates to create, edit, store, and validate dissolution protocols; graphical displays with menus; and icon-based program controls. (Courtesy of Hanson Research).

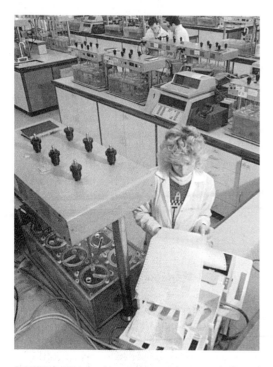

FIGURE 8.17 A modern computer laboratory dedicated to studies of drug dissolution from solid dosage forms. Included are Erweka dissolution baths, Hewlett-Packard computers, and Hewlett-Packard diode assay spectrophotometers. (Courtesy of Elan Corporation, plc.)

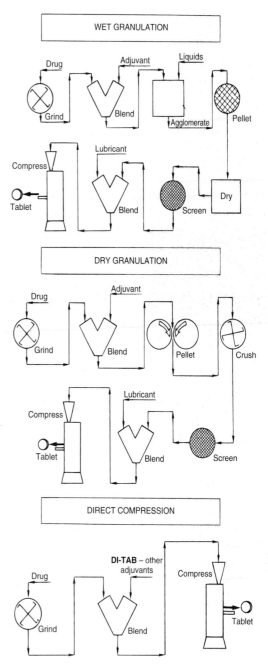

FIGURE 8.18 The three main methods for the preparation of tablets. (Courtesy of Stauffer Chemical Co.)

and *direct compression*. Figure 8.18 presents schematic drawings of each method.

Most powdered medicinal agents require addition of excipients such as diluents, binders, disintegrants, and lubricants to provide the desired characteristics for tablet manufacture and efficacious use. One important requirement in tablet manufacture is that the drug mixture flow freely from the hopper of the tablet press into the dies to enable high-speed compression of the powder mix into tablets. Granulations of powders provide this free flow. Granulations also increase material density, improving powder compressibility during tablet formation.

Wet Granulation

Wet granulation is a widely employed method for production of compressed tablets. The steps required are (*a*) weighing and blending the ingredients, (*b*) preparing a damp mass, (*c*) screening the damp mass into pellets or granules, (*d*) drying the granulation, (*e*) sizing the granulation by dry screening, (*f*) adding lubricant and blending, and (*g*) forming tablets by compression.

Weighing and Blending

Specified quantities of active ingredient, diluent or filler, and disintegrating agent are mixed by mechanical powder blender or mixer until uniform.

Fillers include lactose, microcrystalline cellulose, starch, powdered sucrose, and calcium phosphate. The choice of filler usually is based on the experience of the manufacturer with the material, its relative cost, and its compatibility with the other formulation ingredients. For example, calcium salts must not be used as fillers with tetracycline antibiotics because of an interaction between the two agents that results in reduced tetracycline absorption from the gastrointestinal tract. Among the fillers most preferred are lactose because of its solubility and compatibility, and microcrystalline cellulose, because of its easy compaction, compatibility, and consistent uniformity of supply (11).

Disintegrating agents include croscarmellose, corn and potato starches, sodium starch glycolate, sodium carboxymethylcellulose, polyvinyl polypyrrolidone (PVP), crospovidone, cation exchange resins, alginic acid, and other materials that swell or expand on exposure to moisture and effect the rupture or breakup of the tablet in the gastrointestinal tract. Croscarmellose (2%) and sodium starch glycolate (5%) are often preferred because of their high water uptake and rapid action. One commercial brand of sodium starch glycolate is reported to swell up to 300% of its volume in water (12). When starch is employed, 5 to 10% is usually suitable, but up to about 20% may be used to promote more rapid tablet disintegration. The total amount of disintegrant used is not always added in preparing the granulation. Often a portion (sometimes half) is reserved and added to the finished granulation prior to tablet formation. This results in double disintegration of the tablet. One portion assists in the breakup of the tablet into pieces, and the other portion assists in the breakup of the pieces into fine particles.

Preparing the Damp Mass

A liquid binder is added to the powder mixture to facilitate adhesion of the powder particles. A damp mass resembling dough is formed and used to prepare the granulation. A good binder results in appropriate tablet hardness and does not hinder the release of the drug from the tablet.

Among binding agents are povidone, an aqueous preparation of cornstarch (10–20%), glucose solution (25–50%), molasses, methylcellulose (3%), carboxymethylcellulose, and microcrystalline cellulose. If the drug substance is adversely affected by an aqueous binder, a nonaqueous solution, or dry binder may be used. The amount of binding agent used is part of the operator's art; however, the resulting binder–powder mixture should compact when squeezed in the hand. The binding agent contributes to adhesion of the granules to one another and maintains the integrity of the tablet after compression. However, care must be exercised not to overwet or underwet the powder. Overwetting can result in granules that are too hard for proper tablet formation, and underwetting can result in tablets that are too soft and tend to crumble. When desired, a colorant or flavorant may be added to the binding agent to prepare a granulation with an added feature.

Screening the Damp Mass Into Pellets or Granules

The wet mass is pressed through a screen (usually 6 or 8 mesh) to prepare the granules. This may be done by hand or with special equipment that prepares the granules by extrusion through perforations in the apparatus. The resultant granules are spread evenly on large pieces of paper in shallow trays and dried.

Drying the Granulation

Granules may be dried in thermostatically controlled ovens that constantly record the time, temperature, and humidity (Fig. 8.19).

Sizing the Granulation by Dry Screening

After drying, the granules are passed through a screen of a smaller mesh than that used to prepare the original granulation. The degree to which the granules are reduced depends on the

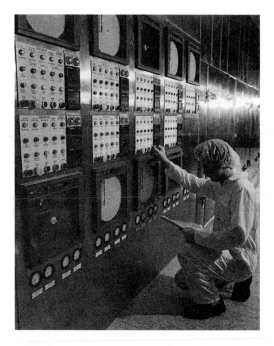

FIGURE 8.19 Temperature-controlled Casburt Drying Oven used in the preparation of granules and controlled release beads. (Courtesy of Elan Corporation, plc.)

size of the punches to be used. In general, the smaller the tablet to be produced, the smaller the granules. Screens of 12- to 20-mesh size are generally used for this purpose. Sizing of the granules is necessary so that the die cavities for tablet compression may be completely and rapidly filled by the free-flowing granulation. Voids or air spaces left by too large a granulation result in production of uneven tablets.

Adding Lubrication and Blending

After dry screening, a dry lubricant is dusted over the spread-out granulation through a fine-mesh screen. Lubricants contribute to preparation of compressed tablets in several ways: They improve the flow of the granulation in the hopper to the die cavity. They prevent adhesion of the tablet formulation to the punches and dies during compression. They reduce friction between the tablet and the die wall during the ejection of the tablet from the machine. They give a sheen to the finished tablet. Among the more commonly used lubricants are magnesium stearate, calcium stearate, stearic acid,

talc, and sodium stearyl fumarate. Magnesium stearate is the most used (11). The quantity of lubricant used varies from one operation to another, but usually ranges from about 0.1% to 5% of the weight of the granulation.

All-in-One Granulation Methods

Technologic advances now allow the entire process of granulation to be completed in a continuous *fluid bed process*, using a single piece of equipment, the fluid bed granulator (Figs. 8.20 and 8.21).

The fluid bed granulator performs the following steps: (*a*) preblending the formulation powder, including active ingredients, fillers, disintegrants, in a bed with fluidized air; (*b*) granulating the mixture by spraying onto the fluidized powder bed, a suitable liquid binder, such as an aqueous solution of acacia, hydroxypropyl cellulose, or povidone; and (*c*) drying the granulated product to the desired moisture content.

Another method, microwave vacuum processing, also allows the powders to be mixed, wetted, agglomerated, and dried within the confines of a single piece of equipment (Fig. 8.22). The wet mass is dried by gentle mixing, vacuum, and microwave. The use of the microwave reduces drying time considerably, often by one-fourth. The total batch production time is usually in the range of 90 minutes. After adding lubricants and screening, the batch is ready for tablet formation or capsule filling.

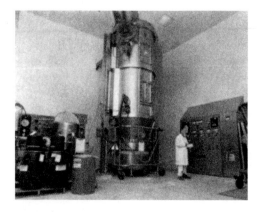

FIGURE 8.20 Fluid bed granulator. (Courtesy of Schering Laboratories.)

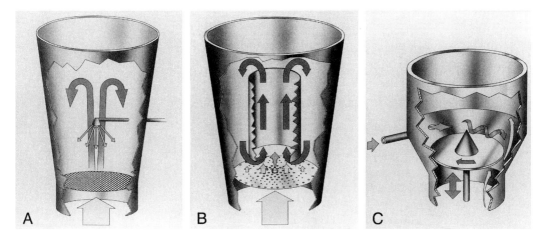

Figure 8.21 Fluid bed coating of solid particles. A. Top spray. **B**. Bottom spray (Wurster). **C**. Tangential spray. (Courtesy of Glatt Air Techniques.)

Dry Granulation

By the dry granulation method, the powder mixture is compacted in large pieces and subsequently broken down or sized into granules

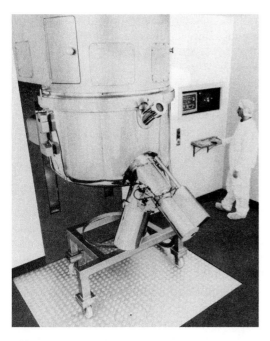

FIGURE 8.22 Microwave vacuum processing in which tablet ingredients are dry-mixed, wetted with a binding liquid, and dried by vacuum and microwave in a single piece of equipment. (Courtesy of GEI Processing.)

(Fig. 8.18). For this method, either the active ingredient or the diluent must have cohesive properties. Dry granulation is especially applicable to materials that cannot be prepared by wet granulation because they degrade in moisture or the elevated temperatures required for drying the granules.

Slugging

After weighing and mixing the ingredients, the powder mixture is slugged, or compressed into large flat tablets or pellets about 1 inch in diameter. The slugs are broken up by hand or by a mill (Fig. 8.23) and passed through a screen of desired mesh for sizing. Lubricant is added in the usual manner, and tablets are prepared by compression. Aspirin, which is hydrolyzed on exposure to moisture, may be prepared into tablets after slugging.

Roller Compaction

Instead of slugging, powder compactors may be used to increase the density of a powder by pressing it between rollers at 1 ton to 6 tons of pressure. The compacted material is broken up, sized, and lubricated, and tablets are prepared by compression in the usual manner. The *roller compaction* method is often preferred to slugging. Binding agents used in roller compaction formulations include methylcellulose or hy-

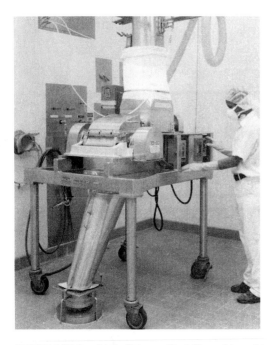

FIGURE 8.23 Frewitt Oscillator or Fitz Mill used to pulverize or granulate. (Courtesy of Eli Lilly and Company.)

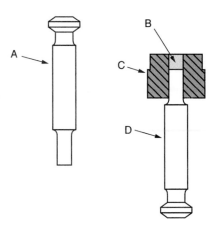

FIGURE 8.24 Punch and die set. **A**. Upper punch. **B**. Die cavity. **C**. Die. **D**. Lower punch. (Courtesy of Cherry-Burrell Corporation.)

droxy methylcellulose (6–12%), which can produce good tablet hardness and friability (13).

Tableting of Granulation

There are a number of types of tablet presses or tableting machines, each varying in productivity but similar in basic function and operation. They all compress a tablet formulation within a steel die cavity by the pressure exerted by the movement of two steel punches, a lower punch and an upper punch (Fig 8.24).

The operation of a single-punch tablet press describes the basic mechanical process. As the lower punch drops, the feed shoe filled with granulation from the hopper is positioned over and fills the die cavity. The feed shoe retracts, scrapes away the excessive granulation, and levels the fill in the die cavity. The upper punch lowers and compresses the fill, forming the tablet. The upper punch retracts as the lower punch rises with the formed tablet to the precise level of the stage. The feed shoe moves over the die cavity, shoves the tablet aside, and once again fills the cavity with granulation to repeat the process. The tablets fall into a collection container. Samples of tablets are assayed and tested for the various quality standards described earlier.

Rotary tablet machines equipped with multiple punches and dies operate via continuous rotating movement of the punches. A single rotary press with 16 stations (16 sets of punches and dies) may produce up to 1150 tablets per minute. Double rotary tablet presses with 27, 33, 37, 41, or 49 sets of punches and dies are capable of producing 2 tablets for each die. Some of these machines can produce 10,000 or more tablets per minute of operation (Fig. 8.25). For such high-speed production, induced die feeders are required to force fill material into the dies to keep up with the rapidly moving punches (Fig. 8.26). A consequence of high-speed production is the increased occurrence of *lamination* (horizontal striations) and tablet *capping*, in which the top of the tablet separates from the whole because the fill material does not have enough time to bond after compression. Reduced speed remedies the problem (14).

Multiple-layer tablets are produced by multiple feed and multiple compression of fill material within a single die. Tablets with an inner core are prepared by machines with a special feed apparatus that places the core tablet precisely within the die for compression with surrounding fill.

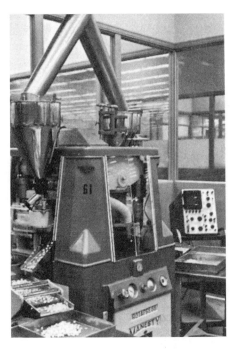

FIGURE 8.25 Manesty Rotapress rotary compression machine. Tablets leaving the machine run over a tablet duster to screen, where they are inspected. Material to be compressed is fed from overhead hopper through yoke to the two compressing machine hoppers. Hardness of tablet is monitored electronically by oscilloscope at right. (Courtesy of Upjohn Company.)

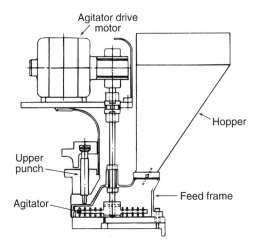

FIGURE 8.26 Induced die feeder. The standard gravity-fed open feed frame can be replaced with an induced die feeder, with which granulation is forced into the die by the rotary action of the agitator. (Courtesy of Cherry-Burrell Corporation.)

Direct Compression Tableting

Some granular chemicals, like potassium chloride, possess free-flowing and cohesive properties that enable them to be compressed directly in a tablet machine without need of granulation. For chemicals lacking this quality, special pharmaceutical excipients may be used to impart the necessary qualities for production of tablets by direct compression. These excipients include *fillers, such as* spray-dried lactose, microcrystals of alpha-monohydrate lactose, sucrose–invert sugar–corn starch mixtures, microcrystalline cellulose, crystalline maltose, and dicalcium phosphate; *disintegrating agents, such as* direct compression starch, sodium carboxymethyl starch, cross-linked carboxymethylcellulose fibers, and cross-linked polyvinylpyrrolidone; *lubricants, such as* magnesium stearate and talc; and *glidants, such as* fumed silicon dioxide.

The capping, splitting, or laminating of tablets is sometimes related to air entrapment during direct compression. When air is trapped, the resulting tablets expand when the pressure of tableting is released, resulting in splits or layers in the tablets. Forced or induced feeders can reduce air entrapment, making the fill powder more dense and amenable to compaction.

Capping also may be caused by punches that are not immaculately clean and perfectly smooth or by a granulation with too much fines, or fine powder. Fine powder, which results when a dried granulation is sized, is generally 10 to 20% of the weight of the granulation. Some fine powder is desired to fill the die cavity properly. However, an excess can lead to tablet softness and capping.

Tablets that have aged or been stored improperly also may exhibit splitting or other physical deformations (Fig. 8.27).

Tablet Dedusting

To remove traces of loose powder adhering to tablets following compression, the tablets are conveyed directly from the tableting machine to a deduster (Fig. 8.28). The compressed tablets may then be coated.

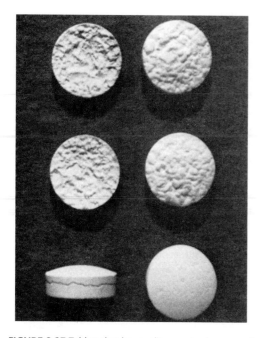

FIGURE 8.27 Tablets that have split on aging because of conditions of manufacture or storage.

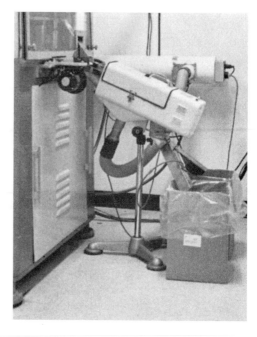

FIGURE 8.28 Model 25 Manesty Tablet Deduster. Tablets leaving tableting machine are dedusted and passed into collection containers. (Courtesy of Eli Lilly and Company.)

Chewable Tablets

Chewable tablets are pleasant-tasting tablets formulated to disintegrate smoothly in the mouth with or without chewing. They are prepared by wet granulation and compression, using only minimal degrees of pressure to produce a soft tablet. Generally, chewable tablets do not contain disintegrants, so patients must be counseled to chew the tablets thoroughly and not swallow them whole.

Mannitol, a white crystalline hexahydric alcohol, is used as the excipient in most chewable tablets. Mannitol is about 70% as sweet as sucrose, with a cool feel in the mouth resulting from its negative heat of solution. Mannitol accounts for 50% or more of the weight of many chewable tablet formulations. Sometimes other sweetening agents, such as sorbitol, lactose, dextrose, crystalline maltose, and glucose, may be substituted for part or all of the mannitol. Xylitol may be used in the preparation of sugar-free chewable tablets. Xylitol is sweeter than mannitol and has the desirable negative heat of solution that provides the cool mouth feel upon dissolution.

Lubricants and binders that do not detract from the texture or desired hardness of the tablet may be used. Colorants and tart or fruity flavorants are commonly employed to enhance the appeal of the tablets. Among the types of products prepared as chewable tablets are antacids (e.g., calcium carbonate), antibiotics (e.g., erythromycin), anti-infective agents (e.g., didanosine), anticonvulsants (e.g., carbamazepine), vasodilators (e.g., isosorbide dinitrate), analgesics (e.g., acetaminophen), various vitamins, and cold–allergy combination tablets. Chewable tablets are particularly useful for children and adults who have difficulty swallowing other solid dosage forms.

The following is a formula for a typical chewable antacid tablet (15):

Per Tablet

Aluminum hydroxide	325.0 mg
Mannitol	812.0 mg
Sodium saccharin	0.4 mg
Sorbitol (10% w/v solution)	32.5 mg
Magnesium stearate	35.0 mg
Mint flavor concentrate	4.0 mg

Preparation: Blend the aluminum hydroxide, mannitol, and sodium saccharin. Prepare a wet granulation with the sorbitol solution. Dry at 49°C (120°F) and screen through a 12-mesh screen. Add the flavor and magnesium stearate, blend, and compress into tablets.

Molded Tablets

Commercial preparation of tablets by molding has been replaced by tablet compression. However, molded tablets, or *tablet triturates*, may be prepared on a small laboratory scale as follows.

The mold is made of hard rubber, hard plastic, or metal. It has two parts, the upper part, or *die* portion, and the lower part, containing squat, flat *punches*. The die portion is a flat plate the thickness of the tablets to be produced with 50 to 200 uniformly drilled and evenly spaced circular holes (Fig. 8.29). The lower part of the mold has corresponding punches that fit the holes precisely. When the die is filled with material and placed atop the punches, the punches gently lift the fill material from the holes to rest upon the punches for drying.

The base for molded tablets is generally a mixture of finely powdered lactose with or without a portion of powdered sucrose (5–20%). The addition of sucrose results in less brittle tablets. In preparing the fill, the drug is mixed uniformly with the base, by geometric dilution when potent drugs are used. The powder mixture is wetted with a 50% mixture of water and alcohol sufficient only to dampen the powder so that is may be compacted. The solvent action of the water on a portion of the lactose or lactose–sucrose base binds the powder mixture upon drying. The alcohol portion hastens drying.

The upper mold is placed on a clean flat glass surface and the damp mass added by a rubbing motion. When each opening is filled completely and smoothed, top and bottom, the mold is fitted on the punch portion of the mold and pressed down, leaving the tablets raised on the pegs to dry.

Before use, the mold should be standardized for the fill material used, since the densities of different formulas result in tablets of different weights. This may be done by preparing a test batch of the formula and weighing and recording the weight of the dry tablets. This weight is used in calculations for production quantities.

Molded tablets are intended to dissolve rapidly in the mouth. They do not contain disintegrants, lubricants, or coatings to slow their rate of dissolution.

AUTHORS' NOTE: *A more complete discussion of the preparation of molded tablets and the standardization of laboratory molds may be found in the fifth edition of this textbook.*

Tablet Coating

Tablets are coated for a number of reasons, including to protect the medicinal agent against destructive exposure to air and/or humidity; to mask the taste of the drug; to provide special characteristics of drug release (e.g., enteric coatings); and to provide aesthetics or distinction to the product.

In a limited number of instances, tablets are coated to prevent inadvertent contact with the drug substance and the effects of drug absorption. For example, Proscar tablets (finasteride, Merck) are coated for just this reason. The drug is used by men in the treatment of benign prostatic hyperplasia. The labeling instructions warn that women who are pregnant or who may become pregnant should not come into contact with it. Drug contact can occur through handling broken tablets. If finasteride is absorbed by a woman who is pregnant with

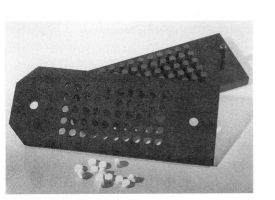

FIGURE 8.29 Laboratory mold for preparation of tablet triturates.

a male baby, the drug has the potential to adversely affect the developing male fetus.

The general methods involved in coating tablets are as follows.

Sugarcoating Tablets

The sugarcoating of tablets may be divided into the following steps: (*a*) waterproofing and sealing if needed, (*b*) subcoating, (*c*) smoothing and final rounding, (*d*) finishing and coloring if desired, and (*e*) polishing. The entire coating process is conducted in a series of mechanically operated acorn-shaped coating pans of galvanized iron, stainless steel, or copper. The pans, which are partially open in the front, have diameters ranging from about 1 to 4 feet and various capacities (Figs. 8.30 and 8.31). The smaller pans are used for experimental, developmental, and pilot plant operations, the larger pans for industrial production. The pans operate at about a 40° angle to contain the tablets while allowing the operator visual and manual access. During operation, the pan is mechanically rotated at moderate speeds, allowing the tablets to tumble over each other while making contact with the coating solutions which are gently poured or sprayed onto the tablets. To allow gradual buildup of the coatings, the solutions are added in portions, with warm air blown in to hasten drying. Each coat is applied only after the previous coat has

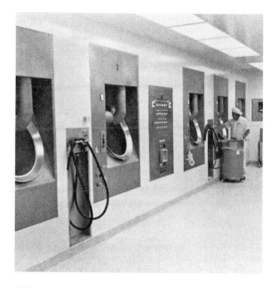

FIGURE 8.31 Modern tablet-coating facility. Air and exhaust ducts to assist drying are automatically operated from central board. (Courtesy of Eli Lilly and Company.)

dried. Tablets intended to be coated are manufactured to be thin-edged and highly convex to allow the coatings to form rounded rather than angular edges.

Waterproofing and Sealing Coats

For tablets containing components that may be adversely affected by moisture, one or more coats of a waterproofing substance, such as pharmaceutical shellac or a polymer, is applied to the compressed tablets before the subcoating application. The waterproofing solution (usually alcoholic) is gently poured or sprayed on the compressed tablets rotating in the coating pans. Warm air is blown into the pan during the coating to hasten the drying and to prevent tablets from sticking together.

Subcoating

After the tablets are waterproofed if needed, three to five subcoats of a sugar-based syrup are applied. This bonds the sugar coating to the tablet and provides rounding. The sucrose and water syrup also contains gelatin, acacia, or polyvinylpyrrolidone (PVP) to enhance coating. When the tablets are partially dry, they are sprinkled with a dusting powder, usually a

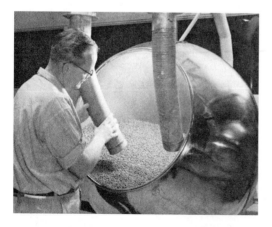

FIGURE 8.30 Tablet coating, an old-style coating pan, showing the warm air supply and the exhaust. (Courtesy of Wyeth Laboratories.)

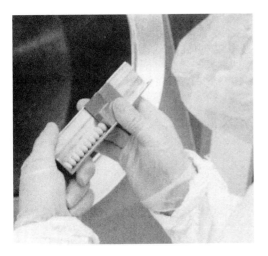

FIGURE 8.32 Gauge used to measure coated tablets. (Courtesy of Eli Lilly and Company.)

mixture of powdered sugar and starch but sometimes talc, acacia, or precipitated chalk as well. Warm air is applied to the rolling tablets, and when they are dry, the process is repeated until the tablets are of the desired shape and size (Fig. 8.32). The subcoated tablets are then scooped out of the coating pan and the excess powder is removed by gently shaking the tablets on a cloth screen.

Smoothing and Final Rounding

After the tablets are subcoated, 5 to 10 additional coatings of a thick syrup are applied to complete the rounding and smooth the coatings. This syrup is sucrose-based, with or without additional components such as starch and calcium carbonate. As the syrup is applied, the operator moves his or her hand through the rolling tablets to distribute the syrup and to prevent the tablets from sticking to one another. A dusting powder is often used between syrup applications. Warm air is applied to hasten the drying time of each coat.

Finishing and Coloring

To attain final smoothness and the appropriate color to the tablets, several coats of a thin syrup containing the desired colorant are applied in the usual manner. This step is performed in a clean pan, free from previous coating materials.

Imprinting

Solid dosage forms may be passed through a special imprinting machine (Fig. 8.33) to impart identification codes and other distinctive symbols. By FDA regulation, effective in 1995, all solid dosage forms for human consumption, including both prescription-only and over-the-counter drug products, must be imprinted with product-specific identification codes. Some exemptions to this requirement are allowed: those used in clinical investigations; those that are extemporaneously compounded in the course of pharmacy practice; radiopharmaceutical drug products; and products that, because of their size, shape, texture, or other physical characteristics, make imprinting technologically not feasible.

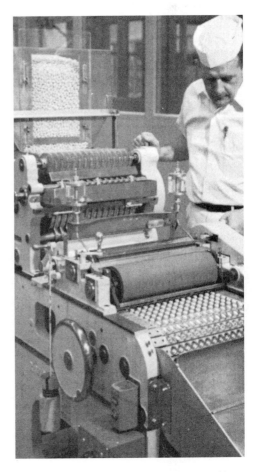

FIGURE 8.33 Branding of coated compression tablets on a Hartnett branding machine. (Courtesy of The Upjohn Company.)

Technically, the imprint may be *debossed*, *embossed*, *engraved*, or printed on the surface with ink. *Debossed* means imprinted with a mark below the surface; *embossed* means imprinted with a mark raised above the surface; and *engraved* means imprinted with a code that is cut into the surface during production.

Polishing

Coated tablets may be polished in several ways. Special drum-shaped pans or ordinary coating pans lined with canvas or other cloth impregnated with carnauba wax and/or beeswax, may be used to polish tablets as they tumble in the pan. Or, pieces of wax may be placed in a polishing pan and the tablets allowed to tumble over the wax until the desired sheen is attained. A third method is light spraying of the tablets with wax dissolved in a nonaqueous solvent. Two or three coats of wax may be applied, depending upon the desired gloss. After each coat has been applied, the addition of a small amount of talc to the tumbling tablets contributes to their high luster (Fig. 8.34).

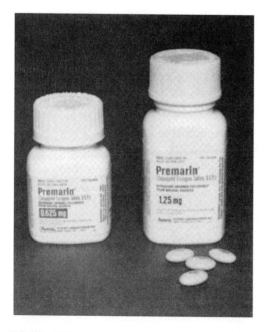

FIGURE 8.34 Coated, polished, and monogrammed tablets. (Courtesy of Wyeth-Ayerst Laboratories.)

Film-Coating Tablets

The sugarcoating process, as described, is not only tedious, time-consuming, and specialized, requiring the expertise of highly skilled technicians; it also results in coated tablets that may be twice the size and weight of the original uncoated tablets. Also, sugarcoated tablets may vary slightly in size from batch to batch and within a batch. All of these factors are important considerations for a manufacturer. From a patient's point of view, large tablets are not as easily swallowed as are small tablets.

The film-coating process, which places a thin, skin-tight coating of a plasticlike material over the compressed tablet, was developed to produce coated tablets having essentially the same weight, shape, and size as the originally compressed tablet. Also, the coating is thin enough to reveal any identifying monograms embossed in the tablet during compression by the tablet punches. Film-coated tablets also are far more resistant to destruction by abrasion than are sugarcoated tablets. However, like sugarcoated tablets, the coating may be colored to make the tablets attractive and distinctive.

Film-coating solutions may be nonaqueous or aqueous. The nonaqueous solutions contain the following types of materials to provide the desired coating to the tablets:

1. A *film former* capable of producing smooth, thin films reproducible under conventional coating conditions and applicable to a variety of tablet shapes. Example: cellulose acetate phthalate.
2. An *alloying substance* providing water solubility or permeability to the film to ensure penetration by body fluids and therapeutic availability of the drug. Example: polyethylene glycol.
3. A *plasticizer* to produce flexibility and elasticity of the coating and thus provide durability. Example: castor oil.
4. A *surfactant* to enhance spreadability of the film during application. Example: polyoxyethylene sorbitan derivatives.
5. *Opaquants* and *colorants* to make the appearance of the coated tablets handsome and distinctive. Examples: Opaquant, tita-

nium dioxide; colorant, FD&C or D&C dyes.

6. *Sweeteners, flavors,* and *aromas* to enhance the acceptability of the tablet to the patient. Examples: sweeteners, saccharin; flavors and aromas, vanillin.

7. A *glossant* to provide luster to the tablets without a separate polishing operation. Example: beeswax.

8. A *volatile solvent* to allow the spread of the other components over the tablets while allowing rapid evaporation to permit an effective yet speedy operation. Example: alcohol mixed with acetone.

Tablets are film-coated by application or spraying of the coating solution on the tablets in ordinary coating pans. The volatility of the solvent enables the film to adhere quickly to the surface of the tablets.

Because of both the expense of the volatile solvents used in the film-coating process and the environmental problem of the release of solvents, pharmaceutical manufacturers generally favor the use of aqueous solutions. One of the problems attendant to these, however, is slow evaporation of the water base compared to the volatile organic solvent–based solutions. One commercial water-based colloidal coating dispersion called Aquacoat (FMC Corporation) contains a 30% ethyl cellulose pseudolatex. Pseudolatex dispersions have a high solids content for greater coating ability and a relatively low viscosity. The low viscosity allows less water to be used in the coating dispersion, requiring less evaporation and reducing the likelihood that water will interfere with tablet formulation. In addition, the low viscosity permits greater coat penetration into the crevices of monogrammed or scored tablets. A plasticizer may be added to assist in the production of a dense, relatively impermeable film with high gloss and mechanical strength. Other aqueous film-coating products use cellulosic materials such as methylcellulose, hydroxypropyl cellulose, and hydroxypropyl methylcellulose as the film-forming polymer.

A typical aqueous film-coating formulation contains the following (16):

1. *Film-forming polymer* (7–18%). Examples: cellulose ether polymers such as hydroxypropyl methylcellulose, hydroxypropyl cellulose, and methylcellulose.

2. *Plasticizer* (0.5–2.0%). Examples: glycerin, propylene glycol, polyethylene glycol, diethyl phthalate, and dibutyl subacetate.

3. *Colorant and opacifier* (2.5–8%). Examples: FD&C or D&C lakes and iron oxide pigments.

4. *Vehicle* (water, to make 100%).

There are some problems attendant on aqueous film coating, including the appearance of small amounts (*picking*) or larger amounts (*peeling*) of film fragments flaking from the tablet surface; roughness of the tablet surface due to failure of spray droplets to coalesce (*orange peel effect*); an uneven distribution of color on the tablet surface (*mottling*); filling-in of the score line or indented logo on the tablet by the film (*bridging*); and disfiguration of the core tablet when subjected for too long to the coating solution (tablet *erosion*). The cause of each of these problems can be determined and the problem rectified through appropriate changes in formulation, equipment, technique, or process.

Enteric Coating

Enteric-coated solid dosage forms are intended to pass through the stomach intact to disintegrate and release their drug content for absorption along the intestines. The design of an enteric coating may be based on the transit time required for passage to the intestines and may be accomplished through coatings of sufficient thickness. However, usually an enteric coating is based on factors of pH, resisting dissolution in the highly acid environment of the stomach but yielding to the less acid environment of the intestine. Some enteric coatings are designed to dissolve at pH 4.8 and greater.

Enteric-coating materials may be applied to either whole compressed tablets or to drug particles or granules used in the fabrication of tablets or capsules. The coatings may be applied in multiple portions to build a thick coating or as a thin film coat. The coating system may be aqueous or organic solvent–based and effective so long as the coating material resists breakdown in the gastric fluid. Among the materials used in enteric coatings are pharmaceutical shellac, hydroxypropyl methylcellulose phthalate, polyvinyl acetate phthalate, diethyl phthalate, and cellulose acetate phthalate.

Fluid Bed or Air Suspension Coating

Fluid bed coating, which uses equipment of the type shown in Figure 8.35, is spray coating of powders, granules, beads, pellets, or tablets held in suspension by a column of air. Fluid bed processing equipment is multifunctional and may also be used in preparing tablet granulations.

In the Wurster process, named after its developer, the items to be coated are fed into a vertical cylinder and are supported by a column of air that enters from the bottom of the cylinder. Within the air stream, the solids rotate both vertically and horizontally. As the coating solution enters the system from the bottom, it is rapidly applied to the suspended, rotating solids, with rounding coats being applied in less than an hour with the assistance of warm air blasts released in the chamber.

In another type of fluid bed system, the coating solution is sprayed downward onto the particles to be coated as they are suspended by air from below. This method is commonly referred to as the *top-spray* method. This method provides greater capacity, up to 1500 kg, than the other air suspension coating methods (17). Both the top-spray and bottom-spray methods may be employed using a modified apparatus used for fluid bed granulation. A third method, the *tangential spray technique*, is used in rotary fluid bed coaters. The bottom, top, and tangential spray methods are depicted in Figure 8.21. Electron microscope images of the results of this process are shown in Fig. 8.36.

The three systems are increasingly used for application of aqueous or organic solvent–based polymer film coatings. The top-spray coating method is particularly recommended for taste masking, enteric release, and barrier films on particles or tablets. It is most effective when coatings are applied from aqueous solutions, la-

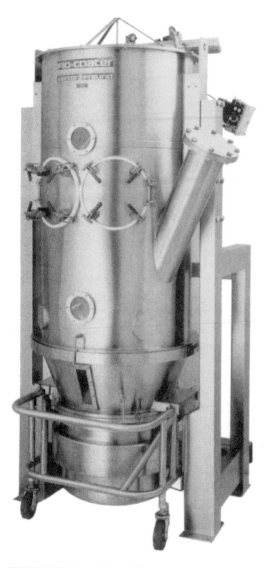

FIGURE 8.35 Vector/Freund Flo-Coater production system. A fluid bed system used to apply coatings to beads, granules, powders, and tablets. Capacity of models ranges from 5 kg to 700 kg. (Courtesy of Vector Corporation.)

texes, or hot melts (17, 18). The bottom-spray method is recommended for sustained-release and enteric-release products; and the tangential method is used for layering coatings and for sustained-release and enteric-coated products (18).

Among the variables requiring control to produce desired and consistent quality are equipment and the method of spraying (e.g., top, bottom, tangential), spray nozzle distance from spraying bed, droplet size, spray rate,

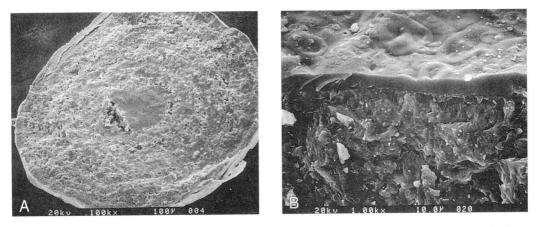

FIGURE 8.36 Scanning electron microscope images of pharmaceutical granules coated through fluid bed technology: **A**. Layered and coated granule. **B**. Cross-section of top-spray enteric-coated granule. (Courtesy of Glatt Air Techniques.)

spray pressure, volume of the air column, batch size, method and time for drying, and air temperature and moisture content in the processing compartment (18).

Compression Coating

In a manner similar to the preparation of multiple compressed tablets having an inner core and an outer shell of drug material, core tablets may be sugarcoated by compression. The coating material, in the form of a granulation or powder, is compressed onto a tablet core of drug with a special tablet press. Compression coating is an anhydrous operation and thus may be safely employed in the coating of tablets containing a drug that is labile to moisture. Compared to sugarcoating using pans, compression coating is more uniform and uses less coating material, resulting in tablets that are lighter, smaller, easier to swallow, and less expensive to package and ship.

Irrespective of the method used in coating, all tablets are visually or electronically inspected for physical imperfections (Fig. 8.37).

Impact of Manufacturing Changes on Solid Dosage Forms

The quality and performance of a solid dosage form may be altered by changes in formulation or by changes in the method of manufacture.

The changes in formulation may arise from (*a*) the use of starting raw materials, including both the active ingredient and pharmaceutical excipients, that have different chemical or physical characteristics (e.g., solubility or particle size) than the standards set for the original components; (*b*) the use of different pharmaceutical

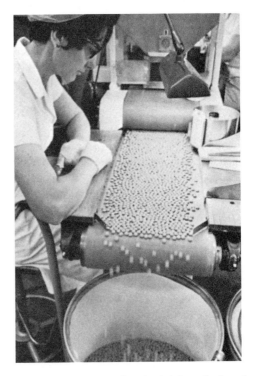

FIGURE 8.37 Checking for physical imperfections in coated tablets. (Courtesy of Smith, Kline & French.)

excipients (e.g., magnesium stearate instead of calcium stearate as the lubricant); (*c*) the use of different quantities of the same excipients in a formulation (e.g., use of a more concentrated wet tablet binder); or (*d*) the addition of a new excipient to a formulation (e.g., a revised tablet coating formula).

The changes in the method of manufacture may be (*a*) use of processing or manufacturing equipment of a different design; (*b*) a change in the steps or order in the process or method of manufacture (e.g. different mixing times); (*c*) different in-process controls, quality tests, or assay methods; (*d*) production of different batch sizes; (*e*) employment of different product reprocessing procedures; or (*f*) employment of a different manufacturing site.

Changes such as these may be proposed or implemented during the product development stage, during scale-up of product manufacture before NDA approval, or after NDA approval and product marketing. In all instances, it is critical to assess any effects of the change in meeting the proposed or established standards for product quality (e.g., dissolution rate and bioavailability). It is necessary for a manufacturer to document the change, validate its effect, and provide the necessary information to the FDA. Some changes are considered minor (e.g., a change in tablet color) and do not affect product quality; they do not require prior FDA approval. Other changes that may affect product quality and performance (e.g., use of a substantially different quantity or grade of an excipient or use of a piece of manufacturing equipment that changes the methodology of manufacture) require prior FDA approval (19).

Official and Commercially Available Tablets

There are hundreds of tablets recognized by the USP and literally thousands of commercially available tablet products from virtually all pharmaceutical manufacturers, in most therapeutic categories, and in various dosage strengths. Examples of a limited number of these are presented in Table 8.1.

Packaging and Storing Tablets

Tablets are stored in tight containers, in places of low humidity, and protected from extremes in temperature. Products that are prone to decomposition by moisture generally are packaged with a desiccant packet. Drugs that are adversely affected by light are packaged in light-resistant containers. With a few exceptions, tablets that are properly stored will remain stable for several years or more.

In dispensing tablets, the pharmacist is well advised to use a similar type of container as provided by the manufacturer of the product. The patient is well advised to keep the drug in the container dispensed. Storage conditions, as recommended for the particular product, should be maintained by the pharmacist and patient alike and expiration dates observed.

The pharmacist should be aware also that the hardness of certain tablets may change upon aging, usually resulting in a decrease in the disintegration and dissolution rates of the product. The increase in tablet hardness can frequently be attributed to the increased adhesion of the binding agent and other formulative components within the tablet. Examples of increased tablet hardening with age have been reported for a number of drugs, including aluminum hydroxide, sodium salicylate, and phenylbutazone (20).

In tablets containing volatile drugs, such as nitroglycerin, the drug may migrate between tablets in the container, resulting in a lack of uniformity among the tablets (21). Also, packing materials, such as cotton and rayon, in contact with nitroglycerin tablets may absorb varying amounts of nitroglycerin, reducing potency of the tablets (22). The USP directs that nitrogen tablets be preserved in tight containers, preferably of glass, at controlled room temperature.

The USP further directs that nitroglycerin tablets be dispensed in the original unopened container, labeled with the following statement directed to the patient. "Warning: to prevent loss of potency, keep these tablets in the original container or in a supplemental nitroglycerin container specifically labeled as being suitable for nitroglycerin tablets. Close tightly immediately after use" (4).

TABLE 8.1 EXAMPLES OF OFFICIAL TABLETS

OFFICIAL TABLET	REPRESENTATIVE COMMERCIAL PRODUCTS	STRENGTH	CATEGORY
Acetaminophen	Tylenol (McNeil)	325, 500 mg	Analgesic, antipyretic
Acyclovir	Zovirax (Glaxo Wellcome)	400, 800 mg	Antiviral
Allopurinol	Zyloprim (Glaxo Wellcome)	100, 300 mg	Antigout and antiurolithic
Amitriptyline HCl	Elavil HCl (Zeneca)	10, 25, 50, 75, 100, 150 mg	Antidepressant
Carbamazepine	Tegretol (Novartis)	200 mg	Anticonvulsant
Chlorambucil	Leukeran (Glaxo Wellcome)	2 mg	Antineoplastic
Cimetidine	Tagamet (SmithKline Beecham)	200, 300, 400 mg	Histamine H_2 receptor antagonist
Ciprofloxacin	Cipro (Bayer)	150, 500, 750 mg	Antibacterial
Conjugated estrogens	Premarin (Wyeth-Ayerst)	0.3, 0.625, 0.9, 1.25, 2.5 mg	Estrogen
Diazepam	Valium (Roche)	2, 5, 10 mg	Sedative, skeletal muscle relaxant
Digoxin	Lanoxin (Glaxo Wellcome)	0.125, 0.25 mg	Cardiotonic
Enalapril	Vasotec (Merck)	2.5, 5, 10, 20 mg	Antihypertensive
Furosemide	Lasix (Hoechst Marion Roussel)	20, 40, 80 mg	Diuretic, antihypertensive
Griseofulvin	Fulvicin (Schering)	250, 500 mg	Antifungal
Haloperidol	Haldol (Ortho McNeil)	0.5, 1, 2, 5, 10, 20 mg	Tranquilizer
Ibuprofen	Motrin (McNeil)	400, 600, 800 mg	Analgesic and antipyretic
Levothyroxine sodium	Synthroid (Knoll)	0.025, 0.05, 0.075, 0.088, 0.1, 0.122, 0.125, 0.137, 0.15, 0.2, 0.3 mg	Thyroid hormone
Loratadine	Claritin (Schering)	10 mg	Antihistamine
Meperidine HCl	Demerol (Sanofi Winthrop)	50, 100 mg	Narcotic analgesic
Methyldopa	Aldomet (Merck)	125, 250, 500 mg	Antihypertensive
Nitroglycerin	Nitrostat (Parke-Davis)	0.3, 0.4, 0.6 mg	Antianginal
Penicillin V	Pen Vee K (Wyeth-Ayerst)	250, 500 mg	Anti-infective
Pergolide Mesylate	Permax (Athena)	0.05, 0.25, 1 mg	Dopamine receptor agonist
Propanolol	Inderal (Wyeth-Ayerst)	10, 20, 40, 60, 80 mg	Antianginal, antiarrhythmic, antihypertensive
Terbutaline Sulfate	Brethine (Novartis)	2.5, 5 mg	Antiasthmatic
Verapamil HCl	Calan (Searle)	40, 80, 120 mg	Antihypertensive
Warfarin sodium	Coumadin (DuPont)	1, 2, 2.5, 4.5, 7.5, 10 mg	Anticoagulant

The pharmacist also should caution patients about handling medication when it poses a risk. For example, as noted earlier, finasteride tablets are taken by men to treat benign prostatic hyperplasia. Finasteride has the potential to harm a male fetus if absorbed by a pregnant woman through either direct contact with finasteride or possibly through semen. Therefore, a woman who is pregnant or who may become pregnant should not handle finasteride tablets or come into contact with finasteride powder. In addition, when the male patient's sexual partner is pregnant or may become pregnant, the patient should avoid exposure of his partner to semen or should discontinue use of the drug.

Other Solid Dosage Forms for Oral Administration

Lozenges

Lozenges can be made by compression or molding. Compressed lozenges are made using a tablet machine and large, flat punches. The machine is operated at a high degree of compression to produce lozenges that are harder than ordinary tablets so that they dissolve or disintegrate slowly in the mouth. Medicinal substances that are heat stable may be molded into a hard sugar candy lozenges by candy-making machines that process a warm, highly concentrated, flavored syrup as the base and form the lozenges by molding and drying.

Lozenges have a special place in the delivery of medication. A number of lozenge dosage forms are available for self-care drugs, including benzocaine, dextromethorphan, phenyl-propanolamine, and zinc, to treat self-limiting cough and cold symptoms and minor sore throat.

Lollipops

The fentanyl Actiq (manufactured by Anesta Corporation and distributed by Abbott Labora-tories) is a raspberry lollipop that differs from the fentanyl Oralet. It is a sugar-based lozenge on a stick and contains fentanyl citrate. It is an off-white color and the stick bears a large Rx mark. Actiq is the first product specifically designed to aid in controlling breakthrough pain in cancer patients. It is indicated only for the management of breakthrough cancer pain in patients with malignancies who are already taking and are tolerant to opioids. Breakthrough cancer pain occurs in about 50% of cancer pain patients and is a component of chronic cancer pain that is particularly difficult to treat because of its severity, rapid onset, and frequent unpredictability. The lollipop provides almost immediate relief as the drug starts being absorbed in the mouth and starts to work within minutes; its effects last for only about 15 minutes, but that is usually long enough to relieve breakthrough pain. The concern about this product being accidentally used by children is addressed by special packaging that requires scissors to open (1).

Pills

By definition, pills are small, round solid dosage forms containing a medicinal agent and intended to be administered orally. Although the manufacture and administration of pills was at one time quite prevalent, today pills have been replaced by compressed tablets and capsules. A procedure for the extemporaneous preparation of pills on a small scale may be found in the first edition of this text.

PHARMACEUTICS CASE STUDY

Subjective Information

A pharmaceutical manufacturer has developed a formula for an antihistamine compressed tablet. During the initial run, the tablets were found to be too friable. What can be done?

Objective Information

The formula for the tablet is as follows:

Antihistamine	50 mg
Directly compressible lactose	150 mg
Magnesium stearate	10 mg
Starch	100 mg
Talc	25 mg

Pharmaceutics Case Study cont.

The tablet is to be compressed, so it has the following characteristics:

Description   8-mm white biconvex bisected tablet
Weight   335 mg
Hardness   8 kg
Dissolution   Medium: 0.01 N hydrochloric acid, 500 mL
Apparatus 2: 50 rpm
Time: 30 minutes

Following the initial run, hardness testing reveals that the tablet's hardness is only 6.5 kg.

Assessment

The tablet's hardness must be increased to meet specifications. There are a couple of different approaches to accomplishing this:

1. Increase the pressure of the upper punch of the tableting machine.
2. Add a tablet binder, such as pregelatinized starch, acacia, or methylcellulose. Some or all of the starch in the tablet formula could be replaced by pregelatinized starch, as it will serve all of the functions of regular starch (diluent, dissolution enhancer) plus serve as a tablet binder.

Plan

Adjust the tableting machine and increase the pressure of the upper punch. Sometimes the simplest solutions are the best.

CLINICAL CASE STUDY

Subjective

HPI: F. L. is a 46-y/o AAM brought to the emergency department (ER) by his wife with chief complaint of "chest pain." His spouse states that F. L. began to feel constant pain in his chest while watching television. The pain radiated to his left arm and back. Spouse noticed excessive sweating on his forehead as he started to "gasp for breath." Immediately she brought him to the ER. At the ER, F. L. describes pain as the "worst pain of his life" and feels like "an elephant's foot is pressuring into my chest." Patient was brought into the ER within an hour of onset of symptoms. F. L. denies any previous episodes of chest pain, sweating, weakness, shortness of breath, syncope, nausea, or vomiting. Patient denies any previous episodes of pain on exertion. He rates pain intensity as 10/10.

PMH: HTN × 12 years
Type II diabetes × 2 years
PSH: Lasik eye surgery, 2002
SH: (−) EtOH: quit drinking in 1996
(−) Tobacco: quit smoking in 1996
(−) Caffeine
(−) Illicit drugs: "none, never"
Patient lives in Hanover Park with wife and 1 daughter and 1 son, no pets
Has own business, works at home
FH: Father died of an asthma attack at 67 y/o
Mother died of an MI at 59 y/o
Sister: asthma

Diet: Eats 3 times a day and 2 or 3 snacks a day. Denies following any low-fat, low-cholesterol diet, low-salt diet. On a low-sugar diet and states he follows it. Eats fast food at

Clinical Case Study cont.

least twice a week. Snacks consist mostly of chips, cookies, and salsa.

Exer: Pt states, "I don't have time to exercise. I've got a business and a family to handle." The extent of patient's exercise is walking up and down the stairs when he needs to get around the house.

All: NKDA

PTA: lisinopril (Zestril) 40 mg PO QHS for HTN

felodipine (Plendil) 10 mg PO QD for HTN

glyburide/metformin (Glucovance) 2.5/500 mg PO TID for Type II diabetes

Adherence

Pt states he adheres to all his medications. He uses a pillbox to help remind him. He checks his blood glucose levels three times a day, alternating before and after meals.

Objective

Ht:	5'8"	**Wt:**	185lb
Pain:	10/10	**BP:**	112/80
Na:	140 mmol/L	**K:**	4.0 mmol/L
Cl:	100 mmol/L	**CO$_2$:**	24 mmol/L
BUN:	4.0 mmol/L	**SrCr:**	70 mmol/L
HgA$_{1c}$:	7	**CK:**	30

Last Accuchecks: After breakfast, 9:30 A.M.: 151

After lunch, 1:00 P.M.: 155

After dinner, 7:00 P.M.: 141

Assessment

Pt is a 46 y/o AAM with a PMH of controlled HTN and type II diabetes who has had his first MI. Pt is at increased risk for MI due to HTN, diabetes, and significant family history. Though patient adheres to his medication regimen, he does not adhere to a healthy diet and exercise plan, which may increase his chances of experiencing a similar episode in the future.

Plan

1. Recommend sustained-release nitroglycerin (NTG) Nitrobid 2.5-mg capsules once a day on an empty stomach with a full glass of water, either 30 minutes before or an hour after meals. Instruct patient to take the medication the same time each day and to swallow the capsule whole. If the patient misses a dose, he should take it as soon as he remembers unless the next scheduled dose is within 2 hours; in that case he should skip the missed dose and take only the next dose.

2. Recommend sublingual nitroglycerin (NTG) NitroQuick 0.30 mg (1/200 gr) tablets. Instruct patient to use the sublingual tablet at the first sign of attack. Instruct patient to wet the tablet with saliva and place under the tongue or between gums or in cheek until tablet dissolves. Do not swallow the tablet. Effects of NTG should be felt within 2 minutes, lasting for up to 30 minutes. If symptoms do not resolve within 5 minutes of the first dose, repeat with a second sublingual tablet. Again, wait 5 minutes and use a third sublingual tablet if symptoms persist. Call for emergency assistance (911) if symptoms continue after three doses of NTG. Inform patient to keep and store sublingual tablets in original glass container, keep them away from heat or light, and keep bottle tightly closed after use.

3. Counsel patient on common side effects of NTG, such as headache, dizziness, drowsiness, and low blood pressure. Recommend acetaminophen (e.g., Tylenol) for relief of headache. Tell patient to avoid alcoholic beverages and medications containing alcohol while using NTG, as their concurrent use may cause severe hypotension and cardiovascular

Clinical Case Study cont.

difficulties. Inform the patient that the use of Sildenafil (Viagra) is dangerous and should be avoided while using this medication, as it may increase the blood pressure–lowering effect of NTG. Instruct patient to check expiration dates of tablets regularly because therapeutic effectiveness of NTG may decrease in tablets older than 6 months. Consult physician before stopping use of NTG because abrupt discontinuation may cause severe chest pain.

4. Educate the spouse and patient to recognize the signs and symptoms of a heart attack (e.g., excessive sweating, chest pain, jaw or back pain). Explain that a "silent" MI can occur without any symptoms. Further education on the condition and how it may be managed and prevented may benefit this patient. Stress

the importance of lifestyle changes such as exercise and dietary modifications (e.g., low-fat, low-salt, low-cholesterol diet). Have patient consult physician before embarking on an exercise regimen. An exercise regimen may include exercising at least 3 or 4 times a week for 15 to 30 minutes or as tolerated by the patient.

5. Monitoring parameters: BP, signs and symptoms of heart attack, frequency of episodes, side effects of the medication. Goal: Increased patient knowledge of condition, improved adherence to diet and exercise regimen, no medication side effects, no second episode. Make sure patient understands importance of follow-up physician visits and exercising caution when purchasing nonprescription and herbal products (i.e., consult a pharmacist).

REFERENCES

1. Physicians' Desk Reference, 57th ed. Montvale NJ: Medical Economics, 2003: 1184, 3018–3020.
2. Product Package. Dimetapp ND. Wyeth Consumer Healthcare, Madison, NJ.
3. Package Insert. Tempra Quicklets, Bristol-Myers Products, New York.
4. The United States Pharmacopeia 26–National Formulary 21. Rockville MD: U.S. Pharmacopeial Convention, 2003.
5. Skoug JW, Halstead GW, Theis DL, Freeman JE, Fagan DT, Rohrs BR. Strategy for the development and validation of dissolution tests for solid oral dosage forms. Pharm Tech 1996;20:58–71.
6. Guidance for industry: dissolution testing of immediate release solid oral dosage forms. Rockville MD: FDA/CDER, 1997.
7. Amidon GL, Lennernas, Shah VP, Crison JR. A theoretical basis for a biopharmaceutic drug classification: the correlation of in vitro drug product dissolution and in vivo bioavailability. Pharm Res 1995;12: 413–420.
8. Swarbrick J. In vitro dissolution, drug bioavailability, and the spiral of science. Pharm Tech 1997;21:68–72.
9. Chowhan ZT. Factors affecting dissolution of drugs and their stability upon aging in solid dosage forms. PharmTech 1994;18:60–73.
10. Hanson R, Swartz ME, Jarnutowski RJ. Pooled dissolution testing: a primer. Dissolution Technologies 1998;5:15–17.
11. Shangraw RF, Demarest DA. A survey of current industrial practices in the formulation and manufacture of tablets and capsules. Pharm Tech 1993;17:32–44.
12. Explotab. Patterson, NY: Mendell, Penmwest Co. 1992.
13. METHOCEL as a granulation binding agent for immediate-release tablet and capsule products. Wilmington, DE: Dow Chemical, 1996.
14. Rubinstein MH. Lubricant behaviour of magnesium stearate. Acta Pharmaceutica Suecica 1987;24:43.
15. Atlas mannitol, USP tablet excipient. Wilmington, DE: ICI Americas, 1973.
16. Mathur LK, Forbes SJ, Yelvigi M. Characterization techniques for the aqueous film coating process. Pharm Tech 1984;8:42.
17. Jones DM. Factors to consider in fluid-bed processing. Pharm Tech 1985;9:50–62.
18. Mehta AM. Scale-up considerations in the fluid-bed process for controlled-release products. Pharm Tech 1988;12
19. Lucisano LJ, Franz RM. FDA proposed guidance for chemistry, manufacturing, and control changes for immediate-release solid dosage forms: a review and industrial perspective. Pharm Tech 1995;19:30–44.
20. Barrett D, Fell JT. Effect of aging on physical properties of phenylbutazone tablets. J Pharm Sci 1975;64: 335.
21. Page DP et al. Stability study of nitroglycerin sublingual tablets. J Pharm Sci 1975;64:140.
22. Fusari SA. Nitroglycerin sublingual tablets I: Stability of conventional tablets. J Pharm Sci 1973;62:122.

Solid Oral Modified-Release Dosage Forms and Drug Delivery Systems

9

Chapter at a glance

This chapter describes solid oral dosage forms and drug delivery systems that by virtue of formulation and product design have modified drug release features. The forecast is for the drug delivery market to grow to about $70 billion by 2005, and the market for oral controlled drug delivery alone is expected to grow at 9% or more every year through 2007 (1). There are two primary driving forces behind this market, namely patient-related factors and market-driven factors (2). The patient-related factors are discussed later in the chapter. The life cycle of a drug includes introduction of the new molecular entity (NME), initial product introduction, and later, possibly a new patent or patents obtained by the introduction of controlled-release formulations of the existing immediate-release products. This and the addition of new therapeutic indications for these products provide an attractive financial option for pharmaceutical companies. Example products include Augmentin XR (GlaxoSmith-Kline) and Cipro XR (Bayer) (2).

In contrast to conventional (immediate release) forms, modified-release products provide either delayed release or extended release of drug. Most *delayed-release* products are enteric-coated tablets or capsules designed to pass through the stomach unaltered, later to release their medication within the intestinal tract. As noted in the previous chapter, enteric coatings are used either to protect a substance from destruction by gastric fluids or to reduce stomach distress caused by irritating drugs. *Extended-release* products are designed to release their medication in a *controlled* manner, at a predetermined rate, duration, and location to achieve and maintain optimum therapeutic blood levels of drug.

Most modified-release products are orally administered tablets and capsules, and therefore these dosage forms are emphasized in this chapter. However, some other modified-release dosage forms and drug delivery systems are also described, including ocular, parenteral, subdermal, and vaginal products. Transdermal patches, which provide rate-controlled drug delivery are touched on here and discussed at length in Chapter 11.

The Rationale for Extended-Release Pharmaceuticals

Some drugs are inherently long lasting and require only once-a-day oral dosing to sustain adequate drug blood levels and the desired therapeutic effect. These drugs are formulated in the conventional manner in immediate-release dosage forms. However, many other drugs are not inherently long lasting and require multiple daily dosing to achieve the desired therapeutic results.

Multiple daily dosing is inconvenient for the patient and can result in missed doses, made-up doses, and noncompliance with the regimen. When conventional immediate-release dosage forms are taken on schedule and more than once daily, they cause sequential therapeutic blood level peaks and valleys (troughs) associated with the taking of each dose (Fig. 9.1). However, when doses are *not* administered on schedule, the resulting peaks and valleys reflect less than optimum drug therapy. For example, if doses are administered too frequently, minimum toxic concentrations (MTC) of drug may be reached, with toxic side effects resulting. If doses are missed, periods of subtherapeutic drug blood levels or those below the minimum effective concentration (MEC) may result, with no benefit to the patient.

Extended-release tablets and capsules are commonly taken only once or twice daily, compared with counterpart conventional forms

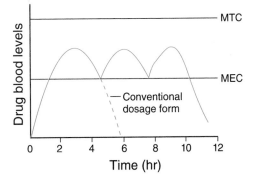

FIGURE 9.1 Hypothetical drug blood level–time curves for a conventional solid dosage form and a multiple-action product.

that may have to be taken three or four times daily to achieve the same therapeutic effect. Typically, extended-release products provide an immediate release of drug that promptly produces the desired therapeutic effect, followed by gradual release of additional amounts of drug to maintain this effect over a predetermined period (Fig. 9.2). The sustained plasma drug levels provided by extended-release products oftentimes eliminates the need for night dosing, which benefits not only the patient but the caregiver as well (3–5). For nonoral rate-controlled drug delivery systems, the drug release pattern ranges in duration from 24 hours for most transdermal patches to 3 months for the estradiol vaginal ring insert (Estring, Pharmacia & Upjohn) to 5 years for

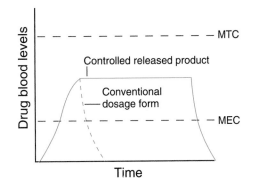

FIGURE 9.2 Hypothetical drug blood level-time curves for a conventional solid dosage form and a controlled-release product.

TABLE 9.1 ADVANTAGES OF EXTENDED-RELEASE DOSAGE FORMS OVER CONVENTIONAL FORMS

ADVANTAGE	EXPLANATION
Less fluctuation in drug blood levels	Controlling rate of release eliminates peaks and valleys of blood levels.
Frequency reduction in dosing	Extended-release products frequently deliver more than a single dose, hence may be taken less often than conventional forms.
Enhanced convenience and compliance	With less frequency of dosing, a patient is less apt to neglect taking a dose; also greater convenience with day and night administration.
Reduction in adverse side effects	Because of fewer blood level peaks outside therapeutic range and into toxic range, adverse side effects are less frequent.
Reduction in overall health care costs	Although initial cost of extended-release dosage forms may be greater than for conventional forms, overall cost of treatment may be less because of enhanced therapeutic benefit, fewer side effects, reduced time for health care personnel to dispense and administer drugs and monitor patients.

levonorgestrel subdermal implants (Norplant System, Wyeth-Ayerst).

Some advantages of extended-release systems are given in Table 9.1. Some disadvantages are the loss of flexibility in adjusting the drug dose and/or dosage regimen and a risk of sudden and total drug release, or dose dumping, due to a failure of technology.

Terminology

Drug products that provide extended or sustained release first appeared as a major new class of dosage form in the late 1940s and early 1950s (6). Over the years, many terms (and abbreviations), such as *sustained release* (SR), *sustained action* (SA), *prolonged action* (PA), *controlled release* (CR), *extended release* (ER), *timed release* (TR), *and long acting* (LA), have been used by manufacturers to describe product types and features. Although these terms often have been used interchangeably, individual products bearing these descriptions may differ in design and performance and must be examined individually to ascertain their respective features. For the most part, these terms are used to describe orally administered dosage forms, whereas the term *rate-controlled delivery* is applied to certain types of drug delivery systems in which the rate of delivery is controlled by features of the device rather than

by physiologic or environmental conditions like gastrointestinal pH or drug transit time through the gastrointestinal tract.

Modified Release

In recent years, *modified release* has come into general use to describe dosage forms having drug release features based on time, course, and/or location that are designed to accomplish therapeutic or convenience objectives not offered by conventional or immediate-release forms (4, 7). The *United States Pharmacopeia* (USP) differentiates modified-release forms as *extended release* and *delayed release* (8).

Extended Release

The U.S. Food and Drug Administration (FDA) defines an extended-release dosage form as one that allows a reduction in dosing frequency from that necessitated by a conventional dosage form, such as a solution or an immediate-release dosage form (4, 9).

Delayed Release

A delayed-release dosage form is designed to release the drug at a time other than promptly after administration. The delay may be time based or based on the influence of environmental conditions, like gastrointestinal pH.

Repeat Action

Repeat-action forms usually contain two single doses of medication, one for immediate release and the second for delayed release. Two-layer tablets, for example, may be prepared with one layer of drug for immediate release with the second layer designed to release drug later as either a second dose or in an extended-release manner.

Targeted Release

Targeted release describes drug release directed toward isolating or concentrating a drug in a body region, tissue, or site for absorption or for drug action.

Extended-Release Oral Dosage Forms

Not all drugs are suited for formulation into extended-release products, and not all medical conditions require treatment with such a product. The drug and the therapeutic indication must be considered jointly in determining whether or not to develop an extended-release dosage form.

Drug Candidates for Extended-Release Products

To be a successful extended-release product, the drug must be released from the dosage form at a predetermined rate, dissolve in the gastrointestinal fluids, maintain sufficient gastrointestinal residence time, and be absorbed at a rate that will replace the amount of drug being metabolized and excreted.

In general, the drugs best suited for incorporation into an extended-release product have the following characteristics.

1. *They exhibit neither very slow nor very fast rates of absorption and excretion.* Drugs with slow rates of absorption and excretion are usually inherently long-acting, and it is not necessary to prepare them in extended-release forms. Drugs with very short half-lives, that is, less than 2 hours, are poor candidates for extended release because of the large quantities of drug required for such a formulation. Also, drugs that act by affecting enzyme systems may be longer acting than indicated by their quantitative half-lives because of residual effects and recovery of the diminished biosystem (10).

2. *They are uniformly absorbed from the gastrointestinal tract.* Drugs prepared in extended-release forms must have good aqueous solubility and maintain adequate residence time in the gastrointestinal tract. Drugs absorbed poorly or at varying and unpredictable rates are not good candidates for extended-release products.

3. *They are administered in relatively small doses.* Drugs with large single doses frequently are not suitable for extended release because the tablet or capsule needed to maintain a sustained therapeutic blood level of the drug would be too large for the patient to swallow easily.

4. *They possess a good margin of safety.* The most widely used measure of the margin of a drug's safety is its therapeutic index, that is, the median toxic dose divided by the median effective dose. For very potent drugs the therapeutic index may be narrow, or very small. The larger the therapeutic index, the safer the drug. Drugs that are administered in very small doses or possess very narrow therapeutic indices are poor candidates for formulation into extended-release formulations because of technologic limitations of precise control over release rates and the risk of dose dumping due to a product defect. Patient misuse (e.g., chewing dosage unit) also could result in toxic drug levels.

5. *They are used in the treatment of chronic rather than acute conditions.* Drugs for acute conditions require greater adjustment of the dosage by the physician than that provided by extended-release products.

Extended-Release Technology for Oral Dosage Forms

For orally administered dosage forms, extended drug action is achieved by affecting the rate at which the drug is released from the dosage form and/or by slowing the transit time of the dosage form through the gastrointestinal tract (4).

The rate of drug release from solid dosage forms may be modified by the technologies described next, which in general are based on (*a*) modifying drug dissolution by controlling access of biologic fluids to the drug through the use of barrier coatings; (*b*) controlling drug diffusion rates from dosage forms; and (*c*) chemical reaction or interaction between the drug substance or its pharmaceutical barrier and site-specific biologic fluids.

Coated Beads, Granules, and Microspheres

In these systems, the drug is distributed onto beads, pellets, granules, or other particulate systems. Using conventional pan coating or air suspension coating, a solution of the drug substance is placed on small inert nonpareil seeds or beads made of sugar and starch or on microcrystalline cellulose spheres. The nonpareil seeds are most often in the range of 425 to 850 μm, whereas the microcrystalline cellulose spheres range from 170 to 600 μm. The microcrystalline spheres are considered more durable during production than sugar-based cores (11).

If the dose of the drug is large, the starting granules of material may be composed of the drug itself. Some of these granules may remain uncoated to provide immediate drug release. Other granules (about two-thirds to three-fourths) receive varying coats of a lipid material like beeswax, carnauba wax, glyceryl monostearate, or cetyl alcohol or a cellulosic material like ethylcellulose. Then granules of different coating thicknesses are blended to achieve a mix having the desired drug-release characteristics. The coating material may be colored to distinguish granules or beads of different coating thicknesses (by depth of color) and to provide distinctiveness to the product. When properly blended, the granules may be placed in capsules or formed into tablets. Various commercial aqueous coating systems use ethyl cellulose and plasticizer as the coating material (e.g., Aquacoat [FMC Corporation] and Surelease [Colorcon]) (12, 13). Aqueous coating systems eliminate the hazards and environmental concerns associated with organic solvent–based systems.

The variation in the thickness of the coats and in the type of coating material used affects the rate at which body fluids penetrate the coating to dissolve the drug. Naturally, the thicker the coat, the more resistant to penetration and the more delayed will be drug release and dissolution. Typically the coated beads are about 1 mm in diameter. They are combined to have three or four release groups among the more than 100 beads contained in the dosing unit (10). This provides the different desired rates of sustained or extended release and the targeting of the coated beads to the desired segments of the gastrointestinal tract. An example of this type of dosage form is the Spansule (SmithKline Beecham) capsule shown in Figure 9.3.

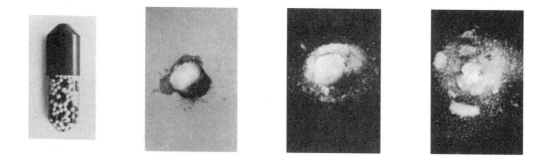

FIGURE 9.3 The Spansule capsule showing the hard gelatin capsule containing hundreds of tiny pellets for sustained drug release and rupture of one of the pellets as occurs in the gastric fluid. (Courtesy of SmithKline Beecham.)

Multitablet System

Small spheroid compressed tablets 3 to 4 mm in diameter may be prepared to have varying drug release characteristics. They then may be placed in gelatin capsule shells to provide the desired pattern of drug release (14). Each capsule may contain 8 to 10 minitablets, some uncoated for immediate release and others coated for extended drug release.

Microencapsulated Drug

Microencapsulation is a process by which solids, liquids, or even gases may be enclosed in microscopic particles by formation of thin coatings of wall material around the substance. The process had its origin in the late 1930s as a cleaner substitute for carbon paper and carbon ribbons as sought by the business machines industry. The ultimate development in the 1950s of reproduction paper and ribbons that contained dyes in tiny gelatin capsules released on impact by a typewriter key or the pressure of a pen or pencil was the stimulus for the development of a host of microencapsulated materials, including drugs. Gelatin is a common wall-forming material, and synthetic polymers, such as polyvinyl alcohol, ethylcellulose, polyvinyl chloride, and other materials also may be used.

The typical encapsulation process usually begins with dissolving the wall material, say gelatin, in water. The material to be encapsulated is added and the two-phase mixture thoroughly stirred. With the material to be encapsulated broken up to the desired particle size, a solution of a second material, usually acacia, is added. This additive material concentrates the gelatin (polymer) into tiny liquid droplets. These droplets (the *coacervate*) form a film or coat around the particles of the substance to be encapsulated as a consequence of the extremely low interfacial tension of the residual water or solvent in the wall material so that a continuous tight film coating remains on the particle (Fig. 9.4). The final dry microcapsules are free-flowing discrete particles of coated material. The wall material usually constitutes 2 to 20% of the total particle weight. Different rates of drug release may be obtained by chang-

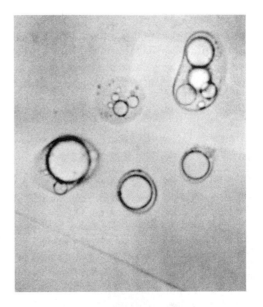

FIGURE 9.4 Microcapsules of mineral oil in a gelatin–acacia coacervate. (Courtesy of James C. Price, PhD, College of Pharmacy, University of Georgia.)

ing the ratio of core to wall, the polymer used for the coating, and the method of microencapsulation (15).

One of the advantages of microencapsulation is that the administered dose of a drug is subdivided into small units that are spread over a large area of the gastrointestinal tract, which may enhance absorption by diminishing local drug concentration (15). An example of a drug commercially available in a microencapsulated extended-release dosage form is potassium chloride (Micro-K Extencaps, A. H. Robins).

Embedding Drug in Slowly Eroding or Hydrophilic Matrix System

The drug substance is combined and made into granules with an excipient material that slowly erodes in body fluids, progressively releasing the drug for absorption. When these granules are mixed with granules of drug prepared without the excipient, the uncombined granules provide the immediate effect, and the drug–excipient granules provide extended action. The granule mix may be formulated as tablets or capsules for oral delivery.

Hydrophilic cellulose polymers are commonly used as the excipient base in tablet matrix systems. The effectiveness of these hydrophilic matrix systems is based on the successive processes of hydration of the cellulosic polymer, gel formation on the polymer's surface, tablet erosion, and the subsequent and continuous release of drug. Hydroxypropyl methylcellulose (HPMC), a free-flowing powder, is commonly used to provide the hydrophilic matrix. Tablets are prepared by thoroughly distributing HPMC in the formulation, preparing the granules by wet granulation or roller compaction, and manufacturing the tablets by compression (16).

After ingestion, the tablet is wetted by gastric fluid and the polymer begins to hydrate. A gel layer forms around surface of the tablet, and an initial quantity of drug is exposed and released. As water permeates further into the tablet, the thickness of the gel layer increases, and soluble drug diffuses through the gel layer. As the outer layer becomes fully hydrated, it erodes from the tablet core. If the drug is insoluble, it is released as such with the eroding gel layer. Thus, the rate of drug release is controlled by diffusion and tablet erosion (17).

For a successful hydrophilic matrix system, the polymer must form a gelatinous layer rapidly enough to protect the inner core of the tablet from disintegrating too rapidly after ingestion. As the proportion of polymer in a formulation increases, so does the viscosity of the gel, with a resultant decrease in the rate of drug diffusion and drug release (17). In general 20% of HPMC results in satisfactory rates of release for an extended-release tablet formulation. However, as with all formulations, consideration must be given to the possible effects of other formulation ingredients, including fillers, tablet binders, and disintegrants. An example of a proprietary product using a hydrophilic matrix base of HPMC for extended drug release is Oramorph SR Tablets (Roxane), which contains morphine sulfate.

When hydrophilic matrix formulations are used in the preparation of extended-release capsules, the same concept applies. When the capsule is ingested, water penetrates the capsule shell, comes in contact with the fill, hydrates the outer layer of powder, and forms a gelatinous plug from which the drug content diffuses gradually over time as hydration continues and the gelatinous plug dissolves.

Manufacturers may prepare two-layer tablets, with one layer containing the uncombined drug for immediate release and the other layer having the drug embedded in a hydrophilic matrix for extended release. Three-layer tablets may be similarly prepared, with both outer layers containing the drug for immediate release. Some commercial tablets are prepared with an inner core containing the extended-release portion of drug and an outer shell enclosing the core and containing drug for immediate release.

Embedding Drug in Inert Plastic Matrix

The drug is granulated with an inert plastic material such as polyethylene, polyvinyl acetate, or polymethacrylate, and the granulation is compressed into tablets. The drug is slowly released from the inert plastic matrix by diffusion. The compression creates the matrix or plastic form that retains its shape during leaching of the drug and during its passage through the alimentary tract. An immediate-release portion of drug may be compressed onto the surface of the tablet. The inert tablet matrix, expended of drug, is excreted with the feces. The primary example of a dosage form of this type is the Gradumet (Abbott).

Complex Formation

Some drug substances, when chemically combined with certain other chemical agents, form complexes that may be only slowly soluble in body fluids, depending on the pH of the environment. This slow dissolution rate provides the extended release of the drug. Salts of tannic acid, tannates, provide this quality in a variety of proprietary products by the trade name Rynatan (Wallace) (10).

Ion Exchange Resins

A solution of a cationic drug may be passed through a column containing an ion exchange resin, forming a complex by the replacement of hydrogen atoms. The resin–drug complex is washed and may be tableted, encapsulated, or suspended in an aqueous vehicle. The release of the drug depends on the pH and electrolyte concentration in the gastrointestinal tract. Release is greater in the acidity of the stomach than in the less acidic environment of the small intestine. Examples of drug products of this type include hydrocodone polistirex and chlorpheniramine polistirex suspension (Tussionex Pennkinetic Extended Release Suspension [CellTech]) and phentermine resin capsules (Ionamin Capsules [CellTech]).

The mechanism of action of drug release from ion exchange resins may be depicted as follows:

In the Stomach
1. Drug resinate + HCl ⇌ acidic resin + drug hydrochloride
2. Resin salt + HCl ⇌ resin chloride + acidic drug

In the Intestine
1. Drug resinate + NaCl ⇌ sodium resinate + drug hydrochloride
2. Resin salt + NaCl ⇌ resin chloride + sodium salt of drug.

This system incorporates a polymer barrier coating and bead technology in addition to the ion exchange mechanism. The initial dose comes from an uncoated portion and the remainder from the coated beads. The coating does not dissolve, and release is extended over 12 hours by ionic exchange. The drug-containing polymer particles are minute and may be suspended to produce a liquid with extended-release characteristics as well as solid dosage forms.

Osmotic Pump

The pioneer *oral osmotic* pump drug delivery system is the *Oros* system developed by Alza. The system is composed of a core tablet surrounded by a semipermeable membrane coating having a 0.4 mm diameter hole produced by laser beam (Fig. 9.5). The core tablet has two layers, one containing the drug (the active layer) and the other containing a polymeric osmotic agent (the push layer). The system operates on the principle of osmotic pressure.

When the tablet is swallowed, the semipermeable membrane permits water to enter from the patient's stomach into the core tablet, dissolving or suspending the drug. As pressure increases in the osmotic layer, it pumps the drug solution out of the delivery orifice on the side of the tablet (Fig. 9.6). Only the drug solution (not the undissolved drug) is capable of passing through the hole in the tablet. The system is designed such that only a few drops of water are drawn into the tablet each hour. The rate of inflow of water and the function of the tablet depends on an osmotic gradient between the contents of the two-layer core and the fluid in the gastrointestinal tract. Drug delivery is essentially constant as long as the osmotic gradient remains constant. The drug release rate may be altered by changing the surface area, thickness or composition of the membrane, and/or diameter of the drug release orifice. The

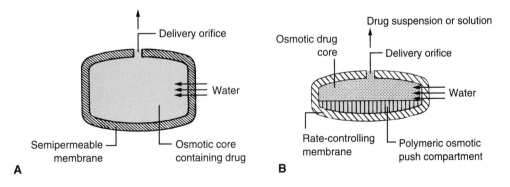

FIGURE 9.5 A. Elementary OROS osmotic pump drug delivery system. **B**. OROS Push-Pull Osmotic System. (Courtesy of Alza Corporation.)

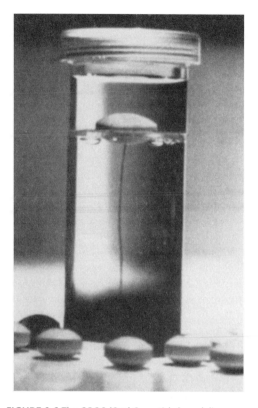

FIGURE 9.6 The OROS (Oral Osmotic) drug delivery system. A tablet core of drug is surrounded by a semipermeable membrane that is pierced by a small laser-drilled hole. After ingestion, water is drawn into the tablet from the digestive tract by osmosis. As water enters the tablet core, the drug gradually goes into solution. The solution is pushed out through the small hole at a controlled rate of about 1 to 2 drops per hour. (Courtesy of Alza Corporation.)

drug release rate is not affected by gastrointestinal acidity, alkalinity, fed conditions, or gastrointestinal motility. The biologically inert components of the tablet remain intact during gastrointestinal transit and are eliminated in the feces as an insoluble shell.

This type of osmotic system, termed the gastrointestinal therapeutic system (GITS [Pfizer]) is employed in the manufacture of Glucotrol XL Extended Release Tablets and Procardia XL Extended Release Tablets. Another example of the osmotic system is the controlled-onset extended release (COER [Searle]) system used in Covera-HS Tablets, in which initial drug is released 4 to 5 hours after tablet ingestion. The delay in drug release is effected by a slowly sol-ubilized coated layer between the active drug core and the outer semipermeable membrane.

Repeat-Action Tablets

Repeat-action tablets are prepared so that an initial dose of drug is released immediately and a second dose follows later. The tablets may be prepared with the immediate-release dose in the tablet's outer shell or coating and the second dose in the tablet's inner core, separated by a slowly permeable barrier coating. In general, the drug from the inner core is exposed to body fluids and released 4 to 6 hours after administration. An example of this type of product is Repetabs (Schering). Repeat-action dosage forms are best suited for treatment of chronic conditions requiring repeated dosing. The drugs should have low dosage and fairly rapid rates of absorption and excretion.

Delayed-Release Oral Dosage Forms

The release of a drug from an oral dosage form may be intentionally delayed until it reaches the intestines for several reasons. The purpose may be to protect a drug destroyed by gastric fluids, to reduce gastric distress caused by drugs particularly irritating to the stomach, or to facilitate gastrointestinal transit for drugs that are better absorbed from the intestines. As stated previously, capsules and tablets specially coated to remain intact in the stomach and to yield their ingredients in the intestines are termed *enteric coated*. The enteric coating may be pH dependent, breaking down in the less acidic environment of the intestine, time dependent, eroding by moisture over time during gastrointestinal transit, or enzyme dependent, deteriorating as a result of the hydrolysis-catalyzing action of intestinal enzymes. Among the many agents used for enteric coating of tablets and capsules are fats, fatty acids, waxes, shellac, and cellulose acetate phthalate.

Examples of modified-release tablets and capsules official in the USP are presented in Table 9.2, and examples of proprietary modified-release oral dosage forms are presented in Table 9.3.

TABLE 9.2 MODIFIED-RELEASE TABLETS AND CAPSULES OFFICIAL IN THE USP

Delayed release
  Aspirin delayed-release tablets
  Dirithromycin delayed-release tablets
  Doxycycline hyclate delayed-release capsules
  Erythromycin delayed-release capsules
  Oxtriphylline delayed-release tablets

Extended Release
  Aspirin extended-release tablets
  Diltiazem extended-release capsules
  Disopyramide phosphate extended-release
    capsules
  Ferrous fumarate and docusate sodium
    extended-release tablets
  Indomethacin extended-release capsules
  Isosorbide dinitrate extended-release tablets and
    capsules
  Lithium carbonate extended-release tablets
  Oxtriphylline extended-release tablets
  Phenylpropanolamine hydrochloride extended-
    release capsules
  Potassium chloride extended-release tablets
  Procainamide hydrochloride extended-release
    tablets
  Propranolol hydrochloride extended-release
    capsules
  Quinidine gluconate extended-release tablets
  Theophylline extended-release capsules

USP Requirements and FDA Guidance for Modified-Release Dosage Forms

The USP contains general chapters and specific tests to determine the drug release capabilities of extended-release and delayed-release tablets and capsules (8).

Drug Release

The USP test for drug release for extended-release and delayed-release articles is based on drug dissolution from the dosage unit against elapsed test time (Fig. 9.7). Descriptions of the various test apparatus and procedures may be found in the USP, Chapter <724> (8). The individual monographs contain specific criteria for compliance with the test and the apparatus and test procedures to be used. For example, for Aspirin Extended-release Tablets, the USP

requires the following aspirin dissolution rate to meet the stated drug release test:

Time (hours)	Amount Dissolved
1.0	15–40%
2.0	25–60%
4.0	35–75%
8.0	not less than 70%

Uniformity of Dosage Units

Modified-release tablets and capsules must meet the USP standard for uniformity as described in Chapter 8 for conventional dosage units. Uniformity of dosage units may be demonstrated by either of two methods, weight variation or content uniformity, as described in USP Chapter <905> (8).

In Vitro–In Vivo Correlations

In vitro–in vivo relationships (IVIVRs) or in vitro–in vivo correlations (IVIVCs) are critical to the development of oral extended-release products. Assessing IVICRs is important throughout product development, clinical evaluation, submission of an application for FDA approval for marketing, and during post approval for any proposed formulation or manufacturing changes (18).

In 1997, the FDA published a guidance document, *Extended Release Oral Dosage Forms: Development, Evaluation, and Application of In Vitro/In Vivo Correlations* (9). It provides guidance to sponsors of new drug applications (NDAs) and abbreviated new drug applications (ANDAs) for extended-release oral products. The guidance provides methods of (*a*) developing an IVIVC and evaluating its predictability, (*b*) using an IVIVC to establish dissolution specifications, and (*c*) applying an IVIVC as a surrogate for in vivo bioequivalence when it is necessary to document bioequivalence during the approval process or during post approval for certain formulation or manufacturing changes.

Three categories of IVIVCs are included in the document:

Level A: A predictive mathematical model for the relationship between the entire in vitro dissolution and release time

TABLE 9.3 PROPRIETARY MODIFIED-RELEASE ORAL DOSAGE FORMS

DRUG PRODUCT AND MANUFACTURER	DOSAGE FORM CHARACTERISTICS
Delayed Release	
E-Mycin (erythromycin) Delayed-Release Tablets (Knoll)	Tablets enteric coated with cellulose acetate phthalate, carnauba wax, and cellulose polymers. Use: antibiotic.
Asacol (mesalamine) Delayed-Release Tablets (Procter & Gamble)	Tablets coated with Eudragit S (methylacrylic acid copolymer B), a resin that bypasses the stomach dissolves in the ileum and beyond. Use: treat ulcerative colitis
Prilosec (omeprazole) Delayed-Release Capsules (Astra-Merck)	Enteric coated granules of omeprazole placed in capsules. Omeprazole is acid labile and is degraded by gastric acid. Use: treatment of duodenal ulcer.
Extended-Release Coated Particles and Beads	
Toprol-XL (metoprolol succinate) Tablets (Astra)	Drug pellets coated with cellulose polymers compressed into tablets. Use: treatment of hypertension.
Indocin SR (indomethacin) Capsules (Merck)	Coated pellets for sustained release. Formulation includes polyvinyl acetate-crotonic acid copolymer and hydroxypropyl methylcellulose. Use: analgesic, anti-inflammatory.
Compazine (prochlorperazine) Spansule Capsules (SmithKline Beecham)	Coated pellets in capsule formulated to release initial dose promptly with additional drug for prolonged release. Use: antinausea, antivomiting.
Extended-Release Inert Matrix	
Desoxyn (methamphetamine HCl) Gradumet Tablets (Abbott)	Drug impregnated in an inert, porous, plastic matrix. Drug leaches out as it passes slowly through the GI tract. Expended matrix is excreted in stool. Use: attention deficit disorder.
Procanbid (procainamide HCl) Tablets (Parke-Davis)	Extended-release tablets with a core tablet of a nonerodible wax matrix coated with cellulose polymers. Use: an antiarrhythmic.
Extended-Release Hydrophilic/Eroding Matrix	
Quinidex (quinidine sulfate) Tablets (Robins)	Extended-release provided by hydrophilic matrix that swells and slowly erodes. Use: antiarrhythmic.
Oramorph SR (morphine sulfate) Tablets (Roxane)	Sustained-release hydrophilic matrix system, based on polymer hydroxypropyl methylcellulose. Use: analgesic for severe pain.
Extended-Release Microencapsulated	
K-Dur Microburst Release System (potassium chloride) Tablets (Key)	Immediately dispersing drug microencapsulated with ethylcellulose and hydroxypropyl cellulose. Use: potassium depletion.
Extended-Release Osmotic	
Glucotrol XL (glipizide) Tablets (Pfizer)	Controlled-release GITS[a] osmotic system. Ingredients include polyethylene oxide, hydroxypropyl cellulose, cellulose acetate. Use: antihyperglycemic.
Covera-HS (verapamil HCl) Tablets (Searle)	A COER[b] osmotic system. Use: antihypertensive, antianginal.

[a]Gastrointestinal therapeutic system.

[b]Controlled onset, extended release.

course and the entire in vivo response time course, for example, the time course of plasma drug concentration or amount of drug absorbed. This is the most common type of correlation submitted.

Level B: A predictive mathematical model of the relationship between summary parameters that characterize the in vitro and in vivo time courses; for example, models that relate the mean in vitro dissolution time to the mean in vivo disso-

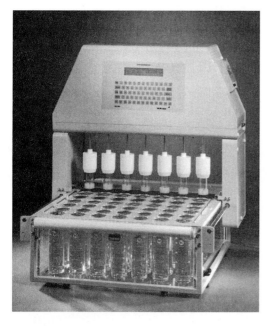

FIGURE 9.7 Varian Biodis Dissolution Apparatus for determining dissolution characteristics of modified release products. (Courtesy of Varian Inc.)

lution time, the mean in vitro dissolution time to the mean residence time in vivo, or the in vitro dissolution rate constant to the absorption rate constant.

Level C: A predictive mathematical model of the relationship between the amount dissolved in vitro at a particular time (or the time required for in vitro dissolution of a fixed percent of the dose, e.g., T_{50}) and a summary parameter that characterizes the in vivo time course (e.g., maximum concentration [C_{max}] or area under the curve [AUC]). The level of IVIVCs may be useful in the early stages of formulation development when pilot formulations are being selected.

The most common process for developing an IVIVC model (level A) is to (*a*) develop formulations with different release rates (e.g., slow, fast, and intermediate) or a single release rate if dissolution is independent of condition; (*b*) obtain in vitro dissolution profiles and in vivo plasma concentration profiles for these formulations, and (*c*) estimate the in vivo absorption or dissolution time course for each formulation and subject using appropriate mathematical approaches.

Among the criteria applicable to the development of IVIVCs are the following (9):

- In determining in vitro dissolution, USP dissolution apparatus, type I (basket) or type II (paddle) is preferred, although type III (reciprocating cylinder) or type IV (flow-through cell) may be applicable in some instances.
- An aqueous medium with a pH not exceeding 6.8 is preferred as the medium for dissolution studies. For poorly soluble drugs, a surfactant (e.g. 1% sodium lauryl sulfate) may be added.
- The dissolution profiles of at least 12 individual dosage units from each lot should be determined.
- For in vivo studies, human subjects are used in the fasted state unless the drug is not well tolerated, in which case the studies may be conducted in the fed state. Acceptable data sets have been shown to be generated with use of 6 to 36 human subjects.
- Crossover studies are preferred, but parallel studies or cross-study analysis may be acceptable using a common reference treatment product, such as an intravenous solution, an aqueous oral solution, or an immediate-release product.

Labeling

The USP indicates labeling requirements for modified-release dosage form articles in addition to general labeling requirements. The requirements are specific to the monograph article. For example, the label of Aspirin Delayed-release Tablets must state that *the tablets are enteric coated*, whereas the labeling for Theophylline Extended-release Capsules must indicate *whether the product is intended for dosing every 12 or 24 hours and state with which in vitro drug release test the product complies* (seven tests are described in the monograph, each with different drug-release times and tolerances).

Clinical Considerations in the Use of Oral Modified-Release Dosage Forms

Patients should be advised of the dose and dosing frequency of modified drug release products and instructed not to use them interchangeably or concomitantly with immediate-release forms of the same drug. Patients stabilized on a modified-release product should not be changed to an immediate-release product without consideration of any existing blood level concentrations of the drug. Also, once stabilized, patients should not be changed to another extended-release product unless there is assurance of equivalent bioavailability. A different product can result in a marked shift in the patient's drug blood level because of differences in drug release characteristics.

Patients should be advised that modified-release tablets and capsules should not be crushed or chewed, since such action compromises their drug release features (19). Patients being fed by enteral nutrition through a nasogastric tube may receive conventional or modified-release medication. For example, coated pellets from inside capsules simply may be mixed with water and poured down the feeding tube (20).

Patients and caregivers should be advised that nonerodible plastic matrix shells and osmotic tablets remain intact throughout gastrointestinal transit and the empty shells or ghosts from osmotic tablets may be seen in the stool. The patient should be assured of the normalcy of this event and that drug absorption has taken place (4).

PHARMACEUTICS CASE STUDY

Subjective

You work in a small but growing pharmaceutical company producing extended-release tablets. Sales have been good, and the pressure is on to increase production by 20% per day. The only way you can accomplish this is to increase the speed at which your rotary machines work, since you are running three shifts of 8 hours each. When you increase the speed of your machine and start production, you start getting reports that the tablets do not produce the proper extended-release dissolution profile and they are not of the proper hardness. Also, the tablets are less potent and weigh less than specifications. No other adjustments have been made to the machine other than to increase the speed. What will you do?

Objective

Your machines are 36-station rotary tablet presses using gravity feed. You produce the tablets, which are oblong, with a hydrophilic matrix system and an oblong punch and die. The optimal speed was established during the scale-up phase of product development and has been used for the past 18 months with no problems.

Assessment

The production of tablets must follow a well-defined set of conditions. If not, the final product may not have the desired characteristics of hardness, disintegration, dissolution, friability, and appearance. It appears that the increase in speed is not allowing the powder blend sufficient time to flow by gravity into the tablet dies, as the increased speed causes the die to pass under the powder feed apparatus faster than before. This results in less powder per tablet in the die, and when they are compressed, the resulting tablets are not as firm; when subjected to a dissolution test, the result is a more rapid release of the drug. This also explains the lighter tablets and the lower quantity of active drug per tablet.

Plan

There are two options here: first, decrease the rate of speed to that at which the production was validated, and second, consider a force-feed system to move the powder into the dies faster. The latter option requires validation of the equipment under the new conditions. A third option may be the most reasonable, and that is to purchase additional machines.

CLINICAL CASE STUDY

Subjective:

CC: K. F. is a 9 y/o WM who arrives at the pediatric clinic with his mother. The mother states that K. F. talks excessively, interrupts others when they speak, rarely follows her directions, and frequently runs around the house. The mother also states that she has heard from the teacher that he leaves the classroom in the middle of the class, often blurts out answers before questions have been completed, has a difficult time waiting his turn (e.g., in the lunchroom), is "fidgety," rarely follows directions or pays attention, and turns in incomplete homework assignments. His teacher has also told the mother that he frequently distracts the other students at school. The mother states, "I would like your help. But I do not want him to be put on a medicine where he has to take it more than once a day because I might forget to give it to him. Also, I do not want him taking any medicine to school."

HPI: The mother states that K. F. has been "this way" since he was 6 y/o. However, it is now at the point where does not complete any of his tasks (e.g., making his bed, doing his homework) and his grades are "slipping." His latest report card showed "many Cs and Ds."

PMH: Otitis media, 4 weeks ago.

Meds: Zithromax Suspension, finished it about 3 weeks ago.

OTC Meds: K. F. (and his mother) deny K. F.'s use of vitamins, herbals, or any other supplements

PSH: None

FH: Mother, DM type II since age 29

SH: (per K. F.)

    (−) Tobacco

    (−) EtOH

    (−) Illicit drugs

    (+) Caffeine: Loves Mountain Dew, drinks a couple of cans (~2–3) per day

Exercise, daily activities: goes to school from 8 A.M. to 3 P.M., after school likes to watch TV, in-line skate, and play basketball.

Timing of meals: Breakfast at 7:30 A.M, lunch at noon, snack at 3:30 P.M., and dinner at 6:30 P.M.

Diet: Chips, candy, peanut butter and jelly sandwiches, pasta, and 2 or 3 cans of Mountain Dew per day

Bedtime: 9:30–10:30 P.M.

Siblings: None

Mother and father are both accountants and each work ~40 hours/week. They have been married for 11 years.

ALL: NKDA

Objective

9 y/o WM

Ht: 4'2"   **Wt:** 71 pounds

BP: 119/75 **P:** 70 **T:** 98.6°F **RR:** 15

Pain: none

The mother presents K. F.'s last report card with grades Cs and Ds along with notes from K. F.'s teacher about his behavior.

Assessment

ADHD: Combined type

Plan

Recommend extended-release methylphenidate HCl (i.e., Concerta) 18mg by mouth once a day with breakfast and a full glass of water, milk, or juice at 7:30 A.M. (to aid with adherence). Inform the mother that the prescription has to be dispensed to her within 7 days after the date it is issued. Concerta has a rapid onset of action to help K. F. focus in the morning at school and a long duration of action, which will be useful during and after school for homework.

    Counsel the mother on possible side effects, such as insomnia, loss of appetite, and weight loss. Inform K. F.'s mother also about a possible decrease in rate of height growth (not final height). Advise her that if her son misses a dose of the drug in the morning not to administer it after school.

Clinical Case Study cont.

Wait until the next morning for the next dose. Do not double the dose the next day. Inform the mother that this product is prepared in a nonabsorbable shell, which means that the empty shell may or may not be observed in the stool. So if K. F. notices something that resembles a tablet in the stool and mentions it to his mother, she can tell him not to worry; the medicine is working. As methylphenidate is a Class II drug, the mother should understand the necessity to secure a new prescription from the physician for every cycle of therapy. This can be done when K. F. returns to the physician's office for routine monitoring (e.g., blood pressure, pulse, height, weight, encountered side effects).

Counsel K. F. and his mother that he should take the tablet with a full glass of water or juice. He should swallow the tablet whole and not to chew it. K. F. and his mother should know that there is no conclusive evidence regarding sugar dietary intake and its effect on ADHD. However, if K. F.'s mother believes that K. F.'s symptoms are worse with sugary foods or drinks, these should be minimized and decreased from his diet. It is a given that the caffeinated soft drink (i.e., Mountain Dew) should be changed for a caffeine-free soft drink. No caffeinated beverages should be ingested by K. F. after 6 P.M.

Goal: Resolution of symptoms (e.g., improved attention, less fidgeting), improvement in grades, no side effects from Concerta. Also, K. F.'s mother should be referred to a child psychologist who can provide K. F. needed behavioral therapy.

www.concerta.net
www.add.org
www.adhd.com

Packaging and Storing Modified-Release Tablets and Capsules

Modified-release tablets and capsules are packaged and stored in the same manner as conventional products as discussed in Chapters 7 and 8.

REFERENCES

1. Drug delivery technologies: innovations and market challenges. New York, NY: Scrip Reports, PJB Publications, 2003.
2. Das NG, Das SK. Controlled-release of oral dosage forms. Formulation, Fill & Finish (Supplement to Pharmaceutical Technology). 2003:10–16.
3. Rogers JD, Kwan KC. Pharmacokinetic requirements for controlled-release dosage forms. In: John Urquhart, ed. Controlled-release pharmaceuticals. Washington: Academy of Pharmaceutical Sciences, American Pharmaceutical Association, 1979; 95–119.
4. Bogner RH. Bioavailability and bioequivalence of extended-release oral dosage forms. US Pharmacist 1997;22(Suppl):3–12.
5. Madan PL. Sustained-release drug delivery systems, part II: preformulation considerations. Pharm Manufact 1985;2:41–45.
6. Madan PL. Sustained-release drug delivery systems, part I: an overview. Pharm Manufact 1985;2:23–27.
7. Scale-up of oral extended-release dosage forms. AAPS/FDA Workshop Committee. Pharm Tech 1995; 19:46–54.
8. United States Pharmacopeia 23–National Formulary 18. U.S. Pharmacopeial Convention, Rockville, MD, 1995.
9. Guidance for industry. Extended release oral dosage forms: development, evaluation, and application of in vitro/in vivo correlations. Rockville, MD: Center for Drug Evaluation and Research, Food & Drug Administration, 1997.
10. Madan PL. Sustained release dosage forms. US Pharmacist 1990;15:39–50.
11. Celphere microcrystalline cellulose spheres. Philadelphia: FMC Corporation, 1996.
12. Aquacoat aqueous polymeric dispersion. Philadelphia: FMC Corporation, 1991.
13. Surelease aqueous controlled release coating system. West Point, PA: Colorcon, 1990.
14. Butler J, Cumming I, Brown J, et al. A novel multiunit controlled-release system. Pharm Tech 1998;22: 122–138.
15. Yazici E, Oner L, Kas HS, Hincal AA. Phenytoin sodium microcapsules: bench scale formulation, process characterization and release kinetics. Pharmaceut Dev Technol 1996;1:175–183.
16. Sheskey PJ, Cabelka TD, Robb RT, Boyce BM. Use of

roller compaction in the preparation of controlled-release hydrophilic matrix tablets containing methylcellulose and hydroxypropyl methylcellulose polymers. Pharm Tech 1994;18:132–150.

17. Formulating for controlled release with methocel premium cellulose ethers. Midland, MI: Dow Chemical, 1995.

18. Devane J, Butler J. The impact of in vitro–in vivo relationships on product development. Pharm Tech 1997; 21:146–159.

19. Mitchell JF. Oral dosage forms that should not be crushed: 1998 update. Hosp Pharm 1998;33:399–415.

20. Beckwith MC, Barton RG, Graves C. A guide to drug therapy in patients with enteral feeding tubes: dosage form selection and administration methods. Hosp Pharm 1997;32:57–64.

Ointments, Creams, and Gels

10

Chapter at a glance

Ointments, creams, and gels are semisolid dosage forms intended for topical application. They may be applied to the skin, placed on the surface of the eye, or used nasally, vaginally, or rectally. Most these preparations are used for the effects of the therapeutic agents they contain. The unmedicated ones are used for their physical effects as protectants or lubricants.

Topical preparations are used for both local and systemic effects. Systemic drug absorption should always be considered when using topical products if the patient is pregnant or nursing, because drugs can enter the fetal blood supply and breast milk and be transferred to the fetus or nursing infant.

Topical applications can be designed for either local effects or systemic absorption. The following distinction is an important one with regard to dermatologic applications. A *topical dermatological* product is designed to deliver drug *into* the skin in treating dermal disorders, *with the skin as the target organ*. A *transdermal* product is designed to deliver drugs *through* the skin (*percutaneous absorption*) to the general circulation for systemic effects, *with the skin not being the target organ* (1).

Ointments

Ointments are semisolid preparations intended for external application to the skin or mucous membranes. Ointments may be medicated or not. Unmedicated ointments are used for the physical effects they provide as protectants, emollients, or lubricants. *Ointment bases*, as described, may by used for their physical effects or as vehicles for medicated ointments.

Ointment Bases

Ointment bases are classified by the USP (2) into four general groups: (*a*) oleaginous bases, (*b*) absorption bases, (*c*) water-removable bases, and (*d*) water-soluble bases.

Oleaginous Bases

Oleaginous bases are also termed *hydrocarbon bases*. On application to the skin, they have an emollient effect, protect against the escape of moisture, are effective as occlusive dressings, can remain on the skin for long periods without drying out, and because of their immiscibility with water are difficult to wash off. Water and aqueous preparations may be incorporated, but only in small amounts and with some difficulty. Petrolatum, white petrolatum, white ointment, and yellow ointment are examples of hydrocarbon ointment bases.

When powdered substances are to be incorporated into hydrocarbon bases, liquid petrolatum (mineral oil) may be used as the levigating agent.

Petrolatum, USP Petrolatum, USP, is a purified mixture of semisolid hydrocarbons obtained from petroleum. It is an unctuous mass, varying in color from yellowish to light amber. It melts at 38° to 60°C and may be used alone or in combination with other agents as an ointment base. Petrolatum is also known as yellow petrolatum and petroleum jelly. A commercial product is Vaseline (Chesebrough-Ponds)

White Petrolatum, USP White Petrolatum, USP, is a purified mixture of semisolid hydrocarbons from petroleum that has been wholly or nearly decolorized. It is used for the same purpose as petrolatum, but because of its lighter color, it is considered more esthetically pleasing by some pharmacists and patients. White petrolatum is also known as white petroleum jelly. A commercial product is White Vaseline (Chesebrough-Ponds)

Yellow Ointment, USP This ointment has the following formula for the preparation of 1000 g:

Yellow wax	50 g
Petrolatum	950 g

Yellow wax is the purified wax obtained from the honeycomb of the bee *Apis mellifera*. The ointment is prepared by melting the yellow wax on a water bath, adding the petrolatum until the mixture is uniform, then cooling and stirring until congealed. Also called simple ointment, it has a slightly greater viscosity than plain petrolatum.

White Ointment, USP This ointment differs from yellow ointment by substitution of white wax (bleached and purified yellow wax) and white petrolatum in the formula.

Absorption Bases

Absorption bases are of two types: (*a*) those that *permit* the incorporation of aqueous solutions resulting in the formation of water-in-oil emulsions (e.g., *hydrophilic petrolatum*), and (*b*) those that *are* water-in-oil emulsions (syn: *emulsion bases*) that permit the incorporation of additional quantities of aqueous solutions (e.g., lanolin). These bases may be used as emollients, although they do not provide the degree of occlusion afforded by the oleaginous bases. Absorption bases are not easily removed from the skin with water washing, since the external phase of the emulsion is oleaginous. Absorption bases are useful as pharmaceutical adjuncts to incorporate small volumes of aqueous solutions into hydrocarbon bases. This is accomplished by incorporating the aqueous solution into the absorption base and then incorporating this mixture into the hydrocarbon base.

Hydrophilic Petrolatum, USP Hydrophilic Petrolatum, USP, has the following formula for the preparation of 1000 g:

Cholesterol	30 g
Stearyl alcohol	30 g
White wax	80 g
White petrolatum	860 g

It is prepared by melting the stearyl alcohol and white wax on a steam bath, adding the cholesterol with stirring until dissolved, adding the white petrolatum, and allowing the mixture to cool while stirring until congealed.

A commercial product, Aquaphor, a variation of hydrophilic petrolatum, has the capacity to absorb up to three times its weight in water.

Lanolin, USP Lanolin, USP, obtained from the wool of sheep (*Ovis aries*), is a purified waxlike substance that has been cleaned, deodorized, and decolorized. It contains not more than 0.25% water. Additional water may be incorporated into lanolin by mixing. *Modified Lanolin, USP*, is lanolin that has been processed to reduce the contents of free lanolin alcohols and any detergent and pesticide residues.

Water-Removable Bases

Water-removable bases are oil-in-water emulsions resembling creams. Because the external phase of the emulsion is aqueous, they are easily washed from skin and are often called water-washable bases. They may be diluted with water or aqueous solutions. They can absorb serous discharges. Hydrophilic Ointment, USP, is an example of this type of base.

Hydrophilic Ointment, USP Hydrophilic Ointment, USP, has the following formula for the preparation of about 1000 g:

Ingredient	Amount (grams)
Methylparaben	0.25
Propylparaben	0.15
Sodium lauryl sulfate	10.00
Propylene glycol	120.00
Stearyl alcohol	250.00
White petrolatum	250.00
Purified water	370.00

The stearyl alcohol and white petrolatum are melted together at about 75°C. The other agents, dissolved in the purified water, are added with stirring until the mixture congeals. Sodium lauryl sulfate is the emulsifying agent, with the stearyl alcohol and white petrolatum constituting the oleaginous phase of the emulsion and the other ingredients the aqueous phase. Methylparaben and propylparaben are antimicrobial preservatives.

Water-Soluble Bases

Water-soluble bases do not contain oleaginous components. They are completely water washable and often referred to as greaseless. Because they soften greatly with the addition of water, large amounts of aqueous solutions are not effectively incorporated into these bases. They mostly are used for incorporation of solid substances. Polyethylene Glycol Ointment, NF, is the prototype example of a water-soluble base.

Polyethylene Glycol Ointment, NF Polyethylene glycol (PEG) is a polymer of ethylene oxide and water represented by the formula $H(OCH_2CH_2)_nOH$, in which n represents the average number of oxyethylene groups. The numeric designations associated with PEGs refer to the average molecular weight of the polymer. PEGs having average molecular weight below 600 are clear, colorless liquids; those with molecular weight above 1000 are waxlike white materials; and those with molecular weight in between are semisolids. The greater the molecular weight, the greater the viscosity. The NF lists the viscosity of PEGs ranging from average molecular weight of 200 to 8000.

The general formula for preparation of 1000 g of polyethylene glycol ointment is

Polyethylene glycol 3350	400 g
Polyethylene glycol 400	600 g

Combining PEG 3350, a solid, with PEG 400, a liquid, results in a very pliable semisolid ointment. If a firmer ointment is desired, the formula may be altered to contain up to equal parts of the two ingredients. When aqueous solutions are to be incorporated into the base, substitution of 50 g of polyethylene glycol 3350 with an equal amount of stearyl alcohol is advantageous in rendering the final product firmer.

Selection of the Appropriate Base

Selection of the base to use in the formulation of an ointment depends on careful assessment of a number of factors, including the following:

Desired release rate of the drug substance from the ointment base
Desirability of topical or percutaneous drug absorption

Desirability of occlusion of moisture from the skin

Stability of the drug in the ointment base

Effect if any of the drug on the consistency or other features of the ointment base

Desire for a base that is easily removed by washing with water

Characteristics of the surface to which it is applied

For example, an ointment is generally applied to dry, scaly skin; a cream is applied to weeping or oozing surfaces, and a lotion is applied to intertriginous areas or where friction may occur, as between the thighs or under the armpit. The base that provides the best combination of the most desired attributes should be selected.

Preparation of Ointments

Ointments are prepared by two general methods, (*a*) incorporation and (*b*) fusion, depending primarily on the nature of the ingredients.

Incorporation

The components are mixed until a uniform preparation is attained (Fig. 10.1). On a small scale, as in extemporaneous compounding, the pharmacist may mix the components using a mortar and pestle, or a spatula may be used to rub the ingredients together on an ointment slab (a large glass or porcelain plate or pill tile). Some pharmacists use nonabsorbent parchment paper to cover the working surface; being disposable, the paper eliminates cleaning the ointment slab. If using an ointment parchment pad, it is best to not allow too long a contact of the ointment with the parchment, as it may soften and tear.

INCORPORATION OF SOLIDS. When preparing an ointment by spatulation, the pharmacist works the ointment with a stainless steel spatula having a long, broad blade and periodically removes the accumulation of ointment on the large spatula with a smaller one. If the components of an ointment react with metal (as does iodine, for example), hard rubber spatulas may be used. The ointment is prepared by thoroughly rubbing and working the components together on the hard surface until the product

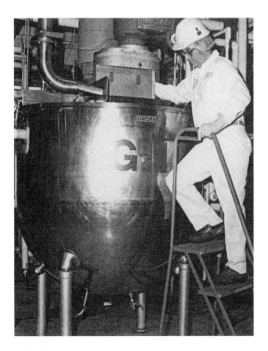

FIGURE 10.1 Creams and ointments in batch sizes up to 1500 kilos are manufactured in this stainless steel tank, which has counter sweep agitation and a built-in homogenizer. (Courtesy of Lederle Laboratories.)

is smooth and uniform. The ointment base is placed on one side of the working surface and the powdered components, previously reduced to fine powders and thoroughly blended in a mortar, on the other side. A small portion of the powder is mixed with a portion of the base until uniform. Geometric dilution is continued until all portions of the powder and base are combined and thoroughly and uniformly blended.

It often is desirable to reduce the particle size of a powder or crystalline material before incorporation into the ointment base so that the final product will not be gritty. This may be done by *levigating*, or mixing the solid material in a vehicle in which it is insoluble to make a smooth dispersion. The levigating agent (e.g., mineral oil for bases in which oils are the external phase or glycerin for bases in which water is the external phase) should be physically and chemically compatible with the drug and base. The levigating agent should be about equal in volume to the solid material. A mortar and pestle are used for levigation. This allows both reduction of particle size and dispersion of the substance in the vehicle. After levigation, the dispersion is incorporated into the ointment base by spatulation or with the mortar and pestle until the product is uniform.

Solids soluble in a common solvent that will affect neither the stability of the drug nor the efficacy of the product may first be dissolved in that solvent (e.g., water or alcohol) and the solution added to the ointment base by spatulation or in a mortar and pestle. The mortar and pestle method is preferred when large volumes of liquid are added, since the liquid is more captive than on an ointment slab.

For incorporating a gummy material, such as camphor, pulverization by intervention can be used. The material is dissolved in a solvent and spread out on the pill tile. The solvent is allowed to evaporate, leaving a thin film of the material onto which the other ingredient or ingredients are spread. The material is then worked into the ingredients by trituration with a spatula.

INCORPORATION OF LIQUIDS. Liquid substances or solutions of drugs, as described above, are added to an ointment only after due consideration of an ointment base's capacity to accept the volume required. For example, as noted previously, only very small amounts of an aqueous solution may be incorporated into an oleaginous ointment, whereas hydrophilic ointment bases readily accept aqueous solutions. When it is necessary to add an aqueous preparation to a hydro*phobic* base, the solution first may be incorporated into a minimum amount of a hydro*philic* base and then that mixture added to the hydrophobic base. However, all bases, even if hydrophilic, have their limits to retain liquids, beyond which they become too soft or semiliquid.

Alcoholic solutions of small volume may be added easily to oleaginous vehicles or emulsion bases. Natural balsams, such as Peru balsam, are usually mixed with an equal portion of castor oil before incorporation into a base. This reduces the surface tension of the balsam and allows even distribution of the balsam throughout the base.

Ointment or roller mills can be used to force coarsely formed ointments through stainless steel or ceramic rollers to produce

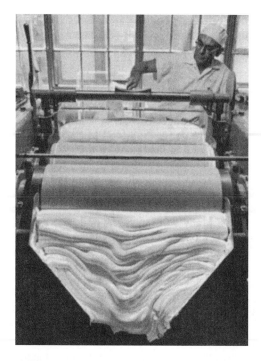

FIGURE 10.2 Day ointment roller mill. Standards of fineness and smoothness require that no grains of material be visible under a 10-power microscope after passage through this machine. (Courtesy of Eli Lilly and Company.)

ointments that are uniform in composition and smooth in texture (Fig. 10.2). Small ointment mills also find use in product development laboratories and in small-batch manufacture or compounding.

Fusion

By the fusion method, all or some of the components of an ointment are combined by being melted together and cooled with constant stirring until congealed. Components not melted are added to the congealing mixture as it is being cooled and stirred. Naturally, heat-labile substances and any volatile components are added last, when the temperature of the mixture is low enough not to cause decomposition or volatilization of the components. Substances may be added to the congealing mixture as solutions or as insoluble powders levigated with a portion of the base. On a small scale, fusion may be conducted in a porcelain dish or glass beaker. On a large scale, it is carried out in large steam-jacketed kettles. Once congealed, the ointment may be passed through an ointment mill (in large-scale manufacture) or rubbed with a spatula or in a mortar to ensure a uniform texture.

Medicated ointments and ointment bases containing components such as beeswax, paraffin, stearyl alcohol, and high-molecular-weight polyethylene glycols, which do not lend themselves well to mixture by incorporation, are prepared by fusion. By this general process, the materials with the highest melting points are heated to the lowest required temperature to produce a melt. The additional materials are added with constant stirring during cooling of the melt until the mixture is congealed. In this way, not all of the components are subjected to the highest temperature. Alternative methods entail melting the component with the lowest melting point first and adding the remaining components in order of their melting points or simply melting all of the components together under slowly increasing temperature. By these methods, a lower temperature is usually sufficient to achieve fusion because of the solvent action exerted by the first melted components on the others.

In preparation of ointments having an emulsion base, the method of manufacture often involves both melting and emulsification. The water-immiscible components such as the oil and waxes are melted together in a steam bath to about 70° to 75°C. Meantime, an aqueous solution of the heat-stable, water-soluble components is prepared and heated to the same temperature as the oleaginous components. Then the aqueous solution is slowly added, with mechanical stirring, to the melted oleaginous mixture. The temperature is maintained for 5 to 10 minutes and the mixture is slowly cooled and stirred until congealed. If the aqueous solution is not the same temperature as the oleaginous melt, some of the waxes will solidify on addition of the colder aqueous solution to the melted mixture.

Compendial Requirements for Ointments (2)

Ointments and other semisolid dosage forms must meet USP tests for *microbial content, min-*

imum fill, packaging, storage, and labeling. As discussed later in this chapter, ophthalmic ointments must also meet tests for *sterility* and *metal particles* content.

Microbial Content

With the exception of ophthalmic preparations, topical applications are not required to be sterile. They must, however, meet acceptable standards for microbial content, and preparations that are prone to microbial growth must contain antimicrobial preservatives. Preparations that contain water tend to support microbial growth to a greater extent than water-free preparations. Among the antimicrobial preservatives used to inhibit microbial growth in topical preparations are methylparaben, propylparaben, phenols, benzoic acid, sorbic acid, and quaternary ammonium salts.

Microbial limits are stated for certain articles in the USP. For example, Betamethasone Valerate Ointment, USP, must *meet the requirements of the tests for absence of* Staphylococcus aureus *and* Pseudomonas aeruginosa. These particular microbes have special importance in dermatologic preparations because of their capacity to infect the skin, which for patients being treated for a skin condition, is already compromised.

In the USP chapter titled "Microbiological Attributes of Nonsterile Pharmaceutical Products," emphasis is placed on strict adherence to environmental control and application of good manufacturing practices to minimize both the type and the number of microorganisms in unsterilized pharmaceutical products (2). This involves the testing of raw materials, use of acceptable water, in-process controls, and final product testing. The USP states that certain products should be routinely tested for microorganisms because of the way they are used. Thus, dermatologic products should be examined for *P. aeruginosa* and *S. aureus*, and those intended for rectal, urethral, or vaginal use should be tested for yeasts and molds, common offenders at these sites of application.

Minimum Fill

The USP's *minimum fill* test is determination of the net weight or volume of the contents of filled containers to ensure proper contents compared with the labeled amount.

Packaging, Storage, and Labeling

Ointments and other semisolid preparations are packaged either in large-mouth ointment jars or in metal or plastic tubes. Semisolid preparations must be stored in well-closed containers to protect against contamination and in a cool place to protect against product separation in heat. When required, light-sensitive preparations are packaged in opaque or light-resistant containers.

In addition to the usual labeling requirements for pharmaceutical products, the USP directs that the labeling for certain ointments and creams include the type of base used (e.g., water soluble or water insoluble).

Additional Standards

In addition to the USP requirements, manufacturers often examine semisolid preparations for viscosity and for in vitro drug release to ensure within-lot and lot-to-lot uniformity (3, 4). In vitro drug release tests include diffusion cell studies to determine the drug's release profile from the semisolid product.

Creams

Pharmaceutical *creams* are semisolid preparations containing one or more medicinal agents dissolved or dispersed in either a water-in-oil emulsion or an oil-in-water emulsion or in another type of water-washable base. The so-called vanishing creams are oil-in-water emulsions containing large percentages of water and stearic acid or other oleaginous components. After application of the cream, the water evaporates, leaving behind a thin residue film of the stearic acid or other oleaginous component. Chapter 14 discusses the types of emulsions, their physical characteristics, and method of manufacture.

Creams find primary application in topical skin products and in products used rectally and vaginally. Many patients and physicians prefer creams to ointments because they are easier to spread and remove. Pharmaceutical manufacturers frequently manufacture topical preparations of a drug in both cream and ointment bases to satisfy the preference of the patient and physician.

Gels

Gels are semisolid systems consisting of dispersions of small or large molecules in an aqueous liquid vehicle rendered jellylike by the addition of a *gelling agent*. Among the gelling agents used are synthetic macromolecules, such as carbomer 934; cellulose derivatives, such as carboxymethylcellulose or hydroxypropyl methylcellulose; and natural gums, such as tragacanth. Carbomers are high-molecular-weight water-soluble polymers of acrylic acid cross-linked with allyl ethers of sucrose and/or pentaerythritol. Their viscosity depends on their polymeric composition. The NF contains monographs for six such polymers, carbomers 910, 934, 934P, 940, 941, and 1342. They are used as gelling agents at concentrations of 0.5 to 2.0% in water. Carbomer 940 yields the highest viscosity, between 40,000 and 60,000 centipoises as a 0.5% aqueous dispersion. Gels are sometimes called *jellies*.

Single-phase gels are gels in which the macromolecules are uniformly distributed throughout a liquid with no apparent boundaries between the dispersed macromolecules and the liquid. A gel mass consisting of floccules of small distinct particles is termed a *two-phase* system, often referred to as a *magma*. Milk of magnesia (or magnesia magma), which consists of a gelatinous precipitate of magnesium hydroxide, is such a system. Gels may thicken on standing, forming a thixotrope, and must be shaken before use to liquefy the gel and enable pouring.

In addition to the gelling agent and water, gels may be formulated to contain a drug substance, solvents, such as alcohol and/or propylene glycol; antimicrobial preservatives, such as methylparaben and propylparaben or chlorhexidine gluconate; and stabilizers, such as edetate disodium. Medicated gels may be prepared for administration by various routes, including the skin, the eye, the nose, the vagina, and the rectum.

Transdermal Preparations

Recent years have seen an increase in the number of topical ointments, creams, and gels designed to delivery a drug systemically. This is often accomplished by addition of penetration enhancers to the topical vehicle. Penetration enhancers include dimethyl sulfoxide (DMSO), ethanol, propylene glycol, glycerin, polyethylene glycol, urea, dimethyl acetamide, sodium lauryl sulfate, the poloxamers, Spans, Tweens, lecithin, terpenes, and many others.

A transdermal preparation commonly compounded is Pluronic lecithin organogel (PLO gel). It consists of a Pluronic (Poloxamer) F127 gel (usually 20% or 30% concentration) mixed at a ratio of approximately 1:5 with a mixture of equal parts of isopropyl palmitate and lecithin. This gel vehicle aids in rapid penetration of many active drugs through the skin.

Miscellaneous Semisolid Preparations: Pastes, Plasters, and Glycerogelatins

Pastes

Pastes are semisolid preparations intended for application to the skin. They generally contain a larger proportion of solid material (such as 25%) than ointments and therefore are stiffer.

Pastes can be prepared in the same manner as ointments, by direct mixing or the use of heat to soften the base prior to incorporating the solids, which have been comminuted and sieved. However, when a levigating agent is to be used to render the powdered component smooth, a portion of the base is often used rather than a liquid, which would soften the paste.

Because of the stiffness of pastes, they remain in place after application and are effectively employed to absorb serous secretions. Because of their stiffness and impenetrability, pastes are not suited for application to hairy parts of the body.

Among the few pastes in use today is zinc oxide paste (Lassar's Plain Zinc Paste), which is prepared by mixing 25% each of zinc oxide and starch with white petrolatum. The product is very firm and is better able to protect the skin and absorb secretions than is zinc oxide ointment.

Plasters

Plasters are solid or semisolid adhesive masses spread on a backing of paper, fabric, moleskin, or plastic. The adhesive material is a rubber base or a synthetic resin. Plasters are applied to the skin to provide prolonged contact at the site. Unmedicated plasters provide protection or mechanical support at the site of application. Adhesive tape used to be official under the title adhesive plaster the use of this material being well known.

Medicated plasters provide effects at the site of application. They may be cut to size to conform to the surface to be covered. Among the few plasters in use today is salicylic acid plaster used on the toes for the removal of corns. The horny layers of skin are removed by the keratolytic action of salicylic acid. The concentration of salicylic acid used in commercial corn plasters ranges from 10 to 40%.

Glycerogelatins

Glycerogelatins are plastic masses containing gelatin (15%), glycerin (40%), water (35%), and an added medicinal substance (10%), such as zinc oxide. They are prepared by first softening the gelatin in the water for about 10 minutes, heating on a steam bath until the gelatin is dissolved, adding the medicinal substance mixed with the glycerin, and allowing the mixture to cool with stirring until congealed.

Glycerogelatins are applied to the skin for the long term. They are melted before application, cooled to slightly above body temperature, and applied to the affected area with a fine brush. Following application, the glycerogelatin hardens, is usually covered with a bandage, and is allowed to remain in place for weeks. The most recent official glycerogelatin was zinc gelatin, used in the treatment of varicose ulcers. It was also known as zinc gelatin boot because of its ability to form a pressure bandage.

Packaging Semisolid Preparations

Topical dermatologic products are packaged in either jars or tubes, whereas ophthalmic, nasal, vaginal, and rectal semisolid products are almost always packaged in tubes.

So-called ointment jars are made of clear or opaque glass or plastic. Some are colored green, amber, or blue. Opaque jars, used for light-sensitive products, are porcelain white, dark green, or amber. Commercially available empty ointment jars vary in size from about 0.5 ounce to 1 pound.

In commercial manufacture and packaging of topical products, the jars and tubes are first tested for compatibility and stability for the intended product. This includes stability testing of filled containers at room temperatures (e.g., 20°C) as well as under accelerated stability testing conditions (e.g., 40 and 50°C).

Tubes used to package topical pharmaceutical products are gaining in popularity. They are light in weight, relatively inexpensive, convenient for use, and compatible with most formulative components, and they provide greater protection against external contamination and environmental conditions than jars (5).

Ointment tubes are made of aluminum or plastic. When the ointment is to be used for ophthalmic, rectal, vaginal, aural, or nasal application, they are packaged with special applicator tips. Tubes of aluminum generally are coated with an epoxy resin, vinyl, or lacquer to eliminate any interactions between the contents and the tube. Plastic tubes are made of high- or low-density polyethylene (HDPE or LDPE) or a blend of each, polypropylene (PP), polyethylene terephthalate (PET), and various plastic, foil, and/or paper laminates, sometimes 10 layers thick.

Each type of plastic offers special features and advantages. For example, LDPE is soft and resilient, and it provides a good moisture barrier. HDPE provides a superior moisture barrier but is less resilient. PP has a high level of heat resistance, and PET offers transparency and a high degree of product chemical compatibility. Laminates provide an excellent moisture barrier because of the foil content, high durability, and product compatibility (5).

These qualities and flexibility make plastic and plastic laminate tubes preferred to metal tubes for packaging of pharmaceuticals.

The cylindrical bodies of plastic tubes are made by extrusion and then joined to the shoulder, neck, and tip piece, which is made by molding. Most multiple-dose tubes used for pharmaceuticals have conventional continuous-thread closures. Single-dose tubes may be prepared with a tearaway tip. Metered-dose, tamper-evident, and child-resistant closures are available (5). Standard sizes of empty tubes have capacities of 1.5, 2, 3.5, 5, 15, 30, 45, 60, and 120 g (6). Ointments, creams, and gels are most frequently packaged in 5-, 15-, and 30-g tubes.

Ophthalmic ointments typically are packaged in small aluminum or collapsible plastic tubes holding 3.5 g (about 0.125 oz) of ointment, as shown in Figure 17.4. The tubes, which are sterilized before being aseptically filled, are fitted with narrow-gauge tips that permit extrusion and placement of narrow bands of ointment on the inner margin of the eyelid, the usual site of application.

Filling Ointment Jars

Ointment jars are filled on a small scale in the pharmacy by carefully transferring the weighed amount of ointment into the jar with a spatula. The ointment is packed on the bottom and along the sides of the jar, avoiding entrapment of air. The jar size should allow the ointment to reach near the top of the jar but not so high as to touch the lid when closed. Through the adept use of the spatula, some pharmacists place a curl in the center of the surface of the ointment. Ointments prepared by fusion may be poured directly into the ointment jar to congeal in it. This must be done cautiously to prevent stratification of the components. In large-scale manufacture of ointments, pressure fillers force the specified amount of ointment into the jars.

Filling Ointment Tubes

Tubes are filled from the open back end of the tube, opposite from the cap end (Fig. 10.3).

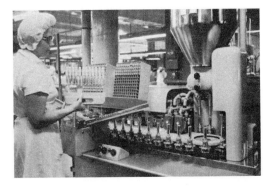

FIGURE 10.3 Arenco tube-filling machine automatically fills 125 tubes a minute with proper amount, tightens cap, orients each tube by electric eye so that label faces forward, then closes and crimps the end. (Courtesy of Eli Lilly and Company.)

Ointments prepared by fusion may be poured while still soft but viscous directly into the tubes with caution to prevent stratification of the components. On a small scale, as in the extemporaneous filling of an ointment in the pharmacy, the tube may be filled manually (Fig. 10.4) or with a small-scale filling machine (Fig. 10.5). The filled tube is closed and sealed. As depicted in Figure 10.4, manual filling of an ointment tube requires a number of steps: (*a*) The prepared ointment, placed on waxed or parchment paper and rolled into a cylindrical shape, is inserted into the open end of the tube and pushed forward as far as allowed. (*b*) With

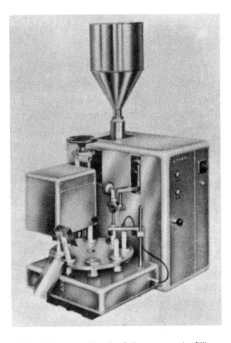

FIGURE 10.5 A small-scale fully automatic filling and crimping machine for collapsible metal tubes. The capacity of the machine is up to 60 units per minute. (Courtesy of Chemical and Pharmaceutical Industry Co.)

a spatula pressing against the lower portion of the tube and making a crease below the ointment fill, the paper is slowly removed, leaving the ointment in the tube. (*c*) The bottom of the tube is flattened, folded, and sealed with a crimping tool or clip.

Industrially, automatic filling, closing, crimping, and labeling machines are used for large-scale tube packaging of semisolid pharmaceuticals (Fig. 10.3). Depending on the model, machines have the capacity to fill about 1000 to 6000 tubes per hour (5, 7). Rotary machines have four stations for tube feeding, cleaning, filling, and closing. Plastic and laminate tubes are closed and sealed by heat and crimping. Metal tubes are sealed by folding and crimping with or without a vinyl, latex, or lacquer sealant (5).

Electronic mortars and pestles can be used to prepare an ointment, cream, or gel in the dispensing container. The ingredients are placed in the container and the cap, which has a stirring rod and blade assembly, put in place. The unit can be programmed for thorough

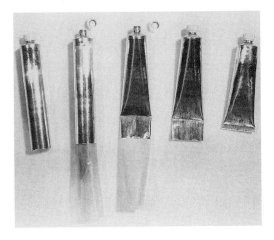

FIGURE 10.4 Steps in the manual filling of ointment tubes.

mixing using different speeds and up and down rates until the product is uniform. The rod is removed and the cap replaced with a dispensing cap. For administration, the bottom of the ointment jar is moved up, forcing the product out of the orifice in the dispensing cap. The small orifice cap is replaced for a tight seal.

Features and Use of Dermatologic Preparations

Among the dosage forms used in the topical treatment of conditions and diseases of the skin are ointments, creams, gels, pastes, and plasters. Other dosage forms include solutions, powders, and transdermal drug delivery systems, discussed elsewhere in this text. Oral therapy also may be used for skin conditions, as in the treatment of poison ivy with prednisone.

In treating skin diseases, the drug in a medicated application should *penetrate* and be *retained* in the skin for a while. Drug penetration into the skin depends on a number of factors, including the physicochemical properties of

the medicinal substance, the characteristics of the pharmaceutical vehicle, and the condition of skin itself. Normal unbroken skin acts as a natural barrier, limiting both the rate and degree of drug penetration.

The skin is divided histologically into the stratum corneum (the outer layer), the living epidermis, and the dermis, collectively a laminate of barriers protecting against permeation by external agents and loss of water from the body. Blood capillaries and nerve fibers rise from the subcutaneous fat into the dermis and up to the epidermis. Sebaceous glands, sweat glands, and hair follicles originating in the dermis and subcutaneous layers rise to the skin's surface (Fig. 10.6). The stratum corneum is the desquamating horny layer, a 10- to 15-μm-thick layer of flat, partially desiccated, dead epidermal cells (8, 9). The stratum corneum is composed of approximately 40% protein (mainly keratin) and 40% water, with the balance being lipid, principally as triglycerides, free fatty acids, cholesterol, and phospholipids. On the surface is a film of emulsified material

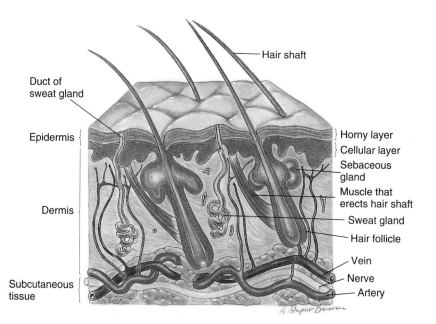

FIGURE 10.6 Stratified organization of the skin. (Reprinted with permission from Bickley LS, Szilagyi P. Bates' guide to physical examination and history taking, 8th ed. Philadelphia: Lippincott Williams & Wilkins, 2003.)

composed of a complex mixture of sebum, sweat, and desquamating epidermal cells.

The film covering the stratum corneum varies in composition, thickness, and continuity as a result of differences in the proportion of sebum and sweat produced and the extent of their removal through washing and sweat evaporation. It offers little resistance to drug penetration. Hair follicles and gland ducts can provide entry for drug molecules, but because their relative surface area is so minute compared to the total epidermis, they are minor factors in drug absorption.

The stratum corneum, being keratinized tissue, behaves as a semipermeable artificial membrane, and drug molecules can penetrate by passive diffusion. The rate of drug movement across this skin layer depends on the drug concentration in the vehicle, its aqueous solubility, and the oil–water partition coefficient between the stratum corneum and the product's vehicle (10). Substances with both aqueous and lipid solubility characteristics are good candidates for diffusion through the stratum corneum. Once through the stratum corneum, drug molecules may pass through the deeper epidermal tissues and into the dermis. If the drug reaches the vascularized dermal layer, it becomes available for absorption into the general circulation.

Whereas drug blood levels achieved by transdermal delivery systems may be measured and equated against desired therapeutic effects, the same is not true for topical *non*systemic dermatologic products. For topical products, the therapeutically effective drug concentration in the skin is not known, so treatment is based on qualitative measures, with clinical efficacy often varying between patients and products.

Differences in emollient and occlusive effects and ease of application and removal between products is a factor of the base used and product type. As noted earlier, oleaginous bases provide greater occlusion and emollient effects than do hydrophilic or water-washable bases. Pastes offer even greater occlusion and are more effective than ointments at absorbing serous discharge. Creams, usually oil-in-water emulsions, spread more easily than ointments and are easier to remove. Water-soluble bases are nongreasy and are easily removed.

Unless otherwise directed, before applying a dermatologic product, the patient should thoroughly clean the affected area with soap and water and dry by patting with a soft cloth. In most instances, a thin layer of medication should be applied to the affected area and spread evenly using gentle pressure with the fingertips. Typically about 1 to 3 mg of ointment or cream is applied per square centimeter of skin (1). Unless there is a specified need for an occlusive dressing to protect the area from excessive contact or contaminants, a bandage should not be used. After application, the hands should be thoroughly washed.

Upon dispensing a prescription or over-the-counter (OTC) product, the pharmacist should be certain that the patient understands the proper method of administration, frequency and duration of use, special warnings (such as those related to pregnancy or nursing), therapeutic goals and anticipated outcomes, signs of adverse response, allergic sensitivity reactions or treatment failure, and reasons to discontinue treatment and seek further professional guidance.

The patient should be advised that if symptoms persist or irritation develops, use of the product should be discontinued and a physician or pharmacist consulted. It is fairly common for patients to have an allergic response, such as a skin rash, to a topical product as a result of sensitivity to the medicinal agent or pharmaceutic ingredient. An alternative product that does not contain the suspected offending agent may be substituted to solve the problem.

Examples of dermatologic ointments, creams, and gels are presented in Tables 10.1 and 10.2.

Features and Use of Ophthalmic Ointments and Gels

Among the dosage forms used in the topical treatment of conditions and diseases of the eye are ointments and gels. Other ophthalmic dosage forms used topically include solutions, suspensions, and inserts, discussed elsewhere in this text. Systemic therapy also may be

TABLE 10.1 DERMATOLOGIC OINTMENTS AND CREAMS BY THERAPEUTIC CATEGORY

PREPARATION	CORRESPONDING COMMERCIAL PRODUCT	USUAL STRENGTH OF ACTIVE INGREDIENT	USE
Adrenocortical Steroids			
Alclometasone dipropionate cream and ointment	Aclovate Cream and Ointment (GlaxoSmithKline)	0.05% cream and ointment	Relief of inflammatory dermatoses
Fluocinolone acetonide cream, ointment	Synalar Cream & Ointment (Roche)	0.025% cream and ointment	Relief of inflammatory dermatoses
Hydrocortisone acetate cream, ointment	Cortaid Cream and Ointment (Pharmacia and Upjohn)	0.5% and 1%	Relief of inflammatory dermatoses
Triamcinolone acetonide cream, ointment	Aristocort A Cream and Ointment (Fujisawa)	0.1% ointment; 0.1%, 0.025%, 0.5% cream	Relief of inflammatory dermatoses
Adrenocorticoid–Antifungal Combination			
Betamethasone, clotrimazole cream	Lotrisone Cream (Schering-Plough)	1% betamethasone, 0.05% clotrimazole	Relief, treatment of inflammatory pruritic manifestations that may be complicated by fungal overgrowth
Analgesic			
Capsaicin cream	Zostrix Cream (Medicis)	0.025%	Relief of arthritic pain
Antiacne			
Tretinoin cream	Retin-A (Ortho McNeil)	0.025%, 0.05%, 0.1%	Derivative of vitamin A for topical treatment of acne vulgaris
Antianginal			
Nitroglycerin ointment	Nitro-Bid Ointment (Hoechst Marion Roussel)	2%	Reduces workload of heart by smooth muscle relaxation of peripheral arteries and veins
Antibacterial/Anti-infectives			
Gentamicin sulfate cream, ointment	Garamycin Cream and Ointment (Schering-Plough)	0.1%	Local treatment of skin infections by susceptible microorganisms
Nystatin cream	Mycostatin Cream (Apothecon)	0.5% 100,000 U/g	Local treatment of skin infections by susceptible microorganisms
Polymyxin B sulfate, bacitracin zinc, neomycin ointment	Neosporin Ointment (GlaxoSmithKline)	5000 U/g polymyxin B; 400 U/g bacitracin zinc; 3.5 mg/g neomycin	Treatment of minor cuts, scrapes.
Antifungals			
Miconazole nitrate cream	Monistat-Derm Cream (Ortho McNeil)	2%	Cutaneous candidiasis, tinea infections of *Trichophyton* spp.
Tolnaftate cream	Tinactin Cream (Schering-Plough)	1%	Topical treatment of tinea pedis, tinea cruris, tinea corporis, tinea manuum.

(continued)

TABLE 10.1 DERMATOLOGIC OINTMENTS AND CREAMS BY THERAPEUTIC CATEGORY

PREPARATION	CORRESPONDING COMMERCIAL PRODUCT	USUAL STRENGTH OF ACTIVE INGREDIENT	USE
Antineoplastic Fluorouracil cream	Efudex Cream (Roche)	5%	Treatment of multiple actinic, solar keratoses
Antipruritic, analgesic Lidocaine ointment	Xylocaine Ointment (Astra)	2.5%	Relief of pain, itching of minor skin irritation, insect bites
Astringent, protectant Zinc oxide ointment	Desitin Ointment (Pfizer)	40%	Topical astringent, protective in skin conditions such as diaper rash
Depigmenting Agents Hydroquinone cream	Eldopaque Cream (ICN)	4%	Temporary bleaching of skin with freckles, old age spots, chloasma
Scabicide Crotamiton cream	Eurax Cream (Westwood-Squibb)	10%	Eradication of scabies, symptomatic treatment of pruritus

undertaken, as in the use of diuretics in the adjunctive treatment of glaucoma.

The application of medication to the eye or conjunctival sac affects the surface of the eye and underlying tissues as the drug penetrates. The major route by which drugs enter the eye is simple diffusion via the cornea. For drugs that are poorly absorbed by the cornea, the conjunctive and sclera provide an alternate route (11). The cornea is a three-layered structure with a lipophilic epithelial layer, a hydrophilic stromal layer, and a less lipophilic endothelial layer on the inside (11). Drug penetration depends on a drug's ability to traverse these three layers. Lipophilic drugs are more capable of penetration than hydrophilic compounds (11).

In general, ocular ophthalmic drug penetration is limited by the short residence time on the surface of the eye because of rapid removal by tearing and other natural mechanisms, the small surface area of the cornea for drug absorption, and the cornea's natural resistance to drug penetration (11). Compared with ophthalmic solutions, ophthalmic ointments and gels provide extended residence time on the surface of the eye, increasing the duration of their surface effects and bioavailability for absorption into the ocular tissues. Ophthalmic ointments are cleared from the eye as slowly as 0.5% per minute, compared with solutions, which can lose up to 16% of their volume per minute (12, 13).

The ointment base selected for an ophthalmic ointment must not be irritating to the eye and must permit the diffusion of the medicinal substance throughout the secretions bathing the eye. Ointment bases used for ophthalmics should have a softening point close to body temperature, both for comfort and for drug release. Most often, mixtures of white petrolatum and liquid petrolatum (mineral oil) are used as the base in medicated and unmedicated (lubricating) ophthalmic ointments. Sometimes a water-miscible agent such as lanolin is added. A gel base of polyethylene glycol and mineral oil is also used; this form permits water and water-insoluble drugs to be retained within the base.

Medicinal agents are added to an ointment base either as a solution or as a finely micronized

TABLE 10.2 EXAMPLES OF TOPICAL GELS

ACTIVE INGREDIENT	PROPRIETARY PRODUCT	GELLING AGENT	ROUTE AND USE
Acetic acid	Aci-Jel (Ortho-McNeil)	Tragacanth, acacia	Vaginal: restoration and maintenance of acidity
Becaplermin	Regranex Gel (Ortho-McNeil)	Sodium CMC	Dermatologic: recombinant human platelet–derived growth factor; promotes healing of diabetic ulcers of lower extremity
Benzoyl peroxide	Desquam-X Gel (Westwood-Squibb)	Carbomer 940	Dermatologic: acne vulgaris
Clindamycin	Cleocin T Topical Gel (Pharmacia & Upjohn)	Carbomer 934P	Dermatologic: acne vulgaris
Clobetasol propionate	Temovate Gel (GlaxoSmithKline)	Carbomer 934P	Dermatologic: antipruritic
Cyanocobalamin	Nascobal (Schwartz Pharma)	Methylcellulose	Nasal: hematologic
Desoximetasone	Topicort Gel (Medicis Dermatologics)	Carbomer 940	Dermatologic: anti-inflammatory, antipruritic
Metronidazole	Metro-Gel Vaginal (Galderma)	Carbomer 934P	Vaginal: bacterial vaginosis
Podofilox	Condylox Gel (Oclassen)	Hydroxypropyl cellulose	Rectal: anogenital warts
Progesterone	Crinone Gel (Serono)	Carbomer 934P	Vaginal: bioadhesive gel for progesterone supplementation and replacement
Timolol Maleate	Timoptic-XE (Merck)	Gelrite gellan gum	Ophthalmic gel-forming solution used in treatment of elevated intraocular pressure
Tretinoin	Retin-A Gel (Ortho McNeil)	Hydroxypropyl cellulose	Dermatologic: acne vulgaris

powder. The ointment is made uniform and smooth by fine milling.

In addition to the previously stated quality standards for ointments, ophthalmic ointments must meet the USP *sterility tests* and the test for *metal particles in ophthalmic ointments*. Rendering an ophthalmic ointment sterile requires special technique and processing. For a number of reasons, the terminal sterilization of a finished ointment by standard methods may be problematic. Steam sterilization or ethylene oxide methods are ineffective because neither is capable of penetrating the ointment base. Although dry heat sterilization can penetrate the ointment base, the high heat required may pose a threat to the stability of the drug substance and introduces the possibility of separating the ointment base from the other components (14). Because of these difficulties,

terminal sterilization generally is not undertaken. Rather, strict methods of aseptic processing are employed as each drug and nondrug component is rendered sterile and then aseptically weighed and incorporated in a final product that meets the sterility requirement (14). When an antimicrobial preservative is needed, among those used are methylparaben (0.05%) and propylparaben (0.01%) combinations, phenylmercuric acetate (0.0008%), chlorobutanol (0.5%), and benzalkonium chloride (0.008%).

The USP test for metal particles is microscopic examination of a heat-melted ophthalmic ointment. Detected metal particles are counted and measured by a calibrated eyepiece micrometer disk. The requirements are met if the total number of particles 50 μm or larger from 10 product tubes does not exceed 50 and if not more than 1 tube contains more than 8 such particles (2).

The USP directs that ophthalmic ointments must be packaged in collapsible ointment tubes. These tubes have an elongated narrow tip to facilitate application of a narrow band of ointment to the eye.

In preparation to apply an ointment to the eye, the patient's or caregiver's hands should be washed and dried thoroughly. Then the ointment tube is held between the thumb and forefinger and the tip placed near the eyelid without touching it. The patient's head should be tilted back, and with the index finger of the opposite hand, the lower eyelid of the affected eye should be gently pulled downward. The tip of the ointment tube should be held slightly above the inside portion of the sack between the lower eyelid and eyeball. Without touching the tip to any part of the eye, a thin ribbon of ointment, approximately 0.25 to 0.5 inch, should be placed along the inside of the lower lid. The patient should face down and slowly close the eye for a few seconds. Then any excess ointment should be wiped from the eyelids and lashes with a clean tissue. To facilitate the procedure, a patient may sit in front of a mirror with elbows stabilized or have another person administer the ointment. After use, the ointment must be capped quickly and tightly.

The patient should be advised that blurred vision will occur as the ointment spreads over the eye and not to be alarmed. If the ointment is to be administered only once daily, it is often preferable to do so at bedtime, when vision impairment will be inconsequential.

It is important to emphasize to the patient that ocular products if handled improperly can become contaminated by bacteria that cause ocular infections, which may lead to serious consequences. Thus every effort must be made to avoid touching the tip of the tube to the eye, eyelid, fingertip, or any other surface, and the ointment should be used by only one person. Examples of ophthalmic ointments and gels are presented in Tables 10.2 and 10.3.

TABLE 10.3 EXAMPLES OF OPHTHALMIC OINTMENTS

OINTMENT	COMMERCIAL PRODUCT	ACTIVE INGREDIENT	CATEGORY
Chloramphenicol ophthalmic	Chloromycetin Ophthalmic Ointment (Parke-Davis)	1%	Antibacterial antibiotic
Dexamethasone sodium phosphate ophthalmic	Decadron Phosphate Ophthalmic Ointment (Merck)	0.05%	Anti-inflammatory adrenocortical steroid
Gentamicin sulfate ophthalmic	Garamycin Ophthalmic Ointment (Schering-Plough)	0.3%	Antibacterial antibiotic
Isoflurophate ophthalmic	Floropryl Sterile Ophthalmic Ointment (Merck)	0.025%	Cholinesterase inhibitor
Polymyxin B–bacitracin ophthalmic	Polysporin Ophthalmic Ointment (Monarch)	per gram: polymyxin B sulfate, 10,000 U; bacitracin zinc, 500 U	Antimicrobial
Polymyxin B–bacitracin–neomycin ophthalmic	Neosporin Ophthalmic Ointment (Monarch)	per gram: polymyxin B sulfate, 5000 U; bacitracin, zinc, 400 U; neomycin sulfate, 5 mg	Antimicrobial
Sulfacetamide sodium ophthalmic	Sodium Sulamyd Ophthalmic Ointment (Schering-Plough)	10, 30%	Antibacterial
Tobramycin ophthalmic	Tobrex Ophthalmic Ointment (Alcon)	0.3%	Antibacterial antibiotic
Vidarabine ophthalmic	Vira-A-Ophthalmic Ointment (Monarch)	3%	Antiviral

Features and Use of Nasal Ointments and Gels

Among the dosage forms used in the topical treatment of the nasal mucosa are ointments and gels. Other dosage forms include inhalants, solutions, and suspensions, discussed elsewhere in this text.

The nose is a respiratory organ, a passageway for air to the lungs. Its surface is coated with a continuous thin layer of mucus produced by subepithelial mucous glands. The ciliated epithelium of the nasal passage facilitates the movement of the mucous layer. The mucus contains lysozyme, glycoproteins, and immunoglobulins that act against bacteria and protect against their entry into the lungs. The ciliary action and the sneeze reflex add further defense against entry (15).

Drugs introduced into the nasal passage are primarily for local effects on the mucous membranes and underlying tissues (e.g., nasal decongestants). However, drug absorption to the general circulation does occur through the rich blood supply feeding the nasal lining. The nasal route of administration is also used for the systemic absorption of a number of drugs, including butorphanol tartrate (Stadol NS, Bristol-Myers Squibb) an analgesic; cyanocobalamin (Nascobal gel, Schwartz) a hematopoietic; narfaralin acetate (Synarel, Searle) for the treatment of endometriosis; and nicotine (Nicotrol NS, McNeil) as an adjunct in smoking cessation. In addition, the nasal route holds great promise for the administration of insulin, vaccines, and a number of other polypeptides and proteins.

Features and Use of Rectal Preparations

Among the dosage forms used in the topical treatment of anorectal conditions are ointments, gels, creams, and creamlike aerosol foams. Other dosage forms are solutions (for enema or irrigation) and suppositories, discussed elsewhere in this text.

Ointments, creams, and gels are used for topical application to the perianal area and for insertion within the anal canal. They largely are used to treat local conditions of anorectal pruritus, inflammation, and the pain and discomfort associated with hemorrhoids. The drugs include astringents (e.g., zinc oxide), protectants and lubricants (e.g., cocoa butter, lanolin), local anesthetics (e.g., pramoxine HCl), and antipruritics and anti-inflammatory agents (e.g., hydrocortisone).

The perianal area is the skin immediately surrounding the anus. The anal canal is approximately 3 cm long and connects to the rectum. Both the anal canal and rectum have mucosal linings. Healthy perianal skin and the mucosa act as barriers to infection.

Substances applied rectally may be absorbed by diffusion into the general circulation via the network of three hemorrhoidal arteries and accompanying veins in the anal canal (16). The rectal route is used for systemic absorption of therapeutic levels of certain drugs (e.g., prochlorperazine as suppositories) when the oral route is unsatisfactory, as during vomiting. However, systemic effects from ointments and creams intended for local action is usually limited by the insolubility of certain agents (e.g., zinc oxide) and absorption of only subtherapeutic amounts of soluble drugs in the formulation.

The bases used in anorectal ointments and creams include combinations of polyethylene glycol 300 and 3350, emulsion cream bases using cetyl alcohol and cetyl esters wax, and white petrolatum and mineral oil. When antimicrobial preservatives are required, methylparaben, propylparaben, benzyl alcohol, and butylated hydroxyanisole (BHA) are frequently used.

Before applying rectal ointments and creams to the perianal skin, the affected area should be cleansed and dried by gentle patting with toilet tissue. Then a portion of the ointment or cream is placed on a tissue and a thin film is gently spread over the affected area. Products having a water-washable base are easier to spread and remove after application and tend to stain clothing less than products having an oleaginous base.

Rectal ointments and creams are packaged with special perforated plastic tips for products to be administered into the anus, primarily in the treatment of the pain and inflammation associated with hemorrhoids (Fig. 10.7). Before

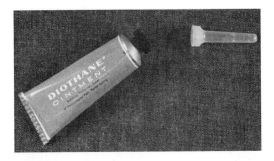

FIGURE 10.7 Rectal ointment with perforated inserter/applicator tip.

use, the rectal tip should be thoroughly cleaned, screwed onto the ointment tube in place of the cap, and lubricated with mineral oil or a lubricating jelly. With the patient lying down on the back or side or in an otherwise comfortable position, the rectal tip is slowly and carefully inserted part way into the anus. Squeezing the tube forces medication through the perforations in the rectal tip and releases it to the inner lining of the anus. The tip is then slowly removed from the anus and any excess ointment or cream removed from the perianal area. The rectal tip should be cleaned thoroughly, the closure cap replaced on the tube, and the hands washed.

Rectal aerosol foam products (e.g., Procto-foam-HC, Schwarz) also are accompanied by applicators to facilitate administration. The applicator is attached to the aerosol container and filled with a measured dose of product. The ap-plicator is then inserted into the anus and the product delivered by pushing the plunger of the applicator. After removal, the applicator and the patient's hands should be thoroughly washed.

Patients should be instructed on the proper use of the product dispensed and in case of rectal bleeding, advised to seek additional medical advice. Examples of rectal ointments and creams are presented in Table 10.4.

Features and Use of Vaginal Preparations

Among the dosage forms used in the topical treatment of conditions and diseases of the vulvovaginal area are ointments, creams, creamlike foams, and gels. Other dosage forms include suppositories, vaginal inserts, transdermal drug delivery systems, and oral forms, discussed elsewhere in this text.

The vaginal surface is lined with squamous epithelium cells and mucus produced by various underlying glands. Topical products are used to treat vulvovaginal infections, vaginitis, conditions of endometrial atrophy, and for contraception with spermatocidal agents.

The usual pathogenic organisms of vulvovaginal infections and vaginitis are *Trichomonas vaginalis*, *Candida* (*Monilia*) *albicans*, and *Haemophilus vaginalis*. Among the anti-infective agents are nystatin, clotrimazole, miconazole, clindamycin, and sulfonamides. Endometrial atrophy may be treated locally with the hor-

TABLE 10.4 EXAMPLES OF RECTAL AND VAGINAL CREAMS AND OINTMENTS

COMMERCIAL PREPARATION	ACTIVE INGREDIENTS	PRODUCT TYPE	PRIMARY USE
Rectal			
Anusol (GlaxoSmithKline)	Starch	Ointment	Hemorrhoid treatment
Tronolane (Ross)	Pramoxine HCl	Cream	Hemorrhoidal analgesic, antipruritic
Vaginal			
Mycelex-7 (Bayer)	Clotrimazole	Cream	Antifungal
AVC (Novavax)	Sulfanilamide	Cream	Vulvovaginitis (*Candida albicans*)
Cleocin (Pharmacia & Upjohn)	Clindamycin PO_4	Cream	Bacterial vaginosis
Terazol 7 (Ortho McNeil)	Terconazole	Cream	Antifungal (*Candida albicans*)
Ogen (Pharmacia & Upjohn)	Estropipate	Cream	Estrogenic for vulvar, vaginal atrophy
Premarin (Wyeth-Ayerst)	Conjugated estrogens	Cream	Atrophic vaginitis, kraurosis vulvae

mones dienestrol and progesterone, which are used to restore the vaginal mucosa to its normal state. Contraceptive preparations containing spermicidal agents such as nonoxynol-9 and octoxynol are used alone or in combination with a cervical diaphragm.

As noted previously, because products intended for use in the vulvovaginal area come into direct contact with tissues prone to infection, it is important that these products be manufactured and tested to be free of offending microorganisms, yeasts, and molds. Because gels are especially subject to bacterial growth, most vaginal gels are preserved with antimicrobial agents.

Ointments, creams, and gels for vaginal use are packaged in tubes; vaginal foams, in aerosol canisters. Although some preparations are applied externally to the vulva (e.g., Mycelex-7 Vaginal Cream, Bayer) most are intended to be delivered to the vagina by means of applicator tips that accompany the products (Fig. 10.8).

In treating external vulvar conditions, the patient squeezes a small amount of product onto the fingers or tissue and gently spreads it over the affected area. For intravaginal treatment, the patient uses a plastic applicator, some of which are prefilled and disposable and others reusable and filled by the patient immediately prior to use.

To fill the applicator, the closure cap is removed from the tube, the applicator screwed on in its place, and the tube gently squeezed until the applicator is filled and the plunger rises to its marked stopping point. The filled applicator is unscrewed from the tube and replaced by the cap. Inserting intravaginal products is best accomplished with the patient lying on her back or in an otherwise comfortable position. The applicator barrel is firmly grasped and inserted into the vagina as far as possible without causing discomfort. The plunger is depressed until it stops, releasing the medication in the vagina. The applicator is carefully withdrawn for washing or discard. The patient should be instructed to wash her hands thoroughly after use.

Aerosol foams are used intravaginally in the same general manner. The aerosol package contains an inserter device that when attached to the canister, may be filled with foam. The filled

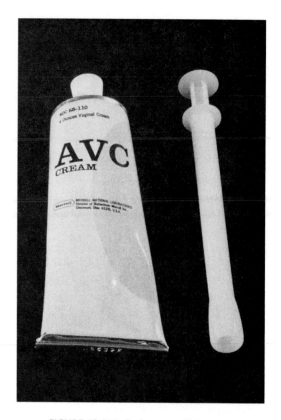

FIGURE 10.8 Vaginal cream with inserter.

inserter is placed in the vagina and the product delivered by pushing the plunger. Vaginal foams are oil-in-water emulsions resembling light creams. They are water miscible and nongreasy.

When once-a-day administration is prescribed, it is best done at bedtime for reasons of medication retention, avoidance of daytime leakage, and lessened soiling of clothing. Creams with water-washable bases are preferred to oleaginous ointments. Patients who are pregnant must not use intravaginal products except with their doctor's approval and supervision. Tampons are not to be used during intravaginal treatment.

Unmedicated lubricant jellies are used by physicians in rectal, urethral, and vaginal examinations. All products should be tightly closed when not in use to prevent contamination. If left unsealed, gels and jellies are particularly prone to dry out. Examples of vaginal ointments, creams, and gels are presented in Tables 10.2 and 10.4.

PHARMACEUTICS CASE STUDY

Subjective

You have received the following prescription:

Rx: Sulfur 2 g
Salicylic acid 2 g
Calamine 5 g
Urea 2 g
Hydrophilic petrolatum qs 100 g

After you prepared the prescription, you observed it to be a granular ointment that is not appropriate for dispensing because it feels very coarse.

Objective

In preparing the ointment, you weighed sublimed sulfur 2 g, salicylic acid 2 g, calamine 5 g, and urea 2 g and mixed the powders together on a pill tile using a spatula. However, you had difficulty with the sulfur, which seemed to be difficult to comminute and blend. Finally, you added the hydrophilic petrolatum and obtained a light pink, quite granular ointment.

Sulfur produces electrostatic charges when mixed on a pill tile using a spatula. It is official as the precipitated sulfur, a very fine powder, and sublimed sulfur, a fine powder. It is practically insoluble in water. Salicylic acid occurs as white crystals, usually in fine needles or a fluffy, white, crystalline powder and is slightly soluble in water and freely soluble in alcohol. Calamine is a fine pink, powder that is insoluble in water. Urea occurs as a white, crystalline powder that is freely soluble in water. It is made up of zinc oxide with a small proportion of ferric oxide.

Assessment

Particle size reduction of sulfur is best accomplished using a levigating agent that is compatible with the base, in this case, hydrophilic petrolatum. Salicylic acid and calamine should pose no real problem in incorporation. Urea can be dissolved, if desired, in a small quantity of water (since it has a solubility of 1 g in 1.5 mL of water, it would take approximately 3 mL of water to dissolve it) and incorporated into the ointment, or, it can be levigated with a small amount of mineral oil prior to incorporation if an anhydrous preparation is desired.

Plan

In this case an anhydrous preparation is desired, so the precipitated sulfur is levigated with about 2 to 3 mL of mineral oil. The urea is levigated with about 2 to 3 mL of mineral oil. The salicylic acid is comminuted to a fine powder, as is the calamine; the two powders are mixed together. The sulfur and urea mixtures are combined and the hydrophilic petrolatum incorporated geometrically. Following this, the salicylic acid and calamine powders are incorporated geometrically and the final preparation thoroughly mixed. This procedure produces a slightly thinner vehicle after the sulfur with urea in mineral oil is incorporated, which makes it easier to incorporate the additional powders. The preparation is then packaged and labeled.

CLINICAL CASE STUDY

A. R. is a 22-y/o WF who comes into the pharmacy complaining of a painful sunburn. She states that she spent most of yesterday, "on the beach with friends" and says she did not use any sunscreen, even though she does occasionally when exposed to the sun. A. R. admits that she did not realize the extent of her sunburn until about 4 hours after her fun on the beach, at which time she began to have pain, chills, and fatigue. Now, she is also itching. When asked, she says she does not have any blisters on her burned skin. When asked if this has happened to her before, A. R. confides that she has had sunburns similar to this about once a summer for approximately the past 5 years. When asked about her pain based on a scale of 1 to 10, she rates her pain as an 8.

PMH: Sunburns many times throughout her life
Moderate acne
Freckles easily, fair complexioned
Red hair
None significant otherwise
SH: None contributory
FH: Mother (−)
Father (−)
Grandfather (+) for melanoma
ALL: NKDA
MEDS: Ortho Tri-Cyclen, 1 tablet po qd
Differin Gel, apply thin layer hs

Pharmaceutical Care Plan

S: Burning, painful, reddened skin, first-degree burn
General fatigue
Chills
Pain 8/10
Itching
O: Bright red skin on face, neck, shoulders, arms, and legs without any evidence of blistering.
A: Patient is a 22 y/o WF with a PMH of sunburns and moderate acne. Patient is at increased risk for sunburns d/t her history of freckling, fair skin, red hair, current medications, and the frequency of past burns. In addition to these characteristics, her FH of melanoma increases her risk of future sunburns and skin cancer.
P: 1. Recommend an oral OTC analgesic to relieve the pain of sunburn. There are many choices, and product selection

often depends on personal preferences. Any NSAID (e.g., ibuprofen 200–400 mg every 4–6 hours prn pain not to exceed 1200 mg per day, naproxen 200 mg every 12 hours prn pain, aspirin 325–650 mg q 3-4 hours prn not to exceed 4 g per day, or acetaminophen 325–650 mg every 4–6 hours prn not to exceed 4 g per day,) would be a good choice. The patient should understand to take these as recommended with a full glass of water and to continue taking them until the pain abates.
2. Applying a clean cloth soaked in cool tap water or taking a cool bath for 10 to 30 minutes will also help to alleviate pain. One can also recommend a topical anesthetic to aid in relieving pain, such as Solarcaine Aloe Extra Burn Relief Cream, Gel, or Spray. A. R. should be instructed that topical anesthetics should not be used more often than 3 or 4 times daily and that continuous pain relief cannot be obtained with these agents. Before and after applying the product, the patient should wash her hands.
3. A W/O topical lotion can provide protection and moisture. These factors are important for sunburned skin because the goal is to replenish skin moisture lost to the sun and protect it from drying out further, which can lead to more irritation and itching. A lotion that could be recommended is Keri. A. R. should apply liberally as needed; however, she should avoid her face, because this lotion contains mineral oil that may exacerbate her acne. Since this lotion has a W/O base, the patient should be told that it will be necessary to use soap and water to remove it.
4) Counsel A. R. on her current medications, especially because the medica-

Clinical Case Study cont.

tions she is using for acne may have played a role in developing the sunburn (i.e., photosensitivity). A. R. should also be told that exposure to the sun can exacerbate her acne. A. R. should avoid excessive sun exposure, especially for the next few weeks, because the skin should have time to heal and will be more susceptible to sunburn during this time. The patient should also be counseled on her many risk factors for skin cancer, including fair skin, red hair, a history of freckling, family history of melanoma, and the frequency of past burns. In the future, A. R. should completely avoid sun exposure. Because this may be unrealis-

tic, she should be told to use a hat and clothing while in the sun to decrease the amount of skin exposed to the sun. If she believes she cannot comply with these suggestions, she should, at least, use a W/O-base sunscreen with an SPF of 30. This will also provide water resistance.

5. Monitoring: The patient should reassess her sunburn in another 24 hours, because the full extent of skin damage may not be initially apparent until 24 to 48 hours after exposure. If she notices any breaks in the skin and/or pain persists or increases, she should seek medical attention from a primary care provider.

REFERENCES

1. Shah VP, Behl CR, Flynn GL, Higuchi WI, Schaefer H. Principles and criteria in the development and optimization of topical therapeutic products. Pharm Res 1992;9:1107–1112.
2. United States Pharmacopeia. 26th ed. Rockville, MD: U.S. Pharmacopeial Convention, 2003.
3. Corbo M, Schulz TW, Wong GK, Van Buskirk GA. Development and validation of in vitro release testing methods for semisolid formulations. Pharm Tech 1993; 17:112–128.
4. Shah VP, Elkins J, Hanus J, Noorizadeh C, Skelly JP. In vitro release of hydrocortisone from topical preparations and automated procedure. Pharm Res 1991;8:55–63.
5. Forcinio H. Tubes: the ideal packaging for semisolid products. Pharm Tech 1998;22:32–36.
6. Montebello Packaging, 124 Madison Street, Oak Park, IL.
7. MG America, Inc., 31 Kulick Rd., Fairfield, NJ.
8. Black CD. Transdermal drug delivery systems. US Pharm 1982;1:49.
9. Walters KA. Percutaneous absorption and transdermal therapy. Pharm Tech 1986;10:30–42.
10. Surber C et al. Optimization of topical therapy: partitioning of drugs into stratum corneum. Pharm Res 1990;7:1320–1324.
11. Lee VHL. Mechanisms and facilitation of corneal drug penetration. J Controlled Release 1990;11:79–90.
12. Compounding ophthalmic preparations. Int J Pharm Compound 1998; 2:184–188.
13. Swanson MW. Ophthalmic disorders. In: Handbook of nonprescription drugs, 12th ed. Washington: American Pharmaceutical Association, 2000; 483–507.
14. Lee JY. Sterilization control and validation for topical ointments. Pharm Tech 1992;16:104–110.
15. Tietze KJ. Disorders related to cold and allergy. In: In: Handbook of nonprescription drugs, 12th ed. Washington: American Pharmaceutical Association, 2000; 179–214.
16. Boyd EL, Berardi RR. Anorectal Disorders. In: In: Handbook of nonprescription drugs, 12th ed. Washington: American Pharmaceutical Association, 2000; 319–336.

Transdermal Drug Delivery Systems

11

Chapter **at a glance**

Transdermal drug delivery systems (TDDSs) facilitate the passage of therapeutic quantities of drug substances through the skin and into the general circulation for their systemic effects. In 1965 Stoughton first conceived of the *percutaneous absorption* of drug substances (1). The first transdermal system, Transderm Scop (Ciba, now Novartis) was approved by the Food and Drug Administration (FDA) in 1979 for prevention of nausea and vomiting associated with travel, particularly by sea.

Evidence of percutaneous drug absorption may be found through measurable blood levels of the drug, detectable excretion of the drug and/or its metabolites in the urine, and clinical response of the patient to the therapy. With transdermal drug delivery, the blood concentration needed to achieve therapeutic efficacy may be determined by comparative analysis of the patient's response to drug blood levels. For transdermal drug delivery, it is considered ideal for the drug to migrate through the skin to the underlying blood supply without

buildup in the dermal layers (2). This is in direct contrast to the types of topical dosage forms discussed in the previous chapter, in which drug residence in the skin, the target organ, is desired.

As discussed in the previous chapter, the skin is composed of the stratum corneum (the outer layer), the living epidermis, and the dermis, which together provide the skin's barrier layers to penetration by external agents (see Fig. 10.6). The film that covers the stratum corneum is composed of sebum and sweat, but because of its varied composition and lack of continuity, it is not a significant factor in drug penetration, nor are the hair follicles and sweat and sebaceous gland ducts, which constitute only a minor proportion of the skin's surface.

Percutaneous absorption of a drug generally results from direct penetration of the drug through the stratum corneum, a 10- to 15-μm-thick layer of flat, partially desiccated nonliving tissue (3, 4). The stratum corneum is composed of approximately 40% protein (mainly keratin) and 40% water, with the balance being lipid, principally as triglycerides, free fatty acids, cholesterol, and phospholipids. The lipid content is concentrated in the extracellular phase of the stratum corneum and forms to a large extent the membrane surrounding the cells. Because a drug's major route of penetration is through the intercellular channels, the lipid component is considered an important determinant in the first step of absorption (5). Once through the stratum corneum, drug molecules may pass through the deeper epidermal tissues and into the dermis. When the drug reaches the vascularized dermal layer, it becomes available for absorption into the general circulation.

The stratum corneum, being keratinized tissue, behaves as a semipermeable artificial membrane, and drug molecules penetrate by passive diffusion. It is the major rate-limiting barrier to transdermal drug transport (6). Over most of the body, the stratum corneum has 15 to 25 layers of flattened corneocytes with an overall thickness of about 10 μm (6). The rate of drug movement across this layer depends on its concentration in the vehicle, its aqueous solubility, and the oil–water partition coefficient between the stratum corneum and the vehicle (7). Substances with both aqueous and lipid solubility characteristics are good candidates for diffusion through the stratum corneum, epidermis, and dermis.

Factors Affecting Percutaneous Absorption

Not all drug substances are suitable for transdermal delivery. Among the factors playing a part in percutaneous absorption are the physical and chemical properties of the drug, including its molecular weight, solubility, partitioning coefficient and dissociation constant (pK_a), the nature of the carrier vehicle, and the condition of the skin. Although general statements applicable to all possible combinations of drug, vehicle, and skin condition are difficult to draw, most research findings may be summarized as follows (2–11).

1. Drug concentration is an important factor. Generally, the amount of drug percutaneously absorbed per unit of surface area per time interval increases with an increase in the concentration of the drug in the TDDS.

2. The larger the area of application (the larger the TDDS), the more drug is absorbed.

3. The drug should have a greater physicochemical attraction to the skin than to the vehicle so that the drug will leave the vehicle in favor of the skin. Some solubility of the drug in both lipid and water is thought to be essential for effective percutaneous absorption. In essence, the aqueous solubility of a drug determines the concentration presented to the absorption site, and the partition coefficient influences the rate of transport across the absorption site. Drugs generally penetrate the skin better in their un-ionized form. Nonpolar drugs tend to cross the cell barrier through the lipid-rich regions (transcellular route), whereas the polar drugs favor transport between cells (intercellular route) (6).

4. Drugs with molecular weights of 100 to 800 and adequate lipid and aqueous solubility can permeate skin. The ideal molecular weight of a drug for transdermal drug delivery is believed to be 400 or less.

5. Hydration of the skin generally favors percutaneous absorption. The TDDS acts as an occlusive moisture barrier through which sweat cannot pass, increasing skin hydration.

6. Percutaneous absorption appears to be greater when the TDDS is applied to a site with a thin horny layer than with a thick one.

7. Generally, the longer the medicated application is permitted to remain in contact with the skin, the greater is the total drug absorption.

These general statements apply to skin in the normal state. Skin that is abraded or cut permits drugs to gain direct access to the subcutaneous tissues and the capillary network, defeating the function of the TDDS.

Percutaneous Absorption Enhancers

There is great interest among pharmaceutical scientists to develop chemical permeation enhancers and physical methods that can increase percutaneous absorption of therapeutic agents.

Chemical Enhancers

By definition, a chemical skin penetration enhancer *increases skin permeability by reversibly damaging or altering the physicochemical nature of the stratum corneum to reduce its diffusional resistance* (12). Among the alterations are increased hydration of the stratum corneum, a change in the structure of the lipids and lipoproteins in the intercellular channels through solvent action or denaturation, or both (4, 13–17).

Some drugs have an inherent capacity to permeate the skin without chemical enhancers. However, when this is not the case, chemical permeation enhancers may render an otherwise impenetrable substance useful in transdermal drug delivery (17). More than 275 chemical compounds have been cited in the literature as skin penetration enhancers; they include acetone, azone, dimethyl acetamide, dimethyl formamide, dimethyl sulfoxide (DMSO), ethanol, oleic acid, polyethylene glycol, propylene glycol, and sodium lauryl sulfate (13–15). The selection of a permeation enhancer should be based not only on its efficacy in enhancing skin permeation but also on its dermal toxicity (low) and its physicochemical and biologic compatibility with the system's other components (16).

Iontophoresis and Sonophoresis

In addition to chemical means, some physical methods are being used to enhance transdermal drug delivery and penetration, namely, iontophoresis and sonophoresis (6, 15, 18–23). *Iontophoresis* is delivery of a charged chemical compound across the skin membrane using an electrical field. A number of drugs have been the subject of iontophoretic studies; they include lidocaine (18); dexamethasone; amino acids, peptides, and insulin (19, 20); verapamil (6); and propranolol (21). There is particular interest to develop alternative routes for delivery of biologically active peptides. At present these agents are delivered by injection because of their rapid metabolism and poor absorption after oral delivery. They are also poorly absorbed by the transdermal route because of their large molecular size and ionic character and the general impenetrability of the skin (20). However, iontophoresis-enhanced transdermal delivery has shown some promise as a means of peptide and protein administration.

Sonophoresis, or high-frequency ultrasound, is also being studied as a means to enhance transdermal drug delivery (22, 23). Among the agents examined are hydrocortisone, lidocaine, and salicylic acid in such formulations as gels, creams, and lotions. It is thought that high-frequency ultrasound can influence the integrity of the stratum corneum and thus affect its penetrability.

Percutaneous Absorption Models

Skin permeability and percutaneous absorption have been the subject of numerous studies to define the underlying principles and to optimize transdermal drug delivery. Although many experimental methods and models have been used, they tend to fall into one of two categories, in vivo or in vitro.

In Vivo Studies

In vivo skin penetration studies may be undertaken for one or more of the following purposes (24):

1. To verify and quantify the cutaneous bioavailability of a topically applied drug
2. To verify and quantify the systemic bioavailability of a transdermal drug
3. To establish bioequivalence of different topical formulations of the same drug substance
4. To determine the incidence and degree of systemic toxicologic risk following topical application of a specific drug or drug product
5. To relate resultant blood levels of drug in human to systemic therapeutic effects

The most relevant studies are performed in humans; however, animal models may be used insofar as they may be effective as predictors of human response. Animal models include the weanling pig, rhesus monkey, and hairless mouse or rat (24, 25). Biologic samples used in drug penetration and drug absorption studies include skin sections, venous blood from the application site, blood from the systemic circulation, and excreta (urine, feces, and expired air) (24–28).

In Vitro Studies

Skin permeation may be tested in vitro using various skin tissues (human or animal whole skin, dermis or epidermis) in a diffusion cell (29). In vitro penetration studies using human skin are limited because of difficulties of procurement, storage, expense, and variation in permeation (30). Excised animal skins may also vary in quality and permeation. Animal skins are much more permeable than human skin. One alternative that has been shown to be effective is shed snakeskin (*Elaphe obsoleta*, black rat snake), which is nonliving, pure stratum corneum, hairless, and similar to human skin but slightly less permeable (30, 31). Also, the product Living Skin Equivalent (LSE) Testskin (Organogenesis, Inc.) was developed as an alternative for dermal absorption studies. The material is an organotypic coculture of human dermal fibroblasts in a collagen-containing matrix and a stratified epidermis composed of human epidermal keratinocytes. The material may be used in cell culture studies or in standard diffusion cells.

Diffusion cell systems are employed in vitro to quantify the release rates of drugs from topical preparations (32). In these systems, skin membranes or synthetic membranes may be employed as barriers to the flow of drug and vehicle to simulate the biologic system. The typical diffusion cell has two chambers, one on each side of the test diffusion membrane. A temperature-controlled solution of the drug is placed in one chamber and a receptor solution in the other chamber. When skin is used as the test membrane, it separates the two solutions. Drug diffusion through the skin may be determined by periodic sampling and assay of the drug content in the receptor solution. The skin may also be analyzed for drug content to show permeation rates and/or retention in the skin (29).

The *United States Pharmacopeia* (USP) describes the apparatus and procedure to determine dissolution (release) of medication from a transdermal delivery system and provides an acceptance table to which the product must conform to meet the monograph standard for a given article (33). Commercial systems use transdermal diffusion cells and automatic sampling systems to determine the release rates of drugs from transdermal systems (34).

Design Features of Transdermal Drug Delivery Systems

TDDSs (also often called transdermal patches) are designed to support the passage of drug substances from the surface of the skin through its various layers and into the systemic circulation. Examples of the configuration and composition of TDDSs are described in the text, presented in Table 11.1 and shown in Figures 11.1 to 11.4. Figures 11.5 to 11.8 depict the manufacture of TDDSs. Technically, TDDSs may be categorized into two types, monolithic and membrane-controlled systems.

Monolithic systems incorporate a drug matrix layer between backing and frontal layers (Fig. 11.3). The drug–matrix layer is composed of a polymeric material in which the drug is dispersed. The polymer matrix controls the rate at which the drug is released for percutaneous absorption. The matrix may be of two types, either with or without an excess of drug with regard to its equilibrium solubility and steady-state concentration gradient at the stratum corneum (21, 35). In types having no excess, drug is available to maintain the saturation of the stratum corneum only as long as the level of drug in the device exceeds the solubility limit of the stratum corneum. As the concentration of drug in the device diminishes below the skin's saturation limit, the transport of drug from device to skin declines (35). In systems with excess drug in the matrix, a drug

TABLE 11.1 EXAMPLES OF TRANSDERMAL DRUG DELIVERY SYSTEMS (40–44, 47–51)

THERAPEUTIC AGENT	TDDS	DESIGN, CONTENTS	COMMENTS
Clonidine	Catapres-TTS (Boehringer Ingelheim)	Four-layer patch: (*a*) backing of pigmented polyester film; (*b*) reservoir of clonidine, mineral oil, polyisobutylene, colloidal silicon dioxide; (*c*) microporous polypropylene membrane controlling rate of delivery; (*d*) adhesive formulation of agents	Transdermal therapeutic system to deliver therapeutic dose of antihypertensive drug at constant rate for 7 days. TDDS generally applied to hairless or shaven area of upper arm or torso.
Estradiol	Estraderm (Novartis)	Four-layer patch: (*a*) transparent polyester film; (*b*) reservoir of estradiol, alcohol gelled with hydroxypropyl cellulose; (*c*) ethylene–vinyl acetate copolymer membrane; (*d*) adhesive formulation of light mineral oil, polyisobutylene	Transdermal system to release 17β-estradiol continuously. Patch is generally applied to trunk, including abdomen and buttocks, alternating sites, twice weekly over 3-week cycle with dosage frequency adjusted as required.
	Vivelle (Novartis)	Three-layer patch: (*a*) translucent ethylene vinyl alcohol copolymer film; (*b*) estradiol in matrix of medical adhesive of polyisobutylene, ethylene vinyl acetate copolymer; (*c*) polyester release liner, removed prior to application.	Use and application similar to Estraderm TDDS.
	Climara (Berlex)	Three-layer system: (*a*) translucent polyethylene film; (*b*) acrylate adhesive matrix containing estradiol; (*c*) protective liner of siliconized or fluoropolymer-coated polyester film, removed prior to use.	Use and application similar to Estraderm TDDS. System may be applied weekly.
Fentanyl	Duragesic (Janssen)	Four-layer patch: (*a*) backing layer of polyester film; (*b*) reservoir of fentanyl, alcohol gelled with hydroxyethyl cellulose; (*c*) rate-controlling ethylene–vinyl acetate copolymer membrane; (*d*) fentanyl-containing silicone adhesive.	Transdermal therapeutic system providing continuous 72-hour systemic delivery of potent opioid analgesic; indicated in patients with chronic pain requiring opioid analgesia.
Nicotine	Habitrol (Novartis Consumer)	Multilayer round patch: (*a*) aluminized backing film; (*b*) pressure-sensitive acrylate adhesive; (*c*) methacrylic acid copolymer solution of nicotine dispersed in pad of nonwoven viscose, cotton; (*c*) acrylate adhesive layer; (*e*) protective aluminized release liner that overlies adhesive layer, removed prior to use.	Transdermal therapeutic systems providing continuous release, systemic delivery of nicotine to aid smoking cessation. Patches vary somewhat in nicotine content and dosing schedules.
	Nicoderm CQ (SmithKline Beecham Consumer)	Multilayer rectangular patch: (*a*) occlusive backing of polyethylene, aluminum, polyester, ethylene–vinyl acetate copolymer; (*b*) reservoir of nicotine in ethylene–vinyl acetate copolymer matrix; (*c*) rate-controlling polyethylene membrane; (*d*) polyisobutylene adhesive; (*f*) protective liner, removed prior to application.	

(continued)

TABLE 11.1 EXAMPLES OF TRANSDERMAL DRUG DELIVERY SYSTEMS (40–44, 47–51)

THERAPEUTIC AGENT	TDDS	DESIGN, CONTENTS	COMMENTS
	Nicotrol (McNeil Consumer)	Multilayer rectangular patch: (a) outer backing of laminated polyester film; (b) rate-controlling adhesive, non-woven material, nicotine; (c) disposable liner, removed prior to use.	
	Prostep (Lederle)	Multilayer round patch: (a) beige foam tape, acrylate adhesive; (b) backing foil, gelatin, low-density polyethylene coating; (c) nicotine gel matrix; (d) protective foil with well; (e) release liner, removed prior to use.	
Nitroglycerin	Deponit (Schwarz Pharma)	Three-layer system: (a) covering foil; (b) nitroglycerin matrix with polyisobutylene adhesive, plasticizer, release membrane; (e) protective foil, removed before use.	
Nitroglycerin	Nitro-Dur (Key)	Nitroglycerin in gel-like matrix of glycerin, water, lactose, polyvinyl alcohol, povidone, sodium citrate sealed in polyester, foil, polyethylene laminate.	
Nitroglycerin	Transderm-Nitro (Novartis)	Four-layer patch: (a) backing layer of aluminized plastic; (b) reservoir of nitroglycerin adsorbed on lactose, colloidal silicon dioxide, ilicone medical sfluid; (c) ethylene–vinyl acetate copolymer membrane; (d) silicone adhesive.	
Scopolamine	Transderm Scop (Novartis Consumer)	Four-layer patch: (a) backing layer of aluminized polyester film; (b) reservoir of scopolamine, mineral oil, polyisobutylene; (c) microporous polypropylene membrane for rate delivery of scopolamine; (d) adhesive of polyisobutylene, mineral oil, scopolamine	Continuous release of drug over 3 days to prevent nausea, vomiting of motion sickness. Patch is placed behind ear. For repeated administration, first patch is removed and second placed behind other ear. Also approved to prevent nausea of certain anesthetics and analgesics used in surgery.
Testosterone	Testoderm (Alza)	Three-layer patch: (a) backing layer of polyethylene terephthalate; (b) matrix film layer of testosterone, ethylene–vinyl acetate copolymer; (c) adhesive strips of polyisobutylene, colloidal silicone dioxide.	Patch is placed on scrotum in treatment of testosterone deficiency.
	Androderm (SmithKline Beecham)	Five-layer patch: (a) backing film of ethylene–vinyl acetate copolymer, polyester laminate; (b) reservoir of testosterone, alcohol, glycerin, glyceryl mono-oleate, methyl laurate gelled with acrylic acid copolymer; (c) microporous polyethylene membrane; (d) acrylic adhesive; (d) adhesive polyester laminate.	Patch is placed on back, abdomen, upper arms, or thighs for treatment of testosterone deficiency.

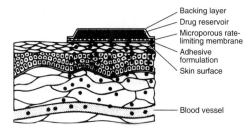

FIGURE 11.1 Four-layer therapeutic transdermal system showing the continuous and controlled amount of medication released from the system, permeating the skin, and entering the systemic circulation (Courtesy of Alza Corporation).

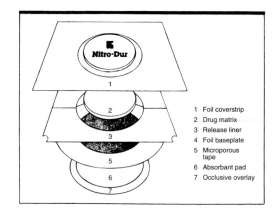

FIGURE 11.3 Nitro-Dur Transdermal Infusion System: construction of the product (Courtesy of Key Pharmaceuticals).

reserve is present to ensure continued saturation at the stratum corneum. In these instances, the rate of drug decline is less than in the type having no reserve.

In the preparation of monolithic systems, the drug and the polymer are dissolved or blended together, cast as the matrix, and dried (21). The gelled matrix may be produced in sheet or cylindrical form, with individual dosage units cut and assembled between the backing and frontal layers. Most TDDSs are designed to contain an excess of drug and thus have drug-releasing capacity beyond the time frame recommended for replacement. This ensures continuous drug availability and absorption as used TDDSs are replaced on schedule with fresh ones.

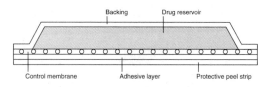

FIGURE 11.2 The Transderm-Nitro Transdermal Therapeutic System (Summit). The patch delivers nitroglycerin through the skin directly into the blood stream for 24 hours. Transderm-Nitro is used to treat and prevent angina. The system consists of a water-resistant backing layer, a reservoir of nitroglycerin, followed by a semipermeable membrane to control precisely and predictably the release of medicine, and an adhesive layer to hold the system onto the skin. The adhesive layer also contains an initial priming dose of nitroglycerin to ensure prompt release and absorption of the medication. (Courtesy of Summit Pharmaceuticals, Novartis).

Membrane-controlled transdermal systems are designed to contain a drug reservoir, or pouch, usually in liquid or gel form, a rate-controlling membrane, and backing, adhesive, and protecting layers (Fig. 11.2). Transderm-Nitro (Novartis) and Transderm-Scop (Novartis) are examples of this technology. Membrane-controlled systems have the advantage over monolithic systems in that as long as the drug solution in the reservoir remains saturated, the release rate of drug through the controlling membrane remains constant (21, 22). In membrane systems, a small quantity of drug is frequently placed in the adhesive layer to initiate prompt drug absorption and pharmacotherapeutic effects on skin placement. Membrane-controlled systems may be prepared by preconstructing the delivery unit, filling the drug reservoir, and sealing or by lamination, a continuous process of construction, dosing, and sealing (Figs. 11.5 to 11.8).

In summary, either the drug delivery device or the skin may serve as the rate-controlling mechanism. If the drug is delivered to the stratum corneum at a rate less than the absorption capacity, the *device* is the controlling factor; if the drug is delivered to the skin area to saturation, the *skin* is the controlling factor. Thus, the rate of drug transport in all TDDSs, monolithic and membrane, is controlled by either artificial or natural (skin) membranes.

Transdermal drug delivery systems may be constructed of a number of layers, including (*a*) an occlusive backing membrane to protect

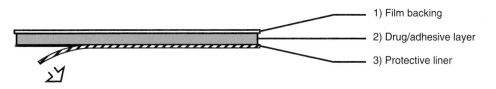

1) Film backing
2) Drug/adhesive layer
3) Protective liner

FIGURE 11.4 Two-layer transdermal drug delivery system, showing removal of the protective liner prior to application.

the system from environmental entry and from loss of drug from the system or moisture from the skin; (*b*) a drug reservoir or matrix system to store and release the drug at the skin site; (*c*) a release liner, which is removed before application and enables drug release; and (*d*) an adhesive layer to maintain contact with the skin after application. Two types of adhesive layers,

the peripheral adhesive and the face adhesive, can be used. The peripheral adhesive contains adhesive around the outer edge of the TDDS, usually in a wide strip surrounding the active drug portion. The face adhesive, which covers the entire face of the TDDS, is very common. TDDSs are packaged in individual sealed packets to preserve and protect them until use.

The backing layer must be occlusive to retain skin moisture and hydrate the site of application, enabling increased drug penetration. Preferred backing materials are approximately 2 to 3 mm thick and have a low moisture vapor transmission rate, less than about 20 g/m^2 in 24 hours (36). Transparent or pigmented films of polypropylene, polyethylene, and polyolefin are in use in TDDSs as backing liners.

The adhesive layer must be pressure sensitive, providing the ability to adhere to the skin with minimal pressure and remain in place for the intended period of wear. The adhesive should be nonirritating, allow easy peel-off after use, permit unimpeded drug flux to the skin, and be compatible with all other system components. The adhesive material is usually safety tested for skin compatibility, including tests for irritation, sensitivity, and cytotoxicity (37). In some TDDSs, the adhesive layer contains the drug. Polybutyl acrylate is commonly

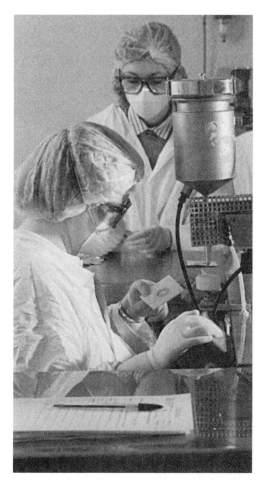

FIGURE 11.5 Pilot-scale manufacture of transdermal patches. (Courtesy of Elan Corporation, plc.)

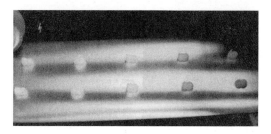

FIGURE 11.6 Measured dose for reservoir, placed on web prior to sealing into the transdermal delivery system. (Courtesy of CIBA Pharmaceutical Company)

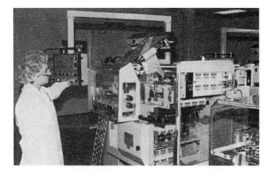

FIGURE 11.7 Equipment used in cutting and packaging transdermal drug delivery patches (Courtesy of Schering Laboratories).

used as the adhesive in TDDSs. The drug release membranes are commonly made of polyethylene, with microporous structures of varying pore sizes to fit the desired specifications of the particular transdermal system.

Included among the design objectives of TDDSs are the following (2,8,35,38–39):

1. Deliver the drug to the skin for percutaneous absorption at therapeutic levels at an optimal rate
2. Contain medicinal agents having the necessary physicochemical characteristics to release from the system and partition into the stratum corneum
3. Occlude the skin to ensure one-way flux of the drug into the stratum corneum
4. Have a therapeutic advantage over other dosage forms and drug delivery systems

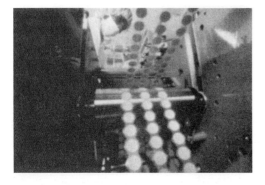

FIGURE 11.8 Rotary die cutting pressure executes the final step in manufacturing Transderm Scop systems prior to packaging (Courtesy of Alza Corporation).

5. Not irritate or sensitize the skin
6. Adhere well to the patient's skin and have size, appearance, and site placement that encourage acceptance

Advantages and Disadvantages of TDDSs

Among the advantages of TDDSs are the following:

1. They can avoid gastrointestinal drug absorption difficulties caused by gastrointestinal pH, enzymatic activity, and drug interactions with food, drink, and other orally administered drugs.
2. They can substitute for oral administration of medication when that route is unsuitable, as with vomiting and diarrhea.
3. They avoid the *first-pass effect*, that is, the initial pass of a drug substance through the systemic and portal circulation following gastrointestinal absorption, possibly avoiding the deactivation by digestive and liver enzymes.
4. They are noninvasive, avoiding the inconvenience of parenteral therapy.
5. They provide extended therapy with a single application, improving compliance over other dosage forms requiring more frequent dose administration.
6. The activity of drugs having a short half-life is extended through the reservoir of drug in the therapeutic delivery system and its controlled release.
7. Drug therapy may be terminated rapidly by removal of the application from the surface of the skin.
8. They are easily and rapidly identified in emergencies (e.g., unresponsive, unconscious, or comatose patient) because of their physical presence, features, and identifying markings.

The disadvantages of TDDSs are as follows:

1. Only relatively potent drugs are suitable candidates for transdermal delivery because of the natural limits of drug entry imposed by the skin's impermeability.
2. Some patients develop contact dermatitis at the site of application from one or more of

the system components, necessitating discontinuation.

Examples of Transdermal Drug Delivery Systems

The following sections briefly describe some of the TDDSs in use. Table 11.1 describes the specific design components of representative examples of these systems.

Transdermal Scopolamine

As noted at the outset of this chapter, transdermal scopolamine was the first TDDS to receive FDA approval. Scopolamine, a belladonna alkaloid, is used to prevent travel-related motion sickness and the nausea and vomiting that result from the use of certain anesthetics and analgesics used in surgery.

The Transderm-Scop system is a circular flat patch 0.2 mm thick and 2.5 cm^2 in area (40). It is a four-layer system described in Table 11.1. The TDDS contains 1.5 mg of scopolamine and is designed to deliver approximately 1 mg of scopolamine at an approximately constant rate to the systemic circulation over the 3-day lifetime of the system. An initial priming dose of 200 μg of scopolamine in the adhesive layer of the system saturates the skin binding sites and rapidly brings the plasma concentration to the required steady-state level. The continuous release of scopolamine through the rate-controlling microporous membrane maintains the plasma level constant. The rate of release is less than the skin's capability for absorption, so the membrane, not the skin, controls the delivery of the drug into the circulation.

The patch is worn in a hairless area behind the ear (Fig. 11.9). Because of the small size of the patch, the system is unobtrusive, convenient, and well accepted by the patient. The TDDS is applied at least 4 hours before the antinausea effect is required. Only one disk should be worn at a time and may be kept in place for up to 3 days. If continued treatment is required, a fresh disk is placed behind the other ear. The most common side effects are dryness of the mouth and drowsiness. Particularly in the geriatric population, use also may

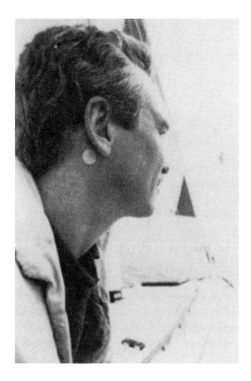

FIGURE 11.9 Transderm Scop (scopolamine) disk provides protection from the nausea and vomiting of motion sickness (Courtesy of Alza Corporation and CIBA Consumer Pharmaceuticals).

interfere with orientation, cognition, and memory. The TDDS is not intended for use in children and should be used with caution during pregnancy.

Transdermal Nitroglycerin

A number of nitroglycerin-containing TDDSs have been developed, including Deponit (Schwarz), Minitran (3M Pharmaceuticals), Nitro-Dur (Key) and Transderm-Nitro (Novartis). The design of each of these systems briefly is described in Table 11.1. Each of these products maintains nitroglycerin drug delivery for 24 hours after application.

Nitroglycerin is used widely in the prophylactic treatment of angina. It has a relatively low dose, short plasma half-life, high peak plasma levels, and inherent side effects when taken sublingually, a popular route. It is rapidly metabolized by the liver when taken orally; this first-pass effect is bypassed by the transdermal route.

The various nitroglycerin TDDSs control the rate of drug delivery through a membrane and/or controlled release from the matrix or reservoir. When a TDDS is applied to the skin, nitroglycerin is absorbed continuously, resulting in active drug reaching the target organs (heart, extremities) before inactivation by the liver. Only a portion of the total nitroglycerin in the system is delivered over the usual 24-hour use period; the remainder serves as the thermodynamic energy source to release the drug and remains in the system. For example, in the Deponit TDDS, only 15% of the nitroglycerin content is delivered after 12 hours of use (41).

The rate of drug release depends on the system. In the Transderm-Nitro system, nitroglycerin 0.02 mg is delivered per hour for every square centimeter of patch, whereas in the Deponit system, each square centimeter delivers approximately 0.013 mg of nitroglycerin per hour (41, 42). Systems of various surface areas and nitroglycerin content are provided to accommodate individual patients' requirements. Because of different release rates, these systems cannot be used interchangeably by a patient.

The Nitro-Dur matrix is in a highly kinetic equilibrium state (43). Dissolved nitroglycerin molecules are constantly exchanging with adsorbed nitroglycerin molecules bound to the surfaces of the suspended lactose crystals. Sufficient nitroglycerin is adsorbed to the lactose in each matrix to maintain nitroglycerin in the fluid phase (aqueous glycerol) at a stable but saturated level (5 mg nitroglycerin/cm^2 matrix). When the matrix is applied to the skin, nitroglycerin molecules migrate by diffusion from solution in the matrix to solution in the skin. To make up for the molecules lost to the body, the equilibrium in the matrix shifts such that more molecules of nitroglycerin leave the crystals than are adsorbed from solution. When balance is restored, the solution is again saturated. Thus, the crystals of lactose act as a reservoir of drug to maintain drug saturation in the fluid phase. The Nitro-Dur matrix in turn acts as a saturated reservoir for diffusive drug input through the skin (43).

Not all nitroglycerin systems have the same construction. For example, the Transderm-Nitro TDDS is a four-layer drug pouch system, as described in Table 11.1 and depicted in Figure 11.2, whereas the Deponit TDDS is a thin two-layer matrix system resembling that shown in Figure 11.4.

Patients should be given explicit instructions regarding the use of nitroglycerin transdermal systems. Generally, these TDDSs are placed on the chest, back, upper arms, or shoulders (Fig. 11.10). The site should be free

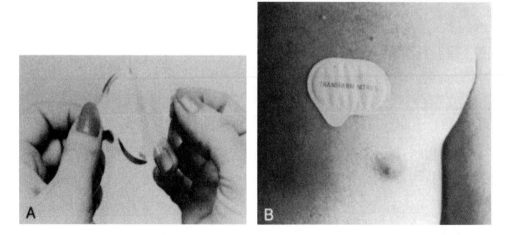

FIGURE 11.10 Transderm-Nitro patch. Before application to the skin a plastic liner is removed, exposing the adhesive side of the patch. Transderm-Nitro delivers nitroglycerin at a constant and predetermined rate through the skin directly into the blood stream. The patch is designed to provide 24-hour protection against angina attacks (Courtesy of Alza Corporation and CIBA Pharmaceuticals, Novartis).

of hair, clean, and dry so that the patch adheres without difficulty. The use of the extremities below the knee or elbow is discouraged, as are areas that are abraded or have lesions or cuts. The patient should understand that physical exercise and elevated ambient temperatures, such as in a sauna, may increase the absorption of nitroglycerin.

Transdermal Clonidine

The first transdermal system for hypertension, Catapres TTS (clonidine transdermal therapeutic system, Boehringer Ingelheim), was marketed in 1985. Clonidine lends itself to transdermal delivery because of its lipid solubility, high volume of distribution, and therapeutic effectiveness in low plasma concentrations. The TDDS provides controlled release of clonidine for 7 days. The product is a four-layer patch as described in Table 11.1.

Catapres TTS is available in several sizes, with the amount of drug released proportional to the patch size. To ensure constant release over the 7-day use period, the drug content is greater than the total amount of drug delivered. The energy of drug release derives from the concentration gradient between a saturated solution of drug in the TDDS and the much lower concentration prevailing in the skin. Clonidine flows in the direction of lower concentration at a constant rate controlled by a membrane (44).

The system is applied to a hairless area of intact skin on the upper outer arm or chest. After application, clonidine in the adhesive layer saturates the skin site. Then clonidine from the reservoir begins to flow through the rate-controlling membrane and the skin to the systemic circulation. Therapeutic plasma clonidine levels are achieved 2 to 3 days after initial application. Application of a new system to a fresh skin site at weekly intervals maintains therapeutic plasma concentrations. If the patch is removed and not replaced with a new system, therapeutic plasma clonidine levels will persist for about 8 hours and then decline slowly over several days. Over this period, blood pressure returns gradually to pretreatment levels. If the patient has local skin irritation before 7 days of use, the

system may be removed and replaced with a new one applied on a fresh skin site (44).

Transdermal Nicotine

Nicotine TDDSs are used as adjuncts (e.g., along with counseling) in smoking cessation programs. They have been shown to be an effective aid in quitting smoking when used according to product-recommended strategies (45). In a blinded study, users of nicotine TDDSs are more than twice as likely to quit smoking as individuals wearing a placebo patch (45).

The nicotine TDDSs provide sustained blood levels of nicotine as nicotine replacement therapy to help the patient establish and sustain remission from smoking (46). Motivation to quit smoking is enhanced through the reduction of withdrawal symptoms and by partially satisfying the nicotine craving and desired sensory feelings provided by smoking (46).

The commercially available patches contain 7 to 22 mg of nicotine for daily application during the course of treatment ranging from about 6 to 12 weeks. Different treatment regimens are used for light versus heavy smokers. Examples of nicotine TDDSs are described in Table 11.1. A nicotine TDDS usually is applied to the arm or upper front torso, with patients advised not to smoke when wearing the system. The TDDS is replaced daily, with sites alternated. Some of the nicotine replacement programs provide a gradual reduction in nicotine dosage (patch strength) during the treatment program. Used TDDSs should be discarded properly, because the retained nicotine is poisonous to children and pets.

Transdermal Estradiol

The estrogen estradiol has been developed for transdermal delivery. The Estraderm (Novartis) TDDS delivers 17β-estradiol through a rate-limiting membrane continuously upon application to intact skin (47). Two systems (10 or 20 cm^2) provide delivery of 0.05 or 0.1 mg estradiol per day. Estraderm is a four-layer TDDS as described in Table 11.1.

Estradiol is indicated for the treatment of moderate to severe vasomotor symptoms associated with menopause, female hypogonadism, female castration, primary ovarian failure, and atrophic conditions caused by deficient endogenous estrogen production, such as atrophic vaginitis and kraurosis vulvae.

Orally administered estradiol is rapidly metabolized by the liver to estrone and its conjugates, giving rise to higher circulating levels of estrone than estradiol. In contrast, the skin metabolizes estradiol only to a small extent. Therefore, transdermal administration produces therapeutic serum levels of estradiol with lower circulating levels of estrone and estrone conjugates than does oral therapy and requires a smaller total dose. Research has demonstrated that postmenopausal women receiving either transdermal or oral therapy will obtain the desired therapeutic effects, that is, lower gonadotropin levels, lower percentages of vaginal parabasal cells, decreased excretion of calcium, and lower ratio of calcium to creatinine, from both dosage forms. Studies have also demonstrated that systemic side effects from oral estrogens can be reduced by using the transdermal dosage form. Because estradiol has a short half-life (about 1 hour), transdermal administration allows a rapid decline in blood levels after the transdermal system is removed, as in a cycling regimen (47).

Therapy is usually administered on a cyclic schedule (3 weeks of therapy followed by 1 week without), especially in women who have not undergone a hysterectomy. The transdermal system is applied to a clean, dry area of the skin on the trunk of the body, either the abdomen or upper quadrant of the buttocks. The patch should not be applied to the waistline, because tight clothing may damage or dislodge it.

The Vivelle (Novartis) and Climara (Berlex) estradiol TDDSs are two-layered matrix systems described in Table 11.1 and resembling that shown in Figure 11.4. The estradiol is contained in the adhesive layer (48, 49). These systems are used in the same general manner as Estraderm TDDS; however, some of these systems are applied every 7 days.

Transdermal Contraceptive System

The Ortho Evra (norelgestromin, ethinyl estradiol) Transdermal System is a combination contraceptive patch with a contact surface area of 20 cm^2; it contains 6 mg of norelgestromin and 0.75 mg of ethyl estradiol. It is released at a rate of norelgestromin 150 μg and ethinyl estradiol 20 μg into the blood stream every 24 hours.

The Ortho Evra is a thin matrix-type transdermal contraceptive patch consisting of three layers, including a two-ply backing layer composed of beige flexible film of low-density polyethylene and a polyester inner ply. The middle layer contains polyisobutylene and polybutene adhesive, crospovidone, nonwoven polyester fabric, and lauryl lactate as inactive components; the norelgestromin and ethinyl estradiol are in this layer. The third layer is the release liner that protects the adhesive layer during storage and is removed just prior to application. It is a transparent polyethylene terephthalate (PET) film with a polydimethylsiloxane coating on the side that is in contact with the middle layer.

Transdermal Testosterone

The testosterone transdermal systems Testoderm (Alza) and Androderm (SmithKline Beecham) are available with various delivery rates as hormone replacement therapy in men who have an absence or deficiency of testosterone (50, 51).

The Testoderm TDDS is a two-layer system as described in Table 11.1. For optimal absorption, it is applied to clean, dry scrotal skin that has been dry-shaved. Scrotal skin is reported to be at least five times as permeable to testosterone as other skin sites (50). The TDDS is placed on the scrotum by stretching the scrotal skin with one hand and pressing the adhesive side of the TDDS against the skin with the other hand, holding it in place for about 10 seconds. The TDDS is applied daily, usually in the morning to mimic endogenous testosterone release (52). Optimum serum levels are reached within 2 to 4 hours after application. The patch is worn 22 to 24 hours daily for 6 to 8 weeks.

The Androderm TDDS is designed to be applied nightly to a clean, dry, unabraded area of the skin of the back, abdomen, upper arms, or thighs. It should not be applied to the scrotum

(51). The five-layer system is described in Table 11.1.

Other Transdermal Therapeutic Systems

Drugs under study for use in TDDSs include diltiazem, isosorbide dinitrate, propranolol, nifedipine, mepindolol and verapamil, cardiovascular agents; levonorgestrel with estradiol for hormonal contraception; physostigmine and xanomeline for Alzheimer's disease therapy; naltrexone and methadone for substance addiction; buspirone for anxiety; bupropion for smoking cessation; and papaverine for male impotence.

General Clinical Considerations in the Use of TDDSs

The patient should be advised of the following general guidelines along with product-specific instructions in the use of TDDSs (53, 54).

1. Percutaneous absorption may vary with the site of application. The preferred general application site is stated in the package insert for each product. The patient should be advised of the importance of using the recommended site and rotating locations within that site. Rotating locations is important to allow the skin beneath a patch to regain its normal permeability after being occluded and to prevent skin irritation. Skin sites may be reused after a week.

2. TDDSs should be applied to clean, dry skin that is relatively free of hair and not oily, irritated, inflamed, broken, or callused. Wet or moist skin can accelerate drug permeation beyond the intended rate. Oily skin can impair adhesion of the patch. If hair is present at the intended site, it should be carefully cut, not wet-shaved, nor should a depilatory agent be used, since the latter can remove the outermost layers of the stratum corneum and affect the rate and extent of drug permeation.

3. Use of skin lotion should be avoided at the application site, because lotions affect skin hydration and can alter the partition coefficient between the drug and the skin.

4. TDDSs should not be physically altered by cutting (as in an attempt to reduce the dose), since this destroys the integrity of the system.

5. A TDDS should be removed from its protective package, with care not to tear or cut into the unit. The protective backing should be removed to expose the adhesive layer with care not to touch the adhesive surface (which sometimes contains drug) to the fingertips. The TDDS should be pressed firmly against the skin site with the heel of the hand for about 10 seconds to ensure uniform contact and adhesion.

6. A TDDS should be placed at a site that will not subject it to being rubbed off by clothing or movement (as the belt line). TDDSs generally may be left on when showering, bathing, or swimming. Should a TDDS prematurely dislodge, an attempt may be made to reapply it or it may be replaced with a fresh system, the replacement being worn for a full period before it is replaced.

7. A TDDS should be worn for the full period stated in the product's instructions. Following that period, it should be removed and replaced with a fresh system as directed.

8. The patient or caregiver should be instructed to cleanse the hands thoroughly before and after applying a TDDS. Care should be taken not to rub the eyes or touch the mouth during handling of the system.

9. If the patient exhibits sensitivity or intolerance to a TDDS or if undue skin irritation results, the patient should seek reevaluation.

10. Upon removal, a used TDDS should be folded in half with the adhesive layer together so that it cannot be reused. The used patch, which contains residual drug, should be placed in the replacement patch's pouch and discarded in a manner safe to children and pets.

PHARMACEUTICS CASE STUDY

Subjective

Working at a large transdermal drug delivery company, you have been given the responsibility of developing an analgesic drug delivery system for use in patients with moderate to severe chronic pain. After development of several prototypes, one is selected that delivers the drug at a rapid rate for the first 12 hours, then at a zero-order rate over the next 36 hours. In clinical trials, however, patients who tended to sweat excessively had to use a new patch about every 6 to 12 hours, as the previous patch would not adhere. They were instructed that if the patch would not adhere after repeated attempts to reapply it, it was to be removed and a new patch applied. These patients had central nervous system depression and respiratory depression as compared to patients who could use a single patch over the 48-hour period. The patients who had to replace the patch early also had blood levels in the toxic range for the drug.

Objective

The release rate of the TDDS was designed to provide a rapid onset of action by providing a high rate of drug transfer after application of the patch from the drug in the adhesive. This high rate of drug flux occurred with repeated application of each new patch. The analgesic

drug is highly lipophilic, and a very low dose (microgram range) is all that is required.

Assessment

There was an initial loading dose of the drug in the adhesive layer and a combination of penetration enhancers in the matrix of the TDDS, including alcohol. The lipophilic nature of the drug apparently resulted in a depot effect of the drug in the fatty tissue of the skin. The drug rapidly moved from the adhesive layer and was followed by the movement of active drug in solution in the alcohol and other penetration enhancers. After the alcohol was depleted in the TDDS matrix, the flux of drug slowed to a near-zero order release.

Plan

Available options include changing the formulation and adding a label caution statement. Changing the formulation would require extensive changes and new in vitro, animal, and clinical studies. A labeling statement could warn against application of a new patch for a preselected time period, such as approximately 12 hours after removal of a patch that would not adhere if it had been applied for less than 24 hours. This would allow for a depletion of the drug buildup in the skin.

CLINICAL CASE STUDY

A. R. is a 20 y/o BF who comes into the pharmacy with concerns because she has missed the last two birth control tablets in week 2 of her cycle. She says, "It's so hard to remember to take the pill every night." She is a student at a local junior college, and her irregular work schedule seems to be the major contributing factor to her lack of adherence. She

expresses concern about the possibility of becoming pregnant and asks for your advice.

PMH: Noncontributory
SH: (+) Smoker (~1 PPD)
       Exercises 3 days per week
FH: Father (+) DM type 2
       Grandmother (+) ovarian cancer

Clinical Case Study cont.

MEDS: Ibuprofen 400 mg po prn cramps
Ortho Tri-Cyclen 1 tablet po qd

Pharmaceutical Care Plan

S: Lack of adherence to birth control pill regimen

O: Smoker
Grandmother (+) ovarian cancer
Father (+) DM type 2

A: A. R. is a 20 y/o BF with a history of lack of adherence to her oral contraceptive regimen. She is a student with an irregular schedule. A. R. smokes about a pack of cigarettes per day and has a family history of diabetes mellitus and ovarian cancer.

P: 1. Suggest to the patient that she contact her physician to change her prescription from an oral contraceptive tablet to a transdermal birth control patch, Ortho Evra.

2. Assuming that the physician concurs and prescribes Ortho Evra, inform the patient that the patch is applied once a week for 3 consecutive weeks, followed by 1 week that is patch free. This should help her compliance because she will have to remember to change the patch only once weekly. However, it will be good to have her write a reminder down somewhere to change the patch on the same day each week. She should not write the date on the patch. It is important for A. R. to know that she should remove the old patch before applying the new patch.

3. When changing over from her oral contraceptive tablet to the transdermal drug delivery system, she should understand to apply the first patch on the first day of her menstrual period. The patch can be applied to her abdomen, buttocks, upper torso (front or back, except the breasts), and the upper outer arm. The patient can rotate the placement of the patch to a different location each week. However, this is not necessary.

4. The patch is to be applied to clean, dry skin. There should be no body lotion or oils on the skin where the patch will be applied. A. R. can shower, bathe, exercise, and swim while the patch is in place. If the patch gets loose or falls off less than 24 hours after application, the patient can reapply it or get a replacement patch at the pharmacy. If a replacement patch is applied, the patient must replace it with the next patch on the original patch change day. However, if it is beyond 24 hours since the initial application of that patch, the patient must start her cycle all over. That is, the patient will start a new 4-week cycle with a new patch change day. In that case, the patient must use backup contraceptive measures, such as condom, spermicide, or diaphragm, for the first week.

5. The patient should be made aware that smoking increases her risk of heart problems, such as blood clots, stroke, and heart attacks, when using a hormonal contraceptive product. A. R. should be encouraged to quit smoking. If the patient agrees that she would like to quit, be prepared to suggest a local wellness program where she can get help and support. Most important, to have an opportunity to quit smoking, she has to make a firm commitment to want to stop smoking.

6. Monitoring: Because the patient has a family history of ovarian cancer, she should be strongly encouraged to have annual Pap smears. In addition, the patient should be advised to continue to exercise regularly and increase her frequency to 4 or 5 days per week. An increase in exercise and a well-balanced diet will be advantageous in the prevention of diabetes mellitus type 2, as her family demonstrates a history of this disease.

REFERENCES

1. Stoughton RD. Percutaneous absorption. Toxicol Appl Pharmacol 1965;7:1–8.
2. Black CD. Transdermal drug delivery systems. US Pharm 1982;1:49.
3. Shah VP, Behl CR, Flynn GL, et al. Principles and criteria in the development and optimization of topical therapeutic products. Pharm Res 1992;9:1107–1111.
4. Walters KA. Percutaneous absorption and transdermal therapy. Pharm Tech 1986;10:30–42.
5. Hadgraft J. Structure activity relationships and percutaneous absorption. J Controlled Release 1991;25: 221–226.
6. Ghosh TK, Banga AK. Methods of enhancement of transdermal drug delivery, part I: physical and biochemical approaches. Pharm Tech 1993;17:72–98.
7. Surber C et al. Optimization of topical therapy: partitioning of drugs into stratum corneum. Pharm Res 1990; 7:1320–1324.
8. Cleary GW. Transdermal concepts and perspectives. Miami: Key Pharmaceuticals, 1982.
9. Melendres JL et al. In vivo percutaneous absorption of hydrocortisone: multiple-application dosing in man. Pharm Res 1992;9:1164.
10. Barr M. Percutaneous absorption. J Pharm Sci 1962; 51:395–409.
11. Idson B. Percutaneous absorption. J Pharm Sci 1975; 64:901–924.
12. Shah VP, Peck CC, Williams RL. Skin penetration enhancement: clinical pharmacological and regulatory considerations. In: Walters KA and Hadgraft J, eds. Pharmaceutical skin penetration enhancement. New York: Dekker, 1993.
13. Osborne DW, Henke JJ. Skin penetration enhancers cited in the technical literature. Pharm Tech 1997;21: 50–66.
14. Idson B. Percutaneous absorption enhancers. Drug Cosmetic Ind 1985;137:30.
15. Rolf D. Chemical and physical methods of enhancing transdermal drug delivery. Pharm Tech 1988;12: 130–139.
16. Ghosh TK, Banga AK. Methods of enhancement of transdermal drug delivery, part IIA: chemical permeation enhancers. Pharm Tech 1993;17:62–90.
17. Ghosh TK, Banga AK. Methods of enhancement of transdermal drug delivery, part IIB: chemical permeation enhancers. Pharm Tech 1993;17:68–76.
18. Riviere JE, Monteiro-Riviere NA, Inman AO. Determination of lidocaine concentrations in skin after transdermal iontophoresis: effects of vasoactive drugs. Pharm Res 1992;9:211–219.
19. Green PG, Hinz RS, Cullander C, Yamane G, Guy RH. Iontophoretic delivery of amino acids and amino acid derivatives across the skin in vitro. Pharm Res 1991;8:1113–1120.
20. Choi HK, Flynn GL, Amidon GL. Transdermal delivery of bioactive peptides: the effect of n-decylmethyl sulfoxide, pH, and inhibitors on enkephalin metabolism and transport. Pharm Res 1990;7:1099–1106.

21. D'Emanuele A, Staniforth JN. An electrically modulated drug delivery device III: factors affecting drug stability during electrophoresis. Pharm Res 1992;9:312–315.
22. Bommannan D, Okuyama H, Stauffer P, Guy RH. Sonophoresis I: the use of high-frequency ultrasound to enhance transdermal drug delivery. Pharm Res 1992;9:559–564.
23. Bommannan D, Menon GK, Okuyama H, Elias PM, Guy RH. Sonophoresis II: examination of the mechanism(s) of ultrasound-enhanced transdermal drug delivery. Pharm Res 1992;9:1043–1047.
24. Shah VP et al. In vivo percutaneous penetration/absorption. Pharm Res 1991;8:1071–1075.
25. Bronaugh RL, Stewart RF, Congdon ER. Methods for in vitro percutaneous absorption studies II. Animal models for human skin. Toxicol Appl Pharmacol 1982;62:481–488.
26. Nugent FJ, Wood JA. Methods for the study of percutaneous absorption. Can J Pharm Sci 1980;15: 1–7.
27. Addicks W et al. Topical drug delivery from thin applications: theoretical predictions and experimental results. Pharm Res 1990;7:1048–1054.
28. Kushla GP, Zatz JL. Evaluation of a noninvasive method for monitoring percutaneous absorption of lidocaine in vivo. Pharm Res 1990;7:1033–1037.
29. Chaisson D. Dissolution performance testing of transdermal systems. Dissolution Technol 1995;2:8–11.
30. Itoh T, Magavi R, Casady RL, Nishihata T, Rytting JH. A method to predict the percutaneous permeability of various compounds: shed snake skin as a model membrane. Pharm Res 1990;7:1302–1306.
31. Itoh T, Wasinger L, Turunen TM, Rytting JH. Effects of transdermal penetration enhancers on the permeability of shed snakeskin. Pharm Res 1992;9: 1168–1172.
32. Rolland A, Demichelis G, Jamoulle JC, Shroot B. Influence of formulation, receptor fluid, and occlusion on in vitro drug release from topical dosage forms, using an automated flow-through diffusion cell. Pharm Res 1992;9:82–86.
33. United States Pharmacopeia, 26th ed. Rockville, MD: U.S. Pharmacopeial Convention, 2003.
34. Microette Transdermal Diffusion Cell Autosampling System. Chattsworth CA: Hanson Research, 1992.
35. Good WR. Transdermal drug-delivery systems. Medical Device Diagnost Ind 1986;8:37–42.
36. Godbey KL. Development of a novel transdermal drug delivery backing film with a low moisture vapor transmission rate. Pharm Tech 1997;21:98–107.
37. 3M transdermal drug delivery components. St. Paul: 3M,1996.
38. Fara JW. Short- and long-term transdermal drug delivery systems. In: Drug delivery systems. Pharm Tech. Springfield, OR: Aster, 1983:33–40.
39. Shaw JE, Chadrasekaran SK. Controlled topical delivery of drugs of systemic action. Drug Metab Rev 1978;8:223.
40. Transderm-Scop Transdermal Therapeutic System: professional literature. Summit, NJ: Novartis Consumer Pharmaceuticals, 1998.

41. Deponit Nitroglycerin Transdermal Delivery System: professional literature. Milwaukee: Schwarz Pharma, 1998.
42. Transderm-Nitro Transdermal Therapeutic System: professional literature. East Hanover, NJ: Novartis Pharmaceuticals, 1998.
43. Nitro-Dur Transdermal Infusion System: professional literature. Kenilworth, NJ: Key Pharmaceuticals, 1998.
44. Catapress-TTS: professional literature. Ridgefield, CT: Boehringer Ingelheim Pharmaceuticals, 1998.
45. Fiore MC, Smith SS, Jorenby DE, Baker TB. The effectiveness of the nicotine patch for smoking cessation. JAMA 1994;271:1940–1947.
46. Wongwiwatthananukit S, Jack HM, Popovich NG. Smoking cessation, part 2: pharmacologic approaches. JAPhA 1998;38:339–353.
47. Estraderm Estradiol Transdermal System: professional literature. East Hanover, NJ: Novartis Pharmaceuticals, 1998.
48. Vivelle Estradiol Transdermal System: professional literature. East Hanover, NJ: Novartis Pharmaceuticals, 1998.
49. Climara Estradiol Transdermal System: professional literature. Wayne, NJ: Berlex Laboratories, 1998.
50. Testoderm Testosterone Transdermal System: professional literature. Palo Alto: Alza Pharmaceuticals, 1998.
51. Androderm Testosterone Transdermal System: professional literature. Philadelphia: SmithKline Beecham Pharmaceuticals, 1998.
52. Levien T, Baker DE. Reviews of transdermal testosterone and liposomal doxorubicin. Hosp Pharm 1996;31:973–988.
53. Black CD. A pharmacist's guide to the use of transdermal medication. Washington: American Pharmaceutical Association, 1996.
54. Berba J, Banakar U. Clinical efficacy of current transdermal drug delivery systems: a retrospective evaluation. Am Pharm 1990;NS30:33–41.

Suppositories and Inserts

12

Chapter at a glance

Suppositories

Suppositories are solid dosage forms intended for insertion into body orifices where they melt, soften, or dissolve and exert local or systemic effects. The derivation of the word *suppository* is from the Latin *supponere*, meaning "to place under," as derived from *sub* (under) and *ponere* (to place) (1). Thus, suppositories are meant both linguistically and therapeutically to be placed under the body, as into the rectum.

Suppositories are commonly used rectally and vaginally and occasionally urethrally. They have various shapes and weights (Fig. 12.1). The shape and size of a suppository must be such that it can be easily inserted into the intended orifice without causing undue distension, and once inserted, it must be retained for the appropriate period. Rectal suppositories are inserted with the fingers, but certain vaginal suppositories, particularly the inserts, or tablets prepared by compression, may be inserted high in the tract with the aid of an appliance.

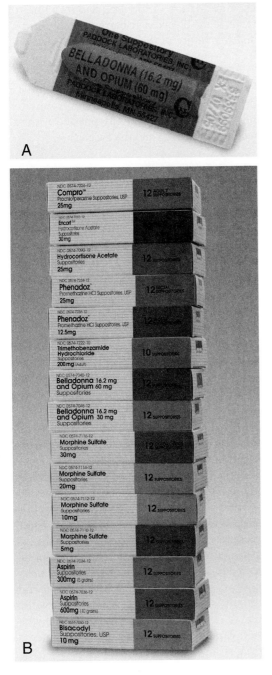

FIGURE 12.1 A, Close-up of a commercial rectal suppository. (Courtesy of Paddock Laboratories) **B**. A variety of commercial rectal suppositories.

Rectal suppositories are usually about 32 mm (1.5 inches) long, are cylindrical, and have one or both ends tapered. Some rectal suppositories are shaped like a bullet, a torpedo, or the little finger. Depending on the density of the base and the medicaments in the suppository, the weight may vary. Adult rectal suppositories weigh about 2 g when cocoa butter (theobroma oil) is employed as the base. Rectal suppositories for use by infants and children are about half the weight and size of the adult suppositories and assume a more pencil-like shape. Vaginal suppositories, also called *pessaries*, are usually globular, oviform, or cone-shaped and weigh about 5 g when cocoa butter is the base. However, depending on the base and the manufacturer's product, the weights of vaginal suppositories may vary widely. Urethral suppositories, also called *bougies*, are slender, pencil-shaped suppositories intended for insertion into the male or female urethra. Male urethral suppositories may be 3 to 6 mm in diameter and approximately 140 mm long, although this may vary. When cocoa butter is employed as the base, these suppositories weigh about 4 g. Female urethral suppositories are about half the length and weight of the male urethral suppository, being about 70 mm long and weighing about 2 g when made of cocoa butter.

Local Action

Once inserted, the suppository base melts, softens, or dissolves, distributing its medicaments to the tissues of the region. These medicaments may be intended for retention within the cavity for local effects, or they may be intended to be absorbed for systemic effects. Rectal suppositories intended for local action are most frequently used to relieve constipation or the pain, irritation, itching, and inflammation associated with hemorrhoids or other anorectal conditions. Antihemorrhoidal suppositories frequently contain a number of components, including local anesthetics, vasoconstrictors, astringents, analgesics, soothing emollients, and protective agents. A popular laxative, glycerin suppositories promote laxation by local irritation of the mucous membranes, probably by the dehydrating effect of the glycerin on those membranes. Vaginal suppositories or inserts intended for local effects are employed mainly as contraceptives, antiseptics in feminine hygiene, and as specific agents to combat an invading pathogen. Most commonly, the drugs used are nonoxynol-9 for contraception and trichomonacides to combat vaginitis caused by *Trichomonas vaginalis, Candida (Monilia) albicans*, and other microorganisms. Urethral suppositories may be antibacterial or a local anesthetic preparative to urethral examination.

Systemic Action

For systemic effects, the mucous membranes of the rectum and vagina permit the absorption of many soluble drugs. Although the rectum is used frequently as the site for the systemic absorption of drugs, the vagina is not as frequently used for this purpose.

Among the advantages over oral therapy of the rectal route for systemic effects are these: (*a*) Drugs destroyed or inactivated by the pH or enzymatic activity of the stomach or intestines need not be exposed to these destructive environments. (*b*) Drugs irritating to the stomach may be given without causing such irritation. (*c*) Drugs destroyed by portal circulation may bypass the liver after rectal absorption (drugs enter the portal circulation after oral administration and absorption). (*d*) The route is convenient for administration of drugs to patients who are unable or unwilling to swallow medication. (*e*) It is an effective route in the treatment of patients with vomiting.

Examples of drugs administered rectally in the form of suppositories for their systemic effects include (*a*) prochlorperazine and chlorpromazine for the relief of nausea and vomiting and as a tranquilizer; (*b*) oxymorphone HCl for opioid analgesia; (*c*) ergotamine tartrate for the relief of migraine syndrome; (*d*) indomethacin, a nonsteroidal anti-inflammatory analgesic and antipyretic; and (*e*) ondansetron for the relief of nausea and vomiting.

Some Factors of Drug Absorption from Rectal Suppositories

The dose of a drug administered rectally may be greater than or less than the dose of the same drug given orally, depending on such factors as the constitution of the patient, the physico-chemical nature of the drug and its ability to traverse the physiologic barriers to absorption, and the nature of the suppository vehicle and its capacity to release the drug and make it available for absorption.

The factors that affect rectal absorption of a drug may be divided into two main groups: (*a*) physiologic factors and (*b*) physicochemical factors of the drug and the base (2, 3).

Physiologic Factors

The human rectum is approximately 15 to 20 cm long. When empty of fecal material, the rectum contains only 2 to 3 mL of inert mucous fluid. In the resting state, the rectum is not motile; there are no villi or microvilli on the rectal mucosa (3). However, there is abundant vascularization of the submucosal region of the rectum wall with blood and lymphatic vessels.

Among the physiologic factors that affect drug absorption from the rectum are the colonic contents, circulation route, and the pH and lack of buffering capacity of the rectal fluids.

Colonic Content

When systemic effects are desired, greater absorption may be expected from a rectum that is void than from one that is distended with fecal matter. A drug will obviously have greater opportunity to make contact with the absorbing surface of the rectum and colon in an empty rectum. Therefore, when deemed desirable, an evacuant enema may be administered and allowed to act before the administration of a suppository of a drug to be absorbed. Other conditions, such as diarrhea, colonic obstruction due to tumorous growths, and tissue dehydration can all influence the rate and degree of drug absorption from the rectum.

Circulation Route

Drugs absorbed rectally, unlike those absorbed after oral administration, bypass the portal circulation during their first pass into the general circulation, thereby enabling drugs otherwise destroyed in the liver to exert systemic effects. The lower hemorrhoidal veins surrounding the colon receive the absorbed drug and initiate its circulation throughout the body, bypassing the liver. Lymphatic circulation also assists in the absorption of rectally administered drugs.

pH and Lack of Buffering Capacity of the Rectal Fluids

Because rectal fluids are essentially neutral in pH (7, 8) and have no effective buffer capacity, the form in which the drug is administered will not generally be chemically changed by the environment.

The suppository base has a marked influence on the release of active constituents. While cocoa butter melts rapidly at body temperature, because of its immiscibility with fluids, it fails to release fat-soluble drugs readily. For systemic drug action using a cocoa butter base, it is preferable to incorporate the ionized (salt) form rather than the un-ionized (base) form of a drug to maximize bioavailability. Although un-ionized drugs more readily partition out of water-miscible bases such as glycerinated gelatin and polyethylene glycol, the bases themselves tend to dissolve slowly and thus retard release of the drug.

Physicochemical Factors of the Drug and Suppository Base

Physicochemical factors include such properties as the relative solubility of the drug in lipid and in water and the particle size of a dispersed drug. Physicochemical factors of the base include its ability to melt, soften, or dissolve at body temperature, its ability to release the drug substance, and its hydrophilic or hydrophobic character.

Lipid–Water Solubility

The lipid–water partition coefficient of a drug (discussed in Chapter 4) is an important consideration in the selection of the suppository base and in anticipating drug release from that base. A lipophilic drug that is distributed in a fatty suppository base in low concentration has less of a tendency to escape to the surrounding aqueous fluids than a hydrophilic substance in a fatty base. Water soluble bases—for example,

polyethylene glycols—that dissolve in the anorectal fluids release for absorption both water-soluble and oil-soluble drugs. Naturally, the more drug a base contains, the more drug will be available for absorption. However, if the concentration of a drug in the intestinal lumen is above a particular amount, which varies with the drug, the rate of absorption is not changed by a further increase in the concentration of the drug.

Particle Size

For undissolved drugs in a suppository, the size of the drug particle will influence its rate of dissolution and its availability for absorption. As indicated many times previously, the smaller the particle, the more readily the dissolution of the particle and the greater the chance for rapid absorption.

Nature of the Base

As indicated earlier, the base must be capable of melting, softening, or dissolving to release its drug for absorption. If the base interacts with the drug to inhibit its release, drug absorption will be impaired or even prevented. Also, if the base irritates the mucous membranes of the rectum, it may initiate a colonic response and prompt a bowel movement, eliminating the prospect of complete drug release and absorption.

In a study of the bioavailability of aspirin from five brands of commercial suppositories, absorption rates varied, and even with the best product, only about 40% of the dose was absorbed when the retention time in the bowel was limited to 2 hours. Thus, the absorption rates were considered exceedingly low, especially when compared with orally administered aspirin, and of dubious dependability (4).

Because of the possibility of chemical and/or physical interactions between the medicinal agent and the suppository base, which may affect the stability and/or bioavailability of the drug, the absence of any drug interaction between the two agents should be ascertained before or during formulation.

Long-acting or slow-release suppositories are also prepared. Morphine sulfate in slow-release suppositories is prepared by compounding pharmacists. The base includes a material such as alginic acid, which will prolong the release of the drug over several hours (5–7).

Suppository Bases

Analogous to the ointment bases, suppository bases play an important role in the release of the medication they hold and therefore in the availability of the drug. Of course, one of the first requisites for a suppository base is that it remain solid at room temperature but soften, melt, or dissolve readily at body temperature so that the drug is fully available soon after insertion. Certain bases are more efficient in drug release than others. For instance, cocoa butter (theobroma oil) melts quickly at body temperature, but because it is immiscible with the body fluids, fat-soluble drugs tend to remain in the oil and have little tendency to enter the aqueous physiologic fluids. For water-soluble drugs in cocoa butter, the reverse is usually true, and good release results. Fat-soluble drugs seem to be released more readily from bases of glycerinated gelatin or polyethylene glycol, both of which dissolve slowly in body fluids. When irritation or inflammation is to be relieved, as in the treatment of anorectal disorders, cocoa butter appears to be the superior base because of its emollient or soothing, spreading action.

Classification of Suppository Bases

For most purposes, it is convenient to classify suppository bases according to their physical characteristics into two main categories and a third miscellaneous group: (*a*) fatty or oleaginous bases, (*b*) water-soluble or water-miscible bases, and (*c*) miscellaneous bases, generally combinations of lipophilic and hydrophilic substances.

Fatty or Oleaginous Bases

Fatty bases are perhaps the most frequently employed suppository bases, principally because cocoa butter is a member of this group of substances. Among the other fatty or oleaginous materials used in suppository bases are many hydrogenated fatty acids of vegetable oils, such as palm kernel oil and cottonseed oil. Also, fat-based compounds containing compounds of glycerin with the higher-molecular-weight fatty acids, such as palmitic and stearic acids, may be found in fatty bases. Such compounds, such as glyceryl monostearate and glyceryl monopalmitate, are examples of this type of agent. The bases in many commercial products employ varied combinations of these types of materials to achieve the desired hardness under conditions of shipment and storage and the desired quality of submitting to the temperature of the body to release their medicaments. Some bases are prepared with the fatty materials emulsified or with an emulsifying agent present to prompt emulsification when the suppository makes contact with the aqueous body fluids. These types of bases are arbitrarily placed in the third, or miscellaneous, group of bases.

Cocoa Butter, NF, is defined as the fat obtained from the roasted seed of *Theobroma cacao*. At room temperature it is a yellowish-white solid having a faint, agreeable chocolate-like odor. Chemically it is a triglyceride (combination of glycerin and one or different fatty acids) primarily of oleopalmitostearin and oleodistearin. Because cocoa butter melts at 30° to 36°C (86°–97°F), it is an ideal suppository base, melting just below body temperature and yet maintaining its solidity at usual room temperatures. However, because of its triglyceride content, cocoa butter exhibits marked *polymorphism*, or existence in several crystalline forms. Because of this, when cocoa butter is hastily or carelessly melted at a temperature greatly exceeding the minimum required temperature and then quickly chilled, the result is a metastable crystalline form (alpha crystals) with a melting point much lower than the original cocoa butter. In fact, the melting point may be so low that the cocoa butter will not solidify at room temperature. However, since the crystalline form is a metastable condition, there is a slow transition to the more stable beta form of crystals having the greater stability and the higher melting point. This transition may require several days. Consequently, if suppositories that have been prepared by melting cocoa butter for the base do not harden soon after molding, they will be useless to the patient and a loss of time, materials, and prestige to the pharmacist. Cocoa butter must be slowly and evenly melted, preferably over a bath of warm water, to avoid formation of the unstable crystalline form and ensure retention in the liquid of the more stable beta crystals that will constitute nuclei upon which the congealing may occur during chilling of the liquid.

Substances such as phenol and chloral hydrate have a tendency to lower the melting point of cocoa butter. If the melting point is low enough that it is not feasible to prepare a solid suppository using cocoa butter alone as the base, solidifying agents like cetyl esters wax (about 20%) or beeswax (about 4%) may be melted with the cocoa butter to compensate for the softening effect of the added substance. However, the addition of hardening agents must not be so excessive as to prevent the base from melting in the body, nor must the waxy material interfere with the therapeutic agent in any way so as to alter the efficacy of the product.

Other bases in this category include commercial products such as Fattibase (triglycerides from palm, palm kernel, and coconut oils with self-emulsifying glyceryl monostearate and polyoxyl stearate) and the Wecobee bases (triglycerides derived from coconut oil), Witepsol bases (triglycerides of saturated fatty acids C12–C18 with varied portions of the corresponding partial glycerides).

Water-Soluble and Water-Miscible Bases

The main members of this group are glycerinated gelatin and polyethylene glycols. Glycerinated gelatin suppositories may be prepared by dissolving granular gelatin (20%) in glycerin (70%) and adding water or a solution or suspension of the medication (10%). A glycerinated gelatin base is most frequently used in preparation of vaginal suppositories, with which prolonged local action of the medicinal agent is usually desired. The glycerinated gelatin base is slower to soften and mix with the physiologic fluids than is cocoa butter and therefore provides a slower release.

Because glycerinated gelatin–based suppositories have a tendency to absorb moisture as a result of the hygroscopic nature of glycerin, they must be protected from atmospheric moisture if they are to maintain their shape and consistency. Also as a result of the hygroscopicity of the glycerin, the suppository may have a dehydrating effect and irritate the tissues upon insertion. The water in the formula for the suppositories minimizes this action; however, if necessary, the suppositories may be moistened with water prior to insertion to reduce the initial tendency of the base to draw water from the mucous membranes and irritate the tissues.

Urethral suppositories may be prepared from a glycerinated gelatin base of a formula somewhat different from the one indicated earlier. For urethral suppositories, the gelatin constitutes about 60% of the weight of the formula, the glycerin about 20%, and the medicated aqueous portion about 20%. Urethral suppositories of glycerinated gelatin are much more easily inserted than those with a cocoa butter base owing to the brittleness of cocoa butter and its rapid softening at body temperature.

Polyethylene glycols are polymers of ethylene oxide and water prepared to various chain lengths, molecular weights, and physical states. They are available in a number of molecular weight ranges, the most commonly used being polyethylene glycol 300, 400, 600, 1000, 1500, 1540, 3350, 4000, 6000, and 8000. The numeric designations refer to the average molecular weight of each of the polymers. Polyethylene glycols having average molecular weights of 300, 400, and 600 are clear, colorless liquids. Those having average molecular weights of greater than 1000 are waxlike white solids whose hardness increases with increase in the molecular weight. Melting ranges for the polyethylene glycols follow:

300	−15 to −18°C
400	4–8°C
600	20–25°C
1000	37–40°C
1450	43–46°C
3350	54–58°C
4600	57–61°C
6000	56–63°C
8000	60–63°C

Various combinations of these polyethylene glycols may be combined by fusion, using two or more of the various types to achieve a suppository base of the desired consistency and characteristics.

Pharmacists have been called on in recent years to prepare progesterone vaginal suppositories extemporaneously. These suppositories, used in premenstrual syndrome, are commonly molded with either a polyethylene glycol base or a fatty acid base. Formulas for these suppositories are presented later in this chapter.

Polyethylene glycol suppositories do not melt at body temperature but rather dissolve slowly in the body's fluids. Therefore, the base need not be formulated to melt at body temperature. Thus it is possible, in fact routine, to prepare suppositories from polyethylene glycol mixtures having melting points considerably higher than that of body temperature. Not only does this property permit a slower release of the medication from the base once the suppository has been inserted, it also permits convenient storage of these suppositories without need for refrigeration and without danger of their softening excessively in warm weather. Their solid nature also permits them to be inserted slowly without fear that they will melt in the fingertips (as cocoa butter suppositories sometimes do). Because they do not melt at body temperature but mix with mucous secretions upon dissolution, polyethylene glycol–based suppositories do not leak from the orifice, as do many cocoa butter–based suppositories. Polyethylene glycol suppositories that do not contain at least 20% water should be dipped in water just before use to avoid irritation of the mucous membranes after insertion. This procedure prevents moisture being drawn from the tissues after insertion and the stinging sensation.

Miscellaneous Bases

In the miscellaneous group of bases are mixtures of oleaginous and water-soluble or water-miscible materials. These materials may be chemical or physical mixtures. Some are preformed emulsions, generally of the water–oil type, or they may be capable of dispersing in aqueous fluids. One of these substances is polyoxyl 40 stearate, a surface-active agent that is employed in a num-

ber of commercial suppository bases. Polyoxyl 40 stearate is a mixture of the monostearate and distearate esters of mixed polyoxyethylene diols and the free glycols, the average polymer length being equivalent to about 40 oxyethylene units. The substance is a white to light tan waxy solid that is water soluble. Its melting point is generally 39° to 45°C (102°–113°F. Other surface-active agents useful in the preparation of suppository bases also fall into this broad grouping. Mixtures of many fatty bases (including cocoa butter) with emulsifying agents capable of forming water–oil emulsions have been prepared. These bases hold water or aqueous solutions and are said to be hydrophilic.

Preparation of Suppositories

Suppositories are prepared by three methods: (a) *molding* from a melt, (b) *compression*, and (c) *hand rolling* and *shaping*. The method most frequently employed both on a small scale and on an industrial scale is molding.

Preparation by Molding

The steps in molding include (a) melting the base, (b) incorporating any required medicaments, (c) pouring the melt into molds, (d) allowing the melt to cool and congeal into suppositories, and (e) removing the formed suppositories from the mold. Cocoa butter, glycerinated gelatin, polyethylene glycol, and most other bases are suitable for preparation by molding.

Suppository Molds

Commercially available molds can produce individual or large numbers of suppositories of various shapes and sizes. Individual plastic molds may be obtained to form a single suppository. Other molds, such as those most commonly found in the community pharmacy, are capable of producing 6, 12, or more suppositories in a single operation (Fig. 12.2). Industrial molds produce hundreds of suppositories from a single batch (Figs. 12.3 and 12.4).

Molds in common use today are made from stainless steel, aluminum, brass, or plastic. The molds, which separate into sections, generally

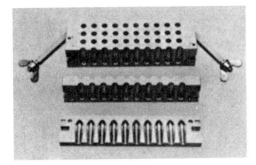

FIGURE 12.2 Partially opened mold capable of producing 50 torpedo-shaped suppositories in a single molding (Courtesy of Chemical and Pharmaceutical Industry Co.).

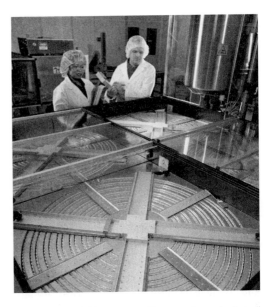

FIGURE 12.4 Highly automated large-scale production of molded suppositories prepared and packaged in strips (Courtesy of Paddock Laboratories).

longitudinally, are opened for cleaning before and after preparation of a batch of suppositories, closed when the melt is poured, and opened again to remove the cold molded suppositories. Care must be exercised in cleaning the molds, as any scratches on the molding surfaces will take away from the desired smoothness of the suppositories. Plastic molds are especially prone to scratching.

Although satisfactory reusable and disposable molds are commercially available for preparation of rectal, vaginal, and urethral suppositories, if necessary temporary molds may be successfully formed by pressing heavy aluminum foil about an object having the shape of the desired suppository, then carefully removing the

object and filling the shaped foil with the melt. For instance, glass stirring rods may be used to form molds for urethral suppositories, round pencils or pens may be used to form molds for rectal suppositories, and any cone-shaped object may be used to form vaginal suppositories.

Lubrication of the Mold

Depending on the formulation, suppository molds may require lubrication before the melt is poured to facilitate clean and easy removal of the molded suppositories. Lubrication is seldom necessary when the base is cocoa butter or polyethylene glycol, as these materials contract sufficiently on cooling to separate from the inner surfaces and allow easy removal. Lubrication is usually necessary with glycerinated gelatin. A thin coating of mineral oil applied with the finger to the molding surfaces usually suffices. However, no material that might irritate the mucous membranes should be employed as a mold lubricant.

Calibration of the Mold

Each individual mold is capable of holding a specific volume of material in each of its openings. Because of the difference in the densities

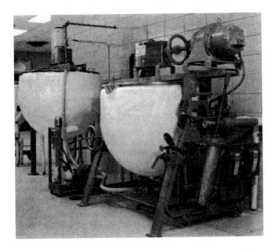

FIGURE 12.3 Large heated tanks for preparation of the melt in commercial production of suppositories by molding (Courtesy of Wyeth-Ayerst Laboratories).

of the materials, if the base is cocoa butter, the weight of the suppositories will differ from the weight of suppositories prepared in the same mold with a base of polyethylene glycols. Similarly, any added medicinal agent alters the density of the base, and the weight of the resulting suppository differs from that of those prepared with base material alone.

The pharmacist should calibrate each suppository mold for the usual base (generally cocoa butter and a polyethylene glycol base) so as to prepare medicated suppositories each having the proper quantity of medicaments.

The first step in calibration of a mold is to prepare molded suppositories from base material alone. After removal from the mold, the suppositories are weighed and the total weight and average weight of each suppository are recorded (for the particular base used). To determine the volume of the mold, the suppositories are carefully melted in a calibrated beaker, and the volume of the melt is determined for the total number as well as for the average of one suppository.

Determination of the Amount of Base Required

In the prescription for medicated suppositories to be prepared extemporaneously by the pharmacist, the prescribing physician indicates the amount of medicinal substance desired in each suppository but leaves the amount of base to the discretion of the pharmacist. Generally, in filling such prescriptions, the pharmacist calculates the amounts of materials needed for the preparation of one or two more suppositories than the number prescribed to compensate for the inevitable loss of some material and to ensure having enough material.

In determining the amount of base to be incorporated with the medicaments, the pharmacist must be certain that the required amount of drug is provided in each suppository. Because the volume of the mold is known (from the determined volume of the melted suppositories formed from the base), the volume of the drug substances subtracted from the total volume of the mold will give the volume of base required. If the added amounts of medicaments

are slight, they may be considered to be negligible, and no deduction from the total volume of base may be deemed necessary. However, if considerable quantities of other substances are to be used, the volumes of these materials are important and should be used to calculate the amount of base actually required to fill the mold. The total volume of these materials is subtracted from the volume of the mold, and the appropriate amount of base is added. Because the bases are solid at room temperature, the volume of base may be converted to weight from the density of the material. For example, if 12 mL of cocoa butter is required to fill a suppository mold and if the medicaments in the formula have a collective volume of 2.8 mL, 9.2 mL of cocoa butter will be required. By multiplying 9.2 mL times the density of cocoa butter, 0.86 g/mL, it may be calculated that 7.9 g of cocoa butter will be required. After adjusting for the preparation of an extra suppository or two, the calculated amount is weighed.

Another method for determination of the amount of base in the preparation of medicated suppositories requires the following steps: (*a*) weigh the active ingredient for the preparation of a single suppository; (*b*) dissolve it or mix it (depending on its solubility in the base) with a portion of melted base insufficient to fill one cavity of the mold, and add the mixture to a cavity; (*c*) add melted base to the cavity to fill it completely; (*d*) allow the suppository to congeal and harden; and (*e*) remove the suppository from the mold and weigh it. The weight of the active ingredients subtracted from the weight of the suppository yields the weight of the base. This amount of base multiplied by the number of suppositories to be prepared in the mold is the total amount of base required.

A third method is to place all of the required medicaments for the preparation of the total number of suppositories (including one extra) in a calibrated beaker, add a portion of the melted base, and incorporate the drug substances. Then add sufficient melted base to reach the required volume of mixture based on the original calibration of the volume of the mold.

A summary of density calculations for molding of suppositories is found in Physical Pharmacy Capsule 12.1.

PHYSICAL PHARMACY CAPSULE 12.1

Density (Dose Replacement) Calculations for Suppositories

In preparation of suppositories, it is generally assumed that if the quantity of active drug is less than 100 mg, then the volume occupied by the powder is insignificant and need not be considered. This is usually based on a 2 gram suppository weight. Obviously, if a suppository mold of less than 2 grams is used, the powder volume may need to be considered.

The density factors of various bases and drugs need to be known to determine the proper weights of the ingredients to be used. Density factors relative to cocoa butter have been determined. If the density factor of a base is not known, it is simply calculated as the ratio of the blank weight of the base and cocoa butter. Density factors for a selected number of ingredients are shown in Table 1.

TABLE 1 DENSITY FACTORS FOR COCOA BUTTER SUPPOSITORIES

Alum	1.7	Morphine HCl	1.6
Aminophylline	1.1	Opium	1.4
Aspirin	1.3	Paraffin	1.0
Barbital	1.2	Peruvian balsam	1.1
Belladonna extract	1.3	Phenobarbital	1.2
Benzoic acid	1.5	Phenol	0.9
Bismuth carbonate	4.5	Potassium bromide	2.2
Bismuth salicylate	4.5	Potassium iodide	4.5
Bismuth subgallate	2.7	Procaine	1.2
Bismuth subnitrate	6.0	Quinine HCl	1.2
Boric acid	1.5	Resorcinol	1.4
Castor oil	1.0	Sodium bromide	2.3
Chloral hydrate	1.3	Spermaceti	1.0
Cocaine HCl	1.3	Sulfathiazole	1.6
Digitalis leaf	1.6	Tannic acid	1.6
Glycerin	1.6	White wax	1.0
Ichthammol	1.1	Witch hazel fluid extract	1.1
Iodoform	4.0	Zinc oxide	4.0
Menthol	0.7	Zinc sulfate	2.8

Three methods of calculating the quantity of base that the active medication will occupy and the quantities of ingredients required are illustrated here: (a) dosage replacement factor, (b) density factor, and (c) occupied volume methods.

DETERMINATION OF THE DOSAGE REPLACEMENT FACTOR METHOD

$$f = \frac{[100\,(E - G)]}{[(G)\,(X)]} + 1$$

where
E is the weight of the pure base suppositories, and
G is the weight of suppositories with X% of the active ingredient.

Physical Pharmacy Capsule 12.1 cont.

Cocoa butter is arbitrarily assigned a value of 1 as the standard base. Examples of other dosage replacement factors are shown in Table 2.

EXAMPLE 1

Prepare a suppository containing 100 mg of phenobarbital (f = 0.81) using cocoa butter as the base. The weight of the pure cocoa butter suppository is 2.0 g. Since 100 mg of phenobarbital is to be contained in an approximately 2.0-g suppository, it will be about 5% phenobarbital. What will be the total weight of each suppository?

$$0.81 = \frac{[100\,(2 - G)]}{[(G)\,(5)] + 1} = 2.019$$

TABLE 2 DOSAGE REPLACEMENT FACTORS FOR SELECTED DRUGS

Balsam peru	0.83	Phenol ·	0.9
Bismuth subgallate	0.37	Procaine HCl	0.8
Bismuth subnitrate	0.33	Quinine HCl	0.83
Boric acid	0.67	Resorcin	0.71
Camphor	1.49	Silver protein, mild	0.61
Castor oil	1.00	Spermaceti	1.0
Chloral hydrate	0.67	White or yellow wax	1.0
Ichthammol	0.91	Zinc oxide	0.15–0.25
Phenobarbital	0.81		

DETERMINATION OF DENSITY FACTOR METHOD

1. Determine the average blank weight, A, per mold using the suppository base of interest.
2. Weigh the quantity of suppository base necessary for 10 suppositories.
3. Weigh 1.0 g of medication. The weight of medication per suppository, B, is equal to 1 g/10 supp = 0.1 g/supp.
4. Melt the suppository base and incorporate the medication, mix, pour into molds, cool, trim, and remove from the molds.
5. Weigh the 10 suppositories and determine the average weight (C).
6. Determine the density factor as follows:

$$\text{Density factor} = \frac{B}{A - C + B}$$

where
A is the average weight of blank,
B is the weight of medication per suppository, and
C is the average weight of medicated suppository.

7. Take the weight of the medication required for each suppository and divide by the density factor of the medication to find the replacement value of the suppository base.
8. Subtract this quantity from the blank suppository weight.
9. Multiply by the number of suppositories required to obtain the quantity of base required for the prescription.

Physical Pharmacy Capsule 12.1 cont.

10. Multiply the weight of drug per suppository by the number of suppositories required to obtain the quantity of active drug required for the prescription.

EXAMPLE 2

Prepare 12 acetaminophen 300 mg suppositories using cocoa butter. The average weight of the cocoa butter blank is 2 g and the average weight of the medicated suppository is 1.8 g.

$$DF = \frac{0.3}{2 - 1.8 + 0.3} = 0.6$$

From step 7:   (0.3 g)/0.6 = 0.5 (the replacement value of the base)
From step 8:   2.0 g–0.5 g = 1.5 g
From step 9:   12 × 1.5 g = 18 g cocoa butter required
From step 10: 12 × 0.3 g = 3.6 g acetaminophen

DETERMINATION OF OCCUPIED VOLUME METHOD

1. Determine the average weight per mold (blank) using the designated base.
2. Weigh out enough base for 10 suppositories.
3. Divide the density of the active drug by the density of the base to obtain a ratio.
4. Divide the total weight of active drug required for the total number of suppositories by the ratio obtained in step 3. This will give the amount of base displaced by the active drug.
5. Subtract the amount obtained in step 4 from the total weight of the prescription (number of suppositories multiplied by the weight of the blanks) to obtain the weight of base required.
6. Multiply the weight of active drug per suppository times the number of suppositories to be prepared to obtain the quantity of active drug required.

EXAMPLE 3

Prepare 10 suppositories, each containing 200 mg of a drug with a density of 3.0. The base has a density of 0.9, and a prepared blank weighs 2.0 g. Using the determination of occupied volume method, prepare the requested suppositories.

From step 1:   The average weight per mold is 2.0 g.
From step 2:   The quantity required for 10 suppositories is 2 g × 10 = 20 g.
From step 3:   The density ratio is 3.0/0.9 = 3.3.
From step 4:   The amount of suppository base displaced by the active drug is 2.0 g/3.3 = 0.6 g.
From step 5:   The weight of the base required is 20 g – 0.6 g = 19.4 g.
From step 6:   The quantity of active drug required is 0.2 g × 10 = 2.0 g.

The required weight of the base is 19.4 g, and the weight of the active drug is 2 g.

Preparing and Pouring the Melt

Using the least possible heat, the weighed suppository base material is melted, generally over a water bath, since no great deal of heat is usually required. A porcelain casserole, that is, a dish with a pouring lip and a handle, is perhaps the best utensil, since it later permits convenient pouring of the melt into the cavities of the mold. Medicinal substances are usually incorporated into a portion of the melted base by mixing on a glass or porcelain tile with a spatula. After incorporation, this material is stirred into the remaining base, which has been allowed to cool almost to its congealing point. Any volatile materials or heat-labile substances should be incorporated at this point with thorough stirring.

The melt is poured carefully and continuously into each cavity of the mold, which has been previously equilibrated to room temperature. If any undissolved or suspended materials in the mixture are denser than the base, so that they have a tendency to settle, constant stirring, even during pouring, is required, else the last filled cavity will contain a disproportionate share of the undissolved materials. The solid materials remain suspended if the pouring is performed just above the congealing point and not when the base is too fluid. If the melt is not near the congealing point when poured, the solids may settle within each cavity of the mold to reside at the tips of the suppositories, with the result that the suppositories may be broken when removed from the mold. Alternatively, a small quantity of silica gel (about 25 mg per suppository) can be incorporated into the formula to aid in keeping the active drug suspended. In filling each suppository cavity, the pouring must be continuous to prevent *layering*, which may lead to a product easily broken on handling. To ensure a completely filled mold upon congealing, the melt is poured excessively over each opening, actually rising above the level of the mold. The excessive material may form a continuous ribbon along the top of the mold above the cavities. This use of extra suppository material prevents formation of recessed dips in the ends of the suppositories and justifies preparation of extra melt. When solidified, the excess material is evenly scraped off of the top of the mold with a spatula warmed by dipping into a beaker of warm water; this will make a smooth surface on the back of the suppository during trimming. The mold is usually placed in the refrigerator to hasten hardening.

When the suppositories are hard, the mold is removed from the refrigerator and allowed to come to room temperature. Then the sections of the mold are separated, and the suppositories are dislodged, with pressure being exerted principally on their ends and only if needed on the tips. Generally little or no pressure is required, and the suppositories simply fall out of the mold when it is opened.

Preparation by Compression

Suppositories may be prepared by forcing the mixed mass of the base and the medicaments into special molds using suppository-making machines. In preparation for compression into the molds, the base and the other formulative ingredients are combined by thorough mixing, the friction of the process softening the base into a pastelike consistency. On a small scale, a mortar and pestle may be used. Heating the mortar in warm water (then drying it) greatly facilitates the softening of the base and the mixing. On a large scale, a similar process may be used, employing mechanical kneading mixers and a warm mixing vessel.

Compression is especially suited for making suppositories that contain heat-labile medicinal substances or a great deal of substances that are insoluble in the base. In contrast to the molding method, compression permits no likelihood of insoluble matter settling during manufacture. The disadvantage to compression is that the special suppository machine is required and there is some limitation as to shapes of suppositories that can be made.

In preparing suppositories with the compression machine, the suppository mass is placed in a cylinder; the cylinder is closed; pressure is applied from one end, mechanically or by turning a wheel; and the mass is forced out of the other end into the mold or die. When the die is filled with the mass, a movable end plate at the back of the die is removed, and when additional pressure is applied to the mass in the cylinder, the formed suppositories are ejected. The end plate is returned and the process is repeated until all of the mass has been used. Various sizes and shapes of dies are available. It is possible to prepare suppositories of uniform circumference by extrusion through a perforated plate and by cutting the extruded mass to the desired length.

Preparation by Hand Rolling and Shaping

With ready availability of suppository molds of accommodating shapes and sizes, there is little requirement for today's pharmacist to shape suppositories by hand. Hand rolling and shaping is a historic part of the art of the pharmacist; a description of it may be found in the third edition of this text or in pharmacy compounding texts.

Rectal Suppositories

Examples of rectal suppositories are presented in Table 12.1. As noted earlier, drugs like aspirin given for pain, ergotamine tartrate for treating migraine headaches, theophylline as a smooth muscle relaxant in treating asthma, and chlorpromazine and prochlorperazine, which act as antiemetics and tranquilizers, are intended to be absorbed into the general circulation to provide systemic effects. The rectal route of administration is especially useful if

the patient is unwilling or unable to take medication by mouth.

Suppositories are also intended to provide local action within the perianal area. Local anesthetic suppositories are commonly employed to relieve *pruritus ani* of various causes and the pain sometimes associated with hemorrhoids. Many commercial hemorrhoidal suppositories contain a number of medicinal agents, including astringents, protectives, anesthetics, lubricants, and others, intended to relieve the discomfort of the condition. Cathartic suppositories are contact-type agents that act directly on the colonic mucosa to produce normal peristalsis. Because the contact action is restricted to the colon, the motility of the small intestine is not appreciably affected. Cathartic suppositories are more rapid acting than

TABLE 12.1 EXAMPLES OF RECTAL SUPPOSITORIES

SUPPOSITORY	COMMERCIAL PRODUCT	ACTIVE CONSTITUENT	TYPE OF EFFECT	CATEGORY AND COMMENTS
Bisacodyl	Dulcolax (Ciba)	10 mg	Local	Cathartic. Base: hydrogenated vegetable oil.
Chlorpromazine	Thorazine (SmithKline Beecham)	25, 100 mg	Systemic	Antiemetic; tranquilizer. Base: glycerin, glyceryl monopalmitate, glyceryl monostearate, hydrogenated fatty acids of coconut and palm kernel oils
Hydrocortisone	Anusol-HC (Warner-Lambert)	25 mg	Local	Pruritus ani, inflamed hemorrhoids, other inflammatory conditions of the anorectum. Base: hydrogenated glycerides.
Hydromorphone	Dilaudid (Knoll)	3 mg	Systemic	Analgesic. Base: Cocoa butter with silicone dioxide.
Mesalamine	Canasa (Axcan Scandipharm)	500 mg	Local	Antiinflammatory. Base: Hard fat.
Oxymorphone	Numorphan (Endo)	5 mg	Systemic	Analgesic. Base: Polyethylene glycols 1000 and 3350.
Prochlorperazine	Compazine (SmithKline Beecham)	2.5, 5, 25 mg	Systemic	Antiemetic. Base: glycerin, monopalmitate, glyceryl monostearate, hydrogenated fatty acids of coconut and palm kernel oils.
Promethazine HCl	Phenergan (Wyeth-Ayerst)	12.5, 25, 50 mg	Systemic	Antihistamine, antiemetic, sedative: used to manage allergic conditions; preoperative or postoperative sedation or nausea and vomiting; motion sickness. Base: cocoa butter, white wax.

orally administered medication. Suppositories of bisacodyl are usually effective in 15 minutes to an hour, and glycerin suppositories usually within a few minutes following insertion.

Some commercially prepared suppositories are available for both adult and pediatric use. The difference is in the shape and drug content. Pediatric suppositories are more narrow and pencil-shaped than the typical bullet-shaped adult suppository. Glycerin suppositories are commonly available in each type.

A formula for glycerin suppositories is as follows:

Glycerin	91 g
Sodium stearate	9 g
Purified water	5 g
To make about	105 g

In preparation of this suppository, the glycerin is heated in a suitable container to about 50°C (120°F). Then the sodium stearate is dissolved with stirring in the hot glycerin, the purified water added, and the mixture immediately poured into the suppository mold. It is recommended that if the mold is metal, it also be heated prior to addition of the glycerin mixture. After cooling to solidification, the suppositories are removed. This formula will prepare about 50 adult suppositories. Approximately the same formulation is used in pharmaceutical and cosmetic stick products, such as deodorants and antiperspirants.

Glycerin, a hygroscopic material, contributes to the laxative effect of the suppository by drawing water from the intestine and from its irritant action on the mucous lining. The sodium stearate, a soap, is the solidifying agent and may also contribute to the laxative action. Because of the hygroscopic nature of glycerin, the suppositories attract moisture and should be maintained in tight containers, preferably at temperatures below 25°C (77°F).

The pharmacist should relate several helpful items of information about the proper use of suppositories. If they must be stored in the refrigerator, suppositories should be allowed to warm to room temperature before insertion. The patient should be advised to rub cocoa butter suppositories gently with the fingers to melt the surface to provide lubrication for insertion. Glycerinated gelatin or polyethylene glycol suppositories should be moistened with water to enhance lubrication. If the polyethylene glycol suppository formulation does not contain at least 20% water, dipping it into water just prior to insertion prevents moisture from being drawn from rectal tissues and decreases irritation. The shape of the suppository determines how it will be inserted. Bullet-shaped rectal suppositories should be inserted pointed end first. The patient who is to use half of a suppository should be told to cut the suppository lengthwise with a clean razor blade. Most suppositories are dispensed in paper, foil, or plastic wrappings, and the patient must be instructed to remove the wrapping completely before insertion.

Urethral Suppositories

Suppositories for urethral administration tend to be thinner and tapered, often about 5 mm in diameter and up to about 60 mm long. They have been used in the treatment of local infections, and a much smaller urethral suppository has been introduced for the administration of alprostadil in the treatment of erectile dysfunction.

Alprostadil Urethral Microsuppository

The MUSE (alprostadil) urethral microsuppository (Vivus, Inc.) is a single-use medicated transurethral system for the delivery of alprostadil to the male urethra. The drug is suspended in a polyethylene glycol 1450 excipient and is formed into a medicated pellet, or microsuppository, measuring 1.4 mm in diameter by 3 mm or 6 mm long. Available strengths are 125, 250, 500, and 1000 µg. The microsuppository resides in the tip of a translucent hollow applicator. It is administered by inserting the applicator tip into the urethra after urination. The pellet is delivered by depressing the applicator button. The polyethylene glycol 1450 vehicle will dissolve in the available fluid, releasing the drug for absorption. The applicator system is composed of medical grade polypropylene; each system is individually foil packaged. The MUSE microsuppository is indicated for the treatment of erectile dysfunction.

Vaginal Suppositories

Examples of vaginal suppository and tablets are presented in Table 12.2. These preparations are employed principally to combat infections in the female genitourinary tract, to restore the vaginal mucosa to its normal state, and for contraception. The usual pathogenic organisms are *Trichomonas vaginalis, Candida (Monilia) albicans* or other species, and *Haemophilus vaginalis.* Among the anti-infective agents in commercial vaginal preparations are nystatin, clotrimazole, butoconazole nitrate, terconazole, and miconazole (antifungals) and triple sulfas, sulfanilamide, povidone iodine, clindamycin phosphate, metronidazole, and oxytetracycline (antibacterials). Nonoxynol-9, a spermicide, is employed for vaginal contraception. Estrogenic substances such as dienestrol are found in vaginal preparations to restore the vaginal mucosa to its normal state.

The most commonly used base for vaginal suppositories consists of combinations of the various molecular weight polyethylene glycols. To this base is frequently added surfactants and preservative agents, commonly the parabens. Many vaginal suppositories and other types of vaginal dosage forms are buffered to an acid pH, usually about pH 4.5, which resembles that of the normal vagina. This acidity discourages pathogenic organisms and provides a favorable environment for eventual recolonization by the acid-producing bacilli normally found in the vagina.

The polyethylene glycol–based vaginal suppositories are water miscible and are generally sufficiently firm for the patient to handle and

insert without great difficulty. However, to make the task easier, many manufacturers provide plastic insertion devices that are used to hold the suppository or tablet for proper placement within the vagina (Fig. 12.5).

As noted earlier, pharmacists frequently are called on to prepare progesterone vaginal suppositories. Formulas for extemporaneous preparation of these suppositories have been presented in the professional literature (8, 9). Micronized progesterone powder is used in a base of polyethylene glycol, although in some formulas cocoa butter is employed. The suppositories are prepared by adding the progesterone to a melt of the base and molding. Some representative formulas:

Rx
Progesterone, micronized powder   q.s.
Polyethylene glycol 400   60%
Polyethylene glycol 8000   40%

Rx
Progesterone, micronized powder   q.s.
Polyethylene glycol 1000   75%
Polyethylene glycol 3350   25%

Rx
Progesterone, micronized powder   q.s.
Cocoa butter   100%

The amount of progesterone per suppository ranges from 25 to 600 mg. The suppositories are used in treating luteal phase defect, premenstrual syndrome, luteal phase spotting, and in preparation of the endometrium for implantation (9).

The pharmacist should share several helpful hints with a woman who is about to use a vaginal suppository. She should first be told to read the instructions with the product. Throughout

TABLE 12.2 EXAMPLES OF VAGINAL SUPPOSITORIES AND TABLETS

PRODUCT (MANUFACTURER)	ACTIVE CONSTITUENTS	CATEGORY AND COMMENTS
AVC Suppositories (Novavax)	Sulfanilamide 1.05 g	For *Candida albicans* infections
Monistat 7 Suppositories (Advanced Care Products)	Miconazole nitrate 200 mg	Antifungal for local vulvovaginal candidiasis (moniliasis)
Mycelex-G Vaginal Tablets (Bayer)	Clotrimazole 500 mg	Vulvovaginal yeast (*Candida*) infections
Semicid Vaginal Contraceptive Inserts (Robins Healthcare)	Nonoxynol-9 100 mg	Nonsystemic reversible birth control

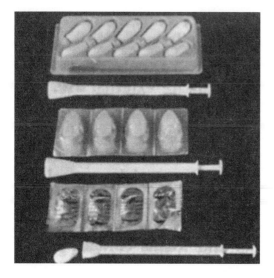

FIGURE 12.5 Dosage forms used intravaginally, including suppositories (*top* and *middle*), vaginal tablets packaged in foil (*bottom*), vaginal cream, and corresponding insert devices.

the course of therapy, the suppository should be inserted high into the vagina with the provided applicator. The patient should not discontinue therapy when the symptoms abate. Furthermore, she should notify her physician if burning, irritation, or any signs of an allergic reaction occur. When vaginal inserts (i.e., compressed tablets) are prescribed, the pharmacist should instruct the woman to dip the tablet into water quickly before insertion. Because these dosage forms are usually administered at bedtime and can be somewhat messy if formulated into an oleaginous base, the pharmacist should suggest that the woman wear a sanitary napkin to protect her nightwear and bed linens.

Quality control procedures listed in the USP 26–NF 21 for manufactured suppositories include identification, assay, and in some cases loss on drying, disintegration, and dissolution. Also, stability considerations in dispensing practice for suppositories include observation for excessive softening and oil stains on packaging (10). Compounded suppositories can be checked for calculations of theoretical and actual weight and weight variation, color, hardness, surface texture, and overall appearance.

Packaging and Storage

Glycerin suppositories and glycerinated gelatin suppositories are packaged in tightly closed glass containers to prevent a change in moisture content. Suppositories prepared from a cocoa butter base are usually individually wrapped or otherwise separated in compartmented boxes to prevent contact and adhesion. Suppositories containing light-sensitive drugs are individually wrapped in an opaque material such as a metallic foil. In fact, most commercial suppositories are individually wrapped in either foil or plastic. Some are packaged in a continuous strip, separated by tearing along perforations. Suppositories are also commonly packaged in slide boxes or in plastic boxes.

Since suppositories are adversely affected by heat, it is necessary to maintain them in a cool place. Cocoa butter suppositories must be stored below 30°C (86°F), and preferably in a refrigerator (2–8°C, or 36–46°F). Glycerinated gelatin suppositories can be stored at controlled room temperature (20–25°C, or 68–77°F). Suppositories made from a base of polyethylene glycol may be stored at usual room temperatures.

Suppositories stored in high humidity may absorb moisture and tend to become spongy, whereas suppositories stored in places of extreme dryness may lose moisture and become brittle.

Vaginal Inserts

Vaginal tablets are more widely used nowadays than are commercial vaginal suppositories; but compounded vaginal suppositories are very widely used. The tablets are easier to manufacture, more stable, and less messy. Vaginal tablets, frequently referred to as *vaginal inserts*, are usually ovoid and are accompanied in their packaging with a plastic inserter, a device for easy placement of the tablet within the vagina. Vaginal tablets contain the same types of anti-infective and hormonal substances as vaginal suppositories. They are prepared by tablet compression and are commonly formulated to contain lactose as the base or filler, a disintegrating agent such as starch, a dispersing agent such as polyvinylpyrrolidone, and a tablet lubricant such as magnesium stearate. The tablets are intended to disintegrate within the vagina, releasing their medication. Examples of vaginal tablets are presented in Table 12.2.

Some vaginal inserts are capsules of gelatin containing medication to be released intravaginally. Capsules may also be used rectally, especially to administer medication to children unwilling or unable to tolerate the drug orally. Capsule insertion into the rectum can be facil-

itated by first lightly wetting the capsule with water. Holes may be punched into these capsules prior to moistening and insertion to facilitate fluid movement into the capsule if desired. Drugs are absorbed from the rectum, but frequently at unpredictable rates and in varying amounts, as previously noted. Drugs that do not dissolve rapidly and that irritate mucous membranes should not be placed in direct contact with such membranes.

PHARMACEUTICS CASE STUDY

Subjective Information

A colleague calls you and asks for help concerning a prescription that was recently compounded. A teenaged boy with epilepsy brought in a prescription for diazepam 10 mg suppositories, and your colleague filled it using a compounded preparation that had been used in the past. However, the boy has been to the emergency room twice now with uncontrolled seizures, even after using the suppositories in an effort to bring the seizures under control. His parents have returned to the pharmacy with questions concerning the use of these suppositories. What should you tell your colleague?

Objective Information

When questioned about the formulation for the suppositories, your colleague provides the following:

For 10 suppositories:

Diazepam Powder, USP   100.0 mg

Cocoa butter   19.9 g

Mix and mold

Assessment

The use of cocoa butter (a fatty acid base) in the formulation for diazepam suppositories may be the problem, because diazepam is a fat-soluble drug. As a result, the drug may remain dissolved in the vehicle and not be released from the dosage form rapidly enough to control the boy's seizures; the tendency for diazepam to diffuse from the lipid suppository base to the aqueous mucosal secretions is low. The use of a water-soluble base such as polyethylene glycol may be a better choice. Another possibility is to use a hollow suppository with a diazepam solution in the cavity.

Plan

Recommend to reformulation of the suppositories using polyethylene glycol as the base.

CLINICAL CASE STUDY

Subjective

HPI: J. R. is a 32 y/o Hispanic female who presents to the oncology clinic for a follow-

up visit 4 days after being discharged from the hospital. At that time, she received her first cycle of cyclophosphamide, doxorubicin, vincristine, and prednisone (CHOP)

Clinical Case Study cont.

chemotherapy for her newly diagnosed large B cell lymphoma. During the administration of CHOP, the patient started a regimen of two antiemetic medications, Compazine 10 mg by mouth every 6 hours as needed and lorazepam 2 mg intravenously every 6 hours as needed, to control her chemotherapy-induced nausea and vomiting (N&V). Upon discharge from the hospital, she was also given a prescription for prochlorperazine 10 mg tablets by mouth every 6 hours as needed for any N&V she might have at home. However, this morning J. R. is complaining of "feeling sick to her stomach" for the past 2 days, and she states, "Yesterday I threw up three times." She took her prochlorperazine tablets. However, twice after taking them she threw them up, and she simply "feels too nauseous now to take anything by mouth." Upon questioning, the patient denies any fever, chills, hematemesis (i.e., bloody vomitus), and diarrhea and otherwise is without complaints except for feeling "a little tired after the chemo."

PMH: large B-cell lymphoma
iron deficiency anemia
PSH: none
MEDS: CHOP regimen (each cycle is 21 days long):
Cyclophosphamide 750 mg/m^2 IV on day 1
Doxorubicin 50 mg/m^2 IV on day 1
Vincristine 1.4 mg/m^2 IV on day 1
Prednisone 100 mg po on days 1–5
Compazine 10 mg tablets po q6h prn N&V
Ferrous sulfate 325 mg tablets po tid
Tylenol 650 mg tablets po q6h prn pain
Allergies: NKDA
SH: (−) Alcohol
(−) Tobacco
(−) Illicit drugs

Pt came to the U.S. from Mexico 2 years ago
FH: Sister with cancer died at age 36

Pharmaceutical Care Plan

S: Chemotherapy-induced N&V uncontrolled by prochlorperazine.

O: Vital Signs: Temp 36.0°, pulse 87, BP 117/76
Na 143, Cl 105, BUN 12, Glu 129
K 3.9, CO$_2$ 30, Cr 0.8

A: A 32 y/o woman with chemotherapy-induced N&V uncontrolled by oral prochlorperazine. Pt is at risk for continued N&V because of the emetogenic potential of the CHOP regimen. Specifically, cyclophosphamide is associated with delayed-onset N&V that can last up to 6 or 7 days after the administration of chemotherapy. Also, J. R. has other characteristics, e.g., female, less than 50 years old, which increase her risk of N&V.

P: Because J. R. cannot take her medication by mouth, the rectal route of administration would be useful for her. Prochlorperazine is available as rectal suppositories, and the recommended dosage for adults for N&V is 25 mg rectally twice daily. J. R. should be counseled to use her prochlorperazine suppositories as needed for N&V.

J. R. should be told that it is not necessary to store the suppositories in the refrigerator. However, they should be kept away from heat. If they are kept in the refrigerator, they should be warmed to room temperature for 5 to 10 minutes before use. Counsel J. R. on the proper administration technique. She should be instructed to remove the foil wrapping before insertion. Advise her to moisten the suppositories with some water to provide lubrication for insertion. Specific instructions are to use her finger to insert the suppository into the rectum about 1

Clinical Case Study cont.

inch and hold the suppository in place for a few moments. Afterwards, the patient should thoroughly wash her hands and then resume her normal activities.

Explain to J. R. the common side effects associated with prochlorperazine use: sedation, restlessness, blurred vision, constipation, dizziness, dry mouth. Caution J. R. about performing activities that require alertness: driving a car, using machinery. Instruct J. R. to avoid alcoholic beverages and prolonged exposure to sunlight because prochlorperazine may cause skin photosensitivity.

J. R. should be monitored for resolution of her N&V. Also, monitor her for any complaint of abnormal body movements associated with long term prochlorperazine use, such as extrapyramidal dyskinesias, tardive dyskinesia.

REFERENCES

1. Merkus FWHM. The correct application of suppositories. Editorial. 1980;December: Pharm Int.
2. Anschel J, Lieberman HA. Suppositories. Drug Cosmetic Ind 1965;97:341.
3. Moolenaar F, Schoonen AJM. Biopharmaceutics of the rectal administration of drugs. Pharm Int 1980;1:444–146.
4. Gibaldi M, Grundhofer B. Bioavailability of aspirin from commercial suppositories. J Pharm Sci 64:1064–1066.
5. Morgan DJ, McCormick Y, Cosolo W, et al. Prolonged release of morphine alkaloid from a lipophilic suppository base in vitro and in vivo. Int J Clin Pharmacol Ther Toxicol 1991;30:576–581.
6. Cole L, Hanning CD, Robertson S, Quinn K. Further development of a morphine hydrogel suppository. Br J Clin Pharmacol 1990;30:781–786.
7. Moolenaar F, Meyuler P, Frijlink E, et al. Rectal absorption of morphine from controlled release suppositories. Int J Pharmaceut 1994;114:170–120.
8. Roffe BD, Zimmer RA, Derewicz HJ. Preparation of progesterone suppositories. Am J Hosp Pharm 1977;34:1334.
9. Allen LV, Stiles ML. Progesterone suppositories: Allen's compounded formulations. Washington: American Pharmaceutical Association, 2003;198–199.
10. United States Pharmacopeia 26–National Formulary 21. Rockville MD: U.S. Pharmacopeial Convention, 2003;2414–2417.

Solutions

13

In physicochemical terms, solutions may be prepared from any combination of solid, liquid, and gas, the three states of matter. For example, a solid solute may be dissolved in another solid, a liquid, or a gas, and the same being true for a liquid solute and for a gas, nine types of homogeneous mixtures are possible. In pharmacy, however, interest in solutions is for the most part limited to preparations of a solid, a liquid, and less frequently a gas solute in a liquid solvent.

In pharmaceutical terms, solutions are "liquid preparations that contain one or more chemical substances dissolved in a suitable solvent or mixture of mutually miscible solvents" (1). Because of a particular pharmaceutical solution's use, it may be classified as oral, otic, ophthalmic, or topical. Still other solutions, because of their composition or use, may be classified as other dosage forms. For example, aqueous solutions containing a sugar are classified as syrups; sweetened hydroalcoholic (combinations of water and ethanol) solutions are termed elixirs; solutions of aromatic materials are termed spirits if the solvent is alcoholic or aromatic waters if the solvent is aqueous. Solutions prepared by extracting active constituents from crude drugs are termed tinctures or fluidextracts, depending on their method of preparation and concentration. Tinctures may also be solutions of chemical substances dissolved in alcohol or in a hydroalcoholic solvent. Certain solutions prepared to be sterile and pyrogen free and intended for parenteral administration are classified as injections. Although other examples could be cited, it is apparent that a solution, as a distinct type of pharmaceutical preparation, is much further defined than the physicochemical definition of the term solution.

Oral solutions, syrups, elixirs, spirits, and tinctures are prepared and used for the specific effects of the medicinal agents they carry. In these preparations, the medicinal agents are intended to provide systemic effects. The fact that they are administered in solution form usually means that they are soluble in aqueous systems and that their absorption from the gastrointestinal tract into the systemic circulation may be expected to occur more rapidly than from suspension or solid dosage forms of the same medicinal agent.

Solutes other than the medicinal agent are usually present in orally administered solutions. These additional agents usually are included to provide color, flavor, sweetness, or stability. In formulating or compounding a pharmaceutical solution, the pharmacist must use information on the solubility and stability of each solute with regard to the solvent or solvent system. Combinations of medicinal or pharmaceutic agents that will result in chemical or physical interactions affecting the therapeutic quality or pharmaceutic stability of the product must be avoided.

For single-solute solutions and especially for multiple-solute solutions, the pharmacist must be aware of the solubility characteristics of the solutes and the features of the common pharmaceutical solvents. Each chemical agent has its own solubility in a given solvent. For many medicinal agents, their solubilities in the usual solvents are stated in the *United States Pharmacopeia–National Formulary* (USP–NF) as well as in other reference books.

Solubility

Attractive forces between atoms lead to the formation of molecules and ions. The intermolecular forces, which are developed between like molecules, are responsible for the physical state (solid, liquid, or gas) of the substance under given conditions, such as temperature and pressure. Under ordinary conditions, most organic compounds, and thus most drug substances, form molecular solids.

When molecules interact, attractive and repulsive forces are in effect. The attractive forces cause the molecules to cohere, whereas the repulsive forces prevent molecular interpenetration and destruction. When the attractive and repulsive forces are equal, the potential energy between two molecules is minimum and the system is most stable.

Dipolar molecules frequently tend to align themselves with other dipolar molecules so that the negative pole of one molecule points toward the positive pole of the other. Large groups of molecules may be associated through these weak attractions, known as dipole–dipole or van der Waals forces. Other attractions also occur between polar and nonpolar molecules and ions. These include ion–dipole forces and hydrogen bonding. The latter is of particular interest. Because of small size and large electrostatic field, the hydrogen atom can move in close to an electronegative atom, forming an electrostatic type of association, a hydrogen bond or hydrogen bridge. Hydrogen bonding involves strongly electronegative atoms such as oxygen, nitrogen, and fluorine. Such a bond exists in water, represented by the dotted lines:

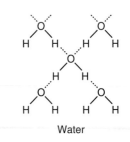

Water

Hydrogen bonds also exist between some alcohol molecules, esters, carboxylic acids, aldehydes, and polypeptides.

When a solute dissolves, the substance's intermolecular forces of attraction must be overcome by forces of attraction between the solute and solvent molecules. This entails breaking the solute–solute forces and the solvent–solvent forces to achieve the solute–solvent attraction.

The solubility of an agent in a particular solvent indicates the maximum concentration to which a solution may be prepared with that agent and that solvent. When a solvent at a given temperature has dissolved all of the solute it can, it is said to be saturated. To emphasize the possible variation in solubility between two chemical agents and therefore in the amounts of each required to prepare a saturated solution, two official aqueous saturated solutions are cited as examples, Calcium Hydroxide Topical Solution, USP, and Potassium Iodide Oral Solution, USP. The first solution, prepared by agitating an excess amount of calcium hydroxide with purified water, contains only about 140 mg of dissolved solute per 100 mL of solution at 25°C, whereas potassium iodide solution contains about 100 g of solute per 100 mL of solution, more than 700 times as much solute as in the calcium hydroxide topical solution. Thus the maximum possible concentration to which a pharmacist may prepare a solution varies greatly and depends in part on the chemical constitution of the solute. Through selection of a different solubilizing agent or a different chemical salt form of the medicinal agent, alteration of the pH of a solution, or substitution in part or in whole of the solvent, a pharmacist can in certain instances dissolve greater quantities of a solute than would otherwise be possible. For example, iodine granules are soluble in water only to the extent of 1 g in about 3000 mL. Using only these two agents, the maximum concentration possible would be approximately 0.03% of iodine. However, through the use of an aqueous solution of potassium iodide or sodium iodide as the solvent, much larger amounts of iodine may be dissolved as the result of the formation of a water-soluble complex with the iodide salt. This reaction is taken advantage of, for example, in Iodine Topical Solution, USP, prepared to contain about 2% iodine and 2.4% sodium iodide.

Temperature is an important factor in determining the solubility of a drug and in preparing its solution. Most chemicals absorb heat when they are dissolved and are said to have a positive heat of solution, resulting in increased solubility with an increase in temperature. A few chemicals have a negative heat of solution and exhibit a decrease in solubility with a rise in temperature. Other factors in addition to temperature affect solubility. These include the various chemical and other physical properties of both the solute and the solvent, pressure, the pH of the solution, the state of subdivision of the solute, and the physical agitation applied to the solution as it dissolves. The solubility of a pure chemical substance at a given temperature and pressure is constant; however, its rate of solution, that is, the speed at which it dissolves, depends on the particle size of the substance and the extent of agitation. The finer the powder, the greater the surface area that comes in contact with the solvent and the more rapid the dissolving process. Also, the greater the agitation, the more unsaturated solvent passes over the drug, and the faster the formation of the solution.

The solubility of a substance in a given solvent may be determined by preparing a saturated solution of it at a specific temperature and determining by chemical analysis the amount of chemical dissolved in a given weight of solution. The amount of solvent required to dissolve the amount of solute can be determined by simple calculation. The solubility may then be expressed as grams of solute dissolving in milliliters of solvent; for example, "1

g of sodium chloride dissolves in 2.8 mL of water." When the exact solubility has not been determined, general expressions of relative solubility may be used. These terms are defined in the USP and presented in Table 13.1 (2).

A great many of the important organic medicinal agents are either weak acids or weak bases, and their solubility depends to a large measure on the pH of the solvent. These drugs react either with strong acids or strong bases to form water-soluble salts. For instance, the weak bases, including many of the alkaloids (atropine, codeine, and morphine), antihistamines (diphenhydramine and tripelennamine), local anesthetics (cocaine, procaine, and tetracaine), and other important drugs are not very water soluble, but they are soluble in dilute solutions of acids. Pharmaceutical manufacturers have prepared many acid salts of these organic bases to enable the preparation of aqueous solutions. However, if the pH of the aqueous solution of these salts is changed by the addition of alkali, the free base may separate from solution unless it has adequate solubility in water. Organic medicinals that are weak acids include the barbiturate drugs (e.g., phenobarbital) and the sulfonamides (e.g., sulfadiazine and sulfacetamide). These and other weak acids form water-soluble salts in basic solution and may separate from solution by a lowering of the pH. Table 13.2 presents the comparative solubilities of some typical examples of weak acids and weak bases and their salts.

TABLE 13.1 RELATIVE TERMS OF SOLUBILITY (2)

DESCRIPTIVE TERM	PARTS OF SOLVENT REQUIRED FOR 1 PART OF SOLUTE
Very soluble	<1
Freely soluble	1–10
Soluble	10–30
Sparingly soluble	30–100
Slightly soluble	100–1000
Very slightly soluble	1000–10,000
Practically insoluble or insoluble	>10,000

TABLE 13.2 WATER AND ALCOHOL SOLUBILITIES OF SOME WEAK ACIDS, WEAK BASES, AND THEIR SALTS

| DRUG | MILLILITERS OF SOLVENT TO DISSOLVE 1 g OF DRUG | |
	WATER	ALCOHOL
Atropine	455.0	2
Atropine sulfate	0.5	5
Codeine	120.0	2
Codeine sulfate	30.0	1,280
Codeine phosphate	2.5	325
Morphine	5,000.0	210
Morphine sulfate	16.0	565
Phenobarbital	1,000.0	8
Phenobarbital sodium	1.0	10
Procaine	200.0	soluble
Procaine hydrochloride	1.0	15
Sulfadiazine	13,000.0	sparingly soluble
Sodium sulfadiazine	2.0	slightly soluble

Although there are no exact rules for predicting unerringly the solubility of a chemical agent in a particular liquid, experienced pharmaceutical chemists can estimate the general solubility of a chemical compound based on its molecular structure and functional groups. The information gathered on a great number of individual chemical compounds has led to the characterization of the solubilities of groups of compounds, and though there may be an occasional inaccuracy with respect to an individual member of a group of compounds, the generalizations nonetheless are useful. As demonstrated by the data in Table 13.2 and other similar data, salts of organic compounds are more soluble in water than are the corresponding organic bases. Conversely, the organic bases are more soluble in organic solvents, including alcohol, than are the corresponding salt forms. Perhaps the most widely written guideline for the prediction of solubility is that like dissolves like, meaning that a solvent having a chemical structure most similar to that of the intended solute will be most likely to dissolve it. Thus,

organic compounds are more soluble in organic solvents than in water. Organic compounds may, however, be somewhat water soluble if they contain polar groups capable of forming hydrogen bonds with water. In fact, the greater the number of polar groups present, the greater will likely be the organic compound's solubility in water. Polar groups include OH, CHO, COH, CHOH, CH_2OH, COOH, NO_2, CO, NH_2, and SO_3H. The introduction of halogen atoms into a molecule tends to decrease water solubility because of an increase in the molecular weight of the compound without a proportionate increase in polarity. An increase in the molecular weight of an organic compound without a change in polarity reduces solubility in water. Table 13.3 demonstrates some of these generalities with specific chemical examples.

As with organic compounds, the pharmacist is aware of some general patterns of solubility that apply to inorganic compounds. For instance, most salts of monovalent cations such as sodium, potassium, and ammonium are water soluble, whereas the divalent cations like calcium, magnesium, and barium usually form water-soluble compounds with nitrate, acetate, and chloride anions but not with carbonate, phosphate, or hydroxide anions. To be sure, certain combinations of anion and cation seem to be similar in makeup but do not have similar solubility characteristics. For instance, magnesium sulfate (Epsom salt) is soluble, but calcium sulfate is only slightly soluble; barium sulfate is very insoluble (1 g dissolves in about 400,000 mL of water) and is used as an opaque medium for x-ray observation of the intestinal tract, but barium sulfide and barium sulfite are more soluble, and their oral use can result in poisoning; mercurous chloride (HgCl) is insoluble and was formerly used as a cathartic, but mercuric chloride ($HgCl_2$) is soluble in water and is a deadly poison if taken internally. In many instances solubilities of drugs and their differentiation from other drugs are critical to the pharmacist for avoidance of compounding failures or therapeutic disasters.

The ability of a solvent to dissolve organic as well as inorganic solutes depends on its effectiveness in overcoming the electronic forces that hold the atoms of the solute together and the corresponding lack of resolute on the part of the

TABLE 13.3 SOLUBILITIES OF SELECTED ORGANIC COMPOUNDS IN WATER AS A DEMONSTRATION OF CHEMICAL STRUCTURE–SOLUBILITY RELATIONSHIP

COMPOUND	FORMULA	MILLILITERS OF WATER REQUIRED TO DISSOLVE 1 g OF COMPOUND
Benzene	C_6H_6	1430.0
Benzoic acid	C_6H_5COOH	275.0
Benzyl alcohol	$C_6H_5CH_2OH$	25.0
Phenol	C_6H_5OH	15.0
Pyrocatechol	$C_6H_4(OH)_2$	2.3
Pyrogallol	$C_6H_3(OH)_3$	1.7
Carbon tetrachloride	CCl_4	2,000.0
Chloroform	$CHCl_3$	200.0
Methylene chloride	CH_2Cl_2	50.0

atoms themselves to resist the solvent action. During dissolution, the molecules of the solvent and the solute become uniformly mixed, and cohesive forces of the atoms are replaced by new forces as a result of the attraction of the solute and solvent molecules for one another.

The student may find the following general rules of solubility useful.

Inorganic Molecules
1. If both the cation and anion of an ionic compound are monovalent, the solute–solute attractive forces are usually easily overcome, and therefore, these compounds are generally water soluble (e.g., NaCl, LiBr, KI, NH_4NO_3, $NaNO_2$).
2. If only one of the two ions in an ionic compound is monovalent, the solute–solute interactions are also usually easily overcome and the compounds are water soluble (e.g., $BaCl_2$, MgI_2, Na_2SO_4, Na_3PO_4).
3. If both the cation and anion are multivalent, the solute–solute interaction may be too great to be overcome by the solute-solvent interaction, and the compound may have poor water solubility (e.g., $CaSO_4$, $BaSO_4$, $BiPO_4$; Exceptions: $ZnSO_4$, $FeSO_4$).
4. Common salts of alkali metals (Na, K, Li, Cs, Rb) are usually water soluble (exception: Li_2CO_3).
5. Ammonium and quaternary ammonium salts are water soluble.
6. Nitrates, nitrites, acetates, chlorates, and

lactates are generally water soluble (exceptions: silver and mercurous acetate).
7. Sulfates, sulfites, and thiosulfates are generally water soluble (exceptions: calcium and barium salts).
8. Chlorides, bromides, and iodides are water soluble (exceptions: salts of silver and mercurous ions).
9. Acid salts corresponding to an insoluble salt will be more water soluble than the original salt.
10. Hydroxides and oxides of compounds other than alkali metal cations and the ammonium ion are generally water insoluble.
11. Sulfides are water insoluble except for their alkali metal salts.
12. Phosphates, carbonates, silicates, borates, and hypochlorites are water insoluble except for their alkali metal salts and ammonium salts.

Organic Molecules
1. Molecules having one polar functional group are usually soluble to total chain lengths of five carbons.
2. Molecules having branched chains are more soluble than the corresponding straight-chain compound.
3. Water solubility decreases with an increase in molecular weight.
4. Increased structural similarity between solute and solvent is accompanied by increased solubility.

It is the pharmacist's knowledge of the chemical characteristics of drugs that permits the selection of the proper solvent for a particular solute. However, in addition to the factors of solubility, the selection is based on such additional characteristics as clarity, low toxicity, viscosity, compatibility with other formulative ingredients, chemical inertness, palatability, odor, color, and economy. In most instances, especially for solutions to be taken orally, used ophthalmically, or injected, water is the preferred solvent because it comes closer to meeting these criteria than other solvents. When water is used as the primary solvent, commonly an auxiliary solvent is also employed to augment the solvent action of water or to contribute to a product's chemical or physical stability. Alcohol, glycerin, and propylene glycol, perhaps the most widely used auxiliary solvents, have been quite effective in contributing to the desired characteristics of pharmaceutical solutions and in maintaining their stability.

Other solvents, such as acetone, ethyl oxide, and isopropyl alcohol, are too toxic to be permitted in pharmaceutical preparations to be taken internally, but they are useful as reagent solvents in organic chemistry and in the preparatory stages of drug development, as in the extraction or removal of active constituents from medicinal plants. For purposes such as this, certain solvents are officially recognized in the compendia. A number of fixed oils, such as corn oil, cottonseed oil, peanut oil, and sesame oil, are useful solvents, particularly in the preparation of oleaginous injections, and are recognized in the official compendia for this purpose.

Some Solvents for Liquid Preparations

The following agents find use as solvents in the preparation of solutions.

Alcohol, USP: Ethyl Alcohol, Ethanol, C_2H_5OH

Next to water, alcohol is the most useful solvent in pharmacy. It is used as a primary solvent for many organic compounds. Together with water it forms a hydroalcoholic mixture that dissolves both alcohol-soluble and water-

soluble substances, a feature especially useful in the extraction of active constituents from crude drugs. By varying the proportion of the two agents, the active constituents may be selectively dissolved and extracted or allowed to remain behind, according to their particular solubility characteristics in the menstruum. Alcohol, USP, is 94.9 to 96.0% C_2H_5OH by volume (i.e., v/v) when determined at 15.56° C, the U.S. government's standard temperature for alcohol determinations. Dehydrated Alcohol, USP, contains not less than 99.5% C_2H_5OH by volume and is used when an essentially water-free alcohol is desired.

Alcohol has been well recognized as a solvent and excipient in the formulation of oral pharmaceutical products. Certain drugs are insoluble in water and must be dissolved in an alternative vehicle. Alcohol is often preferred because of its miscibility with water and its ability to dissolve many water-insoluble ingredients, including drug substances, flavorants, and antimicrobial preservatives. Alcohol is frequently used with other solvents, such as glycols and glycerin, to reduce the amount of alcohol required. It also is used in liquid products as an antimicrobial preservative alone or with parabens, benzoates, sorbates, and other agents.

However, aside from its pharmaceutic advantages as a solvent and preservative, concern has been expressed over the undesired pharmacologic and potential toxic effects of alcohol when ingested in pharmaceutical products, particularly by children. Thus, the U.S. Food and Drug Administration (FDA) has proposed that insofar as possible manufacturers of over-the-counter (OTC) oral drug products restrict the use of alcohol and include appropriate warnings in the labeling. For OTC oral products intended for children under 6 years of age, the recommended alcohol content limit is 0.5%; for products intended for children 6 to 12 years of age, the recommended limit is 5%; and for products recommended for children over 12 years of age and for adults, the recommended limit is 10%.

Diluted Alcohol, NF

Diluted Alcohol, NF, is prepared by mixing equal volumes of Alcohol, USP, and Purified

Water, USP. The final volume of such mixtures is not the sum of the individual volumes of the two components; because the liquids contract upon mixing, the final volume is generally about 3% less than what would otherwise be expected. Thus, when 50 mL of each component is combined, the resulting product measures approximately 97 mL. It is for this reason that the strength of Diluted Alcohol, NF, is not exactly half that of the more concentrated alcohol but slightly greater, approximately 49%. Diluted alcohol is a useful hydroalcoholic solvent in various pharmaceutical processes and preparations.

Alcohol, Rubbing

Rubbing alcohol contains about 70% ethyl alcohol by volume, the remainder consisting of water, denaturants with or without color additives and perfume oils, and stabilizers. Each 100 mL must contain not less than 355 mg of sucrose octa-acetate or 1.4 mg of denatonium benzoate, bitter substances that discourage accidental or abusive oral ingestion. According to the Internal Revenue Service, U.S. Treasury Department, the denaturant employed in rubbing alcohol is formula 23-H, which is composed of 8 parts by volume of acetone, 1.5 parts by volume of methyl isobutyl ketone, and 100 parts by volume of ethyl alcohol. The use of this denaturant mixture makes the separation of ethyl alcohol from the denaturants virtually impossible with ordinary distillation apparatus. This discourages the illegal removal for use as a beverage of the alcoholic content of rubbing alcohol.

The product is volatile and flammable and should be stored in a tight container remote from fire. It is employed as a rubefacient externally and as a soothing rub for bedridden patients, a germicide for instruments, and a skin cleanser prior to injection. It is also used as a vehicle for topical preparations. Synonym: alcohol rubbing compound.

Glycerin, USP (Glycerol), CH₂OH•CHOH•CH₂OH

Glycerin is a clear syrupy liquid with a sweet taste. It is miscible with both water and alcohol. As a solvent, it is comparable with alcohol, but because of its viscosity, solutes are slowly soluble in it unless it is rendered less viscous by heating. Glycerin has preservative qualities and is often used as a stabilizer and as an auxiliary solvent in conjunction with water or alcohol. It is used in many internal preparations.

Isopropyl Rubbing Alcohol

Isopropyl rubbing alcohol is about 70% by volume isopropyl alcohol, the remainder consisting of water with or without color additives, stabilizers, and perfume oils. It is used externally as a rubefacient and soothing rub and as a vehicle for topical products. This preparation and a commercially available 91% isopropyl alcohol solution are commonly employed by diabetic patients in preparing needles and syringes for hypodermic injections of insulin and for disinfecting the skin.

Propylene Glycol, USP, CH₃CH(OH)CH₂OH

Propylene glycol, a viscous liquid, is miscible with water and alcohol. It is a useful solvent with a wide range of applications and is frequently substituted for glycerin in modern pharmaceutical formulations.

Purified Water, USP, H₂O

Naturally occurring water exerts its solvent effect on most substances it contacts and thus is impure, containing varying amounts of dissolved inorganic salts, usually sodium, potassium, calcium, magnesium, and iron; chlorides; sulfates; and bicarbonates, along with dissolved and undissolved organic matter and microorganisms. Water found in most cities and towns where water is purified for drinking usually contains less than 0.1% of total solids, determined by evaporating a 100-mL sample to dryness and weighing the residue (which weighs less than 100 mg). Drinking water must meet the U.S. Public Health Service regulations with respect to bacteriologic purity. Acceptable drinking water should be clear, colorless, odorless, and neutral or only slightly acid or alkaline, the deviation from neutral being due to the nature of the dissolved solids and gases (carbon dioxide contributing to the acidity and ammonia to the alkalinity of water).

Ordinary drinking water from the tap is not acceptable for the manufacture of most aqueous pharmaceutical preparations or for the extemporaneous compounding of prescriptions because of possible chemical incompatibilities between dissolved solids and the medicinal agents being added. Signs of such incompatibilities are precipitation, discoloration, and occasionally effervescence. Its use is permitted in washing, in extraction of crude vegetable drugs, in preparation of certain products for external use, and when the difference between tap water and purified water is of no consequence. Naturally, when large volumes of water are required to clean pharmaceutical machinery and equipment, tap water may be economically employed so long as a residue of solids is prevented by using purified water as the final rinse or by wiping the water dry with a meticulously clean cloth.

Purified Water, USP, is obtained by distillation, ion exchange treatment, reverse osmosis, or other suitable process. It is prepared from water complying with the federal Environmental Protection Agency with respect to drinking water. Purified Water, USP, has fewer solid impurities than ordinary drinking water. When evaporated to dryness, it must not yield more than 0.001% of residue (1 mg of solids per 100 mL of water). Thus, purified water has only 1% as much dissolved solids as tap water. Purified Water, USP, is intended for use in preparation of aqueous dosage forms except those intended for parenteral administration (injections). Water for Injection, USP; Bacteriostatic Water for Injection, USP; or Sterile Water for Injection, USP, is used for injections. These are discussed in Chapter 15.

The main methods used in the preparation of purified water are distillation, ion exchange, and reverse osmosis; these methods are described briefly next.

Distillation Method

Many stills in various sizes and styles with capacities ranging from about 0.5 to 100 gallons of distillate per hour are available to prepare purified water. Generally the first portion of aqueous distillate (about the first 10–20%) must be discarded, since it contains many foreign volatile substances usually found in urban drinking water, the usual starting material. Also, the last portion of water (about 10% of the original volume of water) remaining in the distillation apparatus must be discarded and not subjected to further distillation because distillation to dryness would undoubtedly result in decomposition of the remaining solid impurities to volatile substances that would distill and contaminate the previously collected portion of distillate.

Ion Exchange Method

On a large or small scale, ion exchange for the preparation of purified water offers a number of advantages over distillation. For one thing, the requirement of heat is eliminated and with it costly and troublesome maintenance frequently encountered in the operation of the more complex distillation apparatus. Because of the simpler equipment and the nature of the method, ion exchange permits ease of operation, minimal maintenance, and a more mobile facility. Many pharmacies and small laboratories that purchase large volumes of distilled water from commercial suppliers for use in their work would no doubt benefit financially and in convenience through the installation of an ion exchange demineralizer in the work area.

The ion exchange equipment in use today generally passes water through a column of cation and anion exchangers consisting of water-insoluble synthetic polymerized phenolic, carboxylic, amino, or sulfonated resins of high molecular weight. These resins are mainly of two types: (*a*) the cation, or acid exchangers, which permit the exchange of the cations in solution (in the tap water) with hydrogen ion from the resin; (*b*) the anion, or base exchange resins, which permit the removal of anions. These two processes are successively or simultaneously employed to remove both cations and anions from water. The processes are indicated as follows, with M^+ indicating the metal or cation (as Na^+) and the X^- indicating the anion (as Cl^-).

Cation exchange:

$$\text{H-resin} + M^+ + X^- + H_2O \rightarrow$$
$$\text{M-resin} + H^+ + X^- + H_2O \text{ (pure)}$$

Anion exchange:

$$\text{Resin-NH}_2 + H^+ + X^- + H_2O \rightarrow$$
$$\text{Resin-NH}_2 \cdot HX + H_2O \text{ (pure)}$$

Water purified in this manner, referred to as demineralized or deionized water, may be used in any pharmaceutical preparation or prescription calling for distilled water.

Reverse Osmosis

Reverse osmosis is one of the processes referred to in the industry as cross-flow (or tangential flow) membrane filtration (3). In this process, a pressurized stream of water is passed parallel to the inner side of a filter membrane core. A portion of the feed water, or influent, permeates the membrane as filtrate, while the balance of the water sweeps tangentially along the membrane to exit the system without being filtered. The filtered portion is called the permeate because it has permeated the membrane. The water that has passed through the system is called the concentrate because it contains the concentrated contaminants rejected by the membrane. Whereas in osmosis, the flow through a semipermeable membrane is from a less con-

centrated solution to a more concentrated solution, the flow in this cross-flow system is from a more concentrated to a less concentrated solution; thus the term reverse osmosis. Depending on their pore size, cross-flow filter membranes can remove particles defined in the range of microfiltration (0.1–2 µg, e.g., bacteria); ultrafiltration (0.01–0.1 µg, e.g., virus); nanofiltration (0.001–0.01 µg, e.g., organic compounds in the molecular weight range of 300–1000); and reverse osmosis (particles smaller than 0.001 µg). Reverse osmosis removes virtually all viruses, bacteria, pyrogens, and organic molecules and 90 to 99% of ions (3).

Preparation of Solutions

Most pharmaceutical solutions are unsaturated with solute. Thus the amounts of solute to be dissolved are usually well below the capacity of the volume of solvent employed. The strengths of pharmaceutical preparations are usually expressed in terms of percent strength, although for very dilute preparations, expressions of ratio strength may be used. These expressions and examples are shown in Table 13.4.

The symbol % used without qualification (as with w/v, v/v, or w/w) means percent weight in volume for solutions or suspensions of solids in liquids; percent weight in volume for solutions of gases in liquids; percent volume in volume

TABLE 13.4 COMMON METHODS OF EXPRESSING THE STRENGTHS OF PHARMACEUTICAL PREPARATIONS

EXPRESSION	ABBREVIATED EXPRESSION	MEANING AND EXAMPLE
Percent weight in volume	% w/v	Grams of constituent in 100 mL of preparation (e.g., 1% w/v = 1 g constituent in 100 mL preparation)
Percent volume in volume	% v/v	Milliliters of constituent in 100 mL of preparation (e.g., 1% v/v 1 mL constituent in 100 mL preparation)
Percent weight in weight	% w/w	Grams of constituent in 100 g of preparation (e. g., 1% w/w = 1 g constituent in 100 g preparation)
Ratio strength:weight in volume	–:— w/v	Grams of constituent in stated milliliters of preparation (e.g., 1:1000 w/v = 1 g constituent in 1000 mL preparation)
Ratio strength:volume in volume	–:— v/v	Milliliters of constituent in milliliters of preparation (e.g., 1:1000 v/v = 1 mL constituent in 1000 mL preparation)
Ratio strength:weight in weight	–:— w/w	Grams of constituent in stated number of grams of preparation (e.g., 1:1000 w/w = 1 g constituent in 1000 g preparation)

for solutions of liquids in liquids; and weight in weight for mixtures of solids and semisolids.

Some chemical agents in a given solvent require an extended time for dissolving. To hasten dissolution, a pharmacist may employ one of several techniques, such as applying heat, reducing the particle size of the solute, using a solubilizing agent, or subjecting the ingredients to vigorous agitation. Most chemical agents are more soluble at elevated temperatures than at room temperature or below because an endothermic reaction between the solute and the solvent uses the energy of the heat to enhance dissolution. However, elevated temperatures cannot be maintained for pharmaceuticals, and the net effect of heat is simply an increase in the rate of solution rather than an increase in solubility. An increased rate is satisfactory to the pharmacist, because most solutions are unsaturated anyway and do not require a concentration of solute above the normal capacity of the solvent at room temperature. Pharmacists are reluctant to use heat to facilitate solution, and when they do, they are careful not to exceed the minimally required temperature, for many medicinal agents are destroyed at elevated temperatures, and the advantage of rapid solution may be completely offset by drug deterioration. If volatile solutes are to be dissolved or if the solvent is volatile (as is alcohol), the heat would encourage the loss of these agents to the atmosphere and must therefore be avoided. Pharmacists are aware that certain chemical agents, particularly calcium salts, undergo exothermic reactions as they dissolve and give off heat. For such materials the use of heat would actually discourage the formation of a solution. The best pharmaceutical example of this type of chemical is calcium hydroxide, which is used in the preparation of Calcium Hydroxide Topical Solution, USP. Calcium hydroxide is soluble in water to the extent of 140 mg per 100 mL of solution at 25°C (about 77°F) and 170 mg per 100 mL of solution at 15°C (about 59°F). Obviously the temperature at which the solution is prepared or stored can affect the concentration of the resultant solution.

In addition to or instead of raising the temperature of the solvent to increase the rate of so-

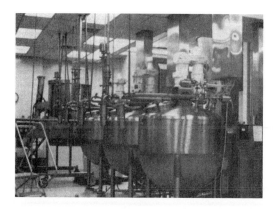

FIGURE 13.1 Large-scale pharmaceutical mixing vessels. (Courtesy of Schering Laboratories.)

lution, a pharmacist may choose to decrease the particle size of the solute. This may be accomplished by comminution (grinding a solid to a fine state of subdivision) with a mortar and pestle on a small scale or industrial micronizer on a large scale. The reduced particle size increases the surface area of the solute. If the powder is placed in a suitable vessel (e.g., a beaker, graduated cylinder, or bottle) with a portion of the solvent and is stirred or shaken, as suited to the container, the rate of solution may be increased by the continued circulation of fresh solvent to the drug's surface and the constant removal of newly formed solution from the drug's surface.

Most solutions are prepared by simple mixing of the solutes with the solvent. On an industrial scale, solutions are prepared in large mixing vessels with ports for mechanical stirrers (Fig. 13.1). When heat is desired, thermostatically controlled mixing tanks may be used.

Oral Solutions and Preparations for Oral Solution

Most solutions intended for oral administration contain flavorants and colorants to make the medication more attractive and palatable. When needed, they may also contain stabilizers to maintain the chemical and physical stability of the medicinal agents and preservatives to prevent the growth of microorganisms in the solution. The formulation pharmacist must be wary of chemical interactions between the various components of a solution that may alter the preparation's stability and/or potency. For instance, esters of p-hydroxybenzoic acid (methyl-, ethyl-, propyl-, and butylparabens), frequently used preservatives in oral preparations, have a tendency to partition into certain flavoring oils (4). This partitioning effect could reduce the effective concentration of the preservatives in the aqueous medium of a pharmaceutical product below the level needed for preservative action.

Liquid pharmaceuticals for oral administration are usually formulated such that the patient receives the usual dose of the medication in a conveniently administered volume, as 5 mL (one teaspoonful), 10 mL, or 15 mL (one tablespoonful). A few solutions have unusually large doses, for example Magnesium Citrate Oral Solution, USP, with a usual adult dose of 200 mL. On the other hand, many solutions for children are given by drop with a calibrated dropper usually furnished by the manufacturer in the product package.

Dry Mixtures for Solution

A number of medicinal agents, particularly certain antibiotics, have insufficient stability in aqueous solution to meet extended shelf life periods. Thus, commercial manufacturers of these products provide them to the pharmacist in dry powder or granule form for reconstitution with a prescribed amount of purified water immediately before dispensing to the patient. The dry powder mixture contains all of the formulative components, including drug, flavorant, colorant, buffers, and others, except for the solvent. Once reconstituted by the pharmacist, the solution remains stable when stored in the refrigerator for the labeled period, usually 7 to 14 days, depending on the preparation. This is a sufficient period for the patient to complete the regimen usually prescribed. However, in case medication remains after the patient completes the course of therapy, the patient should be instructed to discard the remaining portion, which would be unfit for use later.

Examples of dry powder mixtures intended for reconstitution to oral solutions are the following:

Cloxacillin Sodium for Oral Solution, USP (Teva), an anti-infective antibiotic
Penicillin V Potassium for Oral Solution, USP (Pen-Vee K, Wyeth-Ayerst), an anti-infective antibiotic
Potassium Chloride for Oral Solution, USP (K-LOR, Abbott), a potassium supplement

Oral Solutions

The pharmacist may be called on to dispense a commercially prepared oral solution; dilute the concentration of a solution, as in the preparation of a pediatric form of an adult product; prepare a solution by reconstituting a dry powder mixture; or extemporaneously compound an oral solution from bulk components.

In each instance, the pharmacist should be sufficiently knowledgeable about the dispensed product to expertly advise the patient of the proper use, dosage, method of administration, and storage of the product. Knowledge of the solubility and stability characteristics of the medicinal agents and the solvents employed in the commercial products is useful to the pharmacist for informing the patient of the advisability of mixing the solution with juice, milk, or other beverage upon administration. Information regarding the solvents used in each commercial product appears on the product label and in the accompanying package insert. Table 13.5 presents examples of some oral solutions. Some solutions of special pharmaceutical interest are described later in this chapter.

Oral Rehydration Solutions

Rapid fluid loss associated with diarrhea can lead to dehydration and ultimately death in some patients, particularly infants. More than 5 million children younger than 4 years die of diarrhea each year worldwide (5). Diarrhea is characterized by an increased frequency of loose, watery stools, and because of the rapid fluid loss, dehydration can be an outcome. During diarrhea, the small intestine secretes far more than the normal amount of fluid and electrolytes, and this simply exceeds the ability of the large intestine to reabsorb it. This fluid

TABLE 13.5 EXAMPLES OF ORAL SOLUTIONS BY CATEGORY

ORAL SOLUTION	REPRESENTATIVE COMMERCIAL PRODUCTS	CONCENTRATION OF COMMERCIAL PRODUCT	COMMENTS
Antidepressants			
Nortriptyline HCl	Pamelor Oral Solution (Novartis)	10 mg nortriptyline/ 5 mL	Tricyclic antidepressant.
Fluoxetine HCl	Prozac Liquid (Dista)	20 mg fluoxetine/5 mL	For depression, obsessive-compulsive disorder.
Antiperistaltic			
Diphenoxylate HCl, atropine sulfate	Lomotil Liquid (Searle)	2.5 mg diphenoxylate HCl, 0.025 mg atropine sulfate/5 mL	For diarrhea. Diphenoxylate is related structurally and pharmacologically to the opioid meperidine. Atropine sulfate in subtherapeutic amounts discourages (by virtue of side effects) deliberate overdosage.
Loperamide HCl	Imodium A-D Liquid (McNeil Consumer Products)	1 mg loperamide HCl/ 5 mL	For diarrhea in adults and children aged 6 years and older. Structurally related to haloperidol.
Antipsychotics			
Haloperidol Perphenazine	Haloperidol Oral Solution Perphenazine Oral Solution	2 mg haloperidol/mL 16 mg perphenazine/ 5 mL	Primarily for severe neuro-psychiatric conditions when oral medication is preferred and tablets and capsules are impractical. Concentrated solutions used by adding desired amount of concentrate by calibrated dropper to soup or a beverage.
Thiothixene HCl	Navane concentrate (Pfizer)	Equivalent of 5 mg thiothixene/mL	
Bronchodilator			
Theophylline	Theophylline Oral Solution (Roxane)	80 mg theophylline/ 15 mL	Alcohol-free solution for treatment of bronchial asthma and reversible bronchospasm associated with chronic bronchitis and emphysema.
Cathartics			
Magnesium Citrate, USP		Magnesium citrate equivalent to 1.55–1.9 g/100 mL magnesium oxide	Discussed in text
Sodium phosphate	Phospho-Soda (Fleet)	2.4 g monobasic sodium phosphate, 0.9 g dibasic sodium phosphate/5 mL	Works as laxative within 1 hour taken before meals or over-night taken at bedtime. Usual dose is 10–20 mL, best diluted in half-glass of water and followed with full glass of water.
Corticosteroid			
Prednisolone sodium phosphate	Pediapred Oral Solution (Medeva)	5 mg prednisolone (as sodium phosphate)/5 mL	Synthetic adrenocortical steroid with mainly glucocorticoid properties indicated for endocrine, rheumatic, collagen, allergic, and other disorders.

(continued)

TABLE 13.5 EXAMPLES OF ORAL SOLUTIONS BY CATEGORY

ORAL SOLUTION	REPRESENTATIVE COMMERCIAL PRODUCTS	CONCENTRATION OF COMMERCIAL PRODUCT	COMMENTS
Dental caries protectant			
Sodium fluoride	Pediaflor Drops (Boss)	0.5 mg/mL	Prophylaxis of dental caries; for use when community water supply is inadequately fluoridated.
Electrolyte replenisher			
Potassium chloride	KaoChlor 10% Liquid (Adria)	20 mEq KCl/15 mL in flavored aqueous vehicle	For hypopotassemia (low blood level of potassium). Condition may be prompted by severe or chronic diarrhea, low dietary intake of potassium, increased renal excretion of potassium, other causes. Solution is diluted with water or fruit juice.
Fecal softener			
Docusate sodium	Colace Syrup (Shire)	10 mg docusate sodium/mL	Usually 50–200 mg measured by calibrated dropper, mixed with milk, fruit juice, other liquid to mask taste. Softens fecal mass by lowering surface tension, permitting normal bowel habits, particularly in geriatric, pediatric cardiac, obstetric, and surgical patients. Taken for several days or until bowel movements are normal.
Hematinic			
Ferrous sulfate	Fer-In-Sol Drops (Mead Johnson Nutritional)	15 mg/0.6 mL	For prevention and treatment of iron deficiency anemias. Usual prophylactic dose 0.3 or 0.6 mL, measured by calibrated dropper, mixed with water or juice. Dosage form intended primarily for infants and children.
Histamine H_2 antagonist			
Cimetidine HCl	Tagamet HCl Liquid (SmithKline Beecham)	300 mg/5 mL	For peptic ulcer disease, pathologic hypersecretory conditions, e.g., Zollinger-Ellison syndrome.
Opioid agonist analgesic			
Methadone HCl	Methadone HCL (Roxane)	1 or 2 mg/mL	For relief of severe pain; detoxification, maintenance treatment of opioid addiction.
Vitamin D			
Ergocalciferol	Calciferol Drops (Schwarz)	8,000 U/mL	Water-insoluble ergocalciferol (vitamin D_2) in propylene glycol. Usual prophylactic dose about 400 U; therapeutic dose may be as high as 200,000–500,000 U daily in treating rickets.

loss, which occurs mostly from the body's extracellular fluid compartment, can lead to a progressive loss of blood volume culminating in hypovolemic shock.

Diarrhea is a normal physiologic body response to rid itself of a noxious or toxic substance, such as rotavirus or *Escherichia coli*. Thus, the treatment approach is to allow the diarrhea to proceed and not to terminate it too quickly but promptly replace the lost fluid and electrolytes to prevent dehydration. The loss of fluid during diarrhea is accompanied by depletion of sodium, potassium, and bicarbonate ions; if severe, the loss can result in acidosis, hyperpnea, and vomiting as well as hypovolemic shock. If continuous, bouts of vomiting and diarrhea can cause malnutrition as well. Consequently, the goal is to replace lost fecal water with an oral rehydration solution and use nutritional foods, such as soybean formula and bran.

Oral rehydration solutions are usually effective in treatment of patients with mild volume depletion, 5 to 10% of body weight. These are available OTC and are relatively inexpensive, and their use has diminished the incidence of complications associated with parenterally administered electrolyte solutions. Therapy with these solutions is based on the observation that glucose is actively absorbed from the small intestine, even during bouts of diarrhea. This active transport of glucose is advantageous because it is coupled with sodium absorption. Almost in domino fashion, sodium absorption promotes anion absorption, which in turn promotes water absorption to short-circuit dehydration. To produce maximal absorption of sodium and water, studies have demonstrated that the optimal concentrations of glucose and sodium in an isotonic solution are 110 mM (2%) glucose and 60 mEq/L of sodium ion, respectively. Bicarbonate and/or citrate ions are also included in these solutions to help correct the metabolic acidosis caused by diarrhea and dehydration.

A liter of typical oral rehydration solution contains 45 mEq Na^+, 20 mEq K^+, 35 mEq Cl^-, 30 mEq citrate, and 25 g dextrose. These formulations are available in liquid or powder packet form for reconstitution. It is important that the user add the specific amount of water needed to prepare the powder forms. Furthermore, these products should not be mixed with or given with other electrolyte-containing liquids, such as milk or fruit juices. Otherwise, there is no method to calculate how much electrolyte the patient actually received. Commercial ready-to-use oral electrolyte solutions to prevent dehydration or achieve rehydration include Pedialyte Solution (Ross) and Rehydrate Solution (Ross). These products also contain dextrose or glucose. Ricelyte Oral Solution (Mead Johnson) contains electrolytes in a syrup of rice solids. The rice-based formula produces a lower osmotic effect than the dextrose- or glucose-based formulas and is thought to be more effective in reducing stool output and shortening the duration of diarrhea. The pharmacist must discourage the production of homemade versions of electrolyte solutions. The success of the commercial solutions is based on the accuracy of the formulation. If prepared incorrectly, homemade preparations can cause hypernatremia or worsen the diarrhea.

Oral Colonic Lavage Solution

Traditionally, preparation of the bowel for procedures such as a colonoscopy consisted of administration of a clear liquid diet for 24 to 48 hours preceding the procedure, administration of an oral laxative such as magnesium citrate or bisacodyl the night before, and a cleansing enema administered 2 to 4 hours prior to the procedure. Typically, to circumvent hospitalization of the patient the night before the procedure, patients were allowed to perform this regimen at home. However, while the results have been satisfactory, that is, the bowel is cleared for the procedure, poor compliance with and acceptance of this regimen can cause problems during the procedure. Furthermore, additive effects of malnutrition and poor oral intake prior to the procedure can cause more patient problems.

Consequently, an alternative method to prepare the gastrointestinal tract has been devised. This procedure requires less time and dietary restriction and obviates cleansing enemas. This method entails oral administration of a balanced solution of electrolytes with polyethylene glycol (PEG-3350). Before dispensing it to the patient, the pharmacist reconstitutes this powder with water, creating an iso-osmotic solution having a mildly salty taste. The PEG acts as an osmotic agent in the gastrointestinal tract, and the balanced electrolyte concentration results in virtually no net absorption or secretion of ions. Thus, a large volume of this solution can be administered without a significant change in water or electrolyte balance.

The formulation of this oral colonic lavage solution is as follows:

PEG-3350	236.00 g
Sodium sulfate	22.74 g
Sodium bicarbonate	6.74 g
Sodium chloride	5.86 g
Potassium chloride	2.97 g
In 4800 mL disposable container	

The recommended adult dose of this product is 4 L of solution before the gastrointestinal procedure. The patient is instructed to drink 240 mL of solution every 10 minutes until about 4 L is consumed. The patient is advised to drink each portion quickly rather than sipping it continuously. Usually, the first bowel movement will occur within 1 hour. Several regimens are used, and one method is to schedule patients for a midmorning procedure, allowing the patient 3 hours for drinking and a 1-hour waiting period to complete bowel evacuation.

To date, this approach to bowel evacuation has been associated with a low incidence of side effects (primarily nausea, transient abdominal fullness, bloating, and occasionally cramps and vomiting). Ideally, the patient should not have taken any food 3 to 4 hours before beginning to take the solution. In no case should solid foods be taken by the patient for at least 2 hours before the solution is administered. No foods except clear liquids are permitted after this product is administered and prior to the examination. The product must be stored in the refrigerator after reconstitution, and this aids somewhat in decreasing the salty taste of the product.

Magnesium Citrate Oral Solution

Magnesium citrate oral solution is a colorless to slightly yellow clear effervescent liquid having a sweet, acidulous taste and a lemon flavor. It is commonly referred to as citrate or as citrate of magnesia. It is required to contain an amount of magnesium citrate equivalent to 1.55 to 1.9 g of magnesium oxide in each 100 mL.

The solution is prepared by reacting official magnesium carbonate with an excess of citric acid (Equation 13.1), flavoring and sweetening the solution with lemon oil and syrup, filtering with talc, and then carbonating it by the addition of either potassium or sodium bicarbonate (Equation 13.2). The solution may be further carbonated by the use of carbon dioxide under pressure.

$$(MgCO_3)_4 \cdot Mg(OH)_2 + 5H_3C_6H_5O_7 \rightarrow$$
$$5MgHC_6H_5O_7 + 4CO_2 + 6H_2O \quad \text{(Equation 13.1)}$$

$$3KHCO_3 + H_3C_6H_5O_7 \rightarrow$$
$$K_3C_6H_5O_7 + 3CO_2 + 3H_2O \quad \text{(Equation 13.2)}$$

The solution provides an excellent medium for the growth of molds, and any mold spores present during the manufacture of the solution must be killed if the preparation is to remain stable. For this reason, during the preparation of the solution the liquid is heated to boiling (prior to carbonation); boiled water is employed to bring the solution to its proper volume; and boiling water is used to rinse the final container. The final solution may be sterilized.

Magnesium citrate solution has always been troublesome because it has a tendency to deposit a crystalline solid upon standing. Apparently this is due to the formation of some almost insoluble normal magnesium citrate (rather than the exclusively dibasic form, as in Equation 13.1). The cause of the problem has largely been attributed to the indefinite composition of the official magnesium carbonate, which by definition is "a basic hydrated magnesium carbonate or a normal hydrated magnesium carbonate" (Equation 13.1). It contains the equivalent of 40 to 43.5% of magnesium oxide. Apparently, solutions prepared from magnesium carbonates with differing equivalents of magnesium oxide vary in stability, with the most stable ones being prepared from samples of magnesium carbonate having the lower equivalent of magnesium oxide. The formula for the preparation of 350 mL of magnesium citrate solution calls for the use of 15 g of official magnesium carbonate, which corresponds to approximately 6.0 to 6.47 g of magnesium oxide.

In carbonating the solution, the bicarbonate may be added in tablet form rather than as a powder to delay the effervescence resulting from its contact with the citric acid. If the powder were used, the reaction would be immediate and violent, and it would be virtually impossible to close the bottle in time to prevent the loss of carbon dioxide or solution. The solution may be further carbonated by the use of CO_2 under pressure. Most of the magnesium citrate solutions prepared commercially today are packaged in the same type of bottles as soft drinks, or carbonated beverages. The solution is packaged in bottles of 300 mL. Since the solution is carbonated, it loses some of its carbonation if allowed to stand after the container has been opened. Magnesium citrate solution is stored in a cold place, preferably in a refrigerator, keeping the bottle on its side so the cork or rubber liner of the cap is kept moist and swollen, thereby maintaining the airtight seal between the cap and the bottle.

The solution is employed as a saline cathartic, with the citric acid, lemon oil, syrup, carbonation, and the low temperature of the refrigerated solution all contributing to the patient's acceptance of the large volume of medication. For many patients it is a pleasant way of taking an otherwise bitter saline cathartic.

Sodium Citrate and Citric Acid Oral Solution

This official solution contains sodium citrate 100 mg and citric acid 67 mg in each milliliter of aqueous solution. The solution is administered orally in doses of 10 to 30 mL as frequently as four times daily as a systemic alkalinizer. Systemic alkalinization is useful for patients for whom long-term maintenance of an alkaline urine is desirable, such as those with uric acid and cystine calculi of the urinary tract. The solution is also a useful adjuvant when administered with uricosuric agents in gout therapy, since urates tend to crystallize out of an acid urine.

Syrups

Syrups are concentrated aqueous preparations of a sugar or sugar substitute with or without flavoring agents and medicinal substances. Syrups containing flavoring agents but not medicinal substances are called nonmedicated or flavored vehicles (syrups). Some official, previously official, and commercially available nonmedicated syrups are presented in Table 13.6.

TABLE 13.6 EXAMPLES OF NONMEDICATED SYRUPS (VEHICLES)

SYRUP	COMMENTS
Cherry syrup	Sucrose-based syrup with cherry juice about 47% by volume. Tart fruit flavor is attractive to most patients and acidic pH makes it useful as a vehicle for drugs requiring an acid medium.
Cocoa syrup	Suspension of cocoa powder in aqueous vehicle sweetened and thickened with sucrose, liquid glucose, glycerin; flavored with vanilla, sodium chloride. Particularly effective in administering bitter-tasting drugs to children.
Orange syrup	Sucrose-based syrup uses sweet orange peel tincture, citric acid as sources of flavor and tartness. Resembles orange juice in taste; good vehicle for drugs stable in acidic medium.
Ora-Sweet, Ora-Sweet SF	Commercial vehicles for extemporaneous compounding of (Paddock Laboratories) syrups. Both have pH of 4–4.5 and are alcohol free. Ora-Sweet SF is sugar free.
Raspberry syrup	Sucrose-based syrup with raspberry juice about 48% by volume. Pleasant-flavored vehicle to disguise salty or sour taste of saline medicaments.
Syrup	85% sucrose in purified water. Simple syrup may be used as basis for flavored or medicated syrups.

These syrups are intended to serve as pleasant-tasting vehicles for medicinal substances to be added in the extemporaneous compounding of prescriptions or in the preparation of a standard formula for a medicated syrup, which is a syrup containing a therapeutic agent. Due to the inability of some children and elderly people to swallow solid dosage forms, it is fairly common today for a pharmacist to be asked to prepare an oral liquid dosage form of a medication available in the pharmacy only as tablets or capsules. In these instances, drug solubility, stability, and bioavailability must be considered case by case (6, 7). The liquid dosage form selected for compounding may be a solution or a suspension, depending on the chemical and physical characteristics of the particular drug and its solid dosage form. Vehicles are commercially available for this purpose (7).

Medicated syrups are commercially prepared from the starting materials; that is, by combining each of the individual components of the syrup, such as sucrose, purified water, flavoring agents, coloring agents, the therapeutic agent, and other necessary and desirable ingredients. Naturally, medicated syrups are employed in therapeutics for the value of the medicinal agent present in the syrup.

Syrups provide a pleasant means of administering a liquid form of a disagreeable-tasting drug. They are particularly effective in the administration of drugs to youngsters, since their pleasant taste usually dissipates any reluctance on the part of the child to take the medicine. The fact that syrups contain little or no alcohol adds to their favor among parents.

Any water-soluble drug that is stable in aqueous solution may be added to a flavored syrup. However, care must be exercised to ensure compatibility between the drug substance and the other formulative components of the syrup. Also, certain flavored syrups have an acidic medium, whereas others may be neutral or slightly basic, and the proper selection must be made to ensure the stability of any added medicinal agent. Perhaps the most frequently found types of medications administered as medicated syrups are antitussive agents and antihistamines. This is not to imply that other types of drugs are not formulated into syrups; a variety of medicinal substances can be found in syrup form and among the many commercial products. Examples of medicated syrups are presented in Table 13.7.

Components of Syrups

Most syrups contain the following components in addition to the purified water and any medicinal agents present: (*a*) the sugar, usually sucrose, or sugar substitute used to provide sweetness and viscosity; (*b*) antimicrobial preservatives; (*c*) flavorants; and (*d*) colorants. Also, many syrups, especially those prepared commercially, contain special solvents, solubilizing agents, thickeners, or stabilizers.

Sucrose- and Non–Sucrose-Based Syrups

Sucrose is the sugar most frequently employed in syrups, although in special circumstances it may be replaced in whole or in part by other sugars or substances such as sorbitol, glycerin, and propylene glycol. In some instances, all glycogenetic substances (materials converted to glucose in the body), including the agents mentioned earlier, are replaced by nonglycogenetic substances, such as methylcellulose or hydroxy ethylcellulose. These two materials are not hydrolyzed and absorbed into the blood stream, and their use results in an excellent syruplike vehicle for medications intended for use by diabetic patients and others whose diet must be controlled and restricted to nonglycogenetic substances. The viscosity resulting from the use of these cellulose derivatives is much like that of a sucrose syrup. The addition of one or more artificial sweeteners usually produces an excellent facsimile of a true syrup.

The characteristic body that the sucrose and alternative agents seek to impart to the syrup is essentially the result of attaining the proper viscosity. This quality, together with the sweetness and flavorants, results in a type of pharmaceutical preparation that masks the taste of added medicinal agents. When the syrup is swallowed, only a portion of dissolved drug actually makes contact with the taste buds, the remainder of the drug being carried past them and down the throat in the viscous syrup. This type of physical concealment of the taste is not

TABLE 13.7 EXAMPLES OF MEDICATED SYRUPS BY CATEGORY

SYRUP	REPRESENTATIVE COMMERCIAL PRODUCTS	CONCENTRATION OF COMMERCIAL PRODUCT[a]	COMMENTS
Analgesic			
Meperidine HCl	Demerol Syrup (Sanofi)	50 mg/5 mL	Opioid analgesic for relief of moderate to severe pain, adjunct to general anesthesia.
Anticholinergics			
Dicyclomine HCl	Bentyl (Hoechst Marion Roussel)	10 mg/5 mL	Adjunctive therapy in treatment of peptic ulcer.
Oxybutynin chloride	Ditropan Syrup (Alza)	5 mg/5 mL	Relief of symptoms with voiding in patients with uninhibited neurogenic and reflex neurogenic bladder.
Antiemetics			
Chlorpromazine HCl	Thorazine Syrup (SmithKline Beecham)	10 mg HCl/5 mL	Control of nausea and vomiting.
Dimenhydrinate	Children's Dramamine Liquid (Pharmacia & Upjohn)	12.5 mg/5 mL	Control of nausea, vomiting, motion sickness.
Prochlorperazine Edisylate	Compazine Syrup (SmithKline Beecham)	5 mg/5 mL	Control of nausea and vomiting.
Promethazine HCl	Phenergan Syrup (Wyeth-Ayerst)	6.25, 25 mg/5 mL	Control of nausea, vomiting, motion sickness, allergic reactions.
Anticonvulsant			
Sodium valproate	Depakene Syrup (Abbott)	250 mg as sodium salt/5 mL	Sole or adjunctive therapy in simple (petit mal), complex absence seizure disorders.
Antihistamines			
Chlorpheniramine maleate	Chlor-Trimeton Allergy Syrup (Schering-Plough)	2 mg/5 mL	For prevention, treatment of allergic reactions.
Hydroxyzine HCl	Atarax Syrup (Roerig)	10 mg/5 mL	
Antipsychotic			
Citalopram hydrobromide	Celexa	10 mg/5 mL	For depression.
Lithium citrate	Lithium Citrate Syrup (Roxane)	8 mEq/5mL	Management of psychotic disorders.
Risperidone	Risperdal	1 mg/mL	For treatment of schizophrenia.
Antitussives			
Dextromethorphan	Benylin Adult Cough Formula (Warner-Lambert Consumer)	15 mg/5 mL	For relief of cough.
Diphenhydramine	Benadryl Allergy Liquid Medication (Pfizer)	12.5 mg/5 mL	For control of coughs due to colds or allergy.
Antiviral			
Amantadine HCl	Symmetrel Syrup (Endo)	50 mg/5 mL	Prevention of respiratory infections caused by A2 (Asian) viral strains. Treatment of idiopathic Parkinson's disease.
Lamivudine	Epivir Oral Solution	10 mg/mL	Treatment of HIV.

(continued)

TABLE 13.7 EXAMPLES OF MEDICATED SYRUPS BY CATEGORY

SYRUP	REPRESENTATIVE COMMERCIAL PRODUCTS	CONCENTRATION OF COMMERCIAL PRODUCT[a]	COMMENTS
Lopinavir, ritonavir	Kaletra	Lopinavir 80 mg, ritonavir 20 mg/mL	Treatment of HIV.
Ritonavir	Norvir	80 mg/mL	Treatment of HIV.
Bronchodilators			
Albuterol sulfate	Proventil Syrup (Schering) Ventolin Syrup (Allen & Hanburys)	2 mg/5 mL	Relief of bronchospasm of obstructive airway disease; prevention of exercise-induced bronchospasm.
Metaproterenol sulfate	Alupent Syrup (Boehringer Ingelheim)	10 mg/5 mL	
Cathartic			
Lactulose	Chronulac Syrup (Hoechst Marion Roussel)	10 g/15 mL	15–30 mL qd as laxative.
Cholinergic			
Pyridostigmine bromide	Mestinon Syrup (ICN Pharmaceuticals)	60 mg/5 mL	Treatment of myasthenia gravis.
Decongestant			
Pseudoephedrine hydrochloride	Children's Sudafed Liquid (Warner-Lambert)	15 mg/5 mL	Temporary relief of nasal congestion of common cold, hay fever, upper respiratory allergies, sinusitis.
Emetic			
Ipecac	Ipecac Syrup (Roxane)	21 mg ether-soluble alkaloids of ipecac/ 15 mL	To induce vomiting in poisoning. Dose of 15 mL may be repeated in 20 minutes if vomiting does not occur. If after the second dose, vomiting does not occur, the stomach should be emptied by gastric lavage.
Expectorant			
Guaifenesin	Guaifenesin Syrup (Roxane)	100 mg/5 mL	For symptomatic relief of respiratory conditions associated with cough and bronchial congestion.
Fecal softener			
Docusate sodium	Colace Syrup (Roberts)	20 mg/5 mL	Stool softener by surface action.
Gastrointestinal stimulant			
Metoclopramide	Reglan Syrup (Robins)	5 mg/5 mL	Relief of symptoms of diabetic gastroparesis (gastric stasis) and gastroesophageal reflux.
Hemostatic			
Aminocaproic Acid	Amicar Syrup (Immunex)	1.25 g/5 mL	Treatment of excessive bleeding from systemic hyperfibrinolysis, urinary fibrinolysis.

(continued)

TABLE 13.7 EXAMPLES OF MEDICATED SYRUPS BY CATEGORY

SYRUP	REPRESENTATIVE COMMERCIAL PRODUCTS	CONCENTRATION OF COMMERCIAL PRODUCT[a]	COMMENTS
Hypnotic sedative			
Chloral hydrate	Chloral Hydrate Syrup (Pharmaceutical Associates)	500 mg/5 mL	Sedative at 250 mg; hypnotic to induce sleep at 500 mg. Alcoholic beverages should be avoided. Usually diluted with water or other beverage.

[a]A usual single dose unless otherwise stated.

possible for a solution of a drug in an unthickened, mobile aqueous preparation. In the case of antitussive syrups, the thick, sweet syrup has a soothing effect on the irritated tissues of the throat as it passes over them.

Most syrups contain a high proportion of sucrose, usually 60 to 80%, not only because of the desirable sweetness and viscosity of such solutions but also because of their inherent stability in contrast to the unstable character of dilute sucrose solutions. The aqueous sugar medium of dilute sucrose solutions is an efficient nutrient medium for the growth of microorganisms, particularly yeasts and molds. On the other hand, concentrated sugar solutions are quite resistant to microbial growth because of the unavailability of the water required for the growth of microorganisms. This aspect of syrups is best demonstrated by the simplest of all syrups, Syrup, NF, also called simple syrup. It is prepared by dissolving 85 g of sucrose in enough purified water to make 100 mL of syrup. The resulting preparation generally requires no additional preservation if it is to be used soon; in the official syrup, preservatives are added if the syrup is to be stored. When properly prepared and maintained, the syrup is inherently stable and resistant to the growth of microorganisms. An examination of this syrup reveals its concentrated nature and the relative absence of water for microbial growth. Syrup has a specific gravity of about 1.313, which means that each 100 mL of syrup weighs 131.3 g. Because 85 g of sucrose is present, the difference between 85 g and 131.3 g, or 46.3 g, represents the weight of the purified water. Thus, 46.3 g, or mL, of purified water is used to dissolve 85 g of sucrose. The solubility of sucrose in water is 1 g in 0.5 mL of water; therefore, to dissolve 85 g of sucrose, about 42.5 mL of water would be required. Thus, only a very slight excess of water (about 3.8 mL per 100 mL of syrup) is employed in the preparation of syrup. Although not enough to be particularly amenable to the growth of microorganisms, the slight excess of water permits the syrup to remain physically stable in varying temperatures. If the syrup were completely saturated with sucrose, in cool storage some sucrose might crystallize from solution and, by acting as nuclei, initiate a type of chain reaction that would result in separation of an amount of sucrose disproportionate to its solubility at the storage temperature. The syrup would then be very much unsaturated and probably suitable for microbial growth. As formulated, the official syrup is both stable and resistant to crystallization and microbial growth. However, many of the other official syrups and a host of commercial syrups are not intended to be as nearly saturated as Syrup, NF, and therefore must employ added preservative agents to prevent microbial growth and to ensure their stability during their period of use and storage.

As noted earlier, sucrose-based syrup may be substituted in whole or in part by other agents in the preparation of medicated syrups. A solution of a polyol, such as sorbitol, or a mixture of polyols, such as sorbitol and glycerin, are commonly used. Sorbitol Solution, USP, which contains 64% by weight of the polyhydric alcohol sorbitol is employed as shown in the following example formulations for medicated syrups (8):

Antihistamine Syrup

Chlorpheniramine maleate	0.4 g
Glycerin	25.0 mL
Syrup	83.0 mL
Sorbitol solution	282.0 mL
Sodium benzoate	1.0 g
Alcohol	60.0 mL
Color and flavor	q.s.
Purified water, to make	1000.0 mL

Ferrous Sulfate Syrup

Ferrous sulfate	135.0 g
Citric acid	12.0 g
Sorbitol solution	350.0 mL
Glycerin	50.0 mL
Sodium benzoate	1.0 g
Flavor	q.s.
Purified water, to make	1000.0 mL

Acetaminophen Syrup

Acetaminophen	24.0 g
Benzoic acid	1.0 g
Disodium calcium EDTA	1.0 g
Propylene glycol	150.0 mL
Alcohol	150.0 mL
Saccharin sodium	1.8 g
Purified water	200.0 mL
Flavor	q.s.
Sorbitol solution, to make	1000.0 mL

Cough and Cold Syrup

Dextromethorphan hydrobromide	2.0 g
Guaifenesin	10.0 g
Chlorpheniramine maleate	0.2 g
Phenylephrine hydrochloride	1.0 g
Sodium benzoate	1.0 g
Saccharin sodium	1.9 g
Citric acid	1.0 g
Sodium chloride	5.2 g
Alcohol	50.0 mL
Sorbitol solution	324.0 mL
Syrup	132.0 mL
Liquid glucose	44.0 mL
Glycerin	50.0 mL
Color	q.s.
Flavor	q.s.
Purified water, to make	1000.0 mL

All materials used in the extemporaneous compounding and manufacturing of pharmaceuticals should be of USP–NF quality and obtained from FDA-approved sources.

Antimicrobial Preservative

The amount of a preservative required to protect a syrup against microbial growth varies with the proportion of water available for growth, the nature and inherent preservative activity of some formulative materials (e.g., many flavoring oils that are inherently sterile and possess antimicrobial activity), and the capability of the preservative itself. Among the preservatives commonly used in syrups with the usually effective concentrations are benzoic acid 0.1–0.2%, sodium benzoate 0.1–0.2%, and various combinations of methylparabens, propylparabens, and butylparabens totaling about 0.1%. Frequently alcohol is used in syrups to assist in dissolving alcohol-soluble ingredients, but normally it is not present in the final product in amounts that would be considered to be adequate for preservation (15 to 20%). See Physical Pharmacy Capsule 13.1, Preservation of Syrups.

Flavorant

Most syrups are flavored with synthetic flavorants or with naturally occurring materials, such as volatile oils (e.g. orange oil), vanillin, and others, to render the syrup pleasant tasting. Because syrups are aqueous preparations, these flavorants must be water soluble. However, sometimes a small amount of alcohol is added to a syrup to ensure the continued solution of a poorly water-soluble flavorant.

Colorant

To enhance the appeal of the syrup, a coloring agent that correlates with the flavorant employed (i.e., green with mint, brown with chocolate) is used. The colorant is generally water soluble, nonreactive with the other syrup components, and color stable at the pH range and under the intensity of light that the syrup is likely to encounter during its shelf life.

Preparation of Syrups

Syrups are most frequently prepared by one of four general methods, depending on the phys-

Preservation of Syrups

Syrups can be preserved by (a) storage at low temperature, (b) adding preservatives such as glycerin, benzoic acid, sodium benzoate, methyl paraben or alcohol in the formulation, or (c) by the maintenance of a high concentration of sucrose as a part of the formulation. High sucrose concentrations will usually protect an oral liquid dosage form from growth of most microorganisms. A problem arises, however, when pharmacists must add other ingredients to syrups that can result in a decrease in the sucrose concentration. This may cause a loss of the preservative effectiveness of the sucrose. This can be overcome, however, by calculating the quantity of a preservative (such as alcohol) to add to the formula to maintain the preservative effectiveness of the final product.

EXAMPLE

Rx Active drug	5 mL volume occupied
Other drug solids	3 mL volume occupied
Glycerin	15 mL
Sucrose	25 g
Ethanol	95% q.s.
Purified water q.s.	100 mL

How much alcohol would be required to preserve this prescription? We will use the free-water method to calculate the quantity of alcohol required.

Simple syrup contains 85 g sucrose per 100 mL of solution, which weighs 131.3 g (specific gravity, 1.313). It takes 46.3 mL of water to prepare the solution (131.3 − 85 = 46.3), and the sucrose occupies a volume of (100 − 46.3 = 53.7) 53.7 mL.

1. Since this solution is preserved, 85 g of sucrose preserves 46.3 mL of water, and 1 g of sucrose preserves 0.54 mL of water. With 25 g of sucrose present, the amount of water preserved is

$$25 \times 0.54 = 13.5 \text{ mL}$$

2. Since 85 g of sucrose occupies a volume of 53.7 mL, 1 g of sucrose will occupy a volume of 0.63 mL. The volume occupied by the sucrose in this prescription is

$$25 \times 0.63 = 15.75 \text{ mL}$$

3. The active drug and other solids occupy 8 mL (5 + 3) volume.
4. Each mL of glycerin can preserve an equivalent quantity of volume (2 × 15 = 30), so 30 mL would be preserved.
5. The volume taken care of so far is 13.5 + 15.75 + 8 + 30 = 67.25 mL. The quantity of free water remaining is

$$100 - 67.25 = 32.75 \text{ mL}$$

6. Since it requires about 18% alcohol to preserve the water,

$$0.18 \times 32.75 = 5.9 \text{ mL of alcohol (100\%)}$$

would be required.

7. If 95% ethanol is used, 5.9/0.95 = 6.21 mL would be required.

To prepare the prescription, about 6.21 mL of 95% ethanol can be added with sufficient purified water to make 100 mL of the final solution.

ical and chemical characteristics of the ingredients. Broadly stated, these methods are (a) solution of the ingredients with the aid of heat, (b) solution of the ingredients by agitation without the use of heat, or the simple admixture of liquid components, (c) addition of sucrose to a prepared medicated liquid or to a flavored liquid, and (d) percolation of either the source of the medicating substance or of the sucrose. Sometimes a syrup is prepared by more than one of these methods, and the selection may simply be a matter of preference on the part of the pharmacist.

Many of the official syrups have no officially designated method of preparation. This is because most official syrups are available commercially and are not prepared extemporaneously by the pharmacist.

Solution With the Aid of Heat

Syrups are prepared by this method when it is desired to prepare the syrup as quickly as possible and when the syrup's components are not damaged or volatilized by heat. In this method the sugar is generally added to the purified water, and heat is applied until the sugar is dissolved. Then other heat-stable components are added to the hot syrup, the mixture is allowed to cool, and its volume is adjusted to the proper level by addition of purified water. If heat-labile agents or volatile substances, such as volatile flavoring oils and alcohol, are to be added, they are generally added to the syrup after the sugar is dissolved by heat, and the solution is rapidly cooled to room temperature.

The use of heat facilitates rapid solution of the sugar and certain other components of syrups; however, caution must be exercised against becoming impatient and using excessive heat. Sucrose, a disaccharide, may be hydrolyzed into monosaccharides, dextrose (glucose), and fructose (levulose). This hydrolytic reaction is inversion, and the combination of the two monosaccharide products is invert sugar. When heat is applied in the preparation of a sucrose syrup, some inversion of the sucrose is almost certain. The speed of inversion is greatly increased by the presence of acids, the hydrogen ion acting as a catalyst to the reaction.

Should inversion occur, the sweetness of the syrup is altered, because invert sugar is sweeter than sucrose; and the normally colorless syrup darkens because of the effect of heat on the levulose portion of the invert sugar. When the syrup is greatly overheated, it becomes amber colored as the sucrose caramelizes. Syrups so decomposed are more susceptible to fermentation and to microbial growth than the stable, undecomposed syrups. Because of the prospect of decomposition by heat, syrups cannot be sterilized by autoclaving. The use of boiled purified water in the preparation of a syrup can enhance its permanency, and the addition of preservative agents, when permitted, can protect it during its shelf life. Storage in a tight container is a requirement for all syrups.

Solution by Agitation Without the Aid of Heat

To avoid heat-induced inversion of sucrose, a syrup may be prepared without heat by agitation. On a small scale, sucrose and other formulative agents may be dissolved in purified water by placing the ingredients in a vessel larger than the volume of syrup to be prepared, permitting thorough agitation of the mixture. This process is more time consuming than use of heat, but the product has maximum stability. Huge glass-lined or stainless steel tanks with mechanical stirrers or agitators are employed in large-scale preparation of syrups.

Sometimes simple syrup or some other nonmedicated syrup, rather than sucrose, is employed as the sweetening agent and vehicle. In that case, other liquids that are soluble in the syrup or miscible with it may be added and thoroughly mixed to form a uniform product. When solid agents are to be added to a syrup, it is best to dissolve them in a minimal amount of purified water and incorporate the resulting solution into the syrup. When solid substances are added directly to a syrup, they dissolve slowly because the viscous nature of the syrup does not permit the solid substance to distribute readily throughout the syrup to the available solvent and also because a limited amount of available water is present in concentrated syrups.

Addition of Sucrose to a Medicated Liquid or to a Flavored Liquid

Occasionally a medicated liquid, such as a tincture or fluidextract, is employed as the source of medication in the preparation of a syrup. Many such tinctures and fluidextracts contain alcohol-soluble constituents and are prepared with alcoholic or hydroalcoholic vehicles. If the alcohol-soluble components are desired medicinal agents, some means of rendering them water soluble is employed. However, if the alcohol-soluble components are undesirable or unnecessary components of the corresponding syrup, they are generally removed by mixing the tincture or fluidextract with water, allowing the mixture to stand until separation of the water-insoluble agents is complete, and filtering them from the mixture. The filtrate is the medicated liquid to which the sucrose is added in preparation of the syrup. If the tincture or fluidextract is miscible with aqueous preparations, it may be added directly to simple syrup or to a flavored syrup.

Percolation

In the percolation method, either sucrose may be percolated to prepare the syrup, or the source of the medicinal component may be percolated to form an extractive to which sucrose or syrup may be added. This latter method really is two separate procedures: first the preparation of the extractive of the drug and then the preparation of the syrup.

An example of a syrup prepared by percolation is ipecac syrup, which is prepared by adding glycerin and syrup to an extractive of powdered ipecac obtained by percolation. The drug ipecac, which consists of the dried rhizome and roots of *Cephaëlis ipecacuanha*, contains the medicinally active alkaloids emetine, cephaeline, and psychotrine. These alkaloids are extracted from the powdered ipecac by percolation with a hydroalcoholic solvent.

The syrup is categorized as an emetic with a usual dose of 15 mL. This amount of syrup is commonly used in the management of poisoning in children when evacuation of the stomach contents is desirable. About 80% of children given this dose will vomit within a half hour. For a household emetic in event of poisoning, 1-oz. bottles of the syrup are sold without a prescription. Ipecac syrup also has some application as a nauseant expectorant in doses smaller than the emetic dose.

Evidence indicates that many bulimics—most commonly young women in their late teens to early 30s—use syrup of ipecac to bring on attacks of vomiting in an attempt to lose weight (9). Pharmacists must be aware of this misuse of syrup of ipecac and warn these individuals because one of the active ingredients in the syrup is emetine. With continual use of the syrup, emetine builds up toxic levels within body tissues and in 3 to 4 months can do irreversible damage to heart muscles, resulting in symptoms mimicking a heart attack. Shortness of breath is the most common symptom in patients who misuse syrup of ipecac, but some persons describe low blood pressure–related symptoms and irregularities of heartbeat.

Elixirs

Elixirs are clear, sweetened hydroalcoholic solutions intended for oral use and are usually flavored to enhance their palatability. Nonmedicated elixirs are employed as vehicles, and medicated elixirs are used for the therapeutic effect of the medicinal substances they contain. Compared with syrups, elixirs are usually less sweet and less viscous because they contain a lower proportion of sugar and consequently are less effective than syrups in masking the taste of medicinal substances. However, because of their hydroalcoholic character, elixirs are better able than aqueous syrups to maintain both water-soluble and alcohol-soluble components in solution. Also because of their stable characteristics and the ease with which they are prepared (by simple solution), from a manufacturing standpoint, elixirs are preferred to syrups.

The proportion of alcohol in elixirs varies widely, since the individual components of the elixirs have different water and alcohol solubility characteristics. Each elixir requires a specific blend of alcohol and water to maintain all of the components in solution. Naturally, for elixirs containing agents with poor water solubility, the proportion of alcohol required is greater than for elixirs prepared from components having good water solubility. In addition to alcohol and water, other solvents, such as glycerin and propylene glycol, are frequently employed in elixirs as adjunctive solvents.

Although many elixirs are sweetened with sucrose or with a sucrose syrup, some use sorbitol, glycerin, and/or artificial sweeteners. Elixirs having a high alcoholic content usually use an artificial sweetener, such as saccharin, which is required only in small amounts, rather than sucrose, which is only slightly soluble in alcohol and requires greater quantities for equivalent sweetness.

All elixirs contain flavorings to increase their palatability, and most elixirs have coloring agents to enhance their appearance. Elixirs containing more than 10 to 12% of alcohol are usually self-preserving and do not require the addition of an antimicrobial agent.

Although the USP monographs for medicated elixirs provide standards, they do not generally provide official formulas. Formulations are left up to the individual manufacturers. Example formulations for some medicated elixirs are as follows (8):

Phenobarbital Elixir

Phenobarbital	4.00 g
Orange oil	0.25 mL
Propylene glycol	100.00 mL
Alcohol	200.00 mL
Sorbitol solution	600.00 mL
Color	q.s.
Purified water, to make	1000.00 mL

Theophylline Elixir

Theophylline	5.3 g
Citric acid	10.0 g
Liquid glucose	44.0 g
Syrup	132.0 mL
Glycerin	50.0 mL
Sorbitol solution	324.0 mL
Alcohol	200.0 mL
Saccharin sodium	5.0 g
Lemon oil	0.5 g
FDC Yellow No. 5	0.1 g
Purified water, to make	1000.0 mL

Medicated elixirs are formulated so that a patient receives the usual adult dose of the drug in a convenient measure of elixir. For most elixirs, one or two teaspoonfuls (5 or 10 mL) provides the usual adult dose of the drug. One advantage of elixirs over their counterpart drugs in solid dosage forms is the flexibility and ease of dosage administration to patients who have difficulty swallowing solid forms.

A disadvantage of elixirs for children and for adults who choose to avoid alcohol is their alcoholic content. The reader may wish to refer to the discussion of alcohol as a solvent earlier in this chapter for FDA-recommended limits on alcohol content for OTC oral products.

Because of their usual content of volatile oils and alcohol, elixirs should be stored in tight, light-resistant containers and protected from excessive heat.

Preparation of Elixirs

Elixirs are usually prepared by simple solution with agitation and/or by admixture of two or more liquid ingredients. Alcohol-soluble and water-soluble components are generally dissolved separately in alcohol and in purified water, respectively. Then the aqueous solution is added to the alcoholic solution, rather than the reverse, to maintain the highest possible alcoholic strength at all times so that minimal separation of the alcohol-soluble components occurs. When the two solutions are completely mixed, the mixture is made to volume with the specified solvent or vehicle. Frequently the final mixture will be cloudy, principally because of separation of some of the flavoring oils by the reduced alcoholic concentration. If this occurs, the elixir is usually permitted to stand for a prescribed number of hours to ensure saturation of the hydroalcoholic solvent and to permit the oil globules to coalesce so that they may be more easily removed by filtration. Talc, a frequent filter aid in the preparation of elixirs, absorbs the excessive amounts of oils and therefore assists in their removal from the solution. The presence of glycerin, syrup, sorbitol, and propylene glycol in elixirs generally contributes to the solvent effect of the hydroalcoholic vehicle, assists in the dissolution of the solute, and enhances the stability of the preparation. However, the presence of these materials adds to the viscosity of the elixir and slows the rate of filtration.

Nonmedicated Elixirs

Nonmedicated elixirs may be useful to the pharmacist in the extemporaneous filling of prescriptions involving (a) the addition of a therapeutic agent to a pleasant-tasting vehicle and (b) dilution of an existing medicated elixir. In selecting a liquid vehicle for a drug substance, the pharmacist should be concerned with the solubility and stability of the drug substance in water and alcohol. If a hydroalcoholic vehicle is selected, the proportion of alcohol should be only slightly above the amount needed to effect and maintain the drug's solution. When a pharmacist is called on to dilute an existing medicated elixir, the nonmedicated elixir he or she selects as the diluent should have approximately the same alcoholic concentration as the elixir being diluted. Also, the flavor and color characteristics of the diluent should not be in conflict with those of the medicated elixir, and all components should be chemically and physically compatible.

In years past, when pharmacists were called on more frequently than today to compound prescriptions, the three most commonly used nonmedicated elixirs were aromatic elixir, compound benzaldehyde elixir, and isoalcoholic elixir.

Medicated Elixirs

As noted previously, medicated elixirs are employed for the therapeutic benefit of the medicinal agent. Most official and commercial elixirs contain a single therapeutic agent. The main advantage of having only a single therapeutic agent is that the dosage of that single drug may be increased or decreased by simply taking more or less of the elixir, whereas when two or more therapeutic agents are present in the same preparation, it is impossible to increase or decrease the dose one without an automatic and corresponding adjustment in the dose of the other, which may not be desired. Thus, for patients required to take more than a

single medication, many physicians prefer them to take separate preparations of each drug so that if an adjustment in the dosage of one is desired, it may be accomplished without the concomitant adjustment of the other. Table 13.8 presents some examples of medicated elixirs. Some of these are briefly discussed next.

Antihistamine Elixirs

As indicated in Table 13.8, antihistamines are useful primarily in the symptomatic relief of certain allergic disorders. They suppress symptoms caused by histamine, one of the chemical agents released during the antigen–antibody reaction of the allergic response. Although only minor differences exist in the properties of most antihistamines, one or another may be preferred by a prescriber because of experience in managing a specific type of allergic reaction. A prescriber's preference may also be based on the incidence of adverse effects that may be expected to occur. The incidence and severity of these effects do vary somewhat with the drug and the dose. The most common untoward effect is sedation, and patients taking antihistamines should be warned against engaging in activities requiring mental alertness, such as driving an automobile or tractor or operating machinery. Other common adverse effects include dryness of the nose, throat, and mouth; dizziness; and disturbed concentration. Among the most sedating antihistamines are diphenhydramine, doxylamine, and methapyrilene. In fact, diphenhydramine is used as a sleep aid in numerous OTC products for its ability to cause drowsiness.

Most antihistaminic agents are basic amines. By forming salts through interaction with acid, the compounds are rendered water soluble. These salt forms are used in elixirs, so the elixirs of the antihistamines are not required to contain a large proportion of alcohol. Because the acid salts of the antihistamines are used, the pH of these elixirs is on the acid side and must remain so if the drugs are to remain freely soluble in water. A pharmacist should keep this in mind when using one of these elixirs to compound a prescription with other components.

TABLE 13.8 EXAMPLES OF MEDICATED ELIXIRS BY CATEGORY

ELIXIR	REPRESENTATIVE COMMERCIAL PRODUCTS	USUAL ADULT DOSE/ VOLUME OF COMMERCIAL ELIXIR	COMMENTS
Adrenocortical steroid			
Dexamethasone	Dexamethasone Elixir	500 μg/5 mL	Synthetic analogue of hydrocortisone, about 30 times more potent. Commercial elixir is packaged with a calibrated dropper for accurate measurement of small doses; intended primarily for children; also has utility for adults with trouble swallowing tablets. Used for many indications: rheumatoid arthritis, skin diseases, allergies, inflammatory conditions. Commercial product contains 5% alcohol.
Analgesic, antipyretic			
Acetaminophen	Children's Tylenol Elixir (McNeil)	160 mg/5 mL	Reduction of pain and lowering of fever particularly in patients sensitive to or unable to take aspirin. Elixir especially useful for pediatric patients, and is alcohol-free.
Anticholinergic, antispasmodic			
Hyoscyamine sulfate	Levsin Elixir (Schwarz)	0.125 mg/5 mL	Used to control gastric secretion, visceral spasm, hypermotility, abdominal cramps. Commercial product contains 20% alcohol.
Antihistamine			
Diphenhydramine HCl	Diphenhydramine HCl Elixir	12.5 mg/5 mL	Antihistamines are used for a variety of allergic reactions, e.g., perennial and seasonal allergic rhinitis, vasomotor rhinitis, allergic skin manifestations of urticaria, reactions to insect bites. Commercial product contains 5.6% alcohol.
Antipsychotic			
Fluphenazine HCl	Fluphenazine HCl Elixir (Pharmaceutical Associates)	2.5 mg/5 mL	Management of psychotic disorders.
Cardiotonic			
Digoxin	Lanoxin Pediatric Elixir (Glaxo Wellcome)	50 μg/mL	Among other effects, increases force of myocardial contraction. Used in congestive heart failure, atrial fibrillation, other cardiac conditions. Commercial product contains 10% alcohol.
Sedatives, hypnotics			
Butabarbital sodium	Butisol Sodium Elixir (Wallace)	30 mg/5 mL	In low dosage, sedatives; in higher dosage, hypnotics. Butabarbital sodium elixir contains 7% alcohol; phenobarbital elixir contains 14% alcohol.
Phenobarbital	Phenobarbital Elixir (Roxane)	20 mg/5 mL	

Barbiturate Sedative and Hypnotic Elixirs

The barbiturates are sedative and hypnotic agents that are used to produce various degrees of central nervous system depression. As the dose of these drugs is increased, the effects go from sedation to hypnosis to respiratory depression, the last being the cause of death in fatal barbiturate overdosage.

Barbiturates are administered in small doses in the daytime as sedatives to reduce restlessness and emotional tension. The appropriate dose for this purpose is the amount that alleviates anxiety or tension but does not produce drowsiness or lethargy. Greater doses of the barbiturates may be given before bedtime as hypnotics to relieve insomnia.

Barbiturates have been classified according to the duration of their hypnotic effects; that is, long-acting, intermediate-acting, short-acting, or ultrashort-acting agents. The long-acting barbiturates, including phenobarbital, are considered most useful in maintaining daytime sedation and in treating some convulsive states and least useful as hypnotics. The intermediate-acting barbiturates include amobarbital; they are used primarily for short-term daytime sedation and are effective in treating insomnia. The barbiturates classified as short-acting include secobarbital; they are used similarly to the intermediate-acting barbiturates. The ultra–short-acting barbiturates, including thiopental, are given intravenously to induce anesthesia.

The most common untoward effects in patients taking barbiturates are drowsiness and lethargy. Large doses may produce residual sedation resembling the hangover following alcohol intoxication. Prolonged use of barbiturates may lead to psychic or physical dependence. This dependence, in susceptible individuals, leads to compulsive abuse of the drug with severe withdrawal symptoms following abstinence. In heavy chronic users, abrupt withdrawal may lead to convulsions, delirium, and occasionally to coma and death. Some pharmaceutical aspects of phenobarbital elixir are presented below.

Phenobarbital Elixir

Phenobarbital elixir is formulated to contain phenobarbital 0.4%, which provides about 20 mg of drug per teaspoonful (5 mL) of elixir. The elixir is commonly flavored with orange oil, colored red with an FDA-approved colorant, and sweetened with syrup. The official elixir contains about 14% alcohol, which is used to dissolve the phenobarbital. However, this amount is almost the very minimum required to keep the phenobarbital in solution. Therefore, glycerin is often added to enhance the solubility of phenobarbital.

Phenobarbital is a long-acting barbiturate with a duration of action of about 4 to 6 hours, a usual adult dose as a sedative of about 30 mg, and a hypnotic dose of about 100 mg. The strength of the elixir permits convenient adjustment of dosage to achieve the proper degree of sedation in the treatment of infants, children, and certain adults. The elixir is commercially available from a variety of manufacturers under its nonproprietary name.

Digoxin Elixir

No official method of preparation is indicated for Digoxin Elixir, USP; however, it is required to contain 4.5 to 5.25 mg of digoxin per 100 mL of elixir, or about 0.25 mg per 5 mL teaspoonful. The usual oral adult dose of digoxin as a cardiotonic agent is about 1.5 mg on initial therapy and about 0.5 mg for maintenance therapy.

Digoxin is a cardiotonic glycoside obtained from the leaves of *Digitalis lanata*. It is a white crystalline powder that is insoluble in water but soluble in dilute alcohol solutions. The official elixir contains about 10% alcohol. Digoxin is poisonous, and its dose must be carefully determined and administered to each individual patient. Adults generally take digoxin tablets rather than the elixir, which must be measured by the highly variable household teaspoon. The elixir is generally employed for children, and the commercial product available for this purpose is packaged with a calibrated dropper to facilitate accurate dosing.

Digoxin is one of many drugs available in more than a single dosage form. The prescriber frequently has the choice of a solid dosage form—a tablet or capsule—or a liquid. The advantages of each have been noted previously, but it is important to point out again that drugs administered in different dosage forms may exhibit different bioavailability characteristics, with varying patterns of drug release and rates and extents of absorption. Such differences have been noted for digoxin between tablets from different manufacturers and between tablets and oral liquid forms. Figure 13.2 shows the differences noted in one study of the serum digoxin levels following administration of 0.5 mg of digoxin by oral tablet and oral solution having an elixirlike vehicle. It can be readily seen that the serum digoxin levels following administration of the oral solution were considerably greater than from the oral tablet.

A patient taking a drug known to exhibit bioavailability problems and whose therapeutic dosage regimen has been successfully established with a particular drug product should not be changed to another product.

Tinctures

Tinctures are alcoholic or hydroalcoholic solutions prepared from vegetable materials or from chemical substances. They vary in method of preparation, strength of the active ingredient, alcoholic content, and intended use in medicine or pharmacy. When they are prepared from chemical substances (e.g., iodine, thimerosal) tinctures are prepared by simple solution of the chemical agent in the solvent.

Depending on the preparation, tinctures contain alcohol in amounts ranging from approximately 15 to 80%. The alcohol content protects against microbial growth and keeps the alcohol-soluble extractives in solution. In addition to alcohol, other solvents, such as glycerin, may be employed. The solvent mix of each tincture is important in maintaining the integrity of the product. Tinctures cannot be mixed successfully with liquids too diverse in solvent character because the solute may precipitate. For example, compound benzoin tincture, prepared with alcohol as the sole menstruum, contains alcohol-soluble principles that are immediately precipitated from solution upon addition of water.

Because of the alcoholic content, tinctures must be tightly stoppered and not exposed to excessive temperatures. Also, because many of the constituents found in tinctures undergo a photochemical change upon exposure to light, many tinctures must be stored in light-resistant containers and protected from sunlight.

Medicated tinctures taken orally include Paregoric, USP, or camphorated tincture of opium. Usually, patients requiring oral medication nowadays prefer to take a tablet or capsule or a pleasant-tasting elixir or syrup. Tinctures have a rather high alcoholic content, and some physicians and patients alike prefer other forms of medication. Opium Tincture, USP, or laudanum, is much more potent than paregoric,

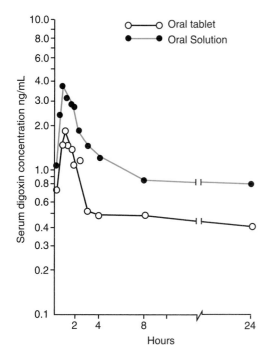

FIGURE 13.2 Serum digoxin concentrations following administration of digoxin 0.5 mg by oral tablet and elixir-like oral solution (Adapted from Huffman DH, Azarnoff DL. Absorption of orally given digoxin preparations. JAMA 1972;222:957).

and the two should not be confused. Any prescription for either one should be carefully evaluated and the dose checked and confirmed.

Proper Administration and Use of Liquid Peroral Dosage Forms

Most of the dosage forms discussed in this chapter are to be administered by mouth. Conveniently, these can be measured in a teaspoon or tablespoon, depending on the desired dosage. Preferably, however, these medicines should be measured out in calibrated devices for administration. These devices ensure that the correct dose will be received, and household flatware can vary dramatically in the volume delivered. Even though these are liquids, it is recommended that the patient follow the administration of the liquid dosage form with a glassful of water.

The pharmacist must be careful in the selection of liquid products, given the patient's history and other concurrent medicines. For example, some syrups contain sucrose or another sugar, and the pharmacist must recall that such syrups would not be suitable for use in an oral prescription intended for a diabetic patient. Similarly, a product that is formulated as an elixir would not be suitable for a patient who receives concurrent medicines that possess an Antabuse-like activity; the patient may get violently ill from the concurrent ingestion of alcohol. Metronidazole and chlorpropamide have been implicated to cause this reaction when mixed with alcohol. Furthermore, if the patient is receiving another drug that causes drowsiness, the pharmacist must consult the prescribing physician to determine whether the prescribed elixir could be harmful to the patient.

Topical Solutions and Tinctures

Generally, the topical solutions employ an aqueous vehicle, whereas the topical tinctures characteristically employ an alcoholic vehicle. As required, cosolvents or adjuncts to enhance stability or the solubility of the solute are employed.

Most topical solutions and tinctures are prepared by simple dissolving. However, certain solutions are prepared by chemical reaction; these in particular are discussed later in this section. Of the tinctures for topical use, one, compound benzoin tincture, is prepared by maceration of the natural components in the solvent; the others are prepared by simple solution.

Because of the nature of the active constituents or the solvents, many topical solutions and tinctures are self-preserved. Those that are not may contain suitable preservatives. Topical solutions and tinctures should be packaged in containers that make them convenient to use. Those that are used in small volume, such as the anti-infectives, are usually packaged in glass or plastic bottles with an applicator tip as a part of the cap assembly or in plastic squeeze bottles that deliver the medication in drops. Many of the anti-infective solutions and tinctures contain a dye to delineate the area of application to the skin. In contrast to aqueous solutions, when the alcoholic tinctures are applied to abraded or broken skin, they sting.

Sprays

Sprays may be defined as aqueous or oleaginous solutions in the form of coarse droplets or as finely divided solids to be applied topically, most usually to the nasopharyngeal tract or to the skin. Many commercial sprays are used intranasally to relieve nasal congestion and inflammation and to combat infection and contain antihistamines, sympathomimetic agents, and antibiotic substances. Because of the noninvasive nature and quickness with which nasal sprays can deliver medication systemically, in the future several drugs that typically have been administered by other routes will be taken nasally. Most notably, insulin and glucagon will be administered in this fashion. Research has demonstrated that the administration of glucagon via a nasal spray can relieve hypoglycemic symptoms within 7 minutes, a definite advantage over conventional emergency intravenous glucose or intramuscular glucagon.

Other sprays that are employed against sunburn and heat burn contain local anesthetics, antiseptics, skin protectants, and antipruritics. Throat sprays containing antiseptics, deodorants, and flavorants may be effectively employed to relieve conditions such as halitosis, sore throat, and laryngitis. Other sprays treat athlete's foot and other fungal infections. Numerous other medicinal and cosmetic uses of sprays are commonly available in pharmacies.

To break up a solution into small particles so that it may be effectively sprayed or to facilitate the spraying of a powder, several mechanical devices are commonly employed. The plastic spray bottle, gently squeezed to issue a spray of its contents, is familiar to most. It is commonly used for nasal decongestant sprays as well as cosmetically, especially for body deodorant products. Recently, one-way pump sprays have been developed to deliver medication into the nose. These sprays are used for both legend, such as Nasalide (Syntex), and nonlegend, such as Nostrilla (Boehringer Ingelheim), medicines. The advantage of these over conventional sprays is that the design prevents drawback contamination of nasal fluids into the bottle after administration, a definite advantage for someone trying to cope with viruses associated with the common cold. Pharmacists are familiar with medicinal atomizers, which emit medication in the form of fine droplets (Fig. 13.3). One type of atomizer has a rubber bulb at the end of the apparatus, which when squeezed causes a flow of air, some of which enters the glass reservoir and some of which exits from the opposite end of

the system. The air forced into the reservoir causes the liquid to rise in a small dip tube, forcing the solution up and into the stream of air exiting the system. The air and the solution are forced through a jet opening and the liquid is broken up into a spray, the droplets being carried by the airstream. In other similar apparatus, the stream of air caused by the depression of the bulb does not enter the reservoir of solution but passes swiftly over it, creating a pressure change and sucking the liquid into the dip tube and into the airstream, in which it exits the system. Examples of solutions and tinctures intended for application to the skin are presented in Tables 13.9 and 13.10. As shown in these tables, most of these preparations are used as anti-infective agents. All medication intended for external use should be clearly labeled FOR EXTERNAL USE ONLY and kept out of the reach of children. In addition to their listing in Table 13.9, the following topical solutions are discussed because of their particular pharmaceutic interest.

Aluminum Acetate Topical Solution

Aluminum acetate is colorless and has a faint acetous odor and a sweetish, astringent taste. It is widely applied topically as an astringent wash or wet dressing after dilution with 10 to 40 parts of water. It is frequently used in various types of dermatologic lotions, creams, and pastes. Commercial premeasured tablets and packets of powders are available for preparation of this solution. Synonym: Burow's solution.

Aluminum Subacetate Topical Solution

The requirement for the amount of acetic acid differentiates aluminum acetate topical solution from aluminum subacetate topical solution. In the subacetate solution, the ratio of aluminum oxide to acetic acid is 1:2.35, whereas in the acetate solution the ratio is 1:3.52. Aluminum subacetate topical solution, the stronger of the two, is used in preparation of aluminum acetate topical solution. Aluminum acetate topical solution, diluted first with 20 to 40 parts of water, is used externally

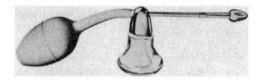

FIGURE 13.3 A common type of atomizer for spray administration of liquid medication. This model has an adjustable tip for directing the spray upward or downward to reach otherwise inaccessible areas of the throat (Courtesy of DeVilbiss Co.).

TABLE 13.9 EXAMPLES OF SOLUTIONS APPLIED TO THE SKIN

SOLUTION	CORRESPONDING COMMERCIAL PRODUCT	ACTIVE CONSTITUENT IN COMMERCIAL SOLUTION	VEHICLE	CATEGORY AND COMMENTS
Aluminum acetate	—	5%	Aqueous	Astringent.
Aluminum subacetate	—	Approx. 2.45% aluminum oxide, 5.8% acetic acid	Aqueous	Astringent.
Calcium hydroxide (limewater)	—	0.14%	Aqueous	Astringent.
Chlorhexidine Gluconate	Hibiclens Skin Cleanser (Stuart)	4%		Skin wound and general skin cleanser, surgical scrub, preoperative skin preparation. Effective for gram-positive and gram-negative bacteria such as *Pseudomonas aeruginosa*.
Clindamycin phosphate	Cleocin T topical Solution (Pharmacia & Upjohn)	1%	Isopropyl alcohol, water	Treatment of acne vulgaris.
Clotrimazole	Lotrimin Solution (Schering)	1%	PEG 400	Antifungal.
Coal tar (liquor carbonis detergens; LCD)	—	20%	Alcohol	Antieczematic; antipsoriatic.
Erythromycin	Erymax Topical Solution (Allergan Herbert)	2%	Polyethylene glycol/ acetone/ alcohol	Treatment of acne vulgaris.
Fluocinolone acetonide	Synalar Topical Solution (Syntex)	0.01%	Propylene glycol	Adrenocortical steroid (topical anti-inflammatory).
Fluorouracil	Efudex Topical Solution (Roche)	2, 5%	Propylene glycol	Antineoplastic (actinic keratoses).
Hydrogen peroxide	—	3%	Aqueous	Topical anti-infective.
Hydroquinone	Melanex Topical Solution (Neutrogena Dermatologies)	3%	Water, alcohol, propylene glycol	Temporary bleaching of hyperpigmented skin, e.g., chloasma, melasma.
Minoxidil	Rogaine Topical Solution (Pharmacia & Upjohn)	2, 5%	Alcohol, water, propylene glycol	Long-term topical treatment of male pattern baldness by stimulating hair regrowth.
Povidone iodine	Betadine Solution (Purdue Frederick)	7.5, 10%	Aqueous	Topical anti-infective.
Tolnaftate	Tinactin Solution (Schering-Plough)	1%	Polyethylene glycol	Topical antifungal.

TABLE 13.10 EXAMPLES OF TINCTURES APPLIED TO THE SKIN

TINCTURE	PERCENT ACTIVE CONSTITUENT IN COMMERCIAL TINCTURE	VEHICLE	CATEGORY AND COMMENTS
Green soap tincture	65%	Alcohol	Detergent. Also contains 2% lavender oil as perfume.
Iodine tincture	2%	Alcohol, water	Topical anti-infective.
Compound benzoin tincture	10% benzoin; 2% aloe; 8% storax; 4% tolu balsam	Alcohol	Topical protectant. Prepared by maceration in alcohol.

as an astringent wash and wet dressing (modified Burow's solution).

Calcium Hydroxide Topical Solution

Calcium hydroxide topical solution, commonly called limewater, must contain not less than 140 mg of $Ca(OH)_2$ in each 100 mL of solution. Calcium hydroxide is less soluble in hot than in cold water, and cool purified water is the solvent. The solution is intended to be saturated with solute, and to ensure saturation, an excess of calcium hydroxide, 300 mg for each 100 mL of solution to be prepared, is agitated with the purified water, vigorously and repeatedly, for 1 hour. After this time, the excess calcium hydroxide is allowed to settle to the bottom of the container. This permits the solution to remain saturated should a portion of the dissolved solute at the solution's surface react with the carbon dioxide of the air to form insoluble calcium carbonate:

$$Ca(OH)_2 + CO_2 \rightarrow CaCO_3 + H_2O$$

The calcium carbonate settles to the bottom of the container and by appearance is indistinguishable from the remaining excess of calcium hydroxide. The calcium hydroxide reserve dissolves as calcium is removed from solution in the form of the carbonate and in this way continually maintains the saturation of the solution. After the solution stands for an appreciable length of time, the undissolved material in the bottom of the container is composed of varying proportions of calcium hydroxide and calcium carbonate. Because of the uncertainty of the residue's composition, one may not prepare additional quantities of calcium hydroxide solution by adding more purified water.

The solution should be stored in well-filled, tightly stoppered containers to deter the absorption of carbon dioxide and should be kept in a cool place to maintain an adequate concentration of dissolved solute. Only the clear supernatant liquid is dispensed. This is best accomplished by the use of a siphon with care not to entrain the residue.

The solution is categorized as an astringent. For this purpose it is generally employed in combination with other ingredients in dermatologic solutions and lotions to be applied topically. Synonyms: limewater, liquor calcis.

Coal Tar Topical Solution

Coal tar topical solution is an alcoholic solution containing 20% coal tar and 5% polysorbate 80. It is prepared by mixing the coal tar with two and a half times its weight of washed sand, adding the polysorbate 80 and most of the alcohol, and then macerating the mixture for 7 days in a closed vessel with frequent agitation followed by filtration and adjustment to the proper volume with alcohol. The final content is 81 to 86% ethyl alcohol.

Coal tar is a nearly black viscous liquid having a characteristic naphthalene-like odor and a sharp, burning taste. It is the tar obtained as a byproduct during the destructive distillation of bituminous coal. It is slightly soluble in water and partially soluble in most organic solvents, including alcohol. In the preparation of the official solution, the coal tar is mixed with the sand to distribute it mechanically and create a large surface area of tar exposed to the solvent action of the alcohol. During the maceration, or soaking, the alcohol-soluble components of the tar dissolve, leaving the undissolved portion clinging to the sand. Filtration removes the sand and the insoluble tar components from the solution. The container in which the solution was prepared should be rinsed with alcohol, and the washings should be passed through the filter paper in the adjustment of the final volume of the solution.

In the extemporaneous compounding of prescriptions and in the therapeutic application of this preparation to the skin, the solution is frequently mixed with aqueous preparations or simply diluted with water. Because coal tar is only slightly soluble in water, it would separate from the solution were it not for the polysorbate 80 in the preparation. This agent, commercially available as Tween 80 (ICI Americas) and as other brand name products, is an oily liquid that is a nonionic surfactant. It is quite effective in dispersing the water-insoluble components of coal tar upon admixture with an aqueous preparation.

Coal tar is a local antieczematic used in external treatment of a wide variety of chronic skin conditions after dilution with about 9 volumes of water, or in combination with other agents in various lotions, ointments or solutions. Synonyms: liquor carbonis detergens; liquor picis carbonis; LCD.

Hydrogen Peroxide Topical Solution

Hydrogen peroxide topical solution contains 2.5 to 3.5% (w/v) hydrogen peroxide, or H_2O_2. Suitable preservatives, totaling not more than 0.05%, may be added.

One method of preparation uses the action of either phosphoric or sulfuric acid on barium peroxide:

$$BaO_2 + H_2SO_4 \rightarrow BaSO_4 + H_2O_2$$

Another method uses electrolytic oxidation of a cold solution of concentrated sulfuric acid to form persulfuric acid, which when hydrolyzed liberates hydrogen peroxide:

$$2H_2SO_4 \rightarrow H_2S_2O_8 + H_2$$

$$H_2S_2O_8 + 2H_2O \rightarrow 2H_2SO_4 + H_2O_2$$

A solution prepared by this method usually contains about 30% hydrogen peroxide and is capable of liberating 100 times its volume of oxygen. A solution of this strength is commonly referred to as 100-volume peroxide. The dilute solution, which contains about 3% hydrogen peroxide and liberates 10 times its volume of oxygen, may be prepared from the concentrated solution.

The solution is a clear, colorless liquid that may be odorless or have the odor of ozone. It usually deteriorates upon long standing, forming oxygen and water. Preservative agents, such as acetanilide, have been found to retard decomposition. Decomposition is enhanced by light and by heat, and for this reason the solution should be preserved in tight, light-resistant containers, preferably at a temperature not exceeding 35°C (95°F). The solution is also decomposed by practically all organic matter and other reducing agents and reacts with oxidizing agents to liberate oxygen and water; metals, alkalis, and other agents can catalyze its decomposition.

Hydrogen peroxide solution is categorized as a local anti-infective for use topically on the skin and mucous membranes. Its germicidal activity is based on the release of nascent oxygen on contact with the tissues. However, because of the short duration of this release, the chief value of the preparation in the reduction of infection is probably its ability to cleanse wounds by mechanical action through the bubbling and frothing caused by the release of oxygen. Synonym: peroxide.

Chlorhexidine Gluconate Solution

Since 1957 chlorhexidine gluconate has been employed extensively as a broad-spectrum antiseptic in clinical and veterinarian medicine. Its spectrum encompasses gram-positive and gram-negative bacteria, including *Pseudomonas aeruginosa*. In a concentration of 4% (Hibiclins, Stuart) it is used as a surgical scrub, hand wash, and skin wound and general skin cleanser. Procedures are established for all of these purposes to maximize the effectiveness of the chlorhexidine. Experience has demonstrated that irritation, dermatitis, and photosensitivity associated with topical use of chlorhexidine are rare.

In 1987, the FDA and the Council of Dental Therapeutics of the American Dental Association approved chlorhexidine gluconate 0.12% (Peridex, Procter & Gamble) as the first prescription-only antiplaque, antigingivitis drug with antimicrobial activity. Microbiologic sampling of plaque has shown a reduction of aerobic and anaerobic bacteria ranging from 54 to 97% through 6 months of use when it is used as a mouth rinse. The oral rinse should be used twice daily for 30 seconds, morning and night, after tooth brushing. Usually a 15-mL dose of undiluted solution is used and expectorated after rinsing. The most common side effect of chlorhexidine is the formation of an extrinsic yellow-brown stain on the teeth and tongue after only a few days of use. The amount of stain depends on the concentration of chlorhexidine and individual susceptibility. Increased consumption of tannin-containing substances, such as tea, red wine, and port wine, will increase the level of discoloration. The developed stain can be periodically removed with dental prophylaxis.

Povidone Iodine Topical Solution

The agent povidone iodine is a chemical complex of iodine with polyvinylpyrrolidone, the latter agent being a polymer having an average molecular weight of about 40,000. The povidone iodine complex contains approximately 10% available iodine and slowly releases it when applied to the skin.

The preparation is employed topically as a surgical scrub and nonirritating antiseptic solution, with its effectiveness directly attributable to the presence and release of iodine from the complex. Commercial product: Betadine Solution (Purdue Frederick).

Thimerosal Topical Solution

Thimerosal is a water-soluble organic mercurial antibacterial agent used topically for its bacteriostatic and mild fungistatic properties. It is used mainly to disinfect skin and as an application to wounds and abrasions. It has been applied to the eye, nose, throat, and urethra in dilutions of 1:5000. It is also used as a preservative for various pharmaceutical preparations, including many vaccines and other biologic products.

Thimerosal topical solution contains 0.1% thimerosal. Also present are ethylene diamine

solution and sodium borate to maintain the alkalinity (usually pH 9.8 to 10.3) required for the solution's stability. Monoethanolamine is used as an additional stabilizer. The solution is affected by light and must be maintained in light-resistant containers. Commercial product: Merthiolate Solution (Lilly).

Vaginal and Rectal Solutions

Vaginal Douches

Solutions may be prepared from powders as indicated earlier or from liquid solutions or liquid concentrates. In using liquid concentrates, the patient is instructed to add the prescribed amount of concentrate (usually a teaspoonful or capful) to a certain amount of warm water (frequently a quart). The resultant solution contains the appropriate amount of chemical agents in proper strength. The agents are similar to the ones described for douche powders. Examples are shown in Figure 13.4.

Powders are used to prepare solutions for vaginal douche, that is, for irrigation cleansing of the vagina. The powders themselves may be prepared and packaged in bulk or as unit packages. A unit package is designed to contain the appropriate amount of powder to prepare the specified volume of douche solution. The bulk powders are used by the teaspoonful or tablespoonful in preparation of the desired solution. The user simply adds the prescribed amount of powder to the appropriate volume of warm water and stirs

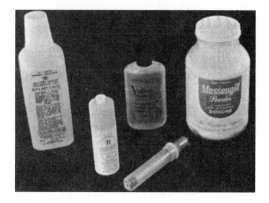

FIGURE 13.4 Products for vaginal use, including solution concentrates, powder, and aerosol foam with insert device.

until dissolved. Among the components of douche powders are the following:

1. Boric acid or sodium borate
2. Astringents, e.g., potassium, alum, ammonium alum, zinc sulfate
3. Antimicrobials, e.g., oxyquinoline sulfate, povidone iodine
4. Quaternary ammonium compounds, e.g., benzethonium chloride
5. Detergents, e.g., sodium lauryl sulfate
6. Oxidizing agents, e.g., sodium perborate
7. Salts, e.g., sodium citrate, sodium chloride
8. Aromatics, e.g., menthol, thymol, eucalyptol, methyl salicylate, phenol

Douche powders are used for their hygienic effects. A few douche powders containing specific therapeutic anti-infective agents such as those mentioned in the discussion of vaginal suppositories are used against monilial and trichomonal infections.

Retention Enemas

A number of solutions are administered rectally for local effects (e.g., hydrocortisone) or for systemic absorption (e.g., aminophylline). In the case of aminophylline, rectal administration minimizes the undesirable gastrointestinal reactions associated with oral therapy. Clinically effective blood levels of the agents are usually obtained within 30 minutes following rectal instillation. Corticosteroids are administered as retention enemas or continuous drip as adjunctive treatment of some patients with ulcerative colitis.

Evacuation Enemas

Rectal enemas are used to cleanse the bowel. Commercially, many enemas are available in disposable plastic squeeze bottles containing a premeasured amount of enema solution. The agents are solutions of sodium phosphate and sodium biphosphate, glycerin and docusate potassium, and light mineral oil.

Instruction from a pharmacist is advantageous to ensure that the patient correctly uses these products. The patient should be advised to gently insert the tip of the product with steady pressure and be told that it is not ab-

solutely necessary to squeeze all of the contents out of the disposable plastic bottle. The patient should be told that the product will most probably work within 5 to 10 minutes.

Topical Tinctures

Examples of tinctures for topical application to the skin are presented in Table 13.10. Those of particular pharmaceutic interest are discussed briefly as follows.

Iodine Tincture

Iodine tincture is prepared by dissolving 2% iodine crystals and 2.4% sodium iodide in an amount of alcohol equal to half the volume of tincture to be prepared and diluting the solution to volume with sufficient purified water. The sodium iodide reacts with the iodine to form sodium triiodide:

$$I_2 + NaI \longleftrightarrow NaI_3$$

This reaction prevents formation of ethyl iodide from the interaction between iodine and alcohol, which would result in the loss of the antibacterial activity of the tincture. An added benefit of the triiodide form of iodine is its water solubility, which is important should the tincture, which contains between 44 and 50% alcohol, be diluted with water during use.

The tincture is a popular local anti-infective agent applied to the skin in general household first aid. The reddish-brown color, which produces a stain on the skin, is useful in delineating the application over the affected skin area. The tincture should be stored in a tight container to prevent loss of alcohol.

Compound Benzoin Tincture

Compound benzoin tincture is prepared by maceration in alcohol of 10% benzoin and lesser amounts of aloe, storax, and tolu balsam totaling about 24% of starting material. The drug mixture is best macerated in a wide-mouthed container, since it is difficult to introduce storax, a sticky semiliquid material into a narrow-mouthed container. Generally, it is advisable to weigh the storax in the container in which it will be macerated to avoid possible loss through a transfer of the material from one container to another.

The tincture is categorized as a protectant. It is used to protect and toughen skin in the treatment of bedsores, ulcers, cracked nipples, and fissures of the lips and anus. It is also commonly used as an inhalant in bronchitis and other respiratory conditions, 1 teaspoonful commonly being added to a pint of boiling water. The volatile components of the tincture travel with the steam vapor and are inhaled by the patient. Because of the incompatibility of the alcoholic tincture and water, the mixture produces a milky product with some separation of resinous material. Alcohol or acetone may be used as necessary to remove the residue from the vaporizer after use.

Compound tincture of benzoin serves as a delivery vehicle of podophyllum in the treatment of venereal warts. It is important that podophyllum not be systemically absorbed because it can cause peripheral neuropathy characterized by paresthesias, loss of sensation, and loss of deep tendon reflexes in the extremities, in addition to neuropathy of the central nervous system including lethargy, confusion, and coma. Second, the podophyllum is teratogenic and should be administered to a pregnant woman only when the risk–benefit ratio is extremely low. Thus, the nonocclusive compound tincture of benzoin is preferred to the occlusive flexible collodion.

Compound benzoin tincture is best stored in tight, light-resistant containers. Exposure to direct sunlight or to excessive heat should be avoided.

The tincture originated in the fifteenth or sixteenth century and through the years probably has acquired more synonyms than any other official preparation. A few of these are friar's balsam, Turlington's drops, Persian balsam, Swedish balsam, Jerusalem balsam, Wade's drops, Turlington's balsam of life.

Thimerosal Tincture

The same general remarks about thimerosal topical solution apply to thimerosal tincture except that sodium chloride and sodium borate are absent from the tincture and the vehicle of

the tincture is water, acetone, and about 50% alcohol. A number of metals, notably copper, cause decomposition of the tincture, and for this reason it must be manufactured and stored in glass or suitably resistant containers. Monoethanolamine and ethylenediamine are used as stabilizers in the official solution and tincture and are thought to be effective because of their chelating action on traces of metallic impurities that may be present at the time of preparation or may later gain access to the preparation.

The commercial preparation is colored orange red and has greenish fluorescence. The red stain it leaves on the skin defines the area of application. It is a commonly used household antiseptic for application to abrasions and cuts and also in preparation of patients for surgery.

Topical Oral (Dental) Solutions

A variety of medicinal substances are employed topically in the mouth for a number of purposes and in a wide range of dosage forms. Among the drugs and preparations included in this group are the following:

Benzocaine: Topical anesthetic. Indicated for temporary relief of pain, soreness, and irritation in the mouth associated with teething, orthodontic appliances, new or poorly fitting dentures, and canker sores.

Camphorated parachlorophenol: Dental anti-infective. A eutectic liquid composed of 65% camphor and 35% parachlorophenol, used in dentistry for sterilization of deep root canals.

Carbamide peroxide topical solution: Dental anti-infective. Acts as a chemomechanical cleansing and debriding agent through the release of bubbling oxygen. The commercial product (Gly-Oxide Liquid, Smith Kline Beecham) contains 10% carbamide in flavored anhydrous glycerin.

Cetylpyridinium chloride solution and cetylpyridinium chloride lozenges: Local anti-infective. Commercial counterparts (Cepacol Mouthwash/Gargle and Cepacol Lozenges) contain 1:2000 w/v and 1:1500 w/v of cetylpyridinium chloride respectively. Used primarily as a freshening mouth cleanser. Lozenges have benzyl alcohol as a local anesthetic in soothing throat irritations.

Erythrosine sodium topical solution and erythrosine sodium soluble tablets: Diagnostic aid (dental disclosing agent). Solution applied to the teeth to reveal plaque left by inadequate brushing. Tablets chewed for the same purpose and are not to be swallowed.

Eugenol: Dental analgesic. Applied topically to dental cavities and dental protectives. Eugenol is a pale yellow liquid having an aromatic odor of clove and a spicy taste.

Lidocaine oral spray: Topical dental anesthetic. Applied through metered spray at 10 mg per spray; 20 mg per quadrant of gingiva and oral mucosa is usually employed (Xylocaine Oral Spray, Astra).

Nystatin oral suspension: Antifungal. May be employed for oral fungal infections by retaining in the mouth as long as possible before swallowing.

Saliva substitutes: Electrolytes in a carboxymethylcellulose base. They are indicated for relief of dry mouth and throat in xerostomia.

Sodium fluoride oral solution and sodium fluoride tablets: Dental caries prophylactic. Solution applied to the teeth; or when drinking water does not contain adequate fluoride, a dilute solution may be swallowed. Tablets containing sodium fluoride 1.1 or 2.2 mg are chewed or swallowed as required.

Sodium fluoride and phosphoric acid gel and sodium fluoride and phosphoric acid topical solution: Dental caries prophylactic. Gel and solution applied to the teeth; each contains 1.23% of fluoride ion and 1% of phosphoric acid.

Triamcinolone acetonide dental paste: Topical anti-inflammatory agent. Applied to the oral mucous membranes as a 0.1% paste.

Zinc oxide–eugenol mixture: Temporary filling mix.

In addition to these drugs and preparations, a host of other products for oral use are commercially available. Some of these products, such as teething lotions and toothache drops, are medicated, whereas others are used for hygienic purposes, such as dentifrices, denture products, and many of the mouthwashes. Among the variety of products is a like variety of physical forms—solutions, emulsions, ointments, pastes, aerosols, and so on, with the manufacture of each following the general procedures outlined in this text. One type of dosage form for oral use, the lozenge, has not been previously described.

Miscellaneous Solutions

Aromatic Waters

Aromatic waters are clear, aqueous solutions saturated with volatile oils or other aromatic or volatile substances. Aromatic waters are no longer in widespread use. In years past, aromatic waters were prepared from a number of volatile substances, including orange flower oil, peppermint oil, rose oil, anise oil, spearmint oil, wintergreen oil, camphor, and chloroform. Naturally, the odors and tastes of aromatic waters are of the volatile substances from which they are prepared.

Most of the aromatic substances in the preparation of aromatic waters have very low solubility in water, and even though a water may be saturated, its concentration of aromatic material is still rather small. Aromatic waters may be used for perfuming and/or flavoring.

Diluted Acids

Diluted acids are aqueous solutions prepared by diluting the corresponding concentrated acids with purified water. The strength of a diluted acid is generally expressed on a percent weight-to-volume (% w/v) basis, that is, the weight in grams of solute per 100 mL of solution, whereas the strength of a concentrated acid is generally expressed in terms of percent weight to weight (% w/w), which indicates the number of grams of solute per 100 g of solution. To prepare a diluted acid from a concentrated one, it is necessary first to calculate the amount of solute required in the diluted product. Then the amount of concentrated acid required to supply the needed amount of solute can be determined.

To illustrate, concentrated hydrochloric acid contains not less than 35 g and not more than 38 g of solute (absolute HCl) per 100 g of acid and therefore is considered to be, on the average, 36.5% w/w in strength. Diluted hydrochloric acid contains 9.5 to 10.5 g of solute per 100 mL of solution and is therefore considered to be approximately 10% w/v in strength. If one wished to prepare 100 mL of the diluted acid from the concentrated acid, one would require 10 g of solute. The amount of concentrated HCl required to supply this amount of solute may be calculated by the following proportion:

$$\frac{36.5 \text{ g (solute)}}{100 \text{ g (conc. acid)}} = \frac{10 \text{ g (solute)}}{\times \text{ (g conc. acid)}}$$

Solving for x:

$$36.5x = 1000 \text{ g}$$
$$x = 27.39 \text{ g (conc. acid)}$$

Thus, 27.39 g of concentrated acid is required to supply 10 g of solute needed for the preparation of 100 mL of the diluted acid. Although the required amount of concentrated acid may be accurately weighed, it is a cumbersome task, and as a rule pharmacists prefer to measure liquids by volume. Therefore, in the preparation of diluted acids, the calculations are generally carried one step further to determine the volume of concentrated acid that corresponds to the calculated weight. Because this additional step requires the use of the concentrated acid's specific gravity, a brief review of specific gravity seems appropriate.

By definition, specific gravity is a ratio, expressed decimally, of the weight of a substance to the weight of an equal volume of a standard, both substances having the same temperature or the temperature of each being known. Water is used as the standard for liquids and solids; hydrogen or air, for gases. In pharmacy, specific gravity calculations mainly involve liquids and solids, and water is an excellent

choice for a standard, because it is readily available and easily purified.

At 4°C, the density of water is 1 g per cubic centimeter. Because the USP states that 1 mL may be considered the equivalent of 1 cc, in pharmacy, water is assumed to weigh 1 g per milliliter. By the following equation used to calculate specific gravity, a substance having a density the same as water would have a specific gravity of 1.0:

$$\text{sp gr} = \frac{\text{weight of a substance}}{\text{weight of an equal volume of water}}$$

In solving this equation, the same units of weight must be used in each part of the ratio. These units cancel out, and the ratio is expressed decimally.

Specific gravity indicates the ratio of the weight of a substance to that of an equal volume of water. For example, say 10 mL of a liquid weighs 20 g. An equal volume of water weighs 10 g, and the ratio in the equation is 20:10, yielding a specific gravity of 2.0. This indicates that the liquid is twice as heavy as water in equal volume. By the same token, a liquid having a specific gravity of 0.5 is half as heavy as water; a liquid with a specific gravity of 0.8 is eight-tenths as heavy as water, and so on.

If both the volume of a liquid and its specific gravity are known, its weight may be calculated. For instance, if concentrated hydrochloric acid has a specific gravity of 1.17, it is that number times as heavy as water, and 100 mL of the acid would weigh 1.17 times as much as 100 mL of water. Since 100 mL of water weighs 100 g, 100 mL of the acid weighs 1.17 times that or 117 g.

If one knows the weight of a liquid and its specific gravity, the volume of the liquid may be determined. For example, a liquid that is twice as heavy as water has a specific gravity of 2.0 and occupies half the volume that an equal weight of water occupies. If one has 100 g of this liquid and substitutes in the equation as indicated next, the volume of the liquid can be arrived at:

$$2.0 = \frac{100 \text{ g}}{\text{weight of an equal volume of water}}$$

$$\text{weight of an equal volume of water} = \frac{100 \text{ g}}{2.0}$$
$$= 50 \text{ g}$$

Since 50 g is the weight of an equal volume of water, it follows that the water must measure 50 mL. Since the volume of the water is an equal volume to the other liquid, that liquid must also measure 50 mL.

The volume represented by 27.39 g of the concentrated hydrochloric acid may be similarly determined by dividing the weight of the concentrated acid by its specific gravity and equating the weight of an equal volume of water to the volume of the acid:

$$\frac{27.39 \text{ g}}{1.17} = 23.41 \text{ g, weight of equal volume of water}$$

Thus, because 23.41 g of water measures 23.41 mL and because it is equal in volume to the concentrated acid, the latter also measures 23.41 mL, and this is the amount required to prepare 100 mL of the 10% w/v diluted acid.

Once the aforementioned is thoroughly understood, the following simplified formula can be used to calculate the amount of a concentrated acid required in the preparation of a specific volume of the corresponding diluted acid:

$$\frac{\text{Percentage strength (w/v) of diluted acid} \times \text{Volume of diluted acid to be prepared}}{\text{Percentage strength of concentrated acid (w/w)} \times \text{Specific gravity of concentrated acid}}$$

$$= \text{volume of concentrated acid to use}$$

Recalculating the preparation of 100 mL of diluted hydrochloric acid from the concentrated acid gives the following:

$$\frac{10 \times 100 \text{ mL}}{36.5 \times 1.17} = \frac{23.41 \text{ mL of concentrated}}{\text{acid to use}}$$

Most diluted acids have a strength of 10% w/v, with the exception of diluted acetic acid, which is 6% w/v. The strengths of these acids are commensurate with the concentrations generally used for medicinal or pharmaceutical purposes. The concentrations of the corresponding concentrated acids vary widely from one acid to another, depending on various properties of the solute such as solubility, stability, and ease of preparation. For instance, concentrated sulfuric acid is generally between 95 and 98% w/w, nitric acid between 69 and 71% w/w, and concentrated phosphoric acid between 85

and 88% w/w. As a result, the amounts of each concentrated acid required to prepare the corresponding diluted acid vary widely and must be calculated on an individual basis.

There is very little use of diluted acids in medicine today. However, because of its antibacterial effects, acetic acid finds application as a 1% solution in surgical dressings, as an irrigating solution to the bladder in 0.25% concentration, and as a spermatocidal in some proprietary contraceptive preparations.

Spirits

Spirits are alcoholic or hydroalcoholic solutions of volatile substances. Generally, the alcoholic concentration of spirits is rather high, usually over 60%. Because of the greater solubility of aromatic or volatile substances in alcohol than in water, spirits can contain a greater concentration of these materials than the corresponding aromatic waters. When mixed with water or with an aqueous preparation, the volatile substances present in spirits generally separate from solution and form a milky preparation.

Spirits may be used pharmaceutically as flavoring agents and medicinally for the therapeutic value of the aromatic solute. As flavoring agents they are used to impart the flavor of their solute to other pharmaceutical preparations. For medicinal purposes, spirits may be taken orally, applied externally, or used by inhalation, depending upon the particular preparation. When taken orally, they are generally mixed with a portion of water to reduce the pungency of the spirit. Depending on the materials, spirits may be prepared by simple solution, solution by maceration, or distillation. The spirits most recently official in the USP–NF are aromatic ammonia spirit, camphor spirit, compound orange spirit, and peppermint spirit.

Nonaqueous Solutions

Liniments

Liniments are alcoholic or oleaginous solutions or emulsions of various medicinal substances intended to be rubbed on the skin. Liniments with an alcoholic or hydroalcoholic vehicle are useful when rubefacient, counterirritant, or penetrating action is desired; oleaginous liniments are employed primarily when massage is desired. By their nature, oleaginous liniments are less irritating to the skin than alcoholic liniments. Liniments are not applied to skin areas that are broken or bruised because excessive irritation might result. The vehicle for a liniment should therefore be selected for the type of action desired (rubefacient, counterirritant, or massage) and also on the solubility of the desired components in the various solvents. For oleaginous liniments, the solvent may be a fixed oil such as almond oil, peanut oil, sesame oil, or cottonseed oil or a volatile substance such as wintergreen oil or turpentine, or it may be a combination of fixed and volatile oils.

All liniments should bear a label indicating that they are suitable only for external use and must never be taken internally. Liniments that are emulsions or that contain insoluble matter must be shaken thoroughly before use to ensure even distribution of the dispersed phase, and these preparations should be labeled SHAKE WELL. Liniments should be stored in tight containers. Depending on their individual ingredients, liniments are prepared in the same manner as solutions, emulsions, or suspensions, as the case may warrant.

Collodions

Collodions are liquid preparations composed of pyroxylin dissolved in a solvent mixture usually composed of alcohol and ether with or without added medicinal substances. Pyroxylin (soluble gun cotton, collodion cotton), obtained by the action of a mixture of nitric and sulfuric acids on cotton, consists chiefly of cellulose tetranitrate. It has the appearance of raw cotton when dry but is harsh to the touch. It is frequently available commercially moistened with about 30% alcohol or other similar solvent.

One part of pyroxylin is slowly but completely soluble in 25 parts of a mixture of 3 volumes of ether and 1 volume of alcohol. It is also soluble in acetone and glacial acetic acid. Pyroxylin is precipitated from solution in these solvents upon the addition of water. Pyroxylin, like collodions, is exceedingly flammable and must be stored away from flame in well-closed containers, protected from light.

Collodions are intended for external use. When applied to the skin with a fine camel's hair brush or glass applicator, the solvent rapidly evaporates, leaving a filmy residue of pyroxylin. This provides an occlusive protective coating to the skin, and when the collodion is medicated, it leaves a thin layer of that medication firmly placed against the skin. Naturally, collodions must be applied to dry tissues to adhere to the skin's surface. The products must be clearly labeled "for external use only" or with words of similar effect.

Collodion

Collodion is a clear or slightly opalescent viscous liquid prepared by dissolving pyroxylin (4% w/v) in a 3:1 mixture of ether and alcohol. The resulting solution is highly volatile and flammable and should be preserved in a tight container remote from fire at a temperature not exceeding 30°C.

The product is capable of forming a protective film on application to the skin and the volatilization of the solvent. The film is useful in holding the edges of an incised wound together. However, its presence on the skin is uncomfortable because of its inflexible nature. The following product, which is flexible, has a greater appeal when a pliable film is acceptable.

Flexible Collodion

Flexible collodion is prepared by adding 2% camphor and 3% castor oil to collodion. The castor oil renders the product flexible, permitting its comfortable use over skin areas that are normally moved, such as fingers and toes. The camphor makes the product waterproof. Physicians frequently apply the coating over bandages or stitched incisions to make them waterproof and to protect them from external stress.

Salicylic Acid Collodion

Salicylic acid collodion is a 10% solution of salicylic acid in flexible collodion. It is used for its keratolytic effects, especially in the removal of corns from the toes. Patients who use such products should be advised about their proper use. The product should be applied one drop at a time on the corn or wart, allowing time to dry before the next drop is added. Because salicylic acid can irritate normal, healthy skin, every attempt must be made to ensure application directly on the corn or wart. A useful preventive measure is to line the adjacent healthy skin with some white petrolatum prior to application of the product. Proper tightening and storage of the product after use are absolutely necessary because of the volatility of the vehicle.

Extraction Methods for Preparing Solutions

Certain pharmaceutical preparations are prepared by extraction, that is, by withdrawal of desired constituents from crude drugs through the use of selected solvents in which the desired constituents are soluble. Crude drugs are vegetable or animal drugs that have undergone no other processes than collection, cleaning, and drying. Because each crude drug contains a number of constituents that may be soluble in a given solvent, the products of extraction, termed extractives, do not contain just a single constituent but rather varying constituents, depending on the drug used and the conditions of the extraction. Tinctures, fluidextracts and extracts are the pharmaceutical products most commonly prepared from extractives.

Plant materials are composed of heterogeneous mixtures of constituents, some of which are pharmacologically active and others, pharmacologically inactive and considered inert. Among the varied plant constituents are sugars, starches, mucilages, proteins, albumins, pectins, cellulose, gums, inorganic salts, fixed and volatile oils, resins, tannins, coloring materials, and a number of very active constituents such as alkaloids and glycosides. The solvent systems used in extraction are selected on the basis of their capacity to dissolve the maximum amount of desired active constituents and the minimum amount of undesired constituents.

In many instances, the active constituents of a plant drug are of the same general chemical type, have similar solubility characteristics, and can be simultaneously extracted with a single solvent or a single solvent mixture. Extraction concentrates the active constituents of a crude drug and removes from it the extraneous matter. In drug extraction, the solvent or solvent mixture is referred to as the menstruum, and the plant residue, which is exhausted of active constituents, is termed the marc.

The selection of the menstruum to use in the extraction of a crude drug is based primarily on its ability to dissolve the active constituents. Although water and alcohol and to a lesser extent glycerin are probably the most frequently employed solvents in drug extraction, acetic acid and organic solvents like ether may be used for special purposes.

Because of its ready availability, cheapness, and good solvent action for many plant constituents, water has some use in drug extraction, particularly in combination with other solvents. However, as a sole solvent it has many disadvantages and is infrequently used alone. For one thing, most active plant constituents are complex organic chemical compounds that are less soluble in water than in alcohol. Although water has a great solvent action on such plant constituents as sugars, gums, starches, coloring principles, and tannins, most of these are not particularly desirable components of an extracted preparation. Water also tends to extract plant principles that separate upon standing in the extractive, leaving an undesired residue. Finally, unless preserved, aqueous preparations serve as excellent growth media for molds, yeasts, and bacteria. When water alone is employed as the menstruum, alcohol is frequently added to the extractive or to the final preparation as an antimicrobial preservative.

Hydroalcoholic mixtures are perhaps the most versatile and most widely employed menstrua. They combine the solvent effects of both water and alcohol, and the complete miscibility of these two agents permits flexible combining of the two agents to form solvent mixtures most suited to the extraction of the active principles from a particular drug. A hydroalcoholic menstruum generally provides inherent protection against microbial contamination and helps to prevent the separation of extracted material on standing. Alcohol is used alone as a menstruum only when necessary because it is more expensive than hydroalcoholic mixtures.

Glycerin, a good solvent for many plant substances, is occasionally employed as a cosolvent with water or alcoholic menstrua because of its ability to extract and then prevent inert materials from precipitating upon standing. It is especially useful in this regard in preventing separation of tannin and tannin oxidation products in extractives. Because glycerin has preservative action, depending on its concentration in the final product, it may contribute to the stability of a pharmaceutical extractive.

Methods of Extraction

The principal methods of drug extraction are maceration and percolation. Generally, the method of extraction selected for a given drug depends on several factors, including the nature of the crude drug, its adaptability to each of the various extraction methods, and the interest in obtaining complete or nearly complete extraction of the drug.

Frequently a combination of maceration and percolation is actually employed in the extraction of a crude drug. The drug is macerated first to soften the plant tissues and to dissolve much of the active constituents, and percolation separates the extractive from the marc.

Maceration

The term maceration comes from the Latin *macerare*, meaning to soak. It is a process in which the properly comminuted drug is permitted to soak in the menstruum until the cellular structure is softened and penetrated by the menstruum and the soluble constituents are dissolved.

In the maceration process, the drug to be extracted is generally placed in a wide-mouth container with the prescribed menstruum, the vessel is stoppered tightly, and the contents are agitated repeatedly over a period usually ranging from 2 to 14 days. The agitation permits the repeated flow of fresh solvent over the entire surface area of the comminuted drug. An alternative to repeated shaking is to place the drug in a porous cloth bag that is tied and suspended in the upper portion of the menstruum, much the same as a tea bag is suspended in water to make a cup of tea. As the soluble constituents dissolve in the menstruum, they tend to settle to the bottom because of an increase in the specific gravity of the liquid due to its added weight. Occasional dipping of the drug bag may facilitate the speed of the extraction. The extractive is separated from the marc by expressing the bag of drug and washing it with additional fresh menstruum, the washings being added to the extractive. If the maceration is performed with the drug loose, the marc may be removed by straining and/or filtration, with the marc being washed free of extractive by the additional passage of menstruum through the strainer or filter into the total extractive.

For drugs containing little or no cellular material, such as benzoin, aloe, and tolu, which dissolve almost completely in the menstruum, maceration is the most efficient method of extraction.

Maceration is usually conducted at a temperature of 15° to 20°C for 3 days or until the soluble matter is dissolved.

Percolation

The term *percolation*, from the Latin *per*, meaning through, and *colare*, meaning to strain, may be described generally as a process in which a comminuted drug is extracted of its soluble constituents by the slow passage of a suitable solvent through a column of the drug. The drug is packed in a special extraction apparatus termed a percolator, with the collected extractive called the percolate. Most drug extractions are performed by percolation, a process whereby coffee is routinely prepared.

In the process of percolation the flow of the menstruum over the drug column is generally downward to the exit orifice, drawn by the force of gravity as well as the weight of the column of liquid. In certain specialized and more sophisticated percolation apparatus, additional pressure on the column is exerted with positive air pressure at the inlet and suction at the outlet or exit.

Percolators for drug extraction vary greatly as to their shape, capacities, composition, and, most important, utility. Percolators employed in the large-scale industrial preparation of extractives are generally stainless steel or glass-lined metal vessels that vary greatly in size and in operation. Percolators used to extract leaves, for instance, may be 6 to 8 feet in diameter and 12 to 18 feet high (Fig. 13.5). Percolators employed to extract other vegetable parts like seeds that are greater in density than leaves and would pack too tightly in percolators of such large dimensions are extracted in much smaller percolators. Some special industrial percolators are designed to percolate with hot menstrua; in others pressure is used to force the menstruum through the drug columns.

Percolation on a small scale generally involves the use of glass percolators of various shapes for extraction of small amounts (perhaps up to 1000 g) of crude drug. The shape of percolators in common laboratory and small-scale use are (*a*) cylindrical, with little if any taper except for the lower orifice; (*b*) roundish, but with a definite taper downward; and (*c*) conical, or funnel-shaped. Each type has a special utility in drug extraction.

The cylindrical percolator is particularly suited to the complete extraction of drugs with a minimal expenditure of menstruum. By the passage of the menstruum over the drug contained in a high, narrow column (rather than in a lower, wider column), each drug particle is more repeatedly exposed to passing solvent. A funnel-shaped percolator is useful for drugs that swell a great deal during maceration, since the large upper surface permits expansion of the drug column with little risk of a too tightly packed column or breakage of a glass percolator.

Example Preparations Prepared by Extraction Processes

Fluidextracts

Fluidextracts are liquid preparations of vegetable drugs prepared by percolation. They contain alcohol as a solvent, preservative, or both and are made so that each milliliter contains the therapeutic constituents of 1 g of the

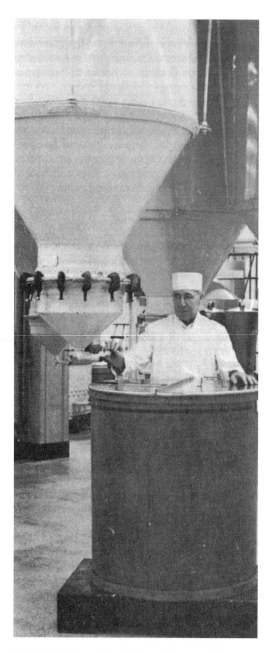

FIGURE 13.5 Large industrial percolators used in extracting crude drugs to make fluidextracts, tinctures, and powdered extracts.

standard drug that it represents. Because of their concentrated nature, many fluidextracts are considered too potent to be safely self-administered, and their use per se is almost nonexistent in medical practice. Also, many fluidextracts are simply too bitter tasting or otherwise unpalatable to be accepted by the patient. Therefore, most fluidextracts today are either modified by the addition of flavoring or sweetening agents before use or are used as the drug source of other liquid dosage forms, such as syrups.

Extracts

Extracts are concentrated preparations of vegetable or animal drugs obtained by removal of the active constituents of the respective drugs with suitable menstrua, evaporation of all or nearly all of the solvent, and adjustment of the residual masses or powders to the prescribed standards.

Extracts are potent preparations, usually between two and six times as potent on a weight basis as the crude drug. They contain primarily the active constituents of the crude drug, with a great portion of the inactive constituents and structural components of the crude drug having been removed. Their function is to provide in small amounts and in convenient, stable physical form the medicinal activity and character of the bulkier plants that they represent. As such, they have use in product formulation.

In the manufacture of most extracts, percolation is employed to remove the active constituents from the drug, with the percolates generally being reduced in volume by distillation under reduced pressure to reduce the degree of heat and to protect the drug substances against thermal decomposition. The extent of removal of the solvent determines the final physical character of the extract. Extracts are made in three forms: (a) semiliquid extracts or those of a syrupy consistency prepared without the intent of removing all or even most of the menstruum, (b) pilular or solid extracts of a plastic consistency prepared with nearly all of the menstruum removed, and (c) powdered extracts prepared to be dry by the removal of all of the menstruum insofar as is feasible or practical. Pilular and powdered extracts differ only by the slight amount of remaining solvent in the former preparation, but each has its pharmaceutical advantage because of its physical form. For instance, the pilular extract is preferred in compounding a plastic dosage form such as an ointment or paste or one in which a pliable material facilitates compounding, whereas the powdered form is preferred in the compounding of such dosage forms as powders, capsules, and tablets.

PHARMACEUTICAL SCIENCE CASE STUDY

Subjective

You have been given the responsibility of formulating a new oral solution containing a nasal decongestant (phenylephrine) and cough suppressant (dextromethorphan) for treating the symptoms of a cold or influenza. The oral solution should have a reasonably pleasant taste and appearance, be stable and preserved, and contain a suitable dose combination so that one or two teaspoonfuls can be used per administration to a 6- to 12-year-old child.

Objective

Phenylephrine hydrochloride ($C_9H_{13}NO_2 \cdot HCl$, molecular weight 203.67) is the salt form selected for this drug. Phenylephrine hydrochloride occurs as white or nearly white odorless crystals with a bitter taste. It melts at 140° to 145°C (284°–293F°). It is freely soluble in water and in alcohol. It is stable in aqueous solution below pH 7. Above pH 7, degradation occurs apparently involving the side chain, with loss of the secondary amine function; the phenolic group remains intact. The presence of heavy metals, especially copper, can catalyze the decomposition. It has two dissociation constant (pK_a) values, one at 8.77 and one at 9.84.

Dextromethorphan ($C_{18}H_{25}NO$, MW 271.40) is a practically white to slightly yellow odorless crystalline powder that melts at 109.5° to 112.5°C (229°–234.5°F). It is prac-

Pharmaceutics Science Case Study cont.

tically insoluble in water. Dextromethorphan hydrobromide ($C_{18}H_{25}NO.HBr.H_2O$, MW 370.32) occurs as practically white crystals or crystalline powder with a faint odor and a melting range of 124° to 126°C (255°–259°F). It is freely soluble in alcohol. It is stable in aqueous and hydroalcoholic solutions.

Assessment

The two drugs should be soluble and stable in a slightly acidic oral solution consisting of water and alcohol. The vehicle should be slightly thickened by a viscosity-increasing additive; it also should be sweetened and flavored. These drugs are bitter, so a flavor that will help mask the bitterness must be selected. The addition of a small amount of menthol may also be considered as a flavor enhancer. An appropriate preservative must be selected.

Plan

An aqueous solution consisting of water, alcohol (low concentration, such as 5%), and glycerin (10%) adjusted to a pH in the range of 4 to 5 should be reasonable. Sucrose can be added as a sweetener (40%) and also for its viscosity-enhancing effect. It can be further thickened with methylcellulose 0.5% or other cellulose polymer commonly used in oral liquids. A small amount of sorbitol (10%) will help give a smooth mouth feel and minimize cap lock of the container. Several flavor combinations can work, but raspberry and marshmallow work nicely to cover bitter tastes of drugs. A blend of 0.05% methylparaben and 0.02% propylparaben can be added as a preservative. The addition of about 0.25% menthol will further enhance the flavoring and also impart an additional aromatic effect.

CLINICAL CASE STUDY

HPI: Late one evening at the local pharmacy, the pharmacist notices a woman searching aimlessly in the nonprescription medication aisle. In hopes of being able to help this customer, the pharmacist approaches the woman and asks if he can help her find anything. The woman replies, "My husband and I are taking a family vacation to Florida tomorrow, and my son gets sick to his stomach when he flies. I was trying to find something that he could take for motion sickness." After asking the woman a few questions, the pharmacist discovers that her 5-year-old son is quite finicky and will not take tablets, including chewables. The pharmacist recalls a similar situation from awhile back for which he compounded an oral solution of dimenhydrinate (Dramamine), and he asked the woman if this

would be a suitable option for her son. The woman expressed much gratitude and asked the pharmacist if he could have the solution ready for her by the morning. The pharmacist said that would be fine, and he obtained the following information about her son, J. M.

PMH: Motion sickness
Recurrent ear infections
SH: None
FH: Mother (−)
Father (+) for hypertension
ALL: NKDA
MEDS: None

Pharmaceutical Care Plan

S: Mother states that her "finicky" son will not take oral tablets, including chewables.

Clinical Case Study cont.

O: Dimenhydrinate, a common nonprescription medication used for motion sickness, is no longer available in liquid form.

A: J. M. is a 5 y/o WM who has motion sickness on airplanes, and his family is leaving on vacation in the morning. Because the patient will not take tablets, the pharmacist plans to compound an oral solution of dimenhydrinate. The patient does not have any present medical conditions or a medication history that would contraindicate the use of dimenhydrinate.

P: 1. The pharmacist decides that to make the compound, he must first review information on the solubility and stability of dimenhydrinate. To do so, he consults Remington (10), where he reads that dimenhydrinate is "slightly soluble in water and freely soluble in alcohol and chloroform."

2. Although the pharmacist has prepared this solution before, he does not remember exactly how he did so. He does, however, remember that in the *US Pharmacist* journal there is a monthly Contemporary Compounding section, which he thinks may be useful. He scans the journal archives in the pharmacy until he finds the article "Oral Solution Stops Motion Sickness" (11). He secures the appropriate issue and reads the article to review how to prepare the dimenhydrinate solution.

3. Following the methods for preparation outlined in this article, the pharmacist prepares the compound from the following formula:

Rx: Dimenhydrinate 12.5mg/5ml Oral Solution

Dimenhydrinate	250 mg
Glycerin	qs
Ora-Plus	50 mL
Ora-Sweet or Ora-Sweet SF	qs 100 mL

4. As the article suggests, the pharmacist packages the solution in a tight, light-resistant container. In addition, he labels the bottle TAKE ONLY AS DIRECTED, KEEP OUT OF THE REACH OF CHILDREN, MAY CAUSE DROWSINESS, and CONTENTS SHOULD BE DISCARDED [6 months from date of preparation].

5. The pharmacist is working the next morning, so he plans to counsel the woman on her son's medication at that time. Based on the dimenhydrinate package directions, a 5-year-old should take one-quarter to one-half a tablet every 6 to 8 hours, not to exceed one and a half tablets in 24 hours or as directed by a doctor. Each manufactured tablet contains dimenhydrinate 50 mg, and the compounded oral solution contains dimenhydrinate 12.5 mg/5 mL. Thus, the pharmacist should instruct the woman to give J. M. 1 to 2 teaspoonfuls by mouth every 6 to 8 hours, not to exceed 5 teaspoonfuls every 24 hours. Because dimenhydrinate's onset of action is approximately 30 minutes, the pharmacist recommends that J. M. take the first dose about 30 minutes prior to the flight departure.

6. In addition to dosage information, the pharmacist counsels the mother on the possible side effects. The most common is drowsiness, which should prove useful in this situation. Other adverse effects include a dry mouth and constipation. However, these can be relieved or prevented by drinking plenty of fluid.

7. Finally, the pharmacist reminds the mother that the solution may be stored at room temperature until the expiration date. After that time, any remaining contents should be discarded. The pharmacist also gives her the directions from the dimenhydrinate package along with the remaining tablets so that the patient and his family have the important product information that should accompany the medication (10, 11).

REFERENCES

1. United States Pharmacopeia 26–National Formulary 21. Rockville, MD: U.S. Pharmacopeial Convention, 2003;2404–2405.
2. United States Pharmacopeia 26–National Formulary 21. Rockville, MD: U.S. Pharmacopeial Convention, 2003;9.
3. Pure water handbook. Minnetonka, MN: Osmonics, 1991.
4. Chemburkar PB, Joslin RS. Effect of flavoring oils on preservative concentrations in oral liquid dosage forms. J Pharm Sci 1975;64:414–441.
5. Gossel TA. Oral rehydration solutions. US Pharmacist 1987;12:90–98.
6. Handbook on extemporaneous formulations. Bethesda, MD: American Society of Hospital Pharmacists, 1987.
7. Pesko LJ. Compounding: oral liquids. Am Druggist 1993;208:49.
8. Oral liquid pharmaceuticals. Wilmington, DE: ICI Americas, 1975.
9. Murphy D. Ipecac misuse by bulimics: APhA launches educational campaign. Am Pharm 1985; NS25:264–265.
10. Gennaro AR. Remington: The science and practice of pharmacy, 20th ed. Philadelphia: Lippincott Williams & Wilkins, 2000.
11. Allen LV Jr. Oral solution stops motion sickness. U.S. Pharmacist 2002;Aug:64–65.

Disperse Systems

14

Chapter at a glance

This chapter includes the main types of liquid preparations containing undissolved or immiscible drug distributed throughout a vehicle. In these preparations, the substance distributed is referred to as the *dispersed phase*, and the vehicle is termed the *dispersing phase* or *dispersion medium*. Together, they produce a *dispersed system*.

The particles of the dispersed phase are usually solid materials that are insoluble in the dispersion medium. In the case of emulsions, the dispersed phase is a liquid that is neither soluble nor miscible with the liquid of the dispersing phase. Emulsification results in the dispersion of liquid drug as fine droplets throughout the dispersing phase. In the case of an aerosol, the dispersed phase may be small air bubbles throughout a solution or an emulsion. Dispersions also consist of droplets of a liquid (solution or suspension) in air.

The particles of the dispersed phase vary widely in size, from large particles visible to the naked eye down to particles of colloidal dimension, falling between 1.0 nm and 0.5 μm. Dispersions containing coarse particles, usually 10 to 50 μm, are referred to as *coarse dispersions*; they include the *suspensions* and *emulsions*. Dispersions containing particles of smaller size are termed *fine dispersions* (0.5–10 μm), and if the particles are in the colloidal range, *colloidal dispersions*. *Magmas* and *gels* are fine dispersions.

Largely because of their greater size, particles in a coarse dispersion have a greater tendency to separate from the dispersion medium than do the particles of a fine dispersion. Most solids in dispersion tend to settle to the bottom of the container because of their greater density than the dispersion medium, whereas most emulsified liquids for oral use are oils, which generally have less density than the aqueous medium in which they are dispersed, so that they tend to rise toward the top of the preparation. Complete and uniform redistribution of the dispersed phase is essential to the accurate administration of uniform doses. For a properly prepared dispersion, this should be accomplished by moderate agitation of the container.

The focus of this chapter is on dispersions of drugs administered orally or topically. The same basic pharmaceutical characteristics apply to dispersion systems administered by other routes. Included among these are ophthalmic and otic suspensions and sterile suspensions for injection, covered in Chapters 17 and 15, respectively.

Suspensions

Suspensions may be defined as preparations containing finely divided drug particles (the *suspensoid*) distributed somewhat uniformly throughout a vehicle in which the drug exhibits a minimum degree of solubility. Some suspensions are available in ready-to-use form, that is, already distributed through a liquid vehicle with or without stabilizers and other additives (Fig. 14.1). Other preparations are available as dry powders intended for suspension in liquid vehicles. This type of product generally is a powder mixture containing the drug and suitable suspending and dispersing agents to be diluted and agitated with a specified quantity of vehicle, generally purified water. Figure 14.2 demonstrates preparation of this type of product. Drugs that are unstable if maintained for extended periods in the presence of an aqueous vehicle (for example, many antibiotic drugs) are most frequently supplied as dry powder mixtures for reconstitution at the time of dispensing. This type of preparation is designated in the USP by a title of the form "for Oral Suspension." Prepared suspensions not requiring reconstitution at the time of dispensing are simply designated as "Oral Suspension."

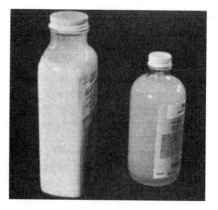

FIGURE 14.1 Commercial oral suspensions.

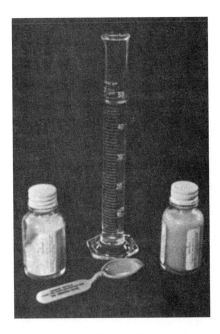

FIGURE 14.2 Commercial antibiotic preparation for oral suspension following reconstitution with purified water. *Left*, dry powder mixture. *Right*, suspension after reconstitution with the specified amount of purified water.

Reasons for Suspensions

There are several reasons for preparing suspensions. For one thing, certain drugs are chemically unstable in solution but stable when suspended. In instances such as this, the suspension ensures chemical stability while permitting liquid therapy. For many patients, the liquid form is preferred to the solid form of the same drug because of the ease of swallowing liquids and the flexibility in administration of a range of doses. This is particularly advantageous for infants, children, and the elderly. The disadvantage of a disagreeable taste of certain drugs in solution form is overcome when the drug is administered as undissolved particles of an oral suspension. In fact, chemical forms of certain poor-tasting drugs have been specifically developed for their insolubility in a desired vehicle for the sole purpose of preparing a palatable liquid dosage form. For example, chloramphenicol palmitate, the water-insoluble ester form of chloramphenicol, was developed to prepare a palatable liquid dosage form of chloramphenicol, the result being the development of Chloramphenicol Palmitate Oral Suspension, USP. Use of insoluble forms of drugs in suspensions greatly reduces the difficult taste-masking problems of developmental pharmacists, and selection of the flavorants to be used in a given suspension may be based on taste preference rather than on a particular flavorant's ability to mask an unpleasant taste. For the most part, oral suspensions are aqueous preparations with the vehicle flavored and sweetened to suit the anticipated taste preferences of the intended patient.

Features Desired in a Pharmaceutical Suspension

There are many considerations in the development and preparation of a pharmaceutically elegant suspension. In addition to therapeutic efficacy, chemical stability of the components of the formulation, permanency of the preparation, and esthetic appeal of the preparation—desirable qualities in all pharmaceutical preparations—a few other features apply more specifically to the pharmaceutical suspension:

1. A properly prepared pharmaceutical suspension should settle slowly and should be readily redispersed upon gentle shaking of the container.
2. The particle size of the suspensoid should remain fairly constant throughout long periods of undisturbed standing.
3. The suspension should pour readily and evenly from its container.

These main features of a suspension, which depend on the nature of the dispersed phase, the dispersion medium, and pharmaceutical adjuncts, will be discussed briefly.

Sedimentation Rate of the Particles of a Suspension

The various factors involved in the rate of settling of the particles of a suspension are embodied in the equation of Stokes' law, which is presented in the Physical Pharmacy Capsule 14.1.

Stokes' equation was derived for an ideal situation in which uniform, perfectly spherical particles in a very dilute suspension settle without producing turbulence, without collid-

PHYSICAL PHARMACY CAPSULE 14.1

Sedimentation Rate and Stokes' Equation

Stokes' Equation:

$$\frac{dx}{dt} = \frac{d^2\,(\rho_i - \rho_e)g}{18\eta}$$

where
  dx/dt is the rate of settling,
  d is the diameter of the particles,
  ρ_i is the density of the particle,
  ρ_e is the density of the medium,
  g is the gravitational constant, and
  η is the viscosity of the medium.

A number of factors can be adjusted to enhance the physical stability of a suspension, including the diameter of the particles and the density and viscosity of the medium. The effect of changing these is illustrated in the following example.

EXAMPLE 1

A powder has a density of 1.3 g/cc and an average particle diameter of 2.5 μg (assuming the particles to be spheres). According to Stokes' equation, this powder will settle in water (viscosity of 1 cps assumed) at this rate:

$$\frac{(2.5 \times 10^{-4})^2\,(1.3 - 1.0)\,(980)}{18 \times 0.01} = 1.02 \times 10^{-4}\ \text{cm/seconds}$$

If the particle size of the powder is reduced to 0.25 μm and water is still used as the dispersion medium, the powder will now settle at this rate:

$$\frac{(2.5 \times 10^{-5})^2\,(1.3 - 1.0)\,(980)}{18 \times 0.01} = 1.02 \times 10^{-6}\ \text{cm/seconds}$$

As is evident, a decrease in particle size by a factor of 10 results in a reduction in the rate of settling by a factor of 100. This enhanced effect is a result of the d factor in Stokes' equation being squared.

If a different dispersion medium, such as glycerin, is used in place of water, a further decrease in settling will result. Glycerin has a density of 1.25 g/mL and a viscosity of 400 cps. The larger particle size powder (2.5 μm) will settle at this rate:

$$\frac{(2.5 \times 10^{-4})^2\,(1.3 - 1.25)\,(980)}{18 \times 4} = 4.25 \times 10^{-8}\ \text{cm/seconds}$$

The smaller particle size (0.25 μm) powder will now settle at this rate:

$$\frac{(2.5 \times 10^{-5})^2\,(1.3 - 1.25)\,(980)}{18 \times 4} = 4.25 \times 10^{-10}\ \text{cm/seconds}$$

A summary of these results is shown in the following table:

CONDITION	RATE OF SETTLING (CM/SECONDS)
2.5 μm powder in water	1.02×10^{-4}
0.25 μm powder in water	1.02×10^{-6}
2.5 μm powder in glycerin	4.25×10^{-8}
0.25 μm powder in glycerin	4.25×10^{-10}

As is evident from this table, a change in dispersion medium results in the greatest change in the rate of settling of particles. Particle size reduction also can contribute significantly to suspension stability. These factors are important in the formulation of physically stable suspensions.

ing with other particles of the suspensoid, and without chemical or physical attraction or affinity for the dispersion medium. Obviously, Stokes' equation does not apply precisely to the usual pharmaceutical suspension in which the suspensoid is irregularly shaped and of various particle diameters, in which the fall of the particles *does* result in both turbulence and collision, and also in which the particles may have some affinity for the suspension medium. However, the basic concepts of the equation do give a valid indication of the factors that are important to suspension of the particles and a clue to the possible adjustments that can be made to a formulation to decrease the rate of sedimentation.

From the equation it is apparent that the velocity of fall of a suspended particle is greater for larger particles than it is for smaller particles, all other factors remaining constant. Reducing the particle size of the dispersed phase produces a slower *rate* of descent of the particles. Also, the greater the density of the particles, the greater the rate of descent, provided the density of the vehicle is not altered. Because aqueous vehicles are used in pharmaceutical oral suspensions, the density of the particles is generally greater than that of the vehicle, a desirable feature, for if the particles were less dense than the vehicle, they would tend to float, and floating particles would be quite difficult to distribute uniformly in the vehicle. The rate of sedimentation may be appreciably reduced by increasing the viscosity of the dispersion medium, and within limits of practicality this may be done. However, a product having too high a viscosity is not generally desirable, because it pours with difficulty and it is equally difficult to redisperse the suspensoid. Therefore, if the viscosity of a suspension is increased, it is done so only to a modest extent to avoid these difficulties.

The viscosity characteristics of a suspension may be altered not only by the vehicle used, but also by the solids content. As the proportion of solid particles in a suspension increases, so does the viscosity. The viscosity of a pharmaceutical preparation may be determined through the use of a viscometer, such as a Brookfield Viscometer, which measures viscosity by the force required to rotate a spindle in the fluid being tested (Fig. 14.3).

For the most part, the physical stability of a pharmaceutical suspension appears to be most appropriately adjusted by an alteration in the dispersed phase rather than through great changes in the dispersion medium. In most instances, the dispersion medium supports the adjusted dispersed phase. These adjustments mainly are concerned with particle size, uniformity of particle size, and separation of the particles so that they are not likely to become greatly larger or to form a solid cake on standing.

Physical Features of the Dispersed Phase of a Suspension

Probably the most important single consideration in a discussion of suspensions is the size of the particles. In most good pharmaceutical suspensions, the particle diameter is 1 to 50 μm.

Particle size reduction is generally accomplished by dry milling prior to incorporation of the dispersed phase into the dispersion medium. One of the most rapid, convenient, and inexpensive methods of producing fine drug powders of about 10 to 50 μm size is *micropulverization*. Micropulverizers are high-speed attrition or impact mills that are efficient in reducing powders to the size acceptable for most oral and topical suspensions. For still finer particles, under 10 μm, *fluid energy* grinding, sometimes referred to as *jet milling* or *micronizing*, is quite effective. By this process, the shearing action of high-velocity compressed airstreams on the particles in a confined space produces the desired ultrafine or micronized particles. The particles to be micronized are swept into violent turbulence by the sonic and supersonic velocity of the airstreams. The particles are accelerated to high velocities and collide with one another, resulting in fragmentation. This method may be employed when the particles are intended for parenteral or ophthalmic suspensions. Particles of extremely small dimensions may also be produced by *spray-drying*. A spray dryer is a cone-shaped apparatus into which a solution of a drug is sprayed and rapidly dried by a current of warm, dry air circulating in the cone. The resulting

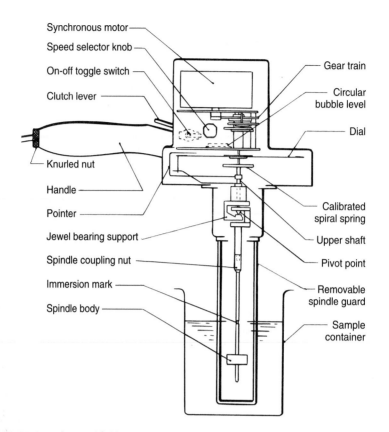

Synchronous motor

Speed selector knob

On-off toggle switch

Clutch lever

Knurled nut

Handle

Pointer

Jewel bearing support

Spindle coupling nut

Immersion mark

Spindle body

Gear train

Circular bubble level

Dial

Calibrated spiral spring

Upper shaft

Pivot point

Removable spindle guard

Sample container

FIGURE 14.3 The Brookfield Viscometer. (Courtesy of Brookfield Engineering Laboratories.)

dry powder is collected. It is not possible for a pharmacist to achieve the same degree of particle-size reduction with such comminuting equipment as the mortar and pestle. However, many micronized drugs are commercially available to the pharmacist in bulk.

As shown by Stokes' equation, the reduction in the particle size of a suspensoid is beneficial to the stability of the suspension because the rate of sedimentation of the solid particles is reduced as the particles are decreased in size. The reduction in particle size produces slow, more uniform rates of settling. However, one should avoid reducing the particle size too much, since fine particles have a tendency to form a compact cake upon settling to the bottom of the container. The result may be that the cake resists breakup upon shaking and forms rigid aggregates of particles that are larger and less suspendable than the original suspensoid. The particle shape of the suspensoid can also affect caking and product

stability. It has been shown that symmetrical barrel-shaped particles of calcium carbonate produced more stable suspensions than did asymmetrical needle-shaped particles of the same agent. The needle-shaped particles formed a tenacious sediment cake on standing that could not be redistributed. whereas the barrel-shaped particles did not cake on standing (1).

To avoid formation of a cake, it is necessary to prevent agglomeration of the particles into larger crystals or into masses. One common method of preventing rigid cohesion of small particles of a suspension is intentional formation of a less rigid or loose aggregation of the particles held together by comparatively weak particle-to-particle bonds. Such an aggregation of particles is termed a *floc* or a *floccule*, with flocculated particles forming a type of lattice that resists complete settling (although flocs settle more rapidly than fine, individual particles) and thus are less prone to compaction than unflocculated particles. The flocs settle to form a higher sediment volume than unflocculated particles, the loose structure of which permits the aggregates to break up easily and distribute readily with a small amount of agitation.

There are several methods of preparing flocculated suspensions, the choice depending on the type of drug and the type of product desired. For instance, in the preparation of an oral suspension of a drug, clays such as diluted bentonite magma are commonly employed as the flocculating agent. The structure of the bentonite magma and of other clays used for this purpose also assists the suspension by helping to support the floc once formed. When clays are unsuitable as agents, as in a parenteral suspension, frequently a floc of the dispersed phase can be produced by an alteration in the pH of the preparation (generally to the region of minimum drug solubility). Electrolytes can also act as flocculating agents, apparently by reducing the electrical barrier between the particles of the suspensoid and forming a bridge so as to link them together. The carefully determined concentration of nonionic and ionic surface-active agents (surfactants) can also induce flocculation of particles in suspension and increase the sedimentation volume.

Dispersion Medium

Oftentimes, as with highly flocculated suspensions, the particles of a suspension settle too rapidly to be consistent with what might be termed a pharmaceutically elegant preparation. The rapid settling hinders accurate measurement of dosage and from an esthetic point of view produces too unsightly a supernatant layer. In many commercial suspensions, suspending agents are added to the dispersion medium to lend it structure. Carboxymethylcellulose, methylcellulose, microcrystalline cellulose, polyvinyl pyrrolidone, xanthan gum, and bentonite are a few of the agents employed to thicken the dispersion medium and help suspend the suspensoid. When polymeric substances and hydrophilic colloids are used as suspending agents, appropriate tests must be performed to show that the agent does not interfere with availability of the drug. These materials can bind certain medicinal agents, rendering them unavailable or only slowly available for therapeutic function. Also, the amount of the suspending agent must not be such to render the suspension too viscous to agitate (to distribute the *suspensoid*) or to pour. The study of flow characteristics is rheology. A summary of the concepts of rheology is found in Physical Pharmacy Capsule 14.2.

Support of the suspensoid by the dispersion medium may depend on several factors: the density of the suspensoid, whether it is flocculated, and the amount of material requiring support.

The solid content of a suspension intended for oral administration may vary considerably, depending on the dose of the drug to be administered, the volume of product to be administered, and the ability of the dispersion medium to support the concentration of drug while maintaining desirable features of viscosity and flow. The usual adult oral suspension is frequently designed to supply the dose of the particular drug in a convenient measure of 5 mL or 1 teaspoonful. Pediatric suspensions are formulated to deliver the appropriate dose of drug by administering a dose-calibrated number of drops. Figure 14.4 shows commonly packaged oral suspensions administered as pediatric drops. Some are accompanied by a calibrated dropper, whereas other packages have the drop capability built into the container. On administration the drops may be placed directly in the infant's mouth or mixed with a small portion of food. Because many of the suspensions of antibiotic drugs intended for pediatric use are

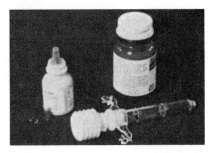

FIGURE 14.4 Oral pediatric suspensions showing package designs of a built-in dropper device and a calibrated dropper accompanying the medication container.

PHYSICAL PHARMACY CAPSULE 14.2

Rheology

Rheology, the study of flow, addresses the viscosity characteristics of powders, fluids, and semisolids. Materials are divided into two general categories, Newtonian and non-Newtonian, depending on their flow characteristics. Newtonian flow is characterized by constant viscosity, regardless of the shear rates applied. Non-Newtonian flow is characterized by a change in viscosity characteristics with increasing shear rates. Non-Newtonian flow includes plastic, pseudoplastic, and dilatant flow.

Newton's law of flow relates parallel layers of liquid, with the bottom layer fixed, when a force is placed on the top layer, the top plane moves at constant velocity, each lower layer moves with a velocity directly proportional to its distance from the stationary bottom layer. The velocity gradient, or rate of shear (dv/dr), is the difference of velocity dv between two planes of liquid separated by the distance dr. The force (F'/A) applied to the top layer that is required to result in flow (rate of shear, G) is called the shearing stress (F). The relationship can be expressed.

$$\frac{F'}{A} = \eta \frac{dv}{dr}$$

where η is the viscosity coefficient, or viscosity. This relationship is often written

$$\eta = \frac{F}{G}$$

where

F = F'/A and
G = dv/dr.

The higher the viscosity of a liquid, the greater the shearing stress required to produce a certain rate of shear. A plot of F versus G yields a rheogram. A Newtonian fluid will plot as a straight line with the slope of the line being η. The unit of viscosity is the *poise*, the shearing force required to produce a velocity of 1 cm/second between two parallel planes of liquid, each 1 cm^2 in area and separated by a distance of 1 cm. The most convenient unit to use is the centipoise, or cp (equivalent to 0.01 poise).

These basic concepts can be illustrated in the following two graphs.

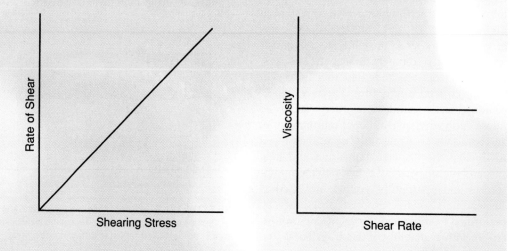

EXAMPLE 1

What is the shear rate when an oil is rubbed into the skin with a relative rate of motion between the fingers and the skin of about 10 cm/seconds and the film thickness is about 0.02 cm?

$$G = \frac{10 \text{ cm/seconds}}{0.02} = 500 \text{ seconds}^{-1}$$

The viscosity of Newtonian materials can be easily determined using a capillary viscometer, such as the Ostwald pipet, and the following relationship:

$$\eta' = ktd$$

where

η' is viscosity,
k is a coefficient, including such factors as the radius and length of the capillary, volume of the liquid flowing, pressure head, and so on,
t is time, and
d is density of the material

The official compendia, the USP and NF, use kinematic viscosity, the absolute viscosity divided by the density of the liquid, as follows:

$$\text{Kinematic viscosity} = \eta'/\rho$$

The relative viscosity of a liquid can be obtained by using a capillary viscometer and comparing data with a second liquid of known viscosity, provided the densities of the two liquids are known, as follows:

$$\eta'/\eta'_o = (\rho t)/(\rho_o t_o)$$

EXAMPLE 2

At 25°C, water has a density of 1 g/cc and a viscosity of 0.895 cps. The time of flow of water in a capillary viscometer is 15 seconds. A 50% aqueous solution of glycerin has a flow time of 750 seconds. The density of the glycerin solution is 1.216 g/cc. What is the viscosity of the glycerin solution?

$$\eta' = \frac{(0.895)\,(750)\,(1.216)}{(1)\,(15)} = 54.4 \text{ cps}$$

EXAMPLE 3

The time of flow between marks on an Ostwald viscometer using water ($\rho = 1$) was 120 seconds at 20°C. The time for a liquid ($\rho = 1.05$) to flow through the same viscometer was 230 seconds. What is the absolute and relative viscosity of the liquid?

$$\eta = (0.01)\,\frac{(1.05)\,(230)}{(1.0)\,(120)}$$

$$\eta = 0.020 \text{ poise} = 2.0 \text{ centipoise}$$

Viscosity is related to temperature thus:

$$\eta' = Ae^{Ev/RT}$$

Physical Pharmacy Capsule 14.2 cont.

where

A is a constant depending on the molecular weight and molar volume of the material,
Ev is the activation energy required to initiate flow between molecules,
R is the gas constant, and
T is the absolute temperature

Viscosity is additive in ideal solutions, as follows:

$$\frac{1}{\eta} = \frac{1}{\eta}V_1 + \frac{1}{\eta}V_2$$

where

η is the viscosity of the solutions and
V_1 and V_2 are the volume fractions of the pure liquids.

EXAMPLE 4

What is the viscosity of the liquid resulting from mixing 300 mL of liquid A (η = 1.0 cp) and 200 mL of liquid B (η = 3.4 cp)?

$$\frac{1}{\eta} = \frac{1\ (0.6)}{1.0} + \frac{1\ (0.4)}{3.4}$$

$$\eta = 1.4\ \text{cps}$$

Non-Newtonian substances are those that fail to follow Newton's equation of flow. Example materials include colloidal solutions, emulsions, liquid suspensions, and ointments. There are three general types of non-Newtonian materials: plastic, pseudoplastic, and dilatant.

Substances that exhibit plastic flow are called *Bingham bodies*. Plastic flow does not begin until a shearing stress corresponding to a certain yield value is exceeded. The flow curve intersects the shearing stress axis and does not pass through the origin. The materials are elastic below the yield value.

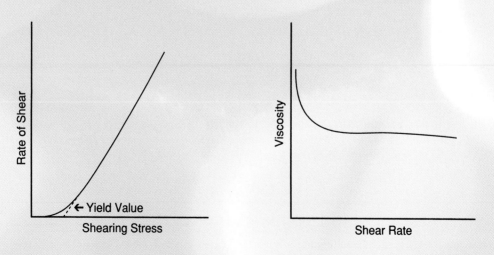

Physical Pharmacy Capsule 14.2 cont.

Pseudoplastic substances begin flow when a shearing stress is applied; therefore, they exhibit no yield value. With increasing shearing stress, the rate of shear increases; consequently, these materials are also called shear-thinning systems. It is postulated that this occurs as the molecules, primarily polymers, align themselves along the long axis and slip or slide past each other.

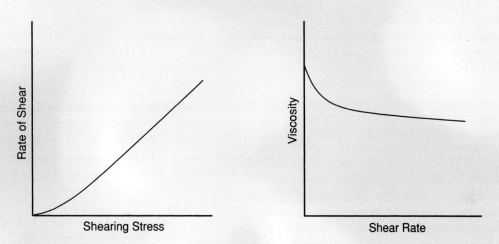

Dilatant materials are those that increase in volume when sheared, and the viscosity increases with increasing shear rate. These are also called shear-thickening systems. Dilatant systems are usually characterized by having a high percentage of solids in the formulation.

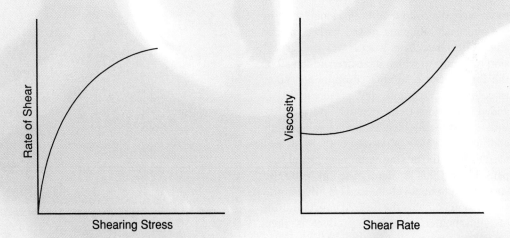

The viscosity of non-Newtonian materials is determined using a viscometer capable of producing differing shear rates, measuring the shear stress, and plotting the results. Other types of flow not detailed here include *thixotropic*, *antithixotropic*, and *rheopexic*. Thixotropic flow is used to advantage in some pharmaceutical formulations. It is a reversible gel–sol transformation. Upon setting, a network gel forms and provides a rigid matrix that will stabilize suspensions and gels. When stressed (by shaking), the matrix relaxes and forms a sol with the characteristics of a liquid dosage form for ease of use. All of these unique flow types can be characterized by studying their respective rheograms.

prepared in a highly flavored, sweetened, colored base, they are frequently referred to by their manufacturers and also popularly as syrups, even though in fact they are suspensions.

Preparation of Suspensions

In the preparation of a suspension, the pharmacist must be acquainted with the characteristics of both the intended dispersed phase and the dispersion medium. In some instances the dispersed phase has an affinity for the vehicle to be employed and is readily wetted by it. Other drugs are not penetrated easily by the vehicle and have a tendency to clump together or to float on the vehicle. In the latter case, the powder must first be wetted to make it more penetrable by the dispersion medium. Alcohol, glycerin, propylene glycol, and other hygroscopic liquids are employed as wetting agents when an aqueous vehicle is to be used as the dispersion phase. They function by displacing the air in the crevices of the particles, dispersing the particles, and allowing penetration of dispersion medium into the powder. In large-scale preparation of suspensions the wetting agents are mixed with the particles by an apparatus such as a colloid mill; on a small scale in the pharmacy, they are mixed with a mortar and pestle. Once the powder is wet, the dispersion medium (to which have been added all of the formulation's soluble components, such as colorants, flavorants, and preservatives) is added in portions to the powder, and the mixture is thoroughly blended before subsequent additions of vehicle. A portion of the vehicle is used to wash the mixing equipment free of suspensoid, and this portion is used to bring the suspension to final volume and ensure that the suspension contains the desired concentration of solid matter. The final product is then passed through a colloid mill or other blender or mixing device to ensure uniformity.

Whenever appropriate, suitable preservatives should be included in the formulation of suspensions to preserve against bacterial and mold contamination.

An example formula for an oral suspension follows (2). The suspensoid is the antacid aluminum hydroxide, the preservatives are methylparaben and propylparaben, and syrup

and sorbitol solution provide the viscosity and sweetness.

Aluminum hydroxide compressed gel	326.8 g
Sorbitol solution	282.0 mL
Syrup	93.0 mL
Glycerin	25.0 mL
Methylparaben	0.9 g
Propylparaben	0.3 g
Flavor	q.s.
Purified water, to make	1000.0 mL

The parabens are dissolved in a heated mixture of the sorbitol solution, glycerin, syrup, and a portion of the water. The mixture is then cooled and the aluminum hydroxide added with stirring. The flavor is added and purified water to volume. The suspension is then homogenized, using a hand homogenizer, homomixer, or colloid mill. A high-speed industrial-size mixer used to prepare dispersions of various types, including suspensions and emulsions, is shown in Figure 14.5. A large

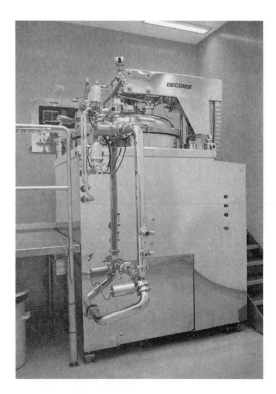

FIGURE 14.5 An industrial mixer for manufacture of disperse systems, including suspensions and emulsions. (Courtesy of Paddock Laboratories.)

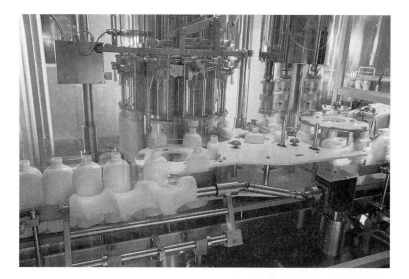

FIGURE 14.6 Liquid filling. Bottles being conveyed after cleaning. As they pass through an indexing worm, the bottles are spaced accurately for filling and capping. (Courtesy of Paddock Laboratories.)

storage holding tank with a liquid filling unit in the process of filling large-mouth suspension bottles is shown in Figure 14.6.

Sustained-Release Suspensions

The formulation of liquid oral suspensions having sustained-release capabilities has had only limited success because of the difficulty of maintaining the stability of sustained-release particles in liquid disperse systems (3). Product development research has centered on the same types of technologies used in preparing sustained-release tablets and capsules (coated beads, drug-impregnated wax matrix, microencapsulation, ion exchange resins). The use of a combination of ion exchange resin complex and particle coating *has* resulted in product success via the so-called Pennkinetic system. By this technique, ionic drugs are complexed with ion exchange resins, and the drug–resin complex particles coated with ethyl cellulose (3). In liquid formulations (suspensions) of the coated particles, the drug remains adsorbed onto the resin but is slowly released by the ion exchange process in the gastrointestinal tract. An example of this product type is hydrocodone polistirex (Tussionex Pennkinetic Extended-Release Suspension, CellTech).

Extemporaneous Compounding of Suspensions

Unfortunately, not all medicines are available in a convenient, easy-to-take liquid dosage form. Consequently, patients who are not able to swallow solid medicines, such as infants and the elderly, may present a special need. Thus the pharmacist may have to use a solid dosage form of the drug and extemporaneously compound a liquid product. A difficulty that confronts the pharmacist is a lack of ready information on stability of a drug in a liquid vehicle. It is known that drugs in liquid form have faster decomposition rates than in solid form, and some are affected by the pH of the medium. Leucovorin calcium when compounded from crushed tablets or the injectable form is most stable in milk or antacid and is unstable in acidic solutions.

To overcome this information gap, the pharmacist can attempt to contact the manufacturer of the solid dosage form to attain stability information. A number of extemporaneous formulations have appeared in the professional literature, such as for prednisone oral suspension (4) and ketoconazole suspension (5), and some manufacturers provide in the package insert a formula for preparation of an oral liquid form, such as Rifadin (rifampin, Hoechst Marion

Roussel). A number of compilations of formulations based upon documented stability data and unpublished data compiled by manufacturers and practitioners are available for pharmacists to use.

Typically, in formation of an extemporaneous suspension, the contents of a capsule are emptied into a mortar or tablets crushed in a mortar with a pestle. The selected vehicle is slowly added to and mixed with the powder to create a paste and then diluted to the desired volume. The selected vehicle can be a commercial product, such as the Ora family of preparations (Ora-Sweet, Ora-Sweet SF, Ora-Plus, Paddock Laboratories).

The extent of the formulation depends upon the patient. For example, a liquid suspension for a neonate should not include preservatives, colorings, flavorings, or alcohol because of the potential for each of these to cause either acute or long-term adverse effects. Because this liquid product will probably be administered through a tube threaded through the mouth into the stomach and because taste is usually underdeveloped in the neonate, a flavoring agent is not required.

In the neonate, alcohol can alter liver function, cause gastric irritation, and effect neurologic depression. So unless it is absolutely necessary, it should be omitted from an extemporaneous formulation. Pharmacists must be cautious, because some vehicles, such as Aromatic Elixir, NF, contain a significant amount of alcohol, 21 to 23%, and are not suitable for use in these patients. The same problem holds for liquid formulations for the elderly or any patient who may be receiving another medication that depresses the central nervous system.

Preservatives have been implicated in adverse effects in preterm infants. Benzyl alcohol should be omitted from neonate formulations because this agent can cause a gasping syndrome characterized by a deterioration of multiple organ systems and eventually death. Propylene glycol has also been implicated in problems such as seizures and stupor in some preterm infants. Thus, formulations for neonates should be kept simple and not compounded to supply more than a few days of medicine.

To minimize stability problems of the extemporaneous product, it should be placed in an air-tight, light-resistant container by the pharmacist and stored in the refrigerator by the patient. Because it is a suspension, the patient should be instructed to shake it well prior to use and watch for any color change or consistency change that might indicate a stability problem.

Packaging and Storage of Suspensions

All suspensions should be packaged in wide-mouth containers having adequate airspace above the liquid to permit thorough mixing by shaking and ease of pouring. Most suspensions should be stored in tight containers protected from freezing, excessive heat, and light. It is important that suspensions be shaken before each use to ensure a uniform distribution of solid in the vehicle and thereby uniform and proper dosage.

Examples of Oral Suspensions

Examples of official and commercial oral suspensions are presented in Table 14.1. Antacid and antibacterial suspensions are briefly discussed next as examples of this dosage form.

Antacid Oral Suspensions

Antacids are intended to counteract the effects of gastric hyperacidity and as such are employed by persons, such as peptic ulcer patients, who must reduce the level of acidity in the stomach. They are also widely employed and sold over the counter (OTC) to patients with acid indigestion, heartburn, and sour stomach. Many patients belch or otherwise reflux acid from the stomach to the esophagus and take antacids to counter the acid in the esophagus and throat.

Most antacid preparations are composed of water-insoluble materials that act within the gastrointestinal tract to counteract the acid and/or soothe the irritated or inflamed linings of the gastrointestinal tract. A few water-soluble agents are employed, including sodium bicarbonate, but for the most part, water-insoluble

TABLE 14.1 ORAL SUSPENSIONS BY CATEGORY

ORAL SUSPENSION	REPRESENTATIVE COMMERCIAL PRODUCTS	DRUG CONCENTRATION IN COMMERCIAL PRODUCT	COMMENTS
Antacids			
Alumina, magnesia, simethicone	Mylanta Liquid (Johnson & Johnson Merck)	Aluminum hydroxide, 200 mg; magnesium hydroxide, 200 mg; and simethicone, 20 mg/5 mL	Counteract gastric hyperacidity, relieve distress in the upper gastrointestinal tract.
Magaldrate	Riopan Oral Suspension (Whitehall)	Hydroxymagnesium aluminate 540 mg (chemical entity of aluminum and magnesium hydroxides)	
Magnesia and alumina	Maalox Suspension (Novartis Consumer Health)	Aluminum hydroxide 225 mg; magnesium hydroxide 200 mg/5 mL	
Aluminum hydroxide, magnesium carbonate	Gaviscon Liquid Antacid (SmithKline Beecham Consumer)	Aluminum hydroxide 95 mg; magnesium carbonate 358 mg/ 15 mL; sodium alginate	
Anthelmintics			
Pyrantel Pamoate	Antiminth Oral Suspension (Pfizer)	250 mg/5 mL	For worm infestations.
Thiabendazole	Mintezol Oral Suspension (Merck)	500 mg/5 mL	
Antibacterials (Antibiotics)			
Erythromycin Estolate	Generic	125, 250 mg/5 mL	Broad-spectrum macrolide antibiotic; bacteriostatic and bacteriocidal activity.
Antibacterials (Nonantibiotic Anti-infectives)			
Methenamine Mandelate	Mandelamine Suspension Forte (Various)	500 mg/5 mL	Oleaginous vehicle; chemical combination of approximately equal parts of methenamine and mandelic acid; destroys most pathogens commonly infecting urinary tract. Acid urine is essential for activity; maximum efficacy at pH 5.5. Methenamine in acid urine is hydrolyzed to ammonia and the bactericidal agent, formaldehyde. Mandelic acid exerts its antibacterial action, contributes to acidification of urine. Usual dose 1 g up to four times a day. Suspension form especially useful for children, adults who do not swallow a tablet (also official and commercially available).

(continued)

TABLE 14.1 ORAL SUSPENSIONS BY CATEGORY

ORAL SUSPENSION	REPRESENTATIVE COMMERCIAL PRODUCTS	DRUG CONCENTRATION IN COMMERCIAL PRODUCT	COMMENTS
Sulfamethoxazole and trimethoprim	Bactrim Suspension (Roche), Septra Suspension (Glaxo Wellcome)	trimethoprim 40 mg, sulfamethoxazole 200 mg/5 mL	For acute middle ear infection (otitis media) in children, urinary tract infections due to susceptible microorganisms.
Sulfamethoxazole	Gantanol Suspension (Roche)	500 mg/5 mL	Bacteriostatic sulfa drug suspensions useful for urinary tract infections. Sulfonamides competitively inhibit bacterial synthesis of folic acid and para-aminobenzoic acid
Sulfisoxazole Acetyl Oral Suspension	Gantrisin Syrup and Gantrisin Pediatric Suspension (Roche)	500 mg/5 mL	
Anticonvulsant			
Primidone	Mysoline Suspension (Wyeth-Ayerst)	250 mg/5 mL	Management of grand mal epilepsy, psychomotor attacks.
Antidiarrheal			
Bismuth subsalicylate	Pepto-Bismol Liquid (Procter & Gamble)	262 mg/15 mL	For indigestion without causing constipation, nausea, control of diarrhea. Unlabeled use for prevention and treatment of traveler's (enterotoxigenic *Escherichia coli*) diarrhea, but not the first line of therapy for either.
Antiflatulent			
Simethicone	Mylicon Drops (Johnson & Johnson Merck)	40 mg/0.6 mL	Symptomatic treatment of gastrointestinal distress due to gas. Reduces surface tension of gas bubbles, enabling them to coalesce and be released through belching or flatus.
Antifungals			
Nystatin	Nystatin Oral Suspension (Teva, Lederle Standard Products)	100,000 U/mL	Antibiotic with antifungal activity. Suspension is held in mouth as long as possible before swallowing in treatment of mouth infections caused by *Candida* (*Monilia*) *albicans*, other *Candida* spp.
Antipsychotics, Sedatives, Antiemetics			
Hydroxyzine Pamoate	Vistaril Oral Suspension (Pfizer)	25 mg/5 mL	Management of anxiety, tension, psychomotor agitation.
Thioridazine	Mellaril-S Oral Suspension (Sandoz)	25 mg/5 mL	Management of psychotic disorders; short-term treatment of moderate to marked depression with variable degrees of anxiety in adults.
Diuretic			
Chlorothiazide	Diuril Oral	250 mg/5 mL	Interferes with renal tubular electrolyte reabsorption; increases sodium, chloride excretion.

(continued)

TABLE 14.1 ORAL SUSPENSIONS BY CATEGORY

ORAL SUSPENSION	REPRESENTATIVE COMMERCIAL PRODUCTS	DRUG CONCENTRATION IN COMMERCIAL PRODUCT	COMMENTS
Nonsteroidal Anti-inflammatory			
Indomethacin	Indocin Oral Suspension (Merck & Co.)	25 mg/5 mL	Active treatment of moderate to severe rheumatoid arthritis (including acute flares of chronic illness), moderate to severe osteoarthritis, acute painful shoulder (bursitis or tendinitis), acute gouty arthritis.

salts of aluminum, calcium, and magnesium are employed; these include aluminum hydroxide, aluminum phosphate, dihydroxyaluminum aminoacetate, calcium carbonate, calcium phosphate, magaldrate, magnesium carbonate, magnesium oxide, and magnesium hydroxide. The ability of each of these to neutralize gastric acid varies with the chemical agent. For instance, sodium bicarbonate, calcium carbonate, and magnesium hydroxide neutralize acid effectively, whereas magnesium trisilicate and aluminum hydroxide do so less effectively and much more slowly. In selecting an antacid, it is also important to consider the possible adverse effects of each agent in relation to the individual patient. Each agent has its own peculiar potential for adverse effects. For instance, sodium bicarbonate can produce sodium overload and systemic alkalosis, a hazard to patients on sodium-restricted diets. Magnesium preparations may lead to diarrhea and are dangerous to patients with diminished renal function because of those patients' inability to excrete all of the magnesium that may be absorbed; the gastric acid converts insoluble magnesium hydroxide to magnesium chloride, which is water soluble and is partially absorbed. Calcium carbonate carries the potential to induce hypercalcemia and stimulation of gastric secretion and acid production, the latter effect known as acid rebound. Excessive use of aluminum hydroxide may lead to constipation and phosphate depletion with consequent muscle weakness, bone resorption, and hypercalciuria.

The use to which an antacid is to be put is a major consideration in its selection. For instance, in the occasional treatment of heartburn or other infrequent episodes of gastric distress, a single dose of sodium bicarbonate or a magnesium hydroxide preparation may be desired. However, for treatment of acute peptic ulcer or duodenal ulcer in which the therapeutic regimen includes frequent administration of antacids, sodium bicarbonate provides too much sodium and magnesium hydroxide induces diarrhea. Thus, in the treatment of ulcerative conditions, a combination of magnesium hydroxide and aluminum hydroxide is frequently used because the latter agent has some constipating effects that counter the diarrhea effects of the magnesium hydroxide.

When frequent dosage administration is required and when gastroesophageal reflux is being treated, liquid antacids generally are preferred to tablet forms. For one thing, the liquid suspensions assert more immediate action, since they do not require time to disintegrate. It is important that an antacid have a reasonably fast onset of action, since gastric emptying may not allow it much time in the stomach. Endoscopic studies have shown that very little antacid remains in the fasting stomach 1 hour after administration. Therefore, the Food and Drug Administration (FDA) requires that antacid tablets not intended to be chewed must disintegrate within 10 minutes in simulated gastric conditions. Frequent food snacks generally prolong the time an antacid remains in the stomach and can prolong its action.

Because many antacids, especially aluminum- and calcium-containing products, interfere with absorption of other drugs, especially the tetracycline antibiotics, pharmacists must caution their patients against taking such drugs concomitantly.

In addition to the suspension forms of antacids, a number of official and commercial liquid antacid preparations of the magma and gel type will be mentioned later in this chapter. These liquid forms are generally pleasantly flavored (usually with peppermint) to enhance their palatability and patient appeal. Because liquid antacid preparations characteristically contain a large amount of solid material, they must be shaken vigorously to redistribute the antacid prior to administration. Also, a large dose of antacid is frequently required. Thus, many patients prefer to swallow one or two tablespoonfuls of a liquid preparation than to swallow whole or chew the corresponding number of tablets (commonly 3 to 6) for the equivalent dose of drug.

Antibacterial Oral Suspensions

The antibacterial oral suspensions include preparations of antibiotic substances (e.g., chloramphenicol palmitate, erythromycin derivatives, and tetracycline and its derivatives), sulfonamides (e.g., sulfamethoxazole and sulfisoxazole acetyl), other anti-infective agents (e.g., methenamine mandelate and nitrofurantoin), or combinations of these (e.g., sulfamethoxazole–trimethoprim).

Many antibiotic materials are unstable when maintained in solution for an appreciable length of time, and therefore, from a stability standpoint, insoluble forms of the drug substances in aqueous suspension or as dry powder for reconstitution (discussed next) are attractive to manufacturers. The antibiotic oral suspensions, including those prepared by reconstitution, provide a convenient way to administer dosages to infants and children and to adult patients who prefer liquid preparations to solid ones. Many of the oral suspensions that are intended primarily for infants are packaged with a calibrated dropper to assist in the delivery of the prescribed dose. Some commercial pediatric antibiotic oral suspensions are pictured in Figure 14.4 and calibrated droppers in Figure 14.7.

The dispersing phase of antibiotic suspensions is aqueous and usually colored, sweetened, and flavored to render the liquid more appealing and palatable. As noted previously, the palmitate form of chloramphenicol was selected for the suspension dosage form not only because of its water insolubility but also because it is flavorless, which eliminates the necessity to mask the otherwise bitter taste of the chloramphenicol base.

Rectal Suspensions

Barium Sulfate for Suspension, USP, may be employed orally or rectally for diagnostic visualization of the gastrointestinal tract. Mesalamine (5-aminosalicylic acid) suspension was introduced to the market in 1988 as Rowasa (Solvay) for treatment of Crohn's disease, distal ulcerative colitis, proctosigmoiditis, and proctitis. It is no longer commercially available but is compounded by pharmacists.

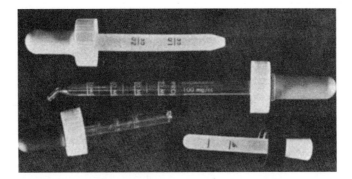

FIGURE 14.7 Calibrated droppers used in the administration of pediatric medications.

Dry Powders for Oral Suspension

A number of official and commercial preparations consist of dry powder mixtures or granules that are intended to be suspended in water or some other vehicle prior to oral administration. As indicated previously, these official preparations have "for Oral Suspension" in their official title to distinguish them from prepared suspensions.

Most drugs prepared as a dry mix for oral suspension are antibiotics. The dry products are prepared commercially to contain the antibiotic drug, colorants (FD&C dyes), flavorants, sweeteners (e.g., sucrose or sodium saccharin), stabilizing agents (e.g., citric acid, sodium citrate), suspending agents (e.g., guar gum, xanthan gum, methylcellulose), and preserving agents (e.g., methylparaben, sodium benzoate) that may be needed to enhance the stability of the dry powder or granule mixture or the liquid suspension. When called on to reconstitute and dispense one of these products, the pharmacist loosens the powder at the bottom of the container by lightly tapping it against a hard surface and then adds the label-designated amount of purified water, usually in portions, and shakes until all of the dry powder has been suspended (Fig. 14.2). It is important to add precisely the prescribed amount of purified water to the dry mixture if the proper drug concentration per dosage unit is to be achieved. Also, the use of purified water rather than tap water is needed to avoid the possibility of adding impurities that could adversely affect the stability of the resulting preparation. Generally, manufacturers provide the dry powder or granule mixture in a slightly oversized container to permit adequate shaking of the contents after the entire amount of purified water has been added. Pharmacists must realize that an oversized bottle is provided with each of these products, and they must carefully measure out the required amount of purified water. They should not "eyeball" the amount of water to be added or fill up the bottle with purified water. Among the official antibiotic drugs for oral suspension are the following:

Amoxicillin for Oral Suspension, USP (Amoxil for Oral Suspension, SmithKline Beecham)

Ampicillin for Oral Suspension, USP (Principen for Oral Suspension Apothecon)

Cefaclor for Oral Suspension, USP (Ceclor for Oral Suspension, Lilly)

Cefixime for Oral Suspension, USP (Suprax Powder for Oral Suspension, Lederle)

Cephradine for Oral Suspension, USP (Velosef for Oral Suspension, Bristol-Myers Squibb)

Cephalexin for Oral Suspension, USP (Keflex for Oral Suspension, Dista)

Dicloxacillin Sodium for Oral Suspension, USP (Pathocil for Oral Suspension, Wyeth-Ayerst)

Doxycycline for Oral Suspension, USP (Vibramycin Monohydrate for Oral Suspension, Pfizer)

Erythromycin Ethylsuccinate for Oral Suspension, USP (E.E.S. Granules for Oral Suspension, Abbott)

Several official antibiotics for oral suspension are also combined with other drugs. For example, erythromycin ethylsuccinate plus acetyl sulfisoxazole granules for oral suspension is indicated for the treatment of acute middle ear infection caused by susceptible strains of *Haemophilus influenzae*. Probenecid is combined with ampicillin for reconstitution and ultimate use for the treatment of uncomplicated infections (urethral, endocervical, or rectal) caused by *Neisseria gonorrhoeae* in adults.

Among the official drugs other than antibiotics prepared as dry powder mixtures for reconstitution to oral suspension are cholestyramine (Questran, Bristol-Myers Squibb), used in the management of high cholesterol levels, and barium sulfate (Barosperse, Mallinckrodt), used orally or rectally as a radiopaque contrast medium to visualize the gastrointestinal tract as an aid to diagnosis. Barium sulfate was introduced into medicine about 1910 as a contrast medium for roentgen ray examination of the gastrointestinal tract. It is practically insoluble in water, and thus its administration even in the large doses required is safe because it is not absorbed from the gastrointestinal tract. The pharmacist must be careful not to confuse barium sulfate with other forms of barium, such as barium *sulfide* and barium *sulfite*, which are soluble salts and *are* poisonous. Barium sulfate is a fine, nongritty odorless and tasteless white powder. When prepared as a suspension and administered orally, it is used to diagnose conditions of the hypopharynx, esophagus, stomach, small intestine, and colon. The barium sulfate renders the gastrointestinal tract opaque to the x-ray so as to reveal any abnormality in the anatomic features of the tract. When administered rectally, barium sulfate allows visualization of the features of the rectum and colon.

Commercially, barium sulfate for diagnostic use is available as a bulk powder containing the required suspending agents for effective reconstitution to an oral suspension or enema. Enema units, which contain prepared suspension in a ready-to-use and disposable bag, are also available.

Emulsions

An emulsion is a dispersion in which the dispersed phase is composed of small globules of a liquid distributed throughout a vehicle in which it is immiscible (Fig. 14.8). In emulsion terminology, the dispersed phase is the *internal phase*, and the dispersion medium is the *external* or *continuous phase*. Emulsions with an

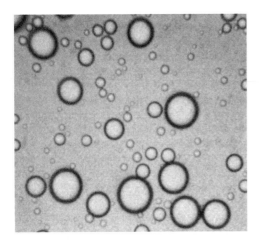

FIGURE 14.8 Mineral oil in water emulsion. The largest oil globule measures approximately 0.04 mm. (Courtesy of James C. Price, PhD, College of Pharmacy, University of Georgia.)

oleaginous internal phase and an aqueous external phase are *oil-in-water* (o/w) emulsions. Conversely, emulsions having an aqueous internal phase and an oleaginous external phase are termed *water-in-oil* (w/o) emulsions. Because the external phase of an emulsion is continuous, an o/w emulsion may be diluted or extended with water or an aqueous preparation and a w/o emulsion, with an oleaginous or oil-miscible liquid. Generally, to prepare a stable emulsion, a third phase, an *emulsifying agent*, is necessary. Depending on their constituents, the viscosity of emulsions can vary greatly, and pharmaceutical emulsions may be prepared as liquids or semisolids. Based on the constituents and the intended application, liquid emulsions may be employed orally, topically, or parenterally; semisolid emulsions, topically. Many pharmaceutical preparations that are actually emulsions are not classified as such because they fit some other pharmaceutical category more appropriately. For instance, emulsions include certain lotions, liniments, creams, ointments, and commercial vitamin drops that are discussed in this book under these various designations.

Purpose of Emulsions and of Emulsification

Emulsification enables the pharmacist to prepare relatively stable and homogeneous mixtures of two immiscible liquids. It permits administration of a liquid drug in the form of minute globules rather than in bulk. For orally administered emulsions, the o/w type permits palatable administration of an otherwise distasteful oil by dispersing it in a sweetened, flavored aqueous vehicle. The reduced particle size of the oil globules may render the oil more digestible and more readily absorbed, or if that is not the intent, more effective in its task, as for example the increased efficacy of mineral oil as a cathartic when emulsified.

Emulsions to be applied to the skin may be o/w or w/o, depending on such factors as the nature of the therapeutic agents, the desirability for an emollient or tissue-softening effect, and the condition of the skin. Medicinal agents that irritate the skin generally are less irritating in the internal phase of an emulsified topical preparation than in the external phase, from which direct contact with the skin is more prevalent. Naturally, the miscibility or solubility in oil and in water of a medicinal agent dictates to a great extent the vehicle, and its nature in turn suggests the phase of the emulsion that the resulting solution should become. On the unbroken skin, a w/o emulsion can usually be applied more evenly, because the skin is covered with a thin film of sebum, and this surface is more readily wetted by oil than by water. A w/o emulsion is also more softening to the skin, because it resists drying and removal by contact with water. On the other hand, if it is desirable to have a preparation that is easily removed from the skin with water, an o/w emulsion is preferred. Also, absorption through the skin (percutaneous absorption) may be enhanced by the diminished particle size of the internal phase. Other aspects of topical preparations are discussed in Chapters 10 and 11.

Theories of Emulsification

Many theories have been advanced in an attempt to explain how emulsifying agents promote emulsification and maintain the stability of the emulsion. Although certain of these theories apply rather specifically to certain types of emulsifying agents and to certain conditions (e.g., the pH of the phases of the system and the nature and relative proportions of the internal and external phases), they may be viewed in a general way to describe the manner in which emulsions may be produced and stabilized. Among the most prevalent theories are the *surface tension theory*, the *oriented-wedge theory*, and the *plastic* or *interfacial film theory*.

All liquids have a tendency to assume a shape having the minimal surface area exposed. For a drop of a liquid, that shape is the sphere. A drop of liquid has internal forces that tend to promote association of the molecules to resist distortion of the sphere. If two or more drops of the same liquid come into contact with one another, the tendency is for them to join or to *coalesce*, making one larger drop having a smaller surface area than the total surface area of the individual drops. This tendency of

liquids may be measured quantitatively, and when the surrounding of the liquid is air, it is referred to as the liquid's surface tension. When the liquid is in contact with a second liquid in which it is insoluble and immiscible, the force causing each liquid to resist breaking up into smaller particles is called interfacial tension. Substances that reduce this resistance encourage a liquid to break up into smaller drops or particles. These tension-lowering substances are *surface active* (surfactant) or *wetting agents*. According to the *surface tension theory* of emulsification, the use of these substances as emulsifiers and stabilizers lowers the interfacial tension of the two immiscible liquids, reducing the repellent force between the liquids and diminishing each liquid's attraction for its own molecules. Thus the surface-active agents facilitate the breaking up of large globules into smaller ones, which then have a lesser tendency to reunite or coalesce.

The *oriented-wedge* theory assumes monomolecular layers of emulsifying agent curved around a droplet of the internal phase of the emulsion. The theory is based on the presumption that certain emulsifying agents orient themselves about and within a liquid in a manner reflective of their solubility in that particular liquid. In a system containing two immiscible liquids, presumably the emulsifying agent is preferentially soluble in one of the phases and is embedded more deeply and tenaciously in that phase than the other. Since many molecules of substances upon which this theory is based (for example, soaps) have a hydrophilic or water-loving portion and a hydrophobic or water-hating portion (but usually lipophilic or oil loving), the molecules position or orient themselves into each phase. Depending on the shape and size of the molecules, their solubility characteristics, and thus their orientation, the wedge shape envisioned for the molecules causes either oil globules or water globules to be surrounded. Generally an emulsifying agent having a greater hydrophilic than hydrophobic character will promote an o/w emulsion, and a w/o emulsion results from use of an emulsifying agent that is more hydrophobic than hydrophilic. Putting it another way, the phase in which the emulsifying agent is more soluble will become the continuous or external phase of the emulsion. Although this theory may not represent a totally accurate depiction of the molecular arrangement of the emulsifier molecules, the concept that water-soluble emulsifiers generally do form o/w emulsions is important and is generally found in practice.

The *plastic* or *interfacial film theory* places the emulsifying agent at the interface between the oil and water, surrounding the droplets of the internal phase as a thin layer of film adsorbed on the surface of the drops. The film prevents contact and coalescing of the dispersed phase; the tougher and more pliable the film, the greater the stability of the emulsion. Naturally, enough of the film-forming material must be available to coat the entire surface of each drop of internal phase. Here again, the formation of an o/w or a w/o emulsion depends on the degree of solubility of the agent in the two phases, with water-soluble agents encouraging o/w emulsions and oil-soluble emulsifiers the reverse.

In actuality, it is unlikely that a single theory of emulsification can explain the means by which the many and varied emulsifiers promote emulsion formation and stability. It is more than likely that even within a given emulsion system, more than one of the aforementioned theories plays a part. For instance, lowering of the interfacial tension is important in the initial formation of an emulsion, but the formation of a protective wedge of molecules or film of emulsifier is important for continued stability. No doubt certain emulsifiers are capable of both tasks.

Preparation of Emulsions

Emulsifying Agents

The initial step in preparation of an emulsion is selection of the emulsifier. To be useful in a pharmaceutical preparation, the emulsifying agent must be compatible with the other formulative ingredients and must not interfere with the stability or efficacy of the therapeutic agent. It should be stable and not deteriorate in the preparation. The emulsifier should be nontoxic with respect to its intended use and the amount to be consumed by the patient. Also, it should possess little odor, taste, or color. Of prime importance is the capability of the emulsifying agent to promote emulsification and to maintain the stability of the emulsion for the intended shelf life of the product.

Various types of materials have been used in pharmacy as emulsifying agents, with hundreds, if not thousands, of individual agents tested for their emulsification capabilities. Although no attempt will be made here to discuss the merits of each of these agents in pharmaceutical emulsions, it would be well to point out the types of materials that are commonly used and their general application. Among the emulsifiers and stabilizers for pharmaceutical systems are the following:

1. Carbohydrate materials, such as the naturally occurring agents acacia, tragacanth, agar, chondrus, and pectin. These materials form hydrophilic colloids when added to water and generally produce o/w emulsions. Acacia is frequently used in the preparation of extemporaneous emulsions. Tragacanth and agar are commonly employed as thickening agents in acacia-emulsified products. Microcrystalline cellulose is employed in a number of commercial suspensions and emulsions as a viscosity regulator to retard particle settling and provide dispersion stability.

2. Protein substances, such as gelatin, egg yolk, and casein. These substances produce o/w emulsions. The disadvantage of gelatin as an emulsifier is that the emulsion frequently is too fluid and becomes more fluid upon standing.

3. High-molecular-weight alcohols, such as stearyl alcohol, cetyl alcohol, and glyceryl monostearate. These are employed primarily as thickening agents and stabilizers for o/w emulsions of certain lotions and ointments used externally. Cholesterol and cholesterol derivatives may also be employed in externally used emulsions to promote w/o emulsions.

4. Wetting agents, which may be anionic, cationic, or nonionic. These agents contain both hydrophilic and lipophilic groups,

with the lipophilic protein of the molecule generally accounting for the surface activity of the molecule. In anionic agents, this lipophilic portion is negatively charged, but in the cationic agent it is positively charged. Owing to their opposing ionic charges, anionic and cationic agents tend to neutralize each other and are thus considered incompatible. Nonionic emulsifiers show no inclination to ionize. Depending on their individual nature, certain of the members of these groups form o/w emulsions and others w/o emulsions. Anionic emulsifiers include various monovalent, polyvalent, and organic soaps, such as triethanolamine oleate, and sulfonates, such as sodium lauryl sulfate. Benzalkonium chloride, known primarily for its bactericidal properties, may be employed as a cationic emulsifier. Agents of the nonionic type include the sorbitan esters and the polyoxyethylene derivatives, some of which appear in Table 14.2.

The ionic nature of a surfactant is a prime consideration. Nonionic surfactants are effective over pH range 3 to 10; cationic surfactants are effective over pH range 3 to 7; and, anionic surfactants require a pH greater than 8 (6).

5. Finely divided solids such as colloidal clays, including bentonite, magnesium hydroxide, and aluminum hydroxide. These generally form o/w emulsions when the insoluble material is added to the aqueous phase if there is a greater volume of the aqueous phase than of the oleaginous phase. However, if the powdered solid is added to the oil and the oleaginous phase volume predominates, a substance like bentonite is capable of forming a w/o emulsion. The relative volume of internal and external phases of an emulsion is important, regardless of the type of emulsifier used. As the internal concentration of an emulsion increases, so does the viscosity of the emulsion to a certain point, after which the viscosity decreases sharply. At this point, the emulsion has undergone *inversion*; that is, it has changed from an o/w emulsion to a w/o, or vice versa. In practice, emulsions may be prepared without inversion with as much as about

TABLE 14.2 HLB VALUES FOR SELECTED EMULSIFIERS

AGENT	HLB
Ethylene glycol distearate	1.5
Sorbitan tristearate (Span 65[a])	2.1
Propylene glycol monostearate	3.4
Triton X-15[b]	3.6
Sorbitan monooleate (Span 80[a])	4.3
Sorbitan monostearate (Span 60[a])	4.7
Diethylene glycol monolaurate	6.1
Sorbitan monopalmitate (Span 40[a])	6.7
Sucrose dioleate	7.1
Acacia	8.0
Amercol L-101[c]	8.0
Polyoxyethylene lauryl ether (Brij 30[a])	9.7
Gelatin	9.8
Triton X-45[b]	10.4
Methylcellulose	10.5
Polyoxyethylene monostearate (Myrj 45[a])	11.1
Triethanolamine oleate	12.0
Tragacanth	13.2
Triton X-100[b]	13.5
Polyoxyethylene sorbitan monostearate (Tween 60[a])	14.9
Polyoxyethylene sorbitan monooleate (Tween 80[a])	15.0
Polyoxyethylene sorbitan monolaurate (Tween 20[a])	16.7
Pluronic F 68[d]	17.0
Sodium oleate	18.0
Potassium oleate	20.0
Sodium lauryl sulfate	40.0

[a]ICI Americas, Wilmington, Delaware.
[b]Rohm and Haas, Philadelphia, Pennsylvania.
[c]Amerchol Corporation, Edison, New Jersey.
[d]BASF-Wyandotte Chemical, Parsippany, New Jersey.

75% of the volume of the product being internal phase.

The HLB System

Generally, each emulsifying agent has a hydrophilic portion and a lipophilic portion, with one or the other being more or less predominant and influencing in the manner already described the type of emulsion. A method has been devised (7) whereby emulsifying or surface-active agents may be categorized on the basis of their chemical makeup as to their hydrophil–lipophil balance, or HLB. By this method, each agent is assigned an HLB value or number indicating the substance's polarity. Although the numbers have been assigned up to about 40, the usual range is between 1 and 20. Materials that are highly polar or hydrophilic have been assigned higher numbers than materials that are less polar and more lipophilic. Generally, surface-active agents having an assigned HLB value of 3 to 6 are greatly lipophilic and produce w/o emulsions, and agents with HLB values of about 8 to 18 produce o/w emulsions. Examples of assigned HLB values for some surfactants are shown in Table 14.2. The type of activity to be expected from surfactants of assigned HLB numbers is presented in Table 14.3.

In the HLB system, in addition to the emulsifying agents, values are assigned to oils and oil-like substances. One selects emulsifying agents having the same or nearly the same HLB value as the oleaginous phase of the intended

TABLE 14.3 ACTIVITY AND HLB VALUE OF SURFACTANTS

ACTIVITY	ASSIGNED HLB
Antifoaming	1–3
Emulsifiers (w/o)	3–6
Wetting agents	7–9
Emulsifiers (o/w)	8–18
Solubilizers	15–20
Detergents	13–16

emulsion. For example, mineral oil has an assigned HLB value of 4 if a w/o emulsion is desired and a value of 10.5 if an o/w emulsion is to be prepared. To prepare a stable emulsion, the emulsifying agent should have an HLB value similar to the one for mineral oil, depending on the type of emulsion desired. When needed, two or more emulsifiers may be combined to achieve the proper HLB value.

Physical Pharmacy Capsule 14.3 summarizes the activities of surfactants and the calculations to determine the quantity of surfactant required for a stable emulsion.

PHYSICAL PHARMACY CAPSULE 14.3

Blending of Surfactants

Wetting agents are surfactants with HLB values of **7** to **9**. Wetting agents aid in attaining intimate contact between solid particles and liquids.

Emulsifying agents are surfactants with HLB values of **3** to **6** or **8** to **18**. Emulsifying agents reduce interfacial tension between oil and water, minimizing surface energy through the formation of globules.

Detergents are surfactants with HLB values of **13** to **16**. Detergents will reduce the surface tension and aid in wetting the surface and the dirt. The soil will be emulsified, and foaming generally occurs and a washing away of the dirt.

Solubilizing agents have HLB values of **15** to **20**.

HLB values are additive, and often surfactants are blended. For example if 20 mL of an HLB of 9.0 is required, two surfactants (with HLB values of 8.0 and 12.0) can be blended in a 3:1 ratio. The following quantities of each will be required:

$$0.75 \times 8.0 = 6.0$$

$$0.25 \times 12.0 = 3.0$$

$$\text{Total HLB} = 9.0$$

Methods of Emulsion Preparation

Emulsions may be prepared by several methods, depending upon the nature of the components and the equipment. On a small scale, as in the laboratory or pharmacy, emulsions may be prepared using a dry Wedgwood or porcelain mortar and pestle, a mechanical blender or mixer, such as a Waring blender or a milkshake mixer, a hand homogenizer (Fig. 14.9), a bench-type homogenizer (Fig. 14.10), or sometimes a simple prescription bottle. On a large scale, large mixing tanks (Fig. 14.5) may be used to form the emulsion through the action of a high-speed impeller. As desired, the product may be rendered finer by passage through a colloid mill, in which the particles are sheared between the small gap separating a high-speed rotor and the stator, or by passage through a large homogenizer, in which the liquid is forced under great pressure through a small valve opening. Industrial homogenizers have the capacity to handle as much as 100,000 L of product per hour.

In the small-scale extemporaneous preparation of emulsions, three methods may be

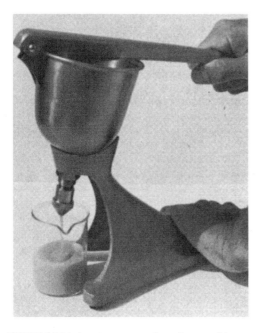

FIGURE 14.9 Laboratory preparation of an emulsion using a hand homogenizer.

used. They are the *continental* or *dry gum method*, the *English* or *wet gum method*, and the *bottle* or *Forbes bottle method*. In the first method, the emulsifying agent (usually acacia) is mixed with the oil before the addition of water. In the second method, the emulsifying agent is added to the water (in which it is soluble) to form a mucilage, and then the oil is slowly incorporated to form the emulsion. The bottle method is reserved for volatile oils or less viscous oils and is a variation of the dry gum method.

Continental or Dry Gum Method

The continental method is also referred to as the 4:2:1 method because for every 4 parts by volume of oil, 2 parts of water and 1 part of gum are added in preparing the initial or *primary emulsion*. For instance, if 40 mL of oil is to be emulsified, 20 mL of water and 10 g of gum would be employed in the primary emulsion, with any additional water or other formulation ingredients added afterward. In this method, the acacia or other o/w emulsifier is triturated with the oil in a perfectly dry Wedgwood or porcelain mortar until thoroughly mixed. A mortar with a rough rather than smooth inner surface must be used to ensure proper grinding action and reduction of the globule size. A glass mortar is too smooth to produce the proper reduction of the internal phase. After the oil and gum have been mixed, the two parts of water are added all at once, and the mixture is triturated immediately, rapidly, and continuously until the primary emulsion is creamy white and produces a crackling sound to the movement of the pestle. Generally, about 3 minutes of mixing is required to produce a primary emulsion. Other liquid formulative ingredients that are soluble in or miscible with the external phase may then be mixed into to the primary emulsion. Solid substances such as preservatives, stabilizers, colorants, and any flavoring material are usually dissolved in a suitable volume of water (assuming water is the external phase) and added as a solution to the primary emulsion. Any substances that might interfere with the stability of the emulsion or the emulsifying agent are

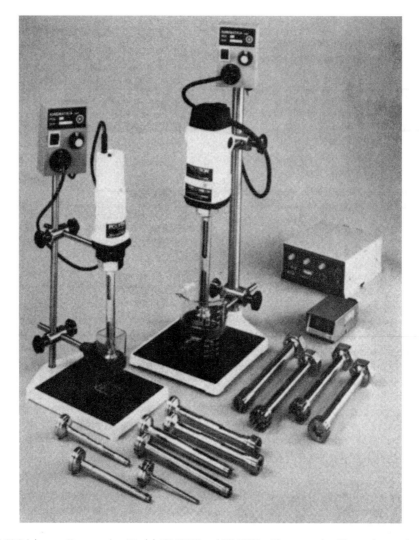

FIGURE 14.10 Brinkmann Homogenizer Models PT 10/35 and PT 45/80 with accessories. The equipment is used for homogenization, dispersion, and emulsification of solids or liquids. Volumes range from 0.5 mL to 25 L. (Courtesy of Brinkmann Instruments, Division of Sybron Corporation.)

added as near last as is practical. For instance, since alcohol has a precipitating action on gums such as acacia, no alcohol or solution containing alcohol should be added directly to the primary emulsion, since the total alcoholic concentration of the mixture would be greater at that point than after other diluents were added. When all necessary agents have been added, the emulsion is transferred to a graduate and made to volume with water previously swirled about in the mortar to remove the last portion of emulsion.

Provided the dispersion of the acacia in the oil is adequate, the dry gum method can almost be guaranteed to produce an acceptable emulsion. Sometimes, however, the amount of acacia must be adjusted upward to ensure that an emulsion can be produced. For example, volatile oils, liquid petrolatum (mineral oil), and linseed oil usually require a 3:2:1 or 2:2:1 ratio for adequate preparation. Rather than use a mortar and pestle, the pharmacist can generally prepare an excellent emulsion using the dry gum method and an electric mixer or blender.

English or Wet Gum Method

By this method, the same proportions of oil, water, and gum are used as in the continental or dry gum method, but the order of mixing is different, and the proportion of ingredients may be varied during the preparation of the primary emulsion as is deemed necessary by the operator. Generally a mucilage of the gum is prepared by triturating in a mortar granular acacia with twice its weight of water. The oil is then added slowly in portions, and the mixture is triturated to emulsify the oil. Should the mixture become too thick, additional water may be blended into the mixture before another portion of oil is added. After all of the oil has been added, the mixture is thoroughly mixed for several minutes to ensure uniformity. Then, as with the continental or dry gum method, the other formulative materials are added, and the emulsion is transferred to a graduate and brought to volume with water.

Bottle or Forbes Bottle Method

The bottle method is useful for the extemporaneous preparation of emulsions from volatile oils or oleaginous substances of low viscosities. Powdered acacia is placed in a dry bottle, two parts of oil are added, and the mixture is thoroughly shaken in the capped container. A volume of water approximately equal to that of the oil is then added in portions and the mixture thoroughly shaken after each addition. When all of the water has been added, the primary emulsion thus formed may be diluted to the proper volume with water or an aqueous solution of other formulative agents.

This method is not suited for viscous oils because they cannot be thoroughly agitated in the bottle when mixed with the emulsifying agent. When the intended dispersed phase is a mixture of fixed oil and volatile oil, the dry gum method is generally employed.

Auxiliary Methods

An emulsion prepared by either the wet gum or the dry gum method can generally be increased in quality by passing it through a hand homogenizer. In this apparatus, the pumping action of the handle forces the emulsion through a very small orifice that reduces the globules of the internal phase to about 5 μm and sometimes less. The hand homogenizer is less efficient in reducing the particle size of very thick emulsions, and it should not be employed for emulsions containing a high proportion of solid matter because of possible damage to the valve.

In Situ Soap Method

The two types of soaps developed by this method are calcium soaps and soft soaps. Calcium soaps are w/o emulsions that contain certain vegetable oils, such as oleic acid, in combination with limewater (synonym: Calcium Hydroxide Solution, USP). They are prepared simply by mixing equal volumes of the oil and limewater. The emulsifying agent in this instance is the calcium salt of the free fatty acid formed from the combination of the two entities. In the case of olive oil, the free fatty acid is oleic acid, and the resultant emulsifying agent is calcium oleate. A difficulty that sometimes arises when preparing this self-emulsifying product is that the amount of free fatty acids in the oil may be insufficient on a 1:1 basis with calcium hydroxide. Typically, to make up for this deficiency a little excess of the olive oil, or even a small amount of oleic acid, is needed to ensure a nice, homogeneous emulsion. Otherwise, tiny droplets of water form on the surface of the preparation. Because the oil phase is the external phase, this formulation is ideal where occlusion and skin softening are desired, such as for itchy, dry skin or sunburned skin. A typical example of this emulsion is calamine liniment:

Calamine	
Zinc oxide aa	80.0 g
Olive oil	
Calcium hydroxide	
solution aa qs ad	1000.0 mL

Microemulsions

Microemulsions are thermodynamically stable, optically transparent isotropic mixtures of a biphasic o/w system stabilized with surfactants.

PHYSICAL PHARMACY CAPSULE 14.4

Surface Area of Globules

The following is a sample calculation for determining the quantity of surfactant required to prepare a stable o/w emulsion.

A surface-active agent will spread itself as a single layer when applied to the surface of still water. The dimensions of a molecule can be determined by their surface orientation. For example, if a micropipet is used to deliver 3 μL of a surfactant to the clean, quiet surface of water, the area over which it spreads, determined experimentally using a film balance, is 12,000 cm². The actual thickness of the film can be calculated by dividing the volume of surfactant applied by the surface area, as follows:

$$\frac{0.003 \text{ cm}^3}{12,000 \text{ cm}^2} = 2.5 \times 10^{-7} \text{ cm}$$

The surfactant has a density of 0.910 g/cc and a molecular weight of 325 g/mole. To calculate the cross-sectional area occupied by each molecule, divide the area of the monomolecular film by the number of molecules in the 3 μL of surfactant comprising the film, as follows:

1. Obtain the weight of the surfactant by multiplying the volume by the density (0.003 mL × 0.910 g/cc = 0.00273 g).
2. To calculate the number of moles present, divide the weight of the surfactant by its molecular weight (0.00273 g/325 g/mole = 8.4×10^{-6} moles).
3. The number of molecules present is the number of moles times Avogadro's number ($8.4 \times 10^{-6} \times 6.02 \times 10^{23} = 5.0568 \times 10^{18}$ molecules).
4. The cross-sectional area can now be calculated by dividing the surface area by the number of molecules (12,000 cm²/$5.0568 \times 10^{18} = 2.373 \times 10^{-15}$ cm² = 23.73×10^{-16}, or approximately 24 square angstroms.

The quantity of surfactant required to emulsify a selected quantity of oil for the preparation of an oil in water emulsion can be calculated as follows.

EXAMPLE

To emulsify 50 mL of oil to an average globular diameter of 1 μg, the volume of each globule is

$$V_i = \frac{4}{3} \pi r^3 = \frac{4}{3} \pi (0.5 \times 10^{-4})^3 = 0.524 \times 10^{-12} \text{ mL}$$

To calculate the number of globules per milliliter, divide 1 mL by the volume of each globule:

$$\frac{1 \text{ mL}}{0.524 \times 10^{-12} \text{ mL/globule}} = 1.91 \times 10^{12} \text{ globules/mL}$$

The surface area (S) of each individual globule will be

$$S = 4\pi r^2 = 4\pi (0.5 \times 10^{-4})^2 = 3.14 \times 10^{-8} \text{ cm}^2$$

and the surface area of all the globules in 1 mL of oil is

$$(1.91 \times 10^{12}) \times (3.14 \times 10^{-8}) = 6 \times 10^4 \text{ cm}^2$$

The number of surfactant molecules that will be adsorbed at the interface of the oil globules and the dispersion medium from 1 mL of oil is equal to the total surface area divided by the cross-sectional area of the surfactant:

Physical Pharmacy Capsule 14.4 cont.

$$\frac{6 \times 10^4 \text{ cm}^2}{2.373 \times 10^{-15} \text{ cm}^2/\text{molecule}} = 2.528 \times 10^{19} \text{ molecules}$$

The number of moles of surfactant required to emulsify 1 mL of oil is equal to the number of molecules adsorbed at the interface divided by Avogadro's number:

$$\frac{2.528 \times 10^{19} \text{ molecules}}{6.02 \times 10^{23} \text{ molecules/mole}} = 4.199 \times 10^{-5} \text{ moles}$$

and the quantity required for 50 mL will be

$$50 \text{ mL} \times 4.199 \times 10^{-5} \text{ moles/mL} = 2.095 \times 10^{-3} \text{ moles}$$

$$2.095 \times 10^{-3} \text{ moles} \times 325 \text{ g/mole} = 0.681 \text{ g, or 681 mg}$$

Therefore, 681 mg of surfactant will be required to emulsify 50 mL of the oil.

The diameter of droplets in a *micro*emulsion may be in the range of 100 Å (10 millimicrons) to 1000 Å, whereas in a *micro*emulsion the droplets may be 5000 Å in diameter (6). Both o/w and w/o microemulsions may be formed spontaneously by agitating the oil and water phases with carefully selected surfactants. The type of emulsion produced depends on the properties of the oil and surfactants.

Hydrophilic surfactants may be used to produce transparent o/w emulsions of many oils, including flavor oils and vitamin oils such as A, D, and E. Surfactants in the HLB range of 15 to 18 have been used most extensively in the preparation of such emulsions. These emulsions are dispersions of oil, not true solutions; however, because of the appearance of the product, the surfactant is commonly said to solubilize the oil. Surfactants commonly used in the preparation of such oral liquid formulations are polysorbate 60 and polysorbate 80.

Among the advantages cited for the use of microemulsions in drug delivery are more rapid and efficient oral absorption of drugs than through solid dosage forms, enhanced transdermal drug delivery through increased diffusion into the skin, and the unique potential application of microemulsions in the development of artificial red blood cells and targeting of cytotoxic drugs to cancer cells (6).

Stability of Emulsions

Generally speaking, an emulsion is considered to be physically unstable if (*a*) the internal or dispersed phase upon standing tends to form aggregates of globules, (*b*) large globules or aggregates of globules rise to the top or fall to the bottom of the emulsion to form a concentrated layer of the internal phase, and (*c*) if all or part of the liquid of the internal phase separates and forms a distinct layer on the top or bottom of the emulsion as a result of the coalescing of the globules of the internal phase. In addition, an emulsion may be adversely affected by microbial contamination and growth and by other chemical and physical alterations.

Aggregation and Coalescence

Aggregates of globules of the internal phase have a greater tendency than do individual particles to rise to the top of the emulsion or fall to the bottom. Such a preparation of the globules is termed the creaming of the emulsion, and provided coalescence is absent, it is a reversible process. The term is taken from the dairy industry and is analogous to creaming, or rising to the top of cream in milk that is allowed to stand. The creamed portion of an emulsion may be redistributed rather homogeneously upon shaking, but if the aggregates are difficult to disassemble or if insufficient shaking is employed before each dose, improper dosage of the internal phase substance may result. Furthermore, a creamed emulsion is not esthetically acceptable to the pharmacist or appealing to the consumer. More important, it increases the risk that the globules will coalesce.

According to Stokes' equation (Physical Pharmacy Capsule 14.1), the rate of separation of the dispersed phase of an emulsion may be related to such factors as the particle size of the dispersed phase, the difference in density between the phases, and the viscosity of the external phase. It is important to recall that the rate of separation is increased by increased particle size of the internal phase, larger density difference between the two phases, and decreased viscosity of the external phase. Therefore, to increase the stability of an emulsion, the globule or particle size should be reduced as fine as is practically possible, the density difference between the internal and external phases should be minimal, and the viscosity of the external phase should be reasonably high. Thickeners such as tragacanth and microcrystalline cellulose are frequently added to emulsions to increase the viscosity of the external phase. Upward creaming takes place in unstable emulsions of the o/w or w/o type in which the internal phase has a lesser density than the external phase. Downward creaming takes place in unstable emulsions in which the opposite is true.

More destructive to an emulsion than creaming is coalescence of the globules of the internal phase and separation of that phase into a layer. Separation of the internal phase from the emulsion is called breaking, and the emulsion is described as being cracked or broken. This is irreversible, because the protective sheath about the globules of the internal phase no longer exists. Attempts to reestablish the emulsion by agitation of the two separate layers are generally unsuccessful. Additional emulsifying agent and reprocessing through appropriate machinery are usually necessary to reproduce an emulsion.

Generally, care must be taken to protect emulsions against extremes of cold and heat. Freezing and thawing coarsen an emulsion and sometimes break it. Excessive heat has the same effect. Because emulsion products may be transported to and used in locations with climates of extremely high or low temperature, manufacturers must know their emulsions' stability before they may be shipped. For most emulsions, the industry performs tests at 5°C, 40°C, and 50°C (41°, 104°, and 122°F) to determine the product's stability. Stability at both 5°C and 40°C for 3 months is considered minimal. Shorter exposure periods at 50°C may be used as an alternative test.

Because other environmental conditions, such as the presence of light, air, and contaminating microorganisms can adversely affect the stability of an emulsion, appropriate formulative and packaging steps are usually taken to minimize such hazards to stability. For light-sensitive emulsions, light-resistant containers are used. For emulsions susceptible to oxidative decomposition, antioxidants may be included in the formulation and adequate label warning provided to ensure that the container is tightly closed to air after each use. Many molds, yeasts, and bacteria can decompose the emulsifying agent, disrupting the system. Even if the emulsifier is not affected by the microbes, the product can be rendered unsightly by their presence and growth and will of course not be efficacious from a pharmaceutical or therapeutic standpoint. Since fungi (molds and yeasts) are more likely to contaminate emulsions than are bacteria, fungistatic preservatives, commonly combinations of methylparaben and propylparaben, are generally included in the aqueous phase of an o/w emulsion. Alcohol in the amount of 12 to 15% based on the external phase volume is frequently added to oral o/w emulsions for preservation.

Examples of Oral Emulsions

Mineral Oil Emulsion

Mineral oil emulsion, or liquid petrolatum emulsion, is an o/w emulsion prepared from the following formula:

Mineral oil	500 mL
Acacia (finely powdered)	125 g
Syrup	100 mL

Vanillin	40 mg
Alcohol	60 mL
Purified water, to make	1000 mL

It is prepared by the dry gum method (4:2:1), mixing the oil with the acacia and adding 250 mL of purified water all at once to make the primary emulsion. To this is slowly added with trituration the remainder of the ingredients, with the vanillin dissolved in the alcohol. A substitute flavorant for the vanillin, a substitute preservative for the alcohol, and a substitute emulsifying agent for the acacia and an alternative method of emulsification may be used as desired.

The emulsion is employed as a lubricating cathartic with a usual dose of 30 mL. The usual dose of plain (unemulsified) mineral oil for the same purpose is 15 mL. The emulsion is much more palatable than is the unemulsified oil. Both are best taken at bedtime. There are a number of commercial preparations of emulsified oil, with many containing additional cathartic agents such as phenolphthalein, milk of magnesia, agar, and others.

Castor Oil Emulsion

Castor oil emulsion is used as a laxative for isolated bouts of constipation and in preparation of the colon for radiography and endoscopic examination. The castor oil in the emulsion works directly on the small intestine to promote bowel movement. This and other laxatives should not be used regularly or excessively, as they can lead to dependence for bowel movement. Overuse of castor oil may cause excessive loss of water and body electrolytes, which can have a debilitating effect. Laxatives should not be used when nausea, vomiting, or abdominal pain is present, since these symptoms may indicate appendicitis, and use of a laxative in this instance could promote rupturing of the appendix.

The amount of castor oil in commercial emulsions varies from about 35 to 67%. The amount of oil influences the dose required. Generally, for an emulsion containing about two-thirds oil, the adult dose is 45 mL, about 3 tablespoonfuls. For children 2 to 6 years of age, 15 mL is usually sufficient, and for children

less than 2 years of age, 5 mL may be given. Castor oil is best taken on an empty stomach, followed with one full glass of water.

Simethicone Emulsion

Simethicone emulsion is a water-dispersible form of simethicone used as a defoaming agent for the relief of painful symptoms of excessive gas in the gastrointestinal tract. Simethicone emulsion works in the stomach and intestines by changing the surface tension of gas bubbles, enabling them to coalesce, freeing the gas for easier elimination. The emulsion in drop form is useful for relief of gas in infants due to colic, air swallowing, or lactose intolerance. The commercial product (Mylicon Drops, Johnson & Johnson Merck) contains 40 mg of simethicone per 0.6 mL. Simethicone is also present in a number of antacid formulations (e.g., Mylanta, Johnson & Johnson Merck) as a therapeutic adjunct to relieve the discomfort of gas.

Examples of Topical Emulsions

Many of the hand and body lotions used to treat dry skin are o/w emulsions. A number of topical emulsions, or lotions, are used therapeutically to deliver a drug systemically. An example is Estrasorb (Novavax, King Pharmaceuticals), which contains estradiol for use in the treatment of hot flashes and night sweats accompanying menopause. It works by replacing the hormones lost during menopause.

Gels and Magmas

Gels are defined as semisolid systems consisting of dispersions made up of either small inorganic particles or large organic molecules enclosing and interpenetrated by a liquid.

Gels are also defined as semirigid systems in which the movement of the dispersing medium is restricted by an interlacing three-dimensional network of particles or solvated macromolecules of the dispersed phase. A high degree of physical or chemical cross-linking may be involved. The increased viscosity caused by the interlacing and consequential internal friction is responsible for the semisolid state. A gel may consist of twisted matted strands often wound together by stronger types of van der Waals forces to form crystalline and amorphous regions throughout the system., such as tragacanth and carboxymethylcellulose.

Some gel systems are as clear as water, and others are turbid, since the ingredients may not be completely molecularly dispersed (soluble or insoluble), or they may form aggregates, which disperse light. The concentration of the gelling agents is mostly less than 10%, usually in 0.5 to 2.0% range, with some exceptions.

Gels in which the macromolecules are distributed so that no apparent boundaries exist between them and the liquid are called *single-phase gels*. When the gel mass consists of floccules of small, distinct particles, the gel is classified as a two-phase system and frequently called a *magma* or a *milk*. Gels and magmas are considered colloidal dispersions, since they contain particles of colloidal dimension.

Colloidal Dispersions

Many of the various types of colloidal dispersions have been given appropriate names. For instance, *sol* is a general term to designate a dispersion of a solid substance in a liquid, solid, or gaseous medium. However, more often than not it is used to describe the solid–liquid dispersion system. To be more descriptive, a prefix such as *hydro-* for water (*hydrosol*) or *alco-* for alcohol (*alcosol*) may be employed to indicate the dispersion medium. The term *aerosol* has similarly been developed to indicate a dispersion of a solid or a liquid in a gaseous phase.

Although there is no precise point at which the size of a particle in a dispersion can be considered to be colloidal, there is a generally accepted size range. A substance is said to be colloidal when its particles fall between 1 nm and 0.5 μm. Colloidal particles are usually larger than atoms, ions, or molecules and generally consist of aggregates of many molecules, although in certain proteins and organic polymers, single large molecules may be of colloidal dimension and form colloidal dispersions. One difference between colloidal dispersions and true solutions is the larger particle size of the disperse phase of the colloidal dispersion. Another difference is the optical prop-

erties of the two systems. True solutions do not scatter light and therefore appear clear, but colloidal dispersions contain opaque particles that do scatter light and thus appear turbid. This turbidity is easily seen, even with dilute preparations, when the dispersion is observed at right angles to a beam of light passed through the dispersion (Tyndall effect). Although reference is made here to dilute colloidal dispersions, most pharmaceutical preparations contain high concentrations of colloidal particles, and in these instances there is no difficulty in observing turbidity. In fact, certain preparations are opaque, depending on the concentration of the disperse phase. Also, the particle size of the dispersed phase in some pharmaceutical preparations is not uniform, and a preparation may contain particles within and outside of the colloidal range, giving the preparation more of an opaque appearance than if all particles were uniformly colloidal.

Particle size is not the only important criterion for establishing the colloidal state. The nature of the dispersing phase with respect to the disperse phase is also of great importance. The attraction or lack of attraction between the disperse phase and the dispersion medium affects both ease of preparation and the character of the dispersion. Certain terminology has been developed to characterize the various degrees of attraction between the phases of a colloidal dispersion. If the disperse phase interacts appreciably with the dispersion medium, it is said to be *lyophilic*, meaning solvent loving. If the degree of attraction is small, the colloid is termed *lyophobic*, or solvent hating. These terms are more suitably used when reference is made to the specific dispersion medium, for a single substance may be lyophobic with respect to one dispersion medium and lyophilic with respect to another. For instance, starch is lyophilic in water but lyophobic in alcohol. Terms such as *hydrophilic* and *hydrophobic*, which are more descriptive of the nature of the colloidal property, have therefore been developed to refer to the attraction or lack of attraction of the substance specifically to water. Generally speaking, because of the attraction to the solvent of lyophilic substances in contrast to the lack of attraction of lyophobic substances, lyophilic colloidal systems are easier to prepare and have greater stability. A third type of colloidal sol, termed an *association* or *amphiphilic colloid*, is formed by grouping or association of molecules that exhibit both lyophilic and lyophobic properties.

Lyophilic colloids are large organic molecules capable of being solvated or associated with the molecules of the dispersing phase. These substances disperse readily upon addition to the dispersion medium to form colloidal dispersions. As more molecules of the substance are added to the sol, the viscosity characteristically increases, and when the concentration of molecules is sufficiently high, the liquid sol may become a semisolid or solid dispersion, termed a *gel*. Gels owe their rigidity to an intertwining network of the disperse phase that entraps and holds the dispersion medium. A change in temperature can cause certain gels to resume the sol or liquid state. Also, some gels become fluid on agitation, only to resume their solid or semisolid state after remaining undisturbed for a period of time, a phenomenon known as *thixotropy*.

Lyophobic colloids are generally composed of inorganic particles. When these are added to the dispersing phase, there is little if any interaction between the two phases. Unlike lyophilic colloids, lyophobic materials do not spontaneously disperse but must be encouraged to do so by special individualized procedures. Their addition to the dispersion medium does not greatly affect the viscosity of the vehicle. Amphiphilic colloids form dispersions in both aqueous and nonaqueous media. Depending on their individual character and the nature of the dispersion medium, they may or may not become greatly solvated. However, they generally increase the viscosity of the dispersion medium with an increase in concentration.

For the most part, the colloidal sols and gels used in pharmacy are aqueous preparations. The various preparations composed of colloidal dispersions are prepared not according to any general method but according to the means best suited to the individual preparation. Some substances, such as acacia, are termed *natural colloids* because they are self-dispersing upon addition to the dispersing medium. Other materials that require special means for prompt dispersion are termed *artificial colloids*. They may require fine pulverization of coarse particles to colloidal size by a colloid mill or a micropulverizer, or colloidal size particles may be formed by chemical reaction under highly controlled conditions.

Terminology Related to Gels

A number of terms are commonly used in discussing some of the characteristics of gels, including imbibition, swelling, syneresis, thixotropy, and xerogel. *Imbibition* is the taking up of a certain amount of liquid without a measurable increase in volume. *Swelling* is the taking up of a liquid by a gel with an increase in volume. Only liquids that solvate a gel can cause swelling. The swelling of protein gels is influenced by pH and the presence of electrolytes. *Syneresis* occurs when the interaction between particles of the dispersed phase becomes so great that on standing, the dispersing medium is squeezed out in droplets and the gel shrinks. Syneresis is a form of instability in aqueous and nonaqueous gels. Separation of a solvent phase is thought to occur because of the elastic contraction of the polymeric molecules; in the swelling process during gel formation the macromolecules become stretched, and the elastic forces increase as swelling proceeds. At equilibrium the restoring force of the macromolecules is balanced by the swelling forces, determined by the osmotic pressure. If the osmotic pressure decreases, as on cooling, water may be squeezed out of the gel. The syneresis of an acidic gel from *Plantago albicans* seed gum may be decreased by the addition of electrolyte, glucose, and sucrose and by increasing the gum concentration. pH has a marked effect on the separation of water. At low pH marked syneresis occurs, possibly as a result of suppression of ionization of the carboxylic acid groups, loss of hydrating water, and the formation of intramolecular hydrogen bonds. This would reduce the attraction of the solvent for the macromolecule. *Thixotropy* is a reversible gel–sol formation with no change in volume or temperature, a type of non-Newtonian flow. A *xerogel* is formed when the liquid is removed from a gel and only the framework remains. Examples include gelatin sheets, tragacanth ribbons, and acacia tears.

Classification and Types of Gels

Table 14.4 is a general classification of gels listing two classification schemes. The first scheme divides gels into inorganic and organic. Most *inorganic hydrogels* are two-phase systems, such as aluminum hydroxide gel and bentonite magma. Bentonite has also been used as an ointment base in about 10 to 25% concentrations. Most *organic gels* are single-phase systems and may include such gelling agents as carbomer and tragacanth and those that contain an organic liquid, such as *Plastibase*.

The second classification scheme divides gels into hydrogels and organogels with some additional subcategories. *Hydrogels* include ingredients that are dispersible as colloidals or soluble in water; they include organic hydrogels, natural and synthetic gums, and inorganic hydrogels. Examples include hydrophilic colloids such as silica, bentonite, tragacanth, pectin, sodium alginate, methylcellulose, sodium carboxymethylcellulose, and alumina, which in high concentration form semisolid gels. Sodium alginate has been used to produce gels that can be employed as ointment bases. In concentrations greater than 2.5% and in the presence of soluble calcium salts, a firm gel, stable between pH 5 and 10, is formed. Methylcellulose, hydroxy ethylcellulose and sodium carboxymethylcellulose are among the commercial cellulose products used in ointments. They are available in various viscosity types, usually high, medium, and low. *Organogels* include the hydrocarbons, animal and vegetable fats, soap base greases, and the hydrophilic organogels. Included in the hydrocarbon type is *Jelene*, or *Plastibase*, a combination of mineral oils and heavy hydrocarbon waxes with a molecular weight of about 1300. Petrolatum is a semisolid gel consisting of a liquid component together with a protosubstance and a crystalline waxy fraction. The crystalline fraction provides rigidity to the structure, while the protosubstance, or gel former, stabilizes the system and thickens the gel. The hydrophilic organogels, or polar organogels, include the polyethylene glycols of high molecular weight, the *carbowaxes*. They are soluble to about 75% in water and are completely washable. The gels look and feel like petrolatum. They are nonionic and stable. *Jellies* are a class of gels in which the structural coherent matrix contains a high proportion of liquid, usually water. They usually are formed by adding a thickening agent such as tragacanth or carboxymethyl cellulose to an aqueous solution of a drug substance. The resultant product is usually clear and uniformly semisolid. Jellies are subject to bacterial contamination and growth,

TABLE 14.4 GENERAL CLASSIFICATION AND DESCRIPTION OF GELS

CLASS	DESCRIPTION	EXAMPLES
Inorganic	Usually two-phase systems	Aluminum hydroxide gel Bentonite magma
Organic	Usually single-phase systems	Carbopol Tragacanth
Hydrogels	Organic hydrogels Natural and synthetic gums Inorganic hydrogels	Pectin paste, Tragacanth jelly Methylcellulose, sodium carboxymethylcellulose, Pluronic Bentonite gel (10–25%), Veegum, silica
Organogels	Hydrocarbon type Animal, vegetable fats Soap base greases Hydrophilic organogels Polar Nonionic	Petrolatum, mineral oil/polyethylene gel (Plastibase) Lard, cocoa butter Aluminum stearate with heavy mineral oil gel Carbowax bases (PEG ointment)

so most are preserved with antimicrobials. Jellies should be stored with tight closure, since water may evaporate, drying out the product.

Some substances, such as acacia, are termed natural colloids because they are self-dispersing in a dispersing medium. Other materials that require special treatment for prompt dispersion are called artificial colloids. The special treatment may involve fine pulverization to colloidal size with a colloid mill or a micropulverizer.

Preparation of Magmas and Gels

Some magmas and gels (inorganic) are prepared by freshly precipitating the disperse phase to achieve a fine degree of subdivision of the particles and a gelatinous character to those particles. The desired gelatinous precipitate results when solutions of inorganic agents react to form an insoluble chemical having a high attraction for water. As the microcrystalline particles of the precipitate develop, they strongly attract water to yield gelatinous particles, which combine to form the desired gelatinous precipitate. Other magmas and gels may be prepared by directly hydrating the inorganic chemical, which produces the disperse phase of the dispersion. In addition to the water vehicle, other agents as propylene glycol, propyl gallate and hydroxypropyl cellulose may be used to enhance gel formation.

Because of the high degree of attraction between the disperse phase and the aqueous medium in both magmas and gels, these preparations remain fairly uniform on standing, with little settling of the disperse phase. However, on long standing a supernatant layer of the dispersion medium develops, but the uniformity of the preparation is easily reestablished by moderate shaking. To ensure uniform dosage, magmas and gels should be shaken before use, and a statement to that effect must be included on the label of such preparations. The medicinal magmas and gels are used orally for the value of the disperse phase.

Examples of Gelling Agents

Gelling agents include acacia, alginic acid, bentonite, carbomer, carboxymethylcellulose sodium, cetostearyl alcohol, colloidal silicon dioxide, ethylcellulose, gelatin, guar gum, hydroxy ethylcellulose, hydroxypropyl cellulose, hydroxypropyl methylcellulose, magnesium aluminum silicate, maltodextrin, methylcellulose, polyvinyl alcohol, povidone, propylene carbonate, propylene glycol alginate, sodium alginate, sodium starch glycolate, starch, tragacanth, and xanthan gum. A few of the more common ones are discussed here.

Alginic acid is obtained from seaweed throughout the world, and the prepared product is a tasteless, practically odorless white to yellowish-white colored fibrous powder. It is used in concentrations of 1 to 5% as a thickening agent in gels. It swells in water to about 200 to 300 times its own weight without dissolving. Cross-linking with increased viscosity occurs upon the addition of a calcium salt, such as calcium citrate. Alginic acid can be dispersed in water vigorously stirred for approximately 30 minutes. Premixing with another powder or with a water-miscible liquid aids dispersion.

Bentonite is discussed later, in the section on preparation of bentonite magma.

Carbomer (Carbopol) resins, first described in the literature in 1955, are ingredients in a variety of dosage systems, including controlled-release tablets, oral suspensions, and topical gels. Carbomer resins are high-molecular-weight allyl pentaerythritol–cross-linked acrylic acid–based polymers modified with C_{10} to C_{30} alkyl acrylates. They are fluffy white dry powders with large bulk density. The 0.5% and 1.0% aqueous dispersions are pH 2.7 to 3.5 and 2.5 to 3.0, respectively. There are many carbomer resins, with viscosity ranges from 0 to 80,000 cps. Carbomers 910, 934, 934P, 940, and 1342 are official in the USP 26–NF 21. Carbomer 910 is effective at very low concentrations when low viscosity is desired and is frequently used for producing stable suspensions. It is the least ion sensitive of these resins.

Carbomer 934 is highly effective in thick formulations such as viscous gels. Carbomer 934P is similar to 934 but is intended for oral and mucosal contact applications and is the most widely used in the pharmaceutical industry. In addition to thickening, suspending, and emulsifying in both oral and topical formulations, the 934 polymer is used in commercial products to provide sustained-release properties in the stomach and intestinal tract. Carbomer 940 forms sparkling clear water or hydroalcoholic gels. It is the most efficient of all the Carbopol resins and has very good nondrip properties.

The addition of alcohol to prepared carbomer gels may decrease their viscosity and clarity. An increase in the concentration of carbomer may be required to overcome the loss of viscosity. Also, gel viscosity depends on the presence of electrolytes and on the pH. Generally, a maximum of 3% electrolytes can be added before a rubbery mass forms. Too much neutralization also will result in decreased viscosity that cannot be reversed by the addition of acid. Maximum viscosity and clarity occur at pH 7, but acceptable viscosity and clarity begin at pH 4.5 to 5.0 and extend to a pH of 11.

Carbomer preparations are primarily used in aqueous systems, although other liquids can be used. In water, a single particle of carbomer will wet very rapidly, but like many other powders, carbomer polymers tend to form clumps of particles when haphazardly dispersed in polar solvents. As the surfaces of these clumps solvate, a layer forms and prevents rapid wetting of the interior of the clumps. When this occurs, the slow diffusion of solvent through this solvated layer determines the mixing or hydration time. To achieve fastest dispersion of the carbomer, it is wise to take advantage of the very small particle size of the carbomer powder by adding it very slowly into the vortex of the liquid while very rapidly stirring it. Almost any device, like a simple sieve, that can sprinkle the powder on the rapidly stirred liquid is useful. The goal is to prevent clumping by slowly sprinkling the very fine powder over the rapidly agitated water.

A neutralizer is added to thicken the gel after the carbomer is dispersed. Sodium hydroxide or potassium hydroxide can be used in carbomer dispersions containing less than 20% alcohol. Triethanolamine will neutralize carbomer resins containing up to 50% ethanol. Other neutralizer agents include sodium carbonate, ammonia, and borax.

Carboxymethylcellulose in concentrations of 4 to 6% of medium viscosity can be used to pro-

duce gels; glycerin may be added to prevent drying. Precipitation can occur below pH 2; it is most stable at pH 2 to 10, and maximum stability is at pH 7 to 9. It is incompatible with ethanol.

Carboxymethylcellulose (CMC) sodium is soluble in water at all temperatures. The sodium salt of CMC can be dispersed with high shear in cold water before the particles can hydrate and swell to sticky gel grains agglomerating into lumps. Once the powder is well dispersed, the solution is heated with moderate shear to about 60°C (140°F) for fastest dissolution. These dispersions are sensitive to pH changes because of the carboxylate group. The viscosity of the product falls markedly below pH 5 or above pH 10.

Colloidal silicon dioxide can be used with other ingredients of similar refractive index to prepare transparent gels. Colloidal silicon dioxide adsorbs large quantities of water without liquefying. The viscosity is largely independent of temperature. Changes in pH may affect the viscosity: it is most effective at pH values up to about 7.5. Colloidal silicon dioxide (fumed silica) will form a gel when combined with 1-dodecanol and n-dodecane. These are prepared by adding the silica to the vehicle and sonicating for about 1 minute to obtain a uniform dispersion and sealing and storing at about 40°C (140°F) overnight to complete gelation. This gel is more hydrophobic than the others.

Gelatin is dispersed in hot water and cooled to form gels. As an alternative, moisten the gelatin with about 3 to 5 parts of an organic liquid that will not swell the polymer, such as ethyl alcohol or propylene glycol followed by the addition of the hot water and cooling.

Magnesium aluminum silicate, or *Veegum*, in concentrations of about 10% forms a firm thixotropic gel. The material is inert and has few incompatibilities but is best used above pH 3.5. It may bind to some drugs and limit their availability.

Methylcellulose is a long-chain substituted cellulose that can be used to form gels in concentrations up to about 5%. Since methylcellulose hydrates slowly in hot water, the powder is dispersed with high shear in about one-third of the required amount of water at 80° to 90°C (176°–194°F). Once the powder is finely dispersed, the rest of the water is added cold or as ice with moderate stirring to cause prompt dissolution. Anhydrous alcohol or propylene glycol may be used to prewet the powders. Maximum clarity, fullest hydration, and highest viscosity will be obtained if the gel is cooled to 0 to 10°C (32°–50°F) for about an hour. A preservative should be added. A 2% solution of methylcellulose 4000 has a gel point about 50°C (122°F). High concentrations of electrolytes will salt out the macromolecules and increase their viscosity, ultimately precipitating the polymer.

Plastibase, or *Jelene*, is a mixture of 5% low-molecular-weight polyethylene and 95% mineral oil. A polymer, it is soluble in mineral oil above 90°C, close to its melting point. When cooled below 90°C, the polymer precipitates and causes gelation. The mineral oil is immobilized in the network of entangled and adhering insoluble polyethylene chains, which probably even associate into small crystalline regions. This gel can be heated to about 60°C (140°F) without substantial loss of consistency.

Poloxamer, or *Pluronic*, gels are made from selected forms of polyoxyethylene–polyoxypropylene copolymers in concentrations ranging from 15 to 50%. Poloxamers generally are waxy white free-flowing granules that are practically odorless and tasteless. Aqueous solutions of poloxamers are stable in the presence of acids, alkalis, and metal ions. Commonly used poloxamers include the 124 (L-44 grade), 188 (F-68 grade), 237 (F-87 grade), 338 (F-108 grade) and 407 (F-127 grade) types, which are freely soluble in water. The "F" designation refers to the flake form. The "L" designation refers to the liquid form. The trade name Pluronic is used in the United States by BASF for pharmaceutical and industrial grade poloxamers. Pluronic F-127 has low toxicity and good solubilizing capacity and optical properties , and it is a good medium for topical drug delivery systems.

Polyvinyl alcohol (PVA) is used at concentrations of about 2.5% in the preparation of various jellies that dry rapidly when applied to the skin. Borax is a good agent that will gel PVA solutions. For best results, disperse PVA in cold water, followed by hot water. It is less soluble in the cold water.

Povidone at the higher molecular weights can be used to prepare gels in concentrations up to about 10%. It has the advantage of being compatible in solution with a wide range of inorganic salts, natural and synthetic resins, and other chemicals. It has also been used to increase the solubility of a number of poorly soluble drugs.

Sodium alginate can be used to produce gels in concentrations up to 10%. Aqueous preparations are most stable at pH 4 to 10; below pH 3, alginic acid is precipitated. Sodium alginate gels for external use should be preserved, for example with 0.1% chloroxylenol or the parabens. If the preparation is acidic, benzoic acid may be used. High concentrations will raise viscosity to the point of salting out the sodium alginate; this occurs at about 4% with sodium chloride.

Tragacanth gum has been used to prepare gels that are most stable at pH 4 to 8. These gels must be preserved with either 0.1% benzoic acid or sodium benzoate or a combination of 0.17% methylparaben and 0.03% propylparaben. These gels may be sterilized by autoclaving. Since powdered tragacanth gum tends to form lumps when added to water, aqueous dispersions are prepared by adding the powder to vigorously stirred water. Also, the use of ethanol, glycerin, or propylene glycol to wet the tragacanth before mixing with water is very effective. If other powders are to be incorporated into the gel, they can be premixed with the tragacanth in the dry state.

Gel Formulation Considerations

In gel preparation, the powdered polymers, when added to water, may form temporary gels that slow dissolution. As water diffuses into these loose clumps of powder, their exterior frequently turns into clumps of solvated particles encasing dry powder. The globs or clumps of gel dissolve very slowly because of their high viscosity and the low diffusion coefficient of the macromolecules.

As a hot colloidal dispersion of gelatin cools, the gelatin macromolecules lose kinetic energy. With reduced kinetic energy, or thermal agitation, the gelatin macromolecules are associated through dipole–dipole interaction into elongated or threadlike aggregates. The size of these association chains increases to the extent that the dispersing medium is held in the interstices among the interlacing network of gelatin macromolecules, and the viscosity increases to that of a semisolid. Gums, such as agar, Irish moss, algin, pectin, and tragacanth form gels by the same mechanism as gelatin.

Polymer solutions tend to cast gels because the solute consists of long, flexible chains of molecular thickness that tend to become entangled, attract each other by secondary valency forces, and even crystallize. Cross-linking of dissolved polymer molecules also causes these solutions to gel. The reactions produce permanent gels, held together by primary valence forces. Secondary valence forces are responsible for reversible gel formation. For example, gelatin will form a gel when lowered to about 30°C, the gel melting point, but aqueous methylcellulose solutions will gel when heated above about 50°C because the polymer, being less soluble in hot water, precipitates. Lower temperatures, higher concentrations, and higher molecular weights promote gelation and produce stronger gels. The reversible gelation of gelatin will occur at about 25°C for 10% solutions, 30°C for 20% solutions and about 32°C for 30% solutions (77°, 86°, and 90°F, respectively). Gelation is rarely observed for gelatin above 34°C (93°F), and regardless of concentration, gelatin solutions do not gel at 37°C (98.6°F). The gelation temperature or gel point of gelatin is highest at the isoelectric point. Water-soluble polymers have the property of thermal gelation, that is, they gel on heating, whereas natural gums gel on cooling. The thermal gelation is reversed on cooling.

Inorganic salts will compete with the water in a gel and cause gelation at lower concentrations. This is usually reversible; upon addition of water, the gels will re-form. Because alcohol is not a solvent or precipitant, it may cause precipitation or gelation, lowering the dielectric constant of the medium and tending to dehydrate the hydrophilic solute. Alcohol lowers the concentrations at which electrolytes salt

out hydrophilic colloids. Phase separation by adding alcohol may cause coacervation.

Aqueous polymer solutions, especially of cellulose derivatives, are stored for approximately 48 hours after dissolution to promote full hydration and maximum viscosity and clarity. Any salts are added at this point rather than dissolving in water prior to adding polymer; otherwise the solutions may not reach their full viscosity and clarity.

Examples of Magmas and Gels

One official magma, Bentonite Magma, NF, used as a suspending agent, finds application in the extemporaneous compounding of prescriptions. Sodium Fluoride and Phosphoric Acid Gel, USP, is applied topically to the teeth as a dental care prophylactic. Other official gels applied topically include Fluocinonide Gel, USP, an anti-inflammatory corticosteroid, and Tretinoin Gel, USP, an irritant that stimulates epidermal cell turnover, causes peeling, and is effective in the treatment of acne. Examples of such drugs and drug products are erythromycin and benzoyl peroxide topical gel (Benzamycin Topical Gel, Dermik Laboratories); clindamycin topical gel (Cleocin T Topical Gel, Pharmacia & Upjohn) and benzoyl peroxide gel (Desquam-X 10 Gel, Westwood-Squibb) used in the control and treatment of acne vulgaris; hydroquinone gel (Solaquin Forte Gel, ICN), a bleach for hyperpigmented skin; salicylic acid gel (Compound W gel, Whitehall), a keratolytic; and desoximetasone gel (Topicort Gel, Medicis Dermatologics), an anti-inflammatory and antipruritic agent.

Other official magmas and gels are employed as antacids: Aluminum Phosphate Gel, USP; Aluminum Hydroxide Gel, USP; and Dihydroxyaluminum Aminoacetate Magma, USP. Some of these preparations are discussed briefly next.

Bentonite Magma, NF

Bentonite magma is a preparation of 5% bentonite, a native colloidal hydrated aluminum silicate, in purified water. It may be prepared mechanically in a blender with the bentonite added directly to the purified water while the machine is running, or it may be prepared by sprinkling the bentonite, in portions, upon hot purified water, allowing each portion to become thoroughly wetted without stirring before another portion is added. By the latter method, the mixture must be allowed to stand for 24 hours before it may be stirred. The standing period ensures complete hydration and swelling of the bentonite. Bentonite, which is insoluble in water, swells to approximately 12 times its volume upon addition to water. The NF monograph for bentonite contains a test for swelling power in which 2 g of a bentonite sample is added in portions to 100 mL water in a 100-mL glass-stoppered cylinder. At the end of a 2-hour period, the mass at the bottom of the cylinder is required to occupy an apparent volume of not less than 24 mL. Other required tests are for gel formation, fineness of powder, and pH, the latter being between 9.5 and 10.5. After bentonite magma has been allowed to stand undisturbed for some time, it sets to a gel. Upon agitation the sol form returns. The process may be repeated indefinitely. As mentioned earlier, this phenomenon is termed *thixotropy*, and bentonite magma is a *thixotropic gel*. The thixotropy occurs only when the bentonite concentration is somewhat above 4%.

Bentonite magma is employed as a suspending agent. Its alkaline pH must be considered, because it is undesirable for certain drugs. Furthermore, because the suspending capacity of the magma is drastically reduced if the pH is lowered to about pH 7, another suspending agent should be selected for drugs requiring a less alkaline medium rather than making bentonite magma more acidic.

Aluminum Hydroxide Gel, USP

Aluminum Hydroxide Gel, USP, is an aqueous suspension of a gelatinous precipitate composed of insoluble aluminum hydroxide and the hydrated aluminum oxide, equivalent to about 4% aluminum oxide. The disperse phase of the gel is generally prepared by chemical reaction, using various reactants. Usually the aluminum source of the reaction is aluminum chloride or aluminum alum, which yields the insoluble aluminum oxide and aluminum hydroxide precipitate. To the gel, the USP permits the addition of peppermint oil, glycerin, sorbitol, sucrose, saccharin, or other flavorants and sweeteners as well as suitable antimicrobial agents.

This antacid preparation is a white, viscous suspension. It is effective in neutralizing a portion of the gastric hydrochloric acid and by virtue of its gelatinous, viscous, and insoluble character, coats the inflamed and perhaps ulcerated gastric surface and is useful in the treatment of hyperacidity and peptic ulcers. The main disadvantage to its use is its constipating effects. The usual dose is 10 mL four or more times a day. The analogous commercial product (Amphojel, Wyeth-Ayerst) at 10 mL has the capacity to neutralize about 13 mEq of acid. The preparation should be stored in a tight container, and freezing should be avoided.

Because it possesses a trivalent cation, aluminum hydroxide interferes with the bioavailability of tetracycline by chelating with the antibiotic in the gastrointestinal tract. Thus, when these two medicines are indicated for patient use, the doses should be staggered to ensure that the patient receives the benefit of both drugs. Aluminum hydroxide gel has also been implicated in decreasing the bioavailability of other drugs by adsorption onto the gel. This is usually illustrated by a decrease in the area under the concentration time curve (AUC) for the concomitantly administered drug. Suffice to say that the clinical significance of the interaction may not be that great, but observation of the patient to ensure the proper therapeutic outcome is important. Thus, for example, if aluminum hydroxide gel is suspected of causing incomplete absorption of the second drug, an upward alteration in the dose of the second drug may be necessary provided the aluminum hydroxide gel administration remains the same.

Milk of Magnesia

Milk of magnesia is a preparation containing 7 to 8.5% magnesium hydroxide. It may be prepared by a reaction between sodium hydroxide and magnesium sulfate (1), diluted solutions being used to ensure a fine, flocculent, gelatinous precipitate of magnesium hydroxide. The precipitate so produced is washed with purified water to remove the sodium sulfate prior to its incorporation with additional purified water to prepare the required volume of product. Commercially, the product is more economically produced by the direct hydration of magnesium oxide.

$$2NaOH + MgSO_4 \rightarrow Mg(OH)_2 + Na_2SO_4$$

$$MgO + H_2O \rightarrow Mg(OH)_2$$

Irrespective of its method of preparation, milk of magnesia is an opaque white viscous preparation from which varying proportions of water separate on standing. For this reason it should be shaken before use. The preparation has a pH of about 10, which may bring about a reaction between the magma and the glass container, imparting a bitter taste to the preparation. To minimize such an occurrence, 0.1% citric acid may be added. Also, flavoring oils at a concentration not exceeding 0.05% may be added to enhance the palatability of the preparation.

Milk of magnesia possesses reasonable acid-neutralizing ability, and a dose of 5 mL will neutralize about 10 mEq of stomach acid. However, to neutralize more acid a higher dose, such as 15 mL, is usually necessary, and this may predispose the patient to the development of diarrhea, a common side effect of this drug. Thus, to circumvent the problem of diarrhea from magnesium hydroxide and the constipating effects of aluminum hydroxide, frequently these two drugs are combined in an antacid preparation. The combination results in a more palatable product with optimum buffering of stomach contents at a pH of 4 to 5 and less of a chance for either diarrhea or constipation to occur. When a laxative effect is desired, a bedtime dose of 30 to 60 mL of milk of magnesia will suffice very nicely by the next morning.

Milk of magnesia is best stored in a tight container, preferably at 0 to 35°C. Freezing results in a coarsening of the disperse phase, and temperatures above 35°C decrease the gel structure.

Starch Glycerite

Starch	100 g
Benzoic acid	2 g
Purified water	200 g
Glycerin	700 g

The starch and benzoic acid are rubbed in the water to a smooth mixture. The glycerin is added and mixed. The mixture is heated to 140°C with constant gentle agitation until a translucent mass forms. The heat ruptures the starch grains and permits the water to reach and hydrate the linear and branched starch molecules, which trap the dispersion medium in the interstices to form a gel. Starch glycerite has been used as a topical vehicle and protectant.

Lubricating Jelly Formula

Methylcellulose, 4000 cps	0.8%
Carbopol 934	0.24%
Propylene glycol	16.7%
Methylparaben	0.015%
Sodium hydroxide, qs ad	pH 7
Purified water, qs ad	100%

Disperse the methylcellulose in 40 mL of hot (80–90°C) water. Chill overnight in a refrigerator to dissolve. Disperse the Carbopol 934 in 20 mL water. Adjust the pH of the dispersion to 7.0 by adding sufficient 1% sodium hydroxide solution (about 12 mL is required) and bring the volume to 40 mL with purified water. Dissolve the methylparaben in the propylene glycol. Mix the methylcellulose, Carbopol 934, and propylene glycol fractions, using caution to avoid incorporating air. Lubricating jellies are used to assist in medical procedures, to aid in insertion of various devices and drugs, including catheters and suppositories, and as vehicles for some drug products, especially in extemporaneous compounding.

Clear Aqueous Gel With Dimethicone

Water	59.8%
Carbomer 934	0.5%
Triethanolamine	1.2
Glycerin	34.2
Propylene glycol	2.0
Dimethicone copolyol	2.3

Prepare the carbomer gel, add the other ingredients, and mix well. Dimethicone copolyol is included to reduce the sticky feel associated with glycerin. These gels are commonly used as vehicles for drug products, especially for those that are extemporaneously compounded.

Poloxamer Gel Base

Pluronic F-127, NF	20–50 g
Purified water/buffer qs	100 mL

Poloxamer gel base is widely used as a vehicle for extemporaneous products. In a combination with isopropyl palmitate and lecithin, it is an absorption-enhancing topical vehicle.

Proper Administration and Use of Disperse Systems

Most dosage forms discussed thus far in this chapter are for oral use. As with the oral solutions discussed in the previous chapter, they can be measured by spoonful or administered dropwise, depending on the appropriate dosage. It is very important that the patient understand the proper quantity of product to use. For example, differences in dosage can occur between product categories, such as OTC antidiarrheal suspensions (tablespoonfuls) versus OTC antacid suspensions (teaspoonfuls). Differences in dosage can also occur within a category, most notably in antacid suspensions. Some are recommended in teaspoon doses because of higher concentration, whereas others are suggested in tablespoon quantities. It is important, therefore, that the pharmacist ensure that the patient knows how much to use, and then use a calibrated device to make sure the right amount is taken.

Many reconstituted products, as mentioned earlier in the chapter, are suspensions. Several problems can emerge if the pharmacist is not careful to counsel the patient about them. Usually the patient or guardian of the patient receives the product in an oversized bottle that allows for the proper shaking of the product prior to its use. To allay fears that the medicine may not all be in the bottle, the pharmacist must make the patient or the guardian aware of this and indicate that this feature enhances the ability to shake it up before administration. Furthermore, some patients do not make the connection that the medicine should be administered by mouth. Oral antibiotic suspensions intended to treat a middle ear infection have been mistakenly administered directly into the ear by some patients or guardians. Thus, the pharmacist should review with the patient the proper route of administration. Lastly, because these are reconstituted with purified water stability problems with the drug usually dictate that it be stored in the refrigerator until it is consumed. The patient has to be informed of this. The consumer may overlook a tiny label directing refrigerator storage. Alternatively, not all suspensions need to be stored in the refrigerator, but because of prior experience with other liquid suspensions that necessitated refrigeration, a patient or guardian may assume this is necessary.

Certain suspensions, such as aluminum hydroxide gel, cholestyramine, and kaolin, by virtue of their active ingredients interfere with absorption of other drugs. For example, cholestyramine has been shown to interfere with and decrease the bioavailability of warfarin, digitoxin, and thyroid hormones. The pharmacist should be aware of this and make recommendations to help avoid this drug interaction whenever possible. The typical suggestion is to stagger the administration of the liquid cholestyramine away from other drug administration by several hours, and giving warfarin at least 6 hours after the cholestyramine reportedly avoids the impaired warfarin bioavailability (8). However, warfarin undergoes enterohepatic recycling in the body, and if cholestyramine is present in the intestine because of earlier administration, it can bind it and decrease warfarin's reabsorption. In this instance, use of one of the two drugs should be discontinued by the physician. However, if concurrent use is necessary, the pharmacist should monitor the patient more frequently for the possibility of an altered anticoagulant response. This is important because if adjustments in warfarin dosage are made on the basis of cholestyramine interference and then the cholestyramine is discontinued, the warfarin dosage also must be decreased according to the patient's prothrombin time.

Aerosols

Pharmaceutical aerosols are pressurized dosage forms that upon actuation emit a fine dispersion of liquid and/or solid materials containing one or more active ingredients in a gaseous medium (Physical Pharmacy Capsule 14.5). Pharmaceutical aerosols are similar to other dosage forms because they require the same types of considerations with respect to formulation, product stability, and therapeutic efficacy. However, they differ from most other dosage forms in their dependence upon the function of the container, its valve assembly, and an added component—the propellant—for the physical delivery of the medication in proper form.

The term *pressurized package* is commonly used when referring to the aerosol container or completed product. Pressure is applied to the aerosol system through the use of one or more liquefied or gaseous propellants. Upon activation of the valve assembly of the aerosol, the pressure exerted by the propellant forces the contents of the package out through the opening of the valve. The physical form in which the contents are emitted depends on the formulation of the product and the type of valve. Aerosol products may be designed to expel their contents as a fine mist; a coarse, wet, or dry spray; a steady stream; or a stable or a fast-breaking foam. The physical form selected for a given aerosol is based on intended use. For instance, an aerosol for inhalation therapy, as in the treatment of asthma or emphysema, must present particles in the form of a fine liquid mist or as finely divided solid particles. Particles less than 6 μm will reach the respiratory bronchioles, and those less than 2 μm will reach the alveolar ducts and alveoli (Fig. 14.11). In contrast, the particle size for a dermatologic spray intended for deposition on the skin is coarser and generally less critical to the therapeutic efficacy of the product. Some dermatologic aerosols present the medication in the form of a powder, a wet spray, a stream of liquid (usually a local anesthetic), or an ointment-like prod-

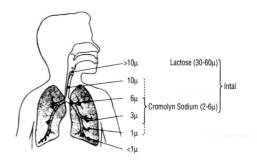

FIGURE 14.11 Relationship of INTAL (cromolyn sodium, Fisons) particle size to airway penetration. (Courtesy of Fisons Corporation.)

uct. Other pharmaceutical aerosols include vaginal and rectal foams.

Aerosols used to provide an airborne mist are termed *space sprays*. Room disinfectants, room deodorizers, and space insecticides characterize this group of aerosols. The particle size of the released product is generally quite small, usually below 50 μm, and must be carefully controlled so that the dispersed droplets or particles remain airborne for a long time. A one-second burst from a typical aerosol space spray will produce 120 million particles, a substantial number of which will remain suspended in the air for an hour.

Aerosols intended to carry the active ingredient to a surface are termed *surface sprays* or *surface coatings*. The dermatologic aerosols can be placed in this group. Also included are a great many cosmetic and household aerosol products, including personal deodorant sprays, hair lacquers and sprays, perfumes and colognes, shaving lathers, toothpaste, surface pesticide sprays, paint sprays, spray starch, waxes, polishes, cleaners, and lubricants. A number of veterinary and pet products have been put into aerosol form, as have such food products as dessert toppings and food spreads. Some of these products are sprays; others, foams; and a few, pastes.

Advantages of the Aerosol Dosage Form

Some features of pharmaceutical aerosols that may be considered advantages over other types of dosage forms are as follows:

PHYSICAL PHARMACY CAPSULE 14.5

Partial Pressure and Aerosol Formulation

Aerosols generally contain an active drug in a liquid gas propellant, in a mixture of solvents with a propellant, or in a mixture with other additives and a propellant. The gas propellants can be formulated to provide desired vapor pressures for enhancing the delivery of the medication through the valve and actuator in accordance with the purpose of the medication. Aerosols are used as space sprays, surface sprays, aerated foams, and for oral inhalation.

Various propellants have properties that may be important including molecular weight, boiling point, vapor pressure, liquid density, and flash point. An example of a calculation to determine the vapor pressure of a certain mixture of hydrocarbon propellants follows.

EXAMPLE 1

What is the vapor pressure of a 60:40 mixture of propane and isobutane? Information on the two propellants is as follows:

PROPERTY	PROPANE	ISOBUTANE
Molecular formula	C_3H_8	C_4H_{10}
Molecular weight	44.1	58.1
Boiling point (°F)	−43.7	10.9
Vapor pressure (psig @ 70°F)	110	30.4
Liquid density (g/mL @ 70°F)	0.50	0.56
Flash point (°F)	−156	−117

1. Assume an ideal solution.
2. For Raoult's law, determine the number of moles of each propellant:

$$n_{propane} = 60/44.1 = 1.36$$

$$n_{isobutane} = 40/58.1 = 0.69$$

3. From Raoult's law, the partial pressure exerted by the propane is

$$P_{propane} = [(n_{propane})/(n_{propane} + n_{isobutane})] P_{propane}$$

$$P_{propane} = [(1.36)/(1.36 + 0.69)] 110 = 72.98 \text{ psi}$$

4. The partial pressure exerted by the isobutane is

$$P_{isobutane} = [(0.69)/(1.36 + 0.69)] 30.4 = 10.23 \text{ psi}$$

5. The vapor pressure exerted by both gases, P_T, is

$$P_T = 72.98 + 10.23 = 83.21 \text{ psi at } 70°F$$

The vapor pressure required for a specific application can be calculated in a similar manner, and different ratios of propellants may be used to obtain that pressure.

1. A portion of medication may be easily withdrawn from the package without contamination or exposure to the remaining material.
2. By virtue of its hermetic character, the aerosol container protects medicinal agents adversely affected by atmospheric oxygen and moisture. Being opaque, the usual aerosol container also protects drugs adversely affected by light. This protection persists during the use and the shelf life of the product. If the product is packaged under aseptic conditions, sterility may also be maintained during the shelf life of the product.
3. Topical medication may be applied in a uniform thin layer to the skin without anything else touching the affected area. This method of application may reduce the irritation that sometimes accompanies mechanical (fingertip) application of topical preparations. The rapid volatilization of the propellant also provides a cooling, refreshing effect.
4. By proper formulation and valve control, the physical form and the particle size of the emitted product may be controlled, which may contribute to the efficacy of a drug, as with the fine controlled mist of an inhalant aerosol. Through the use of *metered valves*, dosage may be controlled.
5. Aerosol application is a clean process, requiring little or no wash-up by the user.

The Aerosol Principle

An aerosol formulation consists of two component parts, the *product concentrate* and the *propellant*. The product concentrate is the active ingredient of the aerosol combined with the required adjuncts, such as antioxidants, surface-active agents, and solvents, to prepare a stable and efficacious product. When the propellant is a liquefied gas or a mixture of liquefied gases, it frequently serves the dual role of propellant and solvent or vehicle for the product concentrate. In certain aerosol systems, compressed gases—carbon dioxide, nitrogen, and nitrous oxide—are employed as the propellant.

For many years, the liquefied gas propellants most used in aerosol products were the chlorofluorocarbons (CFCs). However, these propellants are being phased out and will be prohibited for nonessential use under federal regulations following recognition that they reduce the amount of ozone in the stratosphere, which results in an increase in the amount of ultraviolet radiation reaching the earth, an increase in the incidence of skin cancer, and other adverse environmental effects. Under the law, the FDA has the authority to exempt from the prohibition specific products under the agency's jurisdiction when there is sufficient evidence showing that (*a*) there are no technically feasible alternatives to the use of a CFC propellant in the product; (*b*) the product provides a substantial health or other public benefit unobtainable without the use of the CFC; and (*c*) the use does not involve a significant release of CFCs into the atmosphere or, if it does, the release is warranted by the benefit conveyed. A number of metered-dose pharmaceutical products for oral inhalation have received such essential use exemptions. Among the CFCs used as propellants in pharmaceuticals were dichlorodifluoromethane, dichlorotetrafluoroethane, and trichloromonofluoromethane (Table 14.5).

Fluorinated hydrocarbons are gases at room temperature. They may be liquefied by cooling below their boiling point or by compression at room temperature. For example, dichlorodifluoromethane (Freon 12) will form a liquid when cooled to $-30°C$ ($-22°F$) or when compressed to 70 psig (pounds per square inch gauge) at $21°C$ ($70°F$). Both of these methods for liquefying gases are employed in aerosol packaging, as discussed later in this section.

When a liquefied gas propellant or propellant mixture is sealed within an aerosol container with the product concentrate, equilibrium is quickly established between the portion of propellant that remains liquefied and that which vaporizes and occupies the upper portion of the aerosol container (Fig. 14.12). The vapor phase exerts pressure in all directions—against the walls of the container, the valve assembly, and the surface of the liquid phase, which is composed of the liquefied gas and the product concentrate. It is this pressure that upon actuation of the aerosol valve forces the liquid phase up the dip tube and out of the

TABLE 14.5 PHYSICAL PROPERTIES OF SOME FLUORINATED HYDROCARBON PROPELLANTS

CHEMICAL NAME	CHEMICAL FORMULA	NUMERIC DESIGNATION	VAPOR PRESSURE[a] 70°F	BOILING POINT (1 ATM) °F	LIQUID DENSITY (g/mL) 70°F
Trichloromonofluoromethane	CCl_3F	11	13.4	74.7	1.485
Dichlorodifluoromethane	CCl_2F_2	12	13.4	74.1	1.485
Dichlorotetrafluoroethane	$CClF_2CClF_2$	114	21.6	38.4	1.468
Chloropentafluoroethane	$CClF_2CF_3$	115	17.5	−37.7	1.29
Monochlorodifluoroethane	CH_3CClF_2	142[b]	43.8	15.1	1.119
Difluoroethane	CH_3CHF_2	152[b]	76.4	−11.2	0.911
Octafluorocyclobutane	$CF_2CF_2CF_2CFM_2$ 12	C318	40.1	21.1	1.513

[a]Pounds per square inch absolute, equal to psig + 14.7.

[b]The numeric designations for fluorinated hydrocarbon propellants were designed in the refrigeration industry to simplify communications. The numeric designations are arrived at by the following method: (a) The digit at the extreme right refers to the number of fluorine atoms in the molecule. (b) The second digit from the right is one *greater* than the number of hydrogen atoms in the molecule. (c) The third digit from the right is one *less* than the number of carbon atoms in the molecule; if this number is zero, it is omitted and a two-digit number is used. (d) A capital C before a number indicates the cyclic nature of a compound. (e) The small letters following a number indicate decreasing symmetry of isomeric compounds, with "b" indicating less symmetry than "a," and so forth. The number of chlorine atoms in a molecule may be determined by subtracting the total number of hydrogen and fluorine atoms from the total number of atoms which may be added to the carbon chain.

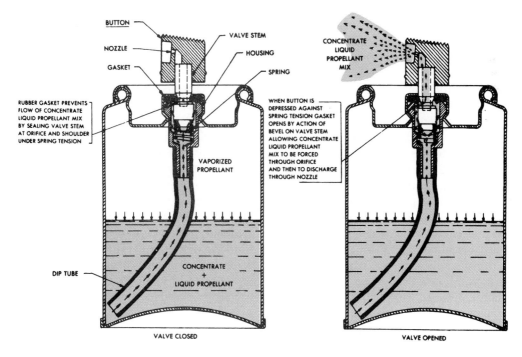

FIGURE 14.12 Cross-section sketches of contents and operation of a typical two-phase aerosol system. (Courtesy of Armstrong Laboratories, , Division of Aerosol Techniques.)

orifice of the valve into the atmosphere. As the propellant meets the air, it expands and evaporates because of the drop in pressure, leaving the product concentrate as airborne liquid droplets or dry particles, depending upon the formulation. As the liquid phase is removed from the container, equilibrium between the propellant remaining liquefied and that in the vapor state is reestablished. Thus, even during expulsion of the product from the aerosol package, the pressure within remains virtually constant, and the product may be continuously released at an even rate and with the same propulsion. However, when the liquid reservoir is depleted, the pressure may not be maintained, and the gas may be expelled from the container with diminishing pressure until it is exhausted.

Aerosol Systems

The pressure of an aerosol is critical to its performance. It can be controlled by (*a*) the type and amount of propellant and (*b*) the nature and amount of product concentrate. Thus, each formulation is unique unto itself, and a specific amount of propellant to be employed in aerosol products cannot be firmly stated, although some general statements may be made. Space sprays generally contain a greater proportion of propellant than do aerosols intended for surface coating; hence they are released with greater pressure, and the resultant particles are projected more violently from the valve. Space aerosols usually operate at 30 to 40 psig at 21°C and may contain as much as 85% propellant. Surface aerosols commonly contain 30 to 70% propellant with pressures between 25 and 55 psig at 21°C. Foam aerosols usually operate between 35 and 55 psig at 21°C and may contain only 6 to 10% propellant.

Foam aerosols may be considered to be emulsions, because the liquefied propellant is partially emulsified with the product concentrate rather than being dissolved in it. Because the fluorinated hydrocarbons are nonpolar organic solvents having no affinity for water, the liquefied propellant does not dissolve in the aqueous formulation. The use of surfactants or emulsifiers in the formulation encourages the mixing of the two components to enhance the emulsion. Shaking of the package prior to use further mixes the propellant throughout the product concentrate. When the aerosol valve is activated, the mixture is expelled to the atmosphere, where the propellant globules vaporize rapidly, leaving the active ingredient in the form of a foam.

Blends of the various liquefied gas propellants are generally used in pharmaceutical aerosols to achieve the desired vapor pressure and to provide the proper solvent features for a given product. Some propellants are eliminated from use in certain products because of their reactivity with other formulative materials or with the proposed container or valve components. For instance, trichloromonofluoromethane tends to form free hydrochloric acid when formulated with systems containing water or ethyl alcohol, the latter a commonly used cosolvent in aerosol systems. The free hydrochloric acid not only affects the efficacy of the product but also corrodes some container components.

The physiologic effect of the propellant must also be considered in formulating an aerosol to ensure safety of the product in its intended use. Even though an individual propellant or propellant blend and the active ingredient of a formulation are nontoxic when tested individually, the use of the combination in aerosol form may have undesirable features. For instance, when an active ingredient ordinarily used in a nasal or oral spray is placed in a fine aerosol mist, it may reach deeper into the respiratory tract than desired and result in irritation. With new dermatologic, vaginal, and rectal aerosol products, the influence of the aerosol form of the drug on the recipient tissue membranes must be evaluated for irritating effects and changes in the absorption of the drug from the site of application. The absorption pattern of a drug may change because of an increased rate of solubility of the fine particles usually produced in aerosol products.

Although the fluorinated hydrocarbons have a relatively low order of toxicity and are generally nonirritating, certain individuals who use an inhalation aerosol may be sensitive to the propellant agent and may exhibit cardiotoxic effects following rapid and repeated use (9).

Two-Phase Systems

As noted previously, the two-phase aerosol system consists of the liquid phase, containing the liquefied propellant and product concentrate, and the vapor phase.

Three-Phase Systems

The three-phase system consists of a layer of water-immiscible liquid propellant, a layer of highly aqueous product concentrate, and the vapor phase. Because the liquefied propellant usually has a greater density than the aqueous layer, it generally resides at the bottom of the container with the aqueous phase floating above it. As with the two-phase system, upon activation of the valve, the pressure of the vapor phase causes the liquid phase to rise in the dip tube and be expelled from the container. To avoid expulsion of the reservoir of liquefied propellant, the dip tube must extend only within the aqueous phase (product concentrate) and not down into the layer of liquefied propellant. The aqueous product is broken up into a spray by the mechanical action of the valve. If the container is shaken immediately prior to use, some liquefied propellant may be mixed with the aqueous phase and be expelled through the valve to facilitate the dispersion of the exited product or the production of foam. The vapor phase within the container is replenished from the liquid propellant phase.

Compressed Gas Systems

Compressed rather than liquefied gases may be used to prepare aerosols. The pressure of the compressed gas in the head space of the aerosol container forces the product concentrate up the dip tube and out of the valve. The use of gases that are insoluble in the product concentrate, as is nitrogen, will result in emission of a product in essentially the same form as it was placed in the container. An advantage of nitrogen as a propellant is its inert behavior toward other formulative components and its protective influence on products subject to oxidation. Also, nitrogen is an odorless and tasteless gas and thus does not contribute adversely to the smell or taste of a product.

Other gases, such as carbon dioxide and nitrous oxide, which are slightly soluble in the liquid phase of aerosol products, may be employed when their expulsion with the product concentrate is desired to achieve spraying or foaming.

Unlike aerosols prepared with liquefied gas propellants, compressed gas–filled aerosols have no reservoir of propellant. Thus higher gas pressures are required in these systems, and the pressure in these aerosols diminishes as the product is used.

Aerosol Container and Valve Assembly

The effectiveness of a pharmaceutical aerosol depends on achieving the proper combination of formulation, container, and valve assembly. The formulation must not chemically interact with the container or valve components so as to interfere with the stability of the formulation or with the integrity and operation of the container and valve assembly. The container and valve must be capable of withstanding the pressure required by the product, it must resist corrosion, and the valve must contribute to the form of the product to be emitted.

Containers

Various materials have been used in the manufacture of aerosol containers, including (a) glass, uncoated or plastic coated; (b) metal, including tin-plated steel, aluminum, and stainless steel; and (c) plastics. The selection of the container for an aerosol product is based on its adaptability to production methods, compatibility with formulation components, ability to sustain the pressure intended for the product, the interest in design and aesthetic appeal on the part of the manufacturer, and cost.

Were it not for their brittleness and danger of breakage, glass containers would be preferred for most aerosols. Glass presents fewer problems with respect to chemical compatibility with the formula than do metal containers, and it is not subject to corrosion. Glass is also more adaptive to creativity in design. On the negative side, glass containers must be precisely engineered to provide the maximum in pressure safety and impact resistance. Plastic coatings are commonly applied to the outer surface of glass containers to render them more resistant to accidental breakage, and in the event of breaking, the plastic coating prevents the scattering of glass fragments. When the total pressure of an aerosol system is below 25 psig and no more than 50% propellant is used, glass containers are considered quite safe. When required, the inner surface of glass containers may be coated to render them more chemically resistant to formulation materials.

Tin-plated steel containers are the most widely used metal containers for aerosols. Because the starting material is in sheets, the completed aerosol cylinders are seamed and soldered to provide a sealed unit. When required, special protective coatings are employed within the container to prevent corrosion and interaction between the container and formulation. The containers must be carefully examined prior to filling to ensure that there are no flaws in the seam or in the protective coating that would render the container weak or subject to corrosion.

Most aluminum containers are manufactured by extrusion or by other methods that make them seamless. They have the advantage over the seam type of container of greater safety against leakage, incompatibility, and corrosion. Stainless steel is employed to produce containers for certain small-volume aerosols in which a great deal of chemical resistance is required. The main limitation of stainless steel containers is their high cost.

Plastic containers have met with varying success in the packaging of aerosols because of their inherent problem of being permeated by the vapor within the container. Also, certain drug–plastic interactions affect the release of drug from the container and reduce the efficacy of the product.

Valve Assembly

The function of the valve assembly is to permit expulsion of the contents of the can in the desired form, at the desired rate, and in the case of metered valves, in the proper amount or dose. The materials used in the manufacture of valves must be inert to the formulations and must be approved by the FDA. Among the materials used in the manufacture of the various valve parts are plastic, rubber, aluminum, and stainless steel.

The usual aerosol valve assembly is composed of the following parts (Fig. 14.13):

1. *Actuator*: The button the user presses to activate the valve assembly for emission of the product. The actuator permits easy opening and closing of the valve. It is through the orifice in the actuator that the product is discharged. The design of the inner chamber and size of the emission orifice of the actuator contribute to the physical form (mist, coarse spray, solid stream, or foam) in which the product is discharged. The type and quantity of propellant used and the actuator design and dimensions control the particle size of the emitted product. Larger orifices (and less propellant) are used for products to be emitted as foams and solid streams than for those intended to be sprays or mists.
2. *Stem*: Supports the actuator and delivers the formulation in the proper form to the chamber of the actuator.
3. *Gasket*: Placed snugly with the stem, pre-

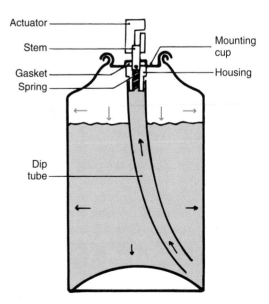

FIGURE 14.13 Valve assembly components.

vents leakage of the formulation when the valve is closed.

4. *Spring:* Holds the gasket in place and is the mechanism by which the actuator retracts when pressure is released, returning the valve to the closed position.

5. *Mounting cup:* Attached to the aerosol can or container, holds the valve in place. Because the underside of the mounting cup is exposed to the formulation, it must receive the same consideration as the inner part of the container with respect to meeting criteria of compatibility. If necessary, it may be coated with an inert material (e.g., an epoxy resin or vinyl) to prevent an undesired interaction.

6. *Housing:* Directly below the mounting cup, the housing links the dip tube and the stem and actuator. With the stem, its orifice helps to determine the delivery rate and the form in which the product is emitted.

7. *Dip tube:* Extends from the housing down into the product; brings the formulation from the container to the valve. The viscosity of the product and its intended delivery rate dictate to a large extent the inner dimensions of the dip tube and housing for a particular product.

The actuator, stem, housing, and dip tube are generally made of plastic, the mounting cup and spring of metal, and the gasket of rubber or plastic resistant to the formulation.

Metered Dose Inhalers

Metering valves are employed when the formulation is a potent medication, as in inhalation therapy (Fig. 14.14). In these metered valve systems, the amount of material discharged is regulated by an auxiliary valve chamber by virtue of its capacity or dimensions. A single depression of the actuator causes evacuation of this chamber and delivery of its contents. The integrity of the chamber is controlled by a dual valve mechanism. When the actuator valve is closed, the chamber is sealed from the atmosphere. However, in this position the chamber is permitted to fill with the contents of the container, to which it is open. Depression of the actuator causes a simultane-

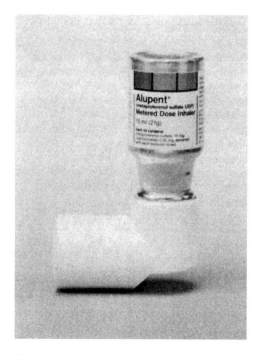

FIGURE 14.14 Metered-dose inhaler. Each metered dose is delivered through the mouthpiece upon actuation of the aerosol unit's valve. (Courtesy of Boehringer Ingelheim.)

ous reversal of positions; the chamber becomes open to the atmosphere, releasing its contents, at the same time becoming sealed from the contents of the container. Upon release of the actuator, the system is restored for the next dose. The USP contains a test to determine quantitatively the amount of medication from a metered valve.

As noted previously, the effectiveness of delivering medication to the lower reaches of the lungs for local or systemic effects depends in part on the particle size of the inhaled drug. Breathing patterns and the depth of respiration also play important roles in the deposition of inhaled aerosols to the lungs. Analysis of dose uniformity (10), particle size distribution patterns (11–13), and the respirable fractions of aerosol-delivered particles (14–15) are areas of research in developing aerosol products for optimal oral inhalation therapy.

A unique translingual aerosol formulation of nitroglycerin (Nitrolingual Spray, Rhône-Poulenc Rorer) permits a patient to spray droplets of nitroglycerin onto or under the tongue for acute relief of an attack or for prophylaxis of angina pectoris due to coronary artery disease. The product is not to be inhaled. At the onset of an attack, two metered spray emissions, each containing 0.4 mg of nitroglycerin, are administered. The product contains 200 doses of nitroglycerin in a propellant mixture of dichlorodifluoromethane and dichlorotetrafluoroethane.

Filling Operations

As explained earlier, fluorinated hydrocarbon gases may be liquefied by cooling below their boiling point or by compressing the gas at room temperature. These two features are used in the filling of aerosol containers with propellant.

Cold Filling

In the cold method, both the product concentrate and the propellant must be cooled to $-34.5°C$ to $-40°C$ ($-30°$–$40°F$). This temperature is necessary to liquefy the propellant gas. The cooling system may be a mixture of dry ice and acetone or a more elaborate refrigeration system. After the chilled product concentrate has been quantitatively metered into an equally cold aerosol container, the liquefied gas is added. The heavy vapors of the cold liquid propellant generally displace the air in the container. However, in the process, some of the propellant vapors are also lost. When sufficient propellant has been added, the valve assembly is inserted and crimped into place. Because of the low temperatures required, aqueous systems cannot be filled by this process, since the water turns to ice. For nonaqueous systems, some moisture usually appears in the final product due to the condensation of atmospheric moisture within the cold containers.

Pressure Filling

By the pressure method, the product concentrate is quantitatively placed in the aerosol container (Fig. 14.15), the valve assembly is inserted and crimped into place, and the liquefied gas, under pressure, is metered into the valve stem from a pressure burette (Fig. 14.16). The desired amount of propellant is allowed to

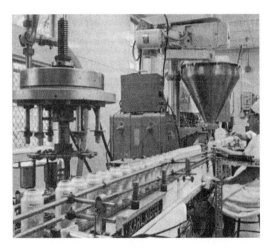

FIGURE 14.15 Filling the aerosol cans with the drug mixture. (Courtesy of Pennwalt Corp.)

enter the container under its own vapor pressure. When the pressure in the container equals that in the burette, the propellant stops flowing. Additional propellant may be added by increasing the pressure in the filling apparatus through the use of compressed air or nitrogen gas. The trapped air in the package may be ignored if it does not interfere with the quality or stability of the product, or it may be evacuated with a special apparatus. After the container is filled with sufficient propellant, the valve actuator is tested for proper function. This spray testing also rids the dip tube of pure propellant prior to consumer use.

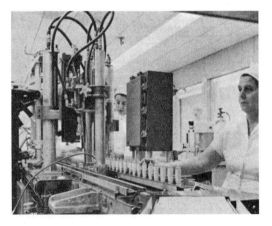

FIGURE 14.16 Pressure filling of aerosol containers. (Courtesy of Pennwalt Corp.)

Pressure filling is used for most pharmaceutical aerosols. It has two advantages over cold filling: there is less danger of moisture contamination of the product, and less propellant is lost in the process.

When compressed gases are employed as the propellant in aerosol systems, the gas is transferred from large steel cylinders into the aerosol containers. Prior to filling, the product concentrate is placed in the container, the valve assembly is crimped into place, and the air is evacuated from the container by a vacuum pump. The compressed gas is then passed into the container through a pressure-reducing valve attached to the gas cylinder; when the pressure within the aerosol container is equal to the predetermined and regulated delivery pressure, the gas flow stops, and the aerosol valve is restored to the closed position. For gases like carbon dioxide and nitrous oxide, which are slightly soluble in the product concentrate, the container is manually or mechanically shaken during the filling operation to achieve the desired pressure in the head space of the aerosol container.

Testing the Filled Containers

After filling by either method, the aerosol container is tested under various environmental conditions for leaks or weakness in the valve assembly or container.

Filled aerosol containers are also tested for proper function of the valve. The *valve discharge rate* is determined by discharging a portion of the contents of a previously weighed aerosol during a period, and calculating, by the difference in weight, the grams of contents discharged per unit of time. As is deemed desirable, aerosols may be tested for their spray patterns, for particle size distribution of the spray, and for accuracy and reproducibility of dosage when using metered valves.

Packaging, Labeling, and Storage

A unique aspect of pharmaceutical aerosols compared to other dosage forms is that the product is actually packaged as part of the manufacturing process. With most other dosage forms, the product is completely manufactured and then placed in the appropriate container.

Most aerosol products have a protective cap or cover that fits snugly over the valve and mounting cup. This protects the valve against contamination with dust and dirt. The cap, which is generally made of plastic or metal, also serves a decorative function.

Medicinal aerosols that are to be dispensed only upon prescription usually are labeled by the manufacturer with plastic peel-away labels or easily removed paper labels so that the pharmacist may easily replace the manufacturer's label with his label containing the directions for use specified by the prescribing practitioner. Most other types of aerosols have the manufacturer's label printed directly on the container or on firmly affixed paper.

In addition to the usual labeling requirements for pharmaceutical products, aerosols have special requirements for use and storage. For example, for safety, labels must warn users not to puncture pressurized containers, not to use or store them near heat or an open flame, and not to incinerate them. Exposure to temperatures above 49°C (120°F) may burst an aerosol container. Most medications in aerosol containers are intended for use at ambient room temperatures. When the canisters are cold, less than the usual spray may result. This may be particularly important to users of metered-dose inhalation sprays. These products are generally recommended for storage between 15°C and 30°C (59°F and 86°F). Pharmaceutical aerosols are labeled with regard to shaking before use, holding at the proper angle and/or distance from the target; there are special detailed instructions for inhaler devices.

Aerosols should be maintained with the protective caps in place to prevent accidental activation of the valve assembly or contamination by dust and other foreign materials. Examples of pharmaceutical aerosols are shown in Figure 14.17 and presented in Table 14.6.

Proper Administration and Use of Pharmaceutical Aerosols

The pharmacist should make every attempt to educate the patient about aerosol dosage

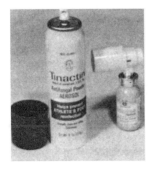

FIGURE 14.17 Pharmaceutical aerosols.

forms, particularly for oral or nasal administration, because these are only effective when properly used. To complement verbal instructions the pharmacist should provide the patient with the written instructions in the product package. It is difficult to predict what percentage of patients will read or understand the printed instruction. Thus, the pharmacist must verbally transmit instruction for proper use. Using the oral metered aerosols as a model, the pharmacist should demonstrate how the inhaler is assembled, stored, and

TABLE 14.6 EXAMPLES OF INHALATION AEROSOLS

AEROSOL	REPRESENTATIVE COMMERCIAL PRODUCTS	CATEGORY AND COMMENTS
Albuterol	Proventil Inhalation Aerosol (Schering) Ventolin Inhalation Aerosol (GlaxoSmithKline)	Beta-adrenergic agonist for prevention and relief of bronchospasm in patients with reversible obstructive airway disease and for relief of exercise-induced bronchospasm.
Beclomethasone dipropionate	Beclovent Inhalation Aerosol (Glaxo Wellcome) Vanceril Inhaler (Schering)	Adrenocortical steroid; aerosol for oral inhalation to control bronchial asthma in patients requiring chronic treatment with corticosteroids plus other therapy, e.g., xanthines, sympathomimetics.
	Beconase Nasal Inhaler (Alien & Hanburys) Vancenase Pockethaler Nasal Inhaler (Schering)	Adrenocortical steroid; aerosol for intranasal relief of seasonal or perennial rhinitis in cases poorly responsive to conventional treatment.
Cromolyn sodium	Intal Inhaler (Rhône-Poulenc Rorer)	Antiasthmatic, antiallergic, mast cell stabilizer; metered dose for oral use to prevent exercise-induced bronchospasm, acute bronchospasm induced by environmental pollutants and known allergens.
Ipratropium bromide	Atrovent Inhalation Aerosol (Boehringer Ingelheim)	Anticholinergic (parasympatholytic) bronchodilator for bronchospasm.
Metaproterenol sulfate	Alupent Inhalation Aerosol (Boehringer Ingelheim)	Sympathomimetic for bronchospasm in patients with reversible obstructive airway disease.
Nedocromil sodium	Tilade Inhaler (Fisons)	Maintenance therapy for mild to moderate bronchial asthma.
Salmeterol xinafoate	Serevent Inhalation Aerosol (Glaxo Wellcome)	Beta-adrenergic agonist for long-term maintenance treatment of asthma, prevention of bronchospasm in patients with reversible obstructive airway disease.
Terbutaline sulfate	Brethine (Novartis)	Beta-adrenergic agonist for relief of bronchospasm.
Triamcinolone acetonide	Azmacort (Aventis)	For patients who require chronic treatment with corticosteroids to control symptoms of bronchial asthma.

cleaned. The patient should be told whether the inhaler requires shaking before use and how to hold it between the index finger and thumb so that the aerosol canister is upside down. The patient should understand that coordination must be achieved between inhalation (after exhaling as completely as possible) and pressing down the inhaler to release one dose. The patient should be instructed to hold the breath for several seconds or as long as possible to gain the maximum benefit from the medication, then remove the inhaler from the mouth and exhale slowly through pursed lips.

Some patients cannot use metered-dose inhalers properly. Thus, after a new prescription is dispensed, it is advisable for the pharmacist to follow up with the patient to make sure the patient can use the inhaler. If the patient cannot use the inhaler, it is advisable for the pharmacist to recommend to the patient or the patient's physician the use of an extender device with the inhaler. Extender devices, or spacers, were originally developed for patients who could not learn to coordinate release of the medication with inhalation. These are now considered an important therapeutic aid because they can effectively assist the delivery of medication despite improper patient inhalation technique. By placing an extender device between the metered-dose inhaler's mouthpiece and the patient's mouth, the patient is permitted to separate activation of the aerosol from inhalation by up to 3 to 5 seconds (a valve in the spacer opens when the patient inhales). Another advantage of the extender is that aerosol velocity is reduced and droplet size is decreased because there is time for evaporation of the fluorohydrocarbon propellant. Thus, extender devices also cause less deposition of medication in the oropharynx. Extender devices can be used with most pressurized canisters, such as Brethancer Inhaler (Geigy) and InspirEase (Schering).

To ensure continuity of therapy it is wise for the pharmacist to share with the patient ways to assess how much medication is left in the canister. This is important to ensure continuity of therapy, especially for those who have respiratory illness and may need their medication on a moment's notice.

For topical administration of aerosol dosage forms, the patient should first clean the affected area gently and pat it dry. Holding the canister with the nozzle pointing toward the body area and about 6 to 8 inches away, the patient should press down the button to deliver enough medication to cover the area. The patient should allow the spray to dry and not cover the area with a bandage or dressing unless instructed to do so by the physician. The patient should avoid accidentally spraying the product into the eyes or mouth. If it is necessary to apply the product to a facial area, the patient should spray the product into the palm of the hand and apply it by this means.

As presented in Table 14.6, a number of drug substances are administered through pressure-packaged *inhalation aerosols* like the type shown in Figure 14.14. For the inhaled drug substance or solution to reach the bronchial tree, the inhaled particles must be just a few microns in size.

Topical Aerosols

Convenient aerosol packages for use on the skin include the anti-infective agents povidone iodine, tolnaftate, and thimerosal; the adrenocortical steroids betamethasone dipropionate and valerate, dexamethasone, and triamcinolone acetonide; and the local anesthetic dibucaine hydrochloride.

The use of topical aerosols provides the patient a means of applying the drug in a convenient manner. The preparation may be applied to the desired surface area without the use of the fingertips, making the procedure less messy than with most other types of topical preparations. Among the disadvantages to the use of topical aerosols are the difficulty in applying the medication to a small area and the greater expense associated with the aerosol package.

Vaginal and Rectal Aerosols

Aerosol foams containing estrogenic substances and contraceptive agents are commercially available. The foams are used intravaginally in the same manner as for creams. The aerosol package contains an inserter that is

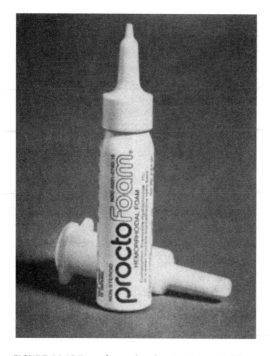

FIGURE 14.18 Foam for anal and perianal use. To fill the applicator, the foam container is shaken vigorously, held upright, and the applicator tip placed on the container opening. With the plunger of the applicator drawn out all the way, pressure is exerted on the container cap and foam fills the applicator tube. (Courtesy of Reed & Carnrick.)

filled with foam and the contents placed in the vagina through activation of the plunger. The foams are generally o/w emulsions resembling light creams. They are water miscible and nongreasy.

Some commercial rectal foams use inserters. One such product, ProctoFoam (Reed & Carnrick), contains pramoxine hydrochloride to relieve inflammatory anorectal disorders (Fig. 14.18).

PHARMACEUTICS CASE STUDY

Subjective

Working for an innovative pharmaceutical company, you have received a request to develop an oral liquid formulation for a new organ rejection drug. The drug must be formulated so that a 5-mg dose can be reasonably easily administered either as the dosage form or immediately after mixing with water or juice. The formulation should be stable and easy to manipulate. The problem is that the drug is not water soluble, but a solution dosage form is desired.

Objective

The drug has a molecular weight of 1015.2 and occurs as a white to off-white powder that is insoluble in water but freely soluble in benzyl alcohol, chloroform, acetone, and acetonitrile.

The drug may be prepared as an aqueous suspension or as a solution in a water-miscible liquid that can be diluted prior to administration. A reasonable dispersant liquid for the insoluble drug may include a blend of lecithin products that would form liposomes upon dilution in an aqueous vehicle. Some commercial blends occur as honey-colored fluids with a typical odor and nutty taste. These can be diluted with water, have densities of approximately 1 to 1.2, and viscosities in the range of 5000 mPas.

It may be wise to add a dispersant such as polysorbate 80 to aid in mixing when this is added to water or juice. Polysorbate 80 (Tween 80, polyoxyethylene 20 sorbitan

Pharmaceutics Case Study cont.

monooleate, $C_{64}H_{124}O_{26}$) has a molecular weight of 1310 and occurs as a yellow oily liquid with a characteristic odor and a warm, somewhat bitter taste. It has a specific gravity of 1.06 to 1.09, and its HLB is 15.0; it forms o/w emulsions. It is stable in the presence of electrolytes, weak acids, and weak bases. It should be stored in a well-closed, light-resistant container in a cool place (5).

Assessment

After viewing the options, you decide to select a solvent system for the drug and prepare it as a solution. The patient can obtain the dose and dilute it immediately prior to administration. This meets the criteria of stability and ease of administration.

You select a commercial dispersant liquid for oral use containing 50% phosphatidylcholine in propylene glycol, sunflower seed oil glycerides, soy acid, alcohol, and ascorbyl palmitate. This product is used as a dispersant, emulsifier, penetrant, and solubilizer for pharmaceuticals, creams, lotions, emulsions, and liposome preparations for dermatology. It is suitable for oral use.

Plan

You formulate the product as a 5-mg dose in 1 mL of the vehicle containing 0.5% polysorbate 80 in the described dispersant liquid. This will provide a stable, easy-to-use product.

For administration, the proper quantity of the oral liquid will be added to approximately 2 to 4 ounces of water or juice. The preparation should be vigorously stirred and taken at once. Various juices can be used depending on the preference of the patient.

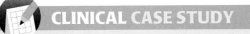

CLINICAL CASE STUDY

HPI: M. H. is a 31 y/o WF who presents to the pharmacy with a prescription for metronidazole. Upon questioning, the patient reveals that she just returned from an appointment with her gynecologist. She has been having symptoms that she describes as "an unusual yellowish smelly discharge with itching and burning." The patient continues, "At first I thought it was just another yeast infection, but the discharge seemed a little different. I did not want to use another OTC product that might not work, so I went to see my doctor." Her gynecologist informed her that she had trichomonas vaginitis, a sexually transmitted disease (STD). When handing the prescription to the pharmacist, she complains that she "hates this medicine. I don't like taking pills even if they aren't big. And they leave an awful taste

in my mouth." The pharmacist knows M. H. as a regular customer and decides to look up her profile to confirm that she had previously taken metronidazole. She also reviews M. H.'s past medical history.

PMH: Asthma since childhood
Vaginal yeast infections about once a year
Bacterial vaginosis in 2001
Miscarriage in 1999

SH: (+) EtOH: Drinks cocktails on weekends, occasionally wine at dinner
(−) Tobacco
(−) Illicit drugs

FH: Mother (+) for breast cancer
Father (+) for hypertension and hypercholesterolemia

Clinical Case Study cont.

Brother (+) for asthma

Allergies: NKDA

Meds: Advair 250/50 1 inhalation bid
Albuterol MDI prn
Gyne-Lotrimin 3 prn yeast
infections

Pharmaceutical Care Plan

S: Patient has vaginal symptoms, including itching, burning, and a yellowish, malodorous discharge. Patient complains about the size of the metronidazole tablets and its metallic taste.

O: The gynecologist has diagnosed trichomonas vaginitis. Previously the patient has been prescribed metronidazole oral tablets for bacterial vaginosis.

A: M. H. is a 31 y/o WF diagnosed with trichomonas vaginitis that is to be treated with oral metronidazole tablets. Although she is in a monogamous relationship, unprotected sex increases the risk of transmitting STDs, such as trichomonas. M. H.'s adherence to the metronidazole regimen is very important, because untreated vaginitis may progress to urethritis and/or cystitis. Worried that the patient may not adhere to her regimen, the pharmacist considers compounding a metronidazole suspension so that the patient will not have to take the tablets and will have an easier dosage form.

P: 1. The pharmacist offers the alternative of a extemporaneously prepared metronidazole suspension in lieu of the oral tablets. The patient agrees to try this option. So the pharmacist calls the patient's physician to seek permission to change the drug delivery system.

2. After securing permission to do so, the pharmacist decides to use metronidazole benzoate powder in lieu of metronidazole HCl, the active ingredient in the oral tablets. The benzoate form is relatively tasteless, which may also be a more suitable option for M. H.

even though the metallic taste will occur from the therapy after administration.

3. The first step in preparation of the suspension is a mathematical calculation to determine the equivalent dose of metronidazole benzoate. The pharmacist confirms that 200 mg of the benzoate ester is equivalent to 125 mg of the HCl salt. The prescribed dose of metronidazole HCl tablets is 250 mg tid for 7 days. Thus, the pharmacist calculates the equivalent metronidazole benzoate dose will be 400 mg tid for 7 days.

4. After weighing the required amount of metronidazole benzoate powder, the pharmacist triturates it in a mortar and pestle to minimize the particle size. The pharmacist selects Ora-Plus as the suspending agent and Ora-Sweet as the flavoring agent. The suspension will be compounded so that the final concentration (w/v) of metronidazole benzoate will be 400 mg/5 mL. With constant mixing, the pharmacist slowly adds Ora-Plus 50 mL to the metronidazole benzoate powder to create a slurry. The resultant suspension is transferred into a graduated cylinder and diluted with enough Ora-Sweet so that the total volume of the suspension is 105 mL. Before bringing the product to final volume, the pharmacist uses some Ora-Sweet to remove as much of the slurry from the mortar as possible.

After stirring the suspension, the contents are transferred into an appropriate-sized plastic bottle and the label with the appropriate information is affixed. The following auxiliary labels should also be affixed to the bottle: KEEP REFRIGERATED, SHAKE WELL BEFORE USING, FINISH THE ENTIRE COURSE OF THERAPY, AVOID ALCOHOLIC BEVERAGES, and TAKE WITH FOOD.

Clinical Case Study cont.

5. When dispensing the metronidazole suspension to the patient, the pharmacist counsels and instructs M. H. M. H. should take 1 teaspoonful by mouth 3 times daily for 7 consecutive days. The daily doses should be taken with food after each meal. The medication should be stored in the refrigerator when not being used, and because it is a suspension, shaken well before each dose. It is assumed that the suspension will be used up before the beyond-use date of 30 days. However, it is necessary for the pharmacist to label the product with the beyond-use date in the event that some is left over.

6. The pharmacist suggests that the medication be taken with food to help prevent stomach upset, nausea, and diarrhea. Although the benzoate form of metronidazole may help to lessen the bitter taste associated with its administration, the metallic taste may still occur after systemic absorption, and the patient should understand this. In addition, M. H. should be told about the interaction (disulfiram reaction) between metronidazole and alcohol. Alcohol must be avoided during therapy and for 72 hours after the last dose. This disulfiram reaction may result in severe flushing, headache, nausea,

vomiting, or chest and abdominal pain. M. H. should also be aware that the medication may darken her urine.

7. Because trichomonas vaginitis is a STD, M. H. must be educated to take certain precautions to prevent transmission and reinfection of herself. During treatment, M. H. should refrain from sexual intercourse. The importance of practicing safe sex (e.g., condom use) should be emphasized to prevent contracting STDs and other serious infections (e.g., HIV, hepatitis). In addition, M. H.'s sexual partner should be treated with metronidazole. Although he may be asymptomatic, there is an elevated risk that he is carrying the trichomonas organism and infecting M. H. during intercourse. Thus, with this prescription, her partner may or may not be treated. If the latter, it is important that the pharmacist tell M. H. not to share her medication with her sexual partner. She is to take a full course of therapy. If there is a primary treatment failure, it is likely that the male sexual partner will also be treated during the second course of therapy. Emphasis will be put on the importance of M. H. completing the full course of metronidazole therapy to prevent resistance, emergence, and recurrent infections.

REFERENCES

1. Heyd A, Dhabhar D. Particle shape effect on caking of coarse granulated antacid suspensions. Drug Cosmet Ind 1979;125:42.
2. Oral Liquid Pharmaceuticals. Wilmington: ICI Americas, 1975.
3. Chang RK. Formulation approaches for sustained-release oral suspensions. Pharm Tech 1992;16:134–136.
4. Allen LV. Prednisone oral suspension. US Pharmacist 1989;14:84.
5. Allen LV. Ketoconazole oral suspension. US Pharmacist 1993;18:98.
6. Bhargava HN, Narurkar A, Lieb LM. Using micro-emulsions for drug delivery. Pharm Tech 1987; 11:46.
7. Griffin WC. J Soc Cosmetics Chemists 1949;1:311; 1954;5:1.
8. Hansten PD, Horn JR. Drug Interactions, 6th ed. Philadelphia: Lea & Febiger, 1989;80.
9. Chiou WL. Aerosol propellants: cardiac toxicity and long biological half-life. JAMA 1974;227:658.
10. Cyr TD et al. Low first-spray drug content in albuterol metered-dose inhalers. Pharm Res 1991;8: 658–660.
11. Miller NC et al. Assessment of the twin impinger for size measurement of metered-dose inhaler sprays. Pharm Res 1992;9:1123–1127.

12. Ranucci JA, Chen FC. Phase Doppler anemometry: a technique for determining aerosol plume-particle size and velocity. Pharm Tech 1993;17:62–73.

13. Ranucci JA, Cooper D, Sethachutkul K. Effect of actuator design on metered-dose inhaler plume-particle size. Pharm Tech 1992;16:84–92.

14. Martonen TB, Katz IM. Deposition of aerosolized drugs within human lungs: effects of ventilatory parameters. Pharm Res 1993;10:871–878.

15. Martonen TB et al. Use of analytically defined estimates of aerosol respirable fraction to predict lung deposition patterns. Pharm Res 1992;9:1634–1639.

Parenterals

15

Chapter at a glance

Considered in this chapter are important pharmaceutical dosage forms with the common characteristic of sterility; that is, they are free from contaminating microorganisms. Among these sterile dosage forms are the various small- and large-volume injectable preparations, irrigation fluids intended to bathe body wounds or surgical openings, and dialysis solutions. Biologic preparations, including vaccines, toxoids, and antitoxins, also among this group are discussed in Chapter 16. Sterility in these preparations is essential because they are placed in direct contact with the internal body fluids or tissues, where infection can easily arise. Ophthalmic preparations, which are also prepared to be sterile, are discussed separately in Chapter 17.

Injections

Injections are sterile, pyrogen-free preparations intended to be administered parenterally. The term *parenteral* refers to the injectable routes of administration. It derives from the Greek words *para* (outside) and *enteron* (intestine) and denotes routes of administration other than the oral route. *Pyrogens*, fever-producing organic substances arising from microbial contamination, are responsible for many of the febrile reactions in patients following intravenous injection. Pyrogens and the determination of their presence in parenteral preparations are discussed later in this chapter. In general, the parenteral routes are used when rapid drug action is desired, as in emergencies; when the patient is uncooperative, unconscious, or unable to accept or tolerate oral medication; or when the drug itself is ineffective by other routes. With the exception of insulin injections, which are commonly *self*-administered by diabetic patients, most injections are administered by the physician, physician's assistant, or nurse in the course of medical treatment. Thus injections are employed mostly in the hospital, extended care facility, and clinic and less frequently in the home. An exception is *home health care* programs, in which health professionals pay scheduled visits to patients at home, providing needed treatment, including intravenous medications. These programs en-

able patients who do not require or are unable to pay for more expensive hospitalization to remain at home while receiving appropriate medical care. The pharmacist supplies injectable preparations to the physician and nurse as required for use in the institutional setting, clinic, office, or home health care program.

Perhaps the earliest injectable drug to receive official recognition was the hypodermic morphine solution, which appeared first in the 1874 addendum to the 1867 *British Pharmacopeia*, and in 1888 in the first edition of the *National Formulary of the United States* (NF). Today, literally hundreds of drugs and drug products are available for parenteral administration.

Parenteral Routes of Administration

Drugs may be injected into almost any organ or area of the body, including the joints (*intra-articular*), joint fluid area (*intrasynovial*), spinal column (*intraspinal*), spinal fluid (*intrathecal*), arteries (*intra-arterial*), and in an emergency, even the heart (*intracardiac*). However, most injections go into a vein (*intravenous, IV*), into a muscle (*intramuscular, IM*), into the skin (*intradermal, ID, intracutaneous*), or under the skin (*subcutaneous, SC, sub-Q, SQ, hypodermic, hypo*) (Fig. 15.1).

Intravenous Route

Intravenous injection of drugs had its scientific origin in 1656 in the experiments of Sir Christopher Wren, architect of St. Paul's Cathedral and amateur physiologist. Using a bladder and quill for a syringe and needle, he injected wine, ale, opium, and other substances into the veins of dogs and studied their effects. Intravenous medication was first given to humans by Johann Daniel Major of Kiel in 1662 but was abandoned for a period because of thrombosis and embolism in the patients so treated. The invention of the hypodermic syringe toward the middle of the 19th century created new interest in intravenous techniques, and toward the turn of the 20th century, intravenous administration of solutions of sodium chloride and glucose became popu-

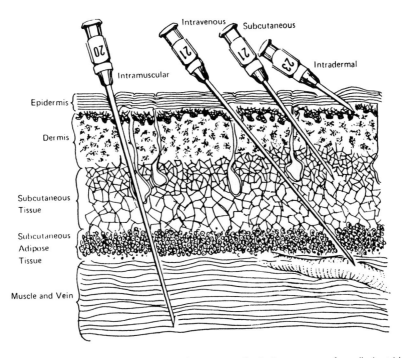

FIGURE 15.1 Routes of parenteral administration. Numbers on needles indicate gauge of needle (outside diameter of shaft). (Reprinted with permission from Turco S, King RE. Sterile dosage forms: their preparation and clinical applications, 3rd ed. Lea & Febiger, 1987.)

lar. Today intravenous administration of drugs is a routine occurrence in the hospital, although recognized dangers are still associated with the practice. Thrombus and embolus formation may be induced by intravenous needles and catheters, and the possibility of particulate matter in parenteral solutions poses a concern.

Intravenous drugs provide rapid action compared with other routes of administration, and because drug absorption is not a factor, optimum blood levels may be achieved with accuracy and immediacy not possible by other routes. In emergencies, intravenous administration of a drug may be lifesaving because of the placement of the drug directly into the circulation and the prompt action that ensues. On the negative side, once a drug is administered intravenously, it cannot be retrieved. In the case of an adverse reaction to the drug, for instance, the drug cannot be easily removed from the circulation, as it could, for example, by induction of vomiting after oral administration of the same drug. Furthermore, the intravenous dose may differ greatly from the oral

dose. Thus, great care must be taken to prevent overdosing or underdosing. The beta-blocker drug class, such as metoprolol, is a perfect example of the vast differences between intravenous (three bolus injections of 5 mg each at about 2-minute intervals) and oral dosing (100 mg/day).

Although most superficial veins are suitable for venipuncture, the veins of the antecubital area (in front of the elbow) are usually selected for direct intravenous injection. The veins in this location are large, superficial, and easy to see and enter. Most clinicians insert the needle with the bevel facing upward, at the most acute angle possible with the vein, to ensure that the direction of flow of the injectable is that of the flow of the blood. Strict aseptic precautions must be taken at all times to avoid risk of infection. Not only are the injectable solutions sterile, the syringes and needles must also be sterilized, and the point of entrance must be disinfected to reduce the chance of carrying bacteria from the skin into the blood via the needle. Before injection, the health care worker must withdraw the plunger of the syringe or squeeze a special bulb found on most intravenous sets to ensure that the needle has been properly seated. A backflow of blood into the administration set or syringe indicates proper placement of the needle in the vein.

Both small and large volumes of drug solutions may be administered intravenously. The use of 1000-mL containers of solutions for intravenous infusion is commonplace in the hospital. These solutions, containing such agents as nutrients, plasma volume expanders, electrolytes, amino acids, and other therapeutic agents, are administered through an indwelling needle or catheter by continuous infusion. The infusion or flow rate may be adjusted according to the needs of the patient. Generally, flow rates for intravenous fluids are expressed in milliliters per hour and range from 42 to 150 mL/hour. Lower rates are used for keep-open (KO, KVO) lines. For intravenous infusion, the needle or catheter is placed in a prominent vein of the forearm or leg and taped firmly to the patient so that it will not slip from place during infusion. The main hazard of intravenous infusion is thrombus formation induced by the catheter or needle touching the wall of the vein. Thrombi are most likely when the infusion solution is irritating to the biologic tissues. A *thrombus* is a blood clot formed within the blood vessel (or heart), usually because of slowing of the circulation or an alteration of the blood or vessel wall. Once such a clot circulates, it becomes an *embolus*, carried by the blood stream until it lodges in a blood vessel, obstructing it and resulting in a block or occlusion referred to as an *embolism*. Such an obstruction may be a critical hazard to the patient, depending on the site and severity of the obstruction.

Intravenous drugs ordinarily must be in aqueous solution; they must mix with the circulating blood and not precipitate from solution. Such an event can lead to pulmonary microcapillary occlusion and blockage of blood flow. Intravenous fat emulsions (e.g., Intralipid, 10, 20, 30%, Clintec; Liposyn II, 10, 20%, Abbott; Liposyn III, 10, 20, 30%, Abbott) have gained acceptance for use as a source of calories and essential fatty acids for patients re-

quiring parenteral nutrition for extended periods, usually more than 5 days. The product contains up to 30% soybean oil emulsified with egg yolk phospholipids in a vehicle of glycerin in water for injection. The emulsion is administered via a peripheral vein or by central venous infusion.

Naturally, the intravenous route is used for blood transfusions, and it also serves as the point of exit for removal of blood from patients for diagnostic work and for donation.

In the late 1980s, automated intravenous delivery systems for intermittent self-administration of analgesics became commercially available. Patient-controlled analgesia (PCA) has been used to control the pain associated with a variety of surgical procedures, labor, sickle cell crisis, and cancer. For patients with chronic malignant pain, PCA allows a greater degree of ambulation and independence (1).

The typical PCA device includes a syringe or chamber that contains the analgesic drug and a programmable electromechanical unit. The unit, which may be compact enough to be worn on a belt or carried in a pocket (e.g., WalkMed PCA, McKinley, Wheat Ridge, CO), controls the delivery of drug by advancing a piston when the patient presses a button. The drug can be loaded into the device by a health care professional or dispensed from preloaded cartridges available from the manufacturer. The devices deliver intravenous bolus injections to produce rapid analgesia, along with slower infusion to produce steady-state concentrations for sustained pain control.

The advantage of the PCA is its ability to provide constant and uniform analgesia. The typical injection of an opioid into a depot muscular site may result in variable absorption, leading to unpredictable blood concentrations. Furthermore, these injections are usually given when needed and are often inadequate to treat the pain. The PCA can prevent pharmacokinetic and pharmacodynamic differences between patients from interfering with the effectiveness of analgesia. Because opioid kinetics differ greatly among patients, the rates of infusion must be tailored (2).

The PCA also permits patients to medicate themselves for breakthrough pain. It eliminates the delay between the perception of pain and receiving the medication. Furthermore, it saves nursing time. Otherwise, the nurse must check analgesic orders given by the physician, sign out the pain reliever from a controlled, locked location, and then administer the medication to the patient.

The PCA also provides better pain control with less side effects by minimizing the variations between suboptimal pain relief and overuse of opioids. When the side effect profile of PCA patients is compared to those of patients maintained on intramuscular opioids, nausea, sedation, and respiratory depression occur less often in the PCA group. Finally, patients accept the PCA as a favorable mode of relief, perhaps because of the sense of being in control and taking an active part in their pain relief.

PCA devices can be used for intravenous, subcutaneous, or epidural administration. Usually, these devices are either *demand dosing* (a fixed dose of drug is injected intermittently) or *constant-rate infusion plus demand dosing* (2). Regardless of type used, the physician or nurse establishes the loading dose, the rate of background infusion, dose per demand, lockout interval (minimum time between demand doses), and maximum dosage over a specified time. Figure 15.2 demonstrates the PCA Plus II (Lifecare 4100) infuser. With this device, the patient pushes a button on a pendant to deliver a prescribed quantity of the analgesic.

Intramuscular Route

Intramuscular injections of drugs provide effects that are less rapid but generally longer lasting than those obtained from intravenous administration (3). Aqueous or oleaginous solutions or suspensions of drug substances may be administered intramuscularly. Depending on the type of preparation, absorption rates vary widely. Drugs in solution are more rapidly absorbed than those in suspension, and drugs in aqueous preparations are more rapidly absorbed than oleaginous preparations. The physical type of preparation is based on the properties of the drug itself and on the therapeutic goals.

Intramuscular injections are performed deep into the skeletal muscles. The point of in-

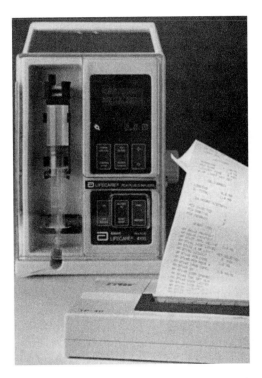

FIGURE 15.2 PCA Plus II (LifeCare 4100): patient-controlled analgesic infuser. (Courtesy of Abbott Hospital Products Division.)

jection should be as far as possible from major nerves and blood vessels. Injuries to patients from intramuscular injection usually are related to the point at which the needle entered and where the medication was deposited. Such injuries include paralysis resulting from neural damage, abscess, cyst, embolism, hematoma, sloughing of the skin, and scarring.

In adults, the upper outer quadrant of the gluteus maximus is the most frequently used site for intramuscular injection. In infants, the gluteal area is small and composed primarily of fat, not muscle. The muscle is poorly developed. An injection in this area may come dangerously close to the sciatic nerve, especially if the child is resisting the injection and squirming or fighting. Thus, in infants and young children, the deltoid muscles of the upper arm or the midlateral muscles of the thigh are preferred. An injection in the upper or lower portion of the deltoid would be well away from the radial nerve. The deltoid may also be used in adults, but the pain is more noticeable here than in the gluteal area. If a series of injections are to be given, the injection site is usually varied. To be certain that a blood vessel has not been entered, the clinician may aspirate slightly on the syringe following insertion of the needle to observe any blood entering the syringe. The volume of medication that may be conveniently administered by the intramuscular route is limited, generally to a maximum of 5 mL in the gluteal region and 2 mL in the deltoid of the arm.

The Z-track technique is useful for intramuscular injections of medications that stain upper tissue, such as iron dextran injection, and those that irritate tissue, such as diazepam, by sealing these medications in the lower muscle. Because of its staining qualities, iron dextran must be injected only into the muscle mass of the upper outer quadrant of the buttock. The skin is displaced laterally prior to injection, then the needle is inserted and syringe aspirated, and the injection performed slowly and smoothly. The needle is then withdrawn and the skin released. This creates a Z pattern that blocks infiltration of medication into the subcutaneous tissue. The injection is 2 to 3 inches deep, and a 20- to 22-gauge needle is used. To reduce further any staining of upper tissue, usually one needle is used to withdraw the iron dextran from its ampul and replaced with another for the injection.

Subcutaneous Route

The subcutaneous route may be used for injection of small amounts of medication. Injection of a drug beneath the skin is usually made in the loose interstitial tissue of the outer upper arm, the anterior thigh, or the lower abdomen. The site of injection is usually rotated when injections are frequently given, as with daily insulin injections. Prior to injection, the skin at the injection site should be thoroughly cleansed. The maximum amount of medication that can be comfortably injected subcutaneously is about 1.3 mL, and amounts greater than 2 mL will most likely cause painful pressure. Syringes with up to 3-mL capacities and 24- to 26-gauge needles are used. These needles have cannula lengths of three-eighths of

an inch to an inch. Most typically, subcutaneous insulin needles are 25 to 30 gauge with length of five-sixteenths to five-eighths of an inch. Upon insertion, if blood appears in the syringe, a new site should be selected.

Irritating drugs and those in thick suspension may produce induration, sloughing, or abscess and may be painful. Such preparations are not suitable for subcutaneous injection.

Intradermal Route

A number of substances may be effectively injected into the corium, the more vascular layer of the skin just beneath the epidermis. These substances include various agents for diagnostic determinations, desensitization, or immunization. The usual site for intradermal injection is the anterior forearm. A short (three-eighths of an inch) and narrow (23- to 26-gauge) needle is usually employed. The needle is inserted horizontally into the skin with the bevel facing up. The injection is made with the bevel just disappearing into the corium. Usually only about 0.1 mL may be administered in this manner.

Specialized Access

When it is necessary to administer repeated injections over time, it is prudent to employ devices that provide continued access and reduce pain associated with administration.

Several types of central venous catheters are used in institutions and on an outpatient basis for a variety of parenteral medications (e.g., cancer chemotherapy, long-term antibiotic therapy, total parenteral nutrition solutions). They can remain in place for a few days to several months. When not in use, they require heparinization to maintain patency of the catheter lumen.

The use of indwelling plastic catheters reduces the need for multiple punctures during intravenous therapy. Composed of polyvinyl chloride, Teflon, and polyethylene, these should be radiopaque to ensure that they are visible on radiographs. Usually, these must be removed within 48 hours after insertion. The choice of catheter depends on several factors, including length of time of the infusion, purpose of the infusion, and condition and availability of the veins. Three types of catheters are available: plain plastic, catheter over needle or catheter outside needle, and catheter inside needle.

Implantable devices provide long-term venous access in various diseases. Broviac and Hickman catheters are notable examples. These do carry a risk of morbidity, including fracture of the catheters, entrance site infection, and catheter sepsis. Developed to overcome catheter complications, they are designed to provide repeated access to the infusion site. The delivery catheter can be placed in a vein, cavity, artery, or the central nervous system. A Huber-point needle allows access through the skin into a self-sealing silicone plug positioned in the center of the portal.

Official Types of Injections

According to the USP, injectable materials are separated into five general types. These may contain buffers, preservatives, and other added substances.

1. *Injection:* Liquid preparations that are drug substances or solutions thereof (e.g., Insulin Injection, USP).
2. *For injection:* Dry solids that upon addition of suitable vehicles yield solutions conforming in all respects to the requirements for injections (e.g., Cefuroxime for Injection, USP).
3. *Injectable emulsion:* Liquid preparation of drug substance dissolved or dispersed in a suitable emulsion medium (e.g., Propofol, USP).
4. *Injectable suspension:* Liquid preparation of solid suspended in a suitable liquid medium (e.g., Methylprednisolone Acetate Suspension, USP).
5. *For injectable suspension:* Dry solid that upon addition of suitable vehicle yields preparation conforming in all respects to the requirements for *injectable suspensions* (e.g., Imipenem and Cilastatin for Injectable Suspension, USP).

The form in which the manufacturer prepares a given drug for parenteral use depends on the nature of the drug itself with respect to its physical and chemical characteristics and on certain therapeutic considerations. Generally, if a drug is unstable in solution, it may be prepared as a dry powder intended for reconstitution with the proper solvent at the time of administration, or it may be prepared as a suspension. If the drug is unstable in water, that solvent may be replaced in part or totally by a solvent in which the drug is insoluble. If the drug is insoluble in water, an injection may be prepared as an aqueous suspension or as a solution in a suitable nonaqueous solvent, such as a vegetable oil. If an aqueous solution is desired, a water-soluble salt form of the insoluble drug is frequently prepared. Aqueous or blood-miscible solutions may be injected directly into the blood stream. Blood-immiscible liquids, such as oleaginous injections and suspensions, can interrupt the normal flow of blood, and their use is generally restricted to other than intravenous administration. The onset and duration of action of a drug may be somewhat controlled by its chemical form, the physical state of the injection (solution or suspension), and the vehicle. Drugs that are very soluble in body fluids generally have the most rapid absorption and onset of action. Thus, drugs in aqueous solution have a more rapid onset of action than do drugs in oleaginous solution. Drugs in aqueous suspension are also more rapid acting than drugs in oleaginous suspension because of the greater miscibility of the aqueous preparation with the body fluids after injection and the more rapid contact of the drug particles with the body fluids. Oftentimes long action is desired to reduce the frequency of injections. These long-acting injections are called repository or depot preparations.

The solutions and suspensions of drugs intended for injection are prepared in the same general manner as solutions (Chapter 13) and disperse systems (Chapter 14), with the following differences:

1. Solvents or vehicles must meet special purity and other standards ensuring their safety by injection.
2. The use of added substances, such as buffers, stabilizers, and antimicrobial preservatives,

fall under specific guidelines of use and are restricted in certain parenteral products. The use of coloring agents is strictly prohibited.

3. Parenteral products are always sterilized, meet sterility standards, and must be pyrogen free.
4. Parenteral solutions must meet compendial standards for particulate matter.
5. Parenteral products must be prepared in environmentally controlled areas, under strict sanitation standards, and by personnel specially trained and clothed to maintain the sanitation standards.
6. Parenteral products are packaged in special hermetic containers of specific and high quality. Special quality control procedures are used to ensure hermetic seal and sterile condition.
7. Each container of an injection is filled to a volume in slight excess of the labeled volume to be withdrawn. This overfill permits ease of withdrawal and administration of the labeled volumes.
8. The volume of injection permitted in multiple-dose containers is restricted, as are the types of containers (single-dose or multiple-dose) that may be used for certain injections.
9. Specific labeling regulations apply to injections.
10. Sterile powders intended for solution or suspension immediately prior to injection are frequently packaged as *lyophilized* or freeze-dried powders to permit ease of solution or suspension upon the addition of the solvent or vehicle.

Solvents and Vehicles for Injections

The most frequently used solvent in the large-scale manufacturer of injections is *Water for Injection, USP*. This water is purified by distillation or by reverse osmosis and meets the same standards for the presence of total solids as does *Purified Water, USP*—that is, not more than 1 mg/100 mL Water for Injection, USP—and may not contain added substances. Although water for injection is not required to be sterile, it must be pyrogen free. The water is intended to be

used in the manufacture of injectable products to be sterilized after preparation. Water for injection should be stored in tight containers at temperatures below or above the range in which microbial growth occurs. Water for injection is intended to be used within 24 hours after collection. Naturally, the water should be collected in sterile and pyrogen-free containers. The containers are usually glass or glass lined.

Sterile Water for Injection, USP, is packaged in single-dose containers not larger than 1 L. As with water for injection, it must be pyrogen free but does have an allowable endotoxin level, not more than 0.25 USP endotoxin units per milliliter. Also, it may not contain any antimicrobial agent or other added substance. This water may contain slightly more total solids than water for injection because of the leaching of solids from the glass-lined tanks during sterilization. This water is intended to be used as a solvent, vehicle, or diluent for already sterilized and packaged injectable medications. The 1-L bottles cannot be administered intravenously because they have no tonicity. Thus, they are used for reconstitution of multiple antibiotics. In use, the water is aseptically added to the vial of medication to prepare the desired injection. For instance, a suitable injection may be prepared from the dry powder Sterile Ampicillin Sodium, USP, by aseptic addition of sterile water for injection.

Bacteriostatic Water for Injection, USP, is sterile water for injection containing one or more suitable antimicrobial agents. It is packaged in prefilled syringes or in vials containing not more than 30 mL of the water. The container label must state the names and proportions of the antimicrobial agent or agents. The water is employed as a sterile vehicle in the preparation of small volumes of injectable preparations. Theoretically, presence of the bacteriostatic agent gives the flexibility for multiple-dose vials. If the first person to withdraw medication inadvertently contaminates the vial contents, the preservative will destroy the microorganism, although there has been debate on how much protection the antimicrobial agent can provide in a multiple-dose vial (4). Because of the presence of antimicrobial agents, the water must be used only in parenterals that are administered in small volumes. Its use in parenterals administered in large volume is restricted by the excessive and perhaps toxic amounts of the antimicrobial agents that would be injected along with the medication. Generally, if more than 5 mL of solvent is required, sterile water for injection rather than bacteriostatic water for injection is preferred. In using bacteriostatic water for injection, due regard must also be given to the chemical compatibility of the bacteriostatic agent or agents with the particular medicinal agent being dissolved or suspended.

USP labeling requirements demand that the label state NOT FOR USE IN NEONATES. This statement was the result of problems encountered with neonates and toxicity of the bacteriostat, that is, benzyl alcohol. This toxicity results from the high cumulative amounts (milligrams per kilogram) of benzyl alcohol and the limited detoxification capacity of the neonate liver. This solution has not been reported to cause problems in older infants, children, or adults.

Benzyl alcohol poisoning is recognized as gasping syndrome. In one study, 10 premature infants developed this clinical syndrome characterized by the development of multiorgan failure and eventually died (5). The typical clinical course included metabolic acidosis, respiratory distress requiring mechanical ventilation, central nervous system dysfunction, hyperactivity, hypotonia, depression of the sensorium, apnea, seizure, coma, intraventricular hemorrhage, hepatic and renal failure, and eventual cardiovascular collapse and death. In the study, the amount of benzyl alcohol received ranged from 99 to 234 mg/kg/day. Based on the concentration of 0.9% benzyl alcohol in the bacteriostatic water for injection and sodium chloride injection, death resulted from as little as 11 mL/kg/day.

Following toxicity reports and the deaths of infants in the early 1980s, the FDA issued a very strong recommendation to stop the use of fluids preserved with benzyl alcohol for use in neonates as a flush solution or to reconstitute medications.

Sodium Chloride Injection, USP, is a sterile isotonic solution of sodium chloride in water for injection. It contains no antimicrobial agents but has approximately 154 mEq each of sodium and chloride ions per liter. It may be used as a sterile vehicle in solutions or suspensions of drugs for parenteral administration.

Besides its use to reconstitute medications for injection, sodium chloride injection is frequently used as a catheter or intravenous line flush to maintain patency. Catheters or intravenous lines are constantly used to infuse fluids and intravenous medications and draw blood for laboratory analysis, among others. Usually 2 mL is used to flush the line after each use or every 8 hours if the line is not used.

Bacteriostatic Sodium Chloride Injection, USP, is a sterile isotonic solution of sodium chloride in water for injection. It contains one or more suitable antimicrobial agents, which must be specified on the labeling. Sodium chloride 0.9% renders the solution isotonic. For the reasons noted for bacteriostatic water for injection, this solution may not be packaged in containers larger than 30 mL. When this solution is used as a vehicle, care must be exercised to ensure compatibility of the added medicinal agent with the preservative or preservatives and with the sodium chloride.

Bacteriostatic sodium chloride injection is also used to flush a catheter or intravenous line to maintain its patency. When used in only small quantities for flushing lines and reconstituting medications, the amount of benzyl alcohol is negligible and safe. But in neonates, especially premature infants with very low birth weights, accumulation of benzoic acid and unmetabolized benzyl alcohol may occur as a result of liver immaturity. Because of their low physical weight, their acute illness and consequent need for medications, and the frequent use of the umbilical catheter for various purposes, these patients may receive much more flush solution relative to their body weight than adults. Thus, bacteriostatic sodium chloride injection also carries the warning NOT FOR USE IN NEONATES.

Suffice it to say that benzyl alcohol may be present in other parenteral medications, and the pharmacist must be vigilant for its inappropriate use in neonates. Generally speaking, however, the amount of benzyl alcohol received through this means is negligible compared to the amount received from flush solutions. Preferably, the medication is available in a preservative-free formulation (i.e., single-use dose), and that should be used. However, if such a formulation is not available and there is no alternative, a medication preserved with benzyl alcohol may still be used if the physician's clinical judgment is that the risk-to-benefit ratio is appropriate.

Ringer's Injection, USP, is a sterile solution of sodium chloride, potassium chloride, and calcium chloride in water for injection. The three agents are present in concentrations similar to those of physiologic fluids. Ringer's is employed as a vehicle for other drugs or alone as an electrolyte replenisher and plasma volume expander. *Lactated Ringer's Injection, USP*, has different quantities of the three salts in Ringer's injection, and it contains sodium lactate. This injection is a fluid and electrolyte replenisher and a systemic alkalizer.

Nonaqueous Vehicles

Although an aqueous vehicle is generally preferred for an injection, it may be precluded by the limited water solubility of a medicinal substance or its susceptibility to hydrolysis. When such physical or chemical factors limit the use of a wholly aqueous vehicle, the pharmaceutical formulator must turn to one or more nonaqueous vehicles.

The selected vehicle must be nonirritating, nontoxic in the amounts administered, and not sensitizing. Like water, it must not exert a pharmacologic activity of its own, nor may it adversely affect the activity of the medicinal agent. In addition, the physical and chemical properties of the solvent or vehicle must be considered, evaluated, and determined to be suitable for the task at hand. Among the many considerations are the solvent's physical and chemical stability at various pH levels, viscosity, which must be such as to allow ease of injection (suitable for use in syringes); fluidity, which must be maintained over a fairly wide temperature range; boiling point, which should be sufficiently high to permit heat sterilization; miscibility with body fluids; low va-

por pressure to avoid problems during heat sterilization; and constant purity or ease of purification and standardization. No single solvent is free of limitations; hence, cross-consideration and assessment of each solvent's advantages and disadvantages help the formulator determine the most appropriate solvent for a given preparation. Among the nonaqueous solvents employed in parenteral products are fixed vegetable oils, glycerin, polyethylene glycols, propylene glycol, alcohol, and a number of less often used agents, including ethyl oleate, isopropyl myristate, and dimethyl acetamide. These and other nonaqueous vehicles may be used provided they are safe in the amounts administered and do not interfere with the therapeutic efficacy of the preparation or with its response to prescribed assays and tests.

The United States Pharmacopeia (USP) specifies restrictions on the fixed vegetable oils in parenteral products. For one thing, they must remain clear when cooled to 10°C (50°F) to ensure the stability and clarity of the injectable product during refrigeration. The oils must not contain mineral oil or paraffin, as these materials are not absorbed by body tissues. The fluidity of a vegetable oil generally depends on the proportion of unsaturated fatty acids, such as oleic acid, to saturated acids, such as stearic acid. Oils to be employed in injections must meet officially stated requirements of iodine number and saponification number.

Although the toxicity of vegetable oils is generally considered to be relatively low, some patients exhibit allergic reactions to specific oils. Thus, when vegetable oils are employed in parenteral products, the label must state the specific oil. The most commonly used fixed oils in injections are corn oil, cottonseed oil, peanut oil, and sesame oil. Castor oil and olive oil have been used on occasion (Physical Pharmacy Capsule 15.1).

By selective employment of solvent or vehicle, a pharmacist can prepare injectable preparations as solutions or suspensions in either an aqueous or nonaqueous vehicle. For the most part, oleaginous injections are administered intramuscularly. They must not be administered

Colligative Properties of Drugs

Drug molecules have properties that are often divided into additive, constitutive, or colligative.

Additive properties depend on the total contribution of the atoms in the molecule or on the sum of the properties of the constituents of the solution. An example is molecular weight.

Constitutive properties depend on the arrangement and to a lesser extent the number and kind of atoms in a molecule. Examples are refraction of light, electrical properties, and surface and interfacial properties.

Colligative properties depend primarily on the number of particles in solution. Example properties include changes in vapor pressure, boiling point, freezing point, and osmotic pressure. These values should be approximately equal for equimolar concentrations of drugs.

LOWERING OF VAPOR PRESSURE

A vapor in equilibrium with its pure liquid at a constant temperature will exert *vapor pressure*. When a solute is added to the pure liquid, it will alter the tendency of the molecules to escape the original liquid. In an ideal solution or one that is very dilute, the partial vapor pressure of one component (p_1) is proportional to the mole fraction of molecules (N_1) of that component in the mixture:

$$p_1 = N_1 p^\circ_1$$

where p°_1 is the vapor pressure of the pure component.

EXAMPLE 1

What is the partial vapor pressure of a solution containing 50 g dextrose in 1000 mL of water? The vapor pressure of water is given as 23.76 mm Hg.

1. (50 g dextrose)/(MW of 180) = 0.28 moles of dextrose
2. (1000 g water)/MW of 18) = 55.56 moles of water
3. 0.28 + 55.56 = 55.84 total moles
4. (55.56)/(55.84) = 0.995 mole fraction of water
5. p_1 = (0.995)(23.76 mm Hg) = 23.64 mm Hg

The vapor pressure of the solution is 23.64 mm Hg. The decrease in vapor pressure by the addition of the 50 g dextrose is 23.76 − 23.64 = 0.12 mm Hg.

INCREASE IN BOILING POINT

The *boiling point* of a liquid is the temperature at which the vapor pressure of the liquid comes into equilibrium with the atmospheric pressure. The vapor pressure is reduced when a nonvolatile solute is added to a solvent, so the solution must reach a higher temperature to reestablish the equilibrium, hence an increase in the boiling point. This is described in the following equation:

$$\Delta T_b = k_b m$$

where

ΔT_b is the change in boiling point,
k_b is the molar elevation constant of water, and
m is the molality of the solute.

Physical Pharmacy Capsule 15.1 cont.

EXAMPLE 2

What is the boiling point elevation of a solution containing 50 g dextrose in 1000 mL of water? The molal elevation constant of water is 0.51.

1. (50 g dextrose)/(MW of 180) = 0.28 moles of dextrose in 1000 mL of water or 0.28 molal solution.
2. ΔT_b = (0.51) (0.28) = 0.143°C.

DECREASE IN FREEZING POINT

The *freezing point* of a pure liquid is the temperature at which the solid and liquid phases are in equilibrium at 1 atmosphere. The freezing point of a solution is the temperature at which the solid phase of pure solvent and the liquid phase of solution are in equilibrium at 1 atmosphere pressure. When a solute is added to a solvent, the decrease in freezing point is proportional to the concentration of the solute. The relationship is described by the following equation:

$$\Delta T_f = k_f m$$

where

ΔT_f is the change in freezing point,
k_f is the molal freezing point depression constant of water, and
m is the molality of the solute.

EXAMPLE 3

What is the decrease in freezing point of a solution containing 50 g dextrose in 1000 mL of water? The molal elevation constant of water is −1.86°C.

1. (50 g dextrose)/(MW of 180) = 0.28 moles of dextrose in 1000 mL of water or 0.28 molal solution.
2. ΔT_f = (−1.86) (0.28) = −0.52°C.

OSMOTIC PRESSURE

The pressure that must be applied to a more concentrated solution to prevent the flow of pure solvent into the solution separated by a semipermeable membrane is called the *osmotic pressure*. This relationship can be expressed as follows:

$$PV = nRT$$

where

P is the pressure (atm),
V is the volume (L),
n is number of moles of solute,
R is the gas constant (0.082 L-atm/mole deg), and
T is the absolute temperature in °C.

EXAMPLE 4

What is the osmotic pressure of 50 g dextrose in 1000 mL of water at room temperature (25°C)?

1. (50 g dextrose)/(MW of 180) = 0.28 moles of dextrose
2. 273°C + 25°C = 298°C

Physical Pharmacy Capsule 15.1 cont.

3. Volume will be 1 L
4. $P = [(0.28)(0.082)(298)]/(1) = 6.84$ atm

Deviations from reality in these ideal examples of colligative properties are explained by the use of the Van't Hoff term i, which considers that electrolytes exert more pressure than nonelectrolytes and is related to the number of ionic species present. These deviations may be caused by ionic interaction, degree of dissociation of weak electrolytes, or associations of nonelectrolytes.

MILLIEQUIVALENTS

An *equivalent weight* is the atomic weight in grams of a material divided by its valence, or charge. Milliequivalents are related to equivalents, which are also considered measures of combining power, chemical activity, or chemical reactivity. Equivalency, or milliequivalency, takes into consideration the total number of ionic charges in solution and the valence of the ions. Normally, plasma contains about 155 milliequivalents of cations and anions in solution. The number of cations is always matched by the number of anions.

A *milliequivalent* is the quantity in milligrams of a solute equal to 1/1000 of its gram-equivalent weight. Consider the following example.

EXAMPLE 5

What is the milliequivalent weight of sodium?

1. The atomic weight of sodium is 23.
2. The valence of sodium is +1.
3. The equivalent weight of sodium is (23 g)/(1) = 23 g.
4. The milliequivalent weight of sodium is (23 g)/1000 = 0.023 g, or 23 mg.
5. Therefore, one milliequivalent of sodium weighs 23 mg.

Milliequivalent calculations are commonly required in pharmacy practice today. The following are some examples.

EXAMPLE 6

How many milliequivalents of potassium chloride are in a solution containing 74.5 mg/mL?

1. The atomic weight of potassium is 39, and that of chloride is 35.5. The combined molecular weight is 74.5.
2. Since the valence is 1 for both potassium and chloride, the equivalent weight for potassium chloride is 74.5 g and the milliequivalent weight is 74.5 mg.
3. The solution contains 74.5 mg/mL, and the milliequivalent weight is 74.5 mg; therefore, there is 1 mEq/mL of potassium chloride in the solution.

EXAMPLE 7

How many milliequivalents of calcium are in 10 mL of 10% calcium chloride ($CaCl_2 \cdot 2 H_2O$) solution?

1. The formula weight for calcium chloride dihydrate is 147.
2. The equivalent weight is 147/2 = 73.5, since calcium is divalent.
3. Therefore, 1 milliequivalent of calcium chloride weighs 73.5 mg.

Physical Pharmacy Capsule 15.1 cont.

4. (10 mL) (10%) = 1 g, or 1000 mg, of calcium chloride dihydrate.
5. (1000 mg)/(73.5 mg) = 13.6 mEq of calcium chloride dihydrate, which also is 13.6 mEq of calcium.

EXAMPLE 8

How many milliequivalents of sodium are contained in a 1-L bag of 0.9% sodium chloride?

1. (1000 mL) (0.009) = 9 g, or 9000 mg.
2. The formula weight for sodium chloride is 23 + 35.5 = 58.5.
3. The milliequivalent weight for sodium chloride is 58.5 mg.
4. (9000)/(58.5) = 153.8 mEq, or 154 mEq.

In these cases, since sodium chloride is monovalent, there is 154 mEq of sodium, 154 mEq of chloride, or 154 mEq of sodium chloride.

OSMOLALITY AND TONICITY

Biologic systems are compatible with solutions having similar osmotic pressures, that is, an equivalent number of dissolved species. For example, red blood cells, blood plasma, and 0.9% sodium chloride solution contain approximately the same number of solute particles per unit volume and are termed iso-osmotic and isotonic.

If solutions contain more (hypertonic) or fewer (hypotonic) dissolved species, it may be necessary to alter the composition of the solution to bring them into an acceptable range.

An osmol (Osm) is related to a mole (gram molecular weight) of the molecules or ions in solution. One mole of glucose (180 g) dissolved in 1000 g of water has an osmolality of 1 Osm, or 1000 mOsm/kg of water. One mole of sodium chloride (23 + 35.5 = 58.5 g) dissolved in 1000 g of water has an osmolality of almost 2000 mOsm, since sodium chloride dissociates into almost two particles per molecule. In other words, a 1-molal solution of sodium chloride is equivalent to a 2-molal solution of dextrose.

Normal serum osmolality values are in the vicinity of 285 mOsm/kg (often expressed as 285 mOsm/L). Ranges may include values from about 275 to 300 mOsm/L. Pharmaceuticals should be close to this value to minimize discomfort on application to the eyes or nose or on injection.

Some solutions are iso-osmotic but not isotonic. This is because the physiology of the cell membranes must be considered. For example, the cell membrane of the red blood cell is not semipermeable to all drugs. It allows ammonium chloride, alcohol, boric acid, glycerin, propylene glycol, and urea to diffuse freely. In the eye, the cell membrane is semipermeable to boric acid, and a 1.9% solution of boric acid is an isotonic ophthalmic solution. But even though a 1.9% solution of boric acid is isotonic with the eye and is iso-osmotic, it is not isotonic with blood—since boric acid can freely diffuse through the red blood cells—and it may cause hemolysis.

Pharmacists are often called upon to calculate the quantity of solute that must be added to adjust a hypotonic solution of a drug to isotonic. This can be done using several methods, including L, sodium chloride equivalent, and cryoscopy.

One of the most frequently used methods for calculating the quantity of sodium chloride necessary to prepare an isotonic solution is the *sodium chloride equivalent method*. A sodium chloride equivalent is the amount of sodium chloride that is osmotically equivalent to 1 g of the drug. For example, the sodium chloride equivalent of ephedrine sulfate is 0.23; that is, 1 g of ephedrine sulfate is equivalent to 0.23 g of sodium chloride.

Physical Pharmacy Capsule 15.1 cont.

EXAMPLE 9

How much sodium chloride is required to make the following prescription isotonic?

> Rx Ephedrine sulfate 2%
> Sterile water, qs   30 mL
> M. isoton with sodium chloride

1. (30 mL) (0.009) = 0.270 g sodium chloride is required if only sodium chloride is present in the 30 mL of solution.
2. (30 mL) (0.02) = 0.6 g ephedrine sulfate is to be present.
3. (0.6 g) (0.23) = 0.138 g is the quantity of sodium chloride represented by the ephedrine sulfate.
4. Since 0.270 g sodium chloride is required if only sodium chloride is used and the quantity of sodium chloride that is equivalent to 0.6 g of ephedrine sulfate is 0.138 g, then 0.270 g − 0.138 g = 0.132 g of sodium chloride required to render the solution isotonic.
5. Therefore, the solution requires ephedrine sulfate 0.6 g, sodium chloride 0.132 g, and sufficient sterile water to make 30 mL.

intravenously, as the oil will occlude the pulmonary microcirculation. Some examples of official injections with oil as the vehicle are presented in Table 15.1.

Added Substances

The USP permits addition of suitable substances to official preparations intended for injection to increase stability or usefulness as long as the substances are not interdicted in the individual monographs, are harmless in the amounts administered, and do not interfere with the therapeutic efficacy of the preparation or with specified assays and tests. Many of these added substances are antibacterial preservatives, buffers, solubilizers, antioxidants, and other adjuncts. Agents employed solely for their coloring effect are strictly prohibited in parenteral products.

The USP requires that one or more suitable substances be added to parenteral products

TABLE 15.1 SOME INJECTIONS IN OIL

INJECTION	OIL	CATEGORY
Dimercaprol	Peanut	Antidote to arsenic, gold, and mercury poisoning
Estradiol cypionate	Cottonseed	Estrogen
Estradiol valerate	Sesame or castor	Estrogen
Fluphenazine decanoate	Sesame	Antipsychotic
Fluphenazine enanthate	Sesame	Antipsychotic
Hydroxyprogesterone caproate	Castor	Progestin
Progesterone in Oil	Sesame or peanut	Progestin
Testosterone cypionate	Cottonseed	Androgen
Testosterone cypionate and estradiol cypionate	Cottonseed	Androgen and estrogen
Testosterone enanthate	Sesame	Androgen
Testosterone enanthate and estradiol valerate	Sesame	Androgen and estrogen

that are packaged in multiple-dose containers to prevent the growth of microorganisms regardless of the method of sterilization employed, unless otherwise directed in the individual monograph or unless the injection's active ingredients are themselves bacteriostatic. Such substances are used in concentrations that prevent the growth of or kill microorganisms. Because many of the usual preservative agents are toxic in large amounts or irritating when parenterally administered, special care must be exercised in the selection of the appropriate preservative agents. For the following preservatives, the indicated maximum limits prevail for use in a parenteral product unless otherwise directed: for agents containing mercury and the cationic surface-active compounds, 0.01%; for agents like chlorobutanol, cresol, and phenol, 0.5%; for sulfur dioxide as an antioxidant or for an equivalent amount of the sulfite, bisulfite, or metabisulfite of potassium or sodium, 0.2%.

In addition to the stabilizing effect of the additives, the air accompanying an injectable product is frequently replaced with an inert gas, such as nitrogen, to enhance the stability of the product by preventing a chemical reaction between oxygen and the drug.

Methods of Sterilization

The term *sterilization*, as applied to pharmaceutical preparations, means destruction of all living organisms and their spores or their complete removal from the preparation. Five general methods are used to sterilize pharmaceutical products:

1. Steam
2. Dry heat
3. Filtration
4. Gas
5. Ionizing radiation

The method is determined largely by the nature of the preparation and its ingredients. However, regardless of the method used, the resulting product must pass a test for sterility as proof of the effectiveness of the method and the performance of the equipment and personnel.

Steam Sterilization

Steam sterilization is conducted in an autoclave and employs steam under pressure. It is usually the method of choice if the product can withstand it (Fig. 15.3).

Most pharmaceutical products are adversely affected by heat and cannot be heated safely to the temperature required for dry heat sterilization (about 150°–170°C, or 302°–338°F). When moisture is present, bacteria are coagulated and destroyed at a considerably lower temperature than when moisture is absent. In fact, bacterial cells with a large percentage of water are generally killed rather easily. Spores, which contain a relatively low percentage of water, are comparatively difficult to destroy. The mechanism of microbial destruction in moist heat is thought to be by denaturation and coagulation of some of the organism's essential protein. It is the hot moisture in the microbial cell that permits destruction at relatively low temperature. Death by dry heat is thought to be by dehydration of the microbial cell followed by slow oxidation. Because it is not possible to raise the temperature of steam above 100°C (212°F) under atmospheric conditions, pressure is employed to achieve higher temperatures. It is the temperature, not the pressure, that destroys the microorganisms, and the application of pressure is solely to increase the temperature of the system.

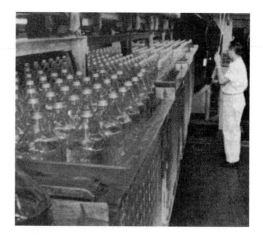

FIGURE 15.3 Autoclaving of intravenous electrolyte solutions. (Courtesy of Abbott Laboratories.)

Time is another important factor in destruction of microorganisms by heat. Most modern autoclaves have gauges to indicate to the operator the internal conditions of temperature and pressure and a timing device to permit the desired exposure time for the load. The usual steam pressures, the temperatures obtainable under these pressures, and the approximate length of time required for sterilization after the system reaches the indicated temperatures are as follows:

10 lb pressure (115.5°C, or 240°F) for 30 minutes
15 lb pressure (121.5°C, or 250°F) for 20 minutes
20 lb pressure (126.5°C, or 260°F) for 15 minutes

As can be seen, the greater the pressure applied, the higher the temperature obtainable and the less the time required for sterilization.

Most autoclaves routinely operate at 121°C (250°F), as measured at the steam discharge line running from the autoclave. The temperature in the chamber of the autoclave must also be reached by the interior of the load being sterilized, and this temperature must be maintained for an adequate time. The penetration time of moist heat into the load varies with the nature of the load, and the exposure time must be adjusted to account for this latent period. For example, a solution packaged in a thin-walled 50-mL ampul may reach 121°C 6 to 8 minutes after that temperature is registered in the steam discharge line, whereas 20 minutes or longer may be required to reach that temperature within a solution packaged in a completely filled thick-walled 1000-mL glass bottle. An estimate of these latent periods must be added to the total time to ensure adequate exposure times. This process depends on moisture and an elevated temperature, so air is removed from the chamber as sterilization begins, because a combination of air and steam yields a lower temperature than does steam alone under the same pressure. For instance, at 15 pounds pressure the temperature of saturated steam is 121.5°C, but a mixture of equal parts of air and steam will reach only about 112°C (234°F).

In general, steam sterilization is applicable to pharmaceutical preparations and materials that can withstand the required temperatures and are penetrated by but not adversely affected by moisture. In aqueous solutions the moisture is already present, and all that is required is elevation of the temperature of the solution for the prescribed period. Thus, solutions in sealed containers, such as ampuls, are readily sterilized by this method. Sealed empty vials can be sterilized by autoclaving only if they contain a small quantity of water. Steam sterilization is also applicable to bulk solutions, glassware, surgical dressings, and instruments. It is not useful for oils, fats, oleaginous preparations, and other preparations not penetrated by the moisture or for exposed powders that may be damaged by the condensed moisture.

Dry Heat Sterilization

Dry heat sterilization is usually carried out in ovens designed for this purpose. The ovens may be heated either by gas or electricity and are generally thermostatically controlled.

Because dry heat is less effective in killing microorganisms than is moist heat, higher temperatures and longer periods of exposure are required. These must be determined for each product with consideration to the size and type of product and the container and its heat distribution characteristics. In general, individual units to be sterilized should be as small as possible, and the sterilizer should be loaded so as to permit free circulation of heated air throughout the chamber. Dry heat sterilization is usually conducted at 150° to 170°C for not less than 2 hours. Higher temperatures permit shorter exposure for a given article; conversely, lower temperatures require longer exposure times. For example, if a particular chemical agent melts or decomposes at 170°C but is unaffected at 140°C (284°F), the lower temperature is used and the exposure time is increased.

Dry heat sterilization is generally employed for substances that are not effectively sterilized by moist heat. Such substances include fixed oils; glycerin; various petroleum products, such as petrolatum, liquid petrolatum (mineral oil), and paraffin; and various heat-stable powders, such as zinc oxide. Dry heat is also an effective method for sterilizing glassware and surgical instruments. Dry heat is the method of choice when dry apparatus or dry containers are required, as in the handling of packaging of dry chemicals or nonaqueous solutions.

Sterilization by Filtration

Sterilization by filtration, which depends on the physical removal of microorganisms by adsorption on the filter medium or by a sieving mechanism, is used for heat-sensitive solutions. Medicinal preparations sterilized by this method must undergo extensive validation and monitoring because the effectiveness of the filtered product can be greatly influenced by the microbial load in the solution being filtered (Fig. 15.4).

Commercially available filters are produced with a variety of pore size specifications. It would be well to mention briefly one type of modern filter, the Millipore filter (Fig. 15.5). The Millipore filter is a thin plastic membrane of cellulosic esters with millions of pores per square inch. The pores are made to be extremely uniform in size and occupy approximately 80% of the membrane's volume, the remaining 20% being the filter material. This high degree of porosity permits flow rates

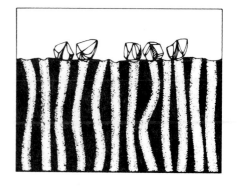

FIGURE 15.5 Membrane filters act as microporous screens that retain all particles and microorganisms larger than the rated pore size on their surface. (Courtesy of Millipore Corporation.)

much in excess of those of other filters having the same particle retention capability. Millipore filters are made from a variety of polymers to be suitable for filtration of almost any liquid or gas system. Also, the filters have various pore sizes, 14 to 0.025 μm, to meet the specific requirements. For comparative purposes, the period that ended the last sentence is approximately 500 μm. The smallest particle visible to the naked eye is about 40 μm, a red blood cell is about 6.5 μm, the smallest bacteria, about 0.2 μm, and a poliovirus, about 0.025 μm.

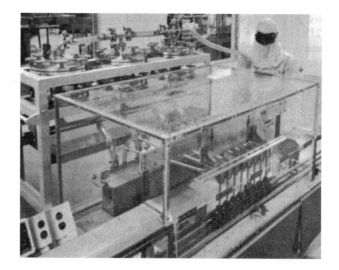

FIGURE 15.4 Sterilization by filtration. An eight-head bottle-filling machine using three large filters in large-scale pharmaceutical production. (Courtesy of Millipore Corporation.)

Although the pore size of a bacterial filter is of prime importance in the removal of microorganisms from a liquid, other factors, such as the electrical charge on the filter and that of the microorganism, the pH of the solution, the temperature, and the pressure or vacuum applied to the system, are also important

The major advantages of bacterial filtration include its speed in the filtration of small quantities of solution, its ability to sterilize thermolabile materials, the relatively inexpensive equipment required, the development and proliferation of membrane filter technology, and the complete removal of living and dead microorganisms and other particulate matter from the solution.

The class of filter medium lends itself to more effective standardization and quality control and also gives the user greater opportunity to confirm the properties of the filter assembly before and after use. The fact that membrane filters are thin polymeric films offers many advantages but also some disadvantages compared to depth filters, such as porcelain or sintered material. Because much of the membrane surface is a void or open space, the properly assembled and sterilized filter offers the advantage of a high flow rate.

One disadvantage is that because the membrane tends to be fragile, it is essential to determine that the assembly was properly made and that the membrane was not ruptured or flawed during assembly, sterilization, or use.

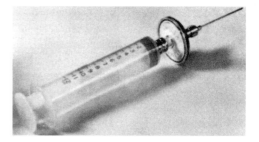

FIGURE 15.6 Luer-Lock syringe adapted with a Millex Filter Unit and hypodermic needle. (Courtesy of Millipore Corporation.)

The housing and filter assemblies should first be validated for compatibility and integrity. This disadvantage is a circumstance not true of methods involving dry or moist heat sterilization, in which the procedures are just about guaranteed to give effective sterilization. Also, filtration of large volumes of liquids requires more time, particularly if the liquid is viscous, than, say, steam sterilization. In essence, bacterial filters are useful when heat cannot be used and also for small volumes of liquids.

Bacterial filters may be used conveniently and economically in the community pharmacy to filter extemporaneously prepared solutions (as ophthalmic solutions) that must be sterile (Figs. 15.6 and 15.7). Furthermore, the membrane filter is the method most commonly used in hospitals. Occasionally, hospitals use the autoclave (moist heat) to sterilize intravenous solutions, such as caffeine citrate.

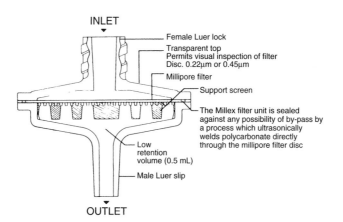

FIGURE 15.7 Cutaway showing composition of the Millex filter unit. (Courtesy of Millipore Corporation.)

To date, information about drug adsorption to membrane filters is limited. Several studies, however, have demonstrated that membrane filters can remove drug from solution (6–9). For example, 0.22-μm filters reduce the in vitro antimicrobial activity of amphotericin B (a colloidal suspension), while filtration of the amphotericin B through 0.85- and 0.45μm filters did not. Butler et al. (10) demonstrated that the potency of drugs administered intravenously and in small doses could be significantly reduced during in-line filtration with a filter containing a cellulose ester membrane. The literature indicates that drugs administered in low doses might present a problem of bonding to the filter. Many filters in clinical use are nitrate or acetate esters of cellulose. These compounds are polar and have residual hydroxyl groups that may adsorb drug. Hydrophobic interactions between hydrocarbon portions of drug molecules being filtered and linear cellulose molecules of filters are also thought to contribute to drug adsorption.

In general, current information suggests that little or no adsorption takes place with membrane filters. However, it is recommended that minute doses of drugs (<5 mg) should not be filtered until sufficient data demonstrate insignificant adsorption. With respect to amphotericin B, to ensure the passage of the antibiotic colloidal dispersion, the filter's mean pore diameter should be more than 1 μm.

Membrane filter media include cellulose acetate, cellulose nitrate, fluorocarbonate, acrylic polymers, polycarbonate, polyester, polyvinyl chloride, vinyl, nylon, polytef, and even metal membranes, and they may be reinforced or supported by an internal fabric.

Gas Sterilization

Some heat-sensitive and moisture-sensitive materials can be sterilized much better by exposure to ethylene oxide or propylene oxide gas than by other means. These gases are highly flammable when mixed with air but can be employed safely when properly diluted with an inert gas such as carbon dioxide or a suitable fluorinated hydrocarbon. Such mixtures are commercially available.

Sterilization by this process requires specialized equipment resembling an autoclave, and many combination steam autoclaves and ethylene oxide sterilizers are commercially available. Greater precautions are required for this method of sterilization than for some of the others, because the variables—for instance, time, temperature, gas concentration, and humidity—are not as firmly quantitated as those of dry heat and steam sterilization. In general, sterilization with gas is enhanced, and the exposure time required is reduced, by increasing the relative humidity of the system (to about 60%) and by increasing the exposure temperature to 50° to 60°C. If the material being sterilized cannot tolerate either the moisture or the elevated temperature, exposure time must be increased. Generally, sterilization with ethylene oxide gas requires 4 to 16 hours of exposure. Ethylene oxide is thought to sterilize by interfering with the metabolism of the bacterial cell.

The great penetrating qualities of ethylene oxide gas make it a useful agent in certain special applications, such as sterilization of medical and surgical supplies and appliances such as catheters, needles, and plastic disposable syringes in their final plastic packaging just prior to shipment. The gas is also used to sterilize certain heat-labile enzyme preparations, certain antibiotics, and other drugs, after testing to ensure absence of chemical reaction and other deleterious effects on the drug substance.

Sterilization by Ionizing Radiation

Techniques are available for sterilization of some types of pharmaceuticals by gamma rays and by cathode rays, but application of such techniques is limited because of the highly specialized equipment required and the effects of irradiation on products and their containers.

The exact mechanism by which irradiation sterilizes a drug or preparation is still subject to investigation. One of the proposed theories is alteration of the chemicals within or supporting the microorganism to form deleterious new chemicals capable of destroying the cell. Another theory proposes that vital structures of the cell, such as the chromosomal nucleoprotein, are disoriented or destroyed. It is probably a combination of irradiation effects that causes the cellular destruction, which is complete and irreversible.

Validation of Sterility

Regardless of the method, pharmaceutical preparations required to be sterile must undergo tests to confirm the absence of microorganisms. The USP contains monographs and standards for biologic indicators of sterilization. A *biologic indicator* is a characterized preparation of specific microorganisms resistant to a particular sterilization process. They may be used to monitor a sterilization cycle and/or periodically to revalidate the process. Biologic indicators are generally of two main forms. In one, spores are added to a carrier, such as a strip of filter paper, packaged to maintain physical integrity while allowing the sterilization effect. In the other, the spores are added to representative units of the product being sterilized, with assessment of sterilization based on these samples. In steam and ethylene oxide sterilization, spores of suitable strains of *Bacillus stearothermophilus* are commonly employed because of their resistance to these modes of sterilization. In dry heat, spores of *Bacillus subtilis* are commonly used. With ionizing radiation, spores of suitable strains of *Bacillus*, including *B. pumilus, B. stearothermophilus*, and *B. subtilis*, have been used.

The effectiveness of thermal sterilization has been quantified through the determination and calculation of *F value* to express the time of thermal death. *Thermal death time* is defined as the time required to kill a particular organism under specified conditions. The F_0 at a particular temperature other than 121°C is the time in minutes required to provide lethality equivalent to that provided at 121°C for a stated time.

Although heat distribution in an autoclave chamber is usually rapid, with 121°C obtained nearly instantaneously throughout the autoclave, the product being sterilized may not achieve identical conditions because of a variety of factors of heat transfer, including the thermal conductivity of the packaging compo-

nents, the viscosity and density of the product, container proximity, passage of steam around containers, and other variables. F values may be computed from biologic data derived from the rate of destruction of known numbers of microorganisms, as shown in the following equation:

$$F_0 = D_{121}(\text{Log A} - \text{Log B})$$

where

D_{121} is the time required for a one-log reduction in the microbial population exposed to a temperature of 121°C,

A is the initial microbial population, and
B is the number of microorganisms that survive after a defined heating time (11).

Pyrogens and Pyrogen Testing

As indicated earlier, *pyrogens* are fever-producing organic substances arising from microbial contamination and responsible for many of the febrile reactions in patients following injection. The causative material is thought to be a lipopolysaccharide from the outer cell wall of the bacteria and endotoxins. Because the material is thermostable and water soluble, it may remain in water even after sterilization by autoclaving or by bacterial filtration.

Manufacturers of water for injection may employ any suitable method for removal of pyrogens from their product. Because pyrogens are organic, one of the more common means of removing them is by oxidizing them to easily eliminated gases or to nonvolatile solids, both of which are easily separated from water by fractional distillation. Potassium permanganate is usually employed as the oxidizing agent, with its efficiency increased by addition of a small amount of barium hydroxide to impart alkalinity to the solution and to make nonvolatile barium salts of any acidic compounds that may be present. These two reagents are added to water that has been distilled several times, and distillation is repeated, the chemical-free distillate being collected under strict aseptic conditions. When properly conducted, this method results in highly pure, sterile, and pyrogen-free water.

However, in each instance the official pyrogen test must be performed to ensure absence of these fever-producing materials.

Pyrogen Test The USP pyrogen test uses healthy rabbits that have been properly maintained in terms of environment and diet before the test. Normal, or control, temperatures are taken for each animal to be used in the test. These temperatures are used as the base for the determination of any temperature increase resulting from injection of a test solution. A given test uses rabbits whose temperatures do not differ by more than 1°C from each other and whose body temperatures are considered not to be elevated. A synopsis of the procedure of the test is as follows.

Render the syringes, needles, and glassware free from pyrogens by heating at 250°C for not less than 30 minutes or by other suitable method. Warm the product to be tested to 37°C ± 2°C.

Inject into an ear vein of each of three rabbits 10 mL of the product per kilogram of body weight, completing each injection within 10 minutes of the start of administration. Record the temperature at 30-minute intervals 1 to 3 hours subsequent to the injection.

If no rabbit shows an individual rise in temperature of 0.5°C or more, the product meets the requirements for the absence of pyrogens. If any rabbit shows an individual temperature rise of 0.5°C or more, continue the test using five other rabbits. If not more than three of the eight rabbits show individual rises in temperature of 0.5°C or more and if the sum of the eight individual maximum temperature rises does not exceed 3.3°C, the material under examination meets the requirements for the absence of pyrogens.

An extract from the blood cells of the horseshoe crab (*Limulus polyphemus*) contains an enzyme and protein system that coagulates in the presence of low levels of lipopolysaccharides. This discovery led to the development of the *Limulus* amebocyte lysate (LAL) test for the presence of bacterial endotoxins. The Bacterial Endotoxins Test, USP, uses LAL and is considered generally more sensitive to endotoxin than the rabbit test. The FDA has endorsed it as a replacement for the rabbit test, and it is used for a number of parenteral products. The USP–NF has specific allowable endotoxin levels for various injections based on the dosage of the individual drugs to keep below a threshold level of administered endotoxins.

Some parenteral products, however, cannot be tested with LAL because the active ingredient interferes with the outcome. Such products include meperidine HCl and promethazine HCl, oxacillin sodium, sulfisoxazole, and vancomycin HCl, among others. These must be tested with the aforementioned Pyrogen Test, USP.

Because the LAL test is so sensitive for the presence of bacterial endotoxins, when the active ingredient of the small-volume parenteral can interfere with the test, a strategy to overcome this interference is to dilute the product more than twofold. Diphenhydramine HCl, ephedrine HCl, meperidine HCl, promethazine HCl, and thiamine HCl, among others, are tested in this manner.

The Industrial Preparation of Parenteral Products

Once the formulation for a particular parenteral product is determined, including selection of the proper solvents or vehicles and additives, the production pharmacist must follow rigid aseptic procedures in preparing the products. In most manufacturing plants the area in which parenteral products are made is maintained bacteria free by use of ultraviolet lights; a filtered air supply; sterile manufacturing equipment, such as flasks, connecting tubes, and filters; and sterilized work clothing (Fig. 15.8).

In preparation of parenteral solutions, the required ingredients are dissolved according to good pharmaceutical practice in water for injection, in another solvent, or in a combination of solvents. The solutions are usually filtered through a membrane until sparkling clear. After filtration, the solution is transferred as rapidly as possible and with the least possible exposure into the final containers. The product is then sterilized, preferably by autoclaving, and samples of the finished product are tested for sterility and pyrogens. If sterilization by autoclaving is impractical because of the nature of

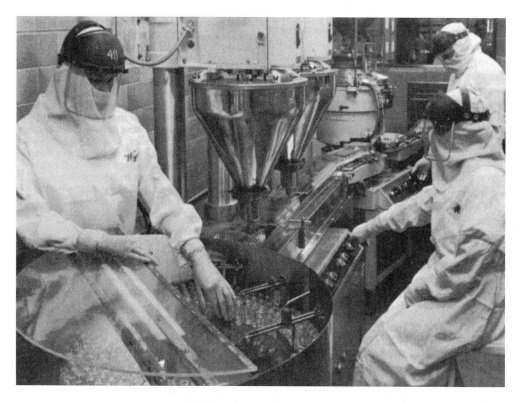

FIGURE 15.8 Sterile filling of vials. (Courtesy of Wyeth Laboratories.)

the ingredients, the individual components of the preparation that are heat or moisture labile may be sterilized by other appropriate means and added aseptically to the sterilized solvent or solution of components that can be autoclaved.

Suspensions of drugs for parenteral use may be prepared by reducing the drug to a very fine powder with a ball mill, micronizer, colloid mill, or other appropriate equipment and then suspending the material in a liquid in which it is insoluble. It is frequently necessary to sterilize separately the individual components of a suspension before combining them, as frequently the integrity of a suspension is destroyed by autoclaving. Autoclaving of a parenteral suspension may alter the viscosity of the product, affecting the suspending ability of the vehicle, or change the particle size of the suspended particles, altering both pharmaceutical and therapeutic characteristics. If a suspension remains unaltered by autoclaving, this method is generally employed to sterilize the final product. Because parenteral emulsions,

which are dispersions or suspensions of a liquid throughout another liquid, are generally destroyed by autoclaving, an alternative method of sterilization must be employed for this type of injectable.

Some injections are packaged as dry solids rather than in conjunction with a solvent or vehicle because the therapeutic agent is unstable in the presence of the liquid component. These dry powders are packaged in the final container to be reconstituted, generally to a solution or less frequently a suspension. The method of sterilization of the powder may be dry heat or another appropriate method. These are examples of sterile drugs prepared and packaged *without* pharmaceutical additives such as buffers, preservatives, stabilizers, and tonicity agents:

Ampicillin sodium
Ceftizoxime sodium
Ceftazidime Sodium
Cefuroxime sodium

Kanamycin sulfate
Nafcillin sodium
Penicillin G benzathine
Streptomycin sulfate
Tobramycin sulfate

Antibiotics are prepared industrially in large fermentation tanks (Fig. 15.9).

Sterile drugs formulated *with* pharmaceutical additives and intended to be reconstituted prior to injection include the following:

Cyclophosphamide
Dactinomycin
Erythromycin lactobionate
Hydrocortisone sodium succinate
Mitomycin
Nafcillin sodium
Oxytetracycline hydrochloride
Penicillin G potassium
Vinblastine sulfate

Sometimes a liquid is packaged along with the dry powder for use at the time of reconstitution (Fig. 15.10). This liquid is sterile and may contain some of the desired pharmaceutical additives, such as the buffering agents. More frequently, the solvent or vehicle is not provided, but the label generally lists suitable solvents. Sodium chloride injection and sterile water for injection are perhaps most frequently employed to reconstitute dry-packaged injections. The dry powders are packaged in containers large enough to permit proper shaking with the liquid component when the latter is aseptically

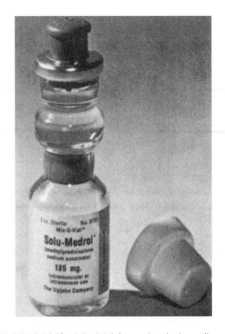

FIGURE 15.10 The Mix-O-Vial contains dry ingredients in the bottom compartment and a liquid diluent in the top, separated by a specially formulated center seal. The bottom compartment can be filled either with a liquid that is frozen and dried to make a lyophilized product or with a powder. The diluent in the top contains a preservative and sometimes one or more active ingredients. To use the vial, the dust cover is removed; pressure is applied with the thumb to the top plunger, which dislodges the center seal; and the vial is shaken well. The top of the plunger is then swabbed with a disinfectant; the syringe needle inserted through the target circle on the plunger; and the contents of the vial withdrawn into the syringe. The Mix-O-Vial offers stability of product until it is activated, convenience, fast operation, and safety as regards the right drug with the proper diluent in the correct proportions. (Courtesy of Pharmacia Company.)

injected through the container's rubber closure during reconstitution. To facilitate dissolution, the dry powder is prevented from caking upon standing by the appropriate means, including lyophilization (Fig. 15.11). Powders so treated form a honeycomb lattice structure that is rapidly penetrated by the liquid, and solution is rapid because of the large surface area of powder exposed.

Pharmacia manufactures the Mix-O-Vial, which incorporates the cover as part of the plunger. Once mixed, the small circle of plastic that covers the injection site is removed. This reduces the touch contamination potential.

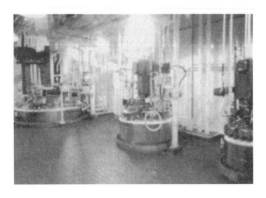

FIGURE 15.9 Fermentation tank for preparation of antibiotics. (Courtesy of Schering-Plough.)

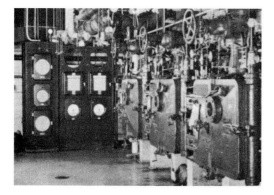

FIGURE 15.11 Antibiotic lyophilizers. (Courtesy of Abbott Laboratories.)

The Abbott ADD-Vantage System IVPB is another example of a ready-to-mix sterile intravenous product designed for intermittent administration of potent drugs that do not have long-term stability in solution. With this system, antibiotics and other drugs do not have to be mixed until just prior to administration. ADD-Vantage consists of two components (Fig. 15.12): a flexible plastic intravenous container partially filled with diluent and a glass vial of powdered or liquid drug. The vials containing the medication and the piggybacks (50–250 mL of dextrose 5% in water injection, 0.45% sodium chloride solution) are specially designed to be used together. The vial locks into a chamber inside the plastic container, and the drug is released by removing the stopper on the vial, allowing the two components to mix. This simple process is performed by external manipulation of the container, preserving the closed, sterile system.

The ADD-Vantage unit may be assembled in a number of locations. Microbiologic tests and sterility tests have been conducted at various intervals following assembly of the units under a laminar flow hood, in a pharmacy on a countertop, and in a patient's hospital room. The final admixtures were sterile, demonstrating that the ADD-Vantage unit can be aseptically assembled under the conditions tested. However, whenever possible, this system should be assembled under a laminar flow hood.

The assembled but not activated ADD-Vantage system can be used within 30 days of

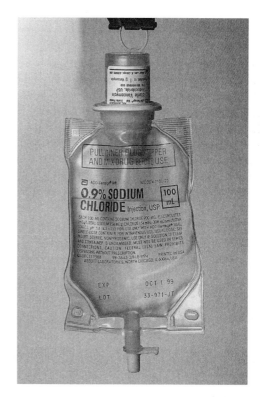

FIGURE 15.12 ADD-Vantage system. (Courtesy of Abbott Laboratories.)

removal of the diluent container from the outer wrapping. ADD-Vantage enables hospitals to reduce drug waste, often caused by canceled or changed prescriptions, and helps the pharmacy conserve labor and reduce material costs.

The Monovial Safety Guard (Becton Dickinson Pharmaceutical Systems) is a new intravenous infusion system for use in preparing extemporaneous small-volume infusions using plastic minibags (Fig. 15.13). When compared to the two traditional methods of preparing small-volume infusions, that is, the transfer needle and vial (TFN) and syringe and vial (SYR) methods, the Monovial system performed quite favorably, saving time, using fewer materials, and costing less (12).

This system is an integrated drug transfer mechanism with a protective shield surrounding the attached transfer needle. Reconstitution and transfer of the drug into an infusion bag are accomplished safely, quickly, and with few materials. The needle is inserted into

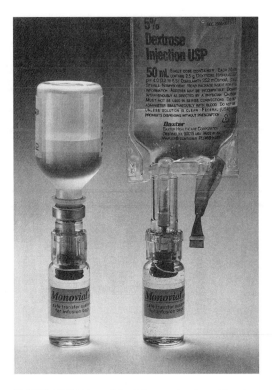

FIGURE 15.13 Monovial safety guard system. (Courtesy of Becton-Dickinson.)

Packaging, Labeling, and Storage of Injections

Containers for injections, including the closures, must not interact physically or chemically with the preparation so as to alter its strength or efficacy (Fig. 15.14). If the container is made of glass, it must be clear and colorless or light amber to permit inspection of its contents. The type of glass suitable for each parenteral preparation is usually stated in the individual monograph. Injections are placed either in single-dose containers or in multiple-dose containers (Figs. 15.15 to 15.17). By definition:

> *Single-dose container:* A hermetic container holding a quantity of sterile drug intended for parenteral administration as a single dose; when opened, it cannot be resealed with assurance that sterility has been maintained.
>
> *Multiple-dose container:* A hermetic container that permits withdrawal of successive portions of the contents without changing the strength, quality, or purity of the remaining portion.

Single-dose containers may be ampuls or single-dose vials. Ampuls (Fig. 15.18) are sealed by fusion of the glass container under aseptic conditions (Figs. 15.19 and 15.20). The glass container is made so as to have a neck that may be easily separated from the body of the

the port of the infusion bag and the transfer set is pushed down toward the vial until it clicks. With the Monovial upright, the infusion bag is squeezed several times to transfer fluid into the Monovial. The Monovial is shaken a few times to reconstitute the drug and inverted. Then the minibag is squeezed and released to transfer the drug back into the infusion bag. This process is repeated until the vial is empty. Diltiazem HCl (Cardizem) for injection is available with the Monovial Safety Guard.

Several manufacturers ship to the hospital pharmacy reconstituted intravenous antibiotic solutions, for example cefazolin sodium, in the frozen state. When thawed, these nonpyrogenic solutions are stable for a finite period. Reconstituted cefazolin is stable for 48 hours at room temperature and for 10 days refrigerated (5°C, or 41°F). The product is packaged in a small plastic bag for piggyback use in intravenous administration.

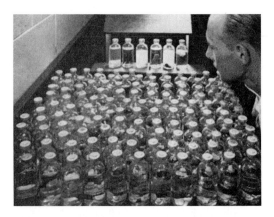

FIGURE 15.14 Testing compatibility of rubber closures with a solution. (Courtesy of Abbott Laboratories.)

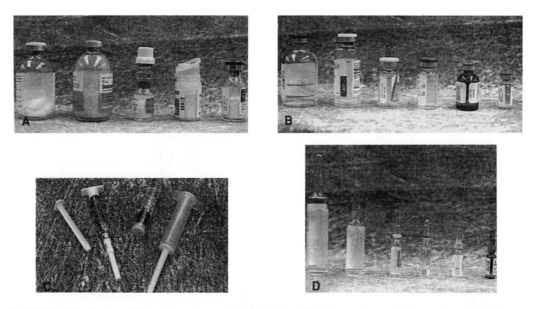

FIGURE 15.15 Packaging of injectable products. **A**. Multiple-dose vials of suspensions and dry powders. **B**. Vials for solutions, including one with light-protective glass. **C**. Unit dose, disposable syringes. **D**. Various sizes of ampuls. (Courtesy of William B. French, PhD.)

container without breaking the glass. After opening, the contents of the ampul should be withdrawn into a syringe with a 5-μm filter needle or straw apparatus. The filter needle is replaced with a regular needle. The filter needle is used to trap any glass particles that entered the sterile solution when the neck of the ampul was broken. If a filter needle is not available, withdrawal of glass can be minimized by holding the ampul upright, tilted slightly,

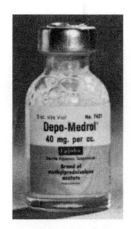

FIGURE 15.16 A typical vial for sterile injectable products, made from type I (borosilicate) glass. The rubber closure has been specially selected for compatibility with the product, desirable physical characteristics, and so on. The overseal holds the closure in place and provides ready access to the contents of the vial. (Courtesy of Pharmacia Company.)

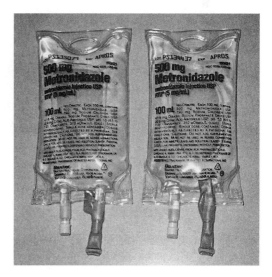

FIGURE 15.17 Two 100-mL single-dose plastic bags for intravenous infusion. (Courtesy of Mr. Akinwale O. Onamade.)

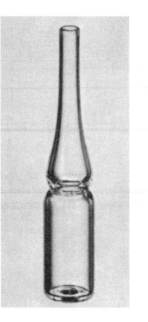

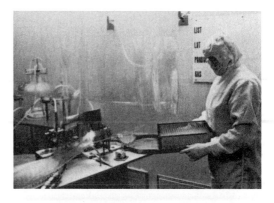

FIGURE 15.19 Ampul filling. (Courtesy of Abbott Laboratories.)

FIGURE 15.18 Ampul before filling and sealing. (Courtesy of Owens Illinois.)

when inserting the needle, and avoiding the outer surface of the neck of the ampul. The needle should not be lowered to the bottom of the ampul but held slightly above to avoid drawing glass into the syringe.

Once opened, the ampul cannot be resealed, and no unused portion may be retained and used later, since the contents would have lost sterility. Some injectable products are packaged in prefilled syringes, with or without special administration devices (Figs. 15.21 to 15.23). The types of glass for parenteral product containers are described in Chapter 5. Types I, II, and III are suitable for parenteral products, with type I being the most resistant to chemical deterioration. The type of glass to be used for a particular injec-

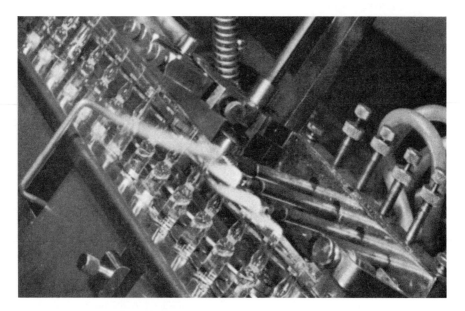

FIGURE 15.20 Ampul sealing. (Courtesy of Abbott Laboratories.)

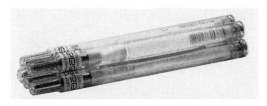

FIGURE 15.21 Medication-containing disposable sterile cartridges compatible with the Carpuject holder. (Courtesy of Abbott Hospital Products Division).

tion is indicated in the individual monograph for that preparation.

One of the prime requisites of parenteral solutions is clarity. They should be sparkling clear and free of all particulate matter; that is, no mobile undissolved substances should be present. Such contaminants include dust, cloth fibers, glass fragments, material leached from

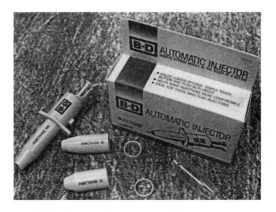

FIGURE 15.23 Inject-Ease automatically inserts the needle of an insulin syringe into the skin when activated. (Courtesy of William B. French, PhD.)

the glass or plastic container or seal, and any other material that may find its way into the product during manufacture or administration or develop during storage.

To keep unwanted particles out of parenteral products, a number of precautions must be taken during manufacture, storage, and use of the products. During manufacture the parenteral solution is usually filtered just before it goes into the container. The containers are carefully selected to be chemically resistant to the solution and of the highest available quality to minimize the chances of container components leaching into the solution. It has been recognized for some time that some particulate matter in parenteral products is leached material from the glass or plastic container. Once the container is selected, it must be carefully cleaned to be free of all extraneous matter (Fig. 15.24). During container filling, extreme care must be exercised to prevent the entrance of airborne dust, lint, or other contaminants. Filtered and directed airflow in production areas reduces the likelihood of contamination. Laminar flow hoods allow for draft-free flow of clean, filtered air over the work area. These hoods are commonly found in hospitals for both manufacture and incorporation of additives into parenteral and ophthalmic products (Fig. 15.25). The personnel who manufacture parenterals must be made acutely aware of the importance of cleanliness and aseptic techniques. They are provided uni-

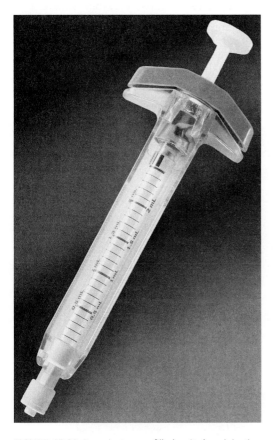

FIGURE 15.22 Carpuject, a prefilled unit dose injection system that includes a reusable clear plastic full-length holder. (Courtesy of Abbott Hospital Products Division.)

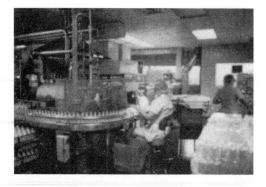

FIGURE 15.24 Production line for preparation of vials for sterilization and filling. (Courtesy of Schering-Plough.)

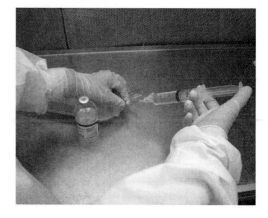

FIGURE 15.26 Pharmacist preparing a parenteral admixture in a laminar flow hood. (Courtesy of Ms. Amy Schuppert Smith)

forms of monofilament fabrics that do not shed lint. They wear face hoods, caps, gloves, and disposable shoe covers to prevent contamination (Fig. 15.26).

After the containers are filled and hermetically sealed, they are visually (Fig. 15.27) or automatically (Fig. 15.28) inspected for particulate matter. Usually an inspector passes the filled container past a light source with a black background to observe for mobile particles.

Particles of approximately 50 μm may be detected in this manner. Reflective particles, such as fragments of glass, may be visualized in smaller size, about 25 μm. Methods to detect smaller particulate matter include microscopic examination and use of sophisticated equipment such as the Coulter Counter, which elec-

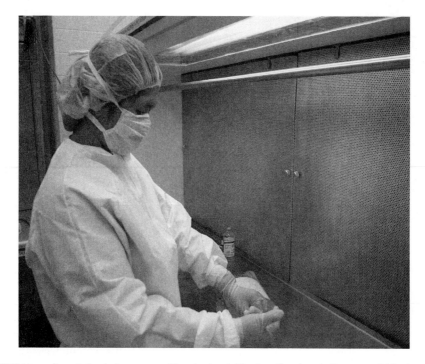

FIGURE 15.25 Hyperalimentation being prepared in a horizontal laminar flow hood. (Courtesy of Ms. Amy Schuppert Smith)

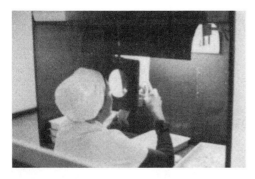

FIGURE 15.27 Industrial inspection of parenteral fluid for particulate matter. (Courtesy of Schering-Plough.)

tronically counts particles in samples. Having passed inspection, the product may be labeled. However, the pharmacist should inspect each parenteral solution for evidence of particulate matter.

Although the total significance of injecting or infusing parenteral solutions containing particulate matter into a patient has not been ascertained, it is apparent that particulate matter has the potential to induce thrombi and vessel blockage, and depending on the chemical composition of the particles, the additional potential to introduce into the patient agents that are undesired and possibly toxic.

In formulating a single-dose parenteral product, the pharmacist must consider not only the physicochemical aspects of the drug

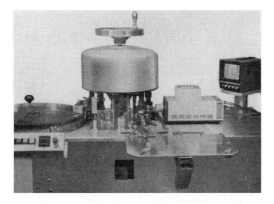

FIGURE 15.28 The Autoskan industrial automatic inspection machine, which detects particulate matter in injectables with a television camera and electronics and automatically rejects them from the production line. (Courtesy of Lakso Company.)

but also the intended therapeutic use of the product. Some single-dose preparations are to be administered rapidly in small volumes, but others infuse slowly into the circulatory system over hours. Most small-volume parenterals are formulated so that a convenient amount of solution, say 0.5 to 2 mL, contains the usual dose of the drug, although larger volumes of more diluted solutions are frequently administered intravenously and intramuscularly. Generally, several strengths of injections of a given drug are marketed to permit a wider dosage selection by the physician without waste, as would be the case if only part of a given single-dose parenteral solution was administered. The large-volume single-dose preparations generally are those used to expand the blood volume or to replenish nutrients or electrolytes and are given by slow intravenous infusion. However, in no instance may a single-dose parenteral container permit withdrawal and administration of more than 1000 mL. In addition, preparations intended for intraspinal, intracisternal, or peridural administration must be packaged only in single-dose containers as a precaution against contamination.

In the hospital, physicians commonly order an additional agent to be placed in a large-volume parenteral solution for infusion. The person filling such an order must be certain that aseptic conditions are employed and that the additive is compatible with the original solution (13). Care must also be exercised not to introduce particulate matter into the solution. Many pharmaceutical companies have developed special devices for aseptic transfer of pharmaceutical additives to large-volume parenterals. An ordinary sterile needle and syringe, preferably with a filtering device, may be effectively employed to transfer solutions from one parenteral product to another (Fig. 15.29). Many hospital pharmacies have established well-controlled *intravenous additive* or *admixture* programs to ensure compatibility, safety, and efficacy of the additive and solution (14).

Multiple-dose containers are affixed with rubber closures to permit penetration of a hypodermic needle without removal or destruction of the closure. Upon withdrawing the needle from the container, the closure reseals and

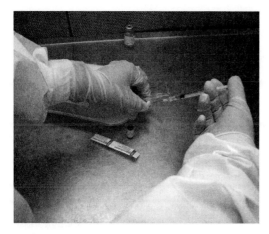

FIGURE 15.29 Use of a filter syringe for aseptic addition of an ingredient to a large-volume parenteral solution. (Courtesy of Ms. Amy Schuppert Smith)

TABLE 15.2 RECOMMENDED OVERAGES FOR OFFICIAL PARENTERAL PRODUCTS IN MILLILITERS

LABELED SIZE	EXCESS VOLUME FOR MOBILE LIQUIDS	EXCESS VOLUME FOR VISCOUS LIQUIDS
0.5	0.10	0.12
1.0	0.10	0.15
2.0	0.15	0.25
5.0	0.30	0.50
10.0	0.50	0.70
20.0	0.60	0.90
30.0	0.80	1.20
50.0 or more	2.00%	3.00%

protects the contents from airborne contamination. The needle may be inserted to withdraw a portion of the prepared liquid injection, or it may be used to introduce a solvent or vehicle to a dry powder for injection. In either instance, the sterility of the injection may be maintained so long as the needle itself is sterile at the time of entry into the container. Unless otherwise indicated in the monograph, multiple-dose injectables are required to contain antibacterial preservatives. Also, unless otherwise specified, multiple-dose containers are not permitted to allow withdrawal of more than 30 mL to limit the number of penetrations into the closure and thus protect against loss of sterility. The limited volume also guards against an excessive amount of antibacterial preservative being inadvertently administered with the drug when unusually large doses of an injection are required, in which case a preservative-free single-dose preparation is advisable. The usual multiple-dose container contains about 10 usual doses of the injection, but quantity may vary greatly with the individual preparation and manufacturer.

Because it is impossible in practice to transfer the entire volume of a single-dose container or the last dose in a multiple-dose container into a hypodermic syringe, a slight excess in volume of the contents of ampuls and vials over the labeled size or volume of the package is permitted. Table 15.2 presents the recommended overages permitted by the USP to allow withdrawal and administration of the labeled volumes.

For labeling purposes, revised injectable product nomenclature became official in the USP 23 on January 1, 1995, and continues. The main points of the revised process are as follows:

I. The term *sterile* was eliminated from the titles of injectable products except appropriate monograph titles for water intended for parenteral use, such as Sterile Water for Injection, USP.
II. For established names of injectable products, all of which are suitable and intended for parenteral administration, USP established the following criteria in determining the product's title:
   A. Liquids
      1. *Injection:* Title for liquid preparations that are drug substances or solutions thereof.
      2. *Injectable suspension:* Title for liquid preparations of solids suspended in a suitable liquid medium.
      3. *Injectable emulsion:* Title for liquid preparations of drug substances dissolved or dispersed in suitable emulsion medium.

B. Solids
  1. *For injection:* Title for dry solids that, upon the addition of suitable vehicles, yield solutions conforming in all respects to the requirements for *Injections.*
  2. *For injectable suspension:* Title for dry solids that, upon the addition of suitable vehicles, yield preparations conforming in all respects to the requirements for *Injectable Suspensions.*

Originally, to facilitate this transition to a new nomenclature, the Center for Drug Evaluation and Research encouraged parenteral drug manufacturers to place a flag, or reminder statement, on the labels of the product for 6 months, alerting practitioners to the changes. The intent was to help practitioners become familiar with the revised rules. An example of a flag: FORMERLY STERILE [DRUG NAME].

In addition, the labels on containers of parenteral products must state the following:

The name of the preparation
For a liquid preparation, the percentage content of drug or the amount of drug in a specified volume
For a dry preparation, the amount of active ingredient present and the volume of liquid to be added to the dry preparation to prepare a solution or suspension
The route of administration
A statement of storage conditions and an expiration date
The name of the manufacturer and distributor
An identifying lot number capable of yielding the complete manufacturing history of the specific package, including all manufacturing, filling, sterilizing, and labeling operations

Injections for veterinary use are labeled so. Preparations intended to be used as dialysis, hemofiltration, or irrigation solutions should meet the requirements for injections except those relating to volume in the containers and should bear a statement indicating that the solution is not intended for use by intravenous infusion. Appropriately labeled containers al-low a sufficient area of the container to remain free of label for its full length or circumference to permit inspection of the contents. Any injection that visual inspection reveals to contain particulate matter other than normally suspended material should be discarded.

Each individual monograph for the official injection states the type of container (single-dose and/or multiple-dose) permitted for the injection, the type of glass preferred for the container, exemptions if any to usual package size limitations, and any special storage instructions. Most injections prepared from chemically pure medicinal agents are stable at room temperature and may be stored without special concern or conditions. However, most biologic products—insulin injection and the various vaccines, toxoids, toxins, and related products—should be stored under refrigeration. Consult the individual monograph to find the proper storage temperature for a particular injection.

Quality Assurance for Pharmacy-Prepared Sterile Products

The American Society of Health-System Pharmacists (formerly the American Society of Hospital Pharmacists) publishes guidelines on quality assurance for pharmacy-prepared sterile products (15). The guidelines were developed to help pharmacists establish quality assurance procedures for preparation of sterile products. The guidelines are appropriate to all practice settings in which pharmacists directly serve patients (e.g., hospitals, community pharmacies, nursing homes, home health care). These are not intended to apply to manufacture of sterile pharmaceuticals as defined in state and federal laws and regulations. Nor are they to apply to preparation of medications by pharmacists, nurses, and physicians intended for immediate administration (minimal delay between preparation and administration) to patients.

The term *sterile products* used within the guidelines refers to sterile or nutritional substances that are prepared (compounded or repackaged) by pharmacy personnel, using aseptic technique and other quality assurance procedures. The objectives of these recommendations are to enable pharmacists to provide the following:

1. Information to pharmacists on quality assurance and quality control activities that may be applied to the preparation of sterile products in pharmacies
2. A scheme to match quality assurance and quality control activities with the risks to patients posed by various types of products

The guidelines define the purpose of these recommendations and encourage pharmacists to participate in quality improvement, risk management, and infection control programs in their organization. In doing so, pharmacists are expected to report findings about quality assurance in sterile products to appropriate staffs or committees and to cooperate with managers of quality improvement, risk management, and infection control to develop optimal sterile product procedures.

Originally, in February 1992, what was then the American Society of Hospital Pharmacists proposed guidelines that formed the basis of the Technical Assistance Bulletin (TAB) (16). This document distinguished between quality control (QC) and quality assurance (QA). By definition, *quality control* is acceptance or rejection of raw materials and packaging components, in-process test materials, and inspections (17). *Quality assurance* is a systematic method to identify problems in patient care that are resolved via administrative, clinical, or educational actions to ensure that final products and outcomes meet applicable specifications (17).

The guidelines classify sterile products into three levels based on risk to the patient. The risk levels range from the least potential risk (level 1) to the greatest potential risk (level 3). The classification system is designed only to assist the pharmacist in selecting sterile preparation procedures. Pharmacists must exercise professional judgment in deciding which risk level applies to a specific product or situation. Factors that increase risk (e.g., multiple system breaks, compounding complexities, high-risk administration sites, immunocompromised patients, microbial growth potential of the prod-

uct, storage conditions) must be weighed by the pharmacist.

Sometimes the pharmacist must make risk–benefit decisions to prepare these products outside of the guidelines (e.g., preparation of a sterile investigational drug in a compassionate-use protocol for a lifesaving effort). The risk assignments listed in Table 15.3 provide a logical template within which to evaluate risk. These do not, however, preclude alternative logical arrangements based on scientific information and professional judgment.

Risk level 1 represents the minimum QA guidelines. In risk levels 2 and 3, products must meet or exceed each of the risk level 1 guidelines. If the risk level assignment is unclear, guidelines for the higher risk level should be followed.

The guidelines delineate the quality assurance components for each risk level. These include policies and procedures; personnel education, training, and evaluation; process validation; storage and handling; facilities and equipment; garb; aseptic technique and product preparation; process evaluation; expiration dating; labeling; end product evaluation; and documentation. Specific recommendations germane to each of these components at each risk level are made in the guidelines; see them for additional information.

The USP 27–NF 22 introduced a new general Chapter <797> "Pharmaceutical Compounding—Sterile Preparations," which establishes standards for aseptic compounding of all sterile dosage forms (18). This chapter explains in detail the various procedures and documentation necessary to prepare and dispense sterile drug products. It includes, among others, validation of sterilization and aseptic processes, personnel training, aseptic techniques, finished product release testing, storage, and beyond-use dating.

Available Injections

Hundreds of injections of various medicinal agents are on the market. Tables 15.4 to 15.7 present some examples of those packaged in small-volume and large-volume containers, the latter for intravenous infusion.

TABLE 15.3 ASHP RISK LEVEL CLASSIFICATION OF PHARMACY-PREPARED STERILE PRODUCTS (15)

RISK LEVEL 1

1. Products
   A. Stored at room temperature and completely administered within 28 hours of preparation
   B. Stored under refrigeration for 7 days or less before complete administration to a patient over a period not to exceed 24 hours
   C. Frozen for 30 days or less before complete administration to a patient over a period not to exceed 24 hours

2. Unpreserved sterile products prepared for administration to one patient or batch-prepared products containing suitable preservatives prepared for administration to more than one patient

3. Products prepared by closed-system aseptic transfer of sterile nonpyrogenic finished pharmaceuticals (e.g., from vials or ampuls) obtained from licensed manufacturer into sterile final containers (e.g., syringes, minibags, elastomeric containers, portable infusion device cassette) obtained from licensed manufacturer

RISK LEVEL 2

1. Products stored beyond 7 days under refrigeration or stored beyond 30 days frozen or administered beyond 28 hours after preparation and storage at room temperature

2. Batch-prepared products without preservatives (e.g., epidural products) intended for use by more than one patient. (Note: Batch-prepared products without preservatives to be administered to multiple patients carry a greater risk to patients than products prepared for a single patient because of the possibility of inaccurate ingredients or product contamination.)

3. Products compounded by complex or numerous manipulations of sterile ingredients obtained from licensed manufacturers in a sterile container or reservoir obtained from a licensed manufacturer by using closed-system aseptic transfer; for example, TPN solutions prepared with an automated compounder.

RISK LEVEL 3
(PRODUCTS EXHIBIT CHARACTERISTIC 1 OR 2)

1. Products compounded from nonsterile ingredients or compounded with nonsterile components, containers, or equipment before terminal sterilization.

2. Products prepared by combining multiple ingredients—sterile or nonsterile—by using an open-system transfer or open reservoir before terminal sterilization.

Small-Volume Parenterals

Table 15.4 presents some commonly employed injections given in small volume. Some of these injections are solutions and others are suspensions.

Premixed intravenous delivery systems have simplified delivery for small-volume parenterals in particular. A distinct advantage of these ready-to-use systems is that they require little or no manipulation to make them patient specific. Thus they are a viable alternative to the traditional labor-intensive method of compounding parenteral medications from individual or multiple doses of intravenous medications and an appropriate parenteral solution. Since the introduction of the first ready-to-use systems in the late 1970s, the availability and variety of systems has increased (e.g., Baxter Healthcare Corporation, Kendall McGaw Laboratories, Abbott Laboratories) (Table 15.5).

The traditional method for preparing small-volume parenteral therapy from a partial-fill drug vial into a minibag can be labor intensive and costly in materials. The savings accrued through ready-to-use systems can be significant (19). Another key advantage of these systems is extended stability dating and reduced wastage. Doses can be put together (but not activated) in cycles, then activated just prior to use and delivered to the nursing station by the pharmacy personnel (19).

The down side of these ready-to-use small parenteral products is that they do not offer

TABLE 15.4 SOME INJECTIONS USUALLY PACKAGED AND ADMINISTERED IN SMALL VOLUME

INJECTION	PHYSICAL FORM	CATEGORY AND COMMENTS
Botulinum toxin type A	Powder for injection	For temporary improvement in appearance of moderate to severe glabellar lines associated with corrugator or procerus muscle activity in adult patients 65 years or younger; administered IM.
Butorphanol tartrate	Solution	Opioid agonist-antagonist analgesic; administered IM or IV for relief of moderate to severe pain, as preoperative or preanesthesia medication.
Chlorpromazine HCl	Solution	Antipsychotic drug with antiemetic (antidopaminergic) effects; should not be administered SQ. Injection should be IM slowly, deep into upper outer quadrant of buttocks. Avoid injecting directly into vein. IV route used ONLY for severe hiccoughs, surgery, tetanus.
Cimetidine HCl	Solution	Histamine H_2 antagonist; IM or IV for pathologic GI hypersecretory conditions or intractable ulcers.
Dalteparin sodium	Solution	Sterile low-molecular-weight heparin for prophylaxis of deep vein thrombosis in patients at risk who are undergoing abdominal surgery. Available in a prefilled syringe; administered SQ.
Dexamethasone sodium phosphate	Solution	Glucocorticoid; IM or IV for cerebral edema, unresponsive shock. Also intra-articular, intralesional, in soft tissue for joints, bursae, and ganglia.
Digoxin	Solution	Cardiotonic given IM (not preferred) or IV with highly individualized and monitored dosage.
Dihydroergotamine mesylate	Solution	Alpha-adrenergic blocking agent specific for migraine, IM or IV.
Diphenhydramine HCl	Solution	Ethanolamine, nonselective antihistamine; IV or IM when PO impractical; indicated for type I (immediate) hypersensitivity reactions, active treatment of motion sickness.
Furosemide	Solution	Loop diuretic; IM or IV slowly for edema or acute pulmonary edema.
Granisetron HCl	Solution	5-HT_3 receptor antagonist for prevention of nausea and vomiting of cancer therapy, including high-dose cisplatin.
Heparin sodium	Solution	Anticoagulant IV or SQ as indicated by activated partial prothrombin time or actuated coagulation time.
Hydromorphone HCl	Solution	Opioid analgesic for relief of moderate to severe pain; SQ, IM, or slow IV.
Ibutilide fumarate	Solution	Antiarrhythmic with predominantly class III (cardiac action potential prolongation) properties according to Vaughn Williams Classification; infused IV undiluted or diluted in 50 mL diluent.
Iron dextran	Solution	Hematinic agent; IV or IM for documented iron deficiency when oral administration is unsatisfactory or impossible.
Isoproterenol HCl	Solution	Adrenergic (bronchodilator) given IM, SQ, or IV.
Ketorolac tromethamine	Solution	NSAID for < 5 days of moderately severe acute pain that requires analgesia at opioid level, usually postoperatively.
Lidocaine HCl	Solution	Cardiac depressant given IV as antiarrhythmic; also local anesthetic epidurally, by infiltration, and in peripheral nerve block.

(continued)

TABLE 15.4 SOME INJECTIONS USUALLY PACKAGED AND ADMINISTERED IN SMALL VOLUME

INJECTION	PHYSICAL FORM	CATEGORY AND COMMENTS
Magnesium sulfate	Solution	Anticonvulsant/electrolyte; IM or direct IV injection, IV infusion, other IV administration for convulsive toxemia of pregnancy, parenteral nutrition therapy, mild magnesium deficiency, severe hypomagnesemia.
Meperidine HCl	Solution	Opioid analgesic given IM, SQ, or slow continuous IV infusion.
Metoclopramide monohydrochloride	Solution	Gastrointestinal stimulant; administered IM, direct IV, or slow IV admixture to prevent chemotherapy emesis.
Midazolam HCl	Solution	Short-acting benzodiazepine CNS depressant; IV or IM; for preoperative sedation, anxiolysis, amnesia.
Morphine sulfate	Solution	Opioid analgesic. IM, IV, PCA.
Nalbuphine HCl	Solution	Opioid agonist-antagonist analgesic; administered SQ, IM, IV for moderate to severe pain, preoperative analgesia.
Naloxone HCl	Solution	Opioid antagonist; prevents or reverses effects of opioids, including respiratory depression, sedation, hypotension; IV, IM, SQ.
Oxytocin	Solution	Oxytocic, given IM (erratic) or IV obstetrically for therapeutic induction of labor.
Phenytoin sodium	Solution	Anticonvulsant; IM (erratic absorption) prophylaxis for neurosurgery or slow IV for status epilepticus.
Phytonadione	Dispersion	Vitamin K (prothrombogenic) for hemorrhage. Aqueous dispersion of phytonadione, a viscous liquid.
Procaine penicillin G	Suspension	Anti-infective; IM for moderately severe infections of penicillin G–sensitive microorganisms.
Prochlorperazine edisylate	Solution	Antidopaminergic; IM or IV for control of severe nausea and vomiting associated with adult surgery.
Propranolol HCl	Solution	Beta-adrenergic receptor blocker for hypertension. Oral dosage (tablets) is usual; IV administration is reserved for life-threatening arrhythmias and those occurring under anesthesia.
Sodium bicarbonate	Solution	Electrolyte; IV, undiluted or diluted for cardiac arrest, less urgent forms of metabolic acidosis.
Sumatriptan succinate	Solution	Selective 5-hydroxytryptamine$_1$ receptor, subtype agonist, for acute migraine with or without aura. Self-administered SQ from unit-of-use syringe, *SELFdose* unit.
Verapamil HCl	Solution	Calcium channel blocker; slow IV over at least 2 minutes for supraventricular tachyarrhythmias.

flexibility in changing the volume or concentration of the product. This may pose a problem to the fluid-restricted patient (19). But the introduction of minibags in volumes of 100 mL, 50 mL, and 25 mL have helped this problem somewhat. Another disadvantage of the ready-to-use products is that some manufacturers' premixed products require thawing. Microwave use for quick thawing poses stability problems for some of these products (e.g., cefazolin). For example, before it was removed from the market, the high energy microwave oven could cause a structural alteration of the cephalothin molecule. Another possibility was that substance would leach from the rubber stopper when frozen ampuls of Neutral Keflin were thawed in the microwave, and oftentimes thawing was not

TABLE 15.5 REPRESENTATIVE MARKETED FROZEN, PREMIXED PRODUCTS ILLUSTRATING STABILITY DATA FROZEN AND AFTER THAWING[a]

DRUG[b]	STRENGTH	DILUENT	FROZEN STABILITY	REFRIGERATED STABILITY	ROOM TEMPERATURE
			EXPIRATION DATING		
Aztreonam	1 g, 2 g	Iso-osmotic in dextrose, 50 ml	12 months	14 days	48 hours
Cefazolin	500 mg, 1 g	Iso-osmotic in dextrose, 50 ml	24 months	30 days	48 hours
Cefotaxime sodium	1 g, 2 g	Iso-osmotic in dextrose, 50 ml	9 months	10 days	24 hours
Cefotetan	1 g, 2 g	Iso-osmotic in dextrose, 50 ml	12 months	21 days	48 hours
Cefoxitin	1 g, 2 g	Iso-osmotic in dextrose, 50 ml	18 months	21 days	24 hours
Ceftazidime sodium	1 g, 2 g	Iso-osmotic in dextrose, 50 ml	9 months	7 days	24 hours
Ceftizoxime	1 g, 2 g	Iso-osmotic in dextrose, 50 ml	12 months	28 days	48 hours
Ceftriaxone	1 g, 2 g	Iso-osmotic in dextrose, 50 ml	15 months	21 days	72 hours
Nafcillin	1 g, 2 g	Iso-osmotic in dextrose, 50 ml, 100 ml	18 months	21 days	72 hours
Oxacillin sodium	1 g, 2 g	Iso-osmotic in dextrose, 50 ml	18 months	21 days	48 hours
Ticarcillin disodium and clavulanate potassium	3.1 g	Iso-osmotic in water, 100 ml	6 months	7 days	24 hours
Vancomycin HCl	500 mg	Iso-osmotic in dextrose, 100 ml	12 months	30 days	72 hours

[a]Stability information provided by Baxter Healthcare Corporation.

[b]Stability data based on packaging drug in a Galaxy[R] container.

even, with the periphery thawed and the central portion still frozen.

General precautions (20) were once published for using a microwave to thaw frozen products. However, this practice is no longer suggested. Instead, many hospital pharmacies use the Sāf-Thaw (MMI of Mississippi, Crystal Springs). This apparatus provides a layer of conditioned air continuously circulating around the frozen product. The thawing surface facili-

TABLE 15.6 INSULIN ACTIVITY PROFILES AND COMPATIBILITY

PREPARATION	ONSET (HR)	PEAK (HR)	DURATION (HR)	COMPATIBLE WITH
Rapid acting				
Insulin Lispro	0.25	0.5–1.0	3	Ultralente; NPH
Insulin Aspart	0.25	0.5–1.0	3	None
Short acting				
Regular insulin	0.5	2–5	5–8	All
Intermediate acting				
Isophane (NPH) insulin	1–2	6–10	16–20	Regular
Insulin zinc (Lente)	1–2	6–12	18–24	Regular, semilente
Long acting				
Insulin zinc extended (Ultralente)	4–6	10–18	24–28	Regular, semilente
Insulin glargine	2	None	>24	None
Mixtures				
Isophane/regular insulin 70/30, 50/500.75	7–12	16–24	—	
NPL/Lispro Mix 75/25	5 min	7–12	1–24	—

TABLE 15.7 SOME INTRAVENOUS INFUSIONS THAT MAY BE ADMINISTERED IN VOLUMES OF 1 L OR MORE, ALONE OR WITH OTHER DRUGS

INJECTION	USUAL CONTENTS	CATEGORY AND COMMENTS
Amino acid	3.5, 5, 5.5, 7, 8.5, 10% crystalline amino acid with or without varying concentrations of electrolytes or glycerin	Fluid and nutrient replenisher
Dextrose Injection, USP	2.5, 5, 10, 20% dextrose, other strengths	Fluid and nutrient replenisher
Dextrose and Sodium Chloride Injection, USP	Dextrose 2.5–10%; NaCl 0.11–0.9% (19–154 mEq sodium)	Fluid, nutrient, electrolyte replenisher
Mannitol Injection, USP	5, 10, 15, 20, 25% mannitol	Diagnostic aid in renal function; diuretic; fluid and nutrient replenisher
Ringer's Injection, USP	147 mEq sodium, 4 mEq potassium, 4.5 mEq calcium, 156 mEq chloride per liter	Fluid and electrolyte replenisher
Lactated Ringer's Injection, USP	2.7 mEq calcium, 4 mEq potassium, 130 mEq sodium, 28 mEq lactate per liter	Systemic alkalinizer; fluid and electrolyte replenisher
Sodium Chloride Injection, USP	0.9% NaCl	Fluid and electrolyte replenisher; isotonic vehicle

tates recirculating the conditioned air in the unit and thereby prevents collection of unconditioned air or moisture from the room where the Sāf-Thaw is operating. The frozen product is placed on the thawing surface, which is approximately 37°C (99°F), warm to the touch when the unit is in operation. Several dozen frozen products can be placed on the thawing surface at one time, depending on their size.

In years past, some manufacturers recommended warming frozen premixed products in a water bath, with a warning not to submerge the product because there was a distinct possibility that water from the bath could enter and contaminate the product. Now manufacturers recommend that the frozen container be thawed at room temperature or in a refrigerator (e.g., for 1 hour) and prohibit the use of a water bath or microwave. Thawed floor stock is usually available for emergency orders. Generally, these are kept in refrigerators and warm up quickly (e.g., 20 minutes) to room temperature.

The ready-to-use systems have not been used much in the pediatric and neonatal population. The unique dosing and fluid requirements of these patients make these systems inappropriate. In some institutions, the unique dosing and fluid requirements of pediatric and neonate patients are addressed by making di-lutions of medications to standardized concentrations, filling and capping individual syringes, and administering these doses through a syringe pump.

Among the most used of the small-volume injections are the various insulin preparations. Insulin, the active principle of the pancreas gland, is primarily concerned with the metabolism of carbohydrates but also influences protein and fat metabolism. Insulin facilitates the cellular uptake of glucose and its metabolism in liver, muscle, and adipose tissue. It increases the uptake of amino acids and inhibits the breakdown of fats and the production of ketones. Insulin is administered to patients with abnormal or absent pancreatic beta cell function to restore glucose metabolism and maintain satisfactory carbohydrate, fat, and protein metabolism. It is used in the treatment of *diabetes mellitus* that cannot be controlled satisfactorily by dietary regulation alone or by oral hypoglycemic drugs. Insulin may also be used to improve the appetite and increase the weight in selected cases of nondiabetic malnutrition and is frequently added to intravenous infusions.

Insulin is administered by needle or jet injection (Figs. 15.30 to 15.32). A system for nasal administration of insulin is under study.

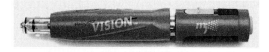

FIGURE 15.30 Medi-Jector II, a jet injection device. The jet injection method uses pressure rather than a needle to provide subcutaneous distribution of medication. This device can be used with U-100 insulin or a combination of insulins and can deliver 2 to 100 units in half-unit increments. (Courtesy of Antares Pharm Inc.)

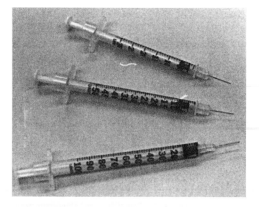

FIGURE 15.31 Insulin syringes calibrated in units. (Courtesy of William B. French, PhD.)

U-100 insulin has been suggested as a replacement for U-40 insulin, with the intention of making U-100 the single strength for in-home use by the patient. In December 1991 Eli Lilly announced that it would cease production of U-40 insulins, and subsequently other insulin manufacturers also decided to cease production of this strength. The basis for this decision was lack of demand (very low numbers of patients using this strength). Recognizing, however, that insulin under 100 U/mL might still be needed, as for small children and veterinary use), Lilly markets a diluting fluid for the Regular, NPH, Lente, and Ultra-Lente insulins of U-100 strength. This fluid can be used to prepare any strength of insulin below 100 U/mL. The diluting solutions are identical to the diluent in the insulin in every way (e.g., preservative agent, buffer, pH) except for the presence of insulin. The recommended storage condition for opened and unopened diluting solutions is controlled room temperature, 25°C (77°F). Once the diluting solutions are opened, the material can be used for a month.

Age-associated sight difficulties and the vision deterioration associated with diabetes can interfere significantly with buying and using insulin products. Therefore, packaging of insulins must make allowances for visual deficits. To facilitate identification of the proper medication at the site of purchase, the arrangement and size of the package lettering must make it easy for the insulin-dependent patient to recognize the type and concentration of the product. In the case of Humulin insulins, an international symbol also appears on the cartons and bottles of all formulations. These symbols help ensure that patients with diabetes secure the correct Humulin formulation anywhere in the world.

The goal of insulin therapy is to achieve tight blood glucose control by mimicking insulin secretion by the normal pancreas. Normal insulin secretion consists of two components, basal and bolus insulin. These components are mimicked by the administration of two types of insulins. Basal insulins are intermediate-acting or long-acting insulins that mimic basal secre-

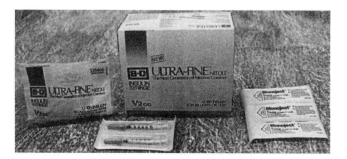

FIGURE 15.32 Packaging of disposable sterile insulin syringes and needles. (Courtesy of William B. French, PhD.)

tion of insulin. This is the small amount that the pancreas secretes continuously. These products help to suppress hepatic glucose production between meals and overnight. Basal insulins provide approximately 50% of a person's daily requirements. Bolus insulins are rapid-acting or short-acting insulins that mimic the extra insulin the pancreas secretes in response to the postprandial rise of blood glucose levels. Postprandial blood glucose values contribute significantly to hemoglobin A_{1C} values and consequently to the long-term complications of diabetes if these blood glucose values are not controlled. Thus, postprandial control of blood glucose is essential for optimal management. Bolus injections are estimated to provide 10 to 20% of a patient's total daily insulin requirement at each meal.

Insulin Injection (Regular)

Insulin injection is a sterile aqueous solution of insulin. Commercially, the solution is prepared from beef or pork pancreas or both or through biosynthetic means (human insulin), discussed in the next section. The source must be stated on the labeling. In 1980, purified pork insulin (Iletin II, pork, Lilly) became available for individuals allergic to or otherwise adversely affected by the mixed pork and beef product. The first insulin developed for clinical use was amorphous. This type has since been replaced by a purer zinc–insulin crystalline product that produces a clear aqueous solution. Originally, insulin injection (regular insulin) was produced at a pH of 2.8 to 3.5. This was necessary because particles formed in the vial when the pH was increased above the acid range. However, changes in manufacturing to produce insulin of greater purity has allowed for insulin injection with a neutral pH. The neutral product is more stable than the acidic product.

Insulin injection is prepared to contain 100 or 500 USP insulin units per milliliter. The labeling must state the potency in USP insulin units per milliliter and the expiration date, which must not be later than 24 months after the date of manufacture. As an added precaution against inadvertent use of the incorrect

strength, the packages are color coded for strength. For instance, all insulins of the various types containing 100 U/mL have orange, and the 500 U/mL preparation has brown with diagonal white stripes. U-500 insulin is indicated for patients with a marked insulin requirement (more than 200 U per day) because a large dose may be administered subcutaneously in a small volume.

Insulin injection is a colorless to straw-colored solution, depending on its concentration; the 500 U/mL product is straw colored. It is substantially free from turbidity. A small amount of glycerin (1.4–1.8%) is added for stability and 0.1 to 0.25% of either phenol or cresol is added for preservation. Insulin remains stable if stored in a cold place, preferably the refrigerator. However, because injection of cold insulin is uncomfortable, the patient may store the vial being used at room temperature (15–30°C or 59–86°F) for up to 1 month. Any insulin remaining in the vial after that time should be discarded. Freezing should be avoided, as this reduces potency.

The various insulin preparations differ as to their onset of action, peak of action, and duration of action (Table 15.6). Insulin injection, being a solution, is categorized as prompt acting. Insulin suspensions are slower acting. Only insulin injection may be administered intravenously; all others, as well as insulin injection, are normally given subcutaneously, usually 30 minutes to 2 hours before a meal so that physiologic effects will parallel absorption of glucose. The dosage is individually determined, with the usual range being 5 to 100 U. The insulin injection containing 500 U/mL is employed in cases of insulin resistance requiring very large doses.

The pharmacist plays a vital role in the education of the diabetes patient, particularly in the proper use of insulin. The insulin dose should always be checked to ensure it is correct. Because it is a solution, regular insulin can be used in emergencies, such as ketoacidosis, to effect a rapid decrease in blood glucose levels. However, with the exception of diabetic ketoacidosis, it is rare for a patient to require a dose of regular insulin greater than 25 U. Typically, diabetes patients combine regular insulin with a modified insulin, such as NPH, to provide daily coverage in two injections (morning, late afternoon) or use premixed preparations. So it is important that the patient understand how much of each to use and in what order to mix them in the syringe. Regular insulin is drawn up first into the syringe.

In an institutional setting the pharmacist must make sure written insulin orders are correctly transcribed or transmitted. Allied health care workers have made errors in insulin dosage. Written orders for 6 U of insulin have been interpreted to mean 60 U, and an order for 4 U has been read as 4 cc. Each of these occurred because the abbreviation U for units was read as a zero or cc.

The patient should be instructed to rotate the site of insulin injections. Rotation of the site will help to avoid lipohypertrophy, a buildup of fibrous tissue. With continual injection into one site, the tissue becomes spongy and avascular. The avascular nature of the site perpetuates the problem because the skin becomes anesthetized and the injection is not felt. This is a particular problem with children who continue to use the same site and do not realize that the absorption of insulin from this site becomes erratic and uncontrollable. Numerous brochures from manufacturers of diabetes supplies demonstrate the appropriate rotation of insulin injection sites over the entire body.

Another problem with insulin injections is the development of lipodystrophy. Generally, this problem appears within 2 months to 2 years following the beginning of insulin therapy and occurs predominantly in women and children. Its cause has been ascribed to injection of refrigerated insulin (not giving enough time for it to warm up prior to injection), to failure to rotate the injection site, and to impurities in the insulin. The result is the formation of a subcutaneous indentation or pothole caused by wasting or atrophy of the lipid tissue. It appears that the greater purity of current insulins has significantly decreased this problem, and a marked improvement in existing atrophic areas has been demonstrated by injection of highly purified pork or human insulin directly into or on the periphery of the atrophic areas.

Prior to use, the patient should be instructed to inspect the insulin carefully. Regular insulin and insulin glargine solutions should appear clear, while the other insulins, which are suspensions, should appear uniformly cloudy. With the suspensions the patient should be instructed how to prepare the insulin: the vial is rotated slowly and gently between the palms of the hands several times before the insulin is drawn into the syringe. This avoids frothing and bubble formation, which would result in an inaccurate dose. The patient should not shake the insulin vial.

Proper storage should also be encouraged. These preparations should be stored in a cool place or a refrigerator. The patient should be warned to avoid allowing the insulin to come into contact with extremes of temperature, that is, freezing, such as overnight in the car in the winter and heat, as in the glove compartment of a car in the summer or in direct sunlight. If this occurs, the patient should discard the insulin and get a new bottle. Any bottle of insulin that appears frosted or clumped should be returned to the pharmacy where the purchase took place. Finally, the patient should use the insulin in a timely fashion, not beyond the expiration date indicated on the insulin vial.

Human Insulin

Biosynthetic human insulin was the first recombinant DNA drug product to receive approval from FDA. This product, Humulin (Lilly), became available in 1983. It is produced by using a special non–disease-forming laboratory strain of *Escherichia coli* and recombinant DNA technology. A recombined plasmid DNA coding for human insulin is introduced into the bacteria, and it is then cultured by fermentation to produce the A and B chains of human insulin. These A and B chains are freed and purified individually before they are linked by the specific disulfide bridges to form human insulin. The insulin produced is chemically, physically, and immunologically equivalent to insulin derived from the human pancreas. The biosynthetic insulin is free of contamination with *E. coli* peptides, and is also free of the pancreatic peptides that are present as impurities in insulin preparations extracted from animal pancreas. These latter impurities include proinsulin and proinsulin intermediates, glucagon, somatostatin, pancreatic polypeptide, and vasoactive intestinal peptide.

Pharmacokinetic studies in some normal subjects and clinical observations in patients indicate that formulations of human insulin have a slightly faster onset of action and a slightly shorter duration of action than their purified pork insulin counterparts. Two formulations of human insulin were initially marketed: neutral regular human insulin (Humulin R, Lilly) and NPH human insulin (Humulin N, Lilly). Neutral regular human insulin consists of zinc insulin crystals in solution. It has a rapid onset of action and a relatively short duration of action at 6 to 8 hours. NPH human insulin is an intermediate-acting turbid preparation with a slower onset of action and longer duration of action (slightly less than 24 hours) than regular human insulin.

Human insulins should be stored as other insulins, in a cold place, preferably a refrigerator. Freezing should be avoided.

Lispro Insulin Solution

Lispro insulin solution consists of zinc insulin lispro crystals dissolved in a clear aqueous fluid. It is created when the amino acids at positions 28 and 29 on the insulin B-chain are reversed.

Lispro insulin solution is rapidly absorbed after subcutaneous administration and demonstrates no significant differences in absorption from abdominal, deltoid, and femoral sites of injection. Its bioavailability mimics that of regular insulin. However, peak serum levels of lispro insulin occur within 0.5 to 1.5 hours and are higher, and it is shorter acting, that is, 6 to 8 hours, than regular insulin. Peak hypoglycemic effects are more pronounced with lispro insulin solution. Thus, hypoglycemia is the primary complication associated with its use. Comparative studies have demonstrated, however, that hypoglycemic episodes have been less frequent with lispro insulin than with regular insulin.

Lispro insulin solution administered 15 minutes before meals has decreased the risk of hypoglycemic episodes and improved postprandial glucose excursions when compared to conventional regular insulin therapy. Some studies have demonstrated a greater impact on the quality of life with lispro insulin solution, and it has been shown to be more effective than regular insulin in reducing hypoglycemia associated with exercise within 3 hours after a meal. Thus, as a new insulin, it offers more flexibility for the diabetes patient and should be added to formularies as an alternative to regular insulin.

Lispro insulin solution should be stored in a refrigerator but not in the freezer. If accidentally frozen, it should not be used. If absolutely necessary, it may be stored at room temperature for up to 28 days, but storage temperature should be as cool as possible. The vial or cartridge should be kept away from direct light and heat. At the end of 28 days, any unused portion of the Lispro insulin solution should be discarded.

Insulin Aspart

Insulin aspart is a recombinant ultra–short-acting insulin using *Saccharomyces cerevisiae* (baker's yeast) as the production organism. It is homologous with regular human insulin except for a single substitution of the amino acid proline by aspartic acid in position B28. This insulin was developed to control postprandial glucose concentrations when administered 5 to 10 minutes before mealtime in a manner similar to that for insulin lispro. The dosage is individualized to the patient's needs.

Insulin aspart demonstrates pharmacokinetics very similar to those of lispro insulin solution in terms of onset of action (0.25 hours), peak effect (0.5–1 hour), and duration of action (3 hours).

Because of its very short duration of action, higher doses of NPH insulin are needed in combination with it than with regular insulin. In a meal-related regimen, 50 to 70% of this requirement may be provided by the insulin aspart and the remainder provided by the intermediate-acting or long-acting insulin. A few studies have demonstrated that patients treated with insulin aspart had better glucose control and fewer nocturnal hypoglycemic episodes than patients using regular insulin. These studies demonstrate that insulin aspart is a viable alternative therapy for patients who use regular insulin.

Mixing insulin aspart with NPH human insulin immediately before injection may produce some attenuation in the peak concentration of the insulin aspart. However, the time to peak concentration and the total bioavailability of the insulin aspart should not be affected. When insulin aspart is mixed with NPH human insulin, the insulin aspart should be drawn up first. This combination should be injected immediately after mixing. Insulin aspart should not be mixed with crystalline zinc insulin preparations because compatibility data are lacking.

Isophane Insulin Suspension (NPH Insulin)

Isophane insulin suspension is a sterile suspension in an aqueous vehicle buffered with dibasic sodium phosphate to pH 7.1 to 7.4. It is prepared from zinc insulin crystals modified by the addition of protamine so that the solid phase of the suspension consists of crystals of insulin, zinc, and protamine. Protamine is prepared from the sperm or the mature testes of fish belonging to the genus *Oncorhynchus* and others. As mentioned in the discussion of the aqueous insulin solutions, suspensions of insulin with a pH on the alkaline side inherently have a longer duration of action than solutions. Insulin is least soluble at pH 7.2.

The rod-shaped crystals of isophane insulin suspension should be approximately 30 μm long and the suspension free of large aggregates of crystals following moderate agitation. This is necessary for it to pass freely through the needle and for absorption of the drug to be consistent from one batch to another. When a portion of the suspension is examined microscopically, the suspended matter is largely crystalline, with only traces of amorphous material. The official injection is required to contain glycerin and phenol for stability and preservation. The specified expiration date is 24 months after the immediate container was filled by the manufacturer. The suspension is packaged in multiple-dose containers having not less than 10 mL of injection. Each milliliter contains 100 U of insulin. The suspension is best stored in a refrigerator, but freezing must be avoided.

As indicated earlier, isophane insulin suspension is an intermediate-acting preparation administered as required mainly as hormonal replacement in diabetes mellitus. The usual dose range subcutaneously is 10 to 80 U. Its effects are comparable with those of a mixture of 2 to 3 parts of regular insulin and 1 part of protamine zinc insulin.

The *NPH* used in some product names stands for neutral protamine Hagedorn, since the preparation is about neutral (pH about 7.2), contains protamine, and was developed by Hagedorn. The term *isophane* is based on the Greek *iso* (equal) and *phane* (appearance) and refers to the equivalent balance between the protamine and insulin.

Isophane Insulin Suspension and Insulin Injection

In years past, patients needing a rapid onset of action and intermediate duration of activity, approximately one day, would routinely mix isophane insulin suspension, an intermediate-acting insulin, with insulin injection, a rapid-acting insulin. Unexpected responses, such as hypoglycemic episodes, were encountered. It was fairly common for the patient to contaminate one of the vials during mixing. Subsequently, a premixed formulation of isophane insulin suspension and insulin injection became available, and now there are two formulations. The 70/30 combination consists of 70% isophane insulin suspension and 30% insulin injection, and the 50/50 combination consists of 50% isophane insulin suspension and 50% insulin injection. These combinations are stable and absorbed as if injected separately.

Humulin 50/50 achieves a higher insulin concentration (C_{max}) and higher maximum glucose infusion rates with more rapid elimination than Humulin 70/30. However, as expected, the cumulative amounts of insulin absorbed (area under the curve, or AUC) and the cumulative effects over 24 hours following injection are identical. Thus, the 70/30 combination provides an initial response tempered with a more prolonged release of insulin. The 50/50 mixture is useful when a greater initial response is required and for patients who have been using extemporaneously compounded insulin mixtures in a 50/50 ratio.

The Humulin 70/30 and 50/50 premixed insulins are cloudy suspensions with a zinc content of 0.01 to 0.04 mg/100 U. These insulins are neutral in pH and phosphate buffered. m-Cresol and phenol are the preservatives for both combinations. Protamine sulfate is the modifying protein salt.

Patients should not attempt to change the ratio of these products by adding NPH or regular insulin. If Humulin N and Humulin R mixtures are prescribed in a different proportion, the individual insulin products should be mixed in the amounts recommended by the physician.

Humalog Mix

Humalog Mix is a manufactured premixed insulin consisting of insulin lispro and neutral protamine lispro (NPL) in a fixed ratio. Humalog Mix 50/50 consists of 50% insulin NPL suspension and 50% insulin lispro injection. Humalog Mix 75/25 contains 75% insulin NPL suspension and 25% insulin lispro injection. It is estimated that these premixed combinations are used by more than 40% of diabetes patients who inject insulin twice daily.

These fixed combinations were developed to give better control for diabetes patients who use a combination of short- and long-acting insulin. In comparison to Humulin 70/30, Humalog Mix 75/25 demonstrated lower postprandial blood glucose levels and no difference between the afternoon and overnight glucose values. Furthermore, insulin NPL suspension was developed as an alternative to combinations employing NPH insulin. NPH insulin was unstable over weeks to months when mixed with lispro insulin.

Insulin Zinc Suspension

Insulin zinc suspension contains zinc chloride, so that the suspended particles consist of a mixture of crystalline and amorphous insulin in a ratio of approximately 7 parts of crystals to 3 parts of amorphous material. The sterile suspension is in an aqueous vehicle buffered with sodium acetate to pH 7.2 to 7.5. In treating insulin with zinc chloride, it is possible to obtain both crystalline and amorphous zinc insulin. The amorphous form has the most prompt hypoglycemic effect, since the particles are the smallest and are absorbed into the system more rapidly after subcutaneous injection than are the crystals. Also, the larger the crystals, the less prompt and the longer-acting will be the suspension. By combining the crystalline and amorphous forms into one preparation, an intermediate-acting suspension is obtained. As noted in Table 15.6, the time activity of insulin zinc suspension is only slightly different from that for isophane insulin suspension. The advantage of the former is that it contains no foreign protein, such as protamine, which may produce local sensitivity reactions. Also, it may be combined as desired with either of the following two suspensions to produce an insulin preparation having the time activity that most closely meets the desires and requirements of the individual. Suspensions contain 100 U/mL in 10-mL vials. The individual crystalline and amorphous particles may be seen microscopically, with the crystals being predominantly 10 to 40 μm in maximum dimension and the amorphous particles no greater than 2 μm.

In addition to the sodium acetate buffer, the suspension contains about 0.7% sodium chloride for tonicity and 0.1% methylparaben for preservation. The expiration date of the suspension is 24 months after the immediate container was filled. The suspension must be stored in a refrigerator without freezing. As with all such preparations, the dose depends on the individual needs of the patient but generally ranges between 10 and 80 U.

Insulin Glargine

Insulin glargine is a long-acting (up to 24 hours) basal insulin preparation intended for once daily subcutaneous administration at bedtime in the treatment of type I diabetes mellitus in adults and children. It can also be used by adults with type II diabetes who require long-acting insulin. It is created when the amino acids at position 21 of human insulin are replaced by glycine and two arginines are added to the C terminus of the B chain.

Insulin glargine is a recombinant human insulin analogue. Formulated at a pH of 4.0, it is completely soluble at that pH. However, once it is injected into subcutaneous tissue, it is neutralized, which causes formation of microspheres. This peakless insulin begins working in 2 hours and mimics basal insulin secretion more closely than other long-acting insulins for 24 hours. This allows for once-daily dosing. Because insulin glargine provides only basal coverage, it is often used in conjunction with other insulins or oral hypoglycemic drugs. However, because of the unique release characteristics of insulin glargine, it should not be mixed with any other insulin. Differences in pH can cause clumping. If it has to be used in combination with a short-acting insulin, the injections must be administered separately.

The unique release characteristics of insulin glargine may help to decrease the number of required injections of long-acting insulin from twice daily to once daily. Clinical studies have demonstrated no relevant differences in insulin glargine absorption after abdominal, deltoid, or thigh administration.

If the patient is changing over to insulin glargine from an intermediate- or long-acting regimen, the dosage may or may not have to be adjusted. When patients are transferred from twice-daily NPH to insulin glargine once daily at bedtime, to reduce the risk of hypoglycemia, the initial dose is usually decreased by approximately 20% from the total daily dose of NPH product for the first week of treatment and then adjusted to the patient's response. However, when patients are transferred from once-daily NPH or ultralente insulin to once-daily insulin glargine, the initial dose is usually not changed.

Extended Insulin Zinc Suspension

Extended insulin zinc suspension is a sterile suspension of zinc insulin crystals in an aqueous medium buffered with sodium acetate to pH 7.2 to 7.5. It also contains 0.7% sodium

chloride for tonicity and 0.1% methylparaben for preservation. Because the suspended matter is composed solely of zinc insulin crystals, which are slowly absorbed, this preparation is classified as long acting. It may be mixed with either insulin zinc suspension or prompt insulin zinc suspension to achieve the proper time activity of an individual patient. The usual dosage range is 10 to 80 U. It is commercially available in 10-mL vials providing 100 U/mL. The suspension must be stored in a refrigerator without freezing. The expiration date of the properly stored injection is not later than 24 months after the immediate container was filled.

Insulin Infusion Pumps

Insulin infusion pumps allow patients to achieve and maintain blood glucose at nearly normal levels on a *constant basis*. Continuous infusion of insulin through use of these small and lightweight pumps eliminates the need for the patient to adhere rigidly to a regimen of multiple daily injections of insulin. This provides convenience, better adherence, and control over the disease process. The main objective of pump therapy is strict control of the blood glucose level at 70 to 140 mg/dL. This is the primary way to avoid complications such as gangrene and diabetic retinopathy.

Early insulin infusion pumps were large bedside units used mainly in hospitals. Today an insulin pump is the size and weight of a personal pager. It is a plastic-encased computer device that can be worn in a pocket or bra or on a belt. A computer chip in the pump allows the patient to program the amount of insulin for the pump to release. Inside the pump, a syringe reservoir holds up to 300 U of U-100 insulin. Unlike conventional insulin therapy, which normally combines rapid-acting and intermediate-acting insulin, the infusion pump delivers either short-acting or rapid-acting insulin. Frequently a rapid-acting insulin, such as aspart (Novolog) or lispro (Humalog) is preferred.

The reservoir delivers insulin through a plastic infusion set, available in 24-inch or 42-inch lengths. The triggering device inserts the infusion set's flexible catheter into the subcutaneous tissue. Once the catheter is inserted, the needle is removed. An alarm can be set to warn of a low battery or to indicate that the insulin was not delivered.

Most patients insert the infusion set into the abdomen. Here the insulin is rapidly and consistently absorbed. It is crucial that the set be inserted subcutaneously and not intramuscularly. Patients should understand not to place it where their clothing may rub against it (e.g., underwear area, waistline, a 4-inch area around the umbilicus) and to make sure to rotate the insertion site.

For optimal working efficiency, the patient should change the infusion site every 2 or 3 days or whenever blood glucose is above 240 mg/dL for two tests in a row. This may indicate that the infusion set is not working properly.

It is very important that patients understand the necessity to monitor their blood glucose so they know to adjust their dosage of insulin. Patients should check their blood glucose level before each meal, at bedtime, and whenever they have symptoms of hypoglycemia (sweating, shakiness, nausea, headache, difficulty concentrating) or hyperglycemia (polyuria, polydipsia, polyphagia, nocturnal enuresis, weakness, fatigue, blurred vision, alteration in mental status).

Infection at the site is a concern and a problem. Prevention is the best treatment; however, if the site becomes infected, the patient's health care provider should be informed and antibiotics ordered to treat it. In the meantime, the infusion set should be moved to another site, or insulin may be administered manually until the infection is cured.

At night, the insulin pump can be placed on the night stand close to the bed, in the bed next to the patient, or in a pajama pocket. When bathing, the patient can place the pump on the bathroom floor and allow the tubing to drape over the side of the tub. For showering, the pump can be placed in a special plastic bag and hung around the patient's neck or on the faucet handle.

Large-Volume Parenterals

Common examples of large volume parenterals in use today are presented in Table 15.7. These solutions are usually administered by intra-

venous infusion to replenish body fluids or electrolytes or to provide nutrition. They are usually administered in volumes of 100 mL to 1 L or more per day by slow intravenous infusion with or without a controlled-rate infusion system (Fig. 15.33). Because of the large volumes administered, these solutions must not contain bacteriostatic agents or other pharmaceutical additives. They are packaged in large single-dose containers (Figs. 15.34 and 15.35).

As indicated previously, electrolytes, vitamins, and antineoplastics are frequently incorporated into large-volume parenterals for coadministration to the patient. It is the responsibility of the pharmacist to understand the physical and chemical compatibility of the

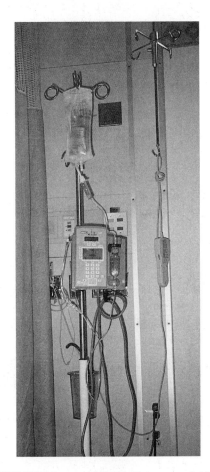

FIGURE 15.33 Accurate delivery of intravenous fluids and medications by use of a controlled-rate infusion system (Alaris Medical Systems) for the drug vial and a volumetric infusion pump for the intravenous fluids. (Courtesy of Mr. Akinwale O. Onamade.)

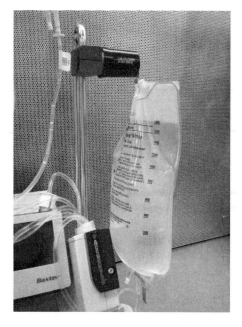

FIGURE 15.34 Intravenous solution packaged in pliable plastic. (Courtesy of Ms. Amy Schuppert Smith)

additive in the solution in which it is placed. Obviously, a combination that results in formation of insoluble material or affects the efficacy or potency of the therapeutic agent of the vehicle is not acceptable.

It is also important to be vigilant for incompatibilities associated with multiple infusions coadministered to a patient. A typical nursing question may be, "Can the dopamine drip be run in with the heparin drip?" To answer these questions, the pharmacist must know about parenteral therapy and be aware of incompatibilities reported in the literature. Numerous

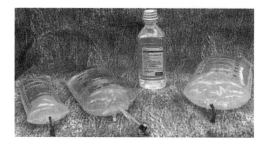

FIGURE 15.35 Peritoneal dialysis and irrigation fluids. (Courtesy of William B. French, PhD.)

references (e.g., *Handbook on Injectable Drugs, King's Guide to Parenteral Admixtures* [King Guide Publications]) are available for sources listing and discussing parenteral incompatibilities. However, the pharmacist should use only the most current edition of these references. Whenever possible, the pharmacist should attempt to answer these important questions and explain the incompatibilities that come to his or her attention as part of the daily routine. Furthermore, the pharmacist should create a file of data and add to it from experience and the literature. Internet-accessible services (e.g., Micromedex) can also be employed to check incompatibilities. These reference the *Handbook on Injectable Drugs* and *King's Guide to Parenteral Admixtures*.

While it is impossible to chart every possible admixture incompatibility, principles can be learned and applied. For example, certain drugs are inactivated or precipitate at either high or low pH values; some drugs (e.g., sympathomimetics) encounter problems when added to intravenous fluids; and certain therapeutic large-volume solutions (e.g., sodium bicarbonate, urea, mannitol) should never contain additives.

Large-volume parenteral solutions are employed in *maintenance therapy* for the patient entering or recovering from surgery and for the patient who is unconscious and unable to take fluids, electrolytes, and nutrition orally. The solutions may also be used in *replacement therapy* for patients who have suffered a heavy loss of fluid and electrolytes.

Maintenance Therapy

When a patient is receiving parenteral fluids for only a few days, simple solutions providing adequate amounts of water, dextrose, and small amounts of sodium and potassium generally suffice. When patients are unable to take oral nutrition or fluids for slightly longer periods, say 3 to 6 days, solutions of higher caloric content may be used. If oral feeding must be deferred for periods of weeks or longer, total parenteral nutrition (TPN) must be implemented to provide all of the essential nutrients to minimize tissue breakdown and to maintain normalcy within the body. Total nutrient admixtures (TNA, three-in-one) include all substrates necessary for nutritional support—carbohydrates, protein, fat, electrolytes, trace elements—mixed in a single plastic intravenous bag for convenient administration.

These admixtures are very useful for chemotherapy, gastrointestinal, and anorexic patients. The use of three-in-one admixtures in pediatrics, especially for neonates, is controversial. The concentrations of calcium, phosphorus, and necessary warm administration for pediatric TPN do not lend themselves to stable preparations. As a result, many pediatric institutions do not compound three-in-one admixtures for their patients but administer the fat emulsion separately.

When using TNA, the pharmacist must consider the order of substrate mixing, differentiate between various brands of substrate and their physicochemical properties, determine the type of plastic bag system that is most appropriate, determine whether (and by what mode) the TNA should be filtered prior to infusion, determine how the product should be stored, and assess any potential complications. For example, the use of "standard" TPN plastic bags may result in plasticizer leaching into the solution and injuring the patient.

In April 1994 the FDA issued a safety alert regarding the hazards of precipitation associated with parenteral nutrition (21). This was in response to two deaths and at least two other cases of respiratory distress associated with the use of three-in-one admixtures. Autopsies revealed diffuse microvascular pulmonary emboli linked to a calcium phosphate precipitate in the admixture. Consequently, the FDA safety alert recommends that a filter be used when infusing either central or peripheral parenteral nutrition admixtures. A 0.22-μm filter containing both a bacterial-retentive and an air-eliminating filter has been recommended for use with lipid-free (two-in-one) parenteral nutrient solutions.

Lipid emulsions and three-in-one parenteral nutrient solutions can be safely filtered at a pore size of at least 1.2 μm. A problem with the lipid emulsion in a three-in-one admixture is that it obscures any precipitate. Thus, if a lipid emulsion is needed, a preferable alternative is to employ a two-in-one admixture with a lipid infused separately via a Y-site.

Replacement Therapy

When the patient has undergone a heavy loss of water and electrolytes, as in severe diarrhea or vomiting, greater than usual amounts of these materials may be initially administered and then maintenance therapy provided. Patients with Crohn's disease, AIDS, burns, or trauma are candidates for replacement therapy.

Water Requirement

In normal individuals, the daily water requirement is the amount needed to replace normal and expected losses. Water is lost daily in the urine and feces and from the skin and respiration. The normal daily requirement of water for adults is about 25 to 40 mL/kg of body weight, or an average of about 2 L/m^2 of body surface area (22). Nomograms for determination of body surface area from height and weight are presented in Figure 2.10. Children and small adults need more water per pound of body weight than do larger adults; water requirements correlate more closely with body surface area than with weight, and a guideline to estimate normal daily requirement for water in these patients is as follows:

1. <10 kg: 100 mL/kg/day
2. 10–20 kg: 1000 mL plus 50 mL/kg/day for weight over 10 kg
3. >20 kg to maximum of 80 kg: 1500 mL plus 20 mL/kg/day for weight over 20 kg

However, in the newborn, the volume administered in the first week or two should be about half that calculated from body surface area.

In water replacement therapy for adults, 70 mL/kg/day may be required in addition to maintenance water requirements; a badly dehydrated infant may require an even greater proportion (22). Thus, a 50-kg patient may require 3500 mL for replacement plus 2400 mL for maintenance. To avoid fluid overload, especially in elderly patients and those with renal or cardiovascular disorders, monitoring of blood pressure is desirable.

Because water administered intravenously as such may cause osmotic hemolysis of red blood cells and because a patient who requires water generally requires nutrition and/or electrolytes, parenteral administration of water is generally as a solution with dextrose or electrolytes with sufficient tonicity (sodium chloride equivalency) to protect the red blood cells from hemolyzing.

Electrolyte Requirement

Potassium, the primary intracellular cation, is particularly important for normal cardiac and skeletal muscle function. The usual daily intake of potassium is about 100 mEq and the usual daily loss is about 40 mEq. Thus, any replacement therapy should include a minimum of 40 mEq plus the amount needed to replace additional losses. Potassium can be lost through excessive perspiration, repeated enemas, trauma (such as severe burns), uncontrolled diabetes, disease of the intestinal tract, surgical operation, and the use of such medications as thiazide and loop diuretics. Poorly nourished people, those using very low-calorie diet products, and victims of anorexia nervosa or acute alcoholism also may have low potassium levels (hypokalemia), because they are not taking in enough of the mineral. Symptoms of potassium loss include a weak pulse, faint heart sounds, falling blood pressure, and general weakness. Severe loss of potassium can lead to death. Too much potassium is not a good thing, either. An excess may cause diarrhea, irritability, muscle cramps, and pain. Hyperkalemia can be caused by kidney failure or excessive consumption of potassium-rich foods. Prescribed potassium supplements, potassium-sparing diuretic therapy, angiotensin-converting enzyme inhibitors (e.g., lisinopril) and the indiscriminate use of OTC salt substitutes have also been implicated to induce hyperkalemia.

In cases of severe potassium deficiency, intravenous electrolyte replacement is usually employed. The pharmacist who receives a prescription for intravenous potassium chloride must be careful and check the amount of potassium chloride in the prescription and the infusion rate. Potassium preparations must be di-

luted with a suitable large-volume parenteral solution, mixed well, and given by slow intravenous infusion. They are not to be administered undiluted. Undiluted potassium chloride administered intravenously has killed people.

The most commonly used concentration of potassium chloride for continuous-infusion maintenance therapy is 20 to 40 mEq/L. With a peripheral line, that concentration may increase to 60 mEq/L, and with a central line, the maximum concentration can be up to 80 mEq/L.

For intermittent potassium replacement therapy in patients with hypokalemia, the usual infusion rate is 10 mEq/hour (maximum recommended rate is 20 mEq/hour). Because of potassium chloride's ability to effect electrocardiographic (ECG) changes (e.g., progressive increase in height and peaking of T waves, lowering of the R wave, decreased amplitude and ultimate disappearance of the P waves), most hospitals establish a maximum infusion rate of 10 mEq/hour if the patient is not monitored by ECG. For patients monitored by ECG, the usual infusion rate is 20 mEq/hour with a maximum infusion rate of 40 mEq/hour, depending on the clinical condition of the patient.

For patients in need of aggressive potassium replacement, the potassium serum level should be assessed every 6 hours during the early intensive phase of therapy and once daily after normal potassium serum levels are achieved. For patients whose serum potassium is more than 2.5 mEq/L, the potassium level should be measured after the first 60 mEq is administered. For patients whose serum potassium is less than 2.5 mEq/L, the potassium level should be measured after the first 80 mEq is administered.

Sodium, the principal extracellular cation, is vital to maintain normal extracellular fluids. Average daily intake of sodium is 135 to 170 mEq (8–10 g). The body is able to conserve sodium when this ion is lost or removed from the diet. When there is sodium loss or a deficit, the daily administration of 3 to 5 g of sodium chloride (51 to 85 mEq) should prevent a negative sodium balance. A low sodium level in the body may result from excessive sweating, use of certain diuretics, or diarrhea. Fatigue, muscle weakness, apprehension, and convulsions are among the symptoms of excessive sodium loss. Sodium concentrations can increase when a person does not drink enough water, especially in hot weather, or if kidney function is impaired. Dry, sticky mucous membranes, flushed skin, elevated body temperature, lack of tears, and thirst are among the symptoms of sodium excess. Sodium has been implicated as a causative factor in about 20% of cases of high blood pressure. Chloride, the principal anion of the extracellular fluid, is usually paired with sodium. Chloride is also important for muscle contraction, balancing the fluid levels inside and outside the cells, and maintaining the acid-base balance of the extracellular fluid. An adequate supply of chloride is necessary to prevent bicarbonate, the second most prevalent anion, from tipping the acid-base balance to the alkaline side. In 1979, a lack of chloride in a brand of infant formula caused metabolic alkalosis in babies who had been exclusively fed that formula. As a result, Congress passed the Infant Formula Act of 1980, which spells out the nutrients that must be in formulas and establishes quality control procedures for the manufacture of these infant foods. Although other electrolytes and minerals, including calcium, magnesium, and iron, are lost from the body, they generally are not required during short-term parenteral therapy.

Caloric Requirements

Generally, patients requiring parenteral fluids are given 5% dextrose to reduce the caloric deficit that usually occurs in patients undergoing maintenance or replacement therapy. The use of dextrose also minimizes ketosis and the breakdown of protein. Basic caloric requirements may be estimated by body weight; in the fasting state, the average daily loss of body protein is approximately 80 g/day for a 70-kg man. Daily ingestion of at least 100 g of glucose reduces this loss by half.

Parenteral Nutrition

Parenteral nutrition is infusion of enough basic nutrients to achieve active tissue synthesis and growth. It is characterized by the long-term intravenous feeding of protein solutions containing high concentrations of dextrose (approximately 20%), electrolytes, vitamins, and in some instances insulin. Among the components used in parenteral nutrition solutions are the following, listed in quantities commonly provided per liter of fluid. The individual components and amounts vary with the patient's needs.

Electrolytes

Sodium	35 mEq
Potassium	30 mEq
Magnesium	5 mEq
Calcium	5 mEq
Chloride	40 mEq
Acetate	35 mEq
Phosphate	15 mM

Vitamins

Vitamin A	3300 IU
Vitamin D	200 IU
Vitamin E	10 IU
Vitamin C	100 mg
Niacin	40 mg
Vitamin B_2	3.6–4.93 mg
Vitamin B_1	3–3.35 mg
Vitamin B_6	4–4.86 mg
Pantothenic acid	15 mg
Folic acid	400 μg
Vitamin B_{12}	5 μg
Biotin	60 μg

Essential Amino Acids

L-Isoleucine	590 mg
L -Leucine	770 mg
L -Lysine acetate	870 mg
(free base	620 mg)
L -Methionine	450 mg
L -Phenylalanine	480 mg
L -Threonine	340 mg
L -Tryptophan	130 mg
L -Valine	560 mg

Nonessential Amino Acids

L -Alanine	600 mg
L -Arginine	810 mg
L -Histidine	240 mg
L -Proline	950 mg
L -Serine	500 mg
Aminoacetic acid	1.19 g

The large proportion of dextrose increases the caloric value of the solution while keeping the volume required to be administered to a minimum. The solution is administered slowly through a large vein, such as the superior vena cava. The superior vena cava is accessed through the subclavian vein immediately beneath the clavicle and near the heart. This permits rapid dilution of the concentrated hyperalimentation fluid and minimizes the risk of tissue or cellular damage due to the hypertonicity of the solution. Generally, final concentrations of dextrose (not more than 10%) can be given peripherally. Solutions containing more than 10% dextrose should be given via the superior vena cava.

Calcium, usually as calcium gluconate, and phosphate, usually as potassium or sodium phosphate, are frequently present in parenteral admixtures. A significant problem associated with their use is the formation of calcium phosphate, an insoluble precipitate. As mentioned earlier in this chapter, formation of calcium phosphate and deposition of its crystals in lung tissue led to the 1994 FDA safety alert (21).

Many factors have been implicated in formation of the insoluble precipitate. Among these are the concentration of the individual ions, the salt form of the calcium, the concentration and type of amino acids, the concentration of the dextrose, the temperature and pH of the TPN, the presence of other additives (e.g., cysteine), and the order of mixing. The potential for calcium phosphate precipitation is especially challenging for compounding neonate and pediatric TPN admixtures because of the small volume they are able to tolerate and the need for aggressive replacement therapy. Thus, pharmacists must be alert to avoid this serious compatibility problem.

Figure 15.36 demonstrates a four-station Nutrimix Macro TPN Compounder. This device can pump four nutritional solutions (dextrose, water, amino acids, fat) simultaneously to compound nutritional admixtures by gravimetric means. The user programs the volume and specific gravity of the fluid to be pumped, and the device calculates the weight of the solution that has to be transferred from the source station to the bag. The fifth load cell

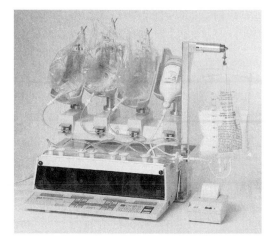

FIGURE 15.36 Nutrimix Macro TPN Compounder. (Courtesy of Abbott Hospital Products Division.)

serves as a confirmation of the weights programmed versus weights delivered. The picture demonstrates big flexible containers and the fat emulsion in glass. Figure 15.37 demonstrates the Nutrimix Micro TPN Compounder. This automatically dispenses small-volume nutritional additives into flexible containers that already contain a base nutritional admixture. The figure depicts 10 stations of small vials.

With the increasing use of parenteral solutions in children, including nutritional solu-

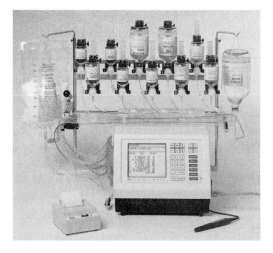

FIGURE 15.37 Nutrimix Micro TPN Compounder. (Courtesy of Abbott Hospital Products Division)

tions, pharmacists are frequently confronted with inquiries concerning the appropriate method of parenteral drug delivery (23). A dilemma with young patients is that they often have a limited fluid capacity caused by disease (e.g., congestive heart failure, renal insufficiency) and limited vascular access. As a consequence, pharmacists are asked whether a medication can be administered along with a parenteral nutrition solution. Although this practice is to be discouraged, it may be the only way to ensure that the patient is receiving adequate nutrition as well as appropriate drug therapy. Furthermore, administering the medication with the nutritive solution, rather than interrupting the feeding to administer medication, makes rebound hypoglycemia less likely. However, the practice of administering medication through a central venous line intended for parenteral nutrition solutions is not without risks. Catheter sepsis and occlusion can result.

Formerly, TPN was prepared 1 L at a time. However, to conserve time, a 24-hour supply is much more efficient and now the norm. Indeed, if a patient encounters a problem necessitating remake of a bag, the cost difference between 1 or 2 1000 mL bags and a 2000 mL bag is not that significant. Waste should not be a consideration because the attending physician should not use the TPN to adjust minutely for a patient's need. Typically, electrolyte requirements exceed the physical compatibilities of the TPN components (e.g., calcium–phosphate compatibilities in lipid-containing TPNs), and when this occurs, the pharmacist should encourage the physician to order a separate infusion to make up the deficiency.

The following abbreviations may be used in the hospital in describing the desired order for parenteral nutrition:

CVTPN (central vein TPN)
TPN (total parenteral nutrition)
PPN (peripheral parenteral nutrition)

Enteral Nutrition

As appropriate, hospitalized and home care patients may receive their nutritional needs through *enteral* rather than *parenteral* means. Enteral nutrition products may be administered orally, via nasogastric tube, via feeding gastrostomy, or via needle–catheter jejunostomy. These products are formulated to contain a variety of vitamins, minerals, carbohydrates, proteins, fats, and caloric requirements to meet the specific needs of patients. While parenteral feeding is appropriate for short-term use in a hospital or long-term care facility or when the gastrointestinal tract is unable to absorb nutrients, enteral feeding is preferable whenever possible. It is just as effective as a source of nutrients, less expensive than parenteral feeding, and has a low potential to cause serious complications.

The defined formula diets may be monomeric or oligomeric (amino acids or short peptides and simple carbohydrates) or polymeric (complex protein and carbohydrates). Modular supplements are used for individual supplementation of protein (ProMod powder, Propac powder), carbohydrate (Moducal powder), or fat (Lipomul liquid) when formulas do not offer sufficient flexibility. For example, a physician may order a powder reconstituted one-quarter strength, half-strength, or full strength for a particular patient and have the preparation administered via a nasogastric tube, a feeding gastrostomy, or a needle–catheter jejunostomy.

There is no single classification system for these products, and there are different criteria for evaluating and categorizing them. Caloric density (generally in the range of 1, 1.5, or 2 kcal/mL) influences the density of other nutrients. Protein content is also a major determinant in these products. For patients with diarrhea and cramping, high-osmolality formulas may present difficulty. Low-fat products should be suggested for patients with significant malabsorption, hyperlipidemia, or exocrine pancreatic insufficiency. Medium-chain triglycerides, while providing a useful source of energy in patients with malabsorption, do not provide essential fatty acids.

Originally, enteral feedings contained lactose and presented problems in lactase-deficient individuals. This ingredient has been eliminated from many of the nutritionally complete enteral formulas. For patients with hepatic or renal disease, the sodium and potassium content of the formulations must be considered. For patients receiving warfarin therapy, consideration should be focused on the content of vitamin K in the formulation. Although many products now have less vitamin K than before, caution is still warranted to avoid hypoprothrombinemic alterations in warfarin therapy.

Specific enteral products are selected according to the patient type they serve. For example, a requirement for less than 2000 calories per day or increased protein typically applies to an elderly, bedfast patient who is not physically active. This level of support is also advocated for postsurgical patients and those with infection or fractured bones. While requiring fewer calories, these individuals still need normal nutrients, including protein. Such products as Ensure HN, Sustacal, and Osmolite HN are appropriate in this circumstance. Most persons, including those with poor appetite or cancer, need 2000 to 3000 calories per day. The last category of patients is those with daily caloric needs that exceed 3000 calories. These individuals usually have high protein losses from severe trauma, such as burns, sepsis, or multiple trauma. As in the first example, there are numerous products for these patient categories.

The pharmacist can help select these products, because they do differ in amounts of carbohydrate, fat, protein, and fiber. Furthermore, these products differ in taste and consumer acceptability criteria, such as mouth feel and cost. Pharmacists may encounter consumers who wish to self-administer an enteral product. If the intent is to supplement calories or protein in an otherwise healthy individual who simply wishes to ensure a balanced dietary intake, a complete formula can be recommended. However, if it is intended to help a person regain weight lost unexpectedly, the individual should be instead referred to a doctor. Sudden weight loss may indicate a serious pathologic problem requiring medical attention.

Pharmacists can also help manage the cost of these products. Composition (oligomeric or polymeric) and form (ready to use vs. powder) influence cost. Generally, the polymeric products are less expensive than the oligomeric products. While powder forms may be less ex-

pensive than ready-to-use formulations, there is an indirect cost of labor required in powder preparation.

Intravenous Infusion Devices

Since the early 1970s, the use of the intravenous route to administer drugs has become increasingly popular. In 1989, it was estimated that about 40% of drugs and fluid used in hospitals was administered intravenously (22). This increase has affected the development and use of mechanical infusion devices. Advances in infusion technology and computer technology have resulted in devices with extremely sophisticated drug delivery capabilities (e.g., multiple-rate programming, pump or controller operation) (24). As a result, these cost-efficient devices provide greater accuracy and reliability of drug delivery than the traditional gravity-flow infusion methods. They also help reduce the fluid volume attributable to the medication infusion and decrease the need for monitoring fluid input, saving nurses' time. Furthermore, multiple-drug dosages can be administered, and incompatible drugs can be administered separately (22).

Originally, the disadvantages associated with these mechanical devices included the initial capital investment and extensive in-service education. Furthermore, the influence of infusion pump devices on the delivery of a drug was not fully recognized by clinicians. For example, intrinsic factors (e.g., operating mechanisms, flow accuracy, flow continuity, occlusion detection) and an extrinsic factor (back pressure) may have altered the rate of drug delivery and the therapeutic response of the patient.

Pumps were classified by their *mechanism of operation* (peristaltic, piston, diaphragm), *frequency or type of drug delivery* (continuous or intermittent, bolus dosing, single solution or multiple solution), or *therapeutic application* (PCA) (25). Current research focuses on the influence of drug delivery by these devices and the creation of new technologies (e.g., implantable pumps, pumps with chronobiologic applications, osmotic pressure devices, and open- or closed-loop systems) (25). Today several features are to be considered in selecting an infusion pump system. Most important is patient safety, then convenience and versatility of the device and cost efficiency.

In terms of enhanced safety, there should be a flow check occlusion alarm system that monitors in-line resistance of incremental back pressure. Also, does the device have a flow rate calculation system that is automatic after the volume and time are selected? Does it protect against inadvertent gravity free flow? Against tampering?

In terms of greater convenience and versatility, does the infusion device possess programmed delivery? Is the system user friendly, easy to understand and use? Does it have an incremental flow rate, and what is the minimum amount that can be delivered incrementally? Some newer infusion devices can deliver 0.1 mL/hour. Does it have an automatic restart feature once an occlusion clears, and can automatic piggybacking be employed to accommodate secondary medications? What is the volume capacity? Some infusion devices can accommodate a range of volumes from 0.1 to 9,999 mL (e.g., Baxter's 6060 Multitherapy Infusion Pump, 0.1–999.9 mL in 0.1-mL increments or 1000–9999 mL in 1-mL increments).

In terms of cost efficiency, can the device be used with standard administration sets? For example, the Baxter Laboratories standard administration sets are compatible with the Flo-Gard 6201 Volumetric Infusion Pump. This eliminates the need for costly disposable sets and reduces the potential for waste.

ALARIS Medical Systems (http://www.alarismed.com/products/infusion_medley.shtml) markets a variety of infusion systems. One of these is the Medley System, which uses modularity, a common user interface, and the Guardrails Safety Software suite of applications, which improve medication safety by using total quality management (TQM) principles for administration at the point of care. Table 15.8 lists several infusion devices used in parenteral nutrition support and features associated with each.

SmartDose, marketed by Pro-Med Medizinische Produktions-und Handels-AG (http://www.smartdose.com/eng/html/pump.shtml),

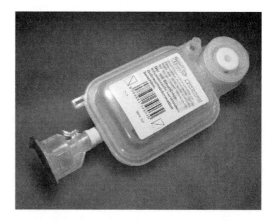

FIGURE 15.38 SmartDose, a portable disposable system for infusion or irrigation therapy. (Courtesy of Pro-Med AG.)

is a portable disposable system for infusion or irrigation therapy that allows the patient a high degree of mobility in a hospital or ambulatory environment (Fig. 15.38). It provides the precision of an electronic pump and the simplicity of an infusion bag. A chemical reaction in the attached power cell creates controlled gas pressure that is applied to dispense the liquid content in an accurate fashion through the dedicated administration set.

Special Considerations Associated With Parenteral Therapy

Look-Alike Products

To prevent mixups in which one drug product is selected in error because of its similarity in appearance to another, storage shelves should be labeled to warn about this possibility. A recent example of a serious medication error occurred when Lupron Depot-Ped 11.25 mg (Leuprolide acetate-TAP), a 1-month gonadotropin-releasing analogue used to treat central precocious puberty, was confused with Lupron Depot 3 Month. The latter is administered every 3 months to women with endometriosis or uterine leiomyomata (fibroids). The product releases its active ingredient over 3 months. Inadvertently, the second product was administered to children and caused them to receive therapy that was too low. It led attending physicians to

TABLE 15.8 SELECTED INFUSION DEVICES USED IN PARENTERAL NUTRITION SUPPORT

PUMP	MANUFACTURER	FEATURES
Breeze Lifecare 175	Abbott	Uses standard Abbott non-cassette gravity tubing. Includes both primary and secondary infusion capability, titration, built-in free-flow protection, adjustable occlusion pressure sensitivity (4 or 8 PSI), alarm history log, and optional flow detector. Air-in-line alarms, proximal and distal occlusion alarms. Indicated for various types of infusion, including parenteral and enteral, TPN, lipids, antibiotics and nitroglycerin therapies.[1]
Colleague 3	Baxter	Micro and macro rate range, basic delivery programming, piggybacking secondary medications, special programming functions for dosing, attachment to a remote nurse call system. A variety of systems exist which enable alert and alarm conditions to be transmitted to a remote location via the communications port on the rear panel assembly of the pump. Auto restart: allows the pump channel to automatically restart if an occlusion is relieved within one minute after detection.[2]
Flo-Gard 6201	Baxter	Flow check occlusion alarm (an in-line resistance display of incremental back pressure), flow rate calculation is automatic after volume and time are selected, slide clamp option offers an additional step to protect against inadvertent gravity free flow, front panel lock-out protects against tampering, automatic restart once occlusion clears, automatic piggybacking of secondary medication, programmed delivery profile allows up to 10 steps, individualizing control of infusion ramping and tapering.[3]
Horizon Nxt	B. Braun	Can deliver fluid from a negative head height (when the I.V. fluid container is lower than the pump), provides clinically accepted volumetric accuracy for all standard I.V. fluids, including blood, lipids and TPN. Profile Delivery mode incorporates a standard ramped delivery regimen, and the Programmable Delivery mode can be set up to sequentially deliver up to nine user-selected volumes of fluid each at a user-selected rate. Both modes are designed for ease of use and can be adapted to home-care settings. Automatically calculates the rate when dose information is entered, or the dose when rate information is entered. Distinct audible and visual alarm signals to indicate KVO, low battery, and actual alarm conditions. alarms: air-in-line, container empty, door open, downstream occlusion, hold time exceeded, low battery, low flow from container, close roller clamp, system error, upstream occlusion.[4]
Sabratek 6060	Baxter	Ambulatory multi-therapy device that can be used for enteral, epidural, subcutaneous, arterial and intravenous applications, using rotary peristaltic operation. It has five different methods of delivery: can be programmed using either milligrams or milliliters, and provides the option of programming using rate (ml/hr.) or time (volume delivered over a specific time period). Memory is indefinite until parameters are changed by the user, and if the pump is stopped during delivery, it will begin at the same point in the infusion when restarted. The pump uses YES/NO response to on-screen questions to facilitate easy programming, also uses a remote bolus cord.[5]

Footnotes

1. http://www.msdistributors.com/biomed/meh/LIFECARE.HTM

2. http://www.ardusmedical.com/products/baxter_colleague.htm

3. http://www.infusingsolutions.com/Assets/FG6201.pdf

4. http://www.ardusmedical.com/products/mcgraw_hor_nxt.htm

5. http://www.ardusmedical.com/products/baxter_6060.htm

believe the drug therapy was a failure. One reason for the confusion was that the pharmacy staff inadvertently selected the wrong computer code during order entry, and this was repeated when, after referencing patients' drug profiles for monthly refills, staff continued to select the 3-month dosage form instead of the monthly pediatric dosage form (26).

The manufacturer actually anticipated the problem and placed a picture of either an adult or a child to help discriminate the products. Unfortunately, price stickers were placed directly over the pictures and obscured the visual cues. To compound the problem, the products were taken to the pediatricians' offices, where the nurses administering the product also failed to note the mistake. The mistake might not have been detected except that a parent of one of the children questioned the pharmacy to ask about the increased prescription cost; Lupron Depot 3-Month costs more than Lupron Depot-Ped.

Adsorption of Drugs

Numerous studies have demonstrated that some drugs are adsorbed to the inner lining of intravenous containers and tubing or administration sets. Some of the drugs that have been implicated in this phenomenon and lost from aqueous solutions during infusion through plastic intravenous delivery systems include the following:

- Chlorpromazine HCl
- Diazepam
- Insulin
- Nitroglycerin
- Promazine HCl
- Promethazine HCl
- Thiopental sodium
- Thioridazine HCl
- Trifluoperazine HCl
- Warfarin sodium

Pharmacists must be cognizant of this and take appropriate steps to prevent it. The significance of the loss is magnified with drugs that are used in small quantities because a small amount lost to adsorption results in a higher percentage loss of the drug delivered to the patient. One method to minimize this is to administer infusions through short lengths of small-diameter tubing made of inert plastics.

Nitroglycerin (NTG), for example, should always be prepared in glass and/or a plastic known to be compatible with it. It is adsorbed (40–80% of total dose) to polyvinyl chloride (PVC), a plastic commonly used in administration components and some infusion solution bags and intravenous tubing. Previously, some manufacturers packaged NTG for intravenous use with special non-PVC tubing to avoid loss (<5%) of the drug into the tubing during administration. However, many manufacturers have discontinued supplying NTG IV in the U.S. market. Baxter Healthcare and Abbott Laboratories still manufacture NTG IV. Baxter Healthcare markets nitroglycerin 25, 50, and 100 mg in a glass bottle, 250 mL in 5% dextrose. However, the administration set, including tubing, is sold separately from the medication.

Special high-density polyethylene administration sets are recommended for NTG IV administration. Hard solid plastics, such as polyethylene and polypropylene, generally do not adsorb NTG. The amount of NTG adsorption depends on such factors as concentration, flow rate (e.g., a slow flow rate and long tubing increase the loss of NTG), surface area of the tubing, and contact time with the tubing.

Intravenous NTG should be regulated by automatic infusion equipment (pumps, controllers) to enhance consistent dose administration. However, infusion pumps may fail to occlude the non-PVC infusion sets completely because the non-PVC tubing is stiffer than standard PVC tubing. Excessive flow at low infusion rate settings may occur, causing alarms or unregulated gravity flow when the infusion pump is stopped. This could lead to overinfusion of NTG.

Some practitioners have responded by using the PVC tubing with the NTG and working around the problem. This is justified by some in that even though a great amount of drug is lost, the amount of drug the patient receives is based on hemodynamic functions. But when the previous set is replaced, retitration of the drug is necessary. To allay this problem, several manufacturers market non–PVC-containing pump administration sets.

The adsorption of insulin onto glassware and tubing depends on several factors, including concentration of insulin, contact time of insulin with glass and tubing, flow rate of the infusion, and presence of negatively charged proteins (human serum albumin). Plastic intravenous infusion sets have reportedly removed up to 80% of a dose, but 20 to 30% is more common. The percent adsorbed is inversely proportional to the insulin concentration and will take place within 30 to 60 minutes. Because this phenomenon cannot be easily and accurately predicted, it is essential to monitor the patient.

Handling and Disposal of Chemotherapeutic Agents for Cancer

In the 1980s health care personnel became aware of environmental contamination from handling cytotoxic agents. Mutagenic and allergic case reports began to emerge in the literature, and in 1985, in response, the then American Society of Hospital Pharmacists (now the American Society of Health-System Pharmacists) published a technical assistance bulletin on handling cytotoxic and hazardous drugs. This bulletin has been updated through the years and is now found in the *Practice Standards of ASHP* (27).

In theory, "correct and perfect preparation and handling techniques will prevent drug particles or droplets from escaping from their containers while they are being manipulated" (27). However, nearly perfect technique is uncommon and perfection is quite impossible. Thus, institutions that use these hazardous drugs must have structured training and quality assurance programs, and the pharmacist must play a vital role in creating and executing them.

At risk for harm are personnel who handle cytotoxic drugs, and steps should be taken to minimize unnecessary exposure by implementing basic steps and following common sense (28). These basic steps include the following:

1. Using vertical laminar flow hoods or bacteriologic glove boxes for preparation and reconstitution of cytotoxic drugs

2. Wearing protective gloves and mask during product preparation
3. Handling and disposing of cytotoxic drugs centrally using specially designed waste containers and incineration
4. Periodic monitoring of personnel who handle admixtures of cytotoxic drugs (e.g., CBC, blood chemistry screen, differential cell count)
5. Informing personnel handling cytotoxic drugs of the risk to their health
6. Specialized labeling of containers to ensure proper handling and disposal of the cytotoxic agent

Other Injectable Products: Pellets or Implants

Historically, pellets or implants were sterile, small, usually cylindrical solid objects about 3.2 mm in diameter and 8 mm long, prepared by compression and intended to be implanted subcutaneously to provide continuous release of medication over time. The pellets, which are implanted under the skin (usually of the thigh or abdomen) with a special injector or by surgical incision, are used for potent hormones. Implantation provides the patient with an economical means of obtaining long-lasting effects (up to many months after a single implantation) and obviates frequent parenteral or oral hormone therapy. The implanted pellet, which may contain 100 times the amount of drug (e.g., desoxycorticosterone, estradiol, testosterone) given by other routes of administration, release the drug slowly into the general circulation.

Pellets were formulated with no binders, diluents, or excipients, to permit total dissolution and absorption of the pellet from the site of implantation. Recently, a levonorgestrel implant contraceptive system was developed. Rather than dissolve entirely, the surgically implanted capsules are intended to be removed by surgery after an appropriate amount of time (up to 5 years).

Levonorgestrel Implants

Levonorgestrel implants are a set of six flexible closed capsules of a dimethylsiloxane–methyl vinyl Siloxane copolymer, each containing 36 mg of the progestin (29). They are found in an insertion kit to facilitate subdermal implantation through a 2-mm incision in the mid upper arm about 8 to 10 cm above the elbow crease. They are implanted in a fanlike pattern about 15° apart for a total of 75°. Appropriate insertion facilitates removal by the end of the fifth year. This system provides long-term (up to 5 years) reversible contraception.

Diffusion of the levonorgestrel through the wall of each capsule provides a continuous low dose of progestin. Initially, the dose of levonorgestrel is about 85 μg/day, declining to about 50 μg/day by 9 months, about 35 μg/day by 18 months, and thereafter to about 30 μg/day. The resulting blood levels are substantially below those generally observed among users of combination oral contraceptives containing the progestins norgestrel or levonorgestrel. Because of the range of blood levels and variation in individual response, blood levels alone are not predictive of the risk of pregnancy in an individual woman (29).

Irrigation and Dialysis Solutions

Solutions for irrigation of body tissues and for dialysis are subject to the same stringent standards as parenteral preparations. The difference is in use. Irrigation and dialysis solutions are not injected into the vein but employed outside of the circulatory system. Because they are generally used in large volumes, they are packaged in large containers, generally of the screw-cap type, which permits rapid pouring. Dialysis solutions generally appear similar to intravenous bags, and irrigation solutions are screw-capped or bagged, so caution is necessary to avoid selecting the wrong product.

Irrigation Solutions

Irrigation solutions are intended to bathe or wash wounds, surgical incisions, or body tissues. Examples are presented in Table 15.9.

TABLE 15.9 EXAMPLES OF IRRIGATION SOLUTIONS

SOLUTION	DESCRIPTION
Acetic Acid Irrigation, USP	0.25% solution applied topically to bladder for irrigation; pH 2.8–3.4, calculated osmolarity 42 mOsm/L; during urologic procedures, washes away blood, surgical debris while maintaining suitable conditions for tissue and permitting unobstructed view.
Neomycin and Polymyxin B Sulfates Solution for Irrigation, USP	Sterile urogenital solution contains 57 mg neomycin sulfate (40 mg neomycin) and polymyxin B sulfate 200,000 U/mL; topical antibacterial in continuous irrigation of bladder; pH 4.5–6; 1 mL added to 1 L 0.9% NaCl, administered via 3-way catheter at 1 L/24 hr (40 mL/hr approx.).
Ringer's Irrigation, USP	NaCl 8.6 g/L, potassium chloride 0.3 g/L, calcium chloride 0.33 g/L in purified water, in same proportions as in Ringer's injection. Sterile and pyrogen free; used topically to irrigate; must be labeled NOT FOR INJECTION; pH 5–7.5, calculated osmolarity 309 mOsm/L.
Sodium Chloride Irrigation, USP	NaCl in water for injection; 77, 154 mEq/L each sodium, chloride in 0.45 and 0.9% solutions, respectively; NaCl irrigation pH 5.3 approx.; 0.45, 0.9% solutions calculated osmolarity 154, 308 mOsm/L, respectively. Employed topically to wash wounds and body cavities where absorption into blood not likely; also employed as enema; for simple evacuation, 150 mL; for colonic flush, 1500 mL may be used.
Sterile Water for Irrigation, USP	Sterilized and suitably packaged. Label designations FOR IRRIGATION ONLY, NOT FOR INJECTION must appear prominently. Must not contain any antimicrobial or other added agent.

Dialysis Solutions

Dialysis is separation of substances from one another in solution by taking advantage of their differing diffusibility through membranes. *Peritoneal dialysis* solutions, allowed to flow into the peritoneal cavity, are used to remove toxic substances normally excreted by the kidney. In cases of poisoning or kidney failure, or in patients awaiting renal transplants, dialysis is an emergency lifesaving procedure. Solutions are commercially available containing dextrose as a major source of calories, vitamins, minerals, electrolytes, and amino acids or peptides as a source of nitrogen. The solutions are made to be hypertonic (with dextrose) to plasma to avoid absorption of water from the dialysis solution into the circulation.

Peritoneal dialysis uses the principles of osmosis and diffusion across the semipermeable peritoneal membrane and includes osmotic and chemical equilibration of the fluid within the peritoneal cavity with that of the extracellular compartment. The semipermeable peritoneal membrane restricts the movement of formed elements (e.g., erythrocytes) and large molecules (e.g., protein) but allows the movement of smaller molecules (e.g., electrolytes, urea, water) in both directions across the membrane according to the concentration on each side of the membrane, with net movement occurring in the direction of the concentration gradient. Intraperitoneal instillation of dialysis solutions containing physiologic concentrations of electrolytes allows for movement of water, toxic substances, and/or metabolites across the membrane in the direction of the concentration gradient, removing these substances from the body following drainage of the solution from the peritoneal cavity (i.e., outflow).

Hemodialysis is employed to remove toxins from the blood. In this method, the arterial blood is shunted through a polyethylene catheter through an artificial dialyzing membrane bathed in an electrolyte solution. Following the dialysis, the blood is returned to the body circulation through a vein.

Various dialysis solutions are available commercially, and the pharmacist may be called upon to provide them or to make adjustments in their composition.

PHARMACEUTICS CASE STUDY

Subjective

You have been asked to prepare progesterone injection 200 mg/mL in sesame oil for a physician's office. How will you formulate it?

Objective

Progesterone is only sparingly soluble in vegetable oils, and cosolvents must be used to obtain the 200 mg/mL concentration. Hormone injections in oil sometimes contain benzyl alcohol and/or benzyl benzoate. Benzyl alcohol, in addition to being a solvent, has preservative and anesthetic properties. Benzyl benzoate can be metabolized to benzyl alcohol and benzoic acid.

Assessment

It is apparent that a cosolvent system must be used, possibly consisting of sesame oil, benzyl alcohol, and benzyl benzoate, similar to other hormone injections. The product must be sterilized and suitably packaged.

Plan

After reviewing the literature and the formulations for other hormone in oil injections, you determine that the formula will consist of benzyl alcohol 20%, benzyl benzoate 20%, and sesame oil 60%. The progesterone will be dissolved in the solvent system and be placed in a suitable container for dry heat sterilization. The dry heat sterilization will be validated but will start with 150° C for 1 hour. After sterilization, the injection will be aseptically packaged and labeled.

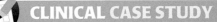

CLINICAL CASE STUDY

M.N. is an 18 y/o AA female diagnosed with type 1 diabetes mellitus 3 months ago. Today she presents to the clinic for her regular checkup. Yesterday, she had her local pharmacist download her blood glucose (BG) levels for the past month from her home monitor. M.N. takes these to her physician for interpretation. M.N. tells her physician that she is "concerned about some of her BG levels, especially in the morning." She notes that her morning BG levels are usually around 160 mg/dL. She also states that she has been waking up from nightmares around 3 A.M. a few times every week. Three nights ago, after waking up, she checked her BG level at 3 A.M. and her value was 192 mg/dL. She repeated the test to ensure that there was no error with her technique, and her reading was 188 mg/dL. Upon further questioning, the physician determines that M.N.'s knowledge of diabetes is increasing. However, the physician believes that M.N. would benefit from further education on diet and exercise. Because M.N. is newly diagnosed, the physician also wants her to review her insulin injection technique "from start to finish."

Meds: Humulin (NPH/Regular) 70/30 18 U before breakfast and 9 U before dinner.

Develop a pharmaceutical care plan addressing the following problems:
Hyperglycemia at 3:00 A.M., 8:00 A.M.
Nutrition and Exercise
Insulin injection technique

Pharmaceutical Care Plan

S: M.N. is seen in the clinic for a regular checkup by her primary care physician. She is concerned with some BG levels that she has recorded over the past month. She says she has had nightmares a few times every week in that time. M.N. has been compliant with her insulin regimen and has requested additional education on insulin injection technique along with nutrition and exercise information.

O: Weight: 120 lb (54.5 kg)
See graph for average BG levels for April.
Current medications:
Humulin (NPH/Regular) 70/30 18 U before breakfast and 9 U before dinner.

A: 1. M.N.'s BG is uncontrolled with hyperglycemia at 3:00 A.M. and 8:00 A.M. Hyperglycemia at these times is most likely because the patient is without appropriate insulin coverage throughout the night. M.N. checked her BG

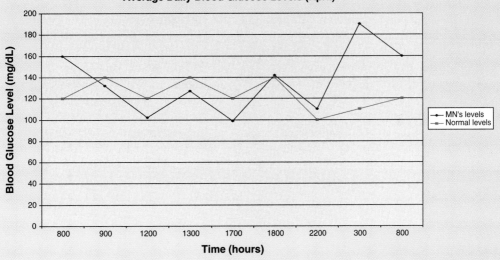

Clinical Case Study cont.

level at 3:00 A.M. after awakening from a nightmare, and the level was found to be elevated. The nightmares are an indication of high BG levels during sleep.

2. M.N. would like to review appropriate insulin injection preparation and administration technique with the pharmacist.

3. M.N. is a newly diagnosed patient and would like further information regarding diet and exercise.

P: 1. Because M.N.'s BG levels at 3:00 A.M. and 8:00 A.M. have been running high, it is appropriate to adjust the dinnertime dose of insulin. With a dinnertime dose of less than 10 U, the UKPDS suggests that the dose of insulin be increased by 1 U (if particular injection dose is more than 10 U, increase by 2 U). Therefore, M.N.'s Humulin 70/30 dose may be increased to 11 U at dinnertime to provide control during the night. M.N. should be instructed to monitor her 8:00 A.M. BG levels and three consecutive 3:00 A.M. BG levels and report these to her physician. If M.N. finds that her BG level after dinner is falling too low, she should increase her meal with one additional carbohydrate exchange.

2. The main points regarding insulin injection technique include in order:
Roll vial of insulin in palms to warm insulin and disperse it evenly.
Swipe the top of the vial once with an alcohol swab.
Swipe the body site for the injection with a different alcohol swab.
Pull air into the syringe. The amount of air pulled in should be equal to the amount of insulin that will be needed for the injection.
Insert the needle into the vial using the anticoring technique (demonstrated to the patient) and push the air into the vial.
While holding onto the vial and the syringe, invert both and remove the desired dose of insulin.
Remove syringe from vial.
At injection site, gather a fold of skin.
Insert needle at 90° angle to injection site.
Inject insulin.
Remove needle from skin.
Discard syringe in designated container for disposal.

3. Refer patient to registered dietitian for tailored meal planning. Some points M.N. should keep in mind:
Eat three scheduled meals per day. Skipping meals can cause BG to be uncontrolled.
Watch for serving sizes and control portion sizes.
Balance diet between carbohydrates, proteins, and fats.
It is important to monitor BG levels regularly.
Instruct patient to make exercise a regular part of her day. Explain that exercise can help lower BG levels and any extra effort can be beneficial (e.g. parking further away from the store, taking the stairs instead of an elevator). Caution: Start off slowly when beginning a new exercise program. For example, the patient may begin walking 3 days per week for 20 minutes and increase as tolerated. Instruct the patient to discuss the exercise regimen with a physician.

REFERENCES

1. Rapp RP, Bivins BA, Littrell RA, Foster, TS. Patient-controlled analgesia: a review of effectiveness of therapy and an evaluation of currently available devices. DICP, Ann Pharmacother 1989;23:899–904.

2. Kwan JW. Use of infusion devices for epidural or intrathecal administration of spinal opioids. Am J Hosp Pharm 1990;47 (Suppl 1):S18–S23.

3. Erstad BL, Meeks ML. Influence of injection site and route on medication absorption. Hosp Pharm 1993; 28:853–856; 858–860; 863–864; 867–868; 871–874; 877–878.

4. Highsmith AK, Greenhood GP, Allen JR. Growth of nosocomial pathogens in multiple-dose parenteral medication vials. J Clin Microbiol 1982;15:1024–1028.

5. Gershanik J, Boecler B, Ensley H, McCloskey S, George W. The gasping syndrome and benzyl alcohol poisoning. N Engl J Med 1982;307:1384–1388.

6. Nema S, Avis KE. Loss of LDH activity during membrane filtration. J Parenter Sci Technol 1993;47:16–21.

7. Sarry C, Sucker H. Adsorption of proteins on microporous membrane filters: Part I. Pharm Technol 1992; 16(Oct):72–82.

8. Sarry C, Sucker H. Adsorption of proteins on microporous membrane filters: Part II. Pharm Technol 1993;17(Jan):60–70.

9. McKinnon BT, Avis KE. Membrane filtration of pharmaceutical solutions. Am J Hosp Pharm 1993;50: 1921–1936.

10. Butler LD, Munson JM, DeLuca PP. Effect of inline filtration on the potency of low-dose drugs. Am J Hosp Pharm 1980;37:935–941.

11. Akers MJ, Attia IA, Avis KE: Understanding and Using F_0 Values. Pharm Tech 1987;11:44–48.

12. Wall DS, Noe LI, Abel SR, Hardwick LI, Plesek SR. A resource use comparison of Monovial with traditional methods of preparing extemporaneous small-volume intravenous infusions. Hosp Pharm 1997;32: 1647–1656.

13. Turco S, Miele WH, Barnoski D. Evaluation of an aseptic technique testing and challenge kit (Attack). Hosp Pharm 1993;28:11–16.

14. Crawford SY, Narducci WA, Augustine SC. National survey of quality assurance activities for pharmacy-prepared sterile products in hospitals. Am J Hosp Pharm 1991;48:2398–2413.

15. ASHP guidelines on quality assurance for pharmacy-prepared sterile products. Am J Health-Syst Pharm 2000;57:1150-1168.

16. ASHP. Draft guidelines on quality assurance for pharmacy-prepared sterile products. Am J Hosp Pharm 1992;49:407–417.

17. Erskine CR, Herzog KA. Quality assurance and control. In Gennaro AR, ed. Remington: the science and practice of pharmacy. 19th ed. Easton, PA: Mack, 1995, 648–652.

18. USP27-NF22. Chapter <797> Pharmaceutical Compounding—Sterile Preparations. Rockville, MD: U.S. Pharmacopeial Conv. Inc., 2004:2350–2370.

19. Maliekal J, Bertch KE, Witte KW. An update on ready-to-use intravenous delivery system. Hosp Pharm 1993;28:970–971, 975–977.

20. Turco S. Parenteral admixtures and incompatibilities. In: Sterile dosage forms. Philadelphia: Lea & Febiger, 1994;11:263.

21. McKinnon BT. FDA Safety alert: hazards of precipitation associated with parenteral nutrition. Nutr Clin Pract 1996;11:59–65.

22. Kwan JW. High-technology IV infusion devices. Am J Hosp Pharm 1989;46:320–335.

23. Munzenberger PJ, Levin S. Home parenteral antibiotic therapy for patients with cystic fibrosis. Hosp Pharm 1993;28:20–28.

24. KITS: Kit for infusion technology self-instruction. Abbott Park, IL: Abbott Laboratories.

25. Keefner KR. Parenteral pumps and controlled-delivery devices. US Pharmacist 1992;17(8):H-3–H-16.

26. Institute for Safe Medication Practices. Look-alike products. Pharmacy Today 2003; (5):20.

27. ASHP technical assistance bulletin on handling cytotoxic and hazardous drugs. Practice Standards of ASHP, 1997–1998. Bethesda, MD: American Society of Health-System Pharmacists, 1997:136–152.

28. Maliekal J, Bertch KE, Witte KW. An update on ready-to-use intravenous delivery system. Hosp Pharm 1993;28:267.

29. Fung S, Ferrill M. Contraceptive update: Subdermal implants. California Pharmacist 1992;40:35–41.

Biologics

16

Chapter at a glance

The Food and Drug Administration (FDA) refers to immunizing agents as biologics. In an encompassing manner, a biologic is a substance produced by a living source; biologics include antibiotics, hormones, and vitamins, among others. The Advisory Committee on Immunization Practices (ACIP) refers to immunizing agents as *immunobiologics*.

According to the *Code of Federal Regulations* (CFR), a biologic product is any virus, therapeutic serum, toxin, antitoxin, or analogous product employed for prevention, treatment, or cure of diseases in humans. The underlying objective of these products is to help develop immunity in the person receiving them. Immunity is defined as natural or acquired resistance to disease.

Provision of immunity through the use of a biologic is immunization. *Vaccination* is the term more commonly used; it refers to the use of a biologic product (a vaccine) to develop active immunity in the patient.

The benefits of these products is apparent when one considers, for example, that the incidence of poliomyelitis fell dramatically after licensure of the inactivated polio vaccine in 1955 and the oral polio vaccine in the 1960s. In the early 1950s there were more than 20,000 cases of polio each year. By 1960 the number of polio cases had dropped to about 3000, and by 1979, the last cases (about 10) of indigenously acquired polio in the United States were reported. Similarly, the largest annual number of cases of rubella, or German measles, an acute viral disease affecting people of all ages, occurred in the United States in 1969 (57,686 cases reported). Following rubella vaccine licensure in 1969, the incidence of this disease fell rapidly, and since 1992 the number of reported cases in the United States has been fewer than 500 per year.

Types of Immunity

Before discussing specific biologics, it is important to understand the different types of immunity. There are two main categories of immunity, natural and acquired.

Natural Immunity

Natural, innate, or native immunity depends on factors that are inborn and can be classified as species immunity, racial immunity, and individual immunity.

Species Immunity

In general, cold-blooded animals are not susceptible to diseases common to warm-blooded animals. Humans are not all susceptible to certain diseases of lower animals, such as chicken cholera. However, a number of infections that occur primarily in animals can be transmitted to humans. Among the most important are anthrax (cattle, sheep, horses), plague (rodents) and rabies (cats, dogs, bats, and others). Correspondingly, many human diseases do not naturally occur in animals. Examples include gonorrhea, typhoid fever, influenza, measles, mumps, and poliomyelitis.

Racial Immunity

Human races differ in susceptibility to common infections (e.g., yellow fever, pneumonia, tuberculosis). Factors that determine racial immunity are elusive and not well known. Racial immunity should not be used synonymously or confused with environmental immunity. Environmental immunity may be the result of resistance to infection among individuals in a community resulting from the degree of acquired immunity and other factors (e.g., nutrition, genetic constitution, fatigue). For example, tuberculosis and smallpox wreaked havoc among the Eskimos and American Indians when these groups were first exposed to them. However, with the course of time, the disease tends to become less severe, and it may eventually reach the same level of incidence and severity as among other races with whom the disease has been endemic for a long time.

Individual Immunity

Apart from any specific immunity to a particular infectious agent, individuals vary in the ability to resist common microbiologic diseases. Some individuals have little capacity to resist skin disorders, the common cold, and other familiar diseases. The natural resistance of the same individual may vary from time to time.

General good health, demonstrated by healthy body tissues, skin, and mucous membranes; leukocytes in plentiful supply; and an active and positive lifestyle (i.e., little or no smoking, alcohol, social drug use), provides adequate barriers to bacterial infiltration. Resident bacteria in the gastrointestinal tract and upper respiratory tract, for example, provide resistance to infection. These play a vital role in resisting invasion by other species of microorganisms capable of producing infection. Also, stomach acid is to a degree capable of destroying ingested bacteria. Intestinal enzymes are also known to provide secondary defense mechanisms.

Acquired Immunity

Acquired immunity is a specific immunity that may be active or passive. *T lymphocytes* regulate cell-mediated immunity and are responsible for controlling certain bacterial and viral infections. These lymphocytes are responsible for mediating graft *versus* host disease, allograft rejection, and delayed hypersensitivity reactions.

T lymphocytes augment the activity of *B lymphocytes*, which are primarily involved with humoral immunity and antibody production. Once an antigen is introduced into the body, *B lymphocytes* differentiate into plasma cells that produce antibodies specific to the invading antigen. These antibodies, known synonymously as immunoglobulins, attach to the invading antigen and cause its destruction by phagocytes and the complement system.

Once exposed to an antigen, the *T* and *B* *lymphocytes* demonstrate memory that allows them to recognize and respond to a specific antigen when exposed again. The second response is far greater in magnitude to the first immunologic response. This memory of an antigen by the immune system allows sensitized individuals to resist infections on subsequent exposure.

Active Immunity

Active immunity develops in response to antigenic substances in the body. This may occur by natural means, as by infection, in which case it is termed *naturally acquired active immunity*, or it may develop in response to administration of a specific vaccine or toxoid, in which case it is *artificially acquired active immunity*. In either case, the body builds up its own defenses in response to the antigen.

Vaccines are administered primarily for prophylactic action, to develop acquired active immunity. Vaccines may contain living attenuated (weakened) or killed microorganisms or fractions of these microorganisms. Toxoids are bacterial toxins modified and detoxified with moderate heat and chemical treatment so that the antigenic properties remain while the substance is rendered nontoxic. Although toxoids do not cause disease, exposure of immunocompetent persons may result in antibody production that will protect the person against disease caused by the natural toxin. A problem with toxoids is that they produce inadequate immunologic responses when administered alone. Therefore, they are often combined with adjuvants (e.g., alum, aluminum phosphate, aluminum hydroxide) that enhance their antigenicity. These agents do so through their insoluble nature, which acts to keep the immunogens in tissue for longer periods and, thus, prolongs the immune response.

A vaccine composed of killed whole bacteria or viruses or substructures of these is known as an inactivated vaccine. Vaccines that contain live but significantly weakened microorganisms are attenuated vaccines. Both types are capable of producing immunity. However, the attenuated vaccines typically have more antigenicity so are more likely to confer permanent immu-

nity. To maintain adequate antibody titers, inactivated vaccines must be administered again over time.

With live vaccines, caution must be exercised with immunocompromised patients. This group of patients includes those with HIV infection, thymic abnormalities, lymphoma, leukemia, generalized malignancy, or advanced debilitating diseases or who are receiving corticosteroids, alkylating agents, antimetabolites, or radiation chemotherapy. These patients are unable to mount immune responses against even weakened microorganisms. The result could be a disseminated bacterial or viral infection. Thus, inactivated vaccines should be employed for these patients.

Immunization during pregnancy is another concern. Live attenuated vaccines should be avoided for pregnant patients because of the danger of transmission of the microorganism to the fetus. For example, measles, mumps, and rubella (MMR) vaccine should not be administered during pregnancy, and pregnancy should be avoided for 1 month following vaccination with monovalent measles vaccine and 4 weeks following MMR or other rubella-containing vaccines.

Passive Immunity

Passive acquired immunity occurs by introduction of the immunoglobulins produced in another individual (human or animal) into the host, who is not involved in their production. In similar fashion to active acquired immunity, passive acquired immunity can be classified as natural or artificial.

Naturally acquired passive immunity occurs by placental transmission of immunoglobulin-gamma (IgG) from the mother to the fetus. Because of the transfer of these immunoglobulins, the infant may have passive immunity to diphtheria, tetanus, measles, mumps, and other infections for the first 4 to 6 months of life.

Several biologic products containing immunoglobulins provide passive immunity. These are limited to provision of temporary prophylaxis to susceptible individuals, for example during an epidemic, and to supplying immediate immunoglobulins for the treatment of infections and toxicities. Notable in this category are the antivenins for treatment of snakebite (e.g., North American coral snake antivenin) and spiders (e.g., black widow spider antivenin).

The acquired passive immunity provided by immunoglobulins is not long lasting, usually1 to 2 weeks. Their important feature is that they offer the susceptible patient protection during a critical period of exposure (e.g., the patient exposed to diphtheria). Immunoglobulins do not last long because their function is to bind to the pathogen as needed. Immunoglobulin is metabolized by the body if not needed for immunologic purposes.

Production of Biologics

Biologics are produced by manufacturers licensed to do so in accordance with the terms of the federal Public Health Service Act (58 Stat. 682) approved July 1, 1944, and each product must meet specified standards as administered by the Center for Biologics Evaluation and Research of the FDA (1). Each lot of a licensed biologic is approved for distribution when it has been determined that the lot meets the specific control requirements for that product. Licensing includes approval of a specific series of production steps and in-process control tests as well as end product specifications that must be met lot by lot.

Generally, each lot of a biologic product must pass rigid control requirements before it may be distributed for general use. Provisions generally applicable to biologic products include tests for potency, general safety, sterility, purity, water (residual moisture), pyrogens, identity, and constituent materials. Constituent materials include preservatives, diluents, and adjuvants, which generally should meet compendial standards; extraneous protein in cell-cultured vaccines (which, if other than serum originating, is excluded); and antibiotics other than penicillin added to the production substrate of viral vaccines, for which compendial monographs on antibiotics and antibiotic substances are available. Additional safety tests on live vaccines and certain other items are also required.

Biologics to be administered by injection are packaged and labeled in the same manner as other injections. In addition, the label of a biologic product must include the title or proper name (the name under which the product is licensed under the Public Health Service Act); the name, address, and license number of the manufacturer; the lot number; the expiration date; and the recommended individual dose for multiple-dose containers. The package label also includes the preservative and its amount; the number of containers if more than one; the amount of product in the container; the recommended storage temperature; a statement, if necessary, that freezing is to be avoided; and such other information as FDA regulations may require to ensure safe and effective use of the product (1).

With few exceptions, most biologics are stored in a refrigerator (2°–8°C, or 35°–46°F), and freezing is avoided. In many instances it is not the biologic substance that is harmed by freezing but rather the container, which may be broken by freezing and expansion of an aqueous vehicle, so that some of the product is lost. Diluents packaged with biologics should not be frozen. Some products are to be held at specified temperatures during shipment.

The expiration date for biologic products varies with the product and the storage temperatures. Most biologic products have an expiration date of a year or longer after the date of manufacture or issue. For biologic products the stated date on each lot determines the dating period, which begins on the date of manufacture and beyond which the product cannot be expected to retain the required safety, purity, and potency. The dating period may comprise an in-house storage period during which the lot is held under prescribed conditions followed by a period after issue. The individual monographs for biologics usually indicate both, the after-issue time frame for use and (in parentheses) the permissible in-house storage period (1).

Storage, Handling, and Shipping of Biologics

Biologics are sensitive to extreme temperatures, and exposure to heat or freezing can decrease their potency and dramatically reduce their effectiveness. Poor storage, handling, and shipping conditions for these products not only wastes the intrinsic value of the products but wastes money as well. Biologics are expensive and can add significantly to one's inventory costs. An inventory of vaccines and other immunologic products can amount to tens of thousands of dollars or more.

A real danger is that if damaged products are administered, the person may get little of the intended benefit The person may not be able to build up immunity and get the infection or may get the disease that the biologic was intended to protect against.

The overriding theme for the pharmacist in storage, handling, and shipping of biologic products is to maintain the cold chain (2). This implies continuity from the manufacturer's refrigerator to one's pharmacy, clinic, or office to administration. If the cold chain is maintained, the pharmacist can be assured that the quality of the product will not be diminished.

In the pharmacy there should be a clear understanding of primary and secondary individuals who are responsible for receiving, handling, and shipping these products. A key ingredient is good storage equipment. Whenever possible, separate commercial refrigerators and freezers should be used for these products. For small-volume biologics, a standard refrigerator-freezer should be used. Frost-free freezers should be used because ice buildup interferes with the freezer's ability to maintain very low temperatures. Also, defrosting requires that product be removed to temporary storage.

Refrigerators and freezers cool by convection. Thus, cool air must have room to circulate around the product. Packing the refrigerator too tightly can lead to small incremental elevations in the temperature of the product.

A separate refrigerator dedicated to biologics is preferable to minimize the times the refrigerator door is opened. The World Health Organization recommends that the door not be opened more frequently than four times per day. Also, doors should be closed as quickly as possible after securing the product, and pharmacists should avoid using the inside of the refrigerator door to store product to avoid unac-

ceptable temperature variations. The door shelving can be used to store diluents or bottles of water. This helps provide insulation and a thermal reserve (2).

If a vaccine must be kept outside of the refrigerator for a few minutes, it is advisable to put the product in an insulated container with coolant packs (thermal packs, blue ice packs, chemical packs) from the freezer. Coolant packs should be kept in the freezer and ready for use in shipping. An additional advantage of freezer packs is that they provide extra insulation and cooling power in the freezer in case of an interruption of electric power or outage.

Coolant packs that contain water have about as much cooling capacity as ethylene glycol packs. An easy way to create a coolant pack is to fill a plastic bottle with water and freeze it. It is important, however, that the product not come in direct contact with these coolant packs because the vial contents may freeze and be damaged. An easy method to separate the product from the coolant pack is to use a towel or sheet of cardboard to separate the two (2).

Periodically, it is advisable for the pharmacist to test the temperature of the refrigerator and freezer. Some adult immunization programs recommend that refrigerator temperature be checked every day and these temperatures recorded in a log. Refrigerator temperatures should range between 2°C and 8°C, and freezers should stay well below 0°C. Usually an optimal temperature is −15°C (5°F).

With respect to personnel, pharmacists should educate and train in good storage and handling procedures every person who will handle biologics. These individuals should understand the importance of reporting any problems or interruption associated with proper handling and storage guidelines. It is far more important to report a breach in handling and storage than to discount and overlook it intentionally. The use of a mishandled or poorly stored biologic could have devastating consequences on the person who receives it.

Store containers of the same vaccine together. To avoid selecting the wrong product or something that has similar packaging, separate the products. A good example of this occurs with pediatric and adult dosage forms (e.g., tetanus–diphtheria toxoids), which could be confused. Keep them separate. Look-alike packaging can easily confuse any conscientious practitioner.

Biologics for Active Immunity

Bacterial Vaccines

A vaccine is a suspension of attenuated (live) or inactivated (killed) microorganisms or fractions thereof that are administered to induce immunity and prevent disease. Originally, the organism is grown in a suitable broth medium in a controlled environment of temperature, pH, and oxygen tension. To reduce the potential for hypersensitivity reactions to the finished product, the medium, whenever possible, should consist of chemically defined ingredients.

Following a suitable amount of time for bacterial growth, the culture is processed in two steps. If the vaccine is to be inactivated microorganisms, the organisms are treated with phenol or formaldehyde. Heat and phenol or heat and acetone are employed for the typhoid fever vaccine. Next, the organisms are separated from the medium through centrifugation and suspended in sterile water or 0.9% sodium chloride for injection. If necessary, the preparation may be further purified by several methods, including dialysis and/or additional centrifugation.

A live attenuated vaccine can also be produced by genetic alteration of the pathogenic organisms. This allows the organism to survive and multiply but not produce the disease. Usually several base pairs of DNA in a key region of the gene structure are eliminated or altered. Thus, the organism is incapable of reverting to its more pathogenic form.

Another way to create a vaccine is to employ purified antigen subunits produced with use of recombinant DNA. With subunit vaccines, the genes that code for the desired antigen are introduced into the nonpathogenic organisms. There is no potential to harm the patient because there is no possibility that a pathogenic organism can be created from only a limited number of components of the original organism. Also, the subunit vaccine can be expected to have a lower incidence of side effects. As an example, the hepatitis B vaccine is produced through recombinant DNA technology by common baker's yeast, into which the gene for the hepatitis B surface antigen (HBsAg) has been inserted.

To date, subunit vaccines have had limited clinical utility because of inability to produce a sufficient specific immune response. However, alternative biotechnologic strategies have been employed to produce subunit vaccine immunogens and adjuvant-active compounds that can be added to enhance the immune response.

The final vaccine may contain one single immunogen (monovalent) or it may contain multiple immunogens (polyvalent, trivalent) to promote immunity against the same disease state. The final product may also be a mixed vaccine. For example, MMR vaccine is a single product with three immunogens for three viral diseases. A mixed biologic may contain a vaccine and a toxoid in the same product, as with diphtheria, tetanus, and pertussis (DTP). Another example of a mixed biologic is the combination vaccine Pediarix (diphtheria and tetanus toxoids and acellular pertussis adsorbed, hepatitis B [recombinant], and inactivated poliovirus vaccine) introduced in late 2002.

The strength of a vaccine may be expressed as total number of organisms, total protective units per milliliter or dose, or micrograms of immunogen in each milliliter or in each dose of vaccine.

Viral Vaccines

Viruses cannot be grown on inanimate media employed to grow bacteria and so are propagated on one of several types of animate media. Examples of animate media include embryonic egg, cell cultures of chick embryo, human diploid cell culture, monkey cell culture, skin of living calves, and intact mice.

In similar fashion to vaccine preparation, after growth of the culture, various techniques are employed to separate the virus from the host cell. Purification steps are taken to reduce the incidence of hypersensitivity reactions to animate media or host cells, most notably embryonic egg. The final viral product may contain a single immunogen (monovalent) or multiple immunogens (polyvalent) to elicit immunity against the same disease.

The vaccine may remain as the whole virion or be further chemically processed to split it into a subvirion vaccine, as is the case with the influenza virus vaccine. This virus is prepared yearly with three virus strains (usually two type A and one type B) chosen on the basis of information provided by a worldwide surveillance network. The information identifies strains most likely to circulate widely during the upcoming season. Strains to be included in the influenza vaccine usually are selected during the preceding January and February because of scheduling requirements for production, quality control, packaging, distribution, and vaccine administration before the onset of the next influenza season.

For 2002 and 2003, the FDA's Vaccines and Related Biologic Products Advisory Committee recommended that the trivalent vaccine for the United States contain A/New Caledonia/20/99-like (H1N1), A/Moscow/10/99-like (H3N2), and B/Hong Kong/330/01-like viruses (3). When there is a good match between the strains in the vaccine and those in the community, inactivated vaccine is 70 to 90% effective in preventing influenza in people under 65 years of age (4–6).

To prolong stimulation of antibodies, the virion may be adsorbed onto aluminum phosphate, as is the case with rabies vaccine (adsorbed). Typically, viral vaccines are available as lyophilized (freeze-dried) products that require reconstitution prior to administration with the provided diluent. Some inactivated vaccines are available in suspensions for injection.

Belshe et al. (7) reported the effectiveness of a live attenuated, cold-adapted, trivalent influenza virus vaccine that was administered intranasally to more than 1000 healthy school-aged children. This placebo-controlled trial demonstrated that children receiving the active vaccine had fewer febrile illnesses, including 30% fewer episodes of febrile otitis media, than the placebo group. This was one significant outcome of the study, because otitis media is a recognized complication of influenza in children, and the influenza virus has been isolated from middle ear fluid in children with influenza and middle ear effusion. The incidence of otitis media increases in the 14-day period after influenza virus infection. Furthermore, administration of inactivated influenza virus vaccine has been shown to reduce outbreaks of otitis media in day care centers (8). Thus, if efforts are employed to immunize more day care children, this might ultimately result in lower incidence of otitis media and less need for prescribed antibiotics.

Historically, the influenza vaccine was strongly recommended annually for children aged 6 months or more with certain risk factors, including but not limited to asthma, cardiac disease, sickle cell disease, HIV, and diabetes. However, as of 2003, all children aged 6 months to 23 months, regardless of risk factors, are recommended to receive this vaccine.

In June 2003, the influenza virus vaccine live intranasal (FluMist, Wyeth; Medimmune) was approved for active immunization against influenza A and B viruses in healthy children aged 5 to 17 and adults 18 to 49 years of age. It is the first vaccine approved in the United States for administration as a nasal mist. The introduction of a nasal vaccine has much implication to help overcome barriers to immunization (fear of side effects, the need for yearly immunizations, perception of low vaccine effectiveness). Widespread use of the nasal vaccine in high-risk children may therefore be more easily achievable than use of injected vaccines. This would be a very effective way to reduce the incidence of influenza in this population. The only downsides initially will be expense (anticipated to be about $55–$60 per patient) and that the cold chain, discussed earlier in this chapter, must be maintained to guarantee adequate stability.

The strength of viral vaccines can be provided in tissue culture infectious doses ($TCID_{50}$), the quantity of virus estimated to infect 50% of inoculated cultures. Also, micrograms of immunogen, international units, D-antigen units, and plaque-forming units for yellow fever vaccine are employed for these products.

Cancer Vaccines

For more than century, the role of the immune system and its relationship to cancer has been researched. It has been only in recent years, however, that the immune response is being clinically explored as a mode to prevent and treat cancer. Cancer vaccines in development are intended to increase recognition of cancer cells by the immune system.

This approach to cancer treatment is exciting, as it offers another modality to complement surgery, radiation therapy, and chemotherapy. Another cause for guarded optimism is that the development of these vaccines may play a role in preventing cancer in patients at high risk because of familial diseases.

For the immune system to recognize and kill a tumor cell, immune cells must recognize antigens on the tumor cell as foreign to the body and receive costimulatory signals. Otherwise, tumor cells go undetected by the immune system and proliferate. Thus, a goal of cancer vaccine development is to increase antigen awareness of the immune cells or increase costimulatory signals that induce an immune response.

T cells, lymphokine-activated killer (LAK) cells, and *natural killer (NK) cells* have antitumor activity. Thus, tumor vaccine development is to stimulate these immune cells instead of antibody-producing cells, the operational model used to protect one from an infection. Tumor-killing cells recognize tumor-associated antigens (TAAs) on the surface of the tumor cells. These antigens have peptide fragments that appear on the cell surface either by the cancer cell or taken up by a phagocytic cell.

TAAs fall into one of three categories. These are patient specific, tumor specific, and shared. Antigens unique to a specific patient are patient specific, such as an antigen expressed on the surface of a B-cell malignancy. A tumor-specific TAA is unique to a particular tumor. Most notable is prostate-specific antigen (PSA), found in prostate tumors. Shared TAAs are created by tumor cells with a common histology. A notable example of this is the carcinoembryonic antigen on adenocarcinoma cells found in colon, ovarian, and lung tumors.

Four types of cancer vaccines are under investigation, and a thorough explanation of each is beyond the scope of this book. Nonetheless, these types are important. They are autologous, allogeneic, anti-idiotypic, and gene therapy–derived vaccines.

Autologous tumor vaccines are developed from antigenic material procured from the tumor of the patient. Tumor cells are isolated from tissue procured during biopsy or surgery. These cells are killed or attenuated and reinfused into the patient. Typically, to enhance immunogenicity, they are combined with an adjuvant, such as bacille Calmette-Guérin (BCG) or c parvum. A major problem with this approach is the work and cost associated with the production of vaccine for the individual patient. Also, some tumors escape the immune system because their antigens are not expressed on the tumor surface.

Allogeneic tumor vaccines use the concept of shared or tumor-specific antigens. These vaccines are produced from cell lines that express tumor-specific or shared TAAs. To induce an immune response, either the fragment of the allogeneic tumor cell or the whole cell is injected. The beneficial aspect of this vaccine is that it can be used in a wide population of patients.

Anti-idiotypic vaccines are three-dimensional immunogenic regions on the antibody that bind antigen. Antibodies that bind TAAs are isolated and injected into mice. The resulting antibodies are harvested and used to vaccinate another mouse. The resulting antibodies have a three-dimensional binding site that mimics the original structure of the TAA. These antibodies are combined with an adjuvant and given as a vaccine. Because the anti-idiotypic antibody closely resembles the antigen, these can be used to induce immune responses (cellular, antibody–antigen) to a given antigen.

Gene therapy allows a DNA template to be placed within a cell, transcribed into messenger RNA, and expressed as a costimulatory protein. One can then induce a cell to synthesize this protein as part of its normal function. A gene that encodes for interleukins or other costimulatory proteins can be placed in cells expressing TAAs. This stimulates the immune response.

Clinical trials are now being undertaken for cancer vaccines for melanoma, colorectal cancer, renal cell carcinoma, breast and ovarian cancers, lung cancer, and cervical cancer. They are being studied also in combination with chemotherapy, surgery, and radiation therapy.

Toxoids

In similar fashion to bacterial vaccines, bacteria are propagated, and after the required growth is achieved, the culture is filtered through a sterilizing membrane filter. The filtrate that contains the toxin (exotoxin) is then processed. Processing involves addition of a concentrated salt solution to precipitate the toxin from the filtrate. After the precipitated toxin is washed and dialyzed to purify it, the toxin is detoxified with formaldehyde.

The detoxified toxin (toxoid) may be plain or contain an adjuvant (e.g., alum, aluminum hydroxide, aluminum sulfate). The product may also contain single, multiple, or mixed immunogens (e.g., tetanus and diphtheria toxoids adsorbed for adult use, which contains two toxoids for active immunization against different toxins). A mixed biologic such as diphtheria and tetanus toxoids and pertussis vaccine adsorbed for pediatric use has two toxoids and a vaccine in a single dosage form for active immunization against different toxicities and infection. Their advantage is broad immunization coverage and minimum number of injections.

These mixtures or types of biologics differ from polyvalent products, which are used for different strains of the same toxicity or infection (e.g., influenza virus vaccine, pneumococcal vaccine polyvalent).

The strength of a toxoid is in flocculating (Lf) units (e.g., tetanus toxoid, 4–5 Lf units/0.5 mL dose). A flocculating unit is the smallest amount of toxin that flocculates most rapidly one unit of standard antitoxin in a series of mixtures containing fixed amounts of antitoxin and varying amounts of toxin.

Biologics for Passive Immunity

Human Immune Sera and Globulins (Homologous Sera)

Human immune sera, or homologous sera, include immunoglobulin and hyperimmune sera for specific diseases. These contain the specific antibodies obtained from the blood of humans and produced as a result of having had the specific disease or having been immunized against it with a specific biologic product. The source of homologous sera is the pooled plasma of adult donors, either from the general population (for immunoglobulin) or from hyperimmunized donors (for immunoglobulins for specific diseases). Thus, these products confer passive immunity.

The pooled plasma from adult donors must be free of hepatitis B antigen and antibodies to HIV. Processing steps include fractional precipitation (e.g., with cold ethanol), maintaining rigorous control of pH and ionic strength. Further purification takes place with a finished biologic product that contains not less than 15% and not more than 18% protein. There are of course exceptions (e.g., Varicella zoster immunoglobulins contain not less than 10% protein).

These preparations are for intramuscular injection and should not be administered intravenously. However, immunoglobulin intravenous (3 to 12% protein) and cytomegalovirus immunoglobulin are administered intravenously.

Sera have the greatest value for the treatment of acute disease, although they are also useful in some instances to prevent illness when immediate protection is needed. Immunity resulting from the injection of an immune serum is brief (a few weeks) because the foreign serum and the antibodies it produces are eliminated from the body within a few weeks.

Animal Immune Sera (Heterologous Sera)

Most commonly employed immune sera are prepared by immunization of horses against the specific immunogen (e.g., toxin, venom). After the plasma is harvested, it is separated by fractional precipitation into two components, immunologically active (immunoglobulins) and immunologically inactive (albumins, clotting factors) ones. The immunologically active component is treated with pepsin to remove the complement-activating component of the molecules and render it less immunogenic. Subsequently, the active component is recovered through dialysis and fractional precipitation or centrifugation.

This category of pharmaceuticals includes antitoxins and antivenins. Antitoxins are produced by inoculating horses with increasing doses of the toxoids and exotoxins. After several injections over weeks or months, the animal is bled with adequate safeguards to avoid contamination and the plasma harvested. Antivenins are produced similarly, by inoculating horses with the venom of selected species and harvesting the plasma.

Before using these products, precautions must be taken to ensure the safety of the patient, who may be sensitive to horse protein. Appropriate measures, including a sensitivity test with suitable controls, should be taken to detect any dangerous hypersensitivity.

Table 16.1 lists representative biologics by category. Although the scope of this book does not permit a thorough description of each according to its intended use, adverse effects, and so on, the list demonstrates the wide applicability of these products to produce active or passive immunity, provide prophylaxis, or serve as a diagnostic tool.

Administration and Toxicity Associated With Biologic Products

Biologics must be dispensed in the original container to avoid contamination and deterioration. They are sterile when packaged and are injected by aseptic techniques. A few are administered by mouth.

Traditional vaccines, often constituted by inactivated whole cells, can cause unwanted side effects. Those developed from selected antigens have demonstrated fewer systemic side effects. Liposomal delivery has decreased side effects while enhancing the vaccine's effectiveness.

Itching, erythema, pain, and tenderness around the injection site occur with subcutaneous, intramuscular, and intradermal administration. Vaccines that contain adjuvants (e.g., BCG) can cause these adverse effects in addition to induration and ulceration at the site. Low-grade fever, myalgia, and arthralgia have occurred in patients who received a BCG-containing biologic product.

These adverse effects are controlled with the use of over-the-counter (OTC) analgesic agents. However, before these are used, the patient's drug history should be obtained to ensure that the use of an analgesic is permissible given a patient's health status and other drug therapy.

The foremost adverse effect of concern with immunization is hypersensitivity, most notably anaphylaxis, ranging from pruritus or urticaria to bronchospasm, respiratory distress, laryngeal edema, circulatory collapse, and death. Life-threatening anaphylaxis is a rarity but quite possible. The risk of an anaphylactic reaction is in the range of one for every 600,000 to 6.4 million doses of vaccine distributed (9).

The immunopathologic classification of allergic drug reactions places anaphylactic reactions in type I. In this situation, initial exposure to an antigen results in production of specific IgE antibodies. Upon reexposure, antigen reacts with antibodies bound to the surface of mast cells or basophils, causing the release of histamine and other mediators. Several weeks is required after initial exposure to antigen and sensitization before an anaphylactic reaction can occur. Once sensitized, however, the patient can demonstrate an attack within minutes of reexposure to small amounts of the drug administered by any route.

Because of the rare nature of anaphylactic reactions, it is difficult to determine whether the patient is allergic to the proteins that make up the active antigenic portion of the vaccine or to the excipients (e.g., thimerosal, neomycin, gelatin, aluminum gels). Several viruses that constitute vaccines are grown in animate media, including embryonic egg and cell cultures of chick embryo. Even though purification techniques decrease dramatically the amount of egg protein in the final product,

TABLE 16.1 EXAMPLES OF OFFICIAL BIOLOGIC PRODUCTS

BIOLOGIC PRODUCT	NATURE OF CONTENTS	ROUTE *	USE
Vaccines and Vaccine Combinations			
Anthrax adsorbed	Toxigenic, nonencapsulated strain of *Bacillus anthracis* culture, protective antigens (proteins common to all harmful strains), aluminum hydroxide as adjuvant to enhance antibody response	Subcutaneous	Active immunizing agent
BCG	Attenuated living culture of BCG strain of *Mycobacterium bovis*.	Percutaneous via multiple-puncture disc	Active immunizing agent
Cholera	Suspension of inactivated *Vibrio cholerae*	IM, SQ	Active immunizing agent
Hepatitis B	Originally, biochemically, biophysically inactivated human HBsAg particles from chronic HBsAg carriers. Now only recombinant vaccines produced in yeast cells are available in the U.S.	IM	Active immunizing agent
Influenza virus	Aqueous suspension of inactivated virus from allantoic fluid of infected chick embryo in phosphate-buffered isotonic NaCl injection.	IM, SQ	Active immunizing agent
Influenza virus	Preservative free, latex free egg-based aqueous solution. Each 0.5 mL contains ~1 × $10^{6.5-7.5}$ tissue culture–infectious doses of virus. Egg base provides protein to increase reproducibility of virus	Intranasal	Active immunizing agent
Measles virus, live	Live attenuated Enders line measles virus from attenuated Edmonston strain in chick embryo cell cultures.	SQ	Active immunizing agent
Measles, mumps, rubella virus, live	Propagated in chick embryo (measles, mumps) and in human diploid cell cultures (rubella)	SQ	Active immunizing agent
Measles, rubella virus, live	Measles virus grown on chicken embryo tissue and rubella virus on duck embryo tissue.	SQ	Active immunizing agent
Mumps virus, live	Live attenuated Jeryl Lynn (B level) strain of virus propagated in chick embryo tissue.	SQ	Active immunizing agent
Plague	Suspension of inactivated 195/P strain of *Yersinia pestis* bacilli in 0.9% NaCl injection.	IM	Active immunizing agent
Pneumococcal, polyvalent	Sterile solution of antigenic capsular polysaccharides from *Streptococcus pneumoniae*. Contains 23 capsular polysaccharide types. Each 0.5-mL dose contains 25 μg of each type of capsule polysaccharide in 0.9% NaCl injection. Also contains phenol or thimerosal preservative.	IM, SQ	Active immunizing agent

(continued)

TABLE 16.1 EXAMPLES OF OFFICIAL BIOLOGIC PRODUCTS

BIOLOGIC PRODUCT	NATURE OF CONTENTS	ROUTE *	USE
Pneumococcal 7-valent conjugate	Sterile 0.5-mL-dose solution of saccharides of capsular antigens of *S. pneumoniae* serotypes 4, 6B, 9V, 14, 18C, 19F, and 23F individually conjugated to diphtheria CRM197 to form glycoconjugate.	IM	Active immunizing agent
Rabies	Inactivated virus from HDCV or RDCV cultures.	HDCV, IM, ID; RDCV, IM only	Active immunizing agent
Rubella virus, live	Live rubella (German measles) virus propagated in human diploid (WI-38) cell culture.	SQ	Active immunizing agent
Rubella and mumps, live	Rubella virus in human diploid cell culture and mumps virus on chicken embryo tissue.	SQ	Active immunizing agent
Smallpox	Dried calf lymph live virus preparation of vaccinia virus	ID	Active immunizing agent
Typhoid	Parenteral form, acetone-killed and dried or heat, phenol-inactivated *Salmonella typhi* of Ty2 strain; oral form, enteric-coated capsules, lyophilized, live *S. typhi* of attenuated Ty21a strain.	SQ or ID; oral	Active immunizing agent
Varicella virus, live	Varicella zoster, Oka/Merck strain, attenuated by multiple passages through cultures of human embryonic lung cell, embryonic guinea pig cell, WI-38 strain of human diploid cell, MRC-5 strain of human diploid cell.	SQ	Active immunizing agent
Yellow fever	Dried frozen attenuated strain of living yellow fever virus cultured in living chick embryo, prepared, processed, freeze-dried, and sealed in nitrogen.	SQ	Active immunizing agent
Toxoids			
Diphtheria and tetanus, adsorbed	Suspension of purified diphtheria toxoid, tetanus toxoid alum precipitated or adsorbed onto aluminum phosphate.	Deep IM	Active immunizing agent
Tetanus	Suspension of formaldehyde-treated tetanus bacillus (*Clostridium tetani*).	IM, SQ	Active immunizing agent
Tetanus, adsorbed	Suspension of toxoid alum precipitated or adsorbed onto aluminum phosphate.	Deep IM	Active immunizing agent
Tetanus, diphtheria adsorbed for adult use	Suspension of toxoids, alum precipitated or adsorbed onto aluminum phosphate.	IM	Active immunizing agent
Antitoxins			
Botulism	Solution of refined, concentrated proteins, chiefly globulins, with antitoxin from blood serum or plasma of healthy horses immunized against toxins produced by type A, B, and E strains of *Clostridium botulinum*.	IM or IV	Passive immunizing agent

(continued)

TABLE 16.1 EXAMPLES OF OFFICIAL BIOLOGIC PRODUCTS

BIOLOGIC PRODUCT	NATURE OF CONTENTS	ROUTE *	USE
Tetanus	Solution of refined, concentrated proteins, chiefly globulins, with antitoxic antibodies from blood serum or plasma of a healthy animal, usually horse, immunized against tetanus toxoid or toxin.	IM or SQ (prophylactic) or IV (therapeutic)	Passive immunizing agent
Immune Sera			
Cytomegalovirus	IgG antibodies from large number of healthy persons who contributed to plasma pools.	IV	Passive for kidney transplant recipients seronegative for CMV who receive kidney from CMV seropositive donor.
Immunoglobulin IM	Nonpyrogenic solution of globulins with many antibodies normally in adult human blood prepared by cold alcohol fractionation of pooled plasma from venous blood of at least 1000 individuals.	IM	Passive immunity to hepatitis A and B, measles, varicella zoster, primary immunodeficiency diseases.
Immunoglobulin IV	Nonpyrogenic solution of globulins with many antibodies normally in adult human blood prepared by cold alcohol fractionation of pooled plasma from venous blood of at least 1000 individuals.	IV	Primary immunodeficiency diseases, HIV, ITP, bone marrow transplant, beta cell CLL.
Rh_o (D) globulin	From plasma or serum of adults with high titer of anti-Rh_o antibody to red blood cell antigen Rh_o (D); contains 10–18% protein; not less than 90% IgG. Commercial solutions contain glycine as a stabilizer and thimerosal as a preservative; pH is adjusted with sodium carbonate or NaCl.	IM	Passive immunizing agent
Tetanus immunoglobulin	Solution of globulins derived from blood plasma of adult human donors hyperimmunized with tetanus toxoid.	IM	Passive immunizing agent
Miscellaneous Biologic Products			
Antivenin (Crotalidae) Polyvalent	Dried frozen solution of specific venom-neutralizing globulins from serum of healthy horses immunized against venoms of four species of pit vipers, *Crotalus atrox, C. adamanteus, C. durissus terrificus,* and *Bothrops atrox.*	IM or IV	Neutralizes venom of crotalids native to the Americas
Candida albicans skin test antigen	From culture filtrate, cells of two strains of *C. albicans.*	ID	Detects reduced cellular hypersensitivity, DTH; assesses diminished cellular immunity in HIV.
Histoplasmin, USP	Standardized culture filtrates of fungus *Histoplasma capsulatum* grown on liquid synthetic medium.	ID	Diagnostic aid (histoplasmosis)

(continued)

TABLE 16.1 EXAMPLES OF OFFICIAL BIOLOGIC PRODUCTS

BIOLOGIC PRODUCT	NATURE OF CONTENTS	ROUTE *	USE
Plasma Protein Fraction, USP	Blood plasma of adult human donors; contains ~5% protein, ~85% albumin; rest alpha and beta globulins.	IV	Blood-volume expansion
Tuberculin, USP	Solution of concentrated soluble products of MTB. Old tuberculin, soluble partially purified product of MTB in special liquid medium free of protein (purified protein derivative).	ID	Diagnostic aid (tuberculosis)

^aThe doses to be administered and the schedule of doses vary widely with the patient's age, exposure, previous record of immunizations, and so on.

BCG, bacille Calmette-Guérin; IM, intramuscular; SQ, subcutaneous; HBsAg, human hepatitis B surface antigen; HDCV, human diploid cell vaccine; RDCV, rhesus diploid cell vaccine; ID, intradermal; ITP, idiopathic thrombocytopenic purpura; CLL, chronic lymphocytic leukemia; IgG, immunoglobulin gamma; DTH, delayed-type hypersensitivity; MTB, *Mycobacterium tuberculosis*

even picograms or nanograms can elicit a response.

Before a vaccination is administered, it is important that a complete and thorough history of previous allergic reactions be taken. This includes the names of the offending agents and the type of reaction. Also, one should determine how long ago the reaction took place. Not only should one inquire about drugs (e.g., neomycin, gelatin) but also foods (e.g., severe allergy to egg products). It may be necessary for an allergist to perform skin testing to determine whether a patient may demonstrate an immediate type I hypersensitivity reaction to a vaccine.

Even though anaphylactic reactions to immunizations are rare, they can occur. Therefore, at the time of immunization adequate safeguards, including proper emergency supplies and adequately trained personnel must be in place to handle such an emergency.

Thimerosal (containing 49.6 w/v%) has been used in vaccines as a preservative since the 1930s. It is effective for killing bacteria in several vaccines and for preventing bacterial contamination, especially in opened multidose vials. Several of the vaccines routinely recommended for children in the United States contain it. In high doses, both forms of organic mercury (methylmercury and ethyl mercury) formed from metabolism of thimerosal can cause neurotoxicity, and definitive information regarding the dose of thimerosal that produces developmental effects in infants is not available. Therefore, in September 1999 the American Academy of Pediatrics (AAP) Committee on Infectious Diseases and Committee on Environmental Health urged government agencies and the pharmaceutical industry to work rapidly toward reducing children's exposure to mercury from all sources, including vaccines. Specifically, these committees urged rapid elimination of thimerosal in vaccines. The academy also issued guidelines to prevent exposure of women of childbearing age to amounts of mercury that might be toxic to the rapidly developing brain of the fetus, which is much more susceptible to toxicity than the adult brain. It also stated that the specific window of highest susceptibility is not known, but exposure after birth should be associated with less toxicity than in *utero* exposure.

When vaccines preserved with thimerosal have been administered in recommended doses, some hypersensitivity reactions have been reported, but no other harmful effects have been noted. However, massive overdoses with thimerosal-containing products have resulted in toxicity expressed in the central nervous system, kidneys, and immune system. Thus, as part of an ongoing review of biologic products in response to the FDA Modernization Act of 1997, the FDA determined that infants who would receive thimerosal-containing vaccines at several visits might be exposed to more mercury than recommended by federal guidelines.

Pichichero et al. (10) demonstrated that mercury does not accumulate in children who receive thimerosal-containing vaccines. After administration of such vaccines, mercury was measured in the urine, blood, and stool samples of 40 term infants less than 6 months old and in 21 control infants who received thimerosal-containing vaccines. The authors concluded from the data at 2 months and at 6 months of age that the amounts of mercury in the blood of infants receiving these vaccines are well below concentrations of mercury associated with toxicity. Thus, the conclusion was that thimerosal in these vaccines poses little risk to term infants, but should not be administered at birth to very low birthweight premature infants.

The AAP also recommended that the benefits and risks of thimerosal-containing vaccines be discussed with parents. It emphasized that the larger risk of not vaccinating the child (e.g., more than 20% will develop pneumonia) far outweigh any known risk of exposure to a thimerosal-containing vaccine. Infants and children who have received vaccines preserved with thimerosal do not need to have blood, urine, or hair tested for mercury because the concentrations of mercury would be quite low and would not require treatment.

All infants need protection against debilitating and potentially harmful childhood diseases as well as consequences from the vaccinations. One concern has been the development of autism in some infants who were administered the MMR vaccination. In a study attempting to resolve the question, Madsen et al. (11) identified more than 537,000 children in Denmark from 1991 to 1998, 82% of whom had received the MMR vaccine. The scientists determined that the relative risk of autistic disorders among vaccinated children was 8% less than among unvaccinated children, not statistically significant. Furthermore, the risk of other autistic spectrum disorders was found to be 17% lower with vaccination, statistically equivalent to the risk of unvaccinated children. In addition, no relationship was identified between the infants' ages at the time of vaccination, time since vaccination, or date of vaccination and the development of the autistic disorder. This study on the possible link between autism and the MMR vaccine should allay the fears of parents, and

the pharmacist should endeavor to educate them on this matter as well as the thimerosal-containing vaccinations.

Administration of Biologics by Health Care Providers

According to the National Childhood Vaccine Injury Act of 1986, health care providers who administer certain vaccines and toxoids are required to keep a permanent record and report any adverse effects resulting from use of a biologic product. Effective October 1, 1988, the act has three primary objectives:

• To avoid future "crises" that could interrupt the national immunization program
• To achieve optimal prevention of adverse reactions to these preparations
• To provide financial compensation for patients who have vaccine-related injuries

The last objective was intended as an alternative to civil litigation under the traditional tort system in that negligence need not be proven. Claims arising from covered vaccines must first be adjudicated through the program before civil litigation can be pursued. This program relies on a vaccine injury table listing the vaccines covered as well as injuries, disabilities, illnesses, and conditions (including death) for which compensation might be awarded.

The act requires that certain specified adverse reactions be reported in detail to the U.S. Department of Health and Human Services (HHS) Vaccine Adverse Event Reporting System (VAERS) to expand knowledge of such reactions. Adverse events that occur within 7 days after administration (e.g., encephalopathy with DPT vaccine) or within such other period as specified for certain vaccines (e.g., paralytic poliomyelitis from oral polio vaccine [OPV] within 30 days of administration) and/or toxoid are to be reported. This is very important, as such an event may be a rarity and one that should be known. For more information about reporting requirements or completion of the reporting forms, health care providers can contact VAERS at 800-822-7967. The act also requires that a surcharge be placed on biologic products to establish a fund to compensate victims.

The act requires that health care providers who administer any vaccine containing measles, mumps, rubella, poliomyelitis, diphtheria, tetanus, or pertussis antigens maintain permanent vaccination records. These records include the type of biologic administered; date of administration; manufacturer and lot number; name, address and title of the person administering the vaccine; and the patient's occupation, lifestyle and history of vaccine-preventable illnesses. Also, information on other vaccines and toxoids administered should be a part of the permanent record. Pharmacists can work with allied health practitioners (e.g., physicians, nurses) to immunize patients, and in 37 states (Alabama, Alaska, Arkansas, California, Colorado, Delaware, Georgia, Hawaii, Idaho, Illinois, Indiana, Iowa, Kansas, Kentucky, Michigan, Minnesota, Mississippi, Missouri, Montana, Nebraska, Nevada, New Mexico, North Carolina, North Dakota, Ohio, Oklahoma, Oregon, Pennsylvania, South Carolina, South Dakota, Tennessee, Texas, Utah, Virginia, Washington, Wisconsin), pharmacists are permitted to give vaccinations. In Massachusetts, pharmacist immunization programs are limited to pilot programs.

The Public Health Service Act (42 U.S.C. § 300aa–26), Section 2126, effective October 1, 1994, mandated that all health care providers who administer any vaccine containing diphtheria, tetanus, pertussis, measles, mumps, rubella, or polio vaccine shall, prior to administration of the vaccine, provide a copy of Vaccine Information Statements

- To any adult to whom the provider intends to administer the vaccine
- To the legal representative (parent, other individual qualified under state law to consent to the immunization of a minor) of any child to whom the vaccine will be administered (12)

Also, the materials are to be supplemented with visual presentation or oral explanations. There is no requirement that the health care provider obtain the signature or initials of the patient or legal representative affirming that the vaccine information materials were provided. Instead, the health care provider is to

make a notation in the patient's permanent medical record indicating that these materials were provided at the time of vaccination (12).

The National Childhood Vaccination Injury Act, effective August 26, 2002, requires all health care providers to give parents or patients copies of Vaccine Instruction Statements before administering each dose of the vaccines listed in the schedule. Additional information is available from state health departments and at http://www.cdc.gov/nip/publications/vis. Detailed recommendations for using vaccines are available from drug manufacturers' package inserts, ACIP statements on specific vaccines, and the 2000 *Red Book*. The ACIP statements for each recommended childhood vaccine can be viewed, downloaded, and printed from the Centers for Disease Control and Prevention (CDC) National Immunization Program at http://www.cdc.gov/nip/publications/acip-list.htm; Instructions on the use of the Vaccine Information Statements are available at http://www.cdc.gov/nip/publications/vis/vis-instructions.pdf.

In addition to complying with the mandatory requirements of the act, the AAP strongly urges health care providers to complete an official immunization record and provide it to the recipient's legal representative. This record should be accorded the status of a birth certificate or passport and retained with other vital documents for subsequent referral. The health care provider should encourage the legal representative to preserve this important record and present it for record keeping with each immunization. This facilitates accurate record keeping and immunization evaluation, particularly for those who move often. This record also documents immunization history for school admission.

Advisory Committee on Immunization Practices

The ACIP, acip@cdc.gov, consists of 15 experts in fields associated with immunization to provide advice and guidance to the secretary of HHS, the assistant secretary for health, and the CDC on the most effective means to prevent vaccine-preventable diseases. The committee also includes nonvoting representatives from more than 20 health professional and pharmaceutical organizations. This committee develops written recommendations for routine vaccine administration schedules, dosages, and contraindications for the childhood and adult populations.

The ACIP is the only federal government entity that makes these recommendations. Its overall goals are to provide advice to assist HHS and the nation reduce the incidence of vaccine-preventable diseases and to increase the safe use of vaccines and related biologic products. Complete minutes of its meetings are published online at www.cdc.gov/nip/ACIP.

National Vaccine Advisory Committee

In 1988, the National Vaccine Advisory Committee (NVAC) was charted to advise and make recommendations to the director of the National Vaccine Program and the assistant secretary for health of HHS on matters related to prevention of infectious diseases through immunization and prevention of adverse reactions to vaccines. NVAC is composed of 15 members from public and private organizations representing vaccine manufacturers, physicians, parents, state and local agencies, and public health organizations. Also, government agency representatives involved in public health care of allied services serve as ex officio members of NVAC (13).

Since its creation, NVAC has developed sets of standards for child and adolescent immunization practices (14) and adult immunization practices (13). These standards constitute the most essential and desirable immunization policies and practices and are directed at health care professionals, an inclusive term for the many people in clinical settings who share in the responsibility for vaccination administration. These standards set forth the most desirable immunization practices to be achieved. The original adult standards were developed in 1990 and the newest revision (13) reflects the experience gained from the 1990s.

The pediatric standards (14) address the following issues:

Availability of vaccines, including vaccination services, coordination of vaccination services with routine well care, identification and minimization of barriers to vaccination, and patient cost considerations

Assessment of vaccination status, including health care professionals reviewing vaccination and health care status of patients and providing appropriate referral and identification of at-risk patients where vaccination is contraindicated

Effective communication, including education of parents and guardians about benefits and risks of vaccination in a culturally appropriate manner

Proper storage and administration of vaccines, including up-to-date written vaccination protocols where vaccines are administered and reporting adverse events after vaccination

Implementation strategies to improve vaccination coverage

The adult standards (13) run parallel to the pediatric standards and include *vaccination availability, assessment of patients' vaccination status, effective communication with patients, proper documentation of vaccine administration, implementation of strategies to improve vaccination rates,* and *establishing partnerships with communities* that are patient oriented and community based.

Childhood Immunization Schedule

Childhood immunization has been shown to be effective and inexpensive. The U.S. Public Health Service's Healthy People 2010: Understanding and Improving Health established a goal of completely immunizing 80% of infants in the United States by 24 months of age (15). In 1998, 73% of children aged 19 to 35 months from the lowest-income households received the combined series of recommended immunizations, compared with 77% of children from higher-income households. These numbers compare favorably to the 41% of infants in this age range immunized in 1991. It is estimated that 4 million children are at risk for serious preventable diseases.

Immunization registries have been created. These are confidential population-based computer information systems that collect vaccination data about children within a geographic area. Providing complete and accurate information on which to base vaccination decisions, registries are key tools to increase and sustain high vaccination coverage. For example, these registries consolidate vaccination records of children from multiple health care providers, identify children who are due or late for vaccinations, generate reminder and recall notices to ensure that children are vaccinated appropriately, and identify provider sites and geographic areas with low vaccination coverage. One of the national health objectives for 2010 is to increase to 95% the proportion of children aged less than 6 years who participate in fully operational population-based immunization registries. In Washington, DC, immunization program staff and school nurses used this registry during the 2000–2001 school year. In do-

ing so, they identified 20,000 children who were not vaccinated according to school requirements.

Residents of rural or large urban areas have particularly low immunization rates. Various ethnic minorities (e.g., Native Americans, Hispanics, African Americans) also have low rates of immunization. It is believed that this low immunization rate in children has been responsible for increased incidence of measles and pertussis. It is hoped that participation in this registry program will help to increase the immunization rates in rural or large urban areas.

In 1995, the CDC's ACIP, the AAP, and the American Academy of Family Physicians (AAFP) announced a unified version of a recommended immunization schedule for children. Subsequently, in late January to February of each year, updated versions of the recommended childhood schedule are published. Figure 16.1 demonstrates the recommended childhood immunization schedule as of January 16, 2004 (16). The intervals demonstrated in Figure 16.1 indicate the range of acceptable

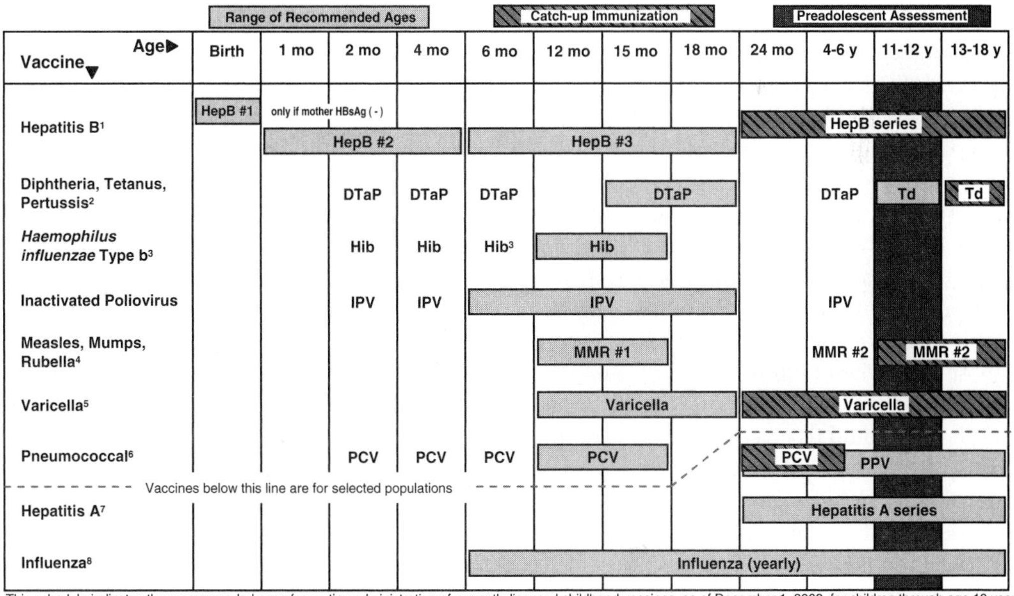

This schedule indicates the recommended ages for routine administration of currently licensed childhood vaccines, as of December 1, 2003, for children through age 18 years. Any dose not given at the recommended age should be given at any subsequent visit when indicated and feasible. ▨ Indicates age groups that warrant special effort to administer those vaccines not previously given. Additional vaccines may be licensed and recommended during the year. Licensed combination vaccines may be used whenever any components of the combination are indicated and the vaccine's other components are not contraindicated. Providers should consult the manufacturers' package inserts for detailed recommendations. Clinically significant adverse events that follow immunization should be reported to the Vaccine Adverse Event Reporting System (VAERS). Guidance about how to obtain and complete a VAERS form can be found on the Internet: http://www.vaers.org/ or by calling 1-800-822-7967.

FIGURE 16.1 Recommended childhood and adolescent immunization schedule for the United States, January to June 2004.

ages for vaccination, including catch-up vaccination and pre-adolescent assessment.

All infants should receive the first dose of hepatitis B vaccine soon after birth and before hospital discharge. Administering the first dose of hepatitis B vaccine soon after birth should minimize the risk of infection caused by errors or delays in maternal hepatitis B surface antigen HBsAg testing or reporting or by exposure to persons with chronic hepatitis B virus infection in the household, and can increase the child's likelihood of completing the vaccination series. Only monovalent hepatitis B vaccine can be used for the birth dose. The first dose may be given by age 2 months if the infants' mother is HBsAg negative. Monovalent or combination vaccine containing hepatitis B immunogen may be used to complete the series. Four doses of vaccine may be administered when a birth dose is given. The second dose should be given at least 4 weeks after the first dose, except for combination vaccines which cannot be administered before 6 weeks of age. The third dose should be given at least 16 weeks after the first dose and at least 8 weeks after the second dose. The last dose in the vaccination series (i.e., third or four dose) should not be administered before age 24 weeks.

Those infants born to HBsAg-positive mothers should receive hepatitis B vaccine and 0.5 mL hepatitis B immunoglobulin (HBIG) within 12 hours of birth at separate sites. The second dose is recommended at age 1 to 2 months, and the last dose should not be administered before 6 months. These infants should be tested for HBsAg and anti-HBs at 9 to 15 months of age to identify those with chronic hepatitis B infection or those who might require revaccination.

Infants born to women whose HBsAg status is unknown should receive the first dose of the hepatitis B series within 12 hours of birth. Maternal blood should be drawn as soon as possible to determine the mother's HBsAg status. If the HBsAg test is positive, the infant should receive HBIG as soon as is possible (no later than age 1 week). The second dose is recommended at age 1 to 2 months. The last dose in the vaccination series should not be administered before age 6 months. Both product strengths are available in 1-mL volumes. Errors can occur

when one product is substituted for another. If, for example, the patient receives the first dose as Engerix-B, 10 μg/mL, the appropriate second dose with Recombivax HB should be 2 mL to deliver the 10 μg needed.

Children and adolescents who have not been vaccinated against hepatitis B in infancy may begin the series during any visit. Those who have not previously received three doses of hepatitis B vaccine should initiate or complete the series during the routine visit to a health care provider at age 11 to 12 years. An unvaccinated older adolescent should be vaccinated whenever possible. The second dose should be administered at least 4 weeks after the first dose, and the third dose should be administered at least 16 weeks after the first dose or at least 8 weeks after the second dose when coverage must be quicker.

In September 1999 the FDA approved an optional two-dose hepatitis B vaccination schedule for adolescents aged 11 to 15 years. The ACIP approved the optional two-dose schedule in October 1999 and recommended to include this schedule in the Vaccines for Children Program in February 2000. Using the two-dose schedule, the adult dose of Recombivax HB (1-mL dose containing 10 μg of HBsAg) is administered to 11- to 15-year-old adolescents. The second dose is administered 4 to 6 months after the first dose.

Diphtheria and tetanus toxoids and acellular pertussis vaccine (DTaP) is the preferred vaccine for all doses in this series, including completion of the series in children who have received one or more doses of whole-cell DTP vaccine.

Clarification was added to the footnotes regarding the timing of the final vaccine doses in the series for DTaP vaccine. The final dose in the DTaP series should be given at more than 4 years (16). Tetanus and diphtheria toxoids, adsorbed, for adult use (Td) is recommended at age 11 to 12 years if at least 5 years has elapsed since the last dose. The age range 13 to 18 years serves as the catch-up interval (16). Subsequent routine Td boosters are recommended every 10 years.

Three *Haemophilus influenzae* type B (HIB) conjugate vaccines are licensed for primary immunization of infants. These vaccines contain type B capsular polysaccharide or capsular polysaccharide oligomers (PRP) that are conjugated to a protein carrier (a more effective antigen) to improve immunogenicity. HbOC (HibTiter), PRP-T (ActHIB, OmniHIB), and PRP-OMP (PedvaxHIB) can be used interchangeably (17). A fourth vaccine, PRP-D (ProHIBiT), is the only one of the HIB conjugate vaccines not licensed for primary immunization of infants. It is licensed as a primary dose only for children aged 15 to 59 months. Any of these four licensed HIB conjugate vaccines is acceptable for use as a booster dose, regardless of which vaccine was used in the primary series.

As mentioned earlier, these three products are now considered interchangeable for primary as well as booster vaccination (17). Excellent immune responses have been achieved when vaccines from different manufacturers have been used interchangeably in the primary series. Children who received the HIB conjugate vaccine (meningococcal protein conjugate [PRP-OMP], PedvaxHIB) demonstrate significant increases in antibody response after a single primary dose at 2 months. However, a two-dose primary series is recommended (another vaccination at 4 months), and a dose at 6 months is not required. Instead, a third dose is administered at 12 months. If PRP-OMP is administered in a series with one of the other two products licensed for infant use, the recommended number of doses to complete the series is determined by the other product, not by PRP-OMP. For example, if PRP-OMP is administered for the first dose at 2 months of age and another vaccine used at 4 months of age, a third dose of any of the three licensed HIB vaccines is recommended at age 6 months to complete the primary series.

Influenza continues to be a major cause of morbidity and mortality in the United States. The U.S. Public Health Service has targeted for elimination HIB in children less than 5 years of age. It is characterized by an abrupt onset of fever, myalgia, headache, severe malaise, cough, sore throat, and rhinitis. Although it resolves within a few days, it can exacerbate chronic conditions (e.g., asthma, diabetes mellitus)

and lead to secondary bacterial pneumonia. The ACIP makes recommendations on a yearly basis concerning the use and composition of the influenza virus vaccine. But in spite of efforts to vaccinate persons at high risk, the annual rate of influenza may reach as high as 40% in children, far above the 10 to 20% encountered in the general population.

Typically, the vaccine is administered parenterally, and it causes concern among parents over the threat of adverse reactions. As mentioned earlier, in June 2003, the first intranasal live attenuated influenza virus (LAIV) vaccine, FluMist was approved for clinical use in the United States. However, its use will be restricted to healthy children aged 5 to 17 and adults aged 18 to 49. For healthy individuals aged 5 to 49, LAIV is an acceptable alternative to the intramuscular trivalent inactivated influenza vaccine (16). The FDA's Vaccines and Related Biological Products Advisory Committee requested that the manufacturer produce more safety data on FluMist administration in young children and later determined that at present the vaccine was not safe for patients under age 5 due to concerns over increased rates of asthma within 6 weeks of vaccination. For patients over 50 years of age, the safe and effective use of FluMist was also not established. Hence, it is restricted from use in this patient population.

FluMist must be used cautiously and never administered parenterally. Patients with a history of anaphylactic reactions to eggs should not generally receive this vaccine. Children and adolescents receiving chronic aspirin therapy, because of the risk of Reye's syndrome, and patients with a history of Guillain-Barré syndrome should not receive FluMist. Pregnant women should not receive FluMist. Whenever the nasal vaccine is administered, epinephrine injection should be available in case of an anaphylactic reaction. The most common adverse effects encountered with FluMist are nasal congestion, runny nose (45%), sore throat (28%), cough (14%) and chills (9%). Serious adverse events occurred at similar rates in patients receiving FluMist and those receiving the placebo dosage form. It is important that suspected adverse events be reported by telephone to the Vaccine Adverse Event Reporting System (800-822-7967).

Each 0.5 mL dose will contain the three viral strains ($1 \times 10^{6.5-7.5}$ median tissue culture infectious doses of each virus) recommended by the U.S. Public Health Service for the upcoming season. The prefilled sprayer will include a Teflon tip equipped with a one-way valve that produces the mist. After 0.25 mL has been delivered into one nostril, the dose divider clip is removed from the plunger, and the remaining 0.25 mL is sprayed into the other nostril (Fig. 16.2). Patients should be advised to clear their nose prior to administration.

Children aged 5 to 8 years need two doses 6 weeks apart the first time they are vaccinated. The vaccine is supplied as a frozen liquid without preservatives in prefilled single use syringelike spray devices. Frost-free freezers are not appropriate for storage unless the vaccine is placed in a freezer box insert available from the manufacturer. It must be stored in a non–frost free freezer at $-15°C$ ($5°F$) or below. The product is to be thawed immediately before it is used by holding the barrel of the sprayer in the palm of the hand. After thawing, it is not to be refrozen. It can be thawed by placing it in a refrigerator, but it must be used within 24 hours.

So now the question that will arise with the availability of an effective intranasal influenza virus vaccine (18) is whether it is more reasonable to vaccinate healthy children, especially those prone to otitis media and those with a high exposure rate to influenza. There will be much appeal to do so, because the administration is not as invasive and the likelihood of adverse effects is less. Certainly, the potential health and economic benefit must be balanced with the challenge to develop and implement such a program and the unpredictable nature of the influenza virus.

Because FluMist is a live vaccine, intramuscular inactivated vaccine is preferred for health care workers and for family members and other close contacts of immunosuppressed patients. The package insert advises FluMist recipients to avoid close contact (e.g., within the same household) with any immunocompromised patients for at least 21 days.

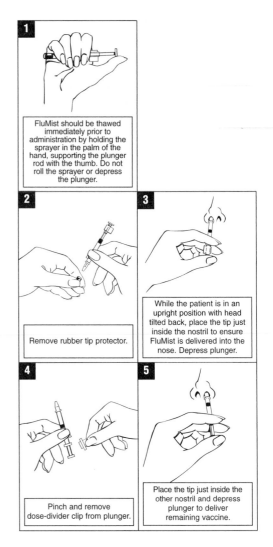

FIGURE 16.2 Instructions for intranasal administration of live attenuated influenza vaccine. (Courtesy of MedImmune Vaccines, Gaithersburg, MD.)

Children aged 6 to 23 months are particularly susceptible to the risk of influenza-related hospitalizations. Thus, vaccination of all children in this age group is encouraged when feasible (3). ACIP has indicated further that beginning in autumn 2004, annual influenza vaccine will be recommended for children 6 to 23 months (16). An updated childhood and adolescent immunization schedule for July to December 2004 will be ultimately released to reflect this change (16).

Influenza vaccination is recommended annually for children over 6 months with certain risk factors (e.g., asthma, cardiac disease, sickle cell disease, HIV, diabetes, household members in groups at high risk) and can be administered to all others wishing to obtain immunity. Children less than 12 years should receive vaccine in a dosage appropriate for their age, that is, 0.25 mL for ages 6 to 35 months and 0.5 mL for ages 3 years and older. Children less than 8 years old who are receiving influenza vaccine for the first time should receive two doses separated by at least 4 weeks.

A new catch-up immunization schedule for children and adolescents who start vaccinations late or who are more than 1 month behind has been published by the CDC (16). Minimum ages and minimum intervals between dosages are provided for each of the routinely recommended childhood and adolescent vaccines. The schedules are divided into two distinct age groupings, ages 4 months to 6 years and ages 7 to 18 years.

One poliovirus vaccine (inactivated poliovirus vaccine [IPV]) is licensed and distributed in the United States. OPV was taken off the U.S. market as of January 1, 2000, to eliminate the risk of vaccine-associated paralytic poliomyelitis. Although no longer available in the United States, OPV remains the vaccine of choice for global polio eradication efforts. An all-IPV schedule for routine childhood poliovirus vaccination has been recommended in the United States since OPV was taken off the market. All children should receive 4 doses of IPV at ages 2, 4, and 6 to 18 months and at age 4 to 6 years. If accelerated protection is warranted, the minimum interval between doses is 4 weeks, although the preferred interval between the second and third doses is 2 months.

For children who received an all-IPV or all-OPV series, a fourth dose is not necessary if the third dose was administered later than age 4 years. If both OPV and IPV were administered as part of a series, a total of four doses should be administered regardless of the child's age. Routine poliovirus vaccination is not generally recommended for persons older than 18 years.

In December 2002, the FDA approved a new vaccine, Pediarix (GlaxoSmithKline) that when administered to infants would result in up to six fewer injections for the infants and consequently reduce pain and discomfort. The new vaccine contains diphtheria and tetanus toxoids and acellular pertussis adsorbed, hepatitis B (recombinant), and inactivated poliovirus vaccine combined. It is to be administered to infants at 2, 4, and 6 months of age for prevention of diphtheria, tetanus, pertussis (whooping cough), hepatitis B, and polio.

This vaccine is unique in that it is the first five-in-one U.S.–licensed vaccine to provide coverage against five serious illnesses in a three-dose regimen, and it makes it easier to comply with the immunization schedule than separately administered vaccines. Currently, children receive approximately 20 injections in the first 2 years of life, and with the development and introduction of new vaccines, that number will continue to increase. Nine injections are recommended to protect the more than 4 million babies born in the United States each year against diphtheria, tetanus, pertussis, hepatitis B, and polio. It has been estimated that the use of this vaccine could result in as many as 24 million fewer injections per year for infants in the United States.

Numerous clinical trials were necessary to demonstrate safety and immunogenicity of the combination vaccine compared to the separate administration of the individual vaccines. More than 20,000 doses of the combination vaccine where administered to more than 7,000 infants. Adverse effects in infants receiving this vaccine included injection site reactions (e.g., pain, redness, swelling), fever, and fussiness. The administration of the vaccine also demonstrated a higher rate of fever than for vaccines administered separately. Consistent with all medications, the vaccine is contraindicated in infants with demonstrated hypersensitivity to any of the product's ingredients, including yeast, neomycin, and polymyxin B.

The first dose of the MMR vaccine should be administered when an infant is 12 to 15 months of age. This single dose induces antibody formation to all three viruses in at least 95% of those vaccinated at this time. Routinely, the second dose of MMR vaccine is recommended at 4 to 6 years of age. It can, however, be administered during any visit, provided at least 4 weeks have elapsed since receipt of the first dose and both doses are administered beginning at or after age 12 months. Those who have not previously received the second dose should complete the schedule no later than the routine visit to a health care provider at age 11 to 12 years.

Varicella virus vaccine live can be administered at any time at or after 12 months of age for susceptible children, that is, those who lack a reliable history of chickenpox. Infants younger that 12 months of age are generally protected from varicella by passive maternal antibody. Routinely, the vaccine is recommended for infants without contraindications at 12 to 18 months of age. Susceptible children aged more than 13 years should receive two doses at least 4 to 8 weeks apart.

Every year there are approximately 5,000 to 9,000 hospitalizations and 100 deaths from chickenpox in the United States. This vaccine has been available in the United States since 1995, and the CDC's ACIP, the AAP, and the AAFP recommend that all children be vaccinated routinely at 12 to 18 months of age and that all susceptible children receive the vaccine before age 13.

Varicella zoster immunoglobulin (VZIG), made from plasma from healthy volunteer blood donors with high levels of antibody to the varicella zoster virus, is recommended after exposure for persons at high risk, that is, immunocompromised patients, pregnant women, infants born at less than 28 weeks' gestation or weighing less than 1 kg (2.2 lb) at birth and premature infants whose mothers are not immune.

In 1998, the FDA approved the first vaccine (RotaShield, Wyeth) to prevent rotavirus gastroenteritis in children. Rotavirus gastroenteritis is the most common cause of severe and sometimes fatal diarrhea in children. Infants and children aged 6 months to about 5 years are most vulnerable to rotavirus infection. The infection causes dehydration and an estimated 1 million deaths worldwide per year. In the United States, this virus causes about 20 to 40 deaths a year and more than 50,000 hospitalizations from severe diarrhea and dehydration.

In July, 1999, the CDC recommended that health care providers and parents postpone the use of tetravalent RotaShield vaccine (19). This action was based on reports of intussusception (the bowel folds in on itself and is obstructed). Intussusception was demonstrated to occur with significantly increased frequency in the first week or two after vaccination with this vaccine, particularly following the first dose. Because of the withdrawal of the vaccine, the ACIP recommends educational efforts toward parents and health care providers to help parents prevent dehydration and to recognize and immediately seek medical care for the treatment of severe diarrhea in children, particularly those aged 5 years or younger.

Adult Immunization Schedule

It is estimated that at least 30,000 to 60,000 individuals die each year of pneumococcal disease, influenza, hepatitis B, and other vaccine-preventable diseases (20). At least 100 times as many adults as children succumb to these illnesses. Many adults do not recognize the need for immunization throughout their lifetime (20). In recent years, the National Adult Immunization Awareness Week (September 26–October 2, 2004) highlights the influenza vaccination season, which typically begins in the early fall (21). This reminds health care providers and public health officials to intensify their effort to vaccinate adults and adolescents according to ACIP recommendations. Besides influenza and pneumococcal vaccines, recommendations also cover diphtheria, hepatitis A and B, measles, mumps, rubella, tetanus, meningococcal disease, and varicella.

Figure 16.3 shows an adult immunization schedule (21). Hepatitis A and B vaccines are recommended for persons who are or will be at increased risk of infection with hepatitis A and B. These high-risk groups include health care personnel, dialysis patients, certain occupations (e.g., morticians, embalmers), immigrants from areas of high hepatitis A or B endemicity, and behavioral predisposition (e.g., homosexually active males, users of illicit injectable drugs, prisoners, and clients in institutions for the mentally retarded). Also included in this group are health professional students who participate in the experiential component

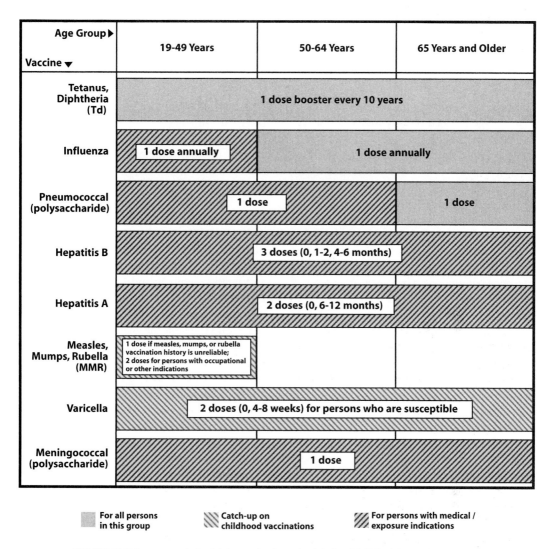

Age Group ▶ Vaccine ▼	19-49 Years	50-64 Years	65 Years and Older
Tetanus, Diphtheria (Td)	1 dose booster every 10 years		
Influenza	1 dose annually	1 dose annually	
Pneumococcal (polysaccharide)	1 dose		1 dose
Hepatitis B	3 doses (0, 1-2, 4-6 months)		
Hepatitis A	2 doses (0, 6-12 months)		
Measles, Mumps, Rubella (MMR)	1 dose if measles, mumps, or rubella vaccination history is unreliable; 2 doses for persons with occupational or other indications		
Varicella	2 doses (0, 4-8 weeks) for persons who are susceptible		
Meningococcal (polysaccharide)	1 dose		

For all persons in this group   Catch-up on childhood vaccinations   For persons with medical / exposure indications

FIGURE 16.3 Recommended adult immunization schedule for the United States, 2003–2004.

of their curricula in health care environments. Hepatitis A vaccine is also indicated for travel anywhere in the world except North America, Western Europe, Scandinavia, Japan, Australia, and New Zealand.

Historically, the influenza virus vaccine was recommended for everyone over age 65 years and for those under 65 who are at special risk to develop complications associated with influenza. Now it is recommended also for those aged 50 to 64, because this group has an increased prevalence of persons with high-risk conditions. Approximately 43 million persons in the United States are in this age group, and

of these 10 million to 14 million have more than one high-risk medical conditions (e.g., diabetes mellitus, cardiovascular disease). Even those in this group without high-risk conditions benefit in terms of decreased influenza illness, less work absenteeism, and decreased need for medical consultation and medications, including antibiotics. For patients aged 19 to 49, one annual dose is recommended to those with medical or occupational indications or household contacts of persons with indications. Research demonstrates that the immunization of high-risk patients is cost effective and reduces complications and death. However, this vaccine is underused in high-risk adults and children. In 1994, for example, vaccination coverage in people over 65 years of age reached only 55% and was only 30% among high-risk adults over 65 years of age. In 1998, vaccination coverage in people over 65 years of age reached 64%—almost double the 1989 rate of 33% (19).

Regrettably, millions of people in the United States get influenza each year. Influenza causes an average of 114,000 hospitalizations and 36,000 deaths annually. Combined with pneumococcal disease, which causes 10,000 to 14,000 deaths annually, this is the sixth leading cause of death in the United States. Anyone can get the flu, and serious problems from influenza can occur at any age. Groups at greatest risk include adults and children with chronic pulmonary and/or cardiovascular diseases that require routine medical examination or hospitalization during the preceding year, including children with asthma. Adults and children who have required regular medical follow-up or hospitalizations during the preceding year because of chronic metabolic diseases (including diabetes mellitus), renal dysfunction, hemoglobinopathies, or immunosuppression (including immunosuppression caused by medications) are also at high risk.

Other groups at high risk to develop influenza-related complications include persons above 65 years of age and residents of nursing homes, extended care facilities, retirement villages, and other chronic care facilities housing patients of any age with chronic medical conditions. Also in this category are those aged 6 months to 18 years who are receiving long-term aspirin therapy and, therefore, are at risk to develop Reye's syndrome after influenza.

Pregnancy can increase the risk of complications in women who contract the flu. These women are more likely to be hospitalized for complications of the flu than those who are not pregnant. Pregnancy can affect the mother's immune system and cardiovascular system and increase the risk of complications.

The influenza vaccine is made from inactivated viruses, and experts consider flu shots safe during any stage of pregnancy. However, miscarriages have been documented, most of-ten in the first trimester of pregnancy. Thus, traditionally women in their second or third trimester of pregnancy during the influenza season should be vaccinated. Also, women who are beyond the first 3 months of their pregnancy during the flu season should receive an inoculation. Those with medical problems that increase their risk of complications if flu is contracted should receive a flu shot prior to the flu season regardless of the stage of their pregnancy.

High-risk individuals who should also be immunized with the influenza virus vaccine include health care workers, employees of nursing homes and chronic care facilities, providers of home care to persons at high risk, and family members and others in close contact with high-risk individuals. These individuals can become clinically or subclinically infected and transmit the virus to persons at high risk whom they care for or live with. Some persons, including the elderly, transplant recipients, and persons with AIDS, can have a low antibody response to the influenza vaccine, and efforts to protect these patients must be made to reduce the likelihood they will contract influenza from their caregivers.

Influenza vaccination is also advocated for individuals who provide vital services to the community (e.g., police, firefighters, emergency medical personnel). Having an inordinate number of these workers out sick with the flu can interrupt the delivery of important services.

The optimum time to administer the influenza vaccine is during October and November. Because of vaccination delays in the past, it is suggested that immunization efforts begin in October with health care workers and those most vulnerable to influenza-related complications. Other groups can begin vaccinations in November. For healthy persons aged 5 to 49 without high risk conditions or occupations, either the inactivated vaccine or the intranasal vaccine may be given (22).

Pneumococcal disease, a vaccine-preventable disease, along with influenza, contributes significantly to the mortality of older persons in the United States. Pneumococcal disease caused approximately 10,000 to 14,000 deaths among persons aged 65 years or older in 1998.

National Health Objectives 2010 include increasing pneumococcal vaccination levels above 90% among persons 65 years of age and older. Health care providers are advised to offer pneumococcal vaccine all year.

To assess progress toward achieving the National Health Objectives 2010, the CDC analyzed data from the 2001 Behavioral Risk Factor Surveillance System (BRFSS), a state-based randomly dialed telephone survey of the civilian population aged 18 years and older who are not institutionalized. The survey is conducted in all 50 states, the District of Columbia, and three U.S. territories. The report summarized findings that the estimated point prevalence of influenza and pneumococcal vaccination were below 80% among persons aged 65 years and older in all reporting areas for influenza vaccine in 2001 and 60% in 2001 for pneumococcal vaccination. The estimated percentages of non-Hispanic blacks (48.1% for influenza, 39.4% for pneumococcal) and Hispanics (55.2% for influenza, 41.6% for pneumococcal) having received both vaccines were less than for non-Hispanic whites (67% for influenza, 63.5% for pneumococcal), demonstrating a statistically significant disparity in vaccination coverage. For all races, a concerted effort must be made to increase vaccination rates yearly to meet the 2010 goals established for influenza and pneumococcal vaccination.

Adults born before 1957 may be considered immune to measles. Adults born after 1957 should receive at least one dose of MMR vaccine unless they have a medical contraindication, documentation of at least one dose, or other acceptable evidence of immunity. A second dose of MMR vaccine is recommended for adults recently exposed to measles or in an outbreak, previously vaccinated with killed measles vaccine, or vaccinated with an unknown vaccine between 1963 and 1967. Students in a postsecondary educational institution, working in a health care facility, and/or planning to travel internationally should also receive a second dose of MMR vaccine (22).

MMR vaccine should not be given to pregnant women or those considering pregnancy within 1 month. These women should also avoid monovalent measles vaccine and any other rubella-containing vaccine for the same period. It is not known whether measles virus can cause fetal harm or affect reproductive capacity. In addition, although mumps virus can infect the placenta and fetus, there is no good evidence that it causes congenital malformations in humans. Attenuated mumps vaccine virus can infect the placenta, but the virus has not been isolated from fetal tissues of susceptible women who were vaccinated and underwent elective abortions. Furthermore, evidence suggests that transmission of attenuated rubella virus to the fetus occurs, although the vaccine is not known to cause fetal harm when administered during pregnancy. Suffice to say that it is prudent not to administer MMR to pregnant women. If postpubertal females are vaccinated, these women should be counseled to avoid pregnancy for 4 weeks after vaccination. Most IgG passage across the placenta occurs during the third trimester.

The Td toxoids are preferred for immunizing adults and children after age 6 years. All persons should maintain tetanus immunity by means of booster doses throughout their lifetime, because tetanus spores are widespread. Tetanus immunity is especially important for military personnel, farm and utility workers, those working with horses, firemen, and all individuals whose occupation or vocation renders them prone to even minor lacerations and abrasions. Similarly, those traveling to developing nations should maintain active tetanus immunization to obviate therapy with equine tetanus antitoxin and avoid its complications.

More than 95% of U.S. citizens are immune to varicella zoster virus. The varicella virus vaccine in adults is intended to cover those who have not had chickenpox and those who do not have a reliable clinical history of varicella infection or serologic evidence of VZV infection who may be at a high risk for exposure or transmission (22). Studies demonstrate that the vaccine is quite effective at blunting breakthrough chickenpox following household exposure, and when chickenpox does occur, reported body lesions are usually far less than normally encountered during a chickenpox attack (300 to 500 maculopapular or vesicular lesions accompanied by fever).

Those who have had chickenpox vaccine may be capable of transmitting the vaccine virus to close contacts. Therefore, vaccine recipients should avoid close association with susceptible high-risk individuals (e.g., newborns, pregnant women, immunocompromised persons). Vaccinated persons should also be warned to avoid the use of salicylates for 6 weeks after vaccination with the varicella vaccine, as Reye's syndrome has been reported following the use of salicylates during natural varicella infections.

Because it is not known whether varicella vaccine can cause fetal harm or affect reproductive ability when administered during pregnancy, it is prudent to avoid vaccination during pregnancy. Natural varicella, however, has sometimes caused fetal harm. In similar fashion to vaccination with MMR, women contemplating pregnancy should be counseled to avoid pregnancy within 4 weeks of vaccination with the chickenpox vaccine.

In December 1998 the FDA licensed the first vaccine for the prevention of Lyme disease (LYMErix, GlaxoSmithKline) and indicated it for active immunization against Lyme disease in individuals aged 15 to 70 years. This vaccine is administered in a series of three 30-µg (0.5 mL) intramuscular doses over a year with injections administered on a 0-, 1-, and 12-month schedule. One dose contains 30 µg of outer surface lipoprotein A (Osp A). Osp A proteins cause vaccine recipients to produce antibodies that kill the Lyme bacterium, a spirochete, *Borrelia burgdorferi*. When the tick ingests the antibodies during the blood meal, the antibodies work to kill the bacteria in the tick's gut. This prevents the spirochete from entering the vaccinee.

To receive the maximum protection, patients must receive the full course of three doses. However, after two injections, there is a 49% efficacy rate in preventing definitive Lyme disease and an 83% efficacy rate in preventing asymptomatic infections.

In clinical trials, LYMEtrix was demonstrated to be 76% effective in preventing Lyme disease infection and entirely effective in preventing asymptomatic infection (23). This vaccine is particularly appropriate for individuals in endemic areas with substantial outdoor exposures related to work (e.g., landscaping, brush clearing, forestry, wildlife management) or hobbies such as fishing, hunting, camping, and gardening. Also, it is advised for people living in or vacationing in endemic areas (e.g., Virginia north to Maine, Wisconsin, Minnesota, northern California). Men are as likely as women to contract Lyme disease, and it also can strike children and adolescents.

The CDC also published a listing of recommended immunizations for adults with certain medical conditions, including pregnancy, diabetes, renal failure, and HIV infection (22) (Fig. 16.4). The footnotes highlight issues unique to chronic disease groups to provide information for providers who are unfamiliar with the dosage of a particular vaccine (e.g., hepatitis A for persons with chronic liver disease) or contraindications (e.g., varicella vaccine in HIV patients).

Several vaccines are undergoing clinical trials. Included is a herpes vaccine designed to prevent all forms of herpes infection, including the sexually transmitted type. Another vaccine that could prevent gum disease is in preclinical testing. The vaccine is being developed to work against *Porphyromonas gingivalis,* the bacterium most associated with gingivitis. The intent is to rid the mouth of *P. gingivalis.*

Vaccination Advocacy From Pharmacists

Perhaps one of the greatest achievements of medical science is the ability to shield individuals from once-common life-threatening diseases by providing immunity via administration of vaccines or antibody-containing solutions. Indeed, the practice of widespread childhood immunizations has reduced dramatically the morbidity and mortality of several infectious diseases and their sequelae. The best examples are the worldwide elimination of smallpox and the virtual elimination of polio from developed countries and the Western Hemisphere.

Preschool immunization programs against measles, mumps, pertussis, and tetanus have resulted in more than 95% reductions in these

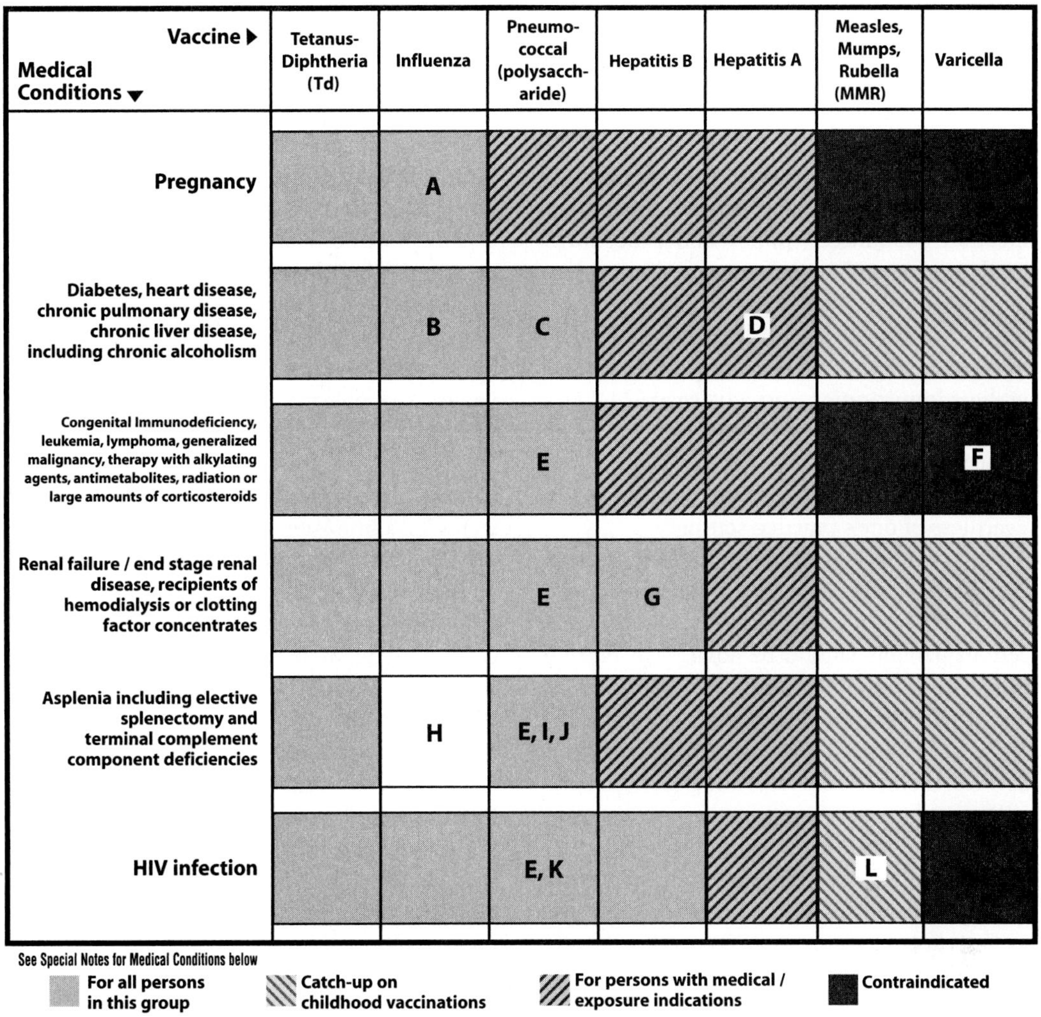

Medical Conditions ▼ / Vaccine ►	Tetanus-Diphtheria (Td)	Influenza	Pneumo-coccal (polysacch-aride)	Hepatitis B	Hepatitis A	Measles, Mumps, Rubella (MMR)	Varicella
Pregnancy		A					
Diabetes, heart disease, chronic pulmonary disease, chronic liver disease, including chronic alcoholism	B		C			D	
Congenital Immunodeficiency, leukemia, lymphoma, generalized malignancy, therapy with alkylating agents, antimetabolites, radiation or large amounts of corticosteroids			E				F
Renal failure / end stage renal disease, recipients of hemodialysis or clotting factor concentrates			E	G			
Asplenia including elective splenectomy and terminal complement component deficiencies	H		E, I, J				
HIV infection			E, K			L	

Legend:
- For all persons in this group
- Catch-up on childhood vaccinations
- For persons with medical / exposure indications
- Contraindicated

See Special Notes for Medical Conditions below

Special Notes for Medical Conditions

A. For women without chronic diseases/conditions, vaccinate if pregnancy will be at 2nd or 3rd trimester during influenza season. For women with chronic diseases/conditions, vaccinate at any time during the pregnancy.

B. Although chronic liver disease and alcoholism are not indicator conditions for influenza vaccination, give 1 dose annually if the patient is ≥ 50 years, has other indications for influenza vaccine, or if the patient requests vaccination.

C. Asthma is an indicator condition for influenza but not for pneumococcal vaccination.

D. For all persons with chronic liver disease.

E. For persons < 65 years, revaccinate once after 5 years or more have elapsed since initial vaccination.

F. Persons with impaired humoral immunity but intact cellular immunity may be vaccinated.
MMWR1999; 48 (RR-06):1-5.

G. Hemodialysis patients: Use special formulation of vaccine (40 ug/mL) or two 1.0 mL 20 ug doses given at one site. Vaccinate early in the course of renal disease. Assess antibody titers to hep B surface antigen (anti-HBs) levels annually. Administer additional doses if anti-HBs levels decline to <10 milliinternational units (mIU)/ mL.

H. There are no data specifically on risk of severe or complicated influenza infections among persons with asplenia. However, influenza is a risk factor for secondary bacterial infections that may cause severe disease in asplenics.

I. Administer meningococcal vaccine and consider Hib vaccine.

J. Elective splenectomy: vaccinate at least 2 weeks before surgery.

K. Vaccinate as close to diagnosis as possible when CD4 cell counts are highest.

L. Withhold MMR or other measles containing vaccines from HIV-infected persons with evidence of severe immunosuppression. MMWR1998; 47 (RR-8):21-22; MMWR2002; 51 (RR-02):22-24.

FIGURE 16.4 Recommended immunizations for adults with medical conditions for the United States, 2003–2004.

diseases. In addition to the vast human savings, a cost benefit accrues. It has been estimated that every $1 spent on immunizing children against measles, mumps, and rubella saves $14 in health care. Unfortunately, however, as mentioned earlier, 50,000 to 70,000 adults die each year of vaccine-preventable diseases and their complications (12). This is at least 100 times the number of children who die of similar afflictions. Adult deaths from hepatitis B and influenza demonstrate that more information must reach adults, among these being that pediatric immunization does not necessarily confer lifetime immunization.

Pharmacists can encourage immunization through (a) formulary management; (b) administrative measures, such as participation on infection committees, policy and procedures development, and advocating standing orders in institutions; (c) participation in administration programs; (d) patient history and screening; (e) counseling and documentation; and (f) public administration and advocacy (24). Depending upon the pharmacist's practice environment, these may not all be possible. However, the key is involvement and advocacy regardless of one's practice setting.

For example, pharmacists should attempt to screen adult patients to determine who may be susceptible to preventable infectious diseases. Certain patients should be advised to receive immunization to influenza (e.g., older than 50 years living in a nursing home), pneumococcus (e.g., alcoholics and those with coexisting diseases, including diabetes and functional impairment of cardiorespiratory, hepatic, or renal systems), or hepatitis (e.g., dialysis patients, homosexually active persons). As an ethnic and racial group, African Americans often are not immunized against or screened for hepatitis A, B, or C because of a variety of social, cultural, and structural barriers. Pharmacists should help educate these patients and support African American communities to conduct prevention strategies and increased emphasis on hepatitis A, B, and C as a serious public health issue and ways to increase immunization rates among this population.

Compliance with established immunization guidelines can also be improved with use of patient profile systems. Incorporation of immunization histories into the patient's pharmacy profile can serve as a reminder when booster immunizations are needed. This is especially important with new patients (e.g., newborns, patients who move into the neighborhood). Indirect passive methods (e.g., posters, buttons, bag stuffers) to communicate the importance of immunizations are somewhat effective. However, it is the direct one-on-one patient contact

and encouragement by the pharmacist that is most important. Shortfalls in immunizations among African Americans, Hispanics, and other racial minorities are not solved merely by pharmacists with these racial backgrounds. Rather, it is accomplished through the dedication and motivation of all pharmacists.

The profession of pharmacy is in an optimal position to become part of a local community immunization effort. Because pharmacists are in residential neighborhoods, people do not have to travel far to reach them, and the convenience of pharmacy open hours makes it an optimal site for immunization awareness and vaccination programs. Also, as mentioned previously, the pharmacist has a legal right in 37 states to administer immunizations. Pharmacists can also have an immunization presence and advocacy in rural areas. Rosenbluth et al. (25) described a pharmacy immunization project in which independent community pharmacies in five contiguous rural counties in West Virginia provided a childhood and adult immunization service.

Professional organizations (e.g., American Pharmacists Association) have resources to assist pharmacists in this endeavor to keep current and provide immunization. The APhA program, for example, helps pharmacists develop immunization clinics for adults. The program includes recommended adult immunization schedules, vaccination administration, techniques, storage, and valuable marketing guidance (26). The program emphasizes that participant pharmacists are not trained to administer immunizations to children. This program is also being taught to clerkship students by some colleges and schools of pharmacy prior to their community clerkship rotations. In addition, the APhA now offers an online immunization and vaccine clinical information service for nonemergency queries only in collaboration with the University of Tennessee Health Center in Memphis. The service is available at www.aphanet.org/forms/immunize-help.asp. It requires pharmacists who submit questions to complete a short form and provide as much information as possible (e.g., age, weight, renal function, immune status, allergies of the patient). Every attempt is made to answer the questions within a reasonable amount of time, and a check box is provided so that inquiring pharmacists can indicate whether an answer is needed by the following day or a date in the future.

Pharmacists must also be attuned to the cost of vaccinations and its implications for the structure and function of state vaccination programs and the children served by those programs. Davis et al. (27) studied childhood vaccine purchase costs in the private sector in terms of past trends and future expectations. The study determined that the cost of vaccine purchase rose from $10 in 1975 to $385 in 2001, and with the recommendation of seven additional vaccines, the cost of vaccination per child could escalate to approximately $1,225 in 2020. So pharmacists must remain as strong advocates for immunizing programs regardless of the cost implications.

Additional Immunization Information Resources

Pharmacists must have contact information for patients with special needs as it relates to immunization information, where to find immunization programs, and issues of travel safety, among others. For example, the National Immunization Hotline (800-232-2522 [English] or 800-232-0233 [Spanish]) allows a person to talk directly to a live person concerning questions about vaccines, securing print-based copies of immunization materials, and information on where to find a local immunization clinic.

The CDC's Fax-Back System for International Travel Information (1-877-FYI-TRIP) can be contacted for a faxed directory of materials, including malaria information. With the directory in hand, the client can call 888-CDC-FAXX and follow the prompts to request specific documents.

For pharmacists seeking education about vaccines and vaccine policies, the IAC Express is coordinated by the Immunization Action Coalition (IAC), St. Paul, Minnesota. Its Web site (www.immunize.org) has a number of patient education tools. Further, the site summarizes new vaccine information and alerts,

among others. To subscribe to the service, pharmacists should forward an e-mail message to express@immunize.org and place the key word *subscribe* in the subject field. The subscriber should *not* enter any message text.

Responding to Bioterrorism

In the wake of the events of September 11, 2001 (9/11), awareness of the necessity for vigilance to illness patterns and diagnostic clues that might indicate an unusual infectious disease outbreak heightened. Pharmacists and allied health professionals were asked to report any indication of suspicious symptoms to local and state health departments. Evidence of intentional release of biologic agents include infection in these groups: (*a*) people in the same location with symptoms that suggest an infectious disease outbreak (e.g. unexplained febrile illness associated with sepsis, pneumonia, respiratory failure, a rash, or a botulism-like syndrome with flaccid muscle paralysis), (*b*) age groups not normally associated with the disease in question, and (*c*) numerous cases of acute flaccid paralysis with prominent bulbar palsies that suggest the release of botulinum toxin.

Pharmacists are also encouraged to participate in their community's disaster preparedness efforts. The pharmacist can bring an important and unique perspective to determining and preparing for health care needs during times of natural disasters or manmade crises. The American Pharmacists Association has attempted to assist involved pharmacists by creating a National Pharmacists Response Team. The 10 teams will assist communities with chemoprophylaxis or vaccinations during times of need. Interested pharmacists can apply for the team online at www.aphanet.org/pharmcare/NPRTform.pdf.

After 9/11, the news media concentrated itself with the threat of an anthrax outbreak without realizing there were other more prominent diseases with greater potential harm to the public. Those listed by the CDC as the biggest biologic threats in addition to anthrax included smallpox and pneumonic plague. Other agents of concern include

Clostridium botulinum toxin (botulism), *Francisella tularensis* (i.e., tularemia), and the hemorrhagic fevers.

Smallpox, caused by variola virus, has initial symptoms that include high fever, fatigue, headache, and backaches. These symptoms are followed by a rash. While most patients recover, up to 30% of cases result in death. This disease is spread by face-to-face contact. Routine vaccination against smallpox ended in 1972, so the level of immunity among persons vaccinated up until this time is unknown. Therefore, all individuals are considered susceptible. In 2002, after evaluating the risk of a bioterrorist attack and the adverse effects of the smallpox vaccine (e.g., lymph node swelling, rash, fever, scarring, severe skin reactions, encephalitis), the ACIP concluded that the risks outweighed the benefits and recommended that the general public not be inoculated against smallpox. It recommended that vaccinations be offered to a total of about 15,000 health care workers around the country who would be designated to investigate smallpox cases and provide direct care at designated hospitals.

In an attempt to determine whether more smallpox vaccine could be made available to the general population given supply questions, a recent study was conducted by the National Institute of Allergy and Infectious Disease (NIAID) (28). The study consisted of 680 adults less than 32 years of age who were never vaccinated for smallpox and who were assigned to three treatment groups. They received vaccine that was undiluted, diluted 1:5, or diluted 1:10 (28). The initial vaccination was successful in 97.8% of all three groups. There were no significant differences in the rate of vesicle formation (the end point demonstrating success of the vaccine) over the range of titers tested. When followed up with a second vaccination, the researchers demonstrated that the two dilutions were both effective against smallpox. The implication was that the 1:10 dilution could protect 10 times as many persons as would be protected by the administration of the undiluted vaccine.

Botulism is a muscle-paralyzing disease caused by the toxin produced by *Clostridium botulinum*. Food-borne botulism is a public health emergency because the contaminated food may still be available to other people. This form of botulism occurs when the preformed toxin is ingested in contaminated food and causes illness within 6 hours to 2 weeks. Symptoms include double vision, blurred vision, drooping eyelids, slurred speech, difficulty swallowing, dry mouth, and muscle weakness that leads to paralysis of the breathing muscles. Botulism is not communicable from one person to the next.

Pneumonic plague occurs when *Y. pestis* infects the lung. The initial symptoms of this illness include fever, headache, weakness, and cough with a bloody or watery sputum. This disease progresses over 2 to 4 days and may cause septic shock. If treatment is not initiated, the result is death. This disease is communicable with face-to-face contact with the infected person. Early treatment with antibiotics (e.g., tetracycline, streptomycin, chloramphenicol) is imperative. There is no vaccine against this disease.

Anthrax has three forms, cutaneous (skin surface is exposed to anthrax particles and skin lesions develop), gastrointestinal (particles are ingested), and inhalation (often fatal). Cutaneous anthrax demonstrates typically on the arms or hands as a swelling of the skin that develops into a central area of ulceration or a depression, and then a dark, blackish-brown scab forms over the area. This manifestation of anthrax can be painless, and a fever may be present. Gastrointestinal anthrax is characterized by an acute inflammation of the intestines, loss of appetite, vomiting, and pain. This is followed by a bout of abdominal pain, vomiting of blood, and severe diarrhea. Initial symptoms of inhalation anthrax resemble the common cold and within a few days progress to severe respiratory problems and shock.

Anthrax cannot be transmitted from one person to another. Treatment is with antibiotics (e.g., penicillin, doxycycline, fluoroquinolones), but only those exposed to this disease should be treated. Initially, with the anthrax scare after 9/11, prescriptions for Cipro, a fluoroquinolone, increased as concerned individuals were stockpiling to protect themselves and their families from the threat of anthrax. This was not a good practice because the drug should be used only by patients exposed to the disease and because storage conditions and validation of expiration dates cannot be ensured.

Diagnostic Skin Antigens

It may be necessary to use antigens *in vivo* as diagnostic tools. Typically, these are injected intradermally and the site inspected for development of a hypersensitivity reaction. A positive reaction is determined by the extent of induration (in millimeters) and degree of reaction, from slight induration to vesiculation and necrosis. These signs demonstrate sensitivity to the antigen and the presence of antibodies due to present or past infection with the particular organism.

The number of diagnostic skin biologics is relatively small. In the late 1970s, many were removed from the market as a result of the recommendations of the FDA Panel on Review of Skin Antigens (29). Specifically, the panel questioned the reliability of skin test antigens for trichinosis, lymphogranuloma venereum, and mumps and recommended that these be withdrawn from the market and not licensed.

Several diagnostic skin antigens are featured in Table 16.1. One of the more recent *in vivo* diagnostic biologics, *Candida albicans* Skin Test Antigen, is useful in the assessment of diminished cellular immunity in persons infected with HIV. Because HIV infection can modify the delayed-type hypersensitivity (DTH) response to tuberculin, it is advisable to skin test HIV-infected patients at high risk for tuberculosis with antigens in addition to tuberculin, to assess their competency to react to tuberculin. Responses to DTH antigens also have prognostic value in patients with cancer.

The Multiple Skin Test Antigens (Multitest CMI, Merieux) is a skin test for multiple antigens consisting of a disposable applicator with eight sterile heads preloaded with seven delayed-hypersensitivity skin test antigens and a glycerin negative control for percutaneous administration. The seven antigens are tetanus toxoid antigen, diphtheria toxoid antigen, streptococcus antigen, old tuberculin, *Candida* antigen, trichophyton antigen, and *Proteus* antigen. The intent of this multiple test is to detect anergy (lack of response to antigens) through delayed hypersensitivity skin testing.

PHARMACEUTICS CASE STUDY

Subjective Information

You are in charge of providing a vaccine for a statewide program to vaccinate a select population of patients at 10 sites throughout the state. The vaccine will go to about 10,000 patients. What will you recommend to the organizing committee to ensure that the vaccine arrives intact, stable, and active?

Objective

The vaccine is a lyophilized vaccine that must be stored in a freezer until it is reconstituted with sterile water for injection and administered. After reconstitution, it is stable for only 1 hour. Prior to reconstitution, it must remain in frozen, and if allowed to reach room temperature prior to reconstitution, it must be discarded after 3 hours.

Assessment

Of the 10 sites for administration, 2 are within 50 miles, 2 more within 100 miles, 3 more within 150 miles, and 3 within approximately 225 miles of your facility.

Plan

The vaccine will be ordered to arrive at your facility, shipped overnight from the manufacturer with sufficient dry ice to keep it frozen, the week before it is to be shipped to the vaccination sites. On Monday of the week of the vaccinations, the vaccines will be packaged in sufficient dry ice and shipped overnight to arrive at each of the 10 sites the next morning (Tuesday). Upon arrival, the vaccine will be placed in freezers until used. The vaccinations can be scheduled for Wednesday through Friday of that week; this will minimize storage and potential handling problems of the vaccine.

CLINICAL CASE STUDY

Vaccines are antigenic substances administered for prophylactic purposes to achieve active immunity. The body's response helps to build up its own immune defenses. Vaccines may be living, attenuated, or killed microorganisms or fractions of microorganisms. They may also be a toxoid, a bacterial toxin that is modified and detoxified by use of moderate heat and chemical treatment. The end result of the processing is considered nontoxic, although the antigenic properties remain. Children and adults are vaccinated, and immunization schedules have been developed for both groups. For example, the pediatric immunization schedule includes 20 immunizations that are administered before the person is 2 years of age.

Pharmaceutical Care Plan

S: J.C. is an 8-week-old female. Her mother brought J. C. to the emergency department at 3:00 P.M. J. C. had been restless and crying inconsolably for the past 4 hours. J. C. was given her 2-month immunization of Pediarix yesterday by her pediatrician. Her mother took a rectal temperature today at 2:00 P.M., and found it to be elevated. J. C. has also had one seizure while in the emergency department.

O: Age, 8 weeks
Temperature (rectal) at 2:00 P.M., 101°F per mother
Currently 105°F in ER

A: The patient is reacting to the immunization Pediarix, a combination of diphtheria and tetanus toxoids and acellular pertussis adsorbed, hepatitis B (recombinant) and inactivated poliovirus vaccine.

J. C. needs these immunizations to protect against many disease states. Diphtheria is an acute toxin-mediated infectious disease caused by toxigenic strains of *Corynebacterium diphtheriae*. Tetanus is a condition of neuromuscular dysfunction as a result of a potent exotoxin released from *Clostridium tetani*. Pertussis, or whooping cough, is a respiratory tract condition caused by *Bordetella pertussis*. Hepatitis B is a condition that affects the liver. Poliomyelitis is a highly contagious disease that can cause paralysis.

J. C. is most likely reacting to the acellular pertussis adsorbed component of Pediarix based on her presenting symptoms of fever above 105° F within 48 hours of Pediarix administration, inconsolable crying for longer than 3 hours within 48 hours of Pediarix administration, and seizure (with or without fever) within 3 days of Pediarix administration.

P: Because J. C. has had a reaction to the pertussis component, she may no longer be a candidate for immunization with Pediarix. Subsequent pertussis vaccinations must be withheld. Her 4-month and 6-month immunizations will have to be individual injections of diphtheria and tetanus toxoid, hepatitis B vaccine, and inactivated poliovirus vaccine.

REFERENCES

1. Biologics. In: U.S. Pharmacopeia, 26th ed. Rockville, MD: U.S. Pharmacopeial Convention, 2003: 2247.
2. Grabenstein JD, Kendal AP, Snyder RH. Storing, handling, and shipping immunologic drugs. Hosp Pharm 1996;31:936–948.
3. CDC. Prevention and Control of Influenza. Recommendations of the ACIP (ACIP). http://www.cdc.gov/ncidod/diseases/flu/fluvirus.htm.
4. Wilde JA, McMillan JA, Serwint J, et al. Effectiveness of influenza vaccine in health care professionals: A randomized trial. JAMA 1999;281:908–913.
5. Bridges CB, Thompson WW, Meltzer MI, et al. Effectiveness and cost-benefit of influenza vaccination in healthy working adults: a randomized controlled trial. JAMA 2000;284:1655–1663.
6. Demicheli V, Jefferson T, Rivett D, et al. Prevention and early treatment of influenza in healthy adults. Vaccine 2000;18:957–1030.
7. Belshe RB, Mendelman PM, Treanor J, et al. The efficacy of live attenuated, cold-adapted, trivalent, intranasal influenzavirus vaccine in children. N Engl J Med 1998;338(20):1405–1412.
8. Clements DA, Langdon L, Bland C, Walter E. Influenza A vaccine decreases the incidence of otitis media in 6- to 30-month old children in day care. Arch Pediatr Adolesc Med 1995;149:1113–1117.
9. Grabenstein JD. Clinical management of hypersensitivities to vaccine components. Hosp Pharm 1997;32(1):77–84.
10. Pichichero ME et al. Mercury concentrations and metabolism in infants receiving vaccines containing thimerosal: a descriptive study. Lancet 2000;360:1737–1741.
11. Madsen et al. A population-based study of measles, mumps, and rubella vaccination and autism. N Engl J Med 2002;347:1477–1482.
12. CDC. General Recommendations on Immunization. MMWR 2002;51(RR-2):25–26.
13. Poland GA et al. Standards for adult immunization practices. Am J Prev Med 2003;25(2):144–150.
14. National Vaccine Advisory Committee. Standards for child and adolescent immunization practices. Pediatrics 2003;112(4):958–963.
15. Healthy health indicators. A critical link to healthy people 2010. Priorities for action. http://www.healthypeople.gov.
16. CDC. Quick Guide. MMWR 2004;53(1):Q1–Q4.
17. Thompson RF. Travel and routine immunizations. Milwaukee: Shoreland. 24–26.
18. Barnett ED. Influenza immunization for children. N Engl J Med 1998;338(20):1459–1461 (editorial).
19. CDC. Morbidity and Mortality Weekly Report. Withdrawal of rotavirus vaccine recommendation. November 5, 1999;48(43):1007.
20. Grabenstein JD. ImmunoFacts: Vaccines and immunologic drugs: Facts and comparisons, revision 26. St. Louis, MO: Woltors Kluwer Co., 2002.
21. CDC. Notice to readers: National adult immunization awareness week. September 26–October 2, 2004. http://www.cdc.gov/search.do?action+search&query-National.
22. CDC. Notice to readers: Recommended adult immunization schedule—United States, 2003–2004. MMWR 2003;52(40):965–969.
23. Steere AC, Sikand VK, Meurice F, et al. Lyme disease vaccine study group. Vaccination against lyme disease with recombinant *Borrelia burgdorferi* outer-surface lipoprotein A with adjuvant. N Engl J Med 1998;339:209–215.
24. ASHP technical assistance bulletin on the pharmacist's role in immunizations. Am J Hosp Pharm 1993; 50:501–505.
25. Rosenbluth SA, Madhavan SS, Borker RD, et al. Pharmacy immunization partnerships: a rural model. JAPhA 2001;41(1):100–107.
26. Hoeben BJ, Dennis MS, Bachman RL, et al. Role of the pharmacist in childhood immunizations. JAPhA 1997;37(5):557–562.
27. Davis M, Freed GL, Zimmerman JL. Childhood vaccine purchase costs in the public sector: past trends, future expectations. Am J Publ Health 2002;92(12):1982.
28. Frey SE et al. Clinical responses to undiluted and diluted smallpox vaccine. N Eng J Med 2002;346:1265–1274.
29. FDA skin test panel report. FDA Drug Bulletin 1978; 8(#2):15–16.

Special Solutions and Suspensions

17

Chapter at a glance

Pharmaceutical dosage forms and drug delivery systems applied topically to the eye, nose, or ear can include solutions, suspensions, gels, ointments, and drug-impregnated inserts. This chapter builds on the general considerations of solutions and suspensions presented in Chapters 13 and 14 by describing additional requirements of these dosage forms when designed specifically for ophthalmic, nasal, or otic use.

Ophthalmic Drug Delivery

Pharmaceutical preparations are applied topically to the eye to treat surface or intraocular conditions, including bacterial, fungal, and viral infections of the eye or eyelids; allergic or infectious conjunctivitis or inflammation; elevated intraocular pressure and glaucoma; and dry eye due to inadequate production of fluids bathing the eye. In treating certain ophthalmic conditions, such as glaucoma, both systemic drug use and topical treatments may be employed.

The normal volume of tear fluid in the cul-de-sac of the human eye is about 7 to 8 μL (1–3). An eye that does not blink can accommodate a maximum of about 30 μL of fluid, but when blinked can retain only about 10 μL (2). Because the capacity of the eye to retain liquid and semisolid preparations is limited, topical applications are administered in small amounts, liquids dropwise and ointments as a thin ribbon applied to the margin of the eyelid. Larger volumes of liquid preparations may be used to flush or bathe the eye.

Excessive liquids, both normally produced and externally delivered, rapidly drain from the eye. A single drop of an ophthalmic solution or suspension measures about 50 µL (based on 20 drops/mL), so much of an administered drop may be lost. The optimal volume to administer, based on eye capacity, is 5 to 10 µL (1). Since microliter-dosing eye droppers are not generally available for personal use, loss of instilled medication using standard eye droppers is a common occurrence.

Because of the dynamics of the lacrimal system, the retention time of an ophthalmic solution on the eye surface is short, and the amount of drug absorbed is usually only a small fraction of the quantity administered. For example, following administration of pilocarpine ophthalmic solution, the solution is flushed from the precorneal area within 1 to 2 minutes, resulting in the ocular absorption of less than 1% of the administered dose (4, 5). This necessitates repeated administration of the solution. Decreased frequency of dosing, increased ocular retention time, and greater bioavailability are achieved by formulations that extend corneal contact time, such as gel systems, liposomes, polymeric drug carriers and ophthalmic suspensions and ointments (6, 7).

Pharmacologic Categories of Ophthalmic Drugs

The major categories of drugs applied topically to the eye:

Anesthetics: Topical anesthetics, such as tetracaine, cocaine, and proparacaine, are employed to provide pain relief preoperatively, postoperatively, for ophthalmic trauma, and during ophthalmic examination.

Antibiotic and antimicrobial agents: Used systemically and locally to combat ophthalmic infection. Among the agents used topically are gentamicin, sulfacetamide, tetracycline, ciprofloxacin, ofloxacin, chloramphenicol, polymyxin B-bacitracin, and tobramycin.

Antifungal agents: Among the agents used topically against fungal endophthalmitis and fungal keratitis are amphotericin B, natamycin, and flucytosine.

Anti-inflammatory agents: Used to treat inflammation of the eye, as allergic conjunctivitis. Among the topical anti-inflammatory steroidal agents are fluorometholone, prednisolone, and dexamethasone salts. Nonsteroidal anti-inflammatory agents include diclofenac, flurbiprofen, ketorolac, and suprofen.

Antiviral agents: Used against viral infections, as that caused by herpes simplex virus. Among the antiviral agents used topically are trifluridine, idoxuridine, and vidarabine.

Astringents: Used in the treatment of conjunctivitis. Zinc sulfate is a commonly used astringent in ophthalmic solutions.

Beta-adrenergic blocking agents: Agents such as betaxolol hydrochloride and timolol maleate are used topically in the treatment of intraocular pressure and chronic open-angle glaucoma.

Miotics and other glaucoma agents: Miotics are used in the treatment of glaucoma, accommodative esotropia, convergent strabismus, and for local treatment of myasthenia gravis. Among the miotics are pilocarpine, echothiophate iodide, and demecarium bromide. Several other types of agents are used in the treatment of glaucoma, including carbonic anhydrase inhibitors, such as acetazolamide (oral); beta-blockers, such as timolol; and an ester prodrug analogue of prostaglandin F2a (latanoprost).

Mydriatics and cycloplegics: Mydriatics allow examination of the fundus by dilating the pupil. Mydriatics having a long duration of action are termed *cycloplegics*. Among the mydriatics and cycloplegics are atropine, scopolamine, homatropine, cyclopentolate, phenylephrine, hydroxyamphetamine, and tropicamide.

Protectants and artificial tears: Solutions employed as artificial tears or as contact lens fluids to lubricate the eye contain agents such as carboxymethyl cellulose, methylcellulose, hydroxypropyl methylcellulose, and polyvinyl alcohol.

Vasoconstrictors and ocular decongestants: Vasoconstrictors applied topically to the mucous membranes of the eye cause transient constriction of the conjunctival blood vessels. They are intended to soothe, refresh, and remove redness due to minor eye irritation. Among the vasoconstrictors used topically are naphazoline, oxymetazoline, and tetrahydrozoline hydrochlorides. Antihistamines, such as pheniramine maleate, are included in some products to provide relief of itching due to pollen, ragweed, and animal dander.

Pharmaceutical Requirements

The preparation of solutions and suspensions for ophthalmic use requires special consideration with regard to sterility, preservation, isotonicity, buffering, viscosity, ocular bioavailability, and packaging.

Sterility and Preservation

Ophthalmic solutions and suspensions must be sterilized for safe use. Although it is preferable to sterilize ophthalmics in their final containers by autoclaving at 121°C (250°F) for 15 minutes, this method sometimes is precluded by thermal instability of the formulation. As an alternative, bacterial filters may be used. Although bacterial filters work with a high degree of efficiency, they are not as reliable as the autoclave. However, since final product testing is used to validate the absence of microbes, sterility may be ensured by either method. One advantage of filtration is the retention of *all* particulate matter (microbial, dust, fiber), the removal of which has substantial importance in the manufacture and use of ophthalmic solutions. Figures 17.1 and 17.2 show bacterial filtration equipment that may be used in the

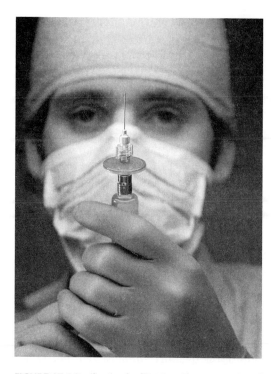

FIGURE 17.1 Sterilization by filtration. The preparation of a sterile solution by passage through a syringe affixed with a microbial filter. (Courtesy of Millipore Corporation.)

extemporaneous preparation of ophthalmic solutions.

To maintain sterility during use, antimicrobial preservatives generally are included in ophthalmic formulations; an exception is for preparations to be used during surgery or in the treatment of traumatized eyes, because some preservatives irritate the eye. These preservative-free preparations are packaged in single-use containers.

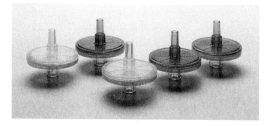

FIGURE 17.2 Examples of sterilizing filters. (Courtesy of Millipore Corporation.)

During preformulation studies, antimicrobial preservatives must demonstrate stability, chemical and physical compatibility with other formulation and packaging components, and effectiveness at the concentration employed. Among the antimicrobial preservatives used in ophthalmic solutions and suspensions and their effective concentrations are benzalkonium chloride, 0.004 to 0.01%; benzethonium chloride, 0.01%; chlorobutanol, 0.5%; phenylmercuric acetate, 0.004%; phenylmercuric nitrite, 0.004%; and, thimerosal, 0.005 to 0.01%. Certain preservatives have limitations; for example, chlorobutanol cannot be autoclaved because it decomposes to hydrochloric acid even in moderate heat. This degradation not only renders a product susceptible to microbial growth but could alter its pH and thereby affect the stability and/or physiologic activity of the therapeutic ingredient.

In concentrations tolerated by the eye, all of the aforementioned preservative agents are *ineffective* against some strains of *Pseudomonas aeruginosa*, which can invade an abraded cornea and cause ulceration and even blindness. However, preservative mixtures of benzalkonium chloride (0.01%) and either polymyxin B sulfate (1000 USP Units/mL) or disodium ethylenediaminetetraacetate (0.01 to 0.1%) *are* effective against most strains of *Pseudomonas*. The latter agent, which is commonly employed as a chelating agent for metals, renders strains of *P. aeruginosa* more sensitive to benzalkonium chloride.

Isotonicity Value

If a solution is placed behind a membrane that is permeable only to solvent molecules and not to solute molecules (a *semipermeable membrane*), *osmosis* occurs as the molecules of solvent traverse the membrane. If a solution-filled membrane is placed in a solution of a higher solute concentration than its own, the solvent, which has free passage in either direction, passes into the more concentrated solution until equilibrium is established on both sides of the membrane and an equal concentration of solute exists on the two sides. The pressure responsible for this movement is termed *osmotic pressure*.

The concentration of a solution with respect to osmotic pressure is concerned with the number of particles of solute in solution. That is, if the solute is not an electrolyte (as with sucrose), the concentration of the solution will depend solely on the number of molecules present. However, if the solute is an electrolyte (as with sodium chloride), the number of particles that it contributes to the solution will depend not only on the concentration of the molecules present but also on their degree of ionization. A chemical that is highly ionized will contribute a greater number of particles to the solution than will the same amount of a poorly ionized substance. The effect is that a solution with a greater number of particles, whether they be molecules or ions, has higher osmotic pressure than does a solution having fewer particles.

Body fluids, including blood and tears, have an osmotic pressure corresponding to that of a 0.9% solution of sodium chloride. Thus, a 0.9% sodium chloride solution is said to be *isosmotic*, or having an osmotic pressure equal to that of physiologic fluids. The term *isotonic*, meaning equal tone, is commonly used interchangeably with isosmotic, although it is correctly used only with reference to a specific body fluid, whereas *isosmotic* is a physicochemical term comparing the osmotic pressure of two liquids that may or may not be physiologic fluids. Solutions with a lower osmotic pressure than body fluids or a 0.9% sodium chloride solution are commonly called *hypotonic*, whereas solutions having a greater osmotic pressure are termed *hypertonic*.

Theoretically, a hypertonic solution added to the body's system will have a tendency to draw water from the body tissues toward the solution in an effort to dilute and establish a concentration equilibrium. In the blood stream, a hypertonic injection can cause *crenation* (shrinking) of blood cells; in the eye, the solution can draw water toward the site of the topical application. Conversely, a hypotonic solution may induce hemolysis of red blood cells or passage of water from the site of an ophthalmic application through the tissues of the eye.

In practice, the isotonicity limits of an ophthalmic solution in terms of sodium chloride or its osmotic equivalent may range from 0.6 to 2.0% without marked discomfort to the eye. Sodium chloride itself does not have to be used to establish a solution's osmotic pressure. Boric acid in a concentration of 1.9% produces the same osmotic pressure as does 0.9% sodium chloride. All of an ophthalmic solution's solutes, including the active and inactive ingredients, contribute to the osmotic pressure of a solution.

The calculations necessary to prepare isosmotic solutions may be made in terms of data relating to the colligative properties of solutions (8). Like osmotic pressure, the other colligative properties of solutions, namely, vapor pressure, boiling point, and freezing point, depend on the number of particles in solution. These properties, therefore, are related, and a change in any one of them will be accompanied by corresponding changes in the others. Although any one of these properties may be used to determine isosmoticity, a comparison of freezing points between the solutions in question is most used.

When 1 g molecular weight of a nonelectrolyte, such as boric acid, is dissolved in 1000 g of water, the freezing point of the solution is about 1.86°C below the freezing point of pure water. By simple proportion, therefore, the weight may be calculated for any nonelectrolyte to be dissolved in each 1000 g of water to prepare a solution isosmotic with lachrymal fluid and blood serum, which have freezing points of −0.52°C.

Boric acid, for example, has a molecular weight of 61.8, so 61.8 g in 1000 g of water should produce a freezing point of −1.86°C. Therefore:

$$\frac{1.86\ (°C)}{0.52\ (°C)} = \frac{61.8\ (g)}{x\ (g)}$$

$$x = 17.3\ g$$

Hence, 17.3 g of boric acid in 1000 g of water theoretically should produce a solution isosmotic with tears and blood.

The calculation employed to prepare a solution isosmotic with tears or blood when using electrolytes is different from the calculation for a nonelectrolyte. Since osmotic pressure de-

pends on the number of particles, substances that dissociate have an effect that increases with the degree of dissociation; the greater the dissociation, the smaller the quantity required to produce a given osmotic pressure. If we assume that sodium chloride in weak solutions is about 80% dissociated, each 100 molecules yield 180 particles, or 1.8 times as many particles as are yielded by 100 molecules of a nonelectrolyte. This dissociation factor, commonly symbolized by the letter i, must be included in the proportion when we seek to determine the strength of an isosmotic solution of sodium chloride (molecular weight, 58.5):

$$\frac{1.86\ (°C) \times 1.8}{0.52\ (°C)} = \frac{58.5\ (g)}{x\ (g)}$$

$$x = 9.09\ g$$

Therefore, 9.09 g of sodium chloride in 1000 g of water should make a solution isosmotic with blood or lacrimal fluid. As indicated previously, a 0.9% (w/v) sodium chloride solution is taken to be isosmotic (and isotonic) with the body fluids.

Simple isosmotic solutions, then, may be calculated by this general formula:

$$\frac{0.52 \times \text{molecular weight}}{1.86 \times \text{dissociation } (i)} = \frac{\text{g of solute per}}{1000\ \text{g of water}}$$

Although the i value has not been determined for every medicinal agent that might be named, the following values may be generally used:

Nonelectrolytes and substances of slight dissociation	1.0
Substances that dissociate into 2 ions	1.8
Substances that dissociate into 3 ions	2.6
Substances that dissociate into 4 ions	3.4
Substances that dissociate into 5 ions	4.2

Since 0.9% sodium chloride is considered to be isosmotic and isotonic with tears, other medicinal substances are compared with regard to their "sodium chloride equivalency." An often-used rule states (8):

Quantities of two substances that are tonicity equivalents are proportional to the molecular weights of each multiplied by the i value of the other.

Using the drug atropine sulfate as an example:

Molecular weight of sodium chloride = 58.5;
$$i = 1.8$$

Molecular weight of atropine sulfate = 695;
$$i = 2.6$$

$$\frac{695 \times 1.8}{58.5 \times 2.6} = \frac{1\ (g)}{x\ (g)}$$

x = 0.12 g of sodium chloride
represented by 1 g of atropine sulfate

Thus, the *sodium chloride equivalent* for atropine sulfate is 0.12 g. To put it one way, 1.0 g of atropine sulfate equals the tonic effect of 0.12 g of sodium chloride. To put it another way, atropine sulfate is 12% as effective as an equal weight of sodium chloride in contributing to tonicity. When a combination of drugs is used in a prescription or formulation to be rendered isotonic, each agent's contribution to tonicity must be taken into consideration. For instance, consider the following prescription:

Atropine sulfate	1%
Sodium chloride	q.s. to isotonicity
Sterile purified water, ad	30.0 mL

To make the 30 mL isotonic with sodium chloride, 30 mL × 0.9% = 0.27 g or 270 mg of sodium chloride would be required. However, since 300 mg of atropine sulfate is to be present, its contribution to tonicity must be taken into consideration. Since the sodium chloride equivalent of atropine sulfate is 0.12, its contribution is calculated as follows:

$$0.12 \times 300\ mg = 36\ mg$$

Thus, 270 mg − 36 mg = 234 mg of sodium chloride required.

Table 17.1 presents a short list of sodium chloride equivalents. A more complete list may be found in pharmaceutical calculations or physical pharmacy textbooks.

As a convenience, some earlier pharmacy reference books list amounts of some common ophthalmic drugs that may be used to prepare isotonic solutions. Some of the drugs and the related values are presented in Table 17.2. The data are used in the following manner. Of each of the drugs listed, 1 g added to purified water will prepare the corresponding volume of an isotonic

TABLE 17.1 SOME SODIUM CHLORIDE EQUIVALENTS

SUBSTANCE	MOLECULAR WEIGHT	IONS	i	SODIUM CHLORIDE EQUIVALENT
Atropine sulfate·H_2O	695.0	3	2.6	0.12
Benzalkonium chloride	360.0	2	1.8	0.16
Benzyl alcohol	108.0	1	1.0	0.30
Boric acid	61.8	1	1.0	0.52
Chlorobutanol	177.0	1	1.0	0.18
Cocaine hydrochloride	340.0	2	1.8	0.17
Ephedrine sulfate	429.0	3	2.6	0.20
Epinephrine bitartrate	333.0	2	1.8	0.18
Ethylmorphine hydrochloride·$2H_2O$	386.0	2	1.8	0.15
Naphazoline hydrochloride	247.0	2	1.8	0.27
Physostigmine salicylate	413.0	2	1.8	0.14
Pilocarpine hydrochloride	245.0	2	1.8	0.24
Procaine hydrochloride	273.0	2	1.8	0.21
Scopolamine hydrobromide·$3H_2O$	438.0	2	1.8	0.13
Tetracycline hydrochloride	481.0	2	1.8	0.12
Zinc sulfate·$7H_2O$	288.0	2	1.4	0.16

TABLE 17.2 ISOTONIC SOLUTIONS PREPARED FROM COMMON OPHTHALMIC DRUGS

DRUG (1.0 G)	VOLUME OF ISOTONIC SOLUTION (ML)
Atropine sulfate	14.3
Boric acid	55.7
Chlorobutanol (hydrous)	26.7
Cocaine hydrochloride	17.7
Colistimethate sodium	16.7
Dibucaine hydrochloride	14.3
Ephedrine sulfate	25.7
Epinephrine bitartrate	20.0
Eucatropine hydrochloride	20.0
Fluorescein sodium	34.3
Homatropine hydrobromide	19.0
Neomycin sulfate	12.3
Penicillin G potassium	20.0
Phenylephrine hydrochloride	35.7
Physostigmine salicylate	17.7
Physostigmine sulfate	14.3
Pilocarpine hydrochloride	26.7
Pilocarpine nitrate	25.7
Polymyxin B sulfate	10.0
Procaine hydrochloride	23.3
Proparacaine hydrochloride	16.7
Scopolamine hydrobromide	13.3
Silver nitrate	36.7
Sodium bicarbonate	72.3
Sodium biphosphate	44.3
Sodium borate	46.7
Sodium phosphate (dibasic, heptahydrate)	32.3
Streptomycin sulfate	7.7
Sulfacetamide sodium	25.7
Sulfadiazine sodium	26.7
Tetracaine hydrochloride	20.0
Tetracycline hydrochloride	15.7
Zinc sulfate	16.7

Adapted from USP XXI, p. 1339.

solution. For instance, 1 g of atropine sulfate will prepare 14.3 mL of isotonic solution. This solution may be diluted with an isotonic vehicle to maintain the isotonicity while changing the strength of the active constituent in the solution to any desired level. For instance, if a 1% isotonic solution of atropine sulfate is desired, 14.3 mL of isotonic solution containing 1 g of atropine sulfate should be diluted to 100 mL (1 g atropine sulfate in 100 mL = 1% w/v solution) with an isotonic vehicle. By using sterile drug, sterile purified water, a sterile isotonic vehicle, and aseptic techniques, a sterile product may be prepared. In addition to being sterile and isotonic, the diluting vehicles generally used are buffered and contain suitable preservative to maintain the stability and sterility of the product.

Buffering

The pH of an ophthalmic preparation may be adjusted and buffered for one or more of the following purposes (9): (*a*) for greater comfort to the eye, (*b*) to render the formulation more stable, (*c*) to enhance the aqueous solubility of the drug, (*d*) to enhance the drug's bioavailability (i.e., by favoring unionized molecular species), and (*e*) to maximize preservative efficacy.

The pH of normal tears is considered to be about 7.4, but it varies; for example, it is more acidic in contact lens wearers (9). Tears have some buffer capacity. The introduction of a medicated solution into the eye stimulates the flow of tears, which attempts to neutralize any excess hydrogen or hydroxyl ions introduced with the solution. Most drugs used ophthalmically are weakly acidic and have only weak buffer capacity. Normally the buffering action of the tears neutralizes the ophthalmic solution and thereby prevents marked discomfort. The eye apparently can tolerate a greater deviation from physiologic pH toward alkalinity (and less discomfort) than toward the acidic range (9). For maximum comfort, an ophthalmic solution should have the same pH as the tears. However, this is not pharmaceutically possible, since at pH 7.4 many drugs are insoluble in water. A few drugs—notably pilocarpine hydrochloride and epinephrine bitartrate—are quite acid and overtax the buffer capacity of the tears.

Most drugs, including many used in ophthalmic solutions, are most active therapeutically at pH levels that favor the undissociated molecule (Physical Pharmacy Capsule 17.1). However, the pH that permits greatest activity may also be the pH at which the drug is least stable. For this reason, a compromise pH is generally selected for a solution and maintained by buffers to permit the greatest activity while maintaining stability.

An isotonic phosphate vehicle prepared at the desired pH (Table 17.3) and adjusted for tonicity may be employed in the extemporaneous compounding of solutions. The desired solution is prepared with two stock solutions, one containing 8 g of monobasic sodium phosphate (NaH_2PO_4) per liter, and the other containing 9.47 g of dibasic sodium phosphate (Na_2HPO_4) per liter, the weights being on an anhydrous basis.

The vehicles listed in Table 17.3 are satisfactory for many ophthalmic drugs, excepting pilocarpine, eucatropine, scopolamine, and homatropine salts, which show instability in the vehicle. The vehicle is used effectively as the diluent for ophthalmic drugs already in isotonic solution, such as those prepared according to the method presented in Table 17.2. When drug substances are added directly to the isotonic phosphate vehicle, the solution becomes slightly hypertonic. Generally, this provides no discomfort to the patient. However, if such a solution is not desired, the appropriate adjustment can be made through calculated dilution of the vehicle with purified water.

Viscosity and Thickening Agents

Viscosity is a property of liquids related to the resistance to flow. The reciprocal of viscosity is *fluidity*. Viscosity is defined in terms of the force required to move one plane surface past another under specified conditions when the space between is filled by the liquid in question. More simply, it can be considered as a relative property, with water as the reference material and all viscosities expressed in terms of the viscosity of pure water at 20°C (68°F). The viscosity of water is given as 1 centipoise (actually 1.0087 cp). A liquid material 10 times as

viscous as water at the same temperature has a viscosity of 10 cp. The centipoise is a more convenient term than the basic unit, the poise; one poise is equal to 100 cp.

Specifying the temperature is important because viscosity changes with temperature; generally, the viscosity of a liquid decreases with increasing temperature. The determination of viscosity in terms of poise or centipoise results in the calculation of *absolute* viscosity. It is sometimes more convenient to use the kinematic scale, in which the units of viscosity are *stokes* and *centistokes* (1 stoke equals 100 centistokes). The kinematic viscosity is obtained from the absolute viscosity by dividing the latter by the density of the liquid at the same temperature:

$$\text{kinematic viscosity} = \frac{\text{absolute viscosity}}{\text{density}}$$

Using water as the standard, these are examples of some viscosities at 20°C:

Ethyl alcohol	1.19 cp
Olive oil	100.00 cp
Glycerin	400.00 cp
Castor oil	1000.00 cp

Viscosity can be determined by any method that will measure the resistance to shear offered by the liquid. For ordinary Newtonian liquids, it is customary to determine the time required for a given sample of the liquid to flow at a regulated temperature through a small vertical capillary tube and to compare this time with that required to perform the same task by the reference liquid. Many capillary tube viscosimeters have been devised, and nearly all are modifications of the Ostwald type. With an apparatus such as this, the viscosity of a liquid may be determined by the following equation:

$$\frac{\eta_1}{\eta_2} = \frac{\rho_1 t_1}{\rho_2 t_2}$$

where

η_1 is the unknown viscosity of the liquid
η_2 is the viscosity of the standard
ρ_1 and ρ_2 are the respective densities of the liquids, and
t_1 and t_2 are the respective flow times in seconds.

pH and Solubility

pH is one of the most important factors in formulation. The effects of pH on solubility and stability are critically important. The effect of pH on solubility is critical in the formulation of liquid dosage forms, from oral and topical solutions to intravenous solutions and admixtures.

The solubility of a weak acid or base is often pH dependent. The total quantity of a monoprotic weak acid (HA) in solution at a specific pH is the sum of the concentrations of both the free acid and salt (A^-) forms. If excess drug is present, the quantity of free acid in solution is maximized and constant because of its saturation solubility. As the pH of the solution is increased, the quantity of drug in solution increases because the water-soluble ionizable salt is formed. The expression is

$$HA \xleftrightarrow{K_a} H^+ + A^-$$

where K_a is the dissociation constant.

At a certain pH level the total solubility (S_T) of the drug solution is saturated with respect to both the salt and acid forms of the drug, that is, the pH_{max}. The solution can be saturated with respect to the salt at pH values higher than this, but not with respect to the acid. Also, at pH values less than this, the solution can be saturated with respect to the acid but not to the salt. This is illustrated in the accompanying figure.

To calculate the total quantity of drug that can be maintained in solution at a selected pH, either of two equations can be used, depending upon whether the product is to be above or below the pH_{max} (figure). The following equation is used when below the pH_{max}:

$$S_T = S_a \left(1 + \frac{K_a}{[H^+]} \right) \quad \textit{(Equation 1)}$$

The next equation is used above the pH_{max}:

$$S_T = S'_a \left(\frac{1 + [H^+]}{K_a} \right) \quad \textit{(Equation 2)}$$

where
  S_a is the saturation solubility of the free acid, and
  S'_a is the saturation solubility of the salt form.

EXAMPLE

A pharmacist prepares a 3.0% solution of an antibiotic as an ophthalmic solution and dispenses it to a patient. A few days later the patient returns the eyedrops to the pharmacist because the product contains a precipitate. The pharmacist, checking the pH of the solution and finding it to be 6.0, reasons that the problem may be pH related. The physicochemical information of interest on the antibiotic includes the following:

Molecular weight	285 (salt) 263 (free acid)
3.0% solution of the drug	0.1053 molar solution
Acid form solubility (S_a)	3.1 mg/mL (0.0118 molar)
K_a	5.86×10^{-6}

Using Equation 1, the pharmacist calculates the quantity of the antibiotic in solution at pH 6.0 (pH $6.0 = [H^+] 1 \times 10^{-6}$)

$$S_T = 0.0118 \left(\frac{1 + 5.86 \times 10^{-6)}}{1 \times 10^{-6}} \right) = 0.0809 \text{ molar}$$

From this the pharmacist knows that at pH 6.0 a 0.0809-molar solution can be prepared. However, the concentration that was to be prepared was 0.1053 molar; consequently, the drug is not in solution at that pH. The pH may have been all right initially but shifted lower over time, resulting in precipitation of the drug. At what pH (hydrogen ion concentration) will the drug remain in solution? This can be calculated using the same equation and the available information . The S_T value is 0.1053 molar.

$$0.1053 = 0.0118 \left(\frac{1 + 5.86 \times 10^{-6}}{[H^+]} \right)$$

$$[H^+] = 7.333 \times 10^{-7}, \text{ or a pH of 6.135}$$

The pharmacist prepares a solution of the antibiotic, adjusting the pH above about 6.2 using a suitable buffer system and dispenses the solution to the patient—with positive results.

An interesting phenomenon concerns the close relationship of pH to solubility. At pH 6.0, only a 0.0809-molar solution could be prepared, but at pH 6.13 a 0.1053-molar solution could be prepared. In other words, a difference of 0.13 pH units resulted in the following:

$$\frac{0.1053 - 0.0809}{0.0809} = 30.1\% \text{ more drug in solution at the higher pH}$$

In other words, a very small change in pH resulted in about 30% more drug going into solution. According to the figure, the slope of the curve would be very steep for this example drug, and a small change in pH (x-axis) results in a large change in solubility (y-axis). From this, it can be reasoned that if one observes the pH–solubility profile of a drug, it is possible to predict the magnitude of the pH change on its solubility.

In recent years, more and more physicochemical information on drugs is being made available to pharmacists in routinely used reference books. This type of information is important for pharmacists in many types of practice, especially those who do compounding and pharmacokinetic monitoring.

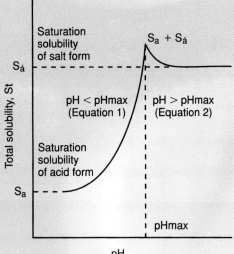

TABLE 17.3 ISOTONIC PHOSPHATE VEHICLE

MONOBASIC SODIUM PHOSPHATE SOLUTION, ML	DIBASIC SODIUM PHOSPHATE SOLUTION, ML	RESULTING BUFFER SOLUTION, PH	SODIUM CHLORIDE REQUIRED FOR ISOTONICITY, G/100 ML
90	10	5.9	0.52
80	20	6.2	0.51
70	30	6.5	0.50
60	40	6.6	0.49
50	50	6.8	0.48
40	60	7.0	0.46
30	70	7.2	0.45
20	80	7.4	0.44
10	90	7.7	0.43
5	95	8.0	0.42

In the preparation of ophthalmic solutions, a suitable grade of methylcellulose or other thickening agent is frequently added to increase the viscosity and thereby aid in maintaining the drug in contact with the tissues to enhance therapeutic effectiveness. Generally, methylcellulose of 4000-cp is used in concentrations of 0.25% and the 25-cp type at 1% concentration. Hydroxypropyl methylcellulose and polyvinyl alcohol are also used as thickeners in ophthalmic solutions. Occasionally a 1% solution of methylcellulose without medication is used as a tear replacement. Viscosity for ophthalmic solutions is considered optimal in the range of 15 to 25 cp.

Ocular Bioavailability

Ocular bioavailability is an important factor in the effectiveness of an applied medication. Physiologic factors that can affect a drug's ocular bioavailability include protein binding, drug metabolism, and lacrimal drainage. Protein-bound drugs are incapable of penetrating the corneal epithelium because of the size of the protein–drug complex (1). Because of the brief time an ophthalmic solution may remain in the eye, the protein binding of a drug substance can quickly negate its therapeutic value by rendering it unavailable for absorption. Normally, tears contain 0.6 to 2.0% of protein, including albumin and globulins, but disease states (e.g., uveitis) can raise these protein lev-

els (1). Although ocular protein binding is reversible, tear turnover results in the loss of both bound and unbound drug (2).

As in the case with other biologic fluids, tears contain enzymes (e.g., lysozyme) capable of metabolic degradation of drug substances. However, only a limited amount of research has been conducted on the ocular metabolism of pharmacologic agents, so the full extent to which drug metabolism occurs and affects therapeutic effectiveness is undetermined (10).

In addition to physiologic factors affecting ocular bioavailability, other factors, such as the physicochemical characteristics of the drug substance and product formulation, are important. Because the cornea is a membrane barrier containing both lipophilic and hydrophilic layers, it is permeated most effectively by drug substances having both lipophilic and hydrophilic characteristics (1).

As discussed previously, ophthalmic suspensions, gels, and ointments mix with lacrimal fluids less readily than do low-viscosity solutions and so remain longer in the cul-de-sac, enhancing drug activity.

Additional Considerations

Ophthalmic solutions must be sparkling clear and free of all particulate matter for comfort and safety. The formulation of an ophthalmic suspension may be undertaken when it is desired to prepare a product with extended corneal contact time, or it may be necessary when the medicinal agent is insoluble or unstable in an aqueous vehicle.

Drug particles in an ophthalmic suspension must be finely subdivided, usually micronized, to minimize eye irritation and/or scratching of the cornea. The suspended particles must not associate into larger particles upon storage and must be easily and uniformly redistributed by gentle shaking of the container prior to use.

Packaging Ophthalmic Solutions and Suspensions

Although a few commercial ophthalmic solutions and suspensions are packaged in small glass bottles with separate glass or plastic droppers, most are packaged in soft plastic containers with a fixed built-in dropper (Figs. 17.3 and 17.4). This type of packaging is preferred both to facilitate administration and to protect the product from external contamination. Ophthalmic solutions and suspensions are commonly packaged in containers holding 2, 2.5, 5, 10, 15, and 30 mL of product.

Patients must be careful to protect an ophthalmic solution or suspension from external contamination. Obviously, the fixed-dropper containers are less likely to acquire airborne contaminants than screw-type bottles, which are fully opened when in use. However, each type is subject to contamination during use by airborne contaminants and by the inadvertent touching of the tip of the dropper to the eye, eyelids, or other surface.

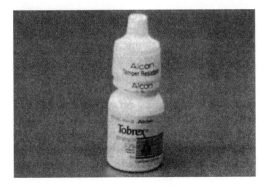

FIGURE 17.3 Commercial ophthalmic solution in a plastic container with built-in dropper device. (Courtesy of Alcon.)

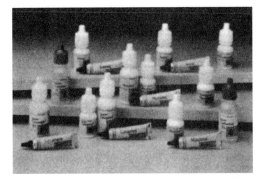

FIGURE 17.4 Ophthalmic product packaging. Liquids are in 5-mL and 15-mL Drop-Tainer dispensers, and ointments are in tubes containing 3.5 g of product. (Courtesy of Alcon.)

Ophthalmic solutions used as eyewashes are generally packaged with an eye cup, which should be cleaned and dried thoroughly before and after each use.

Proper Administration of Ophthalmic Solutions and Suspensions

Prior to the administration of an ophthalmic solution or suspension, the patient or caregiver should be advised to wash the hands thoroughly. If the ophthalmic drops are supplied with a separate dropper, the person should inspect the dropper to make sure it has no chips or cracks. Ophthalmic solutions should be inspected for color and clarity. Out of date or darkened solutions should be discarded. Ophthalmic suspensions should be shaken thoroughly prior to administration to distribute the suspensoid evenly.

The cap of an eyedrop container should be removed immediately prior to use and returned immediately after use. The combined dropper with container as shown in Figure 17.3 is used by holding it between the thumb and middle finger with the index finger on the bottom of the container. One or more drops are delivered by gently squeezing the container. A product packaged with a separate dropper is used by holding the dropper between the thumb and forefinger then drawing up and discharging the medication drop-wise in the usual and familiar manner.

To instill eye drops, the person should tilt the head back and with the index finger of the free hand gently pull downward the lower eyelid of the affected eye to form a pocket or cup. While looking up, and without touching the dropper to the eye, the prescribed number of drops should be instilled into the formed pocket. The lower eyelid should be released and the eye closed to allow the medication to spread over the eye. The eye should be held closed, preferably for a full minute, without blinking, rubbing, or wiping. While the eye is closed, gentle pressure should be applied just under the inner corner of the eye by the nose to compress the nasolacrimal duct to prevent drainage and enhance corneal contact time. Then, any excess liquid may be wiped away with a tissue.

During handling and administration, care must be taken not to touch the dropper to the eye, eyelid, or any other surface. If a separate dropper is used, it should be returned to the container and capped tightly. The dropper should not be rinsed or wiped off. If a combined dropper and container unit is used, the container cap should be returned and tightly closed.

In every case, the patient should be advised about the correct number of drops to instill, the frequency of application, the duration of treatment, proper storage of the medication, and usual side effects specific to the product. Among the side effects encountered with the use of ophthalmic medication are transient stinging or burning, foreign body sensation, itching, tearing, decreased vision, margin crusting, and occasionally a bad (drug) taste.

Examples of some commercially available ophthalmic solutions and suspensions are presented in Table 17.4.

Contact Lenses and Care and Use Solutions

The number of persons wearing contact lenses grows each year. Their popularity and increased use has fostered the development of new types of lenses and lens care products. To counsel patients properly, it is important for pharmacists to know the characteristics and features of the types of contact lenses and the products available for their care and use (11–14).

The three basic types of contact lenses are classified by their chemical composition and physical properties as hard, soft, and rigid gas permeable.

Hard contact lenses provide durability and clear, crisp vision. The lenses are termed *hard* because they are made of a rigid plastic resin, polymethylmethacrylate (PMMA). The lenses are 7 to 10 mm in diameter and are designed to cover only part of the cornea. They float on the tear layer overlying the cornea. Hard lenses require an adaption period sometimes as long as a week for comfort (15). Even then, because of their rigidity, some patients find them difficult to wear. PMMA lenses are practically impermeable to oxygen and moisture (they absorb only about 0.5% water), a disadvantage to corneal epithelial respiration and to comfort. Care must be exercised to prevent the hard lens from resting directly on the corneal surface and causing physical damage to epithelial tissue. To prevent direct contact, solutions are used to wet the lens and provide a cushioning layer between the corneal epithelium and the inner surface of the lens.

Soft contact lenses are more popular than hard lenses because of their greater comfort. They range from about 13 to 15 mm in diameter and cover the entire cornea. Because of their size and coverage, soft lenses are less likely than hard lenses to dislodge spontaneously. They also are less likely to permit irritating foreign particles (e.g., dust or pollen) to lodge beneath them. However for some patients, soft lenses do not provide the same high level of visual acuity as hard lenses. They are less durable than hard lenses and carry some risk of absorbing medication concomitantly applied to the eye.

Soft contact lenses are made of a hydrophilic transparent plastic, hydroxyethyl methacrylate (HEMA), with small amounts of cross-linking agents that provide a hydrogel network (3). Soft lenses contain 30 to 80% water, which enables enhanced permeability to oxygen. There are two general types of soft contact lens: daily wear and extended wear. Whereas daily wear

TABLE 17.4 SOME OPHTHALMIC AGENTS BY CATEGORY

AGENT	COMMERCIAL PRODUCT	ACTIVE INGREDIENT (%)	COMMENTS
Naphazoline HCl	Naphcon-A Ophthalmic Solution (Alcon)	0.025	Topical ocular vasoconstrictor.
Antiallergic			
Cromolyn sodium	Opticrom Ophthalmic Solution (Fisons)	4	For allergic ocular disorders, e.g., vernal conjunctivitis.
Antibacterial			
Ciprofloxacin hydrochloride	Ciloxan Sterile Ophthalmic Solution (Alcon)	0.35	For superficial eye infections due to susceptible microorganisms.
Gentamicin sulfate	Garamycin Ophthalmic Solution (Schering)	0.3	
Tobramycin	Tobrex Ophthalmic Solution (Alcon)]	0.3	
Sulfacetamide sodium	Sodium Sulamyd Ophthalmic Solution (Schering)	10, 30	
Antiviral			
Trifluridine	Viroptic Ophthalmic Solution (Monarch)	1	For herpes simplex keratitis.
Artificial tears			
Dextran 70, Hydroxypropyl Methylcellulose	Tears Naturale II (Alcon)		For relief of dry eyes.
Astringent			
Zinc sulfate	Zincfrin Ophthalmic Solution (Alcon)	0.25	Relief of discomfort, congestion of minor irritations to eyes, such as dust, fatigue, allergies.
Anti-inflammatory			
Dexamethasone sodium phosphate		0.1	Combats inflammation of mechanical, chemical, immunologic causes.
Antibacterial–anti-inflammatory combinations			
Tobramycin and Dexamethasone	TobraDex Sterile Ophthalmic Suspension (Alcon)	0.3 tobramycin, 0.1 dexamethasone	
Beta-adrenergic blocking agents			
Betaxolol HCl	Betoptic Sterile Ophthalmic Solution (Alcon)	0.5	For ocular hypertension, chronic open-angle glaucoma.
Timolol Maleate	Timoptic Sterile Ophthalmic Solution (Merck, Sharpe & Dohme)	0.25, 0.5	For chronic open-angle glaucoma, aphakic patients with glaucoma.
Cholinergic			
Pilocarpine HCl	Isopto Carpine Ophthalmic Solution (Alcon)	0.25–10	Miotic for glaucoma, esp. open-angle; neutralizes mydriasis following ophthalmoscopy or surgery.

(continued)

TABLE 17.4 SOME OPHTHALMIC AGENTS BY CATEGORY

AGENT	COMMERCIAL PRODUCT	ACTIVE INGREDIENT (%)	COMMENTS
Cholinesterase Inhibitor			
Demecarium bromide	Humorsol Sterile Ophthalmic Solution (Merck & Co.)	0.125, 0.25	Intense miosis, ciliary muscle contractions by inhibiting cholinesterase. Used in open-angle glaucoma when shorter-acting miotics inadequate.

lenses must be removed at bedtime, extended wear lenses are designed to be worn for more than 24 hours, with some approved for up to 30 days of continuous wear. However, it is advisable that lenses not be left in the eye for longer than 4 to 7 days without removal for cleaning and disinfection, else the wearer can be predisposed to eye infection.

Disposable soft lenses do not require cleaning and disinfection for the recommended period of use; they are simply discarded and replaced with a new pair. Patients should be advised to resist any temptation to wear the lenses for longer than recommended to avoid risk of eye infection. *Rigid gas permeable (RGP)* contact lenses take advantage of features of both soft and hard lenses. They are oxygen permeable but hydrophobic. Thus, they permit greater movement of oxygen through the lens than hard lenses while retaining the characteristic durability and ease of handling. RGP lenses are more comfortable than hard lenses. The basic type of lens is intended for daily wear; some of the newer super-permeable RGP lenses are suitable for extended wear.

There are advantages and disadvantages associated with each type of contact lens. Hard contact lenses and RGP lenses provide strength, durability, and relatively easy care regimens. They are easy to insert and remove and are relatively resistant to absorption of medications, lens care products, and environmental contaminants. These lenses provide visual acuity superior to that provided by soft contact lenses. On the other hand, hard contact lenses and RGP lenses require a greater adjustment period for the wearer and are more easily dis-

lodged from the eye. Soft contact lenses have a shorter adaption period and may be worn comfortably for longer periods. They do not dislodge as easily or fall out of the eye as readily as the hard lenses. However, they have a shorter life span than hard or RGP lenses, and the wearer must ensure that the lenses do not dry out.

Color Additives to Contact Lenses

Contact lens manufacturers produce clear and colored lenses. The use of color additives in medical devices, including contact lenses, is regulated by the U.S. Food and Drug Administration (FDA) through authority granted by the Medical Device Amendments of 1976. Color additives that come into direct contact with the body for a significant period must be demonstrated to be safe for consumer use. This includes the color additives used in contact lenses. The FDA permits the use of a specific color additive in contact lenses only after reviewing and approving a manufacturer's official *Color Additive Petition*. The petition must contain the requisite chemical, safety, manufacturing, packaging, and product labeling information for FDA review. Many colored contact lenses are prepared as a reaction product, formed by chemically bonding a dye, such as Color Index (CI) Reactive Red 180 (Ciba Vision) to the vinyl alcohol–methyl methacrylate copolymeric lens material.

Care of Contact Lenses

It is important that contact lenses receive appropriate care to retain their shape and optical characteristics and for safe use. Wearers should be instructed in the techniques for insertion and removal of the lenses in methods of cleaning, disinfecting, and storage.

With the exception of disposable soft contact lenses, all soft lenses require a routine care program that includes (*a*) cleaning to loosen and remove lipid and protein deposits, (*b*) rinsing to remove the cleaning solution and material loosened by cleaning, and (*c*) disinfection to kill microorganisms. If the lenses are not maintained at proper intervals, they are prone to deposit buildup, discoloration, and microbial contamination. The moist, porous surface of the hydrophilic lens provides an attractive medium for the growth of bacteria, fungi, and viruses. Thus, disinfection is essential to prevent eye infections and microbial damage to the lens material.

Hard contact lenses require a routine care program that includes (*a*) cleaning to remove debris and deposits from the lens, (*b*) soaking the lens in a storage disinfecting solution while not in use, and (*c*) wetting the lenses to decrease their hydrophobic characteristics.

To achieve the care needs of contact lenses the following types of solutions are used: (*a*) cleaning solutions, (*b*) soaking solutions, (*c*) wetting solutions, and (*d*) mixed-purpose solutions.

Products for Soft Contact Lenses

Cleaners

Because of their porous composition, soft lenses tend to accumulate proteinaceous material that forms a film on the lens, decreasing clarity and serving as a potential medium for microbial growth. The two main categories of cleaners are *surfactants*, which emulsify accumulated oils, lipids, and inorganic compounds, and *enzymatic cleaners*, which break down and remove protein deposits. Surfactant agents are used in a mechanical washing device, by placing several drops of the solution on the lens surface and gently rubbing the lens with the thumb and forefinger, or by placing the lens in the palm of the hand and rubbing gently with a fingertip (about a 20- to 30-second procedure). The ingredients in these cleaners usu-

ally include a nonionic detergent, wetting agent, chelating agent, buffers, and preservatives. Enzymatic cleaning is accomplished by soaking the lenses in a solution prepared from enzyme tablets. This procedure is recommended at least once a week or twice a month in conjunction with regular surfactant cleansing. The enzyme tablets contain either papain, pancreatin, or subtilisin, which causes hydrolysis of protein to peptides and amino acids. Typically these are added to saline solution, but one solution can be prepared using 3% hydrogen peroxide, which combines enzymatic cleaning with disinfection. After the lenses have been soaked for the recommended time they should be thoroughly rinsed.

Rinsing and Storage Solutions

Saline solutions for soft lenses should have a neutral pH and be isotonic with human tears, that is, 0.9% sodium chloride. Besides rinsing the lenses, these solutions are used for storage, because saline maintains their curvature, diameter, and optical characteristics. The solutions also facilitate lens hydration, preventing the lens from drying out and becoming brittle.

Because they are used for storage, some saline solutions contain preservatives, which while inhibiting bacterial growth can induce sensitivity reactions or eye irritation. Thus some manufacturers make available preservative-free saline solutions and package them in aerosol containers or unit-of-use vials. The use of salt tablets to prepare a normal saline solution is discouraged because of the potential for contamination and risk of serious eye infections.

Disinfection and Neutralization

Disinfection can be accomplished by either of two methods, thermal (heat) or chemical (no heat). In the past both methods were equally used; however, with the introduction of hydrogen peroxide systems for chemical disinfection, chemical disinfection has become more popular.

For thermal disinfection, the lenses are placed in a specially designed heating unit with saline solution. The solution is heated sufficiently to kill microorganisms, perhaps for 10 minutes at a minimum of 80°C (176°F). It is important that after disinfection the lenses be stored in the unopened case until ready to be worn. The wearer must also ensure that the lenses have been thoroughly cleaned before using heat disinfection. Otherwise heating can hasten lens deterioration.

In years past chemical disinfection was conducted with products that contained thimerosal in combination with either chlorhexidine or a quaternary ammonium compound. Unfortunately, many wearers had sensitivity reactions, and these products and chemical disinfection fell into disfavor. The introduction of hydrogen peroxide systems for chemical disinfection revitalized this method of disinfection. It is thought that the free radicals chemically released from the peroxide react with the cell wall of the microorganisms, and the bubbling action of the peroxide is thought to promote removal of any remaining debris on the lens.

To prevent eye irritation from residual peroxide after disinfection, it is necessary that the lenses be exposed to one of three types of neutralizing agents: the *catalytic type* (an enzyme catalase or a platinum disk), the *reactive type* (such as sodium pyruvate or sodium thiosulfate), or the *dilution–elution* type.

Chemical disinfection systems may come as two-solution systems, which use separate disinfecting and rinsing solutions, or one-solution systems, which use the same solution for rinsing and storage. It is important that the wearer realize that lenses must not be disinfected by heating when using these solutions.

Products for Hard Contact Lenses

Cleaners

Hard lenses should be cleaned immediately after removal from the eye. Otherwise, oil deposits, proteins, salts, cosmetics, tobacco smoke, and airborne contaminants can build up, interfere with clear vision, and possibly cause irritation upon reinsertion. A surfactant cleaner is used by applying the solution or gel to both surfaces of the lens and then rubbing the lens in the palm of the hand with the index finger for about 20 seconds. Too-vigorous rubbing can scratch or warp the lens.

Soaking and Storage Solutions

Hard lenses are placed in a soaking solution once they are removed from the eye. Soaking solutions contain a sufficient concentration of disinfecting agent, usually 0.01% benzalkonium chloride and 0.01% edetate sodium, to kill surface bacteria. Overnight soaking is advantageous because it keeps the lenses wet and the prolonged contact time helps to loosen deposits that remain after routine cleaning.

Wetting Solutions

Wetting solutions contain surfactants to facilitate hydration of the hydrophobic lens surface and enable the tears to spread evenly across the lens by providing it with temporary hydrophilic qualities. These solutions also provide a cushion between the lens and the cornea and eyelid. Typical ingredients include a viscosity-increasing agent, such as hydroxyethyl cellulose; a wetting agent, such as polyvinyl alcohol; preservatives, such as benzalkonium chloride or edetate disodium; and buffering agents and salts to adjust the pH and maintain tonicity.

Combination Solutions

Combination solutions mix effects, such as cleaning and soaking, wetting and soaking, or cleaning, soaking, and wetting. While they are characterized by ease of use, combination products may lower the effectiveness of cleaning if the concentration of cleaning solution is too low to adequately remove debris from the lens. These combination solutions should be reserved for wearers who have a demonstrated need for simplification of lens care.

Products for RGP Contact Lenses

Care of RGP lenses requires the same general regimen as for hard contact lenses except that RGP-specific solutions must be used. One of two cleaning methods, either hand washing or mechanical washing, may be used. In the first method, the lens may be cleaned by holding the concave side up in the palm of the hand. The lens should not be held between the fingers because the flexibility of the lens may allow it to warp or turn inside out. Mechanical washing is advantageous because the possibility of the lens turning inside out or warping during cleaning is minimized.

After cleansing, the RGP lens should be thoroughly rinsed and soaked in a wetting or soaking solution overnight. After overnight soaking, the lens is rubbed with fresh wetting or soaking solution and inserted into the eye. To facilitate removal of stubborn protein deposits, weekly cleaning with enzymatic cleaners is recommended.

Clinical Considerations in the Use of Contact Lenses

Although most medicated eyedrops may be used in conjunction with the wearing of contact lenses, some caution should be exercised and drug-specific information used, particularly with soft contact lenses, because this type of lens can absorb certain topical drugs and affect bioavailability (12, 14).

Use of ophthalmic suspensions and ophthalmic ointments by contact lens wearers presents some difficulties. The drug particles in ophthalmic suspensions can build up between the cornea and the contact lens, causing discomfort and other undesired effects. Ophthalmic ointments not only cloud vision but may discolor the lens. Thus, an alternative dosage form, such as an ophthalmic solution, may be prescribed or lens wearing deferred until therapy is complete.

Some drugs administered by various routes of administration for systemic effects can find their way to the tears and produce drug–contact lens interactions. This may result in lens discoloration (e.g., orange staining by rifampin), lens clouding (ribavirin), ocular inflammation (salicylates), and refractive changes (acetazolamide) (12). In addition, drugs that cause ocular side effects have the potential to interfere with contact lens use. For example, drugs with anticholinergic effects (e.g., antihistamines, tricyclic antidepressants) decrease tear secretion and may cause lens intolerance and damage to the eye. Isotretinoin, prescribed for severe, recalcitrant acne, can induce marked dryness of the eye and may interfere with the use of contact

lenses during therapy. Drugs that promote excessive lacrimation (e.g., reserpine) or ocular or eyelid edema (e.g., primidone, hydrochlorothiazide, chlorthalidone) also may interfere with lens wear.

Use of ophthalmic vasoconstrictors occasionally causes dilation of the pupil, especially in people who wear contact lenses or whose cornea is abraded. Although this effect lasts only 1 to 4 hours and is not clinically significant, some patients have expressed concern. To allay their concern, the FDA has recommended that patients be advised of this side effect by product labeling stating PUPILS MAY BECOME DILATED (ENLARGED) (15).

The following guidelines should be used by pharmacists in counseling patients: Contact lens wearers should wash their hands thoroughly with a nonabrasive, noncosmetic soap before and after handling lenses. Wearers should not rub the eyes when the lenses are in place, and if irritation develops, the lenses should be removed until these symptoms subside.

Only contact lens care products specifically recommended for the type of lens worn should be used. Also, to avoid differences between products of different manufacturers, it is preferable to use solutions made by a single manufacturer. Cleaning and storing lenses should be performed in the specific solution for that purpose. Lenses should not be stored in tap water, nor should saliva be used to help reinsert a lens into the eye. Saliva is not sterile and contains numerous microorganisms, including *P. aeruginosa*.

As appropriate, contact lens users should be counseled with regard to cosmetic use. It is prudent to purchase makeup in the smallest container, since the longer a container is open and the more its contents are used, the greater the likelihood of bacterial contamination. Mascara and pearlized eye shadow should be avoided by women wearing hard lenses because particles of these products can get into the eye and cause irritation, with corneal damage a possibility. Aerosol hairsprays should be used before the lens is inserted and preferably applied in another room, since airborne particles may attach to the lens during insertion and cause irritation. Lenses should be inserted before makeup application because oily substances on the fingertips can smudge the lenses when they are handled. For similar reasons, lenses should be removed before makeup.

Wearers of contact lenses normally do not have ocular pain. If pain is present, it may be a sign of ill-fitting lenses, corneal abrasion, or other medical condition, and the patient should be advised to consult his or her ophthalmologist (14). Hard or soft contact lenses may occasionally cause superficial corneal changes, which may be painless and not evident to the patient. Thus it is important that all contact lens wearers have their eyes examined regularly to make certain that no damage has occurred.

Nasal Preparations

Most preparations intended for intranasal use contain adrenergic agents and are employed for their decongestant activity on the nasal mucosa. Most of these preparations are in solution form and are administered as nose drops or sprays; however, a few are available as jellies. Examples of products for intranasal use are shown in Figure 17.5 and in Table 17.5.

Nasal Decongestant Solutions

Most nasal decongestant solutions are aqueous, rendered isotonic to nasal fluids (approximately equivalent to 0.9% sodium chloride), buffered to maintain drug stability while approximating the normal pH range of the nasal fluids (pH 5.5 to 6.5), and stabilized and preserved as required. The antimicrobial preservatives are the same as those used in ophthalmic solutions. The concentration of adrenergic

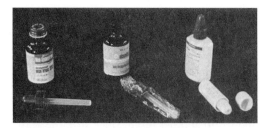

FIGURE 17.5 Commercial packages of nasal solutions, showing drop and spray containers and a nasal inhaler.

agent in most nasal decongestant solutions is quite low, ranging from about 0.05 to 1.0%. Certain commercial solutions are available in adult and pediatric strengths, the pediatric strength being approximately half of the adult strength.

Nasal decongestant solutions are employed in the treatment of rhinitis of the common cold, for vasomotor and allergic rhinitis including hay fever, and for sinusitis. Frequent or prolonged use may lead to chronic edema of the nasal mucosa, that is, rhinitis medicamentosa, aggravating the symptom that they are intended to relieve. Thus, they are best used for short periods (no longer than 3 to 5 days), and the patient should be advised not to exceed the recommended dosage and frequency of use.

The easiest but least comfortable approach to treat rebound congestion is complete withdrawal of the topical vasoconstrictor. Unfortunately, this approach will promptly result in bilateral vasodilation with almost total nasal obstruction. A more acceptable method is to withdraw application of drug in only one nostril, with the patient continuing to use the medication in the other nostril. Once the rebound congestion subsides in the drug-free nostril, after about 1 to 2 weeks, a total withdrawal is instituted. Another approach is substitution of a topical saline solution or spray for the topical vasoconstrictor. This keeps the nasal mucosa moist and provides psychologic assistance to patients who are dependent on placing medication into their nostrils.

Most of the adrenergic drugs used in nasal decongestant solutions are synthetic compounds similar in chemical structure, pharmacologic activity, and side effects to the parent compound, naturally occurring epinephrine. Epinephrine as a pure chemical substance was first isolated from suprarenal gland in 1901 and was called both suprarenin and adrenalin. Synthetic epinephrine was prepared just a few years later.

Most solutions for nasal use are packaged in dropper bottles or in plastic spray bottles, usually containing 15 to 30 mL of medication. The products should be determined to be stable in the container and the package tightly closed while not in use. The patient should be advised

TABLE 17.5 SOME COMMERCIAL NASAL PREPARATIONS

PRODUCT	MANUFACTURER	ACTIVE INGREDIENT	USE/INDICATIONS
Afrin Nasal Spray, Afrin Nose Drops	Schering-Plough	Oxymetazole HCl 0.05%	Adrenergic, decongestant
Beconase AQ Nasal Spray	GlaxoSmithKline	Beclomethasone dipropionate 0.042%	Synthetic corticosteroid for relief of seasonal, perennial allergic, vasomotor rhinitis
Diapid Nasal Spray	Sandoz	Lopressin 0.185 mg/mL	Antidiuretic; control, prevention of diabetes insipidus of deficiency of endogenous posterior pituitary antidiuretic hormone.
Nasalcrom Nasal Spray	Pharmacia & Upjohn	Cromolyn sodium 4%	Prevention and treatment of symptoms of allergic rhinitis
Nasalide Nasal Solution	Dura	Flunisolide 0.025%	Symptoms of seasonal or perennial rhinitis
Neo-Synephrine Nose Drops, Spray	Sanofi-Winthrop	Phenylephrine HCl 0.125 to 1.0%	Adrenergic, decongestant
Neo-Synephrine Maximum Strength 12 Hour	Sanofi-Winthrop	Oxymetazoline HCl 0.05%	Adrenergic, decongestant
Ocean Mist	Fleming	Sodium chloride 0.65%	Restore moisture, relieve dry, crusted, inflamed nasal membranes.
Privine HCl Nasal Solution	Novartis	Naphazoline HCl 0.05%	Adrenergic, decongestant
Syntocinon Nasal Spray	Sandoz	Oxytocin 40 U/mL	Synthetic oxytocin for initial milk let-down preparatory to breast feeding.
Tyzine Pediatric Nose Drops	Key	Tetrahydrozoline HCl (0.05%)	Adrenergic, decongestant

to discard the solution if it becomes discolored or contains precipitated matter.

The patient should also understand that there is a difference in the duration of the effect of topical decongestants. For example, phenylephrine should be used every 3 to 4 hours, whereas oxymetazoline, which is longer acting, should only be used every 12 hours.

Inhalation Solutions

Inhalations are drugs or solutions of drugs administered by the nasal or oral respiratory route. The drugs may be administered for local action on the bronchial tree or for systemic effects through absorption from the lungs. Certain gases, such as oxygen and ether, are administered by inhalation, as are finely powdered drug substances and solutions of drugs administered as fine mists. Sterile Water for Inhalation, USP, and Sodium Chloride Inhalation, USP, may be used as vehicles for inhalation solutions.

As discussed in Chapter 14, a number of drug substances are administered through pressure packaged inhalation aerosols. For the inhaled drug substance or solution to reach the bronchial tree, the inhaled particles must be just a few microns in size.

A widely used instrument capable of producing fine particles for inhalation therapy is the nebulizer. This apparatus, shown in Figure 17.6, contains an atomizing unit in a bulbous glass chamber. A rubber bulb at the end of the apparatus is depressed and the medicated solution is drawn up a narrow glass tube and

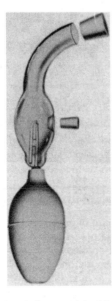

FIGURE 17.6 A nebulizer used in inhalation therapy. (Courtesy of DeVilbiss Co.)

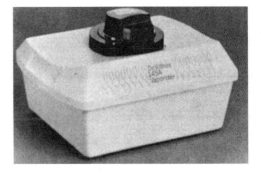

FIGURE 17.7 A commercial vaporizer. (Courtesy of DeVilbiss Co.)

broken into fine particles by the passing airstream. The particles produced range between 0.5 and 5 microns. The larger, heavier droplets of the mist do not exit the apparatus but fall back into the reservoir of medicated liquid. The lighter particles do escape with the airstream and are inhaled by the patient, who operates the nebulizer with the exit orifice in the mouth, inhaling while depressing the rubber bulb.

The pharmacist should advise the patient on the proper technique to use the nebulizer and provide additional instructions, such as not to exceed physician's instructions and to use the smallest amount of product necessary to afford relief. The pharmacist may also advise on how to cope with any dryness of the mouth and should emphasize the need to clean the nebulizer after use and explain how to do it.

The common household vaporizer, like the one depicted in Figure 17.7, produces a fine mist of steam that may be used to humidify a room. When a volatile medication is added to the water in the chamber or to a medication cup, the medication volatilizes and is also inhaled by the patient. Humidifiers, as shown in Figure 17.8, are used to provide a cool mist to the air in a room. Moisture in the air is impor-

tant to prevent mucous membranes of the nose and throat from becoming dry and irritated. Vaporizers and humidifiers are commonly used in the adjunctive treatment of colds, coughs, and chest congestion.

The pharmacist can help a patient select a vaporizer or humidifier according to personal needs. Both devices have advantages and disadvantages. Manufacturing guidelines and legal regulations, such as lock tops, have made vaporizers safer today than in years past, so the possibility of scalding due to an overturned vaporizer is less with newer models. Furthermore, the heat generated in a vaporizer kills any mold and bacteria in the water tank. Humidifiers are more costly but use less electricity than vaporizers. In addition, humidifiers are noisier, can deposit minerals on woodwork and furniture, and can cool down a room by 1° to 3°F (a problem with young children). The

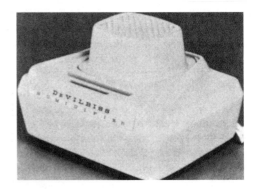

FIGURE 17.8 A commercial humidifier. (Courtesy of DeVilbiss Co.)

patient should learn about these subtle differences from the pharmacist.

Ultrasonic humidifiers are effective and operate at an almost noiseless level, but they apparently pose a health problem. While they are highly efficient at nebulizing water into fine droplets, they are also efficient at nebulizing up to 90% of water contaminants. These contaminants include mold, bacteria, lead, and dissolved organic gases, which could ultimately cause acute respiratory irritation or chronic lung problems in unsuspecting patients. Thus, patients should either be advised to run water through a high-grade demineralization filter before filling their ultrasonic humidifier or buy a humidifier with a built-in filter that works.

Examples of Medicated Inhalation Solutions

A number of inhalations pressure packaged as inhalation aerosols are discussed in Chapter 14. Several other inhalations used in medicine are solutions intended to be administered by nebulizer or other apparatus. Among these are isoetharine inhalation solution (Bronkosol, Sanofi) and isoproterenol inhalation solution (Isuprel Solution, Sanofi), both used to relieve bronchial spasms of bronchial asthma and related conditions.

Inhalants

Inhalants are drugs or combinations of drugs that by virtue of their high vapor pressure can be carried by an air current into the nasal passage, where they exert their effect. The device that holds the drug or drugs and from which they are administered is an inhaler.

Certain nasal decongestants are in the form of inhalants. For instance, propylhexedrine (Benzedrex, Menley & James Labs) is a liquid that volatilizes slowly at room temperature. This quality makes it effective as an inhalant. The inhaler contains cylindrical rolls of fibrous material impregnated with the volatile drug. The medication, which has an amine-like odor, is usually masked with added aromatic agents. The inhaler is placed in the nostril and vapor inhaled to relieve nasal congestion. As with the

other nasal adrenergic agents, excessive or too frequent use can result in nasal edema and increased rather than decreased congestion. The inhalers are effective so long as the volatile drug remains present. To ensure that the drug does not escape during periods of nonuse, the caps on the inhalers should be tightly closed.

Amyl Nitrite Inhalant

Amyl nitrite is a clear yellowish volatile liquid that acts as a vasodilator when inhaled. It is prepared in sealed glass vials that are covered with a protective gauze cloth (Fig. 17.9). Upon use, the glass vial is broken in the fingertips and the cloth soaks up the liquid, from which the vapors are inhaled. The vials generally contain 0.3 mL of the drug substance. The effects of the drug are rapid and are used in the treatment of anginal pain.

Propylhexedrine Inhalant

Propylhexedrine is a liquid adrenergic (vasoconstrictor) agent that volatilizes slowly at room temperature. This quality enables it to be effectively used as an inhalant. The official inhalant consists of cylindrical rolls of suitable fibrous material impregnated with propylhexedrine, usually aromatized to mask its amine-like odor, and contained in a suitable inhaler. The vapor of the drug is inhaled into the nostrils when needed to relieve nasal congestion due to colds and hay fever. It may also be employed to relieve ear block and pressure pain in air travelers.

Each plastic tube of the commercial product contains 250 mg of propylhexedrine with aromatics. The containers should be tightly closed after each opening to prevent loss of the drug vapors. The counterpart commercial product is Benzedrex Inhaler (Menley & James Labs).

Proper Administration and Use of Nasal Drops and Sprays

To minimize the possibility of contamination, the pharmacist should point out to the patient that the nasal product should be used by one person only and kept out of the reach of children. If the nasal product is intended for a child, the directions should be clear to the patient. If

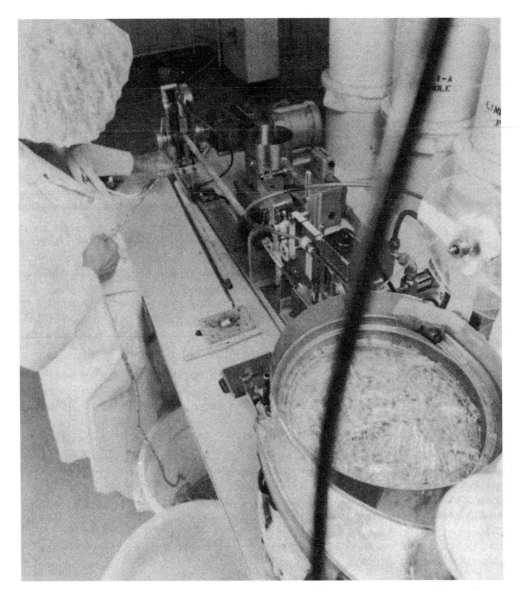

FIGURE 17.9 Silking operation in the production of amyl nitrate Vaporole. (Courtesy of Burroughs Wellcome Company.)

an over-the-counter product is used, the parent should note the directions on the label.

Before using the drops, the patient should be advised to blow the nose gently and wash the hands thoroughly with soap and water. For maximum penetration with drops, a patient should lie down on a flat surface, such as a bed, hanging the head over the edge, and tilting the head back as far as comfortable. The prescribed number of drops are then gently placed in the nostrils, and to allow the medication to spread in the nose, the patient should remain in this position for a few minutes. After this, the dropper should be replaced in the bottle and tightened.

Before using the spray, the patient should gently blow the nose to clear the nostrils and wash the hands thoroughly with soap and water. The patient should be told not to shake the plastic squeeze bottle but be sure to remove the plastic cap. While holding the head upright, the patient should insert the nose piece into the nostril, pointing it slightly backward, and close the other nostril with one finger. The patient should then spray the prescribed or recommended amount, squeezing the bottle sharply and firmly while sniffing. Remove the bottle tip from the nose while maintaining pressure on the bottle sides so as not to aspirate any nasal material into the bottle. Wipe the tip with alcohol or some other appropriate agent, release the pressure on the sides, and repeat the application as necessary. Sprays should always be administered with the patient upright. Spraying medicine into the nostrils should not be performed with the head over the edge of a bed (the preferred procedure for administration of nasal drops) because it could result in systemic absorption of the drug rather than a local effect.

The patient should be advised not to overuse the product. Some decongestant medicines, such as oxymetazoline and xylometazoline, can predispose the patient to rebound congestion if used for more than 3 to 5 consecutive days. The patient should also understand the normal time frame in which to see results and be advised to consult the physician after a certain number of days if relief is not achieved. Finally, patients should not share their medicated spray with another person to prevent the possibility of cross-contamination between individuals. Certain nasal medications, such as beclomethasone dipropionate (Vancenase, Schering), are available for administration through aerosol inhalers.

Nasal Route for Systemic Effects

The nasal route for drug delivery is of interest because of the need to develop a route that is neither oral nor parenteral for newly developed synthetic biologically active peptides and polypeptides (16–21). Polypeptides, such as insulin, that are subject to destruction by the gastrointestinal fluids are administered by injection. However, the nasal mucosa has been shown to be amenable to the systemic absorption of certain peptides, as well as to nonpeptide drug molecules including scopolamine, hydralazine, progesterone, and propranolol (19, 20). The nasal route is advantageous for nonpeptide drugs that are poorly absorbed orally.

The adult nasal cavity has about a 20-mL capacity, with a large surface area (about 180 cm^2) for drug absorption afforded by the microvilli along the pseudostratified columnar epithelial cells of the nasal mucosa (18, 20). The nasal tissue is highly vascularized, providing an attractive site for rapid and efficient systemic absorption. One great advantage to nasal absorption is that it avoids first-pass metabolism by the liver. However, identification of metabolizing enzymes in the nasal mucosa of certain animal species suggests the same possibility in humans and the potential for some intranasal drug metabolism (18).

For some peptides and small molecular compounds, intranasal bioavailability has been comparable to that of injections. However, bioavailability decreases as the molecular weight of a compound increases, and for proteins composed of more than 27 amino acids bioavailability may be low (17). Various pharmaceutic techniques and formulation adjuncts, such as surface-active agents, have been shown to enhance nasal absorption of large molecules (17, 20).

Pharmaceuticals on the market or in various stages of clinical investigation for nasal delivery include lypressin (Diapid, Sandoz), oxytocin (Syntocinon, Sandoz), desmopressin (DDAVP, Rhône-Poulenc Rorer), vitamin B_{12} (Ener-B Gel, Nature's Bounty), progesterone, insulin, calcitonin (Miacalcin, Novartis), propranolol, and butorphanol (Stadol, Mead-Johnson) (16, 17).

Otic Preparations

Otic preparations are sometimes referred to as ear or aural preparations. Solutions are most frequently used in the ear, with suspensions and ointments also finding some application. Ear preparations are usually placed in the ear canal by drops in small amounts for removal of excessive cerumen (earwax) or for treatment of ear infections, inflammation, or pain. Because the outer ear is a skin-covered structure and susceptible to the same dermatologic conditions as other parts of the body's surface, skin conditions are treated using the variety of topical dermatologic preparations discussed in Chapter 10.

Cerumen-Removing Solutions

Cerumen is a combination of the secretions of the sweat and sebaceous glands of the external auditory canal. The secretions, if allowed to dry, form a sticky semisolid that holds shed epithelial cells, fallen hair, dust, and other foreign bodies that make their way into the ear canal. Excessive accumulation of cerumen in the ear may cause itching, pain, and impaired hearing, and it impedes otologic examination. If not removed periodically, the cerumen may become impacted and its removal made more difficult and painful.

Through the years, light mineral oil, vegetable oils, and hydrogen peroxide have been commonly used agents to soften impacted cerumen for its removal. Recently, solutions of synthetic surfactants have been developed for their ability to remove earwax. One of these agents, triethanolamine polypeptide oleate condensate, commercially formulated in propylene glycol, is used to emulsify the cerumen, thereby facilitating its removal (Cerumenex Drops, Purdue Frederick). Another commercial product uses carbamide peroxide in glycerin and propylene glycol (Debrox Drops, SmithKline Beecham). On contact with the cerumen, the carbamide peroxide releases oxygen, which disrupts the integrity of the impacted wax, allowing its easy removal.

Cerumen removal usually involves placing the otic solution in the ear canal with the patient's head tilted at a 45° angle, inserting a cotton plug to retain the medication in the ear for 15 to 30 minutes, followed by gentle flushing of the ear canal with lukewarm water using a soft rubber ear syringe.

Anti-infective, Anti-inflammatory, and Analgesic Ear Preparations

Drugs used topically in the ear for their anti-infective activity include such agents as chloramphenicol, colistin sulfate, neomycin, polymyxin B sulfate, and nystatin, the latter agent used to combat fungal infections. These agents are formulated into eardrops (solutions or suspensions) in a vehicle of anhydrous glycerin or propylene glycol. These viscous vehicles permit maximum contact time between the medication and the tissues of the ear. In addition, their hygroscopicity causes them to draw moisture from the tissues, reducing inflammation and diminishing the moisture available for the life process of the microorganisms. To assist in relieving the pain that frequently accompanies ear infections, a number of anti-infective otic preparations also contain analgesic agents, such as antipyrine, and local anesthetics, such as lidocaine, dibucaine, and benzocaine.

Topical treatment of ear infections is frequently considered adjunctive, with concomitant systemic treatment with orally administered antibiotics.

Liquid ear preparations of the anti-inflammatory agents hydrocortisone and dexamethasone sodium phosphate are prescribed for their effects against the swelling and inflammation that frequently accompany allergic and irritative manifestations of the ear and for the inflammation and pruritus that sometimes follow treatment of ear infections. In the latter instance, some physicians prefer the use of corticosteroids in ointment form, packaged in ophthalmic tubes. These packages allow placement of small amounts of ointment in the ear canal with a minimum of waste. Many commercial products used in this manner are labeled EYE AND EAR to indicate their dual use.

Aside from the antibiotic–steroid combinations that are used to treat otitis externa, or swimmer's ear, acetic acid 2% in aluminum acetate solution and boric acid 2.75% in isopropyl alcohol are used. These drugs help to reacidify the ear canal, and the vehicles help dry the ear canal. Drying the ear canal keeps in check growth of the offending microorganisms, usually *P. aeruginosa*. Pharmacists may also be called on for extemporaneous preparation of a solution of acetic acid 2 to 2.5% in rubbing alcohol (70% isopropyl alcohol or ethanol), propylene glycol, or anhydrous glycerin. The source of the acetic acid can be Glacial Acetic Acid, USP, or Acetic Acid, NF. Boric acid 2 to 5% dissolved in either ethanol or propylene glycol has also been recommended for use in the ear. This substance, however, may be absorbed from broken skin and be toxic. Thus, its use is usually limited, especially in children with burst ear drums.

Pain in the ear frequently accompanies ear infection or inflamed or swollen ear tissue. Frequently the pain is far out of proportion to the actual condition. Because the ear canal is so narrow, even a slight inflammation can cause intense pain and discomfort. Topical analgesic agents generally are employed together with internally administered analgesics, such as aspirin, and other agents, such as anti-infectives, to combat the cause of the problem.

Most topical analgesics for the ear are solutions, and many contain the analgesic antipyrine and the local anesthetic benzocaine in a vehicle of propylene glycol or anhydrous glycerin (Auralgan Otic Solution, Wyeth-Ayerst). Again, these hygroscopic vehicles reduce the swelling of tissues (and thus some pain) and the growth of microorganisms by drawing moisture from the swollen tissues into the vehicle. These preparations are commonly employed to relieve the symptoms of acute otitis media. Examples of some commercial otic preparations are presented in Table 17.6.

As determined on an individual product basis, some liquid otic preparations require preservation against microbial growth. When preservation is required, such agents as chlorobutanol 0.5%, thimerosal 0.01%, and combinations of the parabens are commonly used. Antioxidants, such as sodium bisulfite, and other stabilizers are also included in otic formulations as required. Ear preparations are usually packaged in 5- to-15-mL glass or plastic containers with a dropper.

Otic Suspensions

Subtle differences in the formulation of otic suspensions may be bothersome to the patient. This is so especially as it relates to differences

TABLE 17.6 SOME COMMERCIAL OTIC PREPARATIONS

PRODUCT	MANUFACTURER	ACTIVE INGREDIENT	VEHICLE	USE/INDICATIONS
Americaine Otic	Novartis	Benzocaine	Glycerin, polyethylene glycol 300	Local anesthetic for ear pain, pruritus in otitis media, swimmer's ear, similar conditions
Auralgan Otic Solution	Wyeth-Ayerst	Antipyrine, benzocaine	Dehydrated glycerin	Acute otitis media
Cerumenex Ear Drops	Purdue Frederick	Triethanolamine polypeptide oleate condensate	Propylene glycol	Removes impacted earwax
Chloromycetin Otic	Parke-Davis	Chloramphenicol	Propylene glycol	Anti-infective
Cortisporin Otic Solution	GlaxoSmithKline	Polymyxin B sulfate, neomycin sulfate, hydrocortisone	Glycerin, propylene glycol, water for injection	Superficial bacterial infections
Debrox Drops	Hoechst Marion Roussel	Carbamide peroxide	Anhydrous glycerin	Earwax removal
PediOtic Suspension	GlaxoSmithKline	Polymyxin B sulfate, neomycin sulfate, hydrocortisone	Mineral oil, propylene glycol, water for injection	Superficial bacterial infections
Metreton Ophthalmic, Otic Solution	Schering-Plough	Prednisolone sodium phosphate	Aqueous	Antiinflammatory
Otobiotic Otic Solution	Schering-Plough	Polymyxin B sulfate, hydrocortisone	Propylene glycol, glycerin, water	Superficial bacterial infections
VoSol Otic Solution	Wallace	Acetic acid	Propylene glycol	Antibacterial, antifungal

in inactive or inert ingredients that are considered equivalent on the basis of active ingredients and strength. For example, several suspension combinations of polymyxin B sulfate, neomycin sulfate, and hydrocortisone have been shown to be more acidic at pH 3.0 to 3.5 than the standard product, Cortisporin Otic Suspension (Glaxo Wellcome), whose pH is 4.8 to 5.1. Consequently, there is a risk that when drops are legally substituted, a burning and stinging sensation can occur when the drops are introduced into the ear of young children, especially those with tympanostomies. It has also been demonstrated that with time, the pH of these formulations, including Cortisporin, becomes more acidic, possibly pH 3.0. Thus, if it is stored over time, the acidity may irritate the ear canal on later use. For this reason, this antibiotic–hydrocortisone combination has been formulated into a new suspension product, PediOtic (Glaxo Wellcome), with a minimum pH of 4.1.

Proper Administration and Use of Otic Drops

When eardrops are prescribed, it is important for the pharmacist to determine how the drops are to be used. For example, earwax removal drops should be instilled and then removed with an ear syringe. Drops intended to treat external otitis infection are intended to be instilled and left in the ear.

The pharmacist should make sure the patient or parent understands that administration is intended for the ear and the frequency of application. To facilitate acceptance, the pharmacist should point out that the bottle or container of medication should first be warmed in the hands, and if the product is a suspension, shaken prior to withdrawal into the dropper. The pharmacist should also explain the need to store the medication in a safe place out of the reach of children and away from extremes of temperature.

When instilled into the ear, to allow the drops to run in deeper, the earlobe should be held up and back. For a child, the earlobe should be held down and back. For convenience it is probably easier to have someone other than the patient to administer the drops.

Some eardrops by virtue of their low pH may cause stinging upon administration. Parents and children should be forewarned, especially if a child has tympanostomy tubes in the ear. The patient or parent should also understand how long to use the product. For antibiotic eardrops it is not necessary to finish the entire bottle, because therapy could last 20 to 30 days, depending upon the dosage regimen. Therefore, patients should be instructed to continue using the drops for 3 days after symptoms disappear. Products for otitis externa may take up to 7 to 10 days to demonstrate efficacy.

If a child is prone to develop ear infections as a result of swimming or showering, it might be advisable to recommend the parents to consult a physician for prophylactic medication to use during swimming season and consider using ear plugs that fit snugly in the ear when swimming or showering. After the child emerges from the water or shower, the parents can be advised to use a blow dryer on a low setting to dry the ear quickly without trauma. The dryer should not be held too close to the child's ear.

PHARMACEUTICS CASE STUDY

Subjective

Working as a pharmacist in a local hospital, you receive a prescription for 5 mL of fluorouracil 10 mg/mL ophthalmic solution for topical use in the eye. What is a reasonable technique to compound the preparation so the patient can begin treatment within a couple of hours?

Objective

Fluorouracil is an antineoplastic agent that is used as ancillary treatment of glaucoma,

Pharmaceutics Case Study cont.

pterygium, retinal detachment, and premalignant eye lesions. The 10 mg/mL is often used in the treatment of premalignant lesions of the cornea, conjunctiva, and eyelids.

Fluorouracil occurs as a white to practically white, practically odorless crystalline powder that is sparingly soluble in water and slightly soluble in alcohol. Fluorouracil is commercially available as a solution for injection at a concentration of 50 mg/mL in 10, 20, and 100 mL vials and a 10-mL ampule. The injection has a pH adjusted to approximately 8.6 to 9.4 with sodium hydroxide and hydrochloric acid as needed. It is also available as Fluorouracil Powder, USP, that can be used to compound the preparation.

Assessment

Fluorouracil is water soluble and can be prepared as a sterile, isotonic ophthalmic solution. Two options are available. First,

the commercial injection dosage forms can be diluted with sterile sodium chloride injection to the proper concentration. Second, it can be prepared from the fluorouracil powder in sterile water for injection, adjusted to isotonicity with sodium chloride, and sterile-filtered into a sterile container.

Plan

The physician would like to have this preparation soon, so you select the first option. You obtain a 10-mL vial of fluorouracil 50 mg/mL injection. Using aseptic technique, cytotoxic handling procedures, and an appropriate aseptic clean air environment, you remove 1 mL of the injection, add sufficient sterile 0.9% sodium chloride injection to make 5 mL, and mix well. You package the preparation and add an appropriate label, then dispose of the used materials appropriately for chemotherapy handling and disposal.

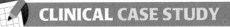

CLINICAL CASE STUDY

HPI: K. P. is a 22 y/o WM who presents to the pharmacy with a prescription for olopatadine hydrochloride (Patanol) for allergic conjunctivitis. K. P. explains to the pharmacist, "My allergies have been so bad this spring that they have been bothering my eyes too. I tried to use Visine, but that just helped with the redness." The patient continues to explain that his eyes are excessively watery, itchy, and burning, and at times he can barely see because the tears make his vision so blurry. He further complains that he has not been able to wear his contacts for almost a week because of his eye problems. K. P. is a college student who just moved to campus and is new to the pharmacy. Before preparing his prescription, the pharmacist takes his medical history.

PMH:	Seasonal allergic rhinitis since high school
	Seasonal allergic conjunctivitis
SH:	(+) EtOH: Drinks 3–4 beers/ night on the weekends
	(−) Tobacco
	(−) Illicit drugs
FH:	Mother (+) for allergic rhinitis
	Father (+) for hypertension
	Sister (+) for asthma
Allergies:	PCN (rash, hives)
Meds:	Loratadine 10 mg po qd
	Visine prn red eyes
	Tylenol 1000 mg po prn headaches
	Centrum 1 tab po qd

Clinical Case Study cont.

Pharmaceutical Care Plan

S: Patient has itching, burning, watery red eyes. Excessive tearing is causing blurred vision.

O: Redness relieved by Visine

A: K. P. is a 22 y/o WM with uncontrolled allergic conjunctivitis. The patient is at high risk for seasonal allergic conjunctivitis because of his history of seasonal allergic rhinitis. K. P. also has a family history significant for allergic rhinitis. Although patient's allergic rhinitis symptoms are controlled by his use of loratadine 10mg po qd, his ocular symptoms persist even though he uses Visine.

P: Based on patient's symptoms and medical and medication histories, olopatadine hydrochloride is an appropriate option for treatment of his allergic conjunctivitis. Thus, after verifying that K. P.'s prescription is complete, the pharmacist dispenses the medication.

The pharmacist should counsel K. P. on his medication. The prescribed dosage is one drop in each affected eye two times daily at an interval of at least 6 to 8 hours (e.g., morning and late afternoon or early evening). To administer the eyedrops, the patient should follow these instructions:

Wash hands thoroughly before using the product.

With the index finger of the free hand, gently pull the lower outer eyelid down and away from the eye to create a pouch.

While tilting the head back, place the dropper over the eye without the tip of the dropper touching the eye.

Just prior to instilling a drop into the eye, look up toward the dropper.

As soon as the drop is instilled into the eye, release the eyelid slowly. Keep the eye closed for a full minute afterward.

While the eye is closed, use a finger to apply gentle pressure over the opening of the tear duct on the innermost (closest to the nose) portion of the eye. This serves to keep the medication in contact with the eye longer.

Excess solution may be gently wiped away with a tissue.

Replace the cap onto the ophthalmic product and keep it tightly closed when not in use.

Advise K. P. against wearing his contact lenses until his eye redness has resolved. Because the preservative in olopatadine hydrochloride may be absorbed by soft contact lenses, K. P. should follow necessary precautions if he decides to resume wearing his contact lenses. K. P. should wait at least 10 minutes after instilling the drops before inserting his contact lenses.

Explain to K. P. the common side effects associated with olopatadine hydrochloride use (e.g., burning or stinging, dry eyes, headache, sinusitis, blurred vision). In addition, K. P. should be instructed to discontinue using Visine while using his prescription.

Remind K. P. to store the eyedrops at room temperature in an upright position with the cap tightly secured. He should follow the expiration date on the bottle. In addition, he should know not to rinse or tamper with the dropper.

REFERENCES

1. Akers HJ. Ocular bioavailability of topically applied ophthalmic drugs. Am Pharm 1983;NS23:33–36.
2. Reddy IK, Ganesan MG. Ocular therapeutics and drug delivery: an overview. In: Reddy IK, ed. Ocular therapeutics and drug delivery. Lancaster, PA: Technomic, 1996;3–29.
3. Reddy IK, Azia W, Sause RB. Artificial tear formulations, irrigating solutions and contact lens products.

In: Reddy IK, ed. Ocular therapeutics and drug delivery. Lancaster, PA: Technomic, 1996;171–211.

4. Lee VHL, Robinson JR. Mechanistic and quantitative evaluation of precorneal pilocarpine distribution in albino rabbits. J Pharm Sci 1979;68:673–684.

5. Shell JW. Pharmacokinetics of topically applied ophthalmic drugs. Surv Ophthalmol 1982;26:207–218.

6. Nadkarni SR, Yalkowski SH. Controlled delivery of pilocarpine 1: in vitro characterization of gelfoam matrices. Pharm Res 1993;10:109–112.

7. Davies NM et al. Evaluation of mucoadhesive polymers in ocular delivery II: polymer-coated vesicles. Pharm Res 1992; 9:1137–1144.

8. Stoklosa MJ, Ansel HC. Pharmaceutical calculations, 10th ed. Baltimore: Williams & Wilkins, 1996.

9. Gangrade NK, Gaddipati NB, Ganesan MG, Reddy IK. Topical ophthalmic formulations: basic considerations. In: Reddy IK, ed. Ocular therapeutics and drug delivery. Lancaster, PA: Technomics, 1996;377–403.

10. Kumar GN. Drug metabolizing enzyme systems in the eye. In: Reddy IK, ed. Ocular therapeutics and drug delivery. Lancaster, PA :Technomics, 1996;149–167.

11. Hind HW, Zuccaro VS. Pharmacist's handbook of contact lenses and contact lens solutions. Sunnyvale, CA: Barnes-Hind, 1986.

12. Engle JP. Assessing and counseling contact lens wearers. Am Pharm 1993;NS33:39–45.

13. Engle JP. Contact lens solutions. Drug Topics 1988;132:56–66.

14. Berkow R, ed. Merck Manual. Rahway, NJ: Merck Sharp & Dohme Research Laboratories, 1987:15:2242–2244.

15. 63 Federal Register 8888–8890 (1998).

16. Nudelman I. Nasal delivery: a revolution in drug administration. Drug Delivery Systems. Eugene, OR: Aster, 1987;43–48.

17. Longenecker JP. New drug delivery systems: intranasal delivery: a novel route for protein therapeutics. Wellcome Trends Pharm 1989;11:7–9.

18. Sarkar MA. Drug metabolism in the nasal mucosa. Pharm Res 1992;9:1.

19. Fu RCC, Whatley JL, Fleitman JS. Intranasal delivery of RS-93522, a dihydropyridine-type calcium-channel antagonist. Pharm Res 1991;8:134–138.

20. Donovan MD, Flynn GL, Amidon GL. The molecular weight of nasal absorption: the effect of absorption enhancers. Pharm Res 1990;8:808–815.

21. Schipper NGM, Verhoef JC, Merkus FWHM. The nasal mucociliary clearance: relevance to nasal drug delivery. Pharm Res 1991;8:812–814.

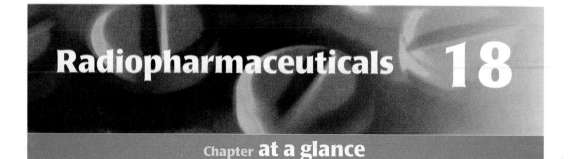

Radiopharmaceuticals 18

Chapter at a glance

By definition, a radiopharmaceutical is a radioactive pharmaceutical agent that is used for diagnostic or therapeutic procedures (1). For a product to be classified as a radiopharmaceutical agent safe for human use, the preparer must satisfy a state agency, the State Board of Pharmacy, and two branches of the federal government whose responsibilities in this category have overlapping jurisdictions. They are the Food and Drug Administration (FDA) and the Nuclear Regulatory Commission (NRC). The extent of oversight by the board of pharmacy differs between states. Because of the stringent regulations of the NRC, some state boards defer and do not have specific rules for nuclear pharmacies. Other state boards have rules within their pharmacy prac-

tice acts that relate to the practice of nuclear pharmacy.

Over the past 3 decades, the discipline of nuclear pharmacy, or radiopharmacy, has become highly specialized and contributed positively to the practice of nuclear medicine. Nuclear pharmacy, the first specialty in pharmacy recognized (in 1978) by the Board of Pharmaceutical Specialties, focuses on the safe and effective use of radioactive drugs or radiopharmaceuticals.

The application of radiopharmaceuticals is divided into two major areas, diagnostic and therapeutic. The diagnostic side is well established, while the therapeutic side of nuclear medicine is evolving. For example, more than 100 radiopharmaceutical products are available, with the largest proportion of these having application in cardiology (e.g., myocardial perfusion), oncology (e.g., tumor imaging and localization), and neurology (e.g., cerebral perfusion). Diagnostically, they are also used for infection imaging and in nephrology. Historically, nuclear medicine has been well established as a therapeutic modality for thyroid cancer, Graves' disease, hyperthyroidism, and bone pain palliation associated with skeletal metastasis. However, recent radiopharmaceuticals (e.g., ^{131}I or ^{125}I labeled MIBG [m-iodobenzylguanidine]) are being used to treat pheochromocytoma and neuroblastoma, and radiolabeled somatostatin analogues are used for the treatment of neuroendocrine tumors (e.g., neuroblastoma) (2). Ongoing investigative studies involving radiopharmaceuticals are being conducted for numerous other diseases (e.g., primary bone cancers, ovarian cancer) using innovative means (e.g., targeting agents) to deliver the drug to the tumor. It is anticipated that many of these radiopharmaceuticals will become available for amelioration of diseases.

A radiopharmaceutical consists of a drug component and a radioactive component. Most radionuclides contain a component that emits *gamma* radiation. Substances that have the same number of protons but have varying numbers of neutrons are called *radionuclides*. Radionuclides may be stable or unstable; those that are unstable are radioactive because their nuclei undergo rearrangement while changing to a stable state, and energy is given off.

An important distinction between radiopharmaceuticals and traditional drugs is lack of pharmacologic activity on the part of radiopharmaceuticals. For intensive purposes, radiopharmaceuticals have been used as tracers of physiologic processes. Their huge advantage is that their radioactivity allows noninvasive external monitoring or targeted therapeutic irradiation with very little effect on the biologic processes in the body. Indeed, radiopharmaceuticals have an excellent safety record, and their incidence of adverse effects is extremely low (3). However, in the past 2 decades, there has been committed interest to developing unsealed radionuclides for treatment of cancers arising from the diversity of newer molecular carriers (e.g., immune-derived molecules, receptor-avid tracers). Technologic advances in molecular pharmacology, combinatorial chemistry, and peptide biochemistry are providing innovative means (e.g., targeting vectors) to enhance radionuclide specificity and targeting cancerous cells in vivo.

Systemic administration of radiopharmaceuticals for site-specific use allows the physician to treat widely disseminated diseases. Optimally, therapeutic radiopharmaceuticals are designed for site specificity even if the actual location of the cancerous tumor is unknown. Ideally, the radiopharmaceutical will cause minimal or tolerable damage to healthy, adjacent tissue. However, a variety of factors related directly to the physical and chemical characteristics of the radiopharmaceutical make this goal difficult to achieve. Research will continue to address problems related to efficient radiopharmaceutical delivery to the target site. For example, the residence time of radioactivity at the target site, the in vivo catabolism and metabolism of the drug, and the optimization of relative rates of radiolabeled drug or drug metabolite clearance from the target site are factors to be determined. Development of an effective radiopharmaceutical for therapeutic use is a complex, difficult undertaking.

Background Information

Not all of the atoms of an unstable radionuclide completely rearrange at the same instant. The time required for a radionuclide to decay to 50% of its original activity is termed its radioactive half-life. Radionuclides range widely in their half-life; for ^{14}C it is 5730 years, whereas for ^{24}Na it is 15 hours, and for ^{81}Kr, 13 seconds.

The activity of radioactive material may be calculated by a decay equation that allows the clinician to predict the activity at any time, earlier or later than the specific assay. The specific decay equation:

$$A_e = A_o\, e^{-\lambda t}$$

where

A_e is the specific activity at time t,
A_o is the initial activity,

λ is the decay constant calculated as $\ln 2$/half-life, and

t is time.

Decay tables have been formulated for various radionuclides by calculating the last portion of the decay equation ($e^{-\lambda t}$). Thus,

$$A_e = A_o \text{ (decay factor)}$$

The activity of a radioactive material is expressed as the number of nuclear transformations per unit of time. Because of decay, all radioactivity decreases with time because fewer atoms remain as the atoms decay. The fraction of nuclei disintegrating with time is always constant, and fewer and fewer atoms are left. The larger the decay constant, the faster the decay, and the shorter the half-life. Thus, as demonstrated by the following, the half-life is inversely proportional to the decay constant:

$$t_{1/2} = \frac{0.69315}{\lambda}$$

where λ is the transformation or decay constant, which has a characteristic value for each radionuclide.

The fundamental unit of radioactivity is the *curie* (Ci), defined as 3.700×10^{10} nuclear transformations per second or disintegrations per second (dps). Multiplying this unit by 60 allows the definition to be expressed as disintegrations per minute (dpm). Multiples and submultiples (e.g., *millicurie* [mCi], *microcurie* [μCi], and *nanocurie* [nCi]) of the curie can be expressed also:

1 millicurie = 10^{-3} curie
1 microcurie = 10^{-6} curie
1 nanocurie = 10^{-9} curie

In July 1974, at the meeting of the International Commission of Radiation Units and Measurements (ICRU), a recommendation was made that within no less than 10 years, the curie would be replaced with a new SI (Système International d'Unites) unit, the reciprocal second (sec^{-1}) (4). The intent was that this new unit be used to express the unit of activity as a function of the rate of spontaneous nuclear transformations of radionuclides, as one per second (dps). It was further recommended that

this new unit of activity be given the name *becquerel*, and bear the symbol *Bq*. The intent was that the becquerel would be equivalent to 1 dps, or approximately 2.703×10^{-11} Ci. For example, a 15 mCi dose of ^{99m}Tc would be referred to as a 555-megabecquerel (MBq) dose. To date, the conversion to SI units in the United States has been slow.

The amount of radiation absorbed by body tissue in which a radioactive substance resides is called the radiation dose. Traditionally, this is measured in rad (*radiation absorbed dose*); 1 rad = 100 ergs of energy absorbed by 1 g of tissue. The Gray (Gy) is the international unit of absorbed dose, equal to 1 joule of energy absorbed in 1 kg of tissue; that is, 1 Gy = 100 rad.

Radiopharmaceutical doses are dispensed to patients in units of activity, typically mCi or μCi. Traditional therapeutic agents are dispensed according to weight-based calculations to determine appropriate activity in millicuries. The pharmacist remains responsible to ensure that the proper prescribed dose is prepared and dispensed. Because of the nature of radiopharmaceuticals, the amount of radioactivity in the unit dose at the time of preparation must be sufficient to allow for decay of radioactivity before the product is administered.

The three main types of radiation decay are alpha particles, beta particles, and gamma photons (or gamma rays). Of the three types alpha particles have the largest mass and charge of radiation, consisting of two protons and two neutrons, identical with the helium nucleus. As an alpha particle loses energy, its velocity decreases. It then attracts electrons and becomes a helium atom. Most alpha particles are unable to pierce the outer layers of skin or penetrate a thin piece of paper. However, because the charge is large, it does cause a great deal of damage to the immediate area by breaking down DNA. Beta particles may be either electrons with negative charge, *negatrons*, or positive electrons, *positrons*. These two particles, β^- and β^+, have a range of more than 100 feet in air and up to about 1 mm in tissue. Beta particles are not as destructive as alpha particles, but they can be used therapeutically. The beta particle possesses a lot of kinetic energy, thousands to millions of electron volts. Nuclear medicine depends mostly on radiopharmaceuticals that decay by gamma emission. Gamma rays are electromagnetic vibrations comparable with light but with much shorter wavelength. Because of their short wavelength and high energy, they are very penetrating.

Auger electrons originate from the orbital electrons rather than from the nucleus. Whenever there is a vacancy in a lower orbital, an electron from a higher orbital falls down into that lower orbital, and the difference in energy between the two orbitals is emitted in the form of a characteristic x-ray. Most of the time, the characteristic x-ray leaves the atom. But sometimes, the characteristic x-ray hits a higher orbital electron of the same atom. Then the transfer of energy from the x-ray to the electron is enough to free it from the atom. This free electron, known as an auger electron, is similar to a beta particle except that it has much less energy, typically only tens to hundreds of electron-volts. In materials with large atomic numbers there are several higher electron orbitals, so several different auger electrons may be produced, each with a different kinetic energy. Thus, the term auger cascade is sometimes used to indicate the production of multiple different auger electrons.

The optimum dose of a radiopharmaceutical is that which allows acquisition of the desired information with the least amount of radiation dose or exposure to the patient. Consequently, the clinical utility of a radiopharmaceutical is determined mainly by the radionuclide's physical properties (e.g., radiation, energy, half-life). Therefore, the best diagnostic images at the lowest radiation dose are attained if the radionuclide has a short half-life and emits only gamma radiation. ^{99m}T is a prime example of a radionuclide with these properties. Its half-life is 6 hours, and gamma emission is in the order of 140 keV, efficiently detected by the gamma camera. For therapeutic use, however, radionuclides should emit particulate radiation (beta particles), which deposits the radiation within the target organ. ^{131}I is a prime example, used for hyperthyroidism and eradication of metastatic disease of the thyroid gland. Because ^{131}I emits both beta and gamma radiation, it can be used diagnostically (gamma rays) and therapeutically (beta particles).

Most radiopharmaceuticals are produced by nuclear activation in a nuclear reactor. In such a reactor, stable atoms are bombarded with excess neutrons in the reactor. The resulting neutron additions to the stable atoms produce unstable atoms and radionuclides. The facilities for the production, use, and storage of radioactive pharmaceuticals are subject to licensing by the NRC or in certain instances to appropriate state agencies. Many states, known as agreement states, have taken over licensing for the NRC. They agree to follow all NRC regulations and in some instances may be more stringent. As for all pharmaceuticals, the FDA enforces strict adherence to good manufacturing practice and proper labeling and use of the products. The Federal Department of Transportation regulates shipment of radiopharmaceuticals, as do state and local agencies.

Radiopharmaceuticals are used to diagnose disease or evaluate the progression of disease following specific therapy intervention. They can also be used to evaluate drug-induced toxicity and to an increasing extent are being used to treat diseased tissue.

The distribution pattern of radiopharmaceuticals can be used for imaging purposes to attain diagnostic information about organs or various body systems (5). Imaging procedures are classified either as *dynamic* or *static*. The dynamic study provides useful information through the rate of accumulation and removal of the radiopharmaceutical from a specific organ. A static study merely provides perfusion and morphologic information, such as assessing adequacy of blood flow; organ size, shape, and position; and any space-occupying lesions.

Diagnostic Imaging

Some radiopharmaceuticals are formulated to be placed within a target organ. ^{131}I is taken up actively by thyroid cells following absorption into the blood stream after oral administration of a capsule or solution. The extent of uptake of the dose by the gland helps assess thyroid function, or an image of the gland can be obtained after administration. Alternatively, when ^{131}I was labeled with orthoiodohippuric acid (^{131}I-orthoiodohippurate, or OIH) and intravenously injected, kidney tubules would actively secrete this agent into urine. Measuring the time course of activity over the kidney with a gamma camera and plotting the rate of radioactivity accumulation and removal versus time yields a measure of kidney function. This dynamic study, termed a *renogram*, is particularly useful to assess renal function in patients with transplanted kidneys. The visualization of the entire kidney anatomically is known as a pyelogram (Fig. 18.1).

There are, however, limitations to the use of ^{131}I-orthoiodohippurate. Because of its beta emissions, the dose must be held to 200 to 400 μCi. The required lower dose with the 364-KeV gamma and beta emissions produces a poorer image than ^{99m}Tc-Mag-3, which has pure gamma emissions of 140 KeV, allowing for a higher dose and enhanced image quality without increasing the total body radiation burden. Mag-3 undergoes both tubular secretion and glomerular filtration in the kidney and provides excellent renograms.

Radiopharmaceuticals are useful to evaluate a patient's response to drug therapy and surgery. These agents can detect early changes in physiologic function that come before morphologic or biochemical end points. An example is perfusion lung imaging using ^{99m}Tc macroaggregated albumin particles to detect pulmonary embolism. Once the embolism is confirmed and thrombolytic and/or anticoagulant therapy initiated, this lung-perfusing agent can be administered again to evaluate its resolution with drug therapy. Cardiac radionuclide ventriculograms using ^{99m}Tc-labeled red blood cells are performed to assess left ventricular function (e.g., ejection fraction, regional wall motion) to evaluate the effect of surgery (e.g., coronary artery bypass graft, valve repair) or the response to drug therapy.

Radiopharmaceuticals also find utility to help monitor drug therapy, including toxicity. For example, the ability of doxorubicin to cause irreversible heart failure is well known, and the cumulative dose of this drug should not exceed 550 mg/m^2. Because there is much variation in the individual response to this drug, serial determinations of left ventricular ejection fraction using ^{99m}Tc are useful to determine the risk of developing doxorubicin-induced heart failure on an individual basis. Also, a ^{99m}Tc ejection fraction study can be performed to assess the benefits of heart medications, such as digoxin.

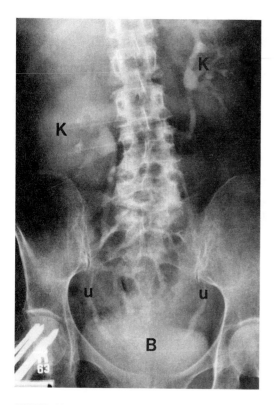

FIGURE 18.1 Intravenous pyelogram in an elderly patient. Note contrast visualization of the kidneys (K), ureters (U), and bladder (B). The patient also has fixation screws in her right hip to stabilize a hip fracture. (Reprinted with permission from Hunter TB, Walsh TK, Hall JN. Agents for diagnostic imaging. In Block JH, Beale JM Jr., eds. Wilson and Gisvold's textbook of organic medicinal and pharmaceutical chemistry, 11th ed. Baltimore: Lippincott Williams & Wilkins, 2004;478.)

Therapeutic Use of Radiopharmaceuticals

Therapeutic radiopharmaceuticals are radiolabeled molecules designed to deliver therapeutic doses of ionizing radiation to specific disease sites, such as cancerous tumors, with high specificity in the body. The design of each radiotherapeutic agent requires optimizing the balance between specific targeting of the disease, such as a cancerous tumor, and the clearance of radioactivity from nontarget radiosensitive tissues; it is also necessary to consider the physical radioactive decay properties of the radionuclide. As mentioned earlier, difficulties in the design and development of a highly selective radiolabeled drug carrier include drug delivery, maximizing the residence time of radioactivity at target sites, in vivo catabolism and metabolism of the drug, and optimization of relative rates of the radiolabeled drug or metabolite clearance from nontarget sites, among others.

Unsealed source radiolabeled agents have been used for treatment of cancers for more than 5 decades. Thyroid disease has been treated with sodium iodide, ^{131}I; polycythemia vera can be treated with sodium phosphate, ^{32}P; peritoneal effusions can be treated with chromic phosphate, ^{32}P; and ^{89}Sr-chloride, ^{153}Sm-EDTMP, and ^{186}Re-HEDP are used for pain relief associated with metastatic bone lesions. The intent is to use beta radiation to destroy diseased tissue selectively. Thus, a minimum sufficient dosage must be administered. In the case of ^{131}I, the therapeutic dose is 5 to 10,000 times the dose used to assess organ function. The major indications for radioiodine therapy include hyperthyroidism (diffuse toxic goiter, or Graves' disease and toxic multinodular goiter) and eradication of metastatic disease (thyroid cancer).

A major focus of current research is to enhance drug targeting to internal target sites (e.g., solid tumors, specific organs). The objective is to enhance the drug by concentrating it at the target site and minimize its effect in (healthy sites. This approach is being investigated for cancer chemotherapy and radioimmunotherapy (RIT). RIT uses antigen-specific monoclonal antibodies (MABs) or their derived reagents to deliver therapeutic radionuclides to tumorous tissue (2). Improved bioengineered delivery vehicles (e.g., humanized and chimeric whole antibodies, Fv fragments, and hypervariable domain region peptides) have reinvigorated RIT, and more and more pretargeting protocols are becoming available (2).

Most chemotherapeutic drugs and radiotherapeutic peptides are small molecules. Consequently, low concentration of drug is obtainable at the target site, largely because of rapid excretion and metabolism by the kidneys and liver. This limits the amount of drug available for localization in the target site from the blood stream. Increasing the dosage of drug is not an option because of the toxicologic implications for one or more body organ systems. Covalent conjugates of MABs were the first generation of drug targeting agents that were employed to attain the concentrating effect in tumors (6).

In 1996, the FDA granted licenses to three manufacturers to market four radiolabeled antibodies for diagnostic imaging. CEA-Scan was a murine MAB fragment linked to ^{99m}Tc. It was reactive with carcinoembryonic antigen, a tumor marker for cancer of the colon and rectum and indicated with other standard diagnostic modalities for the detection of recurrent and/or metastatic colorectal cancer. Cytogen Corporation developed a linker payload system with the attachment of diagnostic (OncoScint Colorectal/Ovarian) or therapeutic substances (cancer cell–killing yttrium in OncoRad Ovarian and OncoRad Prostate systems) on the carbohydrate region of MABs. After injection, the MABs bind to the targeted tumor antigen to facilitate diagnosis or treatment. While tumor targeting was somewhat successful with the large, long circulating radiolabeled MABs, normal organ activity (e.g., blood, kidneys, liver, bone marrow) became problematic.

In the past 2 decades, extensive research for radionuclide therapy has attempted to use ions (molecular weight or MW, 10^2), low-molecular-weight drugs (MW $10^{2–3}$), peptides (MW 10^3), radiolabeled antibody fragments and various proteins (MW 10^4), intact antibodies (MW 10^5), chase molecules, metabolizable linkers, local delivery, antibody-directed enzyme prodrugs, and liposomes for targeting purposes (MW 10^6) (7). The extensive size range demonstrated for a few of these molecules illustrates the several orders of magnitude that these substances cover with respect to molecular weight range (7). Thus, there is much potential for research involving an enormous number of agents with various properties.

One strategy to increase the concentration of a dose-limited, rapidly cleared radionuclide in a tumor was to couple it covalently to a large molecule (e.g., MAB directed against a tumor marker on the surface of the tumor) (8). Because of their large size, these radionuclide conjugates are not rapidly excreted by the kidneys; they are slowly removed from the systemic circulation over several days by the reticuloendothelial system (RES). Still, however, data demonstrate that while the radionuclide has high systemic circulation, very little is localized in the tumor. Thus, getting high tumor uptake with large antibody conjugates has posed a significant challenge. The most popular MAB pretargeting techniques employ either biotin and avidin or the hapten–antibody system and prodrug–enzyme systems or ligand–receptor systems (2). All of these methods employ a long circulating targeting conjugate to get high tumor uptake with a diffusible, rapidly excreted effector molecule. The result is higher ratios of target to normal tissue and consequently less toxicity.

Molecular weight, lipophilicity, and charge of the targeting agents are important properties that influence hepatic and renal excretion. Small water-soluble peptides demonstrate effective excretion, which is beneficial in ridding the body of excess circulating radionuclide labeled compounds. However, if excretion is too rapid, effective levels of the agent reaching the tumor are never achieved.

Creating a targeting agent with a very high molecular weight is thought to reduce the ability of the agent to diffuse through the capillary walls and thereby hinder the ability to target disseminated tumor cells in normally vascularized tissues. Thus, this may only allow tumor targeting in areas of pathologic tumor vasculature of the primary tumor or metastases. The limited passage through the capillary walls may also prolong systemic circulation and cause undesired exposure of normal tissue to radiation. Alternatively, enhanced circulation times may result in higher tumor uptake.

To avoid trapping and degradation of the agents by the RES, therapeutic entities must be designed not to be recognized by the RES (8). Pretherapeutic administration of nonradioac-tive antibodies (preload) can be used to saturate the RES and modify the distribution of the radiolabeled antibody. Pegylation and other preventive modifications have demonstrated some reduction in the RES's ability to uptake macromolecular agents.

In the spring of 2002, the FDA approved a new treatment regimen for low-grade B-cell non-Hodgkin's lymphoma. It was the first regimen that combined a monoclonal antibody with radionuclides. Rituximab is administered in a therapeutic regimen with ibritumomab tiuxetan (Zevalin). This therapy is recommended for patients who have not responded to standard chemotherapeutic treatments or to the prior use of rituximab (Rituxan). Rituximab and ibritumomab tiuxetan target the CD20 antigen on the surface of mature white blood cells (B cells) and B-cell lymphocytes occurring in non-Hodgkin's lymphoma. This is discussed further later in the chapter.

Peptides have been investigated to succeed antibodies as delivery vehicles for linked diagnostic or therapeutic agents. Peptides have the advantage over MABs of being more rapidly cleared from the body, potentially with a lower level of toxicity (6). Further, they provide physiologic evidence of the nature of the disease process or progress of treatment. Radiolabeled peptides are a new class of radiotracers that target a cell or tissue and deliver a diagnostic signal or therapeutic agent to the site of the disease. Peptides are naturally occurring or synthetic compounds that contain one or more amino acid sequences or groups. On their plasma membranes, cells express receptor proteins with high affinity for regulatory peptides, such as somatostatin. Changes in the density of these receptors during disease, such as the overexpression found in many tumors, provide the basis for new imaging and therapeutic applications.

The first peptide analogues successfully applied for visualization of receptor-positive tumors were radiolabeled somatostatin analogues. The next step was to label these analogues with therapeutic radionuclides for peptide receptor radionuclide therapy (PRRT). Results from preclinical and clinical multicenter studies have already shown an effective therapeutic response to radiolabeled somato-statin analogues to treat receptor-positive tumors. Infusion of positively charged amino acids reduces kidney uptake, enlarging the therapeutic window. For PRRT of CCK-B receptor-positive tumors, such as medullary thyroid carcinoma, radiolabeled mini gastrin analogues are being successfully applied (6).

An example of this new class of radiopharmaceuticals is octreotide, a synthetic analogue of the aforementioned peptide hormone, somatostatin, with the ^{111}In-labeled analogue pentetreotide. The resulting product, OctreoScan, became the first radiolabeled peptide approved by the FDA. This agent has made possible the detection of small (0.5–1.0 cm) primary and metastatic tumors, including those of several brain tumor types, pancreatic islet tumors, neuroblastomas, carcinoids, thymomas, and melanomas, among others.

Small antimicrobial peptides are also thought to be candidates to be new antimicrobial agents. Lupetti et al. (9) have developed a scintigraphic approach to studying these pharmacokinetically in animals. These peptides, radiolabeled with ^{99m}Tc, demonstrated rapid accumulation at sites of infection but not at sites of sterile inflammation. This outcome indicated that these radiolabeled antimicrobial peptides could be used in infection detection and allow the effectiveness of antibacterial therapy in animals to be monitored. Another outcome of this research was that the process allowed reliable real-time whole-body imaging and quantitative biodistribution studies without the need to kill animals at each time interval.

Radiopharmaceuticals

The USP 27–NF 22 (10) lists 70 official radioactive pharmaceuticals. Examples are presented in Table 18.1. The following describes some of the radiopharmaceuticals frequently used in daily practice. Several of these radiopharmaceuticals are being used for the delivery of MABs, biotechnologic drugs. For a deeper understanding of these biotechnologic drugs, including terminology, see Chapter 19.

Technetium-99m (^{99m}Tc) possesses a relatively short half-life of 6 hours, which allows administration of higher amounts of activity for faster and clearer images while exposing the patient to a low radiation dose. It offers an abundance of gamma photons for imaging without the hazardous effects of beta particles. Also, its chemistry profile is flexible, which allows it to be used as a binding agent for several pharmaceuticals used for imaging. Kits are available for preparation of various technetium ^{99m}Tc compounds that assist in hepatobiliary imaging (mebrofenin) and ischemic heart disease (sestamibi, tetrofosmin).

^{99m}Tc has also been used as a radiolabel for MABs because of its wide availability in nuclear pharmacies and because it is relatively inexpensive and easy to obtain. It provides low radiation dosimetry and highly efficient detection of photons by planar scintigraphy. Unfortunately, widespread use of this radionuclide in immunoscintigraphy has been hindered by the lack of a simple, efficient, and stable method for attaching the ^{99m}Tc to the antibody molecule.

Strontium-89 Chloride (^{89}Sr) (Metastron), is a sterile, nonpyrogenic aqueous solution for intravenous use and containing no preservative. It decays by beta emission, with a physical half-life of 51 days. This beta emission is very harmful to skeletal tissue, and thus its clinical use is reserved for bone pain palliation associated with primary bone tumors and metastatic involvement (blastic lesions). An advantage of ^{89}Sr is that it is retained and accumulated in metastatic bone lesions much longer and in significantly greater concentration than in normal bone.

Following intravenous administration, strontium compounds demonstrate similar characteristics to calcium analogues. They clear rapidly from the blood stream and selectively localize in bone mineral. The uptake of ^{89}Sr by bone occurs preferentially in sites of osteogenesis imperfecta, a condition characterized by the formation of brittle bones prone to fractures. Thus, as mentioned, it finds utility with primary bone tumors and metastatic bone lesions.

Prior to administration of ^{89}Sr a risk-to-benefit ratio must be determined because of its bone marrow toxicity. It should be used with caution in patients with platelet counts below 60,000 and white cell counts below 2400. After

TABLE 18.1 REPRESENTATIVE RADIOPHARMACEUTICAL DRUGS AND PRIMARY USES

DRUG	TRADE NAME	PRIMARY USES
^{111}In oxyquinoline	Indium-111 Oxine	Radiolabel autologous leukocytes and platelets
^{111}In capromab pendetide	ProstaScint	Monoclonal antibody for imaging prostate cancer
^{111}In pentetreotide	OctreoScan	Imaging of neuroendocrine tumors
^{123}I, sodium iodide	—	Thyroid imaging and uptake
^{131}I, sodium iodide	—	Thyroid imaging, uptake, therapy
^{131}I tositumomab	Bexxar	Treatment of non-Hodgkin's lymphoma
^{131}I-*m*IBG	—	Treatment of neuroendocrine tumors
^{99m}Tc exametazime	Ceretec	Cerebral perfusion, radiolabeling autologous leukocytes
^{99m}Tc macroaggregated albumin	Pulmonite, Macrotec	Pulmonary perfusion
^{99m}Tc mebrofenin	Choletec	Hepatobiliary imaging
^{99m}Tc medronate (MDP)	—	Bone imaging
^{99m}Tc mertiatide	Technescan MAG3	Renal imaging
^{99m}Tc oxidronate (HDP)	OctreoScan HDP	Bone imaging
^{99m}Tc pentetate (DTPA)	Techneplex, Technescan DTPA	Renal imaging and function studies; radioaerosol ventilation imaging
^{99m}Tc pertechnetate	—	Imaging of thyroid, salivary glands, ectopic gastric mucosa, parathyroid glands, dacryocystography, cystography
^{99m}Tc red blood cells	Ultratag	Imaging of gastrointestinal bleeding, cardiac chambers, cardiac first-pass, gated equilibrium imaging
^{99m}Tc sestamibi	Cardiolite, Miraluma	Imaging of myocardial perfusion, breast tumor
^{99m}Tc sulfur colloid		Imaging of reticuloendothelial system, bone marrow, gastric emptying, gastrointestinal bleeding, lymphoscintigraphy, arthrograms
^{99m}Tc tetrofosmin	Myoview	Myocardial perfusion imaging
^{201}Ti	—	Myocardial perfusion imaging; parathyroid and tumor imaging
^{133}Xe	Dupont Xenon, Mallinckrodt Xenon, Nycomed Xenon	Pulmonary ventilation imaging
^{90}Y microspheres	TheraSphere	Therapy for biopsy-proven, unresectable hepatocellular carcinoma
^{90}Y ibitumomab tiuxetan	Zevalin	Non-Hodgkin's lymphoma
^{153}Sm-lexidronam	Quadramet	Palliation of bone pain of skeletal metastases
^{166}Ho-DOTMP	—	Bone cancer therapy
^{186}Re-HEDP	—	Bone cancer therapy

administration of ^{89}Sr, weekly blood tests should be performed and the patient's status monitored. Because the average hematologic recovery time is 6 months of treatment, at least 90 days is required prior to retreatment.

A small percentage of patients receiving ^{89}Sr report a transient increase in bone pain 36 to 72 hours after injection. This is usually mild, self-limiting, and controllable with analgesic therapy. Pain relief from the administration of

[89]Sr typically manifests 7 to 20 days post injection, and a key benefit of its use is a decreased dependence on opioids.

Yttrium-90 (^{90}Y), a trivalent radioactive metal, is a pure beta-emitting radionuclide. It possesses a physical half-life of 64.2 hours (2.68 days) and is frequently used in human studies, in part because of its routine availability from commercial vendors as a sterile, pyrogen-free product with high specific activity (11). Its principal therapeutic application is in RIT of solid large tumors and lymphomas. In addition, it is employed in pain palliation involving soft tissue.

TheraSphere is a therapeutic device approved for use in patients with liver cancer (Fig. 18.2). It is being used for patients with biopsy-proven unresectable hepatocellular carcinoma. It is administered to a conscious patient via a catheter inserted into the femoral artery and is delivered directly into the hepatic artery in an interventional vascular radiology suite to go to the left or right lobe of the liver. Usually, patients receive two treatments to each liver lobe.

Patented in 1988, it consists of microspheres having a mean diameter of 20 to 30 μg (the approximate size of two red blood cells) that are bonded chemically to a radioactive pure beta emitter (^{90}Y). After injection, the product produces radiation to tissue with an average range of 2.5 mm and a maximum range of less than 1 cm. These lodge in end arterioles and capillaries in tumors, which minimizes or prevents delivery of the injected radionuclide to other body organs and tissues.

The sterile, pyrogen-free glass spheres are preformed by incorporating [89]Y oxide into the glass matrix. Subsequently, neutron bombardment is used to convert the [89]Y in the glass to [90]Y. Because the ^{90}Y is embedded in the spheres, it is not leached from the glass or metabolized. This prevents *in vivo* mobilization to distant body tissues and organs (11).

The ^{90}Y decays to stable zirconium-90. Each treatment delivers approximately 150 Gy or 15,000 rad to the liver lobe. Typically, 135 to 540 mCi of [90]Y (5–10 GBq) is delivered in 10 mL of saline that contains 2 million to 8 million microspheres. This is injected over a few minutes into the right or left hepatic artery. Patients are evaluated every month thereafter. Regular blood work that analyzes blood counts and liver function is performed, as is computed tomography (CT) or magnetic resonance imaging (MRI) of the liver.

Thallous-201 Chloride (^{201}Tl) is available as a sterile, nonpyrogenic solution for intravenous administration (Fig. 18.3). It demonstrates a physical half-life of 73.1 hours and decays by electron capture to mercury, [201]Hg. [201]Tl is a potassium analogue that undergoes rapid active transport into the myocardium. Thus, it is an advantageous agent to diagnose and visualize a myocardial infarction or ischemic heart disease. Identified ischemia on ^{201}Tl scanning has been demonstrated to be a strong predictor of long-term mortality in coronary artery disease (12). However, long-term survival after major vascular surgery is improved significantly if patients with moderate to severe ischemia on preopera-

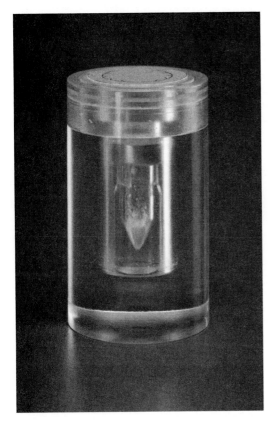

FIGURE 18.2 TheraSphere. (Courtesy of MDS Nordion.)

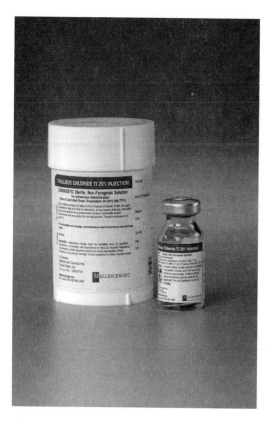

FIGURE 18.3 Product package of Thallous Chloride ^{201}Ti. (Courtesy of Mallinckrodt Medical.)

tive ^{201}Tl scanning undergo selective coronary revascularization (12).

When used in conjunction with exercise stress testing to help differentiate between ischemic and infarcted tissue, ^{201}Tl should be administered at the inception of a period of maximum stress sustained for 30 seconds after injection of the agent. Imaging commences within 10 minutes after administration to obtain maximum target-to-background ratios. If the patient is unable to undergo a treadmill stress exercise because of physical limitation, pharmaceutical agents (e.g., Adenoscan, Persantine) may be used to induce cardiac stress.

^{201}Tl undergoes fast redistribution in normal myocardium. Because of decreased blood flow, the uptake and washout of ^{201}Tl is not quick in ischemic cardiac tissue. If the image demonstrates no uptake, the tissue is classified as infarcted.

Gallium-67 Citrate (^{67}Ga) is available as a sterile, pyrogen-free aqueous solution. Chemically, this drug behaves similarly to ferric ion (Fe^{+3}) and demonstrates a half-life of 78 hours.

^{67}Ga can localize in certain viable primary and metastatic tumors and in focal sites of infection. Investigational studies demonstrate that perhaps ^{67}Ga accumulates in lysosomes and is bound to a soluble intracellular protein. ^{67}Ga may be useful in demonstrating the presence and extent of malignancies associated with Hodgkin's disease, lymphomas, and bronchogenic carcinoma. It can also be useful for localization of focal inflammatory lesions (e.g., sarcoidosis, abscesses, and pyelonephritis). It finds utility in the diagnosis and monitoring of *Pneumocystis carinii* pneumonia of AIDS and can be used as a diagnostic screen in cases of prolonged fever when physical examination, laboratory tests, and other imaging studies have not disclosed the source of the fever (fever of undetermined origin).

Concurrent use of ferric ion can increase ^{67}Ga renal excretion from the body. Although the exact mechanism is not clear, it is thought that elevated serum iron levels may displace ^{67}Ga from plasma protein binding sites and hasten its excretion, resulting in decreased tumor and abscess localization.

The optimal target-to-background concentration ratios are often obtained 48 hours post injection, and delayed imaging is necessary to allow for the ideal target-to-background ratio. However, considerable biologic variation can occur in individuals, and acceptable imaging may be performed 6 to 120 hours after injection. The optimal target-to-background ratios also depend on the area of interest. For example, a lower abdominal scan can be hindered by ^{67}Ga fecal excretion. Thus, the use of laxatives facilitates faster scanning of the patient.

Indium-111 Chloride (^{111}In) has become a popular radionuclide as a label for MABs (Fig. 18.4). The advantage of using ^{111}In for immunoscintigraphy is its long half-life, which allows multiple images to be taken up to 10 to 14 days after administration. In addition, its dual photon peaks provide superior planar and tomographic images. Because it lacks beta

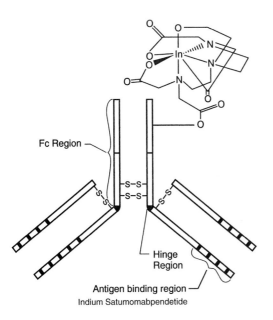

FIGURE 18.4 The indium satumomab pendetide molecule demonstrating attachment to the monoclonal antibody. The antigen-binding region is also depicted. (Reprinted with permission from Hunter TB, Walsh TK, Hall JN. Agents for diagnostic imaging. In Block JH, Beale JM Jr., eds. Wilson and Gisvold's textbook of organic medicinal and pharmaceutical chemistry, 11th ed. Baltimore: Lippincott Williams & Wilkins, 2004;470.)

emission, it can be administered in rather high doses. Lastly, unlike radioiodine complexes, ^{111}In–MAB complexes are relatively stable in the body.

Capromab pendetide (ProstaScint) is a MAB imaging agent linked to ^{111}In. This drug seeks out and attaches itself to prostate cancer and its metastases. ProstaScint images can aid management by helping identify when the cancer has metastasized from the prostate bed to regional lymph nodes or to distant soft tissues. It is also used as a diagnostic imaging agent in postprostatectomy patients with a rising prostate-specific antigen level and a negative or equivocal standard metastatic evaluation in whom there is a high clinical suspicion of occult metastatic disease. This product was approved for use by the FDA in late 1996.

Ibritumomab tiuxetan (Zevalin), approved for use in 2002, is a monoclonal antibody that is labeled with ^{111}In and ^{90}Y in a two-phase regimen for the treatment of refractory low-grade

follicular or transformed B-cell non-Hodgkin's lymphoma, including patients with rituximab-refractory follicular non-Hodgkin's lymphoma (Fig. 18.5). ^{111}In is used for the biodistributive study and administered 1 week prior to the final ibritumomab tiuxetan and ^{90}Y administration. This procedure ensures adequate biodistribution of the test dose. If the biodistribution is deemed unacceptable, the second step of the process is not implemented. This product works like a smart bomb. It is an antibody with a radionuclide attached that seeks and binds to cells with the CD20 receptor. Rituximab is administered prior to Zevalin (an unbound antibody) for both steps to clear most normal B cells and thus reduce the toxicity of the Zevalin.

The therapeutic regimen consists of two steps, as follows:

1. Initially, rituximab is infused in an amount equal to 250 mg/m^2 at 50 mg/hour. The dose is increased by 50 mg/hour every 30 minutes up to a maximum of 400 mg/hour. During the infusion, the patient should be monitored for any hypersensitivity reaction and the infusion stopped if hypersensitivity occurs. If hypersensitivity does occur and is treated, the infusion is resumed at half the previous rate when symptoms improve. After rituximab infusion has been administered, within 4 hours, 5 mCi of ibritumomab tiuxetan is injected over 10 minutes with use of a syringe shield to reduce exposure during administration. The biodistribution of

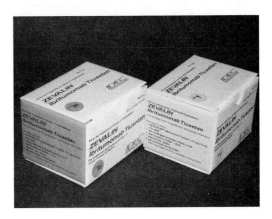

FIGURE 18.5 Product package of Zevalin. (Courtesy of Biogen IDEC.)

the drug is assessed by imaging within 2 to 24 hours and again 48 hours post injection. If the biodistribution is acceptable, the second step is administered after 7 days of initial therapy. Alternatively, if the biodistribution is not acceptable, the therapy does not proceed to the second step.

2. Initiated within 7 to 9 days after step one, the patient receives a rituximab infusion of 250 mg/m^2 at an initial rate of 100 mg/hour. The dosage is increased by 100 mg/hour every 30 minutes to a maximum of 400 mg/hour. Because the most commonly reported adverse effect of this therapy is thrombocytopenia and neutropenia, after the rituximab infusion, if the patient's platelet count is above 150,000 cells/mm^3, a 4-mCi dose of ^{90}Y-labeled ibritumomab tiuxetan is administered. If the patient's platelet count is between 100,000 and 150,000 cells/mm^3, 3 mCi of ^{90}Y-labeled ibritumomab tiuxetan is administered over 10 minutes. If the patient's platelet count is below 100,000 cells/mm^3, the drug is not administered.

The regimen is supplied in two distinct kits (Fig. 18.5) that contain all of the nonradioactive ingredients necessary to create the single doses of ibritumomab tiuxetan labeled with ^{111}In and ^{90}Y. Because ^{90}Y is a pure beta particle–emitting radionuclide, extreme precautions must be taken to protect the caregivers and the patient to keep radiation exposure levels to a minimum.

Sodium Iodide-123 (^{123}I) is available as an oral capsule and is generally preferable to ^{131}I because it delivers lower radiation doses and has better imaging properties. It is used diagnostically to evaluate thyroid function and morphology. ^{123}I emits only gamma rays. In the euthyroid patient, 5 to 30% of the administered dose is concentrated in the thyroid gland at 24 hours and has an effective half-life of 13 hours. The remaining administered activity is distributed within the extracellular fluid and has an effective half-life of 8 hours. Although it is more expensive than ^{99m}Tc, ^{123}I produces a superior image because of its higher target-to-background ratio. Also, it gives a lower radiation dose.

Pharmacists must be aware that concurrently administered drugs can decrease the thyroid uptake of ^{123}I for a variety of reasons. Thus, it is recommended that these medications be withheld for a period prior to the administration of ^{123}I. For example, corticosteroids should be withheld 1 week prior to ^{123}I administration. Benzodiazepines should be withheld up to 4 weeks prior to ^{123}I administration. Vitamins, expectorants, antitussives, and topical medications containing iodine (e.g., clioquinol, Betadine) should be withheld for 2 to 4 weeks prior to the administration of ^{123}I.

Sodium Iodide-131 (^{131}I) is available as a volatile solution that can be purchased from a manufacturer or compounded by the nuclear pharmacist into an oral capsule or solution. In small amounts, it is used for thyroid function studies or thyroid uptake tests by determining the fraction of administered radioiodine activity taken up by the thyroid gland. The thyroid uptake test is used in the diagnosis of hyperthyroidism and in calculating the activity to be administered for radioactive iodine therapy.

Typically, the diagnostic dose of ^{131}I is 2 to 5 mCi. The therapeutic dose is higher, usually 5 to 200 mCi. The upper limit can be calculated to determine just how much radiation a particular patient can withstand. However, more than 200 mCi is usually not given.

^{131}I is also indicated for the evaluation of size; thyroid nodules; carcinoma; and masses in the lingual region, neck, and mediastinum and in the localization of functioning metastatic thyroid tumors. It finds utility in the preoperative and postoperative evaluation of patients with thyroid carcinoma and can be used to assess therapeutic effects in these patients.

The beta emissions from the ^{131}I kill thyroid tissue and in small amounts can be used for diagnostic thyroid imaging. It is not recommended for this use because of its relatively long half-life (8 days), its beta emission, and its poor resolution on gamma camera images. However, if cost is a consideration, ^{131}I is used *in lieu* of ^{123}I. It is also used when availability of ^{123}I is a concern.

The time to radioactivity visualization is generally 18 to 24 hours. However, imaging of functional thyroid metastases is generally performed at 24 to 96 hours to allow maximal uptake and minimal blood pool retention.

Tositumomab with ^{131}I (Bexxar) is a monoclonal antibody product that has a radioactive substance, ^{131}I attached to it. The monoclonal antibody seeks and binds to a protein receptor (CD20) on the surface of normal and malignant cells. It is indicated for treatment of patients with CD20-positive follicular non-Hodgkin's lymphoma, with and without transformation, whose disease is refractory to rituximab and who have relapsed following chemotherapy. Once it is bound to target cells, the product delivers radiation, which enhances the killing effect of the antibody. Normal B cells recover in about 9 months because the parent B cells do not possess the CD20 receptor.

Neuroendocrine tumors, such as neuroblastoma and pheochromocytoma, in adults are treated with ^{131}I-MIBG (11), a structural analogue of guanethidine that has structural similarities to norepinephrine. This drug is selectively taken up by adrenergic neurons, the adrenal medulla, and some neuroendocrine cancer cells by an active uptake mechanism at the cell membrane. It is a good example of how targeted radionuclide therapy can be used for alternative treatment of neuroendocrine tumors, such as neuroblastoma, a heterogeneous pediatric cancer with clinical behavior related to the biologic features of the tumor. It is estimated that 50% of these patients have high-risk disease features, with overall survival rates less than 40%. Most of these children have significant tumor-related pain at the end of life. Often, too, the pain is difficult to treat. In targeted radiotherapy with submyeloablative doses, ^{131}I-MIBG has demonstrated effective palliation in highly refractory neuroblastoma. Most patients showed subjective improvement in pain and/or performance status (13). A retrospective review by Bomanji et al. (14) demonstrated that ^{131}I-MIBG also provides a good therapeutic response in adult patients with metastatic neuroendocrine tumors.

Samarium-153 (^{153}Sm) has a short half-life, 46.3 hours (1.9 days), which can be advantageous for administering repeated doses; the difficulty is manufacturing and delivery. It is a low-energy beta emitter, which is advantageous for treating small clusters of tumorous cells. The range of its beta emissions is short and provides a good bone-to-marrow ratio. Myelotoxicity has been manageable at its approved dose schedule (1 mCi, or 37 MBq, per kilogram) (2).

^{153}Sm is chelated with ethylenediamine tetramethylene phosphonate (^{153}Sm-EDTMP, Quadramet) for the relief of pain in patients with confirmed osteoblastic metastatic bone lesions that enhance on radionuclide bone scan (2). The recommended dose is 1.0 mCi (37 MBq) per kilogram administered intravenously over 1 minute through a secure indwelling catheter and followed with a saline flush. Excretion of this radiolabeled chelate occurs almost exclusively via the kidneys into urine. Within the first 15 minutes of administration of the complex, localization in the kidneys and the skeleton is high to all other organs and tissues. By 30 minutes post administration, most of the non–bone-associated radioactivity is in the urine. The patient should be advised to urinate often after administration of the product to minimize radiation exposure to the bladder.

Several clinical trials have demonstrated significant pain relief in approximately 70 to 80% of patients studied at the standard intravenous dosage of 1 mCi per kilogram. Toxicity is limited to bone marrow suppression manifested by decreased leukocyte counts and thrombocytopenia. The nadir for this is 4 weeks post administration with recovery to normal levels in 6 weeks.

^{153}Sm-labeled monoclonal antibodies are being used in animal research to study angiogenesis, the development of new blood vessels from preexisting ones. Central to this process is the activator vascular endothelial growth factor, and research is being performed in laboratory animals using radiolabeled (^{153}Sm and ^{99m}Tc) antiendothelial monoclonal antibodies that localize in new cancerous vasculature (15).

Holmium-166 (^{166}Ho) when complexed with 1,4,7,10-tetraazacyclododecane-1,4,7,10-tetramethylenephosphonic acid (^{166}Ho-DOTMP) has demonstrated potential to treat multiple myeloma and to ablate bone marrow. It is a bone-seeking complex that emits a high-energy beta particle (E_β (max) = 1.85 MeV). The long range of these beta particles produces excessive marrow suppression and destroys bone marrow cells remote from the surface of the bone where the ^{166}Ho-DOTMP deposits. Thus, it can be used for eradication of multiple myeloma cells and the normal stem cells in the marrow space.

^{166}Ho in a ferric hydroxide macroaggregate complex, (^{166}Ho-FHMA) has been shown experimentally to provide beneficial outcomes for equine metacarpophalangeal and metatarsophalangeal joints. Inflamed equine joints with synovial lining hyperplasia could benefit from ^{166}Ho-FHMA–induced radiation synovectomy if excessive scar tissue formation can be avoided.

Lutetium-177 (^{177}Lu) is being investigated in more than 30 clinical applications, including treatment of colon cancer, metastatic bone cancer, non-Hodgkin's lymphoma, ovarian cancer, and lung cancer. It is estimated that more than 500,000 new cases of these cancers occur each year in the United States and nearly 2 million cases worldwide. ^{177}Lu is a rare earth metal with a physical half-life of 6.75 days and beta emissions (E = 149 keV) that penetrate 0.2 to 0.3 mm in soft tissues. In comparison to ^{90}Y, a higher percentage of ^{177}Lu radiation energy will be absorbed in very small tumors and micrometastases (6).

^{177}Lu also emits two relatively low abundance, low-energy gamma rays (113 and 208 keV) that allow imaging with a gamma camera but pose less radiation risk hazard to health care personnel than ^{131}I. Its most common side effects were delayed transient arthralgia and marrow suppression.

Rhenium-186 (^{186}Re) and **Rhenium-188 ($^{186/188}$Re)** are important radionuclides with therapeutic potential. The availability of ^{186}Re and $^{186/188}$Re provides flexibility in design of radiolabeled agents that are compatible with their *in vivo* applications and pharmacokinetic properties. $^{186/188}$Re has a higher beta particle energy and shorter half-life than ^{186}Re. Thus, it is generally more appropriate for larger tumor targeting and possesses a reasonably fast clearance from the blood and other nontarget tissues. Alternatively, ^{186}Re is a medium-energy beta particle emitter with a 3.7-day half-life, which makes it more appropriate for use with biomolecules that are not cleared from the

blood stream very rapidly. Its lack of availability as a high-specific-activity product limits ^{186}Re use to applications in which high specific activity formulations are not mandatory.

^{188k}**Rhenium-HEDP (hydroxyl ethylene diphosphonate)** is a new radiopharmaceutical for the treatment of metastatic bone pain. It is produced from a (188)W/(188)Re generator. It has a short physical half-life, 16.9 hours, and a maximal beta energy of 2.1 MeV. One study demonstrated a maximum decrease in metastatic bone pain from the third to eighth week after therapy initiation in 76% of the patients with human prostate cancer skeletal metastases. These patients described pain relief without an increase in analgesic intake (16).

Positron Emission Tomography

Since the early 1970s positron emission tomography (PET) has been employed to study cerebral physiology (17). Since that time, it is a rapidly growing noninvasive modality for the diagnosis and management of cancer. PET yields high-quality images that characterize substrate metabolism, cellular proliferation, receptor density, and other parameters used to identify cancer and evaluate its response to treatment (18). Radiolabeled tracers injected in nonpharmacologic doses are used to construct three-dimensional images by computer to demonstrate the location and concentration of the tracer of interest (19). PET allows the physician to secure an image that is essentially a low-resolution autoradiograph showing the regional concentration of a positron-emitting nuclide inside the body (21). It is a method for quantitative imaging of regional function and chemical reactions within various organs of the human body. Imaging applications of PET have shown great use, for instance, in mapping regional blood flow, oxygen metabolism, regional blood volume, rates of use of metabolic substrates, receptor-specific tracer binding, bone remodeling, tumor receptor density, and reporter gene expression (19).

The tracers used in PET imaging are natural biochemicals labeled with radionuclides of carbon, nitrogen, oxygen, and fluorine. This allows analysis in terms of physiology and biochemistry at a level of sophistication beyond that encountered in traditional nuclear medicine. No other technology can image body chemistry with such sensitivity, so that the moment-to-moment change in concentration of a tracer in the blood or tissue can be determined in absolute units. Other imaging modalities, such as CT and MRI, provide predominantly anatomic information. CT is based on portrayal of the distribution of attenuation of x-rays passing through the body. MRI exploits the variation in regional concentrations of hydrogen and nuclear relaxation parameters to generate image contrast and to provide information about free water content, relative blood flow, and the concentration of contrast agents. Clinical PET is being used with CT to combine anatomic information (CT) with functional molecular information (PET) to advance cancer management (19).

Chemical changes occur prior to anatomic changes in most disease states, and PET can detect functional abnormalities before anatomic changes have occurred. PET evolved with its main focus on studies of the brain and heart. However, it has emerged as a valued diagnostic tool for diagnosis and therapy monitoring of patients with lymphoma, as a means to assess estrogen receptors in primary and metastatic breast cancers, and to identify resectable colorectal tumor recurrence. In epilepsy, PET and surface electroencephalography (EEG) are used in concert with clinical assessment of symptoms and signs to try to localize areas of the brain that are the foci of epileptic seizures when surgical intervention is the only remaining method to prevent the seizures.

Tumors have more intermediary metabolism than normal tissue, and PET use is advantageous because it can qualitatively and quantitatively study metabolism. Several processes, including glycolysis, increased membrane glucose transfer capability, and RNA, DNA, and protein synthesis are demonstrated and/or accelerated in tumors. In the 1930s, Warburg demonstrated that glucose was used more in tumorous tissue than in normal tissue, and this remains today as a foundation for PET imaging

in oncology (20). The radiopharmaceutical most widely used for evaluating tumors with PET imaging is $[^{18}F]$-fluorodeoxyglucose, because it has been demonstrated useful for tracing glucose metabolism, for detecting malignant tissue, and for quantifying changes in tumor glycolysis during and after treatment. Thus, it is useful for diagnosis, staging, and monitoring various cancers, including lung, colorectal, melanoma, lymphoma, and head and neck, among others. $[^{18}F]$-FDG has a 110 minute half-life, which is much easier to work with than a 2-minute half-life.

When a radionuclide within the body decays by emission of a positron, that particle travels a very short distance (1–4 mm) in body tissues or water before expending its kinetic energy and combining with an electron. This interaction, one positron annihilation, results in simultaneous emission of two photons, each having a specific energy (511 KeV) and emitted exactly 180° from each other. Therefore, two scintillation detectors are placed, one on either side of the tissue that contains the radionuclide. Detectors are connected to a coincident circuit that provides an output only when a certain level of gamma ray radiation can be simultaneously detected by both. The result is a low-background detector, highly specific for the particular radionuclide and providing excellent resolution.

Radionuclides that undergo positron decay generally have very short half-lives (e.g., ^{15}O; $t_{1/2}$ = 2.04 minutes), which permits administration of large doses of activity without subjecting the patient to excessive radiation exposure. The resulting high count rates facilitate collection of statistically significant images in a very short time and a dynamic study of physiologic processes that produces a quick fluctuation in tissue concentrations of the tracer. The short half-lives also allow repeat image studies within a brief time with no confounding background activity from the prior injection.

It is optimal to label radiopharmaceuticals using radionuclides with the shortest half-life that is compatible with the time scale of the physiologic process to be studied. However, a practical consequence of using short-lived ($t_{1/2}$ < 1 hour) radionuclides in diagnostic medicine is the necessity for the radionuclide production and radiotracer synthesis to occur in the hospital where the imaging procedure will be conducted. Originally, the major production of radionuclides for PET imaging (^{11}C, ^{13}N, ^{15}O, ^{18}F) was generally with in-house biomedical cyclotrons. Today, however, there are numerous commercial cyclotrons nationwide.

For tracers that have demonstrated great utility in PET imaging studies, robotic technique and automated systems have been created for routine radiopharmaceutical synthesis. These systems cannot reduce the personnel needed to supply PET radiopharmaceuticals, but the automated systems encourage frequent syntheses using large amounts of activity to be performed without exposing the personnel to unnecessary or excessive radiation exposure.

PET was once conducted primarily in large medical centers. A prime consideration was that PET radionuclides had short half-lives, often 2 to 20 minutes, which made it difficult to get them from commercial sources. However, commercial dispensing is now possible in certain markets where a PET cyclotron is adjacent to the pharmacy. In other markets, out of necessity, the production facility must be on site, and after rapid synthesis, the pharmaceutical must be purified. Thus, research continues to focus upon sources of PET radionuclides other than cyclotrons, such as radionuclide generators, that would allow PET technology in community-based nuclear medicine and pharmacy environments.

Parent–daughter generator systems are now being investigated as a possible mode to produce PET radionuclides. Potentially, it would free PET imaging from its dependence on cyclotron generation within a hospital. Also, this could make PET a viable clinical diagnosis tool away from the hospital or large medical center. To date, very few positron emitters can be created by these systems, and only two radionuclides, ^{82}Rb and ^{68}Ga, have been extensively reported in the nuclear medicine literature. In late 2003, Ion Beam Applications announced FDA approval of a generator (CardioGen-82) to make ^{82}Rb, a PET agent for the evaluation of coronary artery disease. It is capable of distinguishing normal from abnormal myocardium in

patients with suspected myocardial infarction, and it helps identify patients most likely to benefit from further intervention while reducing the risks of unnecessary medical, radiologic, and/or surgical procedures.

Future studies of new drug entities will include pharmacokinetic determination using PET technology. Further, PET will allow the manufacturer to quantify how much of the drug reaches a specific drug receptor. Thus, comparative PET studies will shed light on which drug, for example, within a therapeutic category can attain the best distribution and concentration at the intended receptor site. It is also conceivable that PET technology will open new vistas for interpretation of drug interactions, particularly where there is competition by two drugs for one receptor site.

Longer-lived PET radionuclides, such as ^{89}Zr ($t_{1/2}$, 78.1 hours), ^{76}Br ($t_{1/2}$, 61.1 hours), ^{124}I ($t_{1/2}$, 4.15 days), and ^{64}Cu ($t_{1/2}$, 12.8 hours) are being investigated as radiolabels for MAB-based PET imaging. Early clinical research has demonstrated that these may be useful for detecting metastases smaller than 1.5 cm. About 2 to 4% of cancer patients have an initial diagnosis of cancer of unknown primary origin (22). In addition to cancer diagnosis, radiolabeled MABs have been used to evaluate cardiovascular disorders. Clinical use of ^{111}In antimyosin include detection of acute myocardial infarct, perioperative myocardial damage assessment, detection of acute myocarditis, diagnosis of rejection and management of patients after heart transplantation, and diagnosis of active rheumatic carditis, among others.

Table 18.2 lists PET radiopharmaceuticals used in common imaging procedures, and the following section highlights a few of the more frequently used PET radiopharmaceuticals.

Carbon-11 Radiopharmaceuticals

^{11}C has been incorporated into a number of organic molecules (e.g., carboxylic acids, alcohols, glucose) for use in diagnostic imaging despite its relatively long half-life (20 minutes). To date palmitic acid is the carboxylic acid used most in PET imaging. As a tracer, it has found utility in the study of myocardial metabolism.

TABLE 18.2 POSITRON-EMITTING RADIOPHARMACEUTICALS USED IN COMMON PET IMAGING PROCEDURES

RADIOPHARMACEUTICAL	APPLICATION	TYPICAL DOSE, PROCEDURE[a]
[^{15}O]-oxygen	Cerebral oxygen extraction, metabolism	50–100 mCi
[^{15}O]-carbon monoxide	Cerebral blood volume Myocardial blood volume	50–100 mCi 50–100 mCi
[^{15}O]-water	Cerebral blood flow Myocardial blood flow	80 mCi 150 mCi
[^{13}N]-ammonia	Myocardial blood flow	15–25 mCi
[^{11}C]-acetate	Myocardial metabolism	30 mCi
[^{11}C]-*N*-methyl spiperone	Dopamine receptor binding	20 mCi
[^{18}F]-fluorodeoxyglucose	Cerebral glucose metabolism Myocardial glucose metabolism Tumor glucose metabolism	5–20 mCi
[^{82}Rb]-Rb$^+$	Myocardial blood flow	10–40 mCi

[a]Many PET studies combine imaging procedures (e.g., measurements of both blood flow and metabolism); the doses given here are typical of those actually used in each procedure of the study. For a single imaging procedure, an allowable dose (a dose that does not lead to excessive radiation exposure) may be significantly higher than these values.

Glucose randomly labeled with ^{11}C has been produced photosynthetically for use in studies of cerebral glucose metabolism. The use of ^{11}C glucose for cerebral glucose metabolism requires imaging less than 5 minutes after injection.

Nitrogen-13 Radiopharmaceuticals

^{13}N ammonia has been used as a tracer for cerebral and myocardial blood flow and demonstrates a half-life of 10 minutes. It undergoes a relatively long extraction into these organs and exhibits prolonged retention, as a major fraction of extractor tracer is metabolically incorporated into amino acids. For study of pulmonary ventilation, ^{13}N gas is superior to the radioactive noble gases because of its lower solubility in blood.

Oxygen-15 Radiopharmaceuticals

^{15}O is the radionuclide of oxygen with the longest half-life, 2.04 minutes. Because very little time is available for tracer synthesis, PET imaging studies employing ^{15}O are restricted to use of a few relatively simple molecules.

Four ^{15}O radiopharmaceuticals are available for clinical use. These are ^{15}O oxygen gas (^{15}OO), ^{15}O carbon monoxide (C^{15}O), ^{15}O carbon dioxide CO^{15}O), and ^{15}O water (H$_2$^{15}O) have been used in hemodynamic studies that take advantage of their short half-life to allow administration of large doses of activity (up to 100 mCi) in imaging studies that can be repeated within 8 to 10 minutes with no carry-over effect.

Labeled oxygen gas, that is, ^{15}OO, can be used directly in studies of oxygen metabolism or can be converted to carbon monoxide, carbon dioxide, or water. C^{15}O can be safely administered via inhalation and serves as a tracer for red blood cell volume upon binding of the C^{15}O to hemoglobin.

H$_2$^{15}O can be used in equilibrium studies of tissue water content and finds its greatest use as a tracer for regional blood flow. Commonly used as a tracer in PET evaluation of cerebral and myocardial perfusion, its 2-minute half-life outweighs its limitation of ability to diffuse freely across the blood-brain barrier at high flow rates.

Fluorine-18 Radiopharmaceuticals

^{18}F has a long half-life, 110 minutes. Compared to radiopharmaceuticals with a shorter half-life, this presents several distinct advantages for synthesis and allows delivery of the radionu-clide to imaging centers a distance from the generating cyclotron.

^{18}F also demonstrates specific activity that makes it attractive for use as a receptor-specific tracer binding. Its major use has expanded beyond the imaging of cerebral, myocardial, and tumor metabolism with 2-[^{18}F]-fluoro-2-deoxy-D-glucose (FDG) to include cancers of the lung and colon and myelomas and lymphomas. In brain-imaging procedures, FDG maps normal brain metabolic activity. In cardiac studies, it identifies ischemic regions in which glucose metabolism increases as a consequence of decreased fatty acid metabolism. As mentioned earlier, glucose metabolism increases in tumor tissue, and FDG localization in that tissue is extremely helpful in the imaging study (23).

Gallium-68 Radiopharmaceuticals

^{68}Ga is rapidly bound by the iron-binding sites of transferrin following intravenous injection of ^{68}Ga citrate and is very useful in studies of regional plasma volume. When combined with a C^{15}O measurement of regional blood cell volume, the ^{68}Ga-transferrin PET study allows calculation of the regional hematocrit. ^{68}Ga-transferrin has also been employed in pulmonary studies of vascular permeability.

Drug Antidote for Radiation Exposure

In October 2003, the FDA approved Prussian blue (ferric hexacyanoferrate, Radiogardase) to treat patients from the harmful levels of ^{137}Cs or thallium radiation exposure and contamination (Fig. 18.6). These are radioactive agents that terrorists might conceivably use to create a dirty bomb that would be inhaled or ingested by victims. The two radioactive substances can cause serious illness and death when they gain entry, as the organs absorb high doses of radiation. At lower doses, these agents can cause cancer. Conventionally, ^{137}Cs is used in a wide range of devices to treat certain cancers. Non-radioactive thallium is used industrially and as a rat poison. In small quantities, radioactive thallium is used for medical imaging.

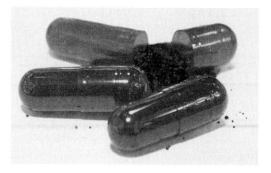

FIGURE 18.6 Radiogardase capsules. (Courtesy of Heyltex Corporation.)

Prussian blue was first manufactured in 1704 as a dye for Prussian military uniforms. To treat cesium and/or thallium radiation exposure, Prussian blue is administered orally in a dose of 3 g three times daily in adults and adolescents. In children aged 2 to 12 years, the dosage is 1 g per day. It works by trapping cesium and thallium ions in the gastrointestinal tract and interrupts their reabsorption back into the systemic circulation. Prussian blue is not absorbed from the gastrointestinal tract to a significant degree. Studies have demonstrated that 99% of the oral dose is excreted in the stool. The duration of treatment depends on the extent of exposure. Preferably, it should be administered as soon as possible after exposure and is continued for 30 days. After this treatment period, the patient should be reassessed.

Counseling a patient prescribed Prussian blue is very important. Food has been demonstrated to increase its effectiveness by stimulating bile secretion. If it is more convenient, as for patients (e.g., young children, geriatric patients) who cannot swallow solid doses, the capsules may be opened and mixed with liquid or bland food. Patients should be forewarned that constipation may occur, and if so, they should increase their dietary fiber. In addition, because the drug is a dye, it may discolor the stool blue, and if it is administered as a liquid or with bland food, it may discolor the lining of the mouth.

It is important that pharmacists help the patient identify the source of the radiation and take appropriate safety measures to minimize exposure to others. Also, men should urinate in a stool rather than a urinal and flush the toilet several times after relieving themselves. Prussian blue is available as an artist's dye, so patients should be forewarned and dissuaded from using that source as a means to treat themselves, as it is not prepared in accordance with pharmaceutical safety procedures.

Nonradioactive Pharmaceutical Use in Nuclear Medicine

The advantage of radiopharmaceutical imaging is that it is a noninvasive modality in the diagnosis and workup of a disease. Generally, radiopharmaceuticals used diagnostically help to monitor a physiologic process without altering it. Sometimes, however, the information gained from the procedure is inadequate to address the clinical questions. To overcome this deficiency, interventional pharmaceutical drugs are used to complement the radiopharmaceutical (24).

These interventional pharmaceutical drugs alter the physiologic process being studied with radiopharmaceuticals. When the interventional drug is used in conjunction with nuclear medicine, the amount of information gained is greatly improved. This intervention improves the information about the process under study and may increase the specificity and sensitivity of the procedure or decrease the time necessary for imaging.

Acetazolamide (Diamox), an agent used to treat glaucoma by diuretic action, has been shown to increase cerebral blood flow following intravenous administration. On average, it can increase cerebral blood flow 23% ± 8% in normal vessels. Its use in cerebral perfusion studies is to enhance the differentiation between normal vessels and diseased vessels, which cannot easily dilate. It is indicated for use in patients with transient ischemic attack, carotid artery disease, or a cerebrovascular accident to help identify areas of the brain that are at risk for an infarct. The drug also is used in other neurologic conditions (e.g., Alzheimer's disease, multi-infarct dementia) with which cerebral perfusion is far from optimal.

Captopril (Capoten) is used to help diagnose renovascular hypertension in hypertensive patients with abdominal bruits, declining renal function, and poorly controlled hypertension with drug therapy. As an angiotensin-converting enzyme inhibitor, this drug blocks conversion of angiotensin I to angiotensin II and prevents vasoconstriction of the efferent arterioles of the kidney. This decreases glomerular filtration pressure in the affected kidney.

Among children, Meckel's diverticulum, a congenital anomaly of the gastrointestinal tract, presents itself in about a quarter of the cases as rectal bleeding and abdominal pain. This diverticulum, an abnormal remnant of the developing gastrointestinal tract, contains gastric mucosa that bleeds abnormally. Within the pediatric population, Meckel's diverticulum, a congenital anomaly of the gastrointestinal tract presents itself in a about a quarter of the cases as rectal bleeding and abdominal pain. This diverticulum is an abnormal remnant of the developing gastrointestinal tract which contains gastric mucosa that bleeds abnormally. This gastric mucosa concentrates ^{99m}Tc-pertechnetate as normal mucosa and cimetidine (i.e., Tagemet) demonstrates usefulness in Meckel's diverticulum imaging by virtue of its action as a histamine-H_2 receptor antagonist. Cimetidine reduces the volume and concentration of stomach acid, and following its administration in a Meckel's study, the cells of the gastric mucosa continue to accumulate ^{99m}Tc-pertechnetate, but secretion of acid into the gastric lumen is reduced or prevented. This allows for continual ^{99m}Tc-pertechnetate accumulation in the gastric mucosa with little transit through the intestinal tract. This results in an enhanced ability to visualize the small area of ectopic gastric mucosa.

Dipyridamole (Persantine) is used as an alternative to a treadmill stress test prior to cardiac imaging. Typically, patients who are candidates to receive pharmaceutical stress as part of the imaging procedure rather than perform the stress test are those with cardiac, respiratory, and/or orthopedic problems, those maintained on beta-blocker or calcium-channel blocker medications, and those with poor motivation. Dipyridamole blocks adenosine deaminase, the enzyme responsible for the degradation of adenosine, a potent coronary vasodilator. Adenosine can increase coronary blood flow up to four to five times resting values. Blood flow through stenosed arteries is less than normal.

Adenosine (Adenocard) is an ideal agent in combination with myocardial perfusion imaging agents. It possesses an ultrashort half-life, less than 10 seconds, and is a potent coronary vasodilator. This drug can increase coronary blood flow four to five times that of rest and can be beneficial as a pharmaceutical stress agent to help diagnose and identify stenosed arteries.

In preparation for the use of adenosine or dipyridamole, theophylline- and caffeine-containing drugs, beverages, and foods must be discontinued and the patient must take nothing by mouth overnight. An advantage of adenosine use over dipyridamole is that adverse effects caused by adenosine (e.g., chest pain, pain in the throat, jaw, or arm, headache, flushing, and dyspnea) generally disappear within 1 to 2 minutes after discontinuation of the infusion. Dipyridamole has a longer half-life (15–30 minutes) with a peak effect 2 to 3 minutes after infusion. When this agent is used, chest pain, headache, and dizziness occur most often.

To reverse the effects of adenosine and dipyridamole, aminophylline can be given intravenously if necessary. Nitroglycerin can be given to relieve the chest pain that follows dipyridamole administration.

Furosemide (Lasix), a loop diuretic, is administered to help confirm or rule out mechanical renal obstruction during renal scintigraphy when significant retention of radioactivity is noted in the renal pelvis. It inhibits the reabsorption of electrolytes, most notably sodium, in the ascending limb of the loop of Henle, and in the proximal and distal tubules. In an obstructed kidney, furosemide diuresis will have little effect on clearance of the radioactivity retained in the kidney. An unobstructed kidney will rapidly clear the radioactivity into the bladder following furosemide administration, and the renograms will show rapid emptying with a steeply declining radioactivity curve.

Schilling's test determines a patient's capability to absorb radioactive vitamin B_{12} from the intestine. Normally, vitamin B_{12} is released from food sources (e.g., meat, eggs, milk) and bound to intrinsic factor in the stomach. Ultimately, this intrinsic factor–vitamin B_{12} complex is absorbed in the ileum and stored in the liver. Once the liver's storage capacity for this complex is exceeded, Vitamin B_{12} is excreted in urine. In cases of Vitamin B_{12} deficiency, it is crucial to determine the cause of the deficiency, either lack of a proper diet or inadequate absorption. For the procedure, 1 mg of nonradioactive vitamin B_{12} is given intramuscularly 2 hours before the ^{57}Co-labeled vitamin B_{12} is administered orally. This large dose is intended to saturate the storage sites and helps flush absorbed radiolabeled B_{12} into the urine. Thus, the excreted radioactivity demonstrates the amount absorbed. Excretion of 5% or less is diagnostic of B_{12} malabsorption. Typical urinary excretion of B_{12} ranges from 15 to 40%.

Practice of Nuclear Pharmacy

As nuclear medicine evolved from a research tool into a mainstream clinical, diagnostic, and therapeutic tool, so has the practice of pharmacy evolved within nuclear medicine. The skills of pharmacists play an important role in the safe and efficient operation of nuclear pharmacies and modern PET facilities. In particular, the role of the pharmacist in PET increases as the use of PET radiopharmaceuticals grows from research to clinical to commercial environments.

Internal dose models and methods in use for many years are well established in nuclear medicine. These allow calculation of radiation doses to stylized models representing reference individuals. In the future, kinetic analyses will have to be carefully planned, and dose conversion factors that are most similar to the subject in question should be chosen to increase patient specificity. The important point is that the pharmacist use his or her expertise to become a part of this and use patient image data to construct individualized models for more detailed and patient-specific dose calculations (25).

The Nuclear Pharmacy Practice Guidelines were created by the American Pharmaceutical (now Pharmacists) Association Academy of Pharmacy Practice and Management (APhA-APPM) Section of Nuclear Pharmacy. They were adopted in 1994, and the Specialty Council on Nuclear Pharmacy of the Board of Pharmaceutical Specialties validated them in 1995.

The Specialty Council surveyed all board-certified nuclear pharmacists about the importance and frequency of each domain, task, and knowledge statement in the guidelines. This validation served as the underpinning for creation of the board examination in nuclear pharmacy. It established the proportion allotted to each of the nine identified domains on the nuclear pharmacy specialty examination (26).

Nuclear pharmacy is a patient-oriented service that embodies the scientific knowledge and professional judgment required to improve and promote health through safe and efficacious use of radioactive drugs for diagnosis and therapy. The pharmacist is expected to understand nuclear medicine procedures and their advantages and disadvantages for diagnostic or therapeutic purposes (27).

Typically, nuclear pharmacy practice occurs primarily in two settings, a large teaching hospital or a centralized commercial operation. Approximately 95% of radiopharmaceuticals are produced in the commercial setting. With practice site differences, activities may not be all-inclusive at each site. The nine general activities encompassing nuclear pharmacy practice are procurement, compounding, quality assurance, dispensing, distribution, health and safety, provision of drug information and consultation, monitoring patient outcomes, and research and development.

Procurement and Storage

Nuclear pharmacists are responsible to secure radiopharmaceuticals, other appropriate drugs, supplies, and materials necessary to effect appropriate outcomes. The effectiveness of some diagnostic radiopharmaceuticals is enhanced or toxicity lessened by coadministration of other drugs. For example, some patients (e.g., elderly, obese, those with orthopedic problems) may not be capable of undergoing an exercise stress test prior to administration of a radiopharmaceutical intended to visualize cardiac perfusion. Thus, as mentioned earlier in this chapter, dipyridamole, a vasodilator, can be used as a substitute for the exercise stress test.

The short half-life of radiopharmaceuticals poses a special problem to the pharmacist in that the traditional pathways (e.g., drug wholesaler) to secure the drug may take longer than the lifetime of the drug. Typically, in the past, the nuclear pharmacist would order the drug directly from the manufacturer, primarily by overnight delivery. Therefore, knowledge of calibration time, shipping and delivery schedules, and radioactive decay associated with the ordered radiopharmaceutical weigh heavily in ordering. Limited quantities also played a vital role in the attempt to obtain products. All of this has led to the rise of centralized radiopharmacies.

Radionuclide storage areas, a laboratory for manipulation and preparation of the radiopharmaceuticals, a counting area for calibration of doses, and a treatment room are among the facilities necessary for this type of practice. In some hospitals, radiopharmaceuticals are dispensed by a hospital pharmacist skilled in working with them. In others, nuclear medicine technologists dispense the drugs. In selection of a counting area in a hospital pharmacy practice, the location of radiographic equipment and other radiation sources must be considered to avoid the background in the counting area from becoming erratic or excessively high. With the advent of precalibrated dosage forms for a significant number of radiopharmaceuticals, elaborate facilities are not required for many diagnostic procedures.

Preparation of the Radiopharmaceutical

Compounding of the radiopharmaceutical can be a simple (e.g., reconstituting reagent kits with ^{99m}Tc sodium pertechnetate) to very complex task (e.g., operating a cyclotron). Aside from the typical compounding procedures with a normal prescription (e.g., receipt of order, validation, safety of dose, supplies and equipment to prepare), the preparation of a radiopharmaceutical is confounded by issues of radioactivity and chemical reactions.

Compounding of a radiopharmaceutical involves chemical reactions to label a molecule with a radionuclide. For most ^{99m}Tc-labeled compounds, stannous chloride is used to reduce Tc(VII) pertechnetate to a lower oxidation state. This then is followed by chelation of the technetium atoms by multidentate ligands. For other radiopharmaceuticals, covalent bonding, transchelation, and coordination complexation reactions are used.

Expense, limited availability, and shipping schedules dictate that radiopharmaceuticals be created on site at a central radiopharmacy using a cyclotron, particularly for PET. Because of this necessary path of preparation, these are usually more expensive than those purchased directly from the manufacturer. A significant number of radiopharmaceuticals use ^{99m}Tc in the form of sodium pertechnetate plus sodium chloride for isotonicity. ^{99m}Tc is formed by decay of ^{99}Mo, a radioactive radionuclide of molybdenum obtained by neutron bombardment of ^{98}Mo. Commonly, a generator or "cow" containing ^{99}Mo (half-life, 67 hours),

produces the sodium pertechnetate ^{99m}Tc at a rate that permits daily elutions of the generator (Fig. 18.7). "Milking the cow" is slang for eluting the generator to obtain the sodium pertechnetate. Other cyclotron-produced radiopharmaceuticals (e.g., ^{111}In, ^{123}I, ^{201}Tl) may be ordered for the next day.

A significant majority of radiopharmaceuticals are produced for parenteral administration. Aseptic technique and methods must be maintained during preparation of the radiopharmaceutical and when radiolabeling biologic products (e.g., MABs, peptides). Further, strict adherence to universal precautions and appropriate infection control handling are a necessity when radiolabeling patient blood cells.

Hung, et al. (28) identified potential deficiencies in manufacturers' product package in-

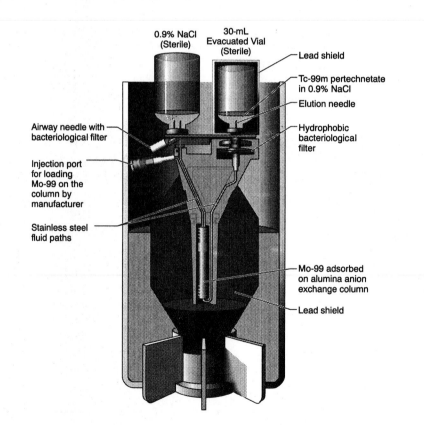

FIGURE 18.7 Cross-section of a radionuclide generator for production of ^{99m}Tc by sterile 0.9% sodium chloride elution of a sterile alumina (Al$_2$O$_3$) column that has ^{99}Mo adsorbed onto it. (Reprinted with permission from Hunter TB, Walsh TK, Hall JN. Agents for diagnostic imaging. In Block JH, Beale JM Jr., eds. Wilson and Gisvold's textbook of organic medicinal and pharmaceutical chemistry, 11th ed. Baltimore: Lippincott Williams & Wilkins, 2004;462. Courtesy of Dupont-Pharma, Billerica, MA.)

sert instructions for the preparation of radiopharmaceutical products. Five categories were identified as follows: (*a*) absent or incomplete instructions, particularly with respect to quality assurance procedures; (*b*) restrictive directions, such as specific instructions for chromatography solvents, counting devices, and reconstitution processes; (*c*) inconsistent instructions, such as different reconstituted volumes for the same final drug product, and unworkable expiration dates; (*d*) impractical directions, such as unrealistically low reconstituted activity limits and dangerously high numbers of radiolabeled particulate matter; and (*e*) vague instructions, such as use of "should," "may," and "recommend." The authors concluded that the manufacturers' instructions for the preparation of these products should be viewed as standard guidance rather than as requirements. They also advocated that nuclear pharmacists be allowed to use alternative validated methods to prepare radiopharmaceutical products as long as they do not conflict with normal pharmacy practice.

Quality Assurance

To ensure the safe use of radiopharmaceuticals in patients, the pharmacist must carry out appropriate tests (e.g., chemical, physical, biologic). USP monographs dictate that radiopharmaceuticals meet delineated specifications, including radionuclide purity, radiochemical purity, chemical purity, pH, particle size, sterility, pyrogenicity (or bacterial endotoxin), and specific activity. When the pharmacist uses an already prepared radionuclide (e.g., ^{201}Tl, ^{123}I, ^{131}I), these qualities are assured by the manufacturer.

Radionuclide purity is the proportion of activity present as the stated nuclide. It can be measured by gamma ray spectroscopy, half-life measurement, and/or other physical measurements that help to detect the presence of extraneous nuclides. Examples of the lack of radionuclide purity are ^{198}Au contaminated with ^{199}Au and ^{99m}Tc contaminated with ^{99}Mo.

Radiochemical purity is the fraction of the stated radionuclide in the stated chemical form. If there are nonradioactive contaminants, the radioactive drug may be radiochemically pure but not chemically pure. Similarly, if there are small amounts of radioactive contaminants, the material may be chemically pure but not radiochemically pure. Column or thin-layer chromatography is useful for purity determination.

Dispensing of a Radiopharmaceutical

A distinct difference between radiopharmaceutical dispensing and the traditional mode by which ordinary prescriptions are dispensed is that radiopharmaceuticals never go directly to the patient; they are provided to trained health care professionals at the hospital or clinic and then administered to the patient. Also, because of the nature of the product, radiopharmaceuticals typically are dispensed in unit doses.

When the radiopharmaceutical is ordered, the dispensing pharmacist must ensure that the ordered dose is safe for the patient. Thus, the pharmacist must weigh and consider patient factors such as age, weight, surface area, and gamma camera sensitivity with each order. Usually prescriptions are ordered and shipped. Therefore, radioactive decay must be considered to accommodate the time from manufacture to administration. Because the product is a radiopharmaceutical, it is subject to special labeling requirements (e.g., standard radiation symbol, CAUTION—RADIOACTIVE MATERIAL). Also, because the radiopharmaceutical is frequently prepared as a parenteral dosage form, aseptic technique is a necessity.

Distribution of Radiopharmaceuticals

Institutional procedures and policies dictate how a radiopharmaceutical is distributed within a health care facility. Generally, a lead-lined syringe container shipped in Department of Transportation–approved and tested cases are used with appropriate identifying information. Some nuclear pharmacies are converting from lead to tungsten containers. Tungsten is lighter, which results in less weight per shipment, and is less hazardous than lead. Local, state (e.g., State Board of Pharmacy), and federal (e.g., Department of Transportation, NRC) regulations are relevant when a radiopharmaceutical is distributed from a central nuclear pharmacy to another institution. Generally, these requirements relate to packaging, labeling, shipping papers, record keeping, shipper and carrier licensing, and personnel training.

Health and Safety

The NRC establishes and enforces radiation safety standards (e.g., limits for radiation doses, levels of radiation in an area, concentrations of radioactivity in air and waste water, waste disposal, precautionary procedures) for the compounding facility. Beyond the radiopharmaceuticals, related aspects of health and safety are a necessity. Hazardous chemicals (e.g., chromatography solvents) must be stored appropriately, handled safely, and disposed of properly. Attention must also be paid to the use of personal protective devices, containers, and the physical environment in which the radiopharmaceuticals are prepared.

Provision of Drug Information and Consultation

It is very important that the nuclear pharmacist possess oral and written communications skills. His or her knowledge and expertise are useful only when they can be conveyed to an allied health professional, the patient, and the patient's caregiver, among others. The nuclear pharmacist must be able to answer inquiries and know where to find requested information.

The type of information can include, among others, the following:

- Biologic effects of radiation
- Radiation physics and protection
- Radiopharmaceutical chemistry, compounding, quality assurance, and products
- Diagnostic and therapeutic applications of radiopharmaceuticals
- Ancillary medications used to enhance radiopharmaceutical procedures
- Drug interactions associated with radiopharmaceuticals (Tables 18.3 to 18.6)
- Precautions associated with the use of radiopharmaceuticals
- Regulatory requirements affecting the use of radiopharmaceuticals

This information can be used for educational purposes (e.g., allied health professionals, consumer groups), for setting policies and procedures, and for diagnostic or therapeutic value in the care of patients.

Monitoring Patient Outcome

Patient safety and optimal outcomes are the goal of the nuclear pharmacist and a central tenet of pharmaceutical care. In that regard the nuclear pharmacist can be instrumental in providing quality patient care. The nuclear pharmacist can, among other things:

- Develop institutional standards for the rationale and appropriate use of radiopharmaceuticals
- Prospectively screen and review patient data to ensure appropriate use of radiopharmaceuticals and ancillary medicines
- Ensure that patients are selected appropriately for radionuclide therapy and monitored after therapy to prevent complications and/or provide necessary therapy
- Evaluate the safety and effectiveness of radiopharmaceuticals and ancillary medications
- Ensure proper preparation of patients prior to administration of the radiopharmaceutical and ancillary medications
- Prevent, minimize, and/or rectify clinical problems associated with the use of radiopharmaceuticals and ancillary medications
- Monitor patients for potential adverse effects following administration of a radiopharmaceutical or interventional medication
- Discontinue incompatible medications before the nuclear medicine study, restart them after the study, and appropriately manage the patient during discontinuation
- Ensure that patients with special needs, problems, or conditions (e.g., pregnancy, nursing mothers, dialysis patients, children, the elderly) are given appropriate consideration before, during, and after radiopharmaceutical administration
- Ensure that information gained from the nuclear medicine procedure is considered

TABLE 18.3 CONCURRENT ADMINISTERED DRUGS KNOWN TO INTERFERE WITH TUMOR AND ABSCESS LOCALIZATION SCINTIGRAPHY

INTERFERING DRUG	EFFECT ON IMAGE
Phenytoin	Localization of RP in mediastinum, pulmonary hilar structures (patients without clinical evidence of lymphadenopathy)
Amiodarone, bleomycin, busulfan, nitrofurantoin, bacille Calmette-Guérin, chemotherapy, lymphangiographic contrast media, addictive drugs of abuse	Diffuse pulmonary localization (sometimes local pulmonary uptake)
Metoclopramide, reserpine, phenothiazines, oral contraceptives, diethylstilbestrol	Localization of RP in breast
Methotrexate, cisplatin, gallium nitrate, mechlorethamine HCl, vincristine, various chemotherapeutic agents, iron	Increased skeletal uptake Increased renal elimination Decreased hepatic accumulation Decreased tumor or abscess uptake
Antibiotics (Clindamycin)	Localization of RP in bowel
Calcium gluconate, IM injections	Soft tissue accumulation of RP
Ampicillin, sulfonamides, sulfinpyrazone, ibuprofen, cephalosporins, hydrochlorothiazide, methicillin, erythromycin, rifampin, pentamidine, phenylbutazone, gold salts, allopurinol, furosemide, phenazone, phenobarbital, phenytoin, phenindione	Increased accumulation of RP in the kidneys
Chemotherapeutic agents, antibiotics	Localization of RP in the thymus

RP, radiopharmaceutical.

TABLE 18.4 DRUGS KNOWN TO INTERFERE WITH BRAIN IMAGING

INTERFERING DRUG	EFFECT ON IMAGE
Cancer chemotherapeutic agents	Patchy increased uptake of RP as a result of chemoneurotoxicity
Corticosteroids	Decreased uptake into brain lesions
Psychotropic drugs	Rapid accumulation of RP in nasopharyngeal area during arterial or capillary phase (cerebral radionuclide angiography)

RP, radiopharmaceutical.

TABLE 18.5 CONCURRENT ADMINISTERED DRUGS KNOWN TO INTERFERE WITH MYOCARDIAL PERFUSION SCINTIGRAPHY

INTERFERING DRUG	EFFECT ON IMAGE
Beta blockers, nitrates, calcium channel blockers	Decreases number and size of exercise-induced ^{201}Tl perfusion defects
Vasopressin	Appearance of myocardial defects in patients without coronary artery disease
Propanolol, cardiac glycosides, procainamide, lidocaine, phenytoin, doxorubicin	Decreased myocardial localization, increased liver localization

TABLE 18.6 DRUGS KNOWN TO INTERFERE WITH RENAL IMAGING

INTERFERING DRUG	EFFECT ON IMAGE
Iodinated contrast agents, aminoglycosides	Decrease in effective plasma flow values; decreased glomerular filtration rate
Cyclosporine, cisplatin	Decreased urinary excretion; decreased tubular function
Furosemide	Misleading renogram and flow curves resulting in false positive/negative studies
Probenecid	Decreased renal accumulation and accumulation

during development of the patient's therapeutic plan
• Perform and enhance the effectiveness of nuclear pharmacy procedures, including administration of therapeutic or diagnostic radiopharmaceuticals and ancillary medications to the patient.

An example of a nuclear pharmacist intervention is use of radiopharmaceuticals in a breast-feeding woman. Specifically, recommendations are made for interruption of breast-feeding in patients who are undergoing a nuclear medicine diagnostic procedure. The nuclear pharmacist should review the patient's data, especially if the woman is of childbearing age. These recommendations include the following:

• Breast-feeding should be noted in the patient history from the attending physician.
• A member of the interdisciplinary team should inquire about the patient's breast-feeding status and notify the nuclear physician when a patient is breast-feeding.
• Breast-feeding should be interrupted for the period during which radioactivity is known to appear in the breast milk.
• Close contact with an infant should be restricted to 5 hours within 24 hours of the procedure for ^{99m}Tc MIBI, ^{99m}Tc-labeled red blood cells, and ^{131}I (>3 mCi) whether or not the mother is breast-feeding [29].

Indirectly, the nuclear pharmacist can provide clinical services that include consultation with other caregivers (e.g., explain a nuclear medicine study), prepare institutional guidelines for the use of radiopharmaceuticals and ancillary medications, provide information and literature reviews related to specific questions or studies, formulate special drugs and/or dosage forms, and conduct drug use evaluation studies or drug use reviews.

Regulatory Process

Pharmacist expertise and experience in the drug regulatory process is very important in nuclear pharmacy practice, and the role of the pharmacist in nuclear medicine is complementary to all health professions practicing within it. The role of the pharmacist will become even more important in the future, with more players entering the marketplace, particularly in the domain of PET. Already there is a variety of corporate and institutional facility partnerships, and with the continual evolution of PET, this should exponentially increase the clinical demand for these agents and increase the role of nuclear pharmacy even further.

PHARMACEUTICS CASE STUDY

Subjective

You are a pharmaceutical researcher assigned to work on a new drug, Radhot-1.

Your project is to determine where Radhot-1 localizes in the body and the rate at which its two major metabolites are eliminated from the body.

Pharmaceutics Case Study cont.

Objective

Radhot-1 contains carbon, hydrogen, sulfur, iodine, and nitrogen; it has been determined that these can be labeled appropriately for the study.

Assessment

To determine its location in the body, you use a gamma-emitting radionuclide. To follow the elimination of the two major metabolites, you label the two different parts of the molecule with two different beta-emitting radionuclides that can be counted separately.

Plan

Radhot-1 will be prepared with a gamma-emitting iodine, beta-emitting carbon in one part of the molecule and a beta-emitting hydrogen in a second part of the molecule, the two parts for beta counting being on the two separate parts of the molecule that split when metabolized. External body counting will be used to determine the source of the iodine localization. Urine samples will be collected and analyzed for the two different beta-emitting isotopes and the data plotted.

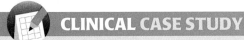

CLINICAL CASE STUDY

M. G. is a 56 y/o woman who presents to her family physician with blood pressure of 210/120. Following thyroid function tests, ultrasound, a nuclear medicine scan, and fine-needle biopsy, she was diagnosed with Hashimoto's thyroiditis and papillary carcinoma of the thyroid gland.

The patient underwent a total thyroidectomy 4 weeks ago and is scheduled today for a 100 mCi radioactive ^{131}I ablation of any residual thyroid tissue. Upon questioning, the patient states that she is allergic to iodine, having had a severe rash following the administration of iodinated contrast medium in the past. The nuclear medicine technologist calls the nuclear pharmacist for advice on how to handle the situation.

Pharmaceutical Care Plan

Subjective

Patient with history of allergy to iodine scheduled to receive ^{131}I ablation.

PMH: HTN 20 years
            Anxiety disorders × 10
            years
            Autoimmune thyroid
            disorder × 1 year
            Thyroidectomy × 4
            weeks

Meps: Calcium carbonate
            (TUMS) 500 mg po qid
            KCl 10 mEq po bid
            Diovan 160/12.5 mg po qd
            Levoxyl 0.175 mg po qd
            Meprobamate 400 mg
            po tid prn
            Calcitriol 0.5 μg po qd
            Diltiazem 240 mg po qd

Family history: Father HTN × 20 years
Social history: (−) smoking
            (−) alcohol
            (−) illicit drugs

Insurance: IPDA
Allergies: Penicillin, iodine

Objective

BP: 134/72   **Ca:** 8.6 (8.7–10.5 mg/dL)
Wt: 195   **Ca, ionized:** 4.5 (4.7–5.2 mg/dL)
Pulse: 67
TSH: 75 (normal 0.35–5.5 ulU/mL) (TSH was 0.275 prior to thyroidectomy)

Clinical Case Study cont.

Pharmaceutical Care Plan

1. Potential allergic reaction to [131]I. The recommended daily allowance is 0.15 mg of dietary iodine per day. The total therapeutic dose given in this situation would be 0.0008 mg of iodine. This amount would not likely cause an allergic reaction to iodine even in the most iodine-allergic patient.
2. Potential pregnancy teratogenicity. The patient is postmenopausal, and no pregnancy test was ordered.
3. Patient education on radioactive ablation

therapy. Patient was educated on procedure and precautions to be taken regarding close contact with other people, particularly children and pregnant women, after radionuclide therapy. Patient was also educated about radioactive ablation therapy, had her questions answered, and written, informed consent was secured.
4. In 4 months, will follow up with endocrinologist who will order a Thyrogen stimulating thyroglobulin test.

Reference: Radiopharmaceuticals in Nuclear Medicine Practice, Kowalski and Perry, 1987.

REFERENCES

1. Nickel RA. Radiopharmaceuticals. In: Early PJ, Sodee DB, eds. Principles and Practice of Nuclear Medicine, 2nd ed. St. Louis: Mosby, 1995;94–117.
2. Srivastava S, Dadachova E. Recent advances in radionuclide therapy. Semin Nucl Med 2001;31:330–341.
3. Silberstein EB, Ryan J, et al. Prevalence of adverse reactions in nuclear medicine. J Nucl Med 1996;37(1):185–192.
4. Early PJ. Methods of radioactive decay. In: Early PJ, Sodee DB, eds. Principles and Practice of Nuclear Medicine, 2nd ed. St. Louis: Mosby, 1995;23–49.
5. Shaw SM. Diagnostic imaging and pharmaceutical care. Am J Pharm Ed 1994;58:190–193.
6. de Jong, Kwekkeboom D, Valkema R, Krenning EP. Radiolabeled peptides for tumour therapy: current status and future directions. Plenary Lecture at the EANM 2002. Eur J Nucl Med Mol Imag 2003;30:463–469.
7. Carlsson J, Aronsson EF, Hietala S-O, et al. Tumour therapy with radionuclides: assessment of progress and problems. Radiother Oncol 2003;66:107–117.
8. Goodwin DA, Meares CF. Advances in pretargeting biotechnology. Biotechnol Adv 2001;19:435–450.
9. Lupetti A, Nibbering PH, Welling MM, Pauwels EKJ. Radiopharmaceuticals: new antimicrobial agents. Trends Biotechnol 2003;21:70–73.
10. U. S. Pharmacopeia 27–National Formulary 22. U.S. Pharmacopeial Convention, Rockville, MD, 2003.
11. Volkert WA, Hoffman TJ. Therapeutic radiopharmaceuticals. Chem Rev 1999;99:2269–2292.
12. Landesberg G, Mosseri M, Wolf YG, et al. Preoperative thallium scanning, selective coronary revascularization, and long-term survival after major vascular surgery. Circulation 2003;108:177–183.
13. Kang TI, Brohpy P, Hickeson M, et al. Targeted radiotherapy with submyeloablative doses of ^{131}I-MIBG is

effective for disease palliation in highly refractory neuroblastoma. J Ped Hematol Oncol 2003;25:769–773.
14. Bomanji JB, Wong W, Gaze MN, et al. Treatment of neuroendocrine tumors in adults with ^{131}I-MIBG therapy. Clin Oncol 2003;15:193–198.
15. Bouziotis P, Fani M, Archimandritis SC, et al. Samarium-153 and technetium-99m-labeled monoclonal antibodies in angiogenesis for tumor visualization and inhibition. Anticancer Res 2003;23:2167–2171.
16. Liepe K, Kropp J, Runge R, Kotzerke J. Therapeutic efficiency of rhenium-188-HEDP in human prostate cancer skeletal metastases. Br J Cancer 2003;89:625–629.
17. Hoffman JM, Hanson MW, Coleman RE. Clinical positron emission tomography imaging. Radiol Clin North Am 1993;31:935–959.
18. Nuclear Pharmacy. Positron Emission Tomography: From production and distribution to drug research and clinical applications. JAPhA 2000;40(5) Supplement 1:S66–S67.
19. Gambhir SS. Molecular imaging of cancer with positron emission tomography. Nature Rev Cancer 2002;2:683–693.
20. Warburg O. The metabolism of tumors. London: A. Constable, 1930;75–327.
21. Green MA, Welch MJ. Radiopharmaceuticals for positron emission tomography (PET). In: Early PJ, Sodee DB, eds. Principles and Practice of Nuclear Medicine, 2nd ed. St. Louis: Mosby, 1995;739–751.
22. Jerusalem G, Hustinx R, Geguin Y, Fillet G. PET scan imaging in oncology. Eur J Cancer 2003;39:1525–1534.
23. Romer W, Schwaiger M. Positron emission tomography in diagnosis and therapy monitoring of patients with lymphoma. Clin Positron Imag 1998;1:101–110.
24. Park HM, Duncan K. Nonradioactive pharmaceuticals in nuclear medicine. J Nucl Med Technol 1994;22:240–248.

25. Stabin MG. Developments in the internal dosimetry of radiopharmaceuticals. Radiat Prot Dosimetry 2003;105:575–580.

26. http://www.bpsweb.org/write.Exam.Questions/Content.Nuclear.shtml.

27. Rhodes BA, Hladik WB III, Norenberg JP. Clinical radiopharmacy: principles and practices. Semin Nucl Med 1996;26(2):77–84.

28. Hung JC, Ponto JA, Gadient KR, Frie JA, et al. Deficiencies of product labeling directions for the preparation of radiopharmaceuticals. JAPhA 2004;44:30–35.

29. Harding LK, Bossuyt A, Pellet S, Talbot JN. Recommendations for nuclear pharmacy physicians regarding breast-feeding mothers. Eur J Nucl Med 1995;22: BP17.

Products of Biotechnology

19

Chapter at a glance

The term *biotechnology* encompasses any technique that uses living organisms (e.g., microorganisms) in the production or modification of products. The classic example of biotechnologic drugs was proteins obtained from rDNA technology. However, biotechnology now encompasses the use of tissue culture, living cells, or cell enzymes to make a defined product. Foremost, recombinant DNA (rDNA) and monoclonal antibody (MAb) technologies are providing exciting opportunities for development of new pharmaceuticals and approaches to the diagnosis, treatment, and prevention of disease.

Biotechnologic products will continue to have a marked impact upon the practice of pharmacy (1). Research will continue to generate potent new medications that require custom dosing for the individual patient and concomitant pharmacists' expertise in the use of and familiarity with sophisticated drug delivery systems.

The revolution in biotechnology is a result of research advancement in intracellular chemistry, molecular biology, rDNA technology, pharmacogenomics, and immunopharmacology. Pharmacogenomics is application of genomic technology to genetic variation in response to pharmaceutical compounds. It is an emerging discipline and an outgrowth of pharmacogenetics that seeks to describe the genetic basis for interindividual differences in drug effectiveness and toxicity, using genome-wide approaches to identify genes that govern an individual's response to specific medications. The initial draft of the human genome has demonstrated that the human genome has more than 1.4 million single-nucleotide polymorphisms, with more than 60,000 of these residing in the coding regions of human genes. Some of these have already been associated with significant changes in metabolism or effects with commonly used medications. Some

genetic polymorphisms (e.g., thiopurine S-methyltransferase, CYP2D6) have a marked effect on drug pharmacokinetics, such that appropriate dosages of drugs are significantly different from traditional dosages. The ultimate goal of pharmacogenomics is to define the contributions of inherited differences in drug disposition and/or targets to drug response and thereby improve safety and effectiveness of medications through genetically guided individualized treatments.

The first of the novel **biotechnologic** pharmaceuticals were proteins, but eventually an increasing number will be smaller molecules, discovered through biotechnology-based methods that will determine just how proteins work. Clearly, biotechnology has established itself as a mainstay in pharmaceutical research and development, and new products will enter the market at an increasing pace in the future.

The transition to molecular medicine has already begun. As biotechnology advances and growing numbers of cancer-related genes are identified and cloned, some predict that therapy with biotechnology products will eventually supplant chemotherapy as the first-line treatment for many malignancies. At this writing, more than 100 gene therapy trials are in progress, and conjugate molecules genetically engineered for specific toxicity to cancer cells are also entering clinical trials.

A vast number of biotechnology-derived medications have been approved and made available since human insulin became the first therapeutic recombinant protein drug in 1982. The commercial success of biotechnology has spurred the entry of many additional products into the development pipelines. In the late 1990s it was estimated that more than 350 biotechnologic drugs were in various stages of development by more than 140 pharmaceutical and biotechnologic companies (2). It was anticipated that patients with hemophilia, serious sepsis, skin ulcers, rheumatoid arthritis, and a number of cancers would benefit in future years as drugs in clinical trials secured market approval. That has been the case, as some of those biotechnologic products are now on the market (e.g., Refacto for hemophilia, Fuzeon for HIV therapy, Kineret for rheumatoid arthritis, Xigris for severe sepsis), and it is anticipated that this trend will continue.

As of 2003, it was estimated that more than 370 biotechnology products were being developed by 144 companies and the National Cancer Institute (3). These products are intended to treat more than 200 disease states, with the largest area of concentration being drug development for cancer and its related conditions. At present, 95 biotechnology medications and vaccines on the U.S. market are benefiting more than 250 million patients (3).

This abundant activity has grown out of entrepreneurism among many small venture-funded, narrowly focused groups. Several of these small companies have by now prospered to the point of becoming fully integrated pharmaceutical companies. More than one-third of biotechnologic drugs in clinical trials are being tested for treatment of cancer, while 29 products are under development for HIV infection, AIDS, and AIDS-related diseases, and 19 other biotechnologic drugs are in development for autoimmune diseases (e.g., rheumatoid arthritis, lupus erythematosus).

Techniques Used to Produce Biotechnologic Products

Numerous techniques are used to create biotechnologic products. These include rDNA technology, MAb technology, polymerase chain reaction, gene therapy, nucleotide blockade or antisense nucleic acids, and peptide technology (4). The following section describes each of these techniques.

Recombinant DNA

DNA, deoxyribonucleic acid, has been called the substance of life. It is DNA that constitutes genes, allowing cells to reproduce and maintain life. Of more than 1 million kinds of plants and animals known today, no two are exactly alike; however, the similarity within families is the result of genetic information stored in cells, duplicated, and passed from cell to cell and from generation to generation. It is DNA that provides this continuity.

DNA was first isolated in 1869. Its chemical composition was determined in the early 1900s, and by the 1940s it had been proved that the genes within cell chromosomes are made of DNA. It was not until the 1950s, when James D. Watson and Francis H. C. Crick postulated the structure of DNA, that biologists began to comprehend the molecular mechanisms of heredity and cell regulation. Watson and Crick described their model of DNA as a double helix, two strands of DNA coiled about themselves like a spiral staircase. It is now known that the two strands of DNA are connected by the bases adenine, guanine, cytosine, and thymine (A, G, C, and T). The order of arrangement of these bases with the two strands of DNA comprise a specific gene for a specific trait. A typical gene has hundreds of bases that are always arranged in pairs. When A occurs on one strand, T occurs opposite it on the other; G pairs with C. A gene is a segment of DNA that has a specific sequence of these chemical base pairs. The pattern constitutes the DNA message for maintaining cells and organisms and building the next generation. To create a new cell or a whole new organism, DNA must be able to duplicate (clone) itself. This is done by unwinding and separating the two strands and attaching new bases to each from within the cell according to the A-T/C-G rule. The result is two new double strands of DNA, each of the same structure and conformation.

DNA also plays an essential role in the production of proteins for cellular maintenance and function. DNA is translated to messenger RNA (mRNA), which contains instructions for production of the 23 amino acids from which all proteins are made. Amino acids can be arranged in a vast number of combinations to produce hundreds of thousands of proteins. In essence, a cell is a miniature assembly plant for production of thousands of proteins. A single

Escherichia coli bacterium is capable of making about 2000 proteins.

The ability to hydrolyze selectively a population of DNA molecules with a number of endonucleases promoted a technique for joining two different DNA molecules: recombinant DNA, or *rDNA*. This technique uses other techniques (replication, separation, identification) that permit production of large quantities of purified DNA fragments. These combined techniques, referred to as *rDNA technology*, allow the removal of a specific piece of DNA out of a larger, more complex molecule. Consequently, rDNAs have been prepared with DNA fragments from bacteria combined with fragments from humans, viruses with viruses, and so forth. The ability to join two different pieces of DNA at specific sites within the molecules is achieved with two enzymes, a restriction endonuclease and a DNA ligase.

With rDNA technology, scientists can use nonhuman cells (e.g., a special strain of *E. coli*) to manufacture proteins identical to those produced in human cells. This process has enabled scientists to produce molecules naturally present in the human body in large quantities previously difficult to obtain from human sources. For example, approximately 50 cadaver pituitary glands were required to treat a single growth hormone–deficient child for 1 year until DNA-produced growth hormone became available through the new technology. Further, the biosynthetic product is freer of viral contamination than the cadaver source. Human growth hormone and insulin were the first rDNA products to become available for patients' use.

DNA probe technology is being used to diagnose disease. It uses small pieces of DNA to search a cell for viral infection or for genetic defects. DNA probes have application in testing for infectious disease, cancer, genetic defects, and susceptibility to disease. Using DNA probes, scientists can locate a disease-causing gene, which in turn can lead to development of replacement therapies. In producing a DNA probe, the initial step is synthesis of the specific strand of DNA with the sequence of nucleotides that matches those of the gene being investigated. For instance, to test for a particular virus, first the DNA strand is developed to

be identical to one in the virus. The second step is to tag the synthetic gene with a dye or radioactive isotope. When introduced into a specimen, the synthetic strand of DNA acts as a probe, searching for a matching or complementary strand. When one is found, the two hybridize, or join together. When the probe is bound to the virus, the dye reveals the location of the viral gene. If the synthetic DNA strand carries a radionuclide isotope, it will bind to the viral strand of DNA and reveal the virus through gamma ray scanning.

Monoclonal Antibodies

When a foreign body or antigen molecule enters the body, an immune response begins. This molecule may contain several different epitopes, and lines of beta lymphocytes will proliferate, each secreting an immunoglobulin (antibody) molecule that fits a single epitope.

In contrast, MAbs are produced as a result of perpetuating the expression of a single beta lymphocyte. Consequently, all of the antibody molecules secreted by a series of daughter cells derived from a single dividing parent beta lymphocyte are genetically identical. Through the development of hybridoma technology emanating from Kohler and Milstein's research (5), it became possible to produce identical monospecific antibodies in almost unlimited quantities. These are constructed by the fusion of beta lymphocytes, stimulated with a specific antigen, with immortal myeloma cells (6). The resultant hybridomas can be maintained in cultures and produce large amounts of antibodies. From these hybrid cells, a specific cell line or clone producing monospecific immunoglobulins can be selected.

A significant number of antibodies now in use belong to the immunoglobulin G (IgG) subclass. The IgG molecule has a molecular weight between 150 and 180 kD and consists of two heavy and two light polypeptide chains connected by disulfide bonds (Fig. 19.1). The heavy and the light chains can be divided into a variable and a constant domain. The constant-domain amino acid sequence is relatively conserved among immunoglobulins of a specific class (e.g., IgG, IgM). The variable domains of

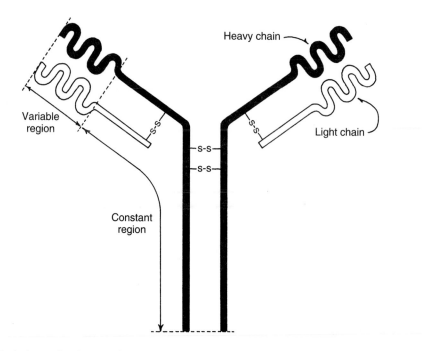

FIGURE 19.1 Basic shape of an immunoglobulin molecule akin to the class IgG, a heterogeneous population of molecules sharing a Y-shaped structure composed of a heavy and light molecular chain linked by disulfide bonds. (Illustration by Alan J. Slade.)

an antibody population are highly heterogeneous. It is the variable domain that gives the antibody its binding specificity and affinity. Thus, the antibody engineer must be cautious to maintain the tertiary structure and orientation of the complementary determining region.

Most of the MAbs in clinical trials have been derived from mice, and patients exposed to them have developed human antimouse antibody responses. This has limited the number of treatments that patients can receive. Typically, patients develop detectable antibody responses against the foreign MAb within 2 to 4 weeks. If the patient receives additional doses of the antibody, a typical allergic reaction is elicited (chills, urticaria, wheezing) and the antibody is rapidly cleared from the serum. In response to this problem, antibody therapy now includes a variety of molecules apart from the conventional immunoglobulin molecule.

Recent advances in understanding of immunoglobulin structure through three-dimensional studies using nuclear magnetic resonance, x-ray crystallography, and increased

computer-assisted molecular modeling capabilities combined with recombinant approaches has led to the evolution of a new class of antibodylike molecules, or *man-made antibodies* (7). Consequently, chimeric and humanized antibodies have been constructed to overcome the lack of intrinsic antitumor activity and the immunogenicity of many murine MAbs. These MAbs retain the binding specificity of the original rodent antibody determined by the variable region but have the potential to activate the human immune system through their human constant region.

As an example, smaller fragments that contain intact immunoglobulin-binding sites, such as F[ab′]$_2$ and Fab′, do not contain the lower binding domain of the molecule (Fig. 19.2). A smaller molecule will tend to be less immunogenic when administered systemically and is more likely to have a greater tumor penetration than a larger structure (8). Also, in diagnostic imaging applications, smaller fragments have demonstrated greater renal, biliary, and colonic uptake at 24 hours than the whole

IgG, because of filtering by the kidneys and excretion via the biliary system of small protein compounds. All three smaller antibody forms have had success at detecting smaller (< 2 cm) lesions not seen on computed tomography (CT) and are superior to the IgC anticarcinoembryonic antigen antibody.

Another example is the smaller Sfv molecule, which contains the heavy and light chains of the binding sites joined by the shorter link (Fig. 19.2). These molecules also have been engineered to attach toxins, cytokines, radiolabeled elements, or genes, thus broadening their ability as delivery vehicles for cancer therapy.

Theoretically, when coupled with a drug molecule, radioactive isotope, or toxin, a MAb can target the desired cells or tissues with great precision. Initially, however, most MAbs did not reach the target tumor cells (e.g., less than 0.1% locates in tumor tissue). A number of barriers impeded antibody distribution within tumors. These include tortuous vasculature, increased hydrostatic pressure within the tumors, and heterogeneity of antigen distribution within tumors. Indeed, if antibodies did reach their intended target, there was little evidence that they could efficiently mediate *in vivo* antibody-dependent cytotoxicity. For this to occur, effector cells, such as macrophages, natural killer cells, or cytotoxic T cells, must be activated by the tumor.

Consequently, one advance has been the engineering and development of bispecific antibodies, which consist of two antibodies with specificity for distinct antigens and immune effector cells. Bispecific antibodies can circumvent the T-cell receptor specificity for one antigen by binding to an activating epitope on the T cell. This provides the T cell with an alternative specificity.

Another approach to activate the immune system is to link the antibody with a superantigen (e.g., staphylococcal enterotoxin A). These toxins are capable of binding directly to macrophages and activating them. For example, if the superantigen is linked to an antibody structure with specificity for a tumor-associated antigen, it targets the activated macrophage to the tumor cell. Both of these research approaches are undergoing Phase I studies.

Polymerase Chain Reaction

Polymerase chain reaction is a biotechnologic process whereby there is substantial amplification (more than 100,000-fold) of a target nucleic acid sequence (a gene). This enzymatic reaction occurs in repeated cycles of a three-step process. First, DNA is denatured to separate the two strands. Next, a nucleic acid primer is hybridized to each DNA strand at a specific location within the nucleic acid sequence. Finally, a DNA polymerase enzyme is added for extension of the primer along the DNA strand to copy the target nucleic acid sequence.

Each cycle duplicates the DNA molecules. This cycle is repeated until sufficient DNA sequence material is copied. For example, 20

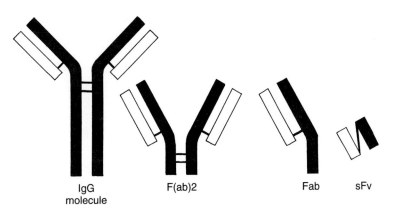

IgG
molecule   F(ab)2   Fab   sFv

FIGURE 19.2 An IgG molecule and its fragments. (Illustration by Alan J. Slade.)

cycles with a 90% success rate will yield 375,000 amplification of a DNA sequence.

Gene Therapy

Gene therapy is a process in which exogenous genetic material is transferred into somatic cells to correct an inherited or acquired gene defect (9). Also, it is intended to introduce a new function or property into cells. These common and life-threatening diseases include cystic fibrosis, hemophilia, sickle cell anemia, and diabetes.

Scientific technology has developed safe and efficient means to transfer genes into cells. Consequently, genetic and molecular delineation of the underlying pathophysiology of many of the primary immunodeficiency disorders has occurred, and gene-based therapy is now a viable option as long as the transferred genetic material can be delivered to the appropriate target cell or tissue.

Controversial ethical considerations over genetic intervention of germ line cells has fostered bioengineering to focus on gene therapy of somatic cells. Because somatic cells are end-stage differentiated cells, research has examined the use of a self-renewing stem cell population for therapeutic transfer of genetic material. Stem cells can renew themselves, and the inserted gene will remain in place through subsequent generations of differentiated cells or tissue populations.

As an example, a patient's cells (e.g., T lymphocytes) are harvested and grown in the laboratory. The cells receive the gene from a viral carrier (e.g., Moloney murine leukemia virus) and start to produce the missing protein necessary to correct the deficiency. These cells with the extra functional gene are then returned to the patient, and the normal protein is produced and released, alleviating the disease.

The genetic cause of numerous primary immunodeficiency disorders has been discovered and described. As a result, gene therapy can now be used as an alternative therapy, particularly in patients for whom bone marrow transplantation may not be suitable (e.g., a bone marrow donor cannot be identified or preparation for transplantation carries sub-stantial risk to the patient). The first primary immunodeficiency disease to be defined was adenosine deaminase deficiency (ADA). The gene encoding for ADA is found on chromosome 20. Gene deletions and point mutations result in a loss or severe reduction in ADA enzymatic activity, leading to a clinical presentation of severe combined immunodeficiency disease (SCID) and often causing death in childhood or adolescence.

The first human protocol for gene therapy was performed in ADA patients in 1990 at the National Institutes of Health. Since that time, the genetic defects of several other primary immunodeficiency disorders have been defined, and the defects have been at least partially corrected by gene therapy using hemopoietic stem cells in vitro. For SCID and other diseases, gene therapy is lifesaving (8).

Nucleotide Blockade/Antisense

Nucleotide blockade and antisense technology focuses on the study of function of specific proteins and intracellular expression. The sequence of a nucleotide chain that contains the information for protein synthesis is called the sense sequence. The nucleotide chain that is complementary to the sense sequence is called the antisense sequence. Antisense drugs recognize and bind to the nucleotide sense sequence of specific mRNA molecules, preventing synthesis of unwanted proteins and actually destroying the sense molecules in the process.

The introduction of antisense nucleic acids into cells has provided new ideas to explore how proteins, whose expression has been selectively repressed in a cell, function within that cell. Another goal is to arrest the expression of dysfunctional mRNA or DNA and control disease processes. Antisense technology is part of a new approach termed *reverse genetics*.

Antisense RNA, for example, can be introduced into the cell by cloning. The specific gene of interest is cloned in an expression vector in the wrong orientation so that complementary mRNA is created to match abnormal mRNA. Then when the two mRNA strands complex together, translation of the mRNA to form disease-producing proteins is prevented. Anti-DNA strands also can be created to complex with DNA to form a triple helix. Oligonucleotides, or short single strands of nucleic acids, instead of the full mRNA also can be employed to block RNA expression. This form of biotechnology is being used for viral disease (e.g., herpes simplex, HIV) and cancer (oncogenes).

Peptide Technology

Peptide technology entails screening for polypeptide molecules that can mimic larger proteins. This is intended to afford relatively simple products that can be stable and easy to produce. These peptides can serve as either protein receptor agonists or antagonists.

Products of Biotechnology

Biotechnologic drugs fall into major classes, such as antisense, clotting factors, hematopoietic factors, hormones, interferons, interleukins, MAbs, tissue growth factors, and vaccines. Biotechnologic drugs are distinguished by whether they are physiologic or nonphysiologic peptides or new biotechnology products.

Physiologic peptides can be further subdivided by intended use. For example, those for substitution include clotting factors, insulin, human growth hormone, and erythropoietin. Biotechnologic products intended for therapeutic purposes in nonphysiologic concentrations include interferons, cytokines, tissue plasminogen activator, and urokinase. Nonphysiologic peptides include mutants of physiologic peptides, vaccines, thrombolytic agents, and antithrombics.

The following sections describe by classification products of biotechnology that have been approved by the FDA or are being developed for submission for approval (Table 19.1). The section describing indication also lists in brackets for some biotechnology drugs and products proposed uses under the Orphan Drug Act. (The FDA Office of Orphan Products Development provides an information packet that includes an overview of the FDA's orphan drug program, a brief description of the orphan products grant program and a current list on designated orphan products.)

Anticoagulant Drug: Lepirudin (Refludan)

Lepirudin (rDNA), a recombinant hirudin derived from yeast cells, is a highly specific direct inhibitor of thrombin. It is the first of the hirudin class of anticoagulants. The polypeptide is composed of 65 amino acids and has a molecular weight of 6979.5 D. Natural hirudin is produced in trace quantity as a family of highly homologous isopolypeptides by the leech *Hirudo medicinalis*. Biosynthetic lepirudin is identical to natural hirudin except for substitution of a leucine molecule for isoleucine at the N-terminal end of the molecule and the absence of a sulfate group on the tyrosine molecule at position 63.

The activity of this anticoagulant is measured in a chromogenic assay. One antithrombin unit (ATU) is the amount of lepirudin that neutralizes one unit of World Health Organization (WHO) preparation 89/588 of thrombin. The specific activity of lepirudin is about 16,000 ATU/mg. One molecule of lepirudin binds to one molecule of thrombin and blocks its activity.

Lepirudin is indicated for heparin-induced thrombocytopenia (HIT) and associated thromboembolic disease to prevent further thromboembolic complications. The formation of antihirudin antibodies have been observed in approximately 40% of HIT patients treated with the drug. This ultimately may increase the anticoagulant effect of the lepirudin because of delayed renal elimination of active lepirudin–antihirudin complexes.

Initial dosage for anticoagulation in patients with HIT and associated thromboembolic disease is 0.4 mg/kg (≤110 kg) slowly intravenously (e.g., over 15–20 seconds) as a bolus dose followed by 0.15 mg/kg (≤110 kg/hour) as a continuous intravenous infusion for 2 to 10 days or longer if clinically necessary. The initial dose depends on the patient's weight and is valid up to 110 kg. For those who weigh more than 110 kg, the dose should not be increased beyond that for 110 kg body weight. The maximum initial bolus dose is 44 mg, and the maximal infusion dose is 16.5 mg/hour.

Therapy with lepirudin is monitored using

TABLE 19.1 REPRESENTATIVE BIOTECHNOLOGY PRODUCTS IN USE IN THE UNITED STATES

GENERIC NAME	TRADE NAME (MANUFACTURER)	INDICATIONS [PROPOSED USE]a
Aldesleukin	Proleukin (Chiron)	Metastatic renal cell carcinoma, melanoma; primary immunodeficiency disease of T-cell defects
Alteplase	Activase (Genentech)	Ischemic stroke
Conjugate vaccine HibTITER	PedvaxHIB	Routine immunization of children aged 2–71 months against HIB
Efavirenz	Sustiva (Dupont)	Treatment of HIV-1 in combination with 2, 3, or 4 other anti-HIV drugs
Epoetin alpha	Epogen (Amgen), Procrit	Certain anemias; chronic renal disease; AIDS; cancer chemotherapy; [anemia associated with end-stage renal disease or HIV infection or treatment; myelodysplastic syndrome; anemia of prematurity in preterm infants]
Filgrastim G-CSF	Neupogen (Amgen)	Decrease incidence of infection (febrile neutropenia) in nonmyeloid malignancies treated with myelosuppressive drugs. Reduce duration of neutropenia, neutropenia-related sequelae in nonmyeloid malignancies treated with myeloablative chemotherapy followed by bone marrow transplant. [Severe chronic neutropenia (absolute neutrophil count $<500/mm^3$); neutropenia of bone marrow transplant; CMV retinitis of AIDS treated with ganciclovir; mobilization of peripheral blood progenitor cells for collection prior to myeloablative or myelosuppressive chemotherapy; reduce duration of neutropenia, fever, antibiotic use, hospitalization following induction, consolidation for acute myeloid leukemia.]
Fomivirsen	Vitravene (Isis/Ciba)	Local treatment of CMV in AIDS patients who are intolerant of or have a contraindication to other treatments for CMV retinitis or have not responded to other treatments for CMV.
Haemophilus B conjugate vaccine	Act-HIB (Connaught)	Routine immunization of children against invasive diseases of HIB
Hepatitis B vaccine	Engerix-B (Smith Kline Beecham), Recombivax HB (MSD)	Hepatitis B prophylaxis
Human growth hormone	Protropin (Genentech), Humatrope (Lilly)	Human growth hormone deficiency in children
Human insulin	Humulin (Lilly), Rapid, Velosulin (Novo Nordisk)	Insulin-dependent diabetes mellitus
Imciromab pentetate	Myoscint (Centocor)	[Detection of early necrosis as indication of rejection of orthotopic cardiac transplant]
Infliximab	Remicade (Centocor)	Active and fistulizing Crohn's disease
Interferon a-2a	Referon A (Hoffman LaRoche)	Hairy cell leukemia, AIDS-related Kaposi's sarcoma
Interferon a-2b	Intron A (Schering-Plough)	Hairy cell leukemia; AIDS-related Kaposi's sarcoma; chronic hepatitis B and C (non-A, non-B); condylomata acuminata

(continued)

TABLE 19.1 REPRESENTATIVE BIOTECHNOLOGY PRODUCTS IN USE IN THE UNITED STATES

GENERIC NAME	TRADE NAME (MANUFACTURER)	INDICATIONS [PROPOSED USE]a
Interferon a-n3	Alferon N (Interferon Sciences)	Condylomata acuminata
Interferon B	Betaseron (Berlex)	Multiple sclerosis
Interferon y-1b	Actimmune	Chronic granulomatous disease
Muromonab-CD3	Orthoclone (Ortho), OKT 3 (Biotech)	Acute allograft rejection in renal transplant patients
Recombinant Factor VIII	Kogenate (Miles), Recombinate (Baxter)	Hemophilia A
Rituximab	Rituxan (IDEC/Genentech)	Relapsed or refractory low-grade or follicular CD20-positive beta-cell non-Hodgkin's lymphoma
Sargramostim (GM-CSF)	Leukine (Immunex), Prokine (Hoechst-Roussel)	Myeloid reconstitution after bone marrow transplantation [Leukine: Neutropenia of bone marrow transplant, graft failure, delay of engraftment, promotion of early engraftment; reduce neutropenia, leukopenia; decrease incidence of death from infection in AML]
Satumomab pendetide	OncoScint CR/OV (Cytogen)	Detection of ovarian carcinoma
Somatropin	Genotropin (Genentech), Humatrope (Lilly), Norditropin (Novo Nordisk),	[Long-term treatment of children with growth failure of inadequate endogenous growth hormone; growth failure in children with inadequate growth hormone; idiopathic or organic growth hormone deficiency in children with growth failure; enhancement of nitrogen retention in hospitalized patients with severe burns; short stature in Turner's syndrome; adults with growth hormone deficiency]
Somatropin for injection	Humatrope (Lilly), Nutropin (Genentech), Serostim (Seronol)	Long-term treatment for growth failure in children who lack endogenous growth hormone secretion. [Long-term treatment of children with growth failure of inadequate secretion of normal endogenous growth hormone; short stature in Turner's syndrome; growth retardation in chronic renal failure; catabolism/weight loss in AIDS; children with AIDS-associated failure to thrive, including wasting; replacement therapy for growth hormone deficiency in adults with epiphyseal closure.]
Tissue plasminogen activator (t-PA, Alteplase)	Activase (Genentech)	Management of acute myocardial infarction (AMI) in adults to improve ventricular function, reduce incidence of CHF, mortality of AMI. Management of acute ischemic stroke in adults to improve neurologic recovery, reduce disability. Management of acute massive PE, lysis of acute PE, defined by obstruction of blood flow to a lobe or multiple segments of the lungs, and for lysis of PE with unstable hemodynamics.
Tissue plasminogen activator (t-PA) [Nonglycosylated deletion mutein]	Retavase (Boehringer-Mannheim)	Management of AMI in adults to improve ventricular function following AMI, reduce incidence of CHF, reduce mortality of AMI.

(continued)

TABLE 19.1 REPRESENTATIVE BIOTECHNOLOGY PRODUCTS IN USE IN THE UNITED STATES

GENERIC NAME	TRADE NAME (MANUFACTURER)	INDICATIONS [PROPOSED USE][a]
Trastuzumab	Herceptin (Genentech)	Treatment of metastatic breast cancer or cancer spread beyond breast and lymph nodes under arm. Used alone in patients with primary failure with other chemotherapies or as a first-line treatment of metastatic disease in combination with paclitaxel

[a]Listing includes proposed uses for orphaned drugs in [brackets]. The Orphan Drug Act defines an orphan drug as a drug or biologic product for the diagnosis, treatment, or prevention of a rare disease or condition. A rare disease is one that affects fewer than 200,000 persons in the United States or more than 200,000 persons but without reasonable expectation that the cost of developing and marketing the drug will be recovered from sales in the United States.

the activated partial thromboplastin time (aPTT) at a given time over a reference value, usually median of the laboratory normal range. The patient's baseline aPTT should be determined prior to administration of the drug because lepirudin should not be given to patients with a baseline aPTT ratio of 2.5 or more to avoid initial overdosing.

Lepirudin powder for injection (Refludan) 50 mg should be reconstituted only with water for injection, 0.9% sodium chloride injection, or 5% dextrose injection. For rapid complete reconstitution, 1 mL of diluent is injected into the vial and the vial shaken gently. After reconstitution, a clear, colorless solution is obtained in no more than 3 minutes.

The reconstituted solution should be used immediately, and it remains stable for 24 hours at room temperature (e.g., during infusion). Prior to administration, it should be warmed to room temperature.

Antisense Drugs

Fomivirsen Sodium (Vitravene)

Fomivirsen sodium injectable is an antisense drug approved for local treatment of cytomegalovirus (CMV) in patients with AIDS who are intolerant of or have a contraindication to other treatments for CMV retinitis. Also, it may be used after other treatment fails.

CMV is an extremely common virus that ultimately infects most people and remains latent (present but not active, as with chickenpox). Although overt disease is uncommon in people

with fully intact immune systems, CMV can be serious in those with impaired immune systems. One of the most serious and debilitating CMV infections is CMV retinitis, which results in gradual destruction of the light-sensitive tissues of the eye. CMV retinitis is the most common cause of blindness in persons with AIDS and other immunosuppressed states.

Fomivirsen sodium, a phosphorothioate oligonucleotide, is administered by direct injection into the vitreous body (the transparent gelatinous mass filling the eyeball behind the lens) of the eye. This oligonucleotide is targeted specifically to the CMV genetic information so that it can shut down the CMV virus but not interfere with the functioning of human DNA.

Two induction doses of the drug are injected into the eye under local anesthesia on days 1 and 15, followed by a monthly injection of 330 μg. This is advantageous for the management of CMV retinitis because it obviates intravenous therapies. Also, it may offer avoidance of surgical implants and their complications and less frequency of intravitreal injections than other antiviral compounds, and it may be a suitable adjunct to oral ganciclovir therapy.

Efavirenz (Sustiva)

Efavirenz is a nonnucleoside reverse transcriptase inhibitor and the first anti-HIV drug to be approved by the FDA for once-daily dosing in combination with other anti-HIV drugs.

Clinical trials demonstrated that efavirenz reduces plasma viral RNA to below quantifiable levels in a majority of HIV-1-infected naive and treatment-experienced individuals in two-, three-, and four-drug combinations.

Efavirenz is available as an oral capsule and can be taken once a day with or without meals. However, it is advised that it not be administered with high-fat meals, since this interaction may increase the drug's systemic absorption.

Clotting Factors

Hemophiliacs bleed internally because of a lack of clotting protein factors. Historically, treatment has been infusions of protein derived from human blood. Now, genetic engineering can create, without donor blood, factors that produce more nearly contaminant free products and therefore expose the patient to fewer contaminants.

Systemic Antihemophilic Factors (Kogenate, Recombinate)

Recombinant antihemophilic factor (AHF) is indicated for treatment of classical hemophilia A, in which there is a demonstrated deficiency of activity of plasma clotting factor (factor VIII). Human recombinant AHF (rAHF) is a sterile, nonpyrogenic concentrate with biologic and pharmacokinetic activity comparable to that of plasma-derived AHF. Additional clinical trials are being conducted to determine whether antibodies to rAHF form more often than with plasma-derived products (10).

rAHF contains albumin as a stabilizer and trace amounts of mouse, hamster, and bovine proteins. These new products are made by modifying hamster cells so that they produce a highly purified version of AHF factor VIII (10).

Each vial of AHF is labeled with the AHF activity expressed in international units (IU). The assignment of potency is referenced to the WHO International Standard. One IU of factor VIII activity, approximately equal to the AHF activity of 1 mL of fresh plasma, increases the plasma concentration of factor VIII by 2%. The specific factor VIII activity ranges from 2 to 200 AHF IU per milligram of total protein.

The dose–response relation is linear, with an approximate yield of a 2% rise in factor VIII activity for each unit of factor VIII per kilogram transfused. The following formulas provide a guide for dosing calculations:

$$\text{Expected factor VIII increase (\% normal)} = \frac{\text{dose AHF/IU administered} \times 2}{\text{body weight (kg)}}$$

$$\text{AHF/IU required} = \text{body weight (kg)} \times \text{desired factor VIII increase (\% normal)} \times 0.5$$

Kogenate is available in strengths of 250 IU (with 2.5 mL sterile water for injection provided as diluent), 500 IU (with 5 mL sterile water for injection provided as diluent), and 1000 IU (with 10 mL sterile water for injection provided as diluent). Each strength contains between 2 and 5 mmol of calcium chloride, 100 to 130 mEq/L of sodium, 100 to 130 mEq/L of chloride, 4 to 10 mg/mL of human albumin, and nanogram quantities of foreign protein (mouse, hamster) per international unit. Kogenate is supplied in a single-dose vial along with the diluent, a sterile filter needle, and a sterile administration set.

Recombinate is available in strengths of 250, 500, and 1000 IU, each with 10 mL sterile water for injection provided as diluent. Each strength contains 12.5 mg/mL of human albumin, 180 mEq/L of sodium, 200 mEq/L of calcium, and a small quantity of foreign protein.

Dry concentrates of rAHF should be stored at 2°C to 8°C (35°–46°F), and the diluent protected from freezing. Kogenate may be stored at room temperatures not exceeding 25°C for 3 months. After reconstitution, the solution should not be refrigerated.

The diluent and dry concentrate should be brought to room temperature (approximately 25°C) prior to reconstitution. These may be allowed to warm to room temperature, or in an emergency warmed via water bath to a range of 30 to 37°C (86°–98.6°F). Once reconstituted, the solution should not be shaken, because shaking could make it foam. The solution should be administered within 3 hours of reconstitution and any partially used vial discarded. This preparation should be administered alone through a separate line, without mixing with other intravenous fluids or medications.

Kogenate may be administered intravenously over 5 to 10 minutes and Recombinate up to 10 mL per minute. The comfort of the patient should guide the rate at which rAHF is administered. If a significant increase in pulse rate occurs, the infusion should be slowed or halted until the pulse rate returns to normal. The risk of an allergic reaction to product proteins (mouse, hamster, bovine) may be present in the MAb-derived and rAHF products.

Recombinant Factor VIII (ReFacto)

Approved for clinical use in March 2000, recombinant factor VIII is indicated for control and prevention of bleeding episodes and surgical prophylaxis to reduce the frequency of spontaneous bleeding episodes (Fig. 19.3). This product is the only factor VIII product indicated for short-term routine prophylaxis.

Hemophilia A is the most common form of hemophilia, an inherited blood disorder. Approximately, 17,000 American patients have a hemophilia A. This form of the disease is the result of deficiency in blood clotting factor VIII.

Recombinant technology allows preparation of clotting factors without human blood or plasma products. This eliminates the risk of blood-borne viral contamination associated with nonrecombinant factor VIII products

prepared from pooled human blood. Also, ReFacto does not contain human serum albumin, whereas previously approved recombinant products (e.g., Kogenate, Bayer) add albumin during the cell culture phase and during the final product formulation. This procedure theoretically increases the possibility of viral contamination in the final product.

Adverse effects of the administration of this product include headache, fever, chills, flushing, nausea, vomiting, lethargy, and allergic reactions. These adverse effects are quite common with intravenously administered recombinant protein products.

Colony-Stimulating Factors

Colony-stimulating factors (CSFs) are four glycoprotein regulators that bind to specific surface receptors and control the proliferation and differentiation of marrow cells into macrophages, neutrophils, basophils, eosinophils, platelets, or erythrocytes (11, 12). These recombinant human CSFs have potential for wide use in oncology (e.g., chemotherapy-induced leukopenia, cancer patients having marrow transplants), inherited disorders (e.g., congenital neutropenia) and infectious disease (e.g., AIDS) (13). Patients with low amounts of endogenous CSFs are prone to secondary infections because of diminished resistance associated with some forms of cancer or more commonly, suppressed marrow function after the use of myelotoxic chemotherapy.

In the absence of pluripotent *stem cells* (an uncommitted cell with the potential to become any cell of the blood), the CSFs cannot be expected to stimulate cell formation and the development of neutrophils. Furthermore, the effectiveness of the CSFs can be expected to be directly related to the absolute numbers of these potential target cells. For example, cancer patients with bone marrow severely depleted by chemotherapy may not respond as well to CSF therapy as cancer patients with normal hemopoietic tissues.

If patients with neutropenia develop an infection, they cannot defend themselves against it because neutrophils are the body's initial defense mechanism. If neutrophils are absent or

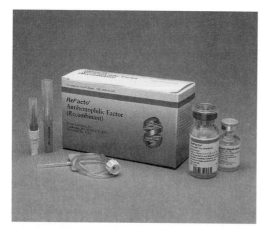

FIGURE 19.3 The product package of ReFacto. (Courtesy of Genetics Institute.)

in very low numbers, the classic signs and symptoms of infection (swelling, pain, redness, heat, purulent discharge) are absent. Neutrophils cause these signs and symptoms, and if they are not present in sufficient numbers, only a fever—with or without sore throat—may signal a serious infection. Thus, a body temperature that exceeds 38°C (100.5°F) is a serious occurrence in a patient who has undergone chemotherapy within the past 3 or 4 weeks.

Granulocyte Colony–Stimulating Factor (Filgrastim)

Produced by rDNA technology, this drug stimulates the production of neutrophils in the bone marrow. It is approved for chemotherapy-related neutropenia and is indicated (to decrease the incidence of infection, as manifested by febrile neutropenia) in patients with nonmyeloid malignancies who are receiving myelosuppressive anticancer drugs and exhibiting severe neutropenia with fever. This drug can also be used as an adjunct to myelosuppressive cancer chemotherapy to help speed the recovery of neutrophils after treatment and to reduce serious infection risk.

For chemotherapy-induced neutropenia, filgrastim is administered intravenously (short infusion, 15–30 minutes), as a subcutaneous bolus or continuous intravenous or subcutaneous injection, in a starting dose of 5 µg/kg once daily, beginning no earlier than 24 hours after administration of the last dose of cytotoxic chemotherapy. This regimen is continued for up to 2 weeks, until the absolute neutrophil count reaches 10,000/mm³ following the *nadir* (the lowest neutrophil count, usually occurring 7–10 days after chemotherapy).

Filgrastim injection contains no preservative and should be stored at 2° to 8°C. It is not to be frozen. Before use, the injection may be allowed to reach room temperature for a maximum of 24 hours, after which time it should be discarded. A clear, colorless solution, it should be inspected visually prior to injection. This product is supplied as a 1-mL or 1.6-mL single-dose vial (Fig. 19.4).

Filgrastim is supplied in boxes containing 10 glass vials, which are packaged in a gel-ice in-

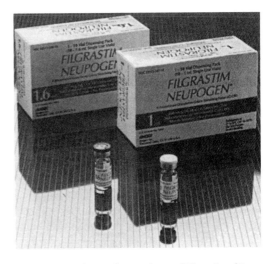

FIGURE 19.4 The product package of Filgrastim. (Courtesy of Amgen, Inc.)

sulating container with a temperature indicator to detect freezing. For convenience and to minimize the risk of breakage, filgrastim should be dispensed to the patient in its original packaging and the patient instructed to refrigerate the product promptly after arriving home.

If the patient has to travel a considerable distance or the outside temperature is high, it may be necessary to place the medication in a small cooler with a gel refrigerant (e.g., blue ice) for transport. It is suggested that the vials be wrapped in a towel to avoid direct contact between them and the blue ice. The drug must be physically separated from the refrigerant to prevent freezing. Dry ice should not be used because of the possibility of freezing the product through inadvertent contact.

It is conceivable that when it is used as an adjunct to cancer chemotherapy, prescriptions for this product will be written for 7 to 10 vials. Indeed, patients may have extra vials of this product at home from previous courses of cancer chemotherapy. The pharmacist should question such patients about having any unexpired, properly stored unused vials from the previous course of therapy. Filgrastim injection repackaged in 1-mL plastic tuberculin syringes stored at 2° to 8° remains sterile for 7 days.

Because granulocyte CSF (G-CSF) is a protein, it can be denatured if severely agitated. If the vial is shaken vigorously, the solution may foam or appear frothy, making withdrawal difficult. Thus, the pharmacist should instruct the patient or caregiver to avoid shaking the vial before use. If it is shaken, the vial should be allowed to stand until the froth diminishes.

If it is necessary to dilute filgrastim, use 5% dextrose injection. When filgrastim is diluted to concentrations ranging between 5 and 15 µg/mL, it should be protected from inadvertent adsorption to plastic materials by the addition of albumin (human) to a final concentration of 2 mg/mL. When diluted in 5% dextrose injection or 5% dextrose plus albumin, filgrastim is compatible with glass bottles, polyvinyl chloride and polyolefin intravenous bags, and polypropylene syringes. Filgrastim should never be diluted with saline at any time, as the product may precipitate.

The manufacturer of filgrastim has developed a step-by-step guide to subcutaneous self-injection. However, the pharmacist should always emphasize the use of proper aseptic technique when preparing and administering the drug, to avoid product contamination and possible infection.

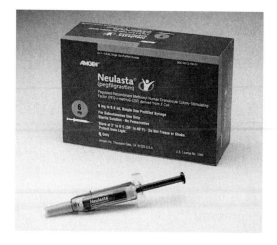

FIGURE 19.5 The product package of Pegfilgrastim. (Courtesy of Amgen, Inc.)

Granulocyte Colony Stimulating Factor and Monomethoxypolyethylene Glycol (Pegfilgrastim)

Pegfilgrastim was approved in late January 2002 by the FDA for use in conjunction with myelosuppressive anticancer drugs to decrease the incidence of infection and neutropenic fever in patients with nonmyeloid malignancies. It is marketed under the trade name of Neulasta (Fig. 19.5). It is derived by adding a 20-kD monomethoxypolyethylene glycol (PEG) molecule to the N-terminal methionine residue of filgrastim. The covalent conjugation of the recombinant human G-CSF filgrastim and PEG alters the pharmacokinetic properties of filgrastim. The pegylation of filgrastim significantly prolongs the drug's half life ($t_{1/2}$, 15–80 hours) over that of filgrastim ($t_{1/2}$, 3–4 hours) by altered clearance. As a result, it is administered as a single fixed dose of 6 mg injected per chemotherapy cycle. This is in comparison to 10 to 14 injections normally needed for filgrastim during a chemotherapy cycle. The signifi-

cantly lower number of injections required with pegfilgrastim is anticipated to increase adherence to the regimen and decrease the demands on medical personnel. Furthermore, early experience suggests that pegfilgrastim may be slightly more effective in reducing febrile neutropenia in breast cancer patients receiving docetaxel and doxorubicin.

Mild to moderate bone pain was the most frequently observed adverse effect (in 25% of patients). Nonopioid analgesics effectively manage this pain. In addition, arthralgias, myalgias, headache, leukocytosis, thrombocytopenia, and elevated function test values and lactic acid dehydrogenase were observed in patients receiving pegfilgrastim.

Pegfilgrastim should not be administered to cancer patients during the 2 weeks prior to the start of chemotherapy. Similarly, cancer patients receiving weekly chemotherapy should not receive pegfilgrastim because it can stimulate the growth of rapidly dividing hematopoietic cells, which are particularly sensitive to the cytotoxic effects of chemotherapy.

Granulocyte Macrophage Colony Stimulating Factor (Sargramostim)

Sargramostim is a recombinant human granulocyte-macrophage CSF (GM-CSF) produced by rDNA technology in a yeast (*Saccharomyces cerevisiae*) expression system. GM-CSF is a growth factor that stimulates proliferation and differentiation of hematopoietic progenitor (precursor) cells into neutrophils and monocytes. It is a glycoprotein composed of 127 amino acids. The sequence of rGM-CSF differs from the natural human GM-CSF at position 23, where leucine is substituted.

This drug is indicated for acceleration of myeloid (marrow) recovery in patients with non-Hodgkin's lymphoma (NHL), acute lymphoblastic leukemia (ALL), and Hodgkin's disease undergoing autologous bone marrow transplantation (a procedure in which the patient's bone marrow is removed, treated to destroy malignant cells, and reinfused into the patient). It is also indicated in failure of bone marrow transplantation or engraftment delay (it takes 3–4 weeks for the new marrow to begin to produce new white blood cells).

GM-CSF accelerates engraftment by promoting the production of white blood cells. Health care costs are controlled, because patients treated with it demonstrate significant earlier increases in white blood cell counts, a reduced need for antibiotics, and a shorter hospitalization. For myeloid reconstitution after autologous bone marrow transplantation, it is administered at 250 μg/m^2/day for 21 days as a 2-hour intravenous infusion beginning 2 to 4 hours after the autologous bone marrow infusion and not less than 24 hours after the last dose of chemotherapy and 12 hours after the last dose of radiation therapy. For bone marrow transplantation failure or engraftment delay, the dose remains the same, but the duration is 14 days, again using a 2-hour intravenous infusion. The dose can be repeated after 7 days of therapy if engraftment has not occurred.

To avoid complications associated with GM-CSF in terms of excessive leukocytosis (white blood cell >50,000 cells/mm^3; absolute neutrophil count, or ANC, >20,000 cells/mm^3), a complete blood count with differential is recommended twice weekly during therapy. When the ANC is above 20,000 cells/mm^3, the administration of GM-CSF should be interrupted or reduced by half.

Sargramostim is manufactured as a powder for injection, lyophilized, in preservative-free single-use vials of 250 or 500 μg. It is reconstituted with 1 mL Sterile Water for Injection, USP (without preservative). The reconstituted solution should appear clear and colorless, and will be isotonic, with a pH of 7.4 ± 0.3. During reconstitution, the Sterile Water for Injection, USP, should be directed at the side of the vial and the contents gently swirled to avoid foaming during dissolution. The product must not be shaken or vigorously agitated. It can also be diluted for intravenous infusion in 0.9% Sodium Chloride Injection, USP. If the final concentration of GM-CSF is below 10 μg/mL, human albumin (0.1%) should be added to the saline before adding GM-CSF. This prevents adsorption of the drug to the components of the drug delivery system. To create a 0.1% albumin solution, the pharmacist should add 1 mg albumin (human) per milliliter 0.9% sodium chloride injection.

An in-line membrane filter for intravenous administration of this drug should not be used. In the absence of compatibility and stability information, other medications should not be admixed to infusion solutions containing sargramostim. Only 0.9% sodium chloride injection should be used to prepare the drug for intravenous infusion.

Because this product is preservative free, it should be administered as soon as possible and within 6 hours following reconstitution or dilution for intravenous infusion.

Erythropoietins

Erythropoietin is a sialic acid–containing glycoprotein that enhances erythropoiesis by stimulating the formation of proerythroblasts and the release of reticulocytes from bone marrow. It is secreted by the kidney in response to hypoxia and transported to the bone marrow in the plasma. It resembles an endocrine hormone more than any other cytokine (14).

Anemia (a deficiency of red blood cell production) is a frequent complication of chronic renal failure, cancer, and cancer therapy. Although it is easily corrected with blood transfusions, erythropoietins are available to treat only the severest forms of anemia and not to maintain the red blood cell mass required for normal activity and well-being. As anemic patients with solid tumors often have lower serum levels of erythropoietin, correction of the erythropoietin deficiency through erythropoietin therapy may be as beneficial for these cancer patients as it has been for uremic patients (14).

Kidney disease also impairs the body's ability to produce this substance and thus results in anemia. In the past, patients received blood transfusions. However, a problem with transfusions was possible exposure to infectious agents (hepatitis, HIV). Now, genetically engineered drugs, such as epoetin alpha and darbepoeitin, are available to stimulate erythropoiesis. Although expensive, these drugs may prove beneficial for patients who require extensive transfusions because of the high cost of transfusions, the risk of infectious disease, and the consequent additional health care costs.

Epoetin Alfa (Epogen, Procrit)

Epoetin alfa, a glycoprotein produced by rDNA technology, contains 165 amino acids in an identical sequence to that of endogenous human erythropoietin. Erythropoietin also effects the release of reticulocytes from the bone marrow into the blood stream, where these mature into erythrocytes. It is approved for anemia related to cancer chemotherapy, chronic dialysis, and zidovudine (AZT) therapy.

Epoetin alfa stimulates erythropoiesis in anemic patients, dialyzed or not. The first evidence of a response to this drug is an increase within 10 days of the reticulocyte count. Coupled with this are subsequent increases in the red blood cell count, hemoglobin and hematocrit, usually within 2 to 6 weeks. Once the hematocrit reaches the suggested target range, 30 to 36%, that level can be sustained in the absence of iron deficiency and concurrent illnesses by epoetin alfa therapy.

Epoetin alfa is administered intravenously or subcutaneously at 50 to 100 IU/kg body weight three times per week. It is given intravenously to patients with available access (e.g., patients who undergo hemodialysis) and either intravenously or subcutaneously to other patients. If after 8 weeks of therapy the hematocrit has not increased at least five to six points

and is still below the target range of 30 to 36%, the dosage may be increased.

Epoetin alfa is available in 1-mL preservative-free single-dose vials (Fig. 19.6) in strengths of 2000, 3000, 4000, 10,000 and 20,000 IU/mL. Each vial contains human albumin 2.5 mg to prevent adsorptive losses. The product should be refrigerated at 2°C to 8°C and protected from freezing. The vial of epoetin alfa, recombinant injection, should not be shaken because this may denature the glycoprotein and render it biologically inactive. Each vial should be used to administer a single dose only, and any unused portion of the solution must be discarded.

The 10,000 U/mL injection is available in 2-mL multidose vials. These are preserved with 1% benzyl alcohol and contain 2.5 mg albumin (human) per milliliter. These vials should be stored at 2° to 8°C after initial entry and between doses and discarded 21 days after initial entry.

Epoetin alfa should not be administered in conjunction with other solutions. However, just before subcutaneous administration, the solution can be admixed in a syringe at a ratio of 1:1 with bacteriostatic 0.9% sodium chloride injection with benzyl alcohol 0.9%. The benzyl alcohol, a local anesthetic, may ameliorate pain associated with subcutaneous injection.

In early 2003, a counterfeit version of epoetin alpha (Procrit) was discovered. It posed a serious health threat because it contained a concentration of the active ingredient one-twentieth of the expected and was contaminated with two types of bacteria. The FDA identified three batches of the fake drug product. Ortho Biotech Products, the manufacturer of the legitimate drug, advised consumers to

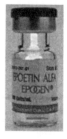

FIGURE 19.6 The product package of Epogen. (Courtesy of Amgen, Inc.)

check for differences on the packaging and vials. For example, the aluminum seal on a vial of real Procrit is smooth, not dented. Also, the closure seals on the outer carton of the real Procrit have writing on the underside and leave a residue when peeled away. In years past, counterfeit drugs were a problem in developing countries. Now, however, these drugs are becoming problematic in the United States, with the FDA investigating more than a half dozen counterfeit drug cases in 2002.

Darbepoetin Alpha (Aranesp)

Darbepoetin alfa, recombinant erythropoietic protein, was first approved for treatment of anemia associated with chronic kidney disease or CRF. It is now approved for the treatment of chemotherapy-induced anemia in patients with nonmyeloid malignancies (Fig. 19.7).

Darbepoetin alfa is an erythropoiesis-stimulating protein that is produced in Chinese hamster ovary cells by rDNA technology. It is administered intravenously or subcutaneously as a single weekly injection. The recommended starting dose for anemia in CRF patients is 0.45 μg/kg body weight. The doses are titrated not to exceed a target hemoglobin concentration of 12 g/dL. Increased hemoglobin levels are not generally observed until 2 to 6 weeks after therapy initiation. Usually, the appropriate maintenance dosage is lower than the starting dose. Once therapy is initiated, hemoglobin should be assessed weekly until it is stabilized and the maintenance dose established. After a dosage adjustment, the hemoglobin should be assessed once weekly for at least 4 weeks until it has been confirmed that the hemoglobin levels have stabilized in response to the dosage adjustment. Thereafter, the hemoglobin levels should be assessed at regular intervals.

When converting patients from epoetin alfa to darbepoetin alfa, the starting weekly dose of darbepoetin is based on the weekly epoetin alfa dose at the time of substitution. Again, the doses are titrated to maintain the target hemoglobin levels. Because of its longer serum half-life of 49 hours (range, 27–89 hours), administration of darbepoetin alfa is less frequent (once per week) compared to epoetin alfa (two to three times per week). If the patient is receiving weekly injections of epoetin alfa, the patient should receive a darbepoetin injection only every 2 weeks.

Dosage with darbepoetin must be individualized to ensure that hemoglobin levels are maintained but not to exceed 12 g/dL. For cancer patients, the recommended starting dose of darbepoetin alfa is 2.25 μg/kg administered as a weekly subcutaneous injection. Again, the dosage is adjusted to achieve and maintain the appropriate hemoglobin level.

Darbepoetin alfa is available as a solution for injection. The injection is preservative free in 1-mL single-dose vials. The polysorbate injection contains polysorbate 80, sodium phosphate monobasic monohydrate, sodium phosphate dibasic anhydrous, and sodium chloride. The albumin solution contains human albumin, sodium phosphate monobasic monohydrate, sodium phosphate dibasic anhydrous, and sodium chloride.

Prior to administration, the vial should be visually inspected for particulate matter and any discoloration. Vials demonstrating particulate matter and/or discoloration should not be used. The vial should not be shaken, as this will denature the darbepoetin and render it inactive. It should not be diluted or administered

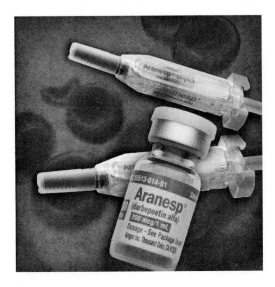

FIGURE 19.7 The product package of Aranesp. (Courtesy of Amgen, Inc.)

with other drug solutions. If there is any unused portion, it should be discarded and not pooled with other unused portions. The product should be stored in a refrigerator (2° to 8° C), not frozen, and protected from light.

Erythropoietic therapies may increase the risk of cardiovascular events, including deaths. This higher risk is associated with increased hemoglobin levels or the higher rates of hemoglobin increase. Darbepoetin alfa should not be administered to patients with uncontrolled blood pressure, as blood pressure may rise during treatment of anemia with either darbepoetin or epoetin. The most frequently reported serious adverse effects with darbepoetin were vascular access thrombosis, congestive heart failure (CHF), sepsis, and cardiac arrhythmia. The most common adverse effects are infection, hypertension, hypotension, myalgia, headache, and diarrhea. The clinician must also keep in mind adverse reactions that occur as a result of a clinical intervention (e.g., discontinuation of darbepoetin therapy, adjustment of dosage). These have included hypotension, hypertension, fever, myalgia, nausea, and chest pain.

Darbepoetin alfa is available in strengths ranging from 25 μg/mL to 500 μg/mL. The lower strengths are available as the polysorbate 80 or human albumin solution. The two highest strengths, 300 and 500 μg/mL, are available only as the albumin formulation. The 150-μg strength is available in a 0.75-mL albumin solution. The pharmacist has to be careful not to miscalculate the dosage required from the latter by assuming that the solution is 1 mL.

Drotrecogin Alfa (activated) (Xigris)

Drotrecogin alfa (activated) is recombinant human activated protein C (rhAPC). Produced naturally in the liver, protein C is converted to activated protein C (APC) through interaction with the thrombin–thrombomodulin complex. APC demonstrates antithrombotic activity through inhibition of factors Va and VIIIa (15).

Approved by the FDA in November 2001, drotrecogin alfa is indicated for a reduction of mortality in patients with severe sepsis associated with acute organ system dysfunction (Fig.

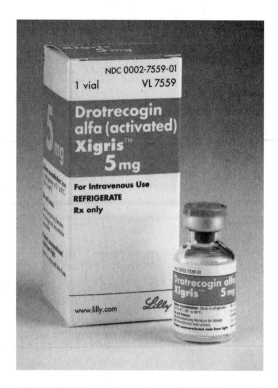

FIGURE 19.8 The product package of Xigris. (Courtesy of Eli Lilly & Co.)

19.8). Sepsis remains a significant cause of death in patients who are critically ill. It has been estimated that more than 750,000 cases of sepsis occur yearly in the United States, with a mortality rate of about 30%.

Drotrecogin alfa (activated) should be administered by continuous intravenous infusion at 24 μg/kg/hour for 96 hours. Because compatibility data are sparse, it should be administered via a dedicated line or dedicated lumen of a multilumen central venous catheter. Administration must be conducted within 12 hours of reconstitution. Periods during which the infusion is interrupted for procedures with an inherent risk of bleeding do not count toward the 96-hour duration of therapy.

Bleeding is the most common adverse effect associated with drotrecogin alfa. The incidence is approximately 3.5% (compared to 2.0% in placebo controls). Therefore, it is contraindicated when bleeding may be associated with a high risk of death (e.g., active internal bleeding, hemorrhagic stroke in the past 3 months, intracranial or intraspinal surgery, or severe head trauma within the past 2 months).

When evaluating the patient's ability to handle drotrecogin alfa (activated) therapy, the potential benefits and risks must be evaluated and carefully considered, especially if one of the following situations is present: concurrent therapeutic heparin therapy, international normalized ratio (INR) > 3.0, platelet count below $30,000 \times 10^6$/L even if the platelet count is increased after transfusions, ischemic stroke in the past 3 months, aspirin more than 650 mg/day, or other platelet inhibitors within the past 7 days.

Drotrecogin alfa (activated) therapy must be considered very carefully, especially in light of the inclusion and exclusion patient criteria, the stability and unique duration of infusion, and the cost of treatment.

Fusion Inhibitors: Enfuvirtide (Fuzeon)

Fusion inhibitors act through a unique mechanism. Enfuvirtide is a 36-amino acid synthetic peptide that corresponds to the C-terminal heptad repeat region (HR2) of the transmembrane subunit of the HIV-1 envelope surface glycoprotein gp41. Enfuvirtide binds to gp41 on the surface of the HIV and prevents the HIV from binding with T cells. Thus, it prevents the virus from infecting healthy cells. Once bound, it inhibits the conformational change in HIV-1 transmembrane glycoprotein gp41 that is required for fusion between HIV-1 and target cell membranes, blocking cell fusion and viral entry into the CD4 cell.

Approved in March 2003, enfuvirtide (known as T-20) is indicated only for patients older than 6 years who have used other anti-HIV medications and have ongoing evidence of viral replication despite ongoing antiretroviral therapy (Fig. 19.9). The dosage of enfuvirtide is 90 mg (1 mL sterile water for injection) subcutaneously twice daily into the upper arm, anterior thigh, or abdomen. Because enfuvirtide is a protein, it must be injected under the skin, making it the first injectable HIV drug. Adherence to the regimen is extremely important, as studies on antiretroviral therapy have demonstrated increased resistance unless nearly every

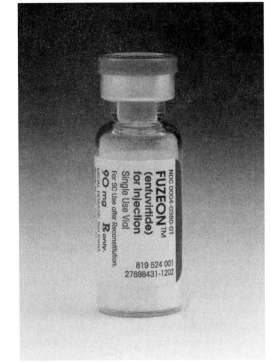

FIGURE 19.9 The product package of Fuzeon. (Courtesy of Roche/Timeris.)

dose is properly administered and on time. The goal is 100% compliance because rates of compliance less than 95% can lead to further resistance (16). If a patient misses a dose, it should be administered as soon as possible, but not if it is almost time for the next dose. In this instance, the patient should know to administer only one dose.

Enfuvirtide is metabolized to its constituent amino acids. Therefore, does not possess a drug interaction problem with other medications, nor will it induce or inhibit microsomal enzyme activity in the liver. Almost all patients (98%) have reactions at the injection site (e.g., pain on injection, erythema, induration, presence of nodules or cysts). This requires prompt discontinuation of the therapy in only 13% of patients. Other common adverse reactions include diarrhea, nausea, and fatigue.

Infections at the injection site are problematic and can be life threatening. Patients should be advised to report to their heath care provider any oozing, increased heat, swelling, redness, and/or pain at the site. Serious allergic reactions are also possible. So patients should be instructed to report any labored breathing, fever with vomiting and a skin rash, blood in the urine, and swelling of the feet.

Patient education including proper injection technique is crucial. For convenience, patients may mix both daily doses at the same time, but the second dose must be refrigerated until shortly before it is to be injected. As with insulin, it should be warmed to room temperature prior to injection. The patient should realize the importance of inspecting the injectable, and if particles are observed floating in the vial after mixing, it should not be used. Other injectable medications should not be mixed with enfuvirtide.

This drug is prescribed for patients with drug-resistant HIV infection, so the patient should understand to take precautions, discarding the syringes and needles into a sharps container. They are not to be discarded into the household garbage.

The manufacturer (Roche) reported that synthesis of this compound took 106 steps, about 10 times as many as to produce a traditional HIV drug. Because of high production costs (estimated to be more than $600 million), there is high expense associated with this product (estimated to be $20,000/year). As expected, there will be a limited supply initially. For the first year at least, the product was to be distributed through a single mail service pharmacy. Once supply demands are met, the distribution was expected to expand to all pharmacies (16).

Growth Factor: Becaplermin (Regranex)

Endogenous platelet-derived growth factor increases the proliferation of cells that repair wounds and form granulation tissue. This factor promotes the chemotactic recruitment and proliferation of cells that participate in wound repair and enhances the formation of granulation tissue.

Becaplermin is a recombinant human platelet-derived growth factor for topical adjunctive treatment of diabetes ulcers, a form of pressure ulcer, of the lower extremities that extend into subcutaneous tissue or beyond and having a sufficient blood supply. It is reasonable to assume that it may find utility as an adjunct to good pressure ulcer care.

A measured quantity of the 0.01% gel formulation is spread evenly over the ulcerated area to yield a thin, continuous sixteenth-inch thickness over the ulcerated area. The prescribed calculated length of the gel is placed on a clean, firm, nonabsorbent surface (e.g., waxed paper). A clean cotton swab, tongue depressor, or similar aid applicator is used to spread the gel over the surface of the ulcer to obtain an even layer and the ulcer is covered with a saline-moistened gauze dressing.

After approximately 12 hours, the ulcer should be gently rinsed with saline or water to remove the residual gel and covered with a saline-moistened gauze dressing without the gel for the remainder of the day. The process is repeated daily until the ulcer has healed. The ulcer should demonstrate size reduction (about 30%) within 10 weeks. If complete healing has not occurred within 20 weeks, the therapy should be reassessed. To facilitate acceptance and convenience, bedtime application can be considered.

Becaplermin gel must be refrigerated for stability but need not be allowed to come to room temperature before it is applied. However, the cold gel may cause discomfort when it is applied. The gel itself has an expiration date of 9 months from the manufacture date, but because one tube lasts for about 2 to 4 weeks, pharmacists can dispense the gel up to a month prior to its expiration date.

Human Growth Hormone

The pituitary gland secretes human growth hormone (hGH), which stimulates growth. It is estimated that approximately 15,000 American children are deficient in hGH and consequently will not achieve normal height as an adult.

In the late 1950s, cadaver pituitaries were harvested to produce hGH and treat these children. Besides the enormous expense, this method exposed the children to the risk of infection from viral contamination of the hormone (17). Genetic engineering now produces highly purified hGH.

Systemic Growth Hormone (Humatrope, Protropin)

Somatrem (Protropin) is a biosynthetic single polypeptide chain of 192 amino acids produced by rDNA in *E. coli*. This drug has one more amino acid (methionine) than natural human growth hormone. Somatropin recombinant (Humatrope), biosynthetically produced by another rDNA process, possesses amino acid sequencing identical to the naturally occurring human growth hormone (191 amino acids).

This hormone stimulates linear growth by affecting the cartilaginous growth areas of long bones. It also stimulates growth by increasing the number and size of skeletal muscle cells, influencing the size of organs, and increasing red cell mass through erythropoietin stimulation.

Somatrem for injection is initially administered intramuscularly or subcutaneously. The dosage, individualized at up to 0.1 mg/kg (0.26 IU/kg), is administered subcutaneously or intramuscularly three times a week. The 5- and 10-mg single-dose vials (Fig. 19.10) are reconstituted using standard aseptic technique with 1 to 5 mL of Bacteriostatic Water for Injection, USP (benzyl alcohol preserved) only. Because of the toxicity of benzyl alcohol in newborns, when administering to this patient population this product should be reconstituted with water for injection. The vial should then be swirled gently to dissolve the contents. If cloudy, the solution should not be used. When prepared with the manufacturer's provided diluent, the reconstituted solution should be stored in the refrigerator and used within 14 days. When water for injection is used to reconstitute this product, each vial should be used for one dose only and the unused portion discarded.

Somatropin, recombinant, for injection, is administered subcutaneously at 0.16 to 0.24 mg/kg body weight per week divided into six or seven subcutaneous injections. This drug is available in various strengths ranging from 1.5 mg (~4 IU/mL) to 10 mg (~30 IU/vial). As Genotropin, for example, the 5.8-mg Intra-Mix two-chamber cartridge (with preservative) is preassembled in a reconstitution device and packaged with a pressure release needle. The front chamber contains 1.5 mg of recombinant somatropin (approximately 4.5 IU), glycine, sodium dihydrogen phosphate anhydrous, and disodium phosphate anhydrous. The rear chamber contains 1.13 mL of water for injection. Depressing the stopper allows the two components to mix. If the diluent and somatropin are in separate vials, aseptic technique must be used to add the desired amount of diluent (1.5–5 mL) provided by the manufacturer, or sterile water for injection to a 5 mg vial. Like Somatrem, Somatropin is stable when refrigerated for up to 14 days following reconstitution with the diluent containing a preservative provided by the manufacturer. When sterile water for injection is used to reconstitute this product, each vial should be refrigerated and used within 24 hours because there is no preservative.

Interferons

In 1957, two British scientists, Alick Isaacs and Jean Lindenmann, found that infected chick embryo cells released a naturally produced glycoprotein that allowed uninfected cells to resist viral infection. They named this factor *interferon* because it appeared "to interfere with the transmission of infection." Later, these researchers demonstrated that interferon does not activate viruses directly but rendered the

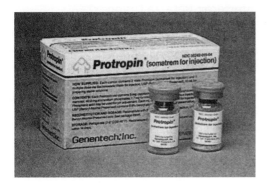

FIGURE 19.10 The product package of Protropin. (Courtesy of Genentech, Inc.)

host cells resistant to viral multiplication. Interferons exert virus-nonspecific but host-specific antiviral activity. By the mid-1970s it appeared that interferon might also curtail the spread of certain types of cancer (e.g., small cell lung cancer, renal cell carcinoma, basal cell carcinoma).

As a class, interferons are a part of the large immune regulatory network within the body that includes lymphokines, monokines, growth factors, and peptide hormones. Interferons are classified into two types, type I, alpha and beta, which share the same molecular receptor, and type II, gamma or immune, which have a different receptor (18).

Interferon Beta-1b (Betaseron)

Interferon beta-1b (IFNB) is a type I interferon made in E. coli using recombinant technology; it differs from natural interferon beta only by the substitution of a serine residue for a cysteine at position 17. This manipulation enhances the stability of the drug while retaining the specific activity of natural interferon beta.

IFNB is effective in the treatment of relapsing and remitting types of multiple sclerosis, an inflammatory demyelinating disease of the central nervous system, at 0.25 mg (8 mIU) injected subcutaneously every other day (19). This form of disease is characterized by recurrent attacks followed by complete or incomplete recovery (20).

The effectiveness of lower doses has not been documented, and there is no evidence of efficacy when this drug is used longer than 2 years.

Lyophilized IFNB (Fig. 19.11) 0.3 mg (9.6 mIU), is reconstituted using a sterile syringe and needle to inject 1.2 mL of supplied diluent (sodium chloride 0.54%) into the vial. The diluent should be added down the side of the vial and the vial then gently swirled, but not shaken, to dissolve the drug completely. After reconstitution with the accompanying diluent, the solution has a strength of 0.25 mg/mL. This product also contains dextrose and albumin (often used in recombinant protein products to prevent sorption of the product to the glass vial, plastic tubing, or syringe). Reconstituted solution 1 mL is withdrawn from the vial into

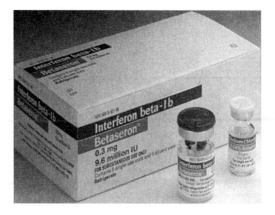

FIGURE 19.11 The product package of Betaseron. (Courtesy of Berlex, Inc.)

a sterile syringe fitted with a 27-gauge needle, and the drug is injected subcutaneously. For purposes of self-injection, the sites may include the arms, abdomen, hips, and thighs.

Because the product has no preservative, the vial is suitable for single use only. Before and after reconstitution, the product should be refrigerated. No more than 3 hours should elapse between reconstitution and use.

IFNB is distributed by a nationwide community pharmacy network called PCS Professional Service Network. The advantage of this system is that it eliminates the pharmacy's inventory and carrying costs, allows the IFNB patient to use a PCS prescription drug card, and pays the participating pharmacy a professional fee for each transaction (20). The cost of therapy was estimated to be approximately $1000 a month initially.

Interferon Beta-1a (Avonex)

Interferon beta-1A was approved for use in multiple sclerosis therapy in 1996, 3 years after interferon beta-1B was approved. It is indicated for treatment of relapsing forms of multiple sclerosis to slow the progression of physical disability and decrease the frequency of clinical exacerbations.

The dosage regimen of interferon beta-1A is 30 μg intramuscularly once per week. Its advantage over interferon beta-1B is less administration during the week. The lyophilized powder for injection is reconstituted with 1.1 mL of diluent and swirled gently to dissolve the active ingredient. The prepared product should be used as soon as possible but no later than 6 hours after reconstitution if stored at 2° to 8°C.

Vials of interferon beta-1A must be refrigerated (2° to 8°C), and if refrigeration is not available, the product can be stored at 25°C (77°F) for up to 30 days.

Interleukins

Originally, interleukins (ILs) were thought to oversee interactions between white blood cells, key components of the immune system. Now, however, it is known that these substances affect a wider variety of cell types. Most clinical interest centers on IL-1, secreted primarily by the monocyte–macrophage that activates T cells and B cells, and IL-2, secreted by the T cell that supports growth and differentiation of T cells and B cells. There are 14 known ILs.

IL-1 was discovered in 1972, and within 7 years its structure and function were delineated. It was first manufactured by rDNA technology in 1984. This substance is a key immune system regulator. It sets into motion a chain reaction that intensifies the immune response. IL-1 responds to the initial presence of an antigen. It activates T cells to mature, proliferate, and produce other *cytokines* (a generic term for soluble substances produced by cells that communicate with other cells to trigger or suppress cellular activity after interaction with an antigen).

IL-1 also intensifies the production of collagenase, prostaglandins, and antibodies. Because of this activity, excessive IL-1 is suspected to be behind many inflammatory disorders (collagenase breaks down connective tissue; prostaglandins are associated with inflammation). Patients with rheumatoid arthritis have an imbalance in which nine times as much IL-1 as IL-1a is present in the synovium. This imbalance favors agonist-derived inflammation and destruction. The cytokine may also be responsible for the fever, headache, fatigue, and weakness of influenza.

IL-2, like other cytokines, was initially greeted with much enthusiasm. Since that time it has been found to be an essential component in the development of antigen-specific and anti-gen-nonspecific immune responses but has found few applications (21). Discovered in 1976, it became available through rDNA technology in 1984. When applied to white blood cells removed from patients and then reinfused as "lymphokine-activated killer cells" along with a booster injection of IL-2, spectacular remissions occurred in some patients with devastating conditions such as advanced malignant melanoma. Unfortunately, highly toxic side effects occurred because appropriate dosing was unknown. A combination of lower doses and physician experience managing its side effects will make IL-2 safer to use in the future.

Other ILs are in the research pipeline. IL-11 is being investigated *in vitro* and in mice to stimulate platelet function. If successful, this substance could help counter the platelet-depleting effects of chemotherapeutic agents. IL-6 (also known as beta-2 interferon) may also be a stimulator of platelet growth, and it is being investigated as an antiproliferative treatment for breast, colon, and skin cancer.

Aldesleukin (Proleukin)

Aldesleukin is synthetically produced by a rDNA process involving genetically engineered *E. coli* containing an analogue of the human IL-2 gene. An expression clone that encodes a modified human IL-2 results from genetic engineering used to modify the human IL-2 gene. Aldesleukin differs from naturally occurring IL-2 in that it is not glycosylated because it is derived from *E. coli*, the molecule has no N-terminal alanine, and the molecule has serine substituted for cysteine at amino acid position 125.

Designated as an orphan drug, aldesleukin is approved for treatment of metastatic renal carcinoma (about 10,000 cases diagnosed annually) in adults (over 18 years), melanomas, and primary immunodeficiency disease associated with T-cell defects. Aldesleukin is being investigated in Phase II clinical trials for efficacy with zidovudine for HIV.

Because of its life-threatening toxicities (drug-related mortality rate is 4%), the physician should consider the benefit-to-risk ratio for the patient. The dosage of IL-2 is usually expressed in units of activity in promoting proliferation in a responsive cell line. Conversion to units from milligrams of protein varies with the source of IL-2. The strength and dosage of commercially available aldesleukin is expressed in international units; 18 million IU equals 1.1 mg protein.

For metastatic renal carcinoma, high-dose therapy involves an intravenous infusion over 15 minutes, 600,000 IU/kg of body weight (0.037 mg/kg body weight) every 8 hours for a total of 14 doses. Following a rest period of 9 days, the schedule is repeated for another 14 doses, for a maximum of 28 doses per course. The manufacturer of aldesleukin recommends that plastic bags be used as the dilution containers (as opposed to glass bottles and polyvinyl chloride bags) for more consistent drug delivery. In-line filters are not recommended because of the risk of adsorption of aldesleukin to the filter.

Each single-use vial contains 22 million IU (1.3 mg of drug) reconstituted for intravenous or subcutaneous injection by addition of 1.2 mL of sterile water for injection. The diluent should be directed to the side of the vial and the contents swirled gently to avoid foaming. The resultant solution should be clear and colorless to slightly yellow. It contains 18 million IU (1.1 mg) per milliliter. The vial should not be shaken. The appropriate dose is withdrawn, diluted in 50 mL of 5% dextrose injection, and infused over 15 minutes. Neither bacteriostatic water for injection nor 0.9% sodium chloride injection should be used to reconstitute this product because of the increased aggregation of the product.

Because the vial has no preservative, the reconstituted and diluted solutions should be refrigerated. However, it should be brought back to room temperature prior to administration. Reconstituted solutions should be used within 48 hours.

Anakinra (Kineret)

Approved in November 2001, anakinra is a recombinant IL-1 receptor antagonist. It competitively binds to the IL-1 receptor, thereby blocking the biologic action of IL-1. Anakinra is an unglycosylated form of human IL-1ra,

which occurs naturally but in insufficient amounts to compete for higher levels of IL-1 in the synovium.

Anakinra is indicated for use in patients 18 years and older who have been treated unsuccessfully with at least one disease-modifying antirheumatic drug (DMARD). It can be used as the sole agent or combined with other DMARDs except the tumor necrosis factor (TNF) α blocking agents. The safety of administering it with the latter agents has not been established.

The recommended dosage of anakinra is 100 mg/day subcutaneously. Clinical trials demonstrated a mild pain sensation at the site of injection and some inflammation, redness, and/or bruising. This drug has been associated with decreased neutrophil count in some patients and an increased incidence of infection, especially when used in conjunction with TNF-blocking agents. Thus, it should not be administered to patients with active infection. Baseline neutrophil counts should be monitored and at monthly intervals for 3 months following initial administration and then on a yearly basis.

Anakinra is packaged in single-use prefilled syringes (Fig. 19.12). These contain no preservatives and should be stored in the refrigerator and protected from light. Patients and caregivers should be educated on the importance of proper disposal and caution against the reuse of needles, syringes, and drug product. The patient should have a puncture-resistant container available for the disposal of used syringes. The cost of the drug is estimated to be $15,000/year.

Oprelvekin (Neumega)

Patients receiving chemotherapy commonly have neutropenia and thrombocytopenia. These hematologic effects make it difficult to maintain the dose and dosing schedule of the chemotherapy regimen. Managing neutropenia became easier with the approval of the CSFs filgrastim and sargramostim. However, before the approval of oprelvekin, the only treatments for chemotherapy-related thrombocytopenia were platelet transfusion or a reduction in chemotherapy dosage.

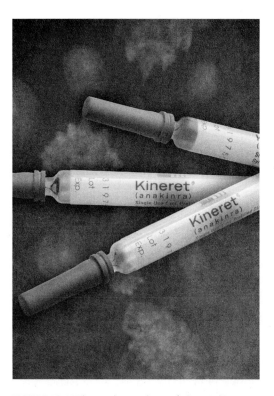

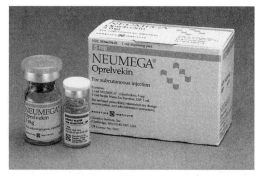

FIGURE 19.13 The product package of Neumega. (Courtesy of Genetics Institute.)

FIGURE 19.12 The product package of Kineret. (Courtesy of Amgen, Inc.)

Oprelvekin is a recombinant human IL-1l (rhIL-1l), a multifunctional cytokine used primarily as a thrombopoietic growth factor. IL-1l interacts with IL-1l receptors on the surface of myeloid progenitor cells to stimulate production of megakaryocytes and platelets.

Oprelvekin was approved specifically for prevention of severe thrombocytopenia and platelet transfusion following myelosuppressive chemotherapy in nonmyeloid malignancy patients (Fig. 19.13). Allowing the maintenance of dose intensity of chemotherapy may increase the probability that cancer patients will remain in remission for 5 years.

Oprelvekin is produced from *E. coli* by rDNA technology. It is supplied as 5 mg of lyophilized powder in a single-use vial. A 5-mL vial of sterile water for injection is supplied for reconstitution, which is confusing, because only 1 mL is needed for reconstitution. Predictably, medication errors have occurred because of overdilution of the product. The man-

ufacturer is attempting to provide a suitable preservative-free 1 mL diluent. When reconstituted appropriately, this provides a daily dose up to 50 μg/kg for a 100-kg patient. There are no preservatives in the vial, as each vial is for single use. The reconstituted solution can be stored in the vial at room temperature or under refrigeration for up to 3 hours.

Oprelvekin is administered subcutaneously as a single daily injection in the abdomen, thigh, hip, or upper arm. Oprelvekin administration should commence 6 to 24 hours after completion of chemotherapy, and platelet counts should be monitored during therapy. The drug should be discontinued when the platelet count reaches more than $50,000/mm^3$ after the nadir. Therapy typically ranges from 10 to 21 days and should be discontinued at least 2 days before the start of the next chemotherapy cycle.

Adverse effects associated with oprelvekin therapy include edema, tachycardia, palpitations, atrial fibrillation and flutter, oral moniliasis, dyspnea, pleural effusion, and conjunctival redness. Edema is a result of drug-associated renal sodium excretion, and diuretics may be used to manage fluid accumulation in some patients.

Monoclonal Antibodies

Historically, MAbs have found use in laboratory diagnostics, site-directed therapies, immunology, and home test kits (e.g., pregnancy, ovulation prediction). In the 1980s, monoclonals were expected to provide a tremendous potential for tumor therapy and immunomodulation. By coupling tracers and toxins to antibodies, tissue-selective or cell-specific targets can be attained.

In the recent past a number of monoclonals have been introduced to clinical practice. These have overcome problems that arose following immediate expectation of many being introduced to the market in the 1990s. However, as of March 1997, only seven MAb products were licensed for *in vivo* use in the United States. The advent of the 21st century has doubled the previous seven. There are three reasons proposed for this low number (22). These included (*a*) insufficient characterization of the product and its performance *in vitro*, (*b*) inadequate preclinical testing, and (*c*) unrealistic expectations of clinical performance, leading to inadequately designed clinical trials (22).

MAbs are purified antibodies produced by a single source or clone of cells (23). These substances are engineered to recognize and bind to a single specific antigen. Thus, a MAb will target a particular protein or cell having the specific matching antigenic feature. When coupled with a drug molecule, radioactive isotope, or toxin, a MAb theoretically can target the desired cells or tissues with great precision. To date, however, most of the MAb does not reach target tumor cells; less than 0.1% locates in tumor tissue.

Diagnostically, the specificity of MAbs helps to detect the presence of endogenous hormones (e.g., luteinizing hormone, human chorionic gonadotropin) in the urine to establish the test results (24). They are also used to detect allergies, anemia, and heart disease, and commercial MAb diagnostic kits are available for drug assays, tissue and blood typing, and infectious diseases including hepatitis, AIDS-related CMV, streptococcal infections, gonorrhea, syphilis, herpes, and chlamydia. When covalently linked with radioisotopes, contrast agents, or anticancer drugs, MAbs can be used to diagnose and treat malignant tumors (6).

Adalimumab (Humira)

Adalimumab was approved by the FDA in early 2003 for reducing signs and symptoms in rheumatoid arthritis patients who have not re-

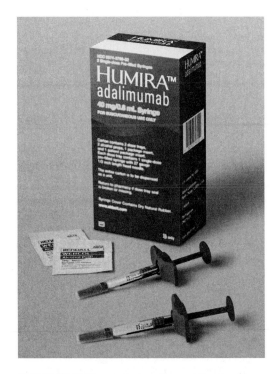

FIGURE 19.14 The product package of Humira. (Courtesy of Abbott Laboratories.)

sponded to previous treatments with methotrexate and other disease modifying anti-rheumatic drugs (DMARDs) (Fig. 19.14). Administered subcutaneously every 2 weeks, this drug now offers an attractive alternative for patients who require TNF-α blocker therapy (25). TNF is responsible for much of the pain and inflammation associated with rheumatoid arthritis.

Adalimumab was approved for monotherapy or combination treatment with methotrexate or other DMARDs. It is available as a prefilled syringe. Compared with other biologic response–modifying rheumatoid arthritis medications, it offers an easier and less frequent dosing regimen. Enbrel, another TNF-α blocker, requires twice weekly injections, and Remicade, another TNF-α blocker, requires an infusion for administration in the physician's office.

Consistent with cautions associated with Enbrel and Remicade, patients who are administered adalimumab should be concerned about serious infections and sepsis. Many problems with this drug have occurred in patients receiving concomitant immunosuppressive therapy. Therefore, it is advisable to administer a tuberculin skin test and initiate therapy for any latent tuberculosis infection before initiating therapy with adalimumab. Furthermore, adalimumab therapy should be discontinued at the first sign of infection. Demyelinating disease is a distinct concern with this type of drug. Adverse effects were similar in patients receiving the drug and placebo. Upper respiratory infection occurred in similar numbers of patients, and injection site reactions occurred more frequently in those receiving active therapy. But the statistical difference occurred only in those receiving the 80-mg dose. Nausea was more common among patients taking adalimumab 20 mg (25).

Adalimumab is packaged in prefilled syringes and vials, and these should be kept refrigerated but not frozen. Patients should inject the entire content (40 mg/0.8 mL) of the prefilled syringes, should rotate injection sites, and should avoid injecting the drug into skin that is inflamed, tender to the touch, bruised, or hard. The medication should also be protected from light and stored in its original carton until it is to be administered. Because the needle's cover on the prefilled syringe contains dry natural rubber, patients who have allergies to rubber and latex should advise their physician and treatment alternatives pursued if deemed necessary.

Basiliximab (Simulect)

Basiliximab is an IL-2 receptor antagonist. It is an example of a chimeric (murine–human) MAb (IgG$_{1K}$) produced by rDNA technology. It functions as an immunosuppressive agent, specifically binding to and blocking the IL-2 receptor alpha chain (IL-2Rα, also known as the CD25 antigen), which is selectively expressed on the surface of activated T-lymphocytes. This high-affinity binding specificity of the drug to IL-2Rα competitively inhibits IL-2-mediated activation of lymphocytes, a critical pathway in the cellular immune response of allograft rejection.

Like Daclizumab, basiliximab is indicated for the prophylaxis of acute organ rejection in patients receiving renal transplants. It is used

as part of an immunosuppressive regimen that includes cyclosporine and corticosteroids.

Basiliximab demonstrates an adverse effect profile similar to that of Daclizumab. Administration of this drug is by central or peripheral intravenous infusion only. The dilute reconstituted basiliximab (20 mg/5 mL) is brought to a 50-mL volume with 0.9% sodium chloride injection or 5% dextrose injection and administered as an intravenous infusion over 20 to 30 minutes.

The recommended regimen for an adult is two doses of 20 mg each. The first dose is administered within 2 hours prior to transplantation surgery. The second dose is administered 4 days after surgery. For children and adolescents aged 2 to 15 years, the recommended regimen is two doses of 12 mg/m^2 each, up to a maximum of 20 mg/dose. The schedule is the same as for an adult.

Daclizumab (Zenapax)

Daclizumab is an immunosuppressive humanized IgG1 MAb produced by rDNA technology that binds specifically to the alpha unit (Tac subunit) of the human high-affinity IL-2 receptor that is expressed on the surface of activated lymphocytes. Daclizumab is a composite of human (90%) and murine (10%) antibody sequences.

Daclizumab is indicated for the prophylaxis of acute organ rejection in patients receiving renal transplants. It is used as part of an immunosuppressive regimen that includes cyclosporine and corticosteroids.

The typical adverse effects associated with the use of Daclizumab were gastrointestinal disorders, including constipation, nausea, diarrhea, vomiting, and abdominal pain, among others. Other side effects include metabolic and nutritional (e.g., peripheral edema, fluid overload), central nervous system (e.g., tremor, headache, dizziness), and genitourinary (e.g., oliguria, dysuria, renal tubular necrosis) effects.

The recommended dose is 1 mg/kg intravenously as part of an immunosuppressive regimen. The calculated volume of Daclizumab is mixed with 50 mL of sterile 0.9% sodium chloride injection and administered via a peripheral or central vein over 15 minutes. The standard course of Daclizumab therapy is five doses. The first dose is administered not more than 24 hours before transplantation, and the remaining four doses are given at intervals of 14 days.

Gemtuzumab Ozogamicin (Mylotarg)

It is estimated that 10% of patients with acute myeloid leukemia (AML) treated with daunorubicin (Cerubidine) and cytarabine (Cytosar-U) have severe, life-threatening prolonged myelosuppression. Most of these patients are more than 60 years of age, and because of this, clinicians are very wary and reluctant to administer this standard treatment. These two drugs indiscriminately wipe out bone marrow.

Gemtuzumab ozogamicin targets myeloid leukemic cells, leaving precursor pluripotent stem cells relatively unscathed and is less toxic than daunorubicin and cytarabine. It was the first drug specifically approved for treating relapsed AML. It is a MAb linked to a highly potent chemotherapeutic agent, calicheamicin. The antibody targets CD33, a glycoprotein on the surface of most AML cells. Thus, it is now also indicated for patients who are older than 60 years and who demonstrate CD33-positive AML and not considered candidates for conventional therapy.

During clinical trials, 47% of patients treated with gemtuzumab ozogamicin developed anemia, and of these 98% demonstrated severe neutropenia and 99%, severe thrombocytopenia. Thus, patients were at severe risk for the development of opportunistic infections and bleeding, and some required transfusion.

The recommended dose is 9 mg/m^2 administered as a 2-hour intravenous infusion followed by a repeat dose 14 days later. This drug can be administered in an ambulatory setting. Treatment causes chills, fever, nausea, and vomiting and less commonly hypotension and dyspnea during the first 24 hours after administration. Vital signs should be monitored for at least 4 hours post administration. Further, it is advised to administer 50 mg diphenhydramine and 650 to 1000 mg acetaminophen 1 hour prior to administration of gemtuzumab ozogamicin to reduce the risk of an infusion reaction. Two additional doses of acetaminophen may be needed.

Ibritumomab Tiuxetan (Zevalin)

Approved by the FDA in February 2002, ibritumomab tiuxetan is the first commercially available radiolabeled antibody for cancer therapy. When infused into the patient, the antibody binds to the surface of the specific cells and delivers radiation directly to the cancer cells. It is indicated for the treatment of relapsed or refractory low-grade follicular or transformed B-cell non-Hodgkins lymphoma (NHL).

Approximately, 55,000 Americans are diagnosed yearly with NHL, and nearly 65% of the cases are the low-grade or follicular subgroup, which has no cure. Patients diagnosed with this disease can remain in remission for years. Ultimately, however, relapses increase in frequency, and as they are treated for subsequent relapses, therapy loses effectiveness. Ibritumomab tiuxetan provides another treatment option when patients in relapse fail to respond to other therapies.

The target for ibritumomab tiuxetan on the surface of NHL cells is the CD20 antibody (human beta lymphocyte-restricted differentiation antigen). This antigen is expressed in 90% of malignant and premalignant and mature beta cells. Because the CD20 antigen does not shed from the cell membrane and does not compete for circulating antibodies, it is an excellent therapeutic target. Thus, an anti-CD20 antibody, rituximab (Rituxan) is covalently linked to tiuxetan. Tiuxetan is a chelator that reacts with ^{111}In or ^{90}Y. ^{111}In decays by electron capture, releasing gamma radiation and an ideal radioisotope for biodistribution imaging of the ibritumomab tiuxetan immunoconjugate because gamma radiation is not very reactive with soft tissue. ^{111}In has a physical half-life of 67.3 hours. Correspondingly, ^{90}Y decays by emission of particles that are heavier and more reactive in human soft tissue than gamma radiation. Thus, it is ideal for bulky, poorly vascularized tumors and tumors of heterogeneous antigen expression. ^{90}Y has a physical half-life of 64.1 hours.

The ibritumomab tiuxetan therapeutic regimen is administered in two steps. On day 1, rituximab (Rituxan) 250 mg/m² is administered intravenously, followed by ¹¹¹In-ibritumomab tiuxetan 5 mCi containing 1.6 mg of the ibritumomab antibody. This initial dose clears peripheral blood of beta cells and maximizes biodistribution of the ibritumomab tiuxetan. Multiple scans are performed to assess whether the antibody is settling in tumor sites and not in other organs. If biodistribution is adequate, the second regimen is administered.

The second step in the ibritumomab regimen, implemented days 7 to 9, consists of a second infusion of rituximab 250 mg/m². This is followed by ⁹⁰Y–ibritumomab tiuxetan 0.4 mCi/kg of actual body weight for patients with a platelet count above 150,000 cells/mm³ and 0.3 mCi/kg of actual body weight for patients whose platelet count is 100,000 to 149,000/mm³. Regardless of actual body weight, the maximum dose of the ⁹⁰Y–ibritumomab tiuxetan component is 32 mCi. This regimen is not implemented in patients demonstrating a platelet count below 100,000 cells/mm³.

Ibritumomab tiuxetan has a black box warning regarding fatal infusion reactions, prolonged and severe cytopenias, and maximum dosing. Hypoxia, pulmonary infiltrates, acute respiratory distress syndrome, myocardial infarction, ventricular fibrillation, and cardiogenic shock characterize fatal infusions. An overwhelming incidence of reactions (80%) occur during the first infusion.

Administration of ibritumomab tiuxetan can also induce prolonged and severe cytopenias. These include thrombocytopenia and neutropenia. Therefore, this drug should be restricted from use in patients who demonstrate more than 25% lymphoma marrow involvement or impaired bone marrow reserve. The most common nonhematologic adverse events include asthenia, nausea, vomiting, chills, fever, dizziness, cough, and dyspnea. Rituximab demonstrated a higher incidence of headache, pruritus, and angioedema compared to ibritumomab.

Because the nuclear pharmacist will be working with a pure beta particle–emitting radionuclide, ⁹⁰Y, extreme care will be necessary when handling the agent to protect fellow employees and patients' radiation exposure and keep it as low as possible.

Infliximab (Remicade)

Infliximab is the only approved drug therapy specifically indicated for the treatment of fistulizing Crohn's disease, an inflammation of the intestine. It is caused by an immune response to infection in which the lining of the intestine ulcerates and form channels of infection. These channels, called fistulas, can spread from the area of ulceration centered in the intestine and tunnel into adjacent tissue, and they may continue until they reach the surface of an organ and/or the skin. These fistulas, contaminated with infection, are capable of spreading the infection that creates them and causing life-threatening conditions such as peritonitis and septicemia.

Approved in 1998, infliximab was originally indicated for short-term treatment. In 2002 this indication was expanded to reduction of the signs and symptoms of and induction and maintenance of clinical remission in patients with moderate to severely active Crohn's disease who demonstrated an inadequate response to conventional therapies. In addition, in 1999, infliximab was approved for the treatment of rheumatoid arthritis, an indication that was expanded in 2002 to include improvement of physical function in patients without an adequate response to methotrexate therapy.

This MAb binds and neutralizes TNF-α, one of the primary cytokines that propagate the inflammatory response in patients with Crohn's disease and rheumatoid arthritis. Thus, infliximab reduces the intestinal inflammation indicative of this disease process. A patient's desire to avoid the adverse effects associated with corticosteroid therapy may influence the switch to infliximab. Correspondingly, a patient's refractiveness to methotrexate therapy may be an indication for a trial with infliximab therapy for rheumatoid arthritis.

Administration of single induction doses of infliximab when patients with Crohn's disease are not receiving immunosuppressive drugs can lead to development of antibodies to the chronic MAb itself. When antibodies to infliximab are present in high concentrations, patients demonstrate shortened duration of benefit, complete loss of response, and/or infusion reactions to the drug itself. Several options are being touted to reduce the immunogenicity of infliximab in patients with Crohn's disease. These include the following:

- Pretreat with an immunosuppressive regimen for a clinically relevant period. These regimens include azathioprine (6-mercaptopurine) for 2 to 3 months or methotrexate for 1.5 to 2 months. Because methotrexate and infliximab may interact (slower elimination rate for the latter during concomitant therapy), some clinicians prefer azathioprine.
- Administer infliximab in an induction regimen with three doses administered at 0, 2, and 6 weeks followed by maintenance doses administered every 8 weeks with moderately to severely active Crohn's disease. However, the role of maintenance infliximab therapy of Crohn's disease remains controversial. Many gastroenterologists elect to retreat patients with infliximab only when they relapse.
- It is advised to pretreat patients with intravenous hydrocortisone administered immediately before infliximab or other immunosuppressive therapy infusion reactions become problematic (26).

Infliximab is supplied in single-use 20-mL vials containing 100 mg of the drug. It has been associated with hypersensitivity reactions, including urticaria, dyspnea, and hypotension, and should be discontinued in case of a severe reaction. Additionally, anti-TNF therapy may result in the formation of autoimmune antibodies and rarely in the development of a lupuslike syndrome. If a patient develops symptoms suggestive of a lupuslike syndrome and is positive for antibodies against double-stranded DNA, infliximab therapy should be discontinued.

Postmarketing surveillance data demonstrated that some patients beginning therapy with infliximab developed tuberculosis, in-cluding presentations of the disease that resulted from infection of tissues other than the lungs (27). This problem occurs most commonly in patients with AIDS and other types of immunosuppression. Patients should be informed that weight loss is the best indicator of tuberculosis and should be reported to the attending physician if it occurs or is noticed. Similarly, malaise, fever, and night sweats occur commonly, especially in patients who are not elderly, and should be reported. The characteristic cough may not be present in many infliximab-associated cases.

There has also been a report of a 45-year-old man who developed a painful pustular rash on the left side of his chest shortly after receiving his third course of infliximab 5 mg/kg for treatment of refractory Crohn's disease (28). Titers of varicella zoster immunoglobulin M were elevated, suggesting an acute zoster infection. The patient was treated with intravenous acyclovir 5 mg/kg every 8 hours for 1 week, and the symptoms were reversed (28).

In addition, infliximab has been associated with worsening heart failure in patients with moderate or severe CHF, especially those taking higher doses of the agent. The manufacturer of Remicade advises that patients with CHF should not be given infliximab for rheumatoid arthritis or Crohn's disease. CHF patients already receiving infliximab should be reevaluated and therapy stopped if CHF worsens or there is no clinical response to the drug.

Patients may have questions about the possibility of problems associated with hydrocortisone doses given before the relatively infrequent infliximab infusions. They should be assured that adverse effects are rare with steroid doses given 8 weeks apart. However, when these do occur, they are much less serious than problems encountered with daily doses.

Muromonab-CD3 (Orthoclone OKT3)

Muromonab-CD3 is a murine MAb that reacts with a T3 (CD3) molecule linked to an antigen receptor on the surface membrane of human T lymphocytes. It blocks both generation and function of the T cells in response to antigenic challenge and is indicated for treatment of organ transplant rejection. Usually it is combined with azathioprine, cyclosporine, and/or corticosteroids to prevent acute rejection of renal transplants. Simultaneously the amount of immunosuppressive drugs a patient must receive has been reduced, effecting better outcomes.

Muromonab-CD3 injection is administered by intravenous push over a period not less than 1 minute. For acute renal allograft rejection it is given at 5 mg/day for 10 to 14 days. To decrease the incidence of reactions resulting from the first injection of muromonab, methylprednisolone sodium succinate 8 mg/kg should be administered intravenously 1 to 4 hours beforehand.

Muromonab-CD3 injection should be drawn into the syringe through a low-protein-binding 0.2- to 0.22-μm filter. The filter should be discarded and the needle for the intravenous bolus injection attached. Because the drug is a protein solution, it may develop a few fine translucent particles that do not affect its potency. This solution has no preservative and so must be used immediately upon opening and the unused portion discarded. As with other protein products, it must not be shaken.

Omalizumab (Xolair)

Omalizumab is the first humanized therapeutic antibody for the treatment of asthma and the first approved therapy designed to target immunoglobulin E (IgE) in the management of asthma. It was approved by the FDA in 2003 for subcutaneous treatment of moderate to severe persistent asthma in patients more than 12 years of age who demonstrate a positive skin test or *in vitro* reaction to a perennial aeroallergen (Fig. 19.15). Another requisite for its use is that the patient is inadequately controlled with inhaled corticosteroids.

Clinical trials demonstrated that when used in conjunction with inhaled corticosteroid therapy, omalizumab reduced mean asthma exacerbations below levels observed in control groups (29). Reduction in asthma exacerbations included symptom scores for nocturnal awakenings and daytime asthma symptoms.

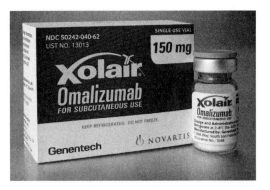

FIGURE 19.15 The product package of Xolair. (Courtesy of Genentech, Inc.)

Omalizumab is administered subcutaneously every 2 to 4 weeks. Dosing is based on the patient's body weight and IgE level and may have to be repeated early in therapy to attain the dose necessary to be effective as a prophylactic agent. The usual dose is 150 to 375 mg, and the doses and frequency are determined by pretreatment serum total IgE levels and body weight using tables available in product labeling. Doses over 150 mg should be divided and administered in multiple sites. Only 150 mg should be injected into one site.

The most serious adverse effects in the omalizumab clinical trials were malignancies (0.5% compared to 0.2% in placebo patients, not statistically significant). The most frequent adverse effects with this drug included pain at the injection site (45% of patients), viral infections (23%), upper respiratory tract infections (20%), sinusitis (16%), headache (15%), and pharyngitis (11%). However, in the trials, these events were observed at similar rates in the omalizumab-treated groups and the control patients.

With any new drug, these events are noteworthy and the patient must be monitored carefully. Further, the patient must understand that this medication is only for prophylaxis and not for treating an acute attack. These patients should also know not to adjust their other asthma medicines on their own. Patients should continue taking their other antiasthmatic medications. They should also understand that this drug does not provide immediate benefit and may take a few weeks to manifest effects.

The intriguing aspect of omalizumab is that it probably will be used off label for seasonal allergic rhinitis and for food allergy because of its unique mechanism of action.

Palivizumab (Synagis)

Palivizumab is a humanized MAb (IgG_{1K}) produced by rDNA technology, directed to the epitope in the A antigenic site of the F protein of respiratory syncytial virus (RSV). It is a composite of human (95%) and murine (5%) antibody sequences.

Palivizumab demonstrates neutralizing and fusion-inhibitory activity against RSV and is used to prevent serious lower respiratory tract disease caused by RSV in children. The safety and efficacy of this drug were established in infants with bronchopulmonary dysplasia (BPD) and infants with a history of prematurity (≤ 35 gestational weeks).

Palivizumab is for intramuscular use only, and the single-use vials of the drug do not contain a preservative. The injection must be administered within 6 hours after reconstitution.

In prophylaxis studies of children with BPD or prematurity, the proportions of subjects in the placebo and palivizumab groups who had adverse side effects were similar. Adverse effects reported in more than 1% of the palivizumab group included cough, wheezing, asthma, dyspnea, and sinusitis, among others.

The recommended dosage of palivizumab is 15 mg/kg intramuscularly in the anterolateral aspect of the thigh (preferable location). The use of the gluteal muscle is not advocated as a site of injection because of the risk of sciatic nerve damage. Patients, including those who develop an RSV infection, should receive monthly doses throughout the RSV season. The first dose is to be administered prior to the onset of the RSV season. In the northern hemisphere, the RSV season commences usually in November and lasts through April. However, it may be earlier or later.

Rituximab (Rituxan)

In November 1997, rituximab was the first MAb approved to treat cancer. It is a chimeric human–murine MoAb directed against the CD20 antigen found on the surface of normal and malignant beta lymphocytes. The Fab domain of rituximab binds to the CD20 antigen on beta lymphocytes, and the Fc domain recruits immune effector functions to mediate beta-cell lysis *in vitro.*

Rituximab is used to treat patients with relapsed or refractory low-grade or follicular CD20 positive beta-cell NHL. The recommended dosage is 375 mg/m² given as an intravenous infusion weekly for 4 doses (days 1, 8, 15, and 22). It may be administered in an outpatient setting.

The first infusion is administered at 50 mg/hour. If no hypersensitivity or infusion-related events occur, the infusion is escalated in 50 mg/hour increments every 30 minutes to a maximum of 400 mg/hour. If hypersensitivity or infusion-related reactions (e.g., fever, chills, nausea, urticaria, fatigue, headache, bronchospasm) develop, the infusion is interrupted or slowed. These reactions generally present within 30 minutes to 2 hours of the first infusion. Subsequent infusions can be administered at a higher rate (100 mg/hour) and increased by 100 mg/hour increments up to a maximum of 400 mg/hour as tolerated.

Premedication with acetaminophen and diphenhydramine may attenuate infusion-related events. Because hypotension may occur during infusion, it is suggested that one consider withholding any antihypertensive medication 12 hours prior to rituximab infusion.

Rituximab (as Rituxan) is available in 10- and 50-mL single-unit vials (10 mg/mL). The required amount of drug is withdrawn and diluted to a final concentration of 1 to 4 mg/mL into an infusion bag containing either 0.9% sodium chloride or 5% dextrose injection. The bag is gently inverted to mix the solution. Any unused portion is discarded.

Satumomab Pendetide (OncoScint CR/OV Kit)

OncoScint CR/OV-In (¹¹¹In satumomab pendetide) is a diagnostic imaging agent that is indicated for determining the extent and location of extrahepatic malignant disease in patients with known colorectal or ovarian carcinoma.

Clinical studies suggest that this imaging agent should be used after completion of standard diagnostic tests, when additional information regarding disease extent could aid in patient management.

Satumomab pendetide is a conjugate produced from the murine MAb CYT-099 (MAb B72.3). MAb B72.3 is a murine MAb of the IgG_{1K} subclass, which is directed to, localizes, and binds with a high-molecular-weight tumor-associated glycoprotein (TAG-72) that is expressed differentially by adenocarcinomas (30). (Adenocarcinoma is a technical name for a malignant tumor derived from a gland or glandular tissue or a tumor whose gland-derived cells form glandlike structures.) *In vitro* immunohistologic studies have reported MAb B72.3 to be reactive with about 83% of colorectal adenocarcinomas, 97% of common epithelial ovarian carcinomas, and most breast, non–small cell lung, pancreatic, gastric, and esophageal cancers evaluated.

OncoScint CR/OV is prepared by site-specific conjugation of the linker-chelator, glycyl tyrosyl-(N,ε-diethylenetriaminepentaacetic acid)-lysine hydrochloride, to the oxidized oligosaccharide component of MAb B72.3. Each kit contains all of the nonradioactive ingredients necessary to produce a single unit dose of OncoScint CR/OV-In for use as an intravenous injection. Each kit contains two vials. A single-dose vial of OncoScint CR/OV, formulated with sterile water for injection, contains 1 mg of satumomab pendetide in 2 mL of sodium phosphate–buffered saline solution adjusted to pH 6 with hydrochloric acid. OncoScint CR/OV is sterile, pyrogen free, clear, and colorless, and it may contain some translucent particles. A vial of sodium acetate buffer contains 136 mg of sodium acetate trihydrate in 2 mL of water for injection adjusted to pH 6 with glacial acetic acid. It is sterile, pyrogen free, clear, and colorless. Neither solution contains a preservative. Each kit also contains one sterile 0.22-μm Millex GV filter, prescribing information, and two identification labels. The kit should be stored upright in a refrigerator (2°–8°C) but not frozen.

Proper aseptic technique and precautions for handling radioactive materials should be employed. Waterproof gloves should be worn during radiolabeling. Consistent with the instructions provided, the sodium acetate buffer solution must be added to the ^{111}In chloride solution to buffer it prior to radiolabeling satumomab pendetide. After radiolabeling with ^{111}In, the immunoscintigraphic agent, OncoScint CR/OV-In (^{111}In satumomab pendetide) is formed.

Trastuzumab (Herceptin)

In September 1998, trastuzumab became the second MAb approved to treat cancer. It is indicated for the treatment of metastatic breast cancer or cancer that has spread beyond the breast and lymph nodes under the arm. The drug is approved for monotherapy in certain patients who have attempted chemotherapy with little success or as a first-line treatment of metastatic disease in combination with paclitaxel (Taxol) in first-line metastatic breast cancer therapy patients whose tumors overexpress the HER2 protein.

Specifically, trastuzumab is a chimeric human–murine MoAb that binds to the HER2 protein found on the surface of normal cells and plays a role in regulating cell growth. In the case of metastatic breast cancer cells, approximately 30% of tumors produce excess amounts of HER2. Thus, only patients who have tumors with this characteristic have shown benefit from trastuzumab. It should be used to treat only tumors that have HER2 protein overexpression. The trastuzumab–paclitaxel cycle is 21 days of treatment for six cycles.

The labeling of trastuzumab contains a black box warning regarding risk of ventricular dysfunction and congestive heart failure. The patient receiving this medicine must be monitored closely.

The recommended loading dose is 4 mg/kg as a 90-minute intravenous infusion along with 175 mg/m²/dose on day 1 of therapy. The weekly maintenance dose is 2 mg/kg over 30 minutes if the loading dose was well tolerated on days 1, 8, and 15 except for day 1 of the first cycle. Herceptin is available in a 440 mg/21 mL multidose vial and can be administered in an outpatient setting.

Tissue Plasminogen Activators

Tissue plasminogen activators are substances produced in small quantity by the inner lining of blood vessels and by the muscular wall of the uterus. They prevent abnormal blood clotting by converting plasminogen, a component of blood, to the enzyme plasmin, which breaks down fibrin, the main constituent of a blood clot.

Genetic engineering has prepared these substances artificially, and they are used as *thrombolytic agents* (agents that dissolve blood clots). They are used for conditions such as heart attack, angina, and occluded arteries. Unlike other anticoagulant drugs, tissue plasminogen activator acts only on the site of the clot.

Recombinant Alteplase (Activase)

Alteplase, a tissue plasminogen activator produced by rDNA, is used in the management of acute myocardial infarction (AMI), acute ischemic stroke, and pulmonary embolism (PE). It is a sterile, purified glycoprotein of 527 amino acids. It is synthesized using the complementary DNA for natural human tissue–type plasminogen activator obtained from a human melanoma cell line.

The biologic activity of alteplase is determined by an *in vitro* clot lysis assay. The activity is expressed in international units as tested against the WHO standard. Its specific activity is 580,000 IU/mg. Alteplase is an enzyme (serine protease) that has the property of fibrin-enhanced conversion of plasminogen to plasmin. It produces limited conversion of plasminogen in the absence of fibrin. When administered, alteplase binds to fibrin in a thrombus and converts the trapped plasminogen to plasmin. This initiates local fibrinolysis with limited systemic proteolysis.

Coronary occlusion due to a thrombus is present in the infarct-related coronary artery in approximately 80% of patients having a transmural myocardial infarction evaluated within 4 hours of onset of symptoms. When administered into the systemic circulation at pharmacologic concentrations, alteplase binds to fibrin in a thrombus. Conversion of the entrapped plasminogen to plasmin initiates the lysis of thrombi that are obstructing coronary arteries, improving ventricular function and reducing the incidence of congestive heart failure.

The goal of the management of acute ischemic stroke is to improve neurologic recovery and reduce the incidence of disability. Therapy with alteplase for this purpose must be within 3 hours after the onset of stroke symptoms and after exclusion of intracranial hemorrhage by cranial CT or other diagnostic imaging of sufficient sensitivity to detect hemorrhage.

Alteplase is indicated for management of massive pulmonary embolism in adults; for lysis of acute pulmonary emboli, defined as an obstruction of blood flow to a lobe or multiple segments of the lung; and for lysis of pulmonary emboli accompanied by unstable hemodynamics (e.g., failure to maintain blood pressure without supportive measures). Unlabeled uses for alteplase are unstable angina pectoris where it may effect coronary thrombolysis and reduction in ischemic events.

An appropriate volume of the accompanying sterile water for injection (without preservatives) is added to the vial containing the lyophilized powder (50 mg or 100 mg) (Fig. 19.16). Reconstitution should be with a large-bore (e.g., 18 gauge) needle and the stream of sterile water for injection directed into the lyophilized cake. A slight foaminess can be expected; when allowed to stand undisturbed, it should dissipate within several minutes. The resultant solution appears as a colorless to pale yellow transparent solution having a pH of approximately 7.3 and containing 1 mg/mL.

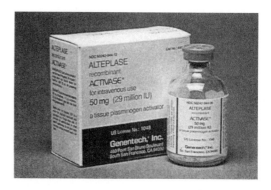

FIGURE 19.16 The product package of Alteplase. (Courtesy of Genentech, Inc.)

There are no antibacterial preservatives in the product, so it should be prepared just before use. Because the alteplase molecule is large, it cannot easily diffuse across biologic membranes and must be administered parenterally, usually intravenously. The solution may be used for direct intravenous administration within 8 hours of reconstitution when stored at 2° to 30°C (36°–86°F). Before diluting or administering the product, it is necessary to inspect it visually for particulate matter and discoloration whenever the solution and container permit.

This product may be administered as reconstituted at 1 mg/mL, or the reconstituted solution may be diluted further immediately preceding administration with an equal volume of 0.9% sodium chloride injection or 5% dextrose injection. Alteplase is stable for up to 8 hours in these solutions at room temperature, and either polyvinyl chloride bags or glass bottles are acceptable. Light exposure has no influence upon stability.

Recombinant Reteplase (Retavase)

Reteplase is a nonglycosylated deletion mutein of tissue plasminogen activator (tPA) containing 355 of the 527 amino acids of native tPA. It is produced by rDNA in *E. coli*. Its mechanism of action is the same as that of alteplase.

Reteplase is indicated for management of AMI in adults, improvement of ventricular function following an AMI, reduction of the incidence of CHF, and reduction in mortality associated with an AMI.

Reteplase is for intravenous administration only. It is administered as a 10 + 10 U double-bolus injection. Each bolus is administered intravenously over 2 minutes. The second bolus is given 30 minutes after initiation of the first bolus injection. An important requirement is that the bolus injection be given via a line in which no other medication is being injected or infused. If reteplase must be injected through an intravenous line containing heparin, the health professional should flush the line with 0.9% sodium chloride injection or 5% dextrose injection before and after reteplase administration.

The lyophilized powder for injection of reteplase should be reconstituted only with sterile water for injection (without preservatives) immediately before use. A colorless solution should be created containing 1 U/mL. A slight foaminess at this point is fairly common, and allowing the solution to stand undisturbed for a few minutes will allow dissipation of any large bubbles.

Reteplase (as Retavase) is available in kits. Each kit contains a two single-use reteplase vials of 10.8 U (18.8 mg), two single-use diluent vials for reconstitution (10 mL sterile water for injection), two sterile 10 mL syringes with 20-gauge needle attached, two sterile dispensing pins, two sterile 20-gauge needles for dosage administration, and two alcohol swabs.

Recombinant Tenecteplase (TNKase)

This new thrombolytic agent is marketed with a needleless administration set that can be used to deliver the medication with just one dose in only 5 seconds. It is packaged in a-10 mL syringe, a dual-cannula device, and a 10-mL vial of sterile water for injection. Doses are calculated on the basis of body weight. After reconstitution of the lyophilized powder, patients will receive 6 to 10 mL. The agent is administered via an intravenous line with saline, as dextrose may cause precipitation. This product contains no bacteriostatic agent and so must be prepared immediately before administration. However, if it is not used immediately, it can be refrigerated for use within 8 hours.

Produced in Chinese hamster ovary cells using rDNA technology, it demonstrated comparable effectiveness (demonstrated mortality rates) and safety (intracranial hemorrhage, major bleeding episodes) as an accelerated infusion of recombinant alteplase in the AS-SENT-2 (ASsessment of the Safety and Efficacy of a New Thrombolytic agent) trial. The tenecteplase protein is a modified form of natural tPA. The three letters in the name derive from amino acid substitutions at three regions of the tPA protein. These substitutions have provided a prolonged half-life that enables single bolus dosing, an enhanced specificity for fibrin (which reduces the agent's disruption of other parts of the coagulation system), and an increased level of resistance to plasminogen activator inhibitor, which can otherwise interfere with the drug's therapeutic action.

To be effective, tenecteplase, like the other clot busters, must be used within the first hours of a heart attack. Thus, patients have to be told to seek medical attention if chest pain occurs. But this drug class is not indicated for patients with conditions that predispose them to bleeding. This includes patients with active internal bleeding, a history of cerebrovascular accidents, intracranial or intraspinal surgery or trauma within 2 months, intracranial neoplasms or aneurysm, known bleeding diathesis (e.g., clotting defects, compromised blood vessels) or severe uncontrolled hypertension.

Tyrosine Kinase Inhibitor

The Philadelphia (Ph) chromosome, a truncated chromosome 22, was the first consistent chromosomal abnormality identified in human malignancy (31). Improved chromosome banding techniques demonstrated that this chromosome was the result of a reciprocal translocation between the long arms of chromosomes 9 and 22. The molecular consequences causes the fusion of the c-Abl oncogene (chromosome 9) and the Bcr sequence (chromosome 22) into the Bcr-Abl gene. This fusion catalyzes the phosphorylation of tyrosine residues from adenosine triphosphate (ATP). Ultimately, this activates several other multiple signaling pathways that affect cell growth, adhesion, and proliferation.

The size of the protein generated by this fusion gene depends on the breakpoint in the Bcr region. For example, 95% of patients with chronic myelogenous leukemia (CML) and up to approximately 20% of adult patients with ALL will demonstrate a 210-kDa fusion protein (p210). Alternatively, a 185-kDa fusion protein (p185) is observed in 10% of adult patients with ALL and is the predominant Bcr-Abl fusion protein in Ph chromosome–positive children with ALL. The product of this fusion gene is a constitutively active tyrosine kinase with markedly enzymatic activity when compared to the Abl kinase. Because all of these events (cell growth, adhesion, proliferation) depend on the increased tyrosine kinase activity of the

fusion protein, it is apparent that inhibition of the enzymatic activity of Bcr-Abl would be an effective treatment of CML. Bcr-Abl is present in most patients with CML, and the causative abnormality of the disease and its kinase activity are central for transformation.

CML is a progressive disorder with three phases. The diagnosis is often made during the chronic phase. The accelerated phase is characterized by white blood cell counts of the patient that become unresponsive to therapy. The blast crisis phase is characterized by rapid proliferation of blast cells and a very poor response to therapy. Hematopoietic stem cell transplantation is a primary therapy for newly diagnosed CML. However, in patients who are not suitable candidates for this procedure (>60 years of age, no suitable donor), imatinib mesylate (Gleevec) is becoming a viable alternative. With an estimated 5000 Americans diagnosed annually with CML and a 68% mortality rate, the FDA reviewed Novartis's

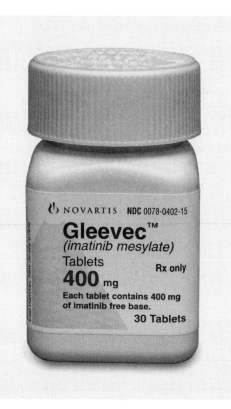

FIGURE 19.17 The product package of Gleevec. (Courtesy of Novartis, Inc.)

application for approval of imatinib mesylate and granted approval of it within 2.5 months.

Imatinib Mesylate (Gleevec)

Imatinib mesylate demonstrates potent and selective inhibitory activity *in vivo* against Abl tyrosine kinases, such as Bcr-Abl, through competitive inhibition at the ATP binding site (32) (Fig. 19.17). It does so without any significant effect on normal cells or other cells affected by the tyrosine oncogenes. Phase I clinical trials of the drug (as ST1571) conducted in June 1998 demonstrated significant activity against CML even in patients who were interferon refractory. A significant finding was that the drug is most advantageous when used early in the disease, in the chronic phase. Thus, some experts have proposed a treatment algorithm that calls for all CML patients to receive imatinib while transplantation is being evaluated. In patients whose condition responded to imatinib and for whom the risk of death from transplantation is higher (all except the youngest patients with sibling donors), the procedure could be withheld or deferred.

A study of 1106 newly diagnosed CML patients randomly received either imatinib mesylate (400 mg by mouth once daily; may be increased to 400 mg bid) or a combination therapy consisting of gradually increasing doses of interferon alfa up to a target dose of 5 million U/day plus subcutaneous cytarabine 20 mg/m^2/day (with a maximum dose of 40 mg) for 10 to 15 days every month. The imatinib demonstrated significantly more hematologic and cytogenetic responses and fewer adverse effects than did the combination therapy (33). At 18 months, 87.1% of patients receiving the imatinib mesylate had major cytogenic responses compared to 34.7% of combination therapy patients. With imatinib mesylate therapy, 96.7% of patients were free from progression of the disease to the accelerated phase or blast crisis. This was a significant difference from the 91.5% of patients who received the combination therapy.

Imatinib mesylate has been shown to be effective against other targets, such as platelet-derived growth factor receptor (PDGF-R) and the c-kit and Arg tyrosine kinases. PDGF-R is known to be associated with chronic myelomonocytic leukemia by forming an active Tel-PDGF-R fusion protein tyrosine kinase and has shown effect *in vivo* against glioblastoma, dermatofibrosarcoma protuberans, and angiogenesis. C-kit is associated with a rare form of a gastrointestinal stromal tumor. It is not likely, however, that these malignant transformations are a result of a single protein kinase, with the exception of the Bcr-Abl. Therefore, it is predicted that to be more efficacious, tyrosine kinase inhibitors will be a component of combination chemotherapy.

The chronic phase dosage is 400 to 600 mg daily. The accelerated phase or blast crisis dosage ranges from 600 to 800 mg daily. The patient should be instructed to take this medication with food and a large glass of water because of mild gastrointestinal effects. Serum concentrations of imatinib are affected by medications that inhibit or induce the CYP 3A4 enzyme. Other common adverse effects include edema, muscle cramps, hemorrhage, and musculoskeletal pain. But these have been mild compared with those of other chemotherapeutic agents.

It is anticipated that monthly cost of therapy with this drug will exceed $2000, and patients are expected to take it for at least a year, or essentially as long as they continue to respond to imatinib. The drug manufacturer, Novartis, has established a patient assistance program designed to help low-income patients without health insurance to secure the medication. After receiving the prescription from the physician, the patient should be instructed to contact the Gleevec Reimbursement Hotline (1-877-GLEEVEC) to determine qualification for financial assistance (34).

Vaccines

Genetically engineered vaccines use a synthetic copy of the protein coat of a virus to fool the body's immune system into mounting a protective response. This avenue avoids the use of live viruses and minimizes the risk of causing the disease the vaccine was intended to prevent. Further, these vaccines will all but eliminate concern about the natural vaccine, which could be derived from blood donor carriers who may harbor the AIDS virus.

The first genetically engineered vaccine for use in the United States was approved by the FDA in 1986 for hepatitis B, a widespread liver infection. This vaccine has now replaced the plasma-derived vaccine.

Hepatitis B Vaccine Recombinant (Engerix-B, Recombivax HB)

The plasma-derived hepatitis B vaccine is no longer being produced in the United States, and its use is limited to hemodialysis patients, other immunocompromised patients, and persons with known allergies to yeast. Recombinant hepatitis B vaccine has demonstrated an ability to induce antibody to hepatitis B surface antigen (anti-HBs) that is biochemically and immunologically comparable to antibody induced by the plasma-derived hepatitis B vaccine. Studies demonstrate that the two are interchangeable in use.

Hepatitis B recombinant vaccine is indicated for immunization of persons of all ages against infection caused by all types of hepatitis B virus. A dialysis formulation (Recombivax HB Dialysis Formulation) is indicated for immunization of adult predialysis and dialysis patients. The vaccine should be administered by intramuscular injection into the deltoid muscle (outer aspect of the upper arm) for immunization of adults and older children. The anterolateral thigh is recommended for infants and younger children. For patients with a risk of hemorrhage following intramuscular injection, the vaccine may be administered subcutaneously, although the subsequent antibody titer may be lower and there may be an increased risk of a local reaction.

The vaccine is administered in a three-dose schedule, Recombivax HB at 0, 1, and 6 months. Ideally, immunization with the vaccine for international travelers and military personnel should be 6 months before traveling to allow completion of the full three-dose vaccine series. If 6 months before travel is not possible, an alternative four-dose schedule, Engerix-B at 0, 1, 2 prior to travel and a dose for prolonged maintenance of protective titers is suggested at 12 months. It is assumed that the four-dose schedule provides a more rapid induction of immunity. However, there is no demonstrated evidence that this schedule provides greater protection than the standard three-dose schedule.

Haemophilus B Conjugate Vaccine (HibTITER, PedvaxHIB, ProHIBiT)

Prior to the introduction of *Haemophilus B* conjugate vaccines, *Haemophilus influenzae* type B (HIB) was the most frequent cause of bacterial meningitis and leading cause of serious systemic bacterial disease among children worldwide. HIB disease occurred primarily in children less than 5 years of age in the United States prior to the initiation of a vaccine program and was estimated to account for nearly 20,000 cases of invasive infections annually, about 12,000 of which were meningitis. The mortality rate from HIB meningitis is about 5%. Among children, the most prevalent cause of *H. influenzae* meningitis is by the capsular strains of type B. In addition to meningitis, *Haemophilus B* is responsible for numerous other invasive disease processes (e.g., epiglottitis, sepsis, septic arthritis, osteomyelitis, pericarditis).

Peak incidence of HIB occurs at ages 6 to 11 months. The disease is also prevalent in populations at risk (e.g., day care attendees, household contacts of cases, Native Americans, African Americans, individuals with low socioeconomic status, whites who lack the G2m [n or 23] immunoglobulin allotype, individuals with asplenia, sickle cell disease, or antibody deficiency syndromes).

HIB conjugate vaccines use a new technology, covalent bonding of the capsular polysaccharide of *Haemophilus influenzae* type B to diphtheria toxoid, diphtheria CRM_{197} protein, or an outer membrane protein complex (OMPC) of *Neisseria meningitidis,* to produce an antigen that is postulated to convert the T-independent antigen to a T-dependent antigen. The protein carries both its own antigenic determinants and those of the covalently bound polysaccharide. Thus, the polysaccharide is theorized to be presented as a T-dependent antigen, resulting in both an enhanced antibody response and an immunologic memory.

HbOC (HibTiter), PRP-T (ActHIB, Omni-HIB), and PRP-OMP (PedvaxHIB) can be used interchangeably. A fourth vaccine, PRP-D (Pro-HIBIT) is the only one of the HIB conjugate vaccines not licensed for the primary immunization of infants. Preferably, the same conjugate vaccine should be used throughout the course of immunization. However, it is likely that on occasion the vaccine provider does not know which vaccine was previously used. Under these circumstances, it is prudent for vaccine providers to ensure that at a minimum an infant 2 to 6 months of age receives a primary series of three doses of conjugate vaccine.

Liquid PedvaxHIB is available as an injection of 7.5 μg *Haemophilus B* PRP, 125 μg *Neisseria meningitidis* OMPC, and 225 μg aluminum (as aluminum hydroxide) per 0.5 mL in a single-dose vial. HibTITER is also available as an injection of 10 μg purified *Haemophilus B* saccharide capsular oligosaccharide and about 25 μg diphtheria CRM_{197} protein/5 mL in 1- and 10-mL dose vials. The HibTITER multidose vials contain thimerosal (1:10,000) as a preservative. ActHIB is available as a lyophilized powder for injection containing 10 μg purified *Haemophilus B* capsular polysaccharide and 24 μg tetanus toxoid/5 mL. This is available in single-dose vials with 7.5- mL vials of diphtheria and tetanus toxoids and pertussis vaccine as diluents or with 0.6 mL vial containing 0.4% sodium chloride diluent.

Other Drugs

This section includes drugs that do not fall conveniently into the preceding categories of biotechnology drugs. Nonetheless, it is important for the pharmacist to know about them.

Goserelin (Zoladex)

Goserelin is indicated for palliative monotherapy of advanced prostatic carcinoma. It is a synthetic luteinizing hormone–releasing hormone analogue. Administration of this drug stimulates the release of luteinizing hormone (LH) and follicle-stimulating hormone (FSH) from the anterior pituitary, which transiently increases testosterone concentrations in males. However, continual ad-

ministration of goserelin in the treatment of prostatic carcinoma suppresses the secretion of LH and FSH, causes a fall in testosterone concentrations, and produces medical castration. This drug offers an alternative treatment of prostatic cancer when *orchiectomy* (removal of one or both testes) or estrogen administration is not indicated or not acceptable to the patient.

In 1998, the FDA approved the combination of Zoladex (3.6- and 10.8-mg goserelin acetate depots) and Eulexin (flutamide) for the management of locally confined stage B2 to C prostate carcinoma. The treatment is initiated 8 weeks prior to radiation therapy and continued during radiation therapy. The treatment regimen used uses one goserelin 3.6-mg depot, followed in 28 days by one 10.8-mg depot.

Goserelin is also indicated for the management of endometriosis, for pain reduction or relief and reduction of endometriotic lesions during therapy. This drug has been demonstrated to be as effective as danazol in relieving the clinical symptoms (dysmenorrhea, dyspareunia, pelvic pain) and signs (pelvic tenderness) of endometriosis and decreasing the size of endometrial lesions. At present, the duration of therapy is recommended to be no longer than 6 months because there are no clinical data on the effect of treatment of benign gynecologic conditions with goserelin for periods greater than 6 months.

Goserelin is administered as a subcutaneous implant. Along with leuprolide acetate (Lupron Depot) it was one of the first polymer systems to receive FDA approval for controlled release of a peptide. This drug is available in a 3.6-mg biodegradable and biocompatible sterile white to cream-colored cylinder about the size of a grain of rice, which is implanted every 28 days into the upper abdominal wall (Fig. 19.18). The drug is dispersed in a matrix of D,L-lactic acid and glycolic acids copolymer. For additional information on this type of dosage form, see Chapter 20.

Leuprolide Acetate (Lupron, Lupron Depot-Ped, Lupron Depot-3)

Leuprolide is a synthetic gonadotropin-releasing hormone analogue. Like the naturally oc-

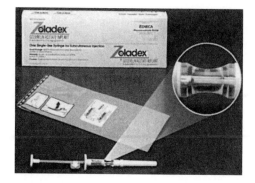

FIGURE 19.18 The product package of Zoladex, which demonstrates the innovative delivery system for the continuous release of goserelin acetate from an injectable pellet. (Courtesy of Zeneca Pharmaceuticals Group.)

curring luteinizing hormone-releasing hormone, initial and intermittent administration of this drug stimulates the release of LH and FSH from the anterior pituitary. As with goserelin, continuous administration of leuprolide suppresses the secretion of LH and FSH, with a concomitant drop in testosterone concentrations and subsequent medical castration.

The usual adult dose for prostatic carcinoma is a subcutaneous injection of 1 mg/day. There is also a monthly (every 28 to 33 days) depot intramuscular injection. The 7.5-mg strength is used for prostatic carcinoma. The powder for intramuscular injection is reconstituted with a special diluent composed of D-mannitol, purified gelatin, D,L-lactic and glycolic acids copolymer, polysorbate 80, and acetic acid.

Lupron should be refrigerated until dispensed, but patients may store the product at room temperature (no more than 30°C, or 86°F). The product should be protected from light and the vial stored in the carton until use. Following reconstitution, the suspension is stable for 1 day. However, because the product has no preservative, it should be discarded if not used immediately.

Lupron Depot-Ped 11.25 and Lupron Depot-3 Month are available in a kit with a prefilled dual-chamber syringe. Because their packages look much alike, they were interchanged mistakenly and children received the adult product. The doses were too low and treatment for central precocious puberty was considered to have failed some of them. This incident was reported in Chapter 16.

Rasburicase (Elitek)

Rasburicase is a recombinant urate oxidase enzyme produced by a genetically modified *S. cerevisiae* strain. In humans, uric acid is the final step in the catabolic pathway of purines. Rasburicase catalyzes enzymatic oxidation of uric acid into an inactive and soluble metabolite, allantoin. Rasburicase is active only at the end of the purine catabolic pathway.

Rasburicase is indicated for initial management of elevated plasma uric acid levels in children with leukemia, lymphoma, and solid tumor malignancies who are receiving oncologic therapy expected to result in tumor lysis.

The recommended dosage of rasburicase is 0.15 or 0.2 mg/kg as a single daily dose for 5 days. Because the safety and effectiveness of the drug have not been determined for more than one administration or beyond five days, more than one course of therapy is not recommended. The chemotherapy regimen is implemented 4 to 24 hours after the first dose of rasburicase. The drug is administered as an intravenous infusion over 30 minutes.

The labeling of rasburicase has several black box warnings about anaphylaxis, hemolysis (in patients deficient in glucose-6-phosphate dehydrogenase, African or Mediterranean descent), methemoglobinemia, and interference with uric acid measurements. Adverse reactions associated with the drug include fever (46%), neutropenia with fever (5%), respiratory distress, sepsis, neutropenia (2%), and mucositis (15%).

Recombinant Human DNase I (Pulmozyme)

In 1989 the cystic fibrosis gene was discovered, and it has helped to lay the groundwork for new therapies to treat this disease, which is the most common inherited fatal disease affecting whites. Cystic fibrosis transmembrane conductance regulator, the protein product of the cystic fibrosis gene, is defective in its ability to facilitate ion transport across the airway epithelial cells in the lung. This defective regulator allows excessive absorption of sodium and adequate amounts of chloride across the cell membrane. Consequently, water from the mucus of the lung gets absorbed into the cell and the mucus dries out, resulting in a thick, tenacious mucus that accumulates in the small airways of the lung. This leads to a domino effect of chronic infection and inflammation, followed by chronic lung disease, pulmonary hypertension, and heart failure.

DNase (recombinant human deoxyribonuclease I), or Dornase alfa, is a DNA enzyme indicated for the treatment of symptoms of cystic fibrosis. This enzyme specifically cleaves extracellular DNA, such as that found in the thick, sticky, mucous secretions of cystic fibrosis patients (35). As a result, airflow in the lung improves and the risk of bacterial infection may decrease. This drug offers hope for breaking the cycle of chronic lung infection and inflammation associated with cystic fibrosis disease, and it demonstrates no effect upon the DNA of intact cells.

DNase showed successful efficacy data from more than 1100 patients in Phase II and Phase III testing. The drug improved the quality of life for the cystic fibrosis patient with mild to moderate pulmonary dysfunction by reducing the need for intravenous antibiotics, hospitalizations, and time missed from school, work, and everyday activities. The risk of respiratory infections was reduced by 27% for patients receiving 2.5 mg once daily in clinical trials, and hospital days were reduced from 7.6 days (untreated patients) to 6.2 days (for treated patients) (36).

Indicated to treat cystic fibrosis in patients aged 5 years and older, DNase is available in 2.5-mL single-use polyethylene ampuls for use with compressed air nebulizers (Fig. 19.19). Three nebulizer systems are recommended, and the safety and efficacy of the administration of DNase with other nebulizer systems have not been demonstrated. Clinical trials have been performed with the Marquest Acorn II nebulizer; the Hudson T Updraft II nebulizer powered by a DeVilbiss Pulmo-aide Compressor; and the Pari LC nebulizer driven

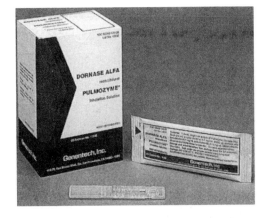

FIGURE 19.19 The product package of Pulmozyme (Courtesy of Genentech, Inc.)

by the Pari Proneb Compressor. Each of these systems delivers approximately 25% of the dose.

Portable jet models and ultrasonic nebulizers should not be used to administer DNase. The ultrasonic nebulizers may heat the protein enough to alter its structure. The portable jet nebulizers simply may not be capable of generating enough force or appropriate particle size to ensure optimal delivery of the drug into the lung.

To make administration efficient, it may be tempting to coadminister other compounds (e.g., albuterol, tobramycin) with DNase. However, no other medication should be mixed in the nebulizer system with this drug because of the possibility that a pH change could alter the DNase protein structure. Bronchodilator and antimicrobial agents that are delivered via nebulizer should be administered to patients sequentially, not mixed together. To date, no literature suggests the optimal sequence for all of these drugs to be administered.

The ampuls have an 18-month expiration date when stored in the refrigerator at 2° to 8°C and should be protected from light. The product cannot be exposed to room temperatures for more than 24 hours. The patient or caregiver should discard the solution if it is cloudy or discolored and should be told to make sure that the product is within the expiration date on the ampul. Unused ampuls should be placed in their protective foil pouch and refrigerated.

The Future of Biotechnology Products

The future will see the development of more protein-based pharmaceuticals as a result of modern biotechnologic strategies, including the development of artificial genes. These protein-based drugs present unique challenges because of intrinsic instability, multifaceted metabolic properties, and limited gastrointestinal absorption (37). Their problems include variable tissue penetration (because of the size of the molecules) and toxicity related to the stimulation of an immune or allergic reaction (37).

A distinct advantage of these biotechnologic proteins over proteins from natural sources is enhanced purity. Hepatitis B virus and the HIV are capable of contaminating proteins and enzymes from human plasma. If their presence is known, they can be isolated or neutralized. However, sometimes their presence has been confirmed only after disastrous results. Products derived from recombinant technology will not have coextracted contaminants.

Research is also directed toward the discovery of new methods of delivery for these agents. Delivery systems being explored include transdermal and nasal routes, other forms of injectables, and oral tablets for smaller proteins. Few protein biopharmaceutical products can be administered orally because of their instability in the strong acid environment of the stomach and the low systemic absorption through gastrointestinal mucosa. A challenge is to deliver regulatory proteins (e.g., insulin, growth hormone) to distant organs or tissue without biotransformation. One strategy that is bearing fruit is encapsulating the protein-based compound in a lipid complex (liposome).

Liposomes are typically composed of some combination of phosphatidylcholine, cholesterol, phosphatidylglycerol, other glycolipids, and/or phospholipids. These are water-filled vesicular structures composed of several phospholipid layers surrounding an aqueous core, with the outer shell capable of providing direction to specific target cells (e.g., tumors). Typically, liposomes concentrate the drug in cells of the reticuloendothelial system of the liver and spleen and reduce drug intake in the heart, kidney, and gastrointestinal tract. For example, use of liposome-associated doxorubicin reduces cardiotoxicity, and liposome-associated amphotericin-B reduces nephrotoxicity and other adverse effects (38). Doxil is doxorubicin produced within microscopic pegylated lipid spheres that are grafted to the liposome surface. The pegylated liposomal shell protects the inner compartment. A single lipid bilayer membrane composed of hydrogenated soy phosphatidyl choline and cholesterol separates this internal aqueous compartment from the external medium. In essence, the drug, doxorubicin, is encapsulated within this internal compartment by the pegylated polymer layer, which protects the drug from rapid capture and clearance from the blood stream by the liver, spleen, and bone marrow (39). It is theorized that the long residence times and stability of pegylated doxorubicin in plasma are related to a steric stabilization effect provided by the PEG coating (39).

Liposomes are popular among particulate carriers because of their relatively low toxicity and the versatility of their release characteristics and disposition *in vivo,* which can be altered by changing preparation techniques and bilayer constituents. Depending on their size, charge, and bilayer rigidity, among other characteristics, liposomes circulate only for a short time (minutes) in the circulation before degradation and uptake by macrophages of the mononuclear phagocyte system. Sometime, their residence in the systemic circulation can be for hours and even days if they are stable and not recognized as foreign bodies by the mononuclear phagocyte system. New design features involve liposome modification by covalent attachment of a hydrophilic polymer group to the liposome surface such as that previously mentioned with pegylated doxorubicin. The polyethylene coating reduces mononuclear phagocyte system uptake and provides long plasma residence times and plasma stability.

Insoluble polymers composed of PEG are now used to form a protective sheath around a drug, inhibiting its degradation (39). Other hydrophilic polymers that are grafted to liposomes and demonstrate increased circulation times include poly(acryloylmorpholine), poly(vinyl pyrrolidone) and poly(2-oxazoline) (39).

Research has also demonstrated that liposome size is critical to the effective delivery of encapsulated drugs when the desired outcome requires deposition of liposomes outside of the capillary bed (39). Most solid tumors exhibit unique features (e.g., extensive angiogenesis, hyperpermeable and defective vasculature, impaired lymphatic drainage, increased production of mediators that enhance vascular permeability). Liposomes extravasate in solid tumors through gaps in the normally continuous vascular endothelium. The gaps in these solid tumors have been found to be no larger than 0.6 µg. If the liposome is too big, it will not be able to extravasate through defects in the capillary endothelium. However, if it is too small, the liposome may have an inadequate amount of drug encapsulated to be effective.

A third strategy delivers extremely toxic proteins to tumor cells. In this prodrug approach, antibodies with specific sensitivities (e.g., MAbs) are fused to toxic proteins (e.g., ricin, *Pseudomonas* exotoxin) and then administered intravenously (40). The fused protein is delivered directly to the specified cancer cells, where one released functional molecule can effect cell death. The most widely studied plant toxin is ricin, a natural product of beans from the plant *Ricinus communis* (41). An example of this strategy is Anti-B4-blocked ricin (Oncolysin B) being tested for B-cell leukemias and lymphomas. Ricin, with a protein structure and a molecular weight of 66 kD, has been the prime target for MAb conjugation. This unmodified compound is extremely cytotoxic, as it enzymatically blocks intracellular protein synthesis at the ribosomal level. It and other immunotoxins have demonstrated antitumor activity against cultured melanoma cells and melanoma tumors growing in mice. Unfortunately, to date these complexes still have limited target-cell specificity, and uptake and sequestration by the liver remain a problem. Further, inside the cell, the toxin must translocate across membranes into the cytosol, where it can inhibit protein synthesis (41).

It is entirely feasible that in the future engineered protein complexes will combine a transporting protein with one that encodes the gene sequence to produce a therapeutic protein in the target tissue. In this instance, the gene will become functional only in certain tissue, decreasing delivery to an unintended site.

There is also a growing knowledge base and research about signaling transduction pathways. This has led to the creation of antibodies that target receptors, enzymes or other growth-regulating molecules.

The future will also see the creation of more diagnostic products for in-home testing. MAb-based diagnostic tests that are now restricted to physician use are under development for home testing. These include products for infectious disease processes (e.g., AIDS, *Chlamydia trachomatis*, streptococcal throat infections). In addition, it is anticipated that MAb-based tests will also be available to assay blood or plasma concentrations of a number of drugs (e.g., digoxin, phenytoin, theophylline).

FDA Office of Biotechnology

In 1989, the FDA Office of Biotechnology was created. The office did not evaluate submissions to the FDA for approval of clinical investigations or for product marketing approvals; these functions were executed by the appropriate FDA centers. Nor was this office intended to perform laboratory research or mandate research priorities to the FDA centers. Instead, it was created to serve a central coordinating, problem-solving, and advisory role within the Office of the Commissioner. It was to become an effective point of contact with the FDA for those outside of the agency on issues related to new biotechnology.

Originally, the FDA Office of Biotechnology had the following responsibilities:

1. It was to advise and assist the commissioner and other central officials about scientific issues related to biotechnology policy, direction, and long-range goals.
2. It represented the FDA on biotechnologic issues to other governmental agencies and intergovernmental groups, state and local governments, industry, consumer organizations, Congress, national and international organizations, and the scientific community.

3. It provided leadership and direction on scientific and regulatory issues related to biotechnology through an agencywide coordinating group, the Biotechnology Coordinating Committee, to promote communication and consistency on biotechnology matters across organizational lines.
4. It provided a problem-solving function for individuals, companies, associations, and organizations with concerns, questions, or complaints about biotechnology policies or procedures or about product jurisdiction and other aspects of product regulation.
5. It coordinated and facilitated guidance on cross-cutting or controversial biotechnology program policies.

The Office of Biotechnology is no longer in existence. In its place, two divisions relating to biotechnologic products (divisions of monoclonal antibodies and therapeutic proteins) were created under the aegis of the Office of Therapeutics Research and Review, Center for Biologics Evaluation and Research of the Food and Drug Administration (42). This agency, at 1401 Rockville Pike, Rockville, MD 20852-1448, has a voice information system at 800-835-4709 with the option of direct access to a consumer safety officer or public affairs specialist. Information can also be found at www.fda.gov/cber.

Patient Information From the Pharmacist

For products that can be parenterally self-administered, the pharmacist should instruct patients in the use of aseptic technique. Appropriate verbal instruction that reinforces the printed information sheet should also be provided when the product requires reconstitution. It is desirable to perform the first injection under the supervision of an appropriately qualified health care professional to ensure that the patient understands the technique and can perform the injection. Some products (e.g., Betaseron) come with a training video that demonstrates reconstitution and self-administration techniques.

Patients who self-administer these products must be taught how to prepare (Fig. 19.20) and give the injection and how to rotate injection sites (Fig. 19.21). Some products provide a schematic illustration of this on the patient information sheet. Patients should understand that changing sites each time helps avoid injection reactions and gives the site opportunity to bounce back from the previous injection. It is important that the patient understand not to administer an injection into the same area as the prior injection or in areas that are tender, red, or hard. The pharmacist should provide a method for the patient to record where previous injections were made. One simple way is to suggest that the patient note the injection site on a calendar.

Patients should be advised about the proper disposal of needles and syringes. In this day of the cost-conscious consumer, patients must be advised against reusing needles and syringes. It is advantageous to provide the patient with a puncture-resistant container for disposal of used needles and syringes along with instruction for the safe disposal of full containers.

The patient should understand that periodic injection site reactions may occur. These may be transient (as in the case of interferon beta-1b) and not require discontinuation of the therapy. It is advisable, however, periodically to reevaluate the patient's understanding and use of aseptic self-administration technique and procedures.

It is very important for the patient to understand that these products should not be agitated or shaken. Otherwise, there is the possibility of product (protein) denaturation and resultant ineffectiveness. Much like the suspension forms of insulin, which should be rolled (or rotated) in the palms of the hands, these products should be gently swirled to dissolve their contents.

Whenever possible, pharmacists must emphasize the need for compliance with dosage regimens. Betaseron, for example, is administered every other day. A calendar reminder system may be helpful for a patient using this medication.

PREPARING THE INJECTION

1. Remove the needle guard of the 1 mL syringe and pull back the plunger to the 1 mL mark.

2. Insert the needle of the 1 mL syringe through the stopper of the vial of Betaseron solution.

3. Gently push the plunger all the way down to inject air into the vial (leave the needle in the vial).

4. Turn the vial of Betaseron (Interferon beta-1b) solution upside down.

NOTE: Keep the needle tip in the liquid.

5. Pull back the plunger to withdraw 1 mL of liquid into the syringe.

6. Hold the syringe with the needle pointing upward.

7. Tap the syringe gently until any air bubbles that formed rise to the top of the barrel of the syringe.

8. Carefully push in the plunger to eject ONLY THE AIR through the needle.

9. Remove the needle/syringe from the vial.

10. Recap the needle on the syringe.

NOTE: The injection should be administered immediately after mixing (if the injection is delayed, refrigerate the solution and inject it within 3 hours). Do not freeze.

11. Throw away unused portion of the solution remaining in the vial.

FIGURE 19.20 Preparing Betaseron for injection. (Courtesy of Berlex, Inc.)

Pharmacist Self-help With Biotechnology Drugs

The advent of biotechnology drugs poses a real dilemma to some pharmacists. They may be reluctant to stock these medications because of their high cost and special storage and handling requirements and because of poor understanding of the drug's therapeutics (including side effects and counseling information required) and/or the difficult issue of reimbursement (43). These products also are far more expensive than ordinary pharmaceuticals.

Unfortunately, pharmacists cannot assume that the responsibility for dispensing these products will automatically fall to them (1). Indeed, the profession's failure to accept responsibility for the radioactive pharmaceutical products used for diagnosis and treatment of disease has resulted in others managing them. Similarly, the profession was not positioned to accept responsibility for patient-controlled analgesia and ultimately lost control to anesthesia departments in many hospitals. Although few biotechnologic products for chronic conditions are currently available in community pharmacies (except insulin, diagnostic tests, vaccines), drugs initially used exclusively in hospitals, as well as newly developed agents (e.g., Betaseron) will soon work their way into community practice (1).

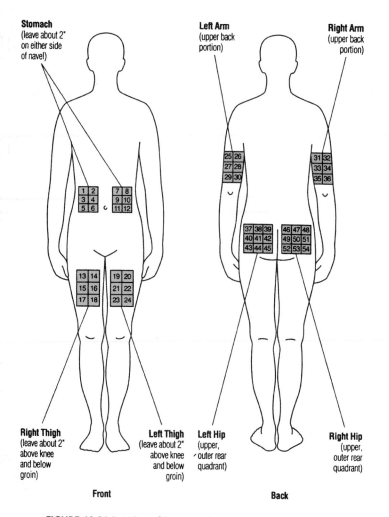

FIGURE 19.21 Rotation of injection sites. (Courtesy of Berlex, Inc.)

It is advisable that pharmacists continue their education on these products, and there are numerous programs to do so. Some are available directly from the manufacturer or through professional associations (e.g., "Biotechnology Update," *Journal of the American Pharmacists Association*) and cover basic biotechnology and/or therapeutic applications of specific products. Pharmacists should realize that various manufacturers of biotechnology products and professional associations provide support services for the profession. Typically, manufacturer services fall into one of three broad categories, professional services, educational materials, and reimbursement support. While the professional services may differ among companies, many have toll-free telephone numbers for obtaining information on biotechnology products.

Pharmacists should take advantage of these programs, realizing that complete knowledge of biotechnology drugs' synthesis and manufacture is not necessary. Pharmacists should, however, understand protein chemistry (as it relates to drug stability and structure) and immunology. Many programs cover basic biotechnology and therapeutic review of individual drugs. Programs can be very helpful—for example, a real danger with these products is that the pharmacist may confuse products with similar names. Many approved and investigational interferons (e.g., alfa-n3, alfa-2b, gamma-1b) differ greatly in activity and indications for use (43).

Most biotechnologic drugs must be administered parenterally, which poses a threat to some pharmacists, who are wary of this administration route and cognizant of their limitations in counseling the patients in appropriate technique. Suffice it to say that the pharmacist should assume the professional responsibility to secure educational materials (videotapes, print) from the manufacturer. Self-injection products contain instruction sheets that offer a step-by-step guide for preparing and administering the injection at home.

Aside from being knowledgeable about such things as therapeutic use, side effects, precautions, and drug interactions, the pharmacist must also be able to identify monitoring parameters to ensure safety and efficacy. For physiologic peptide molecules used for substitution therapy (e.g., insulin, clotting factors, erythropoietin), therapeutic drug monitoring (measurement of serum drug concentrations) is not indicated because alternative methods are routinely available to assess the efficacy and toxicity of these compounds (4). As an example, in insulin-dependent diabetes mellitus patients routinely monitor insulin through the use of blood glucose measurements and glycosylated hemoglobin measurements. For clotting factors, efficacy is assessed by measuring the specific factor being monitored or prothrombin time or partial thromboplastin time.

The pharmacist should be aware of drugs that are administered in conjunction with these agents to reduce the incidence and severity of side effects (e.g., acetaminophen and indomethacin started immediately before aldesleukin therapy to reduce fever; methylprednisolone sodium succinate intravenously prior to first injection of muromonab-CD3).

Medical and product information services are available from the manufacturers for biotechnology drugs, just as for traditional drugs. In addition to answering conventional questions about drug use, indications, adverse effects, and so on, this service helps answer difficult questions (e.g., what to do if a product requiring refrigeration has been left at room temperature for an extended period) and helps to facilitate quick replacement of defective products.

Reimbursement issues are not fully addressed here. However, manufacturers do have support staff who will help the pharmacist deal with third-party payers, particularly if there is a reimbursement issue or problem. Manufacturer reimbursement assurance programs are designed to remove reimbursement barriers when reimbursement has been denied (e.g., if the drug has been used for an unlabeled indication or used in the home rather than in a hospital or physician's office). Many companies also have a long-standing tradition of providing prescription medications free of charge to those who might not otherwise have access to necessary medicines. Physicians can secure these on behalf of their patients; the pharmacist can refer patients and their families to pharmaceutical companies who have cost-sharing or financial assistance programs. The Pharmaceutical Research and Manufacturers of America (PhRMA) has a directory of programs for patients in need. Up-to-date information can be secured by a health care professional by calling the PhRMA (800-PMA-INFO [800-762-4636]) or through the Internet (www.pharma.org/patients).

The Pharmaceutical Research and Manufacturers of America periodically disseminates *Biotechnology Medicines in Development,* which demonstrates biotechnology medicines that have reached the clinical marketplace or are in development. Those desiring to receive this regularly are asked to write to the Editor, Biotechnology Medicines in Development, Communications Division, Pharmaceutical Research and Manufacturers of America, 1100 15th Street, NW, Washington, DC 20005.

PHARMACEUTICS CASE STUDY

Subjective

Working for an up-and-coming biotechnology company, you have been assigned to formulate a new granulocyte macrophage colony–stimulating factor product called CSF-110.

Objective

CSF-110 is a glycoprotein consisting of 143 amino acids and a dose of 100 to 200 μg. It is stable for only 24 hours in aqueous solution at a pH in the range of 6.5 to 7.5 and less stable outside this pH range. It is adsorbed to the interior of glass vials in aqueous solution. A reasonable shelf life is required so the drug can be commercially marketed.

Assessment

This product will be marketed as a dry powder for reconstitution; the powder may be simply preblended or lyophilized. Due to the difficulty of maintaining uniform blends during packaging of a product containing particles of different densities, it may be best to prepare the solutions and lyophilize them in the vials in which they are dispensed. This may also be supported by the coating action of human serum albumin on the interior of the vials in solution form to minimize sorption of the drug to the vial after reconstitution.

Plan

A lyophilized product that can be reconstituted with sterile water for injection prior to use may be feasible. The product could include the drug, a 0.05-M phosphate buffer system at pH 7.0, 0.1% human albumin to minimize sorption, and sodium chloride for tonicity adjustment. The solution will be prepared, poured into vials, lyophilized, labeled, and packaged.

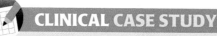

CLINICAL CASE STUDY

Subjective

CC: J.S. is a 31y/o WF who arrives at the clinic with her husband. He explains that J. S. has been feeling depressed ever since she started her new drug therapy a year ago. He is extremely concerned because she doesn't have any interest in the activities that she normally enjoyed to do.

HPI: J.S. was diagnosed with multiple sclerosis a year ago, when she had complaints of blurred vision, fatigue, and tingling sensations in her right leg. She received intravenous corticosteroid therapy for her acute exacerbation. Since then, J.S. has been receiving interferon therapy (Betaseron).

PMH: MS diagnosed 1 year ago
DM type I since 5 y/o
Pneumonia 2 months ago, treated and resolved
Upper neck injury and concussion during rugby game at 22y/o
Automobile accident at age 17 (concussion and shattered left elbow)

Meds: Insulin regular 30u SQ q12h for DM, started at age 5
Interferon beta-1b (Betaseron) 0.25mg QOD (powdered vial) for MS, started 1 year ago

OTC: patient denies taking herbal, homeopathic medications, other supplements

Clinical Case Study cont.

PSH: Left elbow replacement surgery at age 17

FH: Father: H/o DM (type unknown), died of stroke at age 57
Mother: HTN since 55 y/o
Brother: DM type I

SH: (+) Tobacco: smoked for 5 years, quit 6 years ago
(−) ETOH
(−) Caffeine
(−) Illicit drugs

Exercise/daily activities: Used to run and lift weights 2–3×/week, hiking and mountain biking during summers

Diet: Eats fast food and snacks on chips and candy, meal timing varies

Patient used to play professional rugby in Europe. Now she is a sales manager for Nike. Patient lives with husband, married for 5 years

ALL: NKA

MS: Patient reports that blurred vision, fatigue, and tingling sensations have subsided after Betaseron therapy. No allergic reactions or injection site reactions have been reported. Patient has been very compliant with therapy. Patient complains of difficulty in reconstituting the Betaseron.

DM: Patient reports no s/s of hyperglycemia or hypoglycemia. Patient is not aware of recommended American Diabetic Association (ADA) diet. Patient also reports compliance with insulin shots but denies any glucose monitoring at home. Patient made an effort to exercise 3×/wk, but after interferon therapy patient does no exercise anymore.

Objective

31 y/o WF

Ht: 5'8   **Wt:** 63.6 kg

BP: 121/78   **P:** 72   **T:** 98°   **RR:** 19

Pain: none

137 \   104 \   13 / 112
4.3 /   25 /   0.8 \
6.3 \ 13.1 / 269
/ 40 \

HgbA1c: 6.5

LFT: wnl

Assessment

Betaseron therapy is effective in reducing recurrence of symptoms and exacerbations, but patient has depression induced by Betaseron therapy. Studies indicate that interferon in Betaseron is responsible for the depression by suppressing circulating tryptophan and therefore serotonin synthesis. According to patient's husband, the depression is interfering with patient's quality of life.

Based on patient's blood glucose and HgbA1c levels, patient's diabetes is controlled.

Plan

Recommend cessation of Betaseron therapy and substitute with glatiramer acetate (Copaxone). Although there are reports that using serotonin-specific reuptake inhibitors (SSRIs) (citalopram, paroxetine) may treat depression associated with interferon therapy, J.S. states having trouble reconstituting vials, and Copaxone comes as a prefilled syringe and is not associated with depression. In addition, follow-up on depression may be time consuming and cost money, and the side effects associated with SSRIs is another reason not to continue patient on Betaseron. Evaluate therapy at each clinic visit by monitoring side effects, signs and symptoms (s/s) of disease progression, and magnetic resonance imaging should be done at least once a year to assess the reduction of neuronal lesions. Check complete blood count, perform a neurologic examination, and monitor patient's compliance at each clinic visit. Monitor resolution of depression at next visit and encourage patient to exercise regularly and to begin hobbies and activities (avoid activities that put patient at high risk for trauma).

Clinical Case Study cont.

Continue insulin therapy. Recommend J. S. to obtain a glucose monitor and monitor blood glucose daily at home. Also recommend keeping a glucose diary (Goal Fasting Blood Glucose (FBG): 60–110mg/dL, goal HgbA1c: 4–6%). Educate patient on the importance of eating a healthy diet and following a consistent daily meal schedule. Recommend J. S. to start an 1800-calorie ADA diet.

Also recommend patient to check foot and skin daily, teeth and gums every 6 months, and to get an annual eye and foot examination. Monitor for s/s of hypoglycemia and hyperglycemia at each clinic visit and perform urinary analysis (U/A) every 6 months. Recommend patient to obtain a medical bracelet in case of emergency. Encourage J. S. to slowly begin exercising again.

REFERENCES

1. Wade DA, Levy RA. Biotechnology: an opportunity for pharmacists. Am Pharm 1992;NS32(9):33–37.
2. Piascik P. Recent biotechnology drug approvals. JAPhA 1998;38:502–505.
3. Piascik P. New biotechnology approvals for 2002. JAPhA 2003;43:116–117.
4. Wolf BA. Overview of therapeutic drug monitoring and biotechnologic drugs. Ther Drug Monit 1996;18:402–404.
5. Kohler G, Milstein C. Continuous culture of fused cells secreting antibody of predefined specificity. Nature 1975;256:495–497.
6. Vermeij P, Blok D. New peptide and protein drugs. Pharm World Sci 1996;18(3):87–93.
7. Peterson NC. Recombinant antibodies: Alternative strategies for developing and manipulating murine-derived monoclonal antibodies. Lab Anim Sci 1996;46(1):8–14.
8. Jurcic JG, Scheinberg DA, Houghton AN. Monoclonal antibody therapy for cancer. In: Pinedo HM, Longo DL, Chabner BA, eds. Cancer chemotherapy and biological response modifiers annual 17. Edinburgh, UK: Elsevier Science BV: 1997;195–216.
9. Ballow M, Nelson R. Immunopharmacology: Immunomodulation and immunotherapy. JAMA 1997;278:2008–2017.
10. FDA Medical Bulletin. 1993; 23(2):4.
11. Sahai J, Louis SG. Overview of the immune and hematopoietic systems. Am J Hosp Pharm 1993;50 (Suppl 3):S4–S18.
12. Metcalf D. The colony stimulating factors. Cancer 1990;65:2185–2195.
13. Blackwell S, Crawford J. Colony-stimulating factors: clinical applications. Pharmacotherapy 1992;12(2, part 2):20S–31S.
14. Oettgen HF. Cytokines in clinical cancer therapy. Curr Opin Immunol 1991;3:699–705.
15. Erickson A. Droterecogin alfa (activated) has potential to save thousands of sepsis patients annually. Pharmacy Today 2002;8(1):1, 7.
16. Posey LM. FDA approves first fusion inhibitor for HIV. Pharmacy Today 2003;9(4):8.
17. Bagley JL. Biotech. Am Druggist 1986;195(7):57–63.
18. Wordell CJ. Use of beta interferon in multiple sclerosis. Hosp Pharm 1993;28:802–807.
19. Piascik P. A new treatment for multiple sclerosis. Am Pharm 1993; NS33(12):25–26.
20. Piascik P. Administering Betaseron for MS. Am Pharm 1994;NS34(1):21–22
21. Giedlin MA, Zimmerman RJ. The use of recombinant human interleukin-2 in treating infectious diseases. Curr Opin Biotechnol 1993;4:722–726.
22. Stein KE. Overcoming obstacles to monoclonal antibody product development and approval. Trends Biotechnol 1997;15(3):88–90.
23. Tami JA, Parr MD, Brown SA, Thompson JS. Monoclonal antibody technology. Am J Hosp Pharm 1986;43:2816–2826.
24. Newton GD. Monoclonal antibody-based self-testing products. Am Pharm 1993;NS33(9):22–23.
25. Weinblatt ME, Keystone EC, Furst DE, et al. Adalimumab, a fully human anti-tumor necrosis factor alpha monoclonal antibody, for the treatment of rheumatoid arthritis in patients taking concomitant methotrexate: the ARMADA trial. Arthritis Rheum 2003;48:35–45.
26. Farrell RJ, Alsahli M, Jeen YT, et al. Intravenous hydrocortisone premedication reduces antibodies to infliximab in Crohn's disease: a randomized controlled trial. Gastroenterology 2003;124:917–924.
27. Keane J. Tuberculosis associated with infliximab, a tumor necrosis factor α-neutralizing agent. N Engl J Med 2001;345:1098–1104.
28. Baumgart DC, Dignass AU. Shingles following infliximab infusion. Ann Rheum Dis 2002;61:661.
29. Busse WW, Lemanske RF. Asthma. N Engl J Med 2001;344:350–362.
30. Berkower I. The promise and pitfalls of monoclonal antibody therapeutics. Curr Opin Biotechnol 1996 7:622–628.
31. Nowell PC, Hungerford DA. A minute chromosome in human chorionic granulocytic leukemia. Science 1960;132:1497–1501.

32. Buchdunger E, O'Reilly T, Wood J. Pharmacology of imatinib (ST1571). Eur J Cancer 2002;38 Suppl 5:S28–36.

33. OBrien SG, Guilhot F, Larson RA, et al. Imatinib compared with interferon and low-dose cytarabine for newly diagnosed chronic-phase myeloid leukemia. N Engl J Med 2003;348:994–1004.

34. Benz JD. Imatinib opens oncology door to community pharmacists. Pharm Today 2001;7(6):6.

35. Sindelar RE. Biotech products on the horizon. Am Pharm 1993;NS33(11):27–28.

36. Ramsey B. A summary of the results of the phase III multi-center clinical trial: aerosol administration of recombinant human DNase reduces the risk of respiratory infections and improves pulmonary function in patients with cystic fibrosis. Pediatric Pulmonol 1993;9(suppl):12–153.

37. Reddy IK, Banga AK. Biotechnology drug delivery: oral vs. alternate routes. Pharm Times 1993;59(11):92–98.

38. Hudson RA, Black CD. Novel delivery for protein drugs. Am Pharm 1993;NS33(5):23–24.

39. Martin FJ, Huang T. STEALTH liposomal technology: current therapies and future directions. Drug Deliv Technol 2003;3(5):66–73.

40. Houston LL. Targeted delivery of toxins and enzymes by antibodies and growth factors. Curr Opin Biotechnol 1993;4:739–744.

41. Houghton AN, Coit DG. Therapy of metastatic melanoma with monoclonal antibodies. New Perspect Cancer Diagnosis Manag 1993;1(3):65–70.

42. http://www.fda.gov/cber/transfer/transfer.htm.

43. Piascik P. Getting information about biotechnology products. Am Pharm 1993;NS33(4):18–19.

Novel Dosage Forms and Drug Delivery Technologies

20

Chapter at a glance

This chapter discusses novel drug delivery systems that are modifications of those previously presented, are relatively new on the market, or do not fit into categories in previous chapters. They may be relatively new, use new or relatively new delivery systems, or use unique delivery systems or unique devices before, during, or after administration. Dramatic changes have been introduced, with new technology and new devices now on the market. In some cases, traditional capsules and ointments have been replaced by osmotic pumps, wearable ambulatory pumps, electrically assisted drug delivery, and a host of other delivery methods based on various polymer technologies. Feedback mechanisms are now feasible: actual drug delivery may be a response to a sensor detecting variations in certain body chemicals and prompting infusion of a drug to correct the imbalance.

Changes are coming about as new technologies are developed and reduce the limitations of existing therapies. In some cases, the new drugs require new delivery systems because the traditional systems are inefficient or ineffective; this may be true especially of some of the recombinant DNA and gene therapies of the future. We may soon be manipulating genes as active drugs and as drug delivery systems and even work in nanotechnology (nanopharmacy) in the future. Some therapies may become very site specific and require very high concentrations of drugs in selected sites of the body, as more controlled drug delivery systems will be available in the very near future. Traditional oral medications may not be as effective in some of these cases.

New drug delivery system development is largely based on promoting the therapeutic effects of a drug and minimizing its toxic effects by increasing the amount and persistence of a drug in the vicinity of a target cell and reducing the drug exposure of nontarget cells. This is still largely based on Paul Ehrlich's magic bullet concept.

Benefits: New drug delivery systems can provide improved or unique clinical benefits, such as (*a*) improvement of patients' compliance, (*b*) improved outcomes, (*c*) reduction of adverse effects, (*d*) improvement of patients' acceptance of the treatment, (*e*) avoidance of costly interventions such as laboratory services, (*f*) allowing patients to receive medication as outpatients, and possibly (*g*) a reduction in the overall use of medicinal resources.

Mechanisms: Novel drug delivery systems can include those based on physical mechanisms and those based on biochemical mechanisms. Physical mechanisms, also referred to as controlled drug delivery systems, include osmosis, diffusion, erosion, dissolution, and electrotransport. Biochemical mechanisms include monoclonal antibodies, gene therapy and vector systems, polymer drug abducts, and liposomes.

Therapeutic benefits of some of the new drug delivery systems include optimization of the duration of action of the drug, decreasing dosage frequency, controlling the site of release, and maintaining constant drug levels. Safety benefits include reducing adverse effects, decreasing the number of concomitant medications a patient must take, decreasing the need for interventions, and reducing the number of emergency department visits. Economic benefits of novel drug delivery systems include simplifying administration regimens, enhancing patients' compliance, and an overall reduction of health care costs.

Composition

Associated with the various mechanisms that are characteristic of or the basis of the newer drug delivery systems, their composition can be quite variable; ranging from naturally derived substances, such as gelatin and sugars, to the more complex polymers. New drug delivery systems also incorporate mechanical, electronic, and computer components.

The therapeutic efficacy of selected products can be enhanced and in some cases the toxicity can be decreased by incorporating novel polymer technology. For example, degradable bonds can be used to attach an active drug to a synthetic or naturally occurring polymer. Upon delivery to the target site and in the presence of certain enzymes or through hydrolysis or a comparable mechanism the product can be cleaved, releasing the active drug at a specific site of action. Oral, topical, parenteral, and implantable drugs have the potential to be used with this approach.

A number of release profiles using polymers are possible, as are actual penetration into specific tissues and selection of specific target sites. Potential problems of polymers include the following: (*a*) Their high molecular weight may cause them to be very slowly excreted from the body. (*b*) Because of their size, permeability through various membranes may be slow. (*c*) Immunologic or toxic reactions may occur. (*d*) Since they are complex, they may be labor intensive and expensive to develop. Novel drug delivery systems will be discussed in the general categories of topical, oral, vaginal, implanted, ophthalmic, and parenteral preparations.

Topical Administration

The basis for the development of transdermal drug delivery systems (patches) involves percutaneous absorption. See Chapters 10 and 11 for background information on transdermal systems and penetration enhancers. Novel topical systems also include iontophoresis (IP) and phonophoresis.

Iontophoresis

IP is an electrochemical method that enhances the transport of some solute molecules by creating a potential gradient through the skin with an applied electrical current or voltage. It induces increased migration of ionic drugs into the skin by electrostatic repulsion at the active electrode: negative ions are delivered by the cathode and positive ions by the anode. A typical iontophoresis device consists of a battery, microprocessor controller, drug reservoir, and electrodes.

Advantages of IP include (*a*) control of the delivery rates by variations of current density, pulsed voltage, drug concentration, and ionic strength; (*b*) eliminating gastrointestinal incompatibility, erratic absorption, and first-pass metabolism; (*c*) reducing side effects and variation among patients; (*d*) avoiding the risks of infection, inflammation, and fibrosis associated with continuous injection or infusion; and (*e*) enhancing compliance with a convenient and noninvasive therapeutic regimen.

The main disadvantage of IP is skin irritation at high current densities; this can be eliminated or minimized by reducing the current.

IP is gaining increasing acceptance in the pharmaceutical industry with small, efficient iontophoretic patches projected to be on the market within the next few years. Miniaturization is now possible with smaller, more powerful batteries and electronics. The next generation of iontophoresis patch may also include an electronic record of the date, time, and quantity of each dose delivered, providing information for determining patient compliance. Currently, however, iontophoresis involves the use of an iontophoretic device attached to electrodes containing a solution of the drug.

As previously mentioned, iontophoresis involves the use of small amounts of physiologically acceptable electric current to move charged, or ionized, drugs through the skin. Placing an ionized solution of the drug in an electrode of the same charge and applying a current repels the drug from the electrode into the skin. This method of drug delivery has been around for at least 100 years. Since the 1930s, iontophoresis of pilocarpine has been used to induce sweating in the diagnosis of cystic fibrosis. More recently, iontophoresis has been used in the topical delivery of fluoride to the teeth, dexamethasone as an anti-inflammatory into joints, and lidocaine as a topical anesthetic. Drugs such as corticosteroids, nonsteroidal anti-inflammatory agents, and anesthetics are commonly delivered via iontophoresis. Other drugs under study include a number of analgesics, nicotine, anti-AIDS drugs, cancer drugs,

insulin, and proteins. Iontophoresis is also useful in veterinary medicine.

In the iontophoresis process, the current, beginning at the device, is transferred from the electrode through the ionized drug solution as ionic flow. The drug ions move to the skin, where the repulsion continues, moving the drug through whatever pathways are available, namely pores and possibly through a disrupted stratum corneum. The drug-containing electrode is termed the active electrode, and the other electrode, the passive electrode, is placed elsewhere on the body. Current densities up to $0.5 \ mA/cm^2$ can be tolerated with little or no discomfort. The larger the electrode surface, the greater the current the device must supply to provide a current density for moving the drug.

The delivery of a drug iontophoretically is quite complex, depending on the interactions between the drug and the vehicle electrolyte or buffer, partitioning of the drug between the vehicle and the skin, and then diffusion through a highly heterogeneous membrane under the influence of both a chemical and electrical potential gradient.

The movement of ions across the skin is described by the relationship known as the Nernst-Planck equation:

$$J_i = -D_I \, dC_i/dx - z_i \, m \, F \, C_i \, dE/dx$$

where

$-J_i$ is flux,
D_i is diffusivity,
dC_i/dx is concentration gradient,
z_i is valence of the species I,
m is mobility,
F is Faraday's constant,
C_I is concentration, and
dE/dx is electrostatic potential gradient.

Variables affecting iontophoresis include aspects of the current, the physicochemical properties of the drug, formulation factors, biologic factors, and electroendosmotic flow.

The *current* can be direct, alternate, or pulsed and can have various waveforms, including square, sinusoidal, triangular, and trapezoidal. There may not be much advantage to the more complex forms, as direct current is most commonly used at this time.

Physicochemical variables include the charge, size, structure, and lipophilicity of the drug. The drug should be water soluble, low dose, and ionizable with a high charge density. Smaller molecules are more mobile, but large molecules are also usable.

Formulation factors include drug concentration, pH, ionic strength, and viscosity. Increasing drug concentration usually results in greater drug delivery to a certain degree. Buffer ions in a formula will compete with the drug for the delivery current, decreasing the quantity of drug delivered, especially since buffer ions are generally smaller and more mobile than the larger active drug. The pH of solutions can be adjusted and maintained by larger molecules, such as ethanolamine: ethanolamine HCl rather than the smaller hydrochloric acid and sodium hydroxide. An increase in ionic strength of the system will also increase the competition for the available current, especially since the active drugs are generally potent and present in a small concentration as compared to these extraneous ions.

Biologic factors pertain to the skin to which the electrodes are applied; its thickness, permeability, presence of pores, and so on.

Electroendosmotic flow results when a voltage difference is applied across a charged porous membrane, resulting in a bulk fluid flow in the same direction as the flow of counter ions. This fluid flow can actually carry a drug with it into the skin, especially positively charged, cationic, drugs. Neutral drugs can also be carried via electroendosmotic flow.

Iontophoretic devices have changed remarkably over the years, ranging from the galvanometers of the past to the small, specially designed units of today. Iontophoresis devices available from various companies are listed in Table 20.1.

Iontophoretic units will soon be sized similarly to today's transdermal patches. They will be slightly thicker to accommodate the power source and small microprocessor controllers. The future may include IP patches capable of sampling and testing (e.g. glucose levels) and adjusting the delivery rate of a drug (e.g. insulin), all in the same IP system. Reverse iontophoresis can be used to extract chemicals or

TABLE 20.1 IONTOPHORESIS EQUIPMENT, INCLUDING DEVICES AND ELECTRODES

COMPANY	BRAND
Empi (St. Paul)	Dupel Relion (Veterinary-Equine)
General Medical (Los Angeles)	Lectro Patch
Iomed (Salt Lake City)	Phoresor II
LifeTech (Houston)	Iontophor 150
Wescor (Logan, UT)	Macroduct Sweat Collection System Nanoduct Sweat Testing System

drugs from the body for testing. Many types of patches with electrodes may require pharmacists to add the drug prior to dispensing, as is done today in filling reservoirs for parenteral administration. Drugs currently administered using iontophoresis are listed in Table 20.2. Since most solutions designed specifically for iontophoresis are not commercially available, they must be compounded. It is best to have only the drug and water present to minimize competition for the active ions.

A new iontophoresis system called Numby Stuff (IOMED) is used to achieve local anesthesia of the skin and is promoted as a painless, needleless system.

Iontophoretic administration is also used in veterinary pharmacy, using drugs such as those listed in Table 20.3. Because of the difference in the size and anatomy of the animal patient, different electrodes may be required.

Phonophoresis

Phonophoresis (ultrasound, sonophoresis, ultrasonophoresis, ultraphonophoresis) is the transport of drugs through the skin using ultrasound; it is a combination of ultrasound therapy with topical drug therapy to achieve therapeutic drug concentrations at selected sites in the skin. It is widely used by physiotherapists. In this technique, the drug is generally mixed with a coupling agent, usually a gel but sometimes a cream or ointment, that transfers ultrasonic energy

TABLE 20.2 DRUGS USED IN IONTOPHORESIS

DRUG SOLUTION	CONCENTRATION (%)	USE/INDICATION	POLARITY
Acetic acid	2–5	Calcium deposits, calcified tendonitis	Negative
Atropine sulfate	0.001–0.01	Hyperhidrosis	Positive
Calcium chloride	2	Myopathy, myospasm, immobile joints	Positive
Sodium chloride	2	Sclerolytic, scar tissue, adhesions, keloids	Negative
Copper sulfate	2	Astringent, fungus infection	Positive
Dexamethasone sodium phosphate	0.4	Tendonitis, bursitis, arthritis, tenosynovitis, Peyronie's disease	Negative
Estriol	0.3	Acne scars	Positive
Fentanyl citrate		Analgesic	Positive
Fluoride sodium	2	Desensitize teeth	Positive
Gentamicin sulfate	0.8	Ear chondritis	Positive
Glycopyrronium bromide	0.05	Hyperhidrosis	Positive
Hyaluronidase	150 U/mL solution	Absorption enhancement, edema, scleroderma, lymphedema	Positive
Idoxuridine	0.1	Herpes simplex	Negative
Iodine ointment	4.7	Sclerolytic, antimicrobial, fibrosis, adhesions, scar tissue, trigger finger	Negative
Iron/titanium oxide		Skin pigmentation	Positive
Lidocaine hydrochloride	4 (with or without epinephrine 1:50,000–1:100,000)	Skin anesthesia, trigeminal neuralgia	Positive
Lithium chloride	2	Gouty arthritis	Positive
Magnesium sulfate	2	Muscle relaxant, vasodilator, myalgias, neuritis, deltoid bursitis, low back spasm	Positive
Mecholyl chloride	0.25	Vasodilator, muscle relaxant, radiculitis, varicose ulcers	Positive
Meladinine sodium	1	Vitiligo	Negative
Methylphenidate hydrochloride		Attention deficit disorder	Positive
Morphine sulfate	0.2–0.4	Analgesic	Positive
Pilocarpine hydrochloride		Sweat test for cystic fibrosis	Positive
Poldine methyl sulfate	0.05–0.5	Hyperhidrosis	Negative
Potassium iodide	10	Scar tissue	Negative
Sodium salicylate	2	Analgesic, sclerolytic, plantar warts, scar tissue, myalgias	Negative
Tretinoin		Acne scars	Positive
Water	100	Palmar, plantar, axillary hyperhidrosis	Both
Zinc oxide suspension	20	Antiseptic, ulcers, dermatitis, wound healing	Positive

from the phonophoresis device to the skin. The ultrasonic unit has a sound transducer head emitting energy at 1 MHz at 0.5 to 1 W/cm². Although the exact mechanism is not known, it may involve a disruption of the stratum corneum lipids, allowing the drug to pass through the skin.

Originally, the drug-containing coupling agent was applied to the skin and immediately

TABLE 20.3 DRUGS USED IN VETERINARY IONTOPHORESIS

DRUG SOLUTION	COMMERCIAL CONCENTRATION (MG/ML)	TOTAL/6 ML ELECTRODE (MG)	POLARITY
NSAIDs			
Phenylbutazone	200	1200	Negative
Flunixin meglumine	50	300	Negative
Ketoprofen	100	600	Negative
Corticosteroids, anti-inflammatory agents			
Dexamethasone sodium phosphate	2 or 4	12 or 24	Negative
Betamethasone	4	24	Negative
Prednisolone sodium succinate	10 or 50	60 or 300	Negative
Antibiotics			
Gentamicin sulfate	50 or 100	300 or 600	Positive
Amikacin sulfate	50	300	Positive
Ceftiofur sodium	50	300	Negative
Local anesthetic			
Lidocaine hydrochloride	20	120	Positive

Adapted from product information 801419. St. Paul: Empi, 1996.

followed by the ultrasound unit. Today, the product is applied to the skin and some time is allowed for the drug to begin absorption into the skin; then the ultrasound unit is applied. The ultrasound emitted from the unit is actually sound waves outside the normal human hearing range. As ultrasound waves, they can be reflected, refracted, and absorbed by the medium, just as regular sound waves can. Consequently, these are factors that must be considered as affecting phonophoresis efficiency.

Three effects of ultrasound are cavitation, microstreaming, and heat generation. Cavitation is formation and collapse of very small air bubbles in a liquid in contact with ultrasound waves. Microstreaming, closely associated with cavitation, results in efficient mixing by inducing eddies in small-volume elements of a liquid; this may enhance dissolution of suspended drug particles, resulting in a higher concentration of drug near the skin, for absorption. Heat results from the conversion of ultrasound energy to heat energy and can occur at the surface of the skin as well as in deeper layers of the skin.

The vehicle containing the drug must be formulated to provide good conduction of the ultrasonic energy to the skin. The product must be smooth and not gritty, as it will be rubbed into the skin by the head of the transducer. The product should have relatively low

viscosity for ease of application and ease of movement of the transducer head. Gels work very well as a medium. Emulsions have been used, but the oil–water interfaces in emulsions can disperse the ultrasonic waves, reducing the intensity of the energy reaching the skin. It may also cause some local heat. Air should not be incorporated into the product, as air bubbles may disperse the ultrasound waves, resulting in heat at the liquid–air interface.

Hydrocortisone is the drug most often administered, in concentrations ranging from 1 to 10%.

Oral Administration

Chewable Dispersible Tablets

Lamotrigine (Lamictal Chewable Dispersible Tablets) for oral administration contains 2, 5, or 25 mg of lamotrigine and the following inactive ingredients: black currant flavor, calcium carbonate, low-substituted hydroxypropyl cellulose, magnesium aluminum silicate, magnesium stearate, povidone, saccharin sodium, and sodium starch glycolate (1).

Lamotrigine is also available as standard swallow tablets for oral administration in strengths of 25, 100, 150, and 200 mg, also containing lactose, magnesium stearate, microcrystalline cellulose, povidone, sodium starch glycolate, and various coloring agents for the different strengths. Lamotrigine is an antiepileptic drug chemically unrelated to existing drugs in this therapeutic class. The swallow tablets should be swallowed whole, as chewing may leave a bitter taste. The chewable tablets may be swallowed whole, chewed, or mixed in water or diluted fruit juice. If they are chewed, a small amount of water or diluted fruit juice will aid in swallowing. If the tablet is to be dispersed before it is taken, it can be added to a small amount of liquid (1 teaspoonful or sufficient to cover the medication in a glass or spoon), and approximately 1 minute later when the tablet is completely dispersed, it is mixed and administered immediately.

Didanosine (Videx) is available in three dosage forms: a chewable dispersible buffered tablet, buffered powder for oral solution, and a pediatric powder for oral solution (2). Videx is a synthetic purine nucleoside analogue active against HIV. The chewable dispersible buffered tablets are for oral administration in strengths of 25, 50, 100, 150, and 200 mg. Each tablet is buffered with calcium carbonate and magnesium hydroxide. Also contained in the tablet matrix are aspartame, sorbitol, microcrystalline cellulose, polyplasdone, mandarin orange flavor, and magnesium stearate.

Didanosine (2′,3′-dideoxyinosine) is unstable in acidic solutions; at a pH less than 3 at body temperature, 10% of didanosine decomposes to hypoxanthine in less than 2 minutes. This is the reason for the buffering agents in the chewable tablets and in one of the oral solutions. It is also available as an enteric-coated formulation (Videx EC Delayed-Release Capsules) to protect it from the acidic contents of the stomach.

Mucoadhesive System

The Striant mucoadhesive testosterone buccal system is designed to adhere to the gum or inner cheek to provide a controlled and sustained release of testosterone through the buccal mucosa (3). Using a Striant system twice daily, morning and evening, provides continuous systemic delivery of testosterone to the patient. Each Striant buccal system contains 30 mg of testosterone, along with the inactive ingredients anhydrous lactose, carbomer 934P, hypromellose, magnesium stearate, lactose monohydrate, polycarbophil, colloidal silicon dioxide, starch, and talc. When used as directed in hypogonadal males, the circulating testosterone levels should approximate the physiologic levels in healthy men at 300 to 1050 ng/dL.

When applied, Striant begins hydrating, and testosterone is absorbed through the gum and cheek surfaces that are in contact with it. Venous drainage from the mouth is to the superior vena cava, which circumvents first-pass (hepatic) metabolism. Following initial application, the serum testosterone concentration rises to a maximum within 10 to 12 hours; steady-state levels are usually obtained after the first two Striant systems are used. When removed and not reapplied, the serum testosterone levels fall below normal range within 2 to 4 hours.

What is the effect of food when using Striant? No specific studies were reported in the package literature. The effects of toothbrushing, mouth washing, chewing gum, and alcoholic beverages on the use and absorption of testosterone from the Striant system were not specifically studied but were allowed in the Phase 3 clinical studies, and no significant effect was attributed to these activities.

Osmotic Pump

Numerous drug delivery devices now use osmosis as the driving force. The Alzet (Alza osmotic minipump) is used in research laboratories to provide constant-rate delivery and programmed delivery of a drug. It consists of a flexible impermeable diaphragm surrounded by a sealed layer containing an osmotic agent that is enclosed within a semipermeable membrane. A stainless steel or polyethylene tube or catheter is inserted into the inner chamber from which the drug is channeled. When the unit is subjected to an aqueous medium, the water flows through the rate-controlling semipermeable membrane and dissolves the osmotic agent, which provides the pressure on the flexible lining and forces the drug through the tube or catheter. The unit can be presterilized and prefilled using a filling tube.

With the Alzet pump, the drug reservoir is a liquid solution inside an impermeable collapsible polyester bag coated with a layer of an osmotically active salt. It is sealed within a rigid structure coated with a semipermeable membrane. As the salt dissolves, it creates an osmotic pressure gradient, and the drug compartment is reduced in volume, forcing the drug solution out. The delivery rate can be changed by changing the drug concentration (4).

Oral Inhalation

Advair Diskus 100/50, 250/50, and 500/50 contains fluticasone propionate 100, 250, and 500 μg, respectively, along with salmeterol 50 μg in a powder for inhalation. Fluticasone propionate is a corticosteroid, and salmeterol xinafoate is a highly selective beta$_2$-adrenergic bronchodilator. The Advair Diskus is a specially designed plastic device containing a double-foil blister strip of a powder formulation of fluticasone propionate and salmeterol xinafoate intended for oral inhalation only. Each blister in the device contains 100, 250, or 500 μg of microfine fluticasone propionate and 72.5 μg of microfine salmeterol xinafoate salt, the equivalent of 50 μg of salmeterol base, in 12.5 mg of formulation also containing lactose. Each blister contains 1 complete dose of medication. The blister is opened by activating the device and the medication is dispersed into the airstream created by the patient inhaling through the mouthpiece(5).

Fluticasone propionate inhalation powder is available alone as Flovent Rotadisk 50, 100, and 250 μg marketed to be used with the Diskhaler Inhalation Device. Each double-foil Rotadisk contains 4 blisters; each blister contains 50, 100, or 250 μg of fluticasone propionate blended with lactose to a total weight of 25 mg per blister. When the Rotadisk is placed in the Diskhaler, a blister containing the medication is pierced and the fluticasone propionate is dispersed into the airstream as with the Advair Diskus unit (6).

The Foradil Aerolizer is a capsule dosage form for oral inhalation only in the Aerolizer inhaler. The capsule contains a dry powder formulation of 12 μg of formoterol fumarate and 25 mg of lac- tose as a carrier. Formoterol fumarate is a long-acting selective beta$_2$-adrenergic receptor agonist acting locally in the lung as a bronchodilator. To use this delivery system, the capsule is placed inside the well of the Aerolizer inhaler and the capsule is pierced by pressing and releasing the buttons on the side of the device. The patient inhales rapidly and deeply through the mouthpiece, dispersing the formoterol fumarate formulation into the air for inhalation (7).

Zanamivir for inhalation (Relenza) is used to treat influenza. It is a neuraminidase inhibitor. Relenza is packaged in Rotadisks and is administered using a Diskhaler, as previously described. For Relenza, the usual dose is 2 inhalations (1 blister per inhalation) twice daily for 5 days; therefore, four blisters will be used each day. Relenza should be stored at room temperature; it is not a childproof container (8).

Vaginal Administration

Intravaginal Drug Delivery System

Vaginal administration of drugs, especially hormones, has several advantages, including self-insertion and removal, continuous drug administration at an effective dose level, and good patient compliance. The continuous release and local absorption of drug minimizes systemic toxicity that may result from oral peak-and-valley drug administration.

In a polymeric vaginal drug delivery system, such as a resilient medicated vaginal ring, shown in Figure 20.1 or a copper-containing intrauterine contraceptive device, the drug may be uniformly distributed throughout the polymeric matrix. Upon administration and when in contact with vaginal fluids, the drug will slowly dissolve and migrate out of the device. Drug inside the device will diffuse toward the surface along a concentration gradient, resulting in a long-acting drug delivery system.

Intrauterine Progesterone Drug Delivery System

The Progestasert System (Alza Corporation) shown in Figures 20.2 and 20.3 slowly releases an average of 60 μg of progesterone per day for

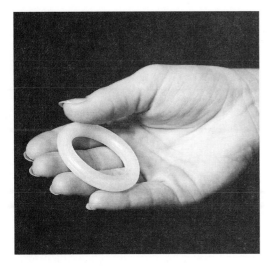

FIGURE 20.1 The Estring (Pharmacia & Upjohn), a polymeric vaginal drug delivery system. (Courtesy of Pharmacia & Upjohn.)

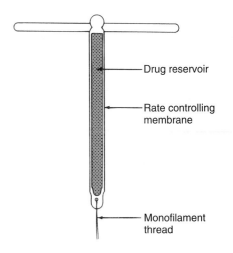

FIGURE 20.3 Schematic of the Progestasert intrauterine drug delivery system. (Courtesy of Alza Corporation.)

1 year after insertion. The continuous release of progesterone into the uterine cavity provides local rather than systemic action. Two hypotheses for the contraceptive action have been offered: progesterone-induced inhibition of sperm capacity for survival and alteration of the uterine milieu so as to prevent nidation. The intrauterine device contains 38 mg of progesterone, a much smaller amount than would be taken by other routes over the same period for the same purpose. The intrauterine device is replaced annually for the maintenance of contraception (9).

The Progestasert provides contraception without the need for daily self-medication and has the advantages of (*a*) using a natural hormone; (*b*) containing no estrogens; (*c*) using a T-shaped delivery device to ensure comfort, safety, and retention, which minimizes mechanically induced irritation; and (*d*) confining the hormonal action to the uterus.

The device contains the progesterone suspended in silicone oil; barium sulfate is added to make it radiopaque. The EVA membrane surrounding the drug core controls the rate of drug release. Titanium dioxide is added to the EVA for a white color. At the end of a year, the device will contain approximately 14 mg of progesterone, the excess being required to maintain the thermodynamic activity of the drug reservoir.

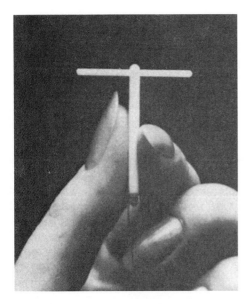

FIGURE 20.2 Progestasert intrauterine progesterone contraceptive system enables prevention of pregnancy in women for a year or more after each insertion. This small, flexible unit releases the natural hormone progesterone directly into the uterus. (Courtesy of Alza Corporation.)

Dinoprostone Vaginal Insert

Dinoprostone (Cervidil, Forest Pharmaceuticals) is a thick, flat rectangular polymeric slab

enclosed in a pouch of a knitted polyester retrieval system. The buff-colored semitrans-
parent polymeric hydrogel slab contains 10
mg of dinoprostone. The retrieval system is in
the shape of a long knitted tape that is used to
retrieve, or remove, the unit after the dosing
interval is complete. The product is designed
to release dinoprostone in vivo at a rate of
about 0.3 mg/hour. The unit contains 10 mg
of dinoprostone in 236 mg of a cross-linked
polyethylene oxide–urethane polymer slab
that measures 29 mm by 9.5 mm and is 0.8
mm thick. When placed in a moist environment, the unit absorbs water, swells, and releases dinoprostone.

It is indicated for initiation and/or continu-
ation of cervical ripening in patients at or near
term when there is medical or obstetrical indication for labor induction.

The product is dosed at 10 mg of dinoprostone (1 unit) inserted vaginally and removed
upon onset of active labor or 12 hours after
insertion. After administration, the patient
should remain supine for 2 hours but may be
ambulatory after that time.

This product should be stored in a freezer at
$-20°$ to $-10°C$ ($-4°–14°F$); it is packaged in
foil and is stable in the freezer for 3 years. After opening and upon exposure to humidity, it
is hygroscopic, and the release characteristics
of the dinoprostone may be altered if it is improperly stored (10). An example is shown in
Figure 20.4.

Estring

A unique method of administering estradiol is
through the use of the estradiol vaginal ring
(Estring, Pharmacia & Upjohn) shown in Figure 20.1. The core of the ring contains a reservoir of estradiol, which is released immediately and then at a continuous rate of 75 μg/24
hours over 90 days. The ring, composed of silicone polymers and barium sulfate, has an
outer diameter of 55 mm and a core diameter
of 2 mm. The ring is inserted into the upper
third of the vaginal vault and is worn continuously for the treatment of urogenital symptoms associated with postmenopausal atrophy
of the vagina.

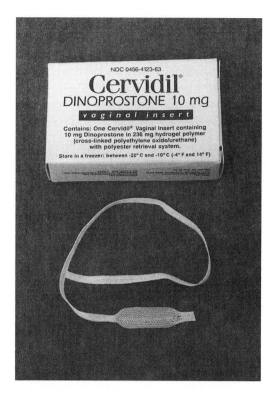

FIGURE 20.4 Cervidil (dinoprostone) vaginal insert. The
polymeric slab containing the dinoprostone is encased in
a pouch of a knitted polyester delivery and retrieval system. (Courtesy of Forest Pharmaceuticals.)

Crinone Gel

Another type of vaginal product with extended action is the bioadhesive vaginal gel
Crinone Gel (Wyeth-Ayerst), which contains
micronized progesterone and the polymer
polycarbophil in an oil-in-water emulsion
system. The polymer, which is insoluble in
water, swells within the vagina and forms a
bioadhesive gel coating on the walls of the
vagina. This allows the absorption of progesterone through the vaginal tissue over 25 to
50 hours. The product is used to assist in reproduction.

Ophthalmics

One of the problems associated with the use
of ophthalmic solutions is the rapid loss of
administered drug due to the blinking of the
eye and the flushing effect of lacrimal fluids.
Up to 80% of an administered dose may be lost

through tears and the action of nasolacrimal drainage within 5 minutes of installation (11). Extended periods of therapy may be achieved by formulations that increase the contact time between the medication and the corneal surface. This may be accomplished through use of agents that increase the viscosity of solutions; by ophthalmic suspensions in which the drug particles slowly dissolve; by slowly dissipating ophthalmic ointments; or by the use of ophthalmic inserts.

Gels

Although ophthalmic dosage forms are discussed at length in Chapter 17, it is useful to note here certain preparations designed to extend drug action. The following are but two examples of proprietary products that use viscosity-increasing agents to increase corneal contact time. Pilocarpine (Pilopine HS Gel, Alcon) employs carbopol 940, a synthetic high-molecular-weight cross-linked polymer of acrylic acid. Timolol maleate (Timoptic-XE, Merck) employs gellan gum (Gelrite), which forms a gel upon contact with the precorneal tear film.

Ophthalmic Inserts

Lacrisert

Lacrisert (Merck) is a rod-shaped water-soluble form of hydroxypropyl cellulose. The insert is placed in the inferior cul-de-sac of the eye once or twice daily for the treatment of dry eyes. The inserts soften and slowly dissolve, thickening the precorneal tear film and prolonging the tear film breakup.

Pilocarpine Insert

Pilocarpine is available in a membrane-controlled reservoir system that is used in the treatment of glaucoma. Pilocarpine is sandwiched between two ethylene vinyl acetate membranes. It also contains alginic acid, a seaweed carbohydrate, that serves as a carrier for pilocarpine. The small, clear device has a white annular border made of ethylene vinyl acetate copolymer impregnated with titanium dioxide (pigment) that makes it easier

for the patient to see. The insert is placed in the cul-de-sac, where it will float with the tears. The pilocarpine will diffuse from the device and exert its pharmacologic effect (Figs. 20.5 and 20.6).

The tear fluid penetrates the microporous membrane, dissolving the pilocarpine. The release rate of pilocarpine is in the range of 20 or 40 μg/hour for 4 to 7 days. One advantage to this system is enhanced compliance, as the patient does not have to remember to instill the drops and has no blurred vision or slight discomfort that occurs when applying drops to the eyes.

The release rate of pilocarpine from the EVA system:

$$dm/dt = \frac{ADK\varDelta C}{h}$$

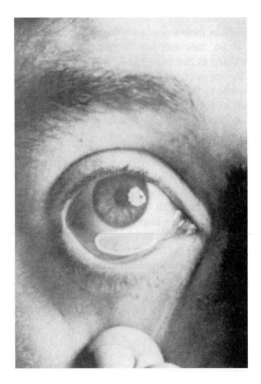

FIGURE 20.5 Ocusert ocular therapeutic systems are thin, flexible wafers placed under the eyelid to provide a week's dose of pilocarpine in the treatment of glaucoma. Ocusert systems cause less blurring of vision than conventional pilocarpine eye drops, which must be administered 4 times daily. (Courtesy of Alza Corporation.)

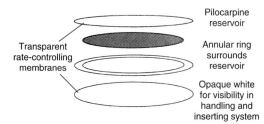

FIGURE 20.6 Construction of the Ocusert ocular therapeutic system containing pilocarpine between transparent rate-controlling membranes. (Courtesy of Alza Corporation.)

where

> dm/dt is the release rate,
> D is the diffusion coefficient of the drug in the membrane,
> K is the partition coefficient that is the ratio of drug concentration at equilibrium inside the membrane to that outside the membrane,
> ΔC is the difference of the drug concentration between the inside and the outside walls of the membrane, and
> A and h are the area and thickness of the system, respectively.

Under routine conditions, the concentration of the drug in the tears is negligible (2–3 μg/mL) compared to that inside the membrane, which is essentially the solubility of the drug, so the equation can be rewritten:

$$dm/dt = \frac{ADKS}{h}$$

The systems are designed to release at 20 or 40 μg/hour for 1 week. Over a week's time, the total drug released by the system is 3.4 or 6.7 mg, for the 20 or 40 μg/hour units, respectively. The units contain either 5 mg or 11 mg of drug initially and are designed to retain about 40% of the initial quantity of drug to provide for a constant delivery rate and a safety margin of an extra day's delivery of drug.

Parenteral Administration

Long-Acting Parenteral Systems

Extended rates of drug action following injection may be achieved in a number of ways, in-cluding the use of crystal or amorphous drug forms having prolonged dissolution characteristics, slowly dissolving chemical complexes of the drug entity, solutions or suspensions of drug in slowly absorbed carriers or vehicles (e.g., oleaginous vehicle), large particles of drug in suspension, or injection of slowly eroding microspheres of drug (12). The duration of action of the various forms of insulin, for example, is based in part on its physical form (amorphous or crystalline), complex formation with added agents, and dosage form (solution or suspension) (13).

Matrix carrier systems based on biodegradable materials for parenteral application have been examined as a potential means of delivering peptides and proteins (22). In such systems, a material such as purified insoluble collagen is used as a matrix that releases the drug contents through controlled diffusion and enzymatic matrix degradation.

In addition to these means of achieving extended drug action, the rate and duration of drug delivery may be controlled mechanically using controlled-rate drug infusion pumps.

Examples of proprietary parenteral products having long-acting features are presented in Table 20.4. Conventional parenteral products and methods of administration are discussed in Chapter 15.

Liposomes

Liposomes are composed of small vesicles of a bilayer of phospholipid encapsulating an aqueous space ranging from about 0.03 to 10 μm in diameter. They are composed of one or many lipid membranes enclosing discrete aqueous compartments. The enclosed vesicles can encapsulate water-soluble drugs in the aqueous spaces, and lipid-soluble drugs can be incorporated into the membranes. Liposomes can be administered parenterally, topically, by inhalation, and possibly by other routes of administration. Current products are administered parenterally.

The following is an oversimplification but will serve to illustrate the preparation of liposomes. Prepare a solution of a lipid (lecithin) in an organic solvent (acetone, chloroform) in a beaker. Allow the solvent to evaporate, leav-

TABLE 20.4 EXAMPLES OF PROPRIETARY EXTENDED ACTION PARENTERAL PRODUCTS

PRODUCT	CONTENTS AND COMMENTS
Bicillin C-R Injection (Wyeth-Ayerst)	Contains penicillin G benzathine, penicillin G procaine, which have low solubility, are slowly released from IM injection sites. Hydrolyze to penicillin G. Hydrolysis plus slow absorption results in prolonged blood serum levels. Usual dose interval, 2–3 days.
Decadron-LA Sterile Suspension (Merck)	Contains dexamethasone acetate, very insoluble ester of dexamethasone. Repository IM injection may be repeated as needed at 1–3 weeks.
Depo-Provera Contraceptive Injection (Pharmacia & Upjohn)	Medroxyprogesterone acetate, water-insoluble, in aqueous suspension. Single IM dose is repeated q3mo.
Abelcet Amphotericin B Lipid Complex Injection (Liposome Company)	Suspension of amphotericin B complexed with two phospholipids administered by IV infusion qd.
Lupron Depot for Suspension (TAP Pharmaceuticals)	Sterile lyophilized microspheres; mixed with diluent, form IM injection suspension q3–4mo.

IM, intramuscular; IV, intravenous.

ing a thin film of the lipid on the walls of the container. Add an aqueous solution of the drug to the beaker and place it in an ultrasonic bath. As the lipid is displaced from the beaker walls, it forms spheres or cylinders, trapping the aqueous solution inside. The liposomes can be collected, sized, and used.

Numerous configurations are possible for liposomes, including spheres and cylinders. Spherical liposomes can be unilamellar (only one layer) or multilamellar (many layers). They are often designated LUV (large unilamellar vesicle), SUV (small unilamellar vesicle) and MLV (multilamellar vesicle). The smaller vesicles, or liposomes, generally range in size from 0.02 μm to 0.2 μm and the large vesicles from about 0.2 μm to more than 10 μm. The MLVs may have an onionskin structure of several layers.

The phospholipids composing liposomes are amphipathic, possessing both a hydrophilic or polar head and a hydrophobic or nonpolar tail. This is similar to the hydrophil–lipophil balance (HLB) and wedge orientation theories of emulsification. The hydrophobic tail is composed of fatty acids containing generally 10 to 24 carbon atoms, and the polar end may contain phosphoric acid bound to a water-soluble portion; the composition may vary considerably. Lecithin (phosphatidylcholine) is a back-

bone structure that has been studied extensively. When these phospholipids are exposed to water and line up, they do so in a manner that the fatty acid tails associate together as the lipophilic phase and the polar head groups associate toward the bulk water phase. Depending on the system and the water solubility of the drug, the drug may be in the aqueous compartments (if water soluble) or in the lipophilic bilayers (if oil soluble).

Some liposomes are unique because they can be selectively absorbed by tissues rich in reticuloendothelial cells, such as the liver, spleen, and bone marrow. This can serve as a targeting mechanism, but it also removes liposomes from the circulation rather rapidly. To extend the half-life of liposomes in the body, "stealth liposomes" have been developed by coating the liposomes with materials, such as the polymer polyethylene glycol, enabling liposomes to evade detection through the components of the body's immune system. This extends their half-life and may also alter their biodistribution.

Advantages of liposomes include the following: (*a*) Liposome-encapsulated drugs are delivered intact to various tissues and cells and can be released when the liposome is destroyed, enabling site-specific and targeted drug delivery. (*b*) Liposomes can be used for both hydrophilic and lipophilic drugs without chemical modification. (*c*) Other tissues and cells of the body are protected from the drug until it is released by the liposomes, decreasing the drug's toxicity. (*d*) The size, charge, and other characteristics can be altered depending on the drug and the intended use of the product.

Disadvantages of liposomes include their tendency to be taken up by cells of the reticuloendothelial system and the slow release of the drug when the liposomes are taken up by phagocytes through endocytosis, fusion, surface adsorption, or lipid exchange.

Many advances in liposome preparation, including composition, sizing, classification, and enhancing stability, have been made. Stability has been a problem, but stable liposomes can now be prepared. Liposomes have been investigated for a number of years as potential drug delivery systems and now are on the market.

One product is Abelcet Injection (Liposome Company). It is a sterile, pyrogen-free suspension for intravenous infusion consisting of amphotericin B complexed with two phospholipids in a 1:1 drug-to-lipid molar ratio. The two phospholipids, L-alpha-dimyristoyl phosphatidylcholine (DMPC) and L-alpha-dimyristoyl phosphatidylglycerol (DMPG) are present in a 7:3 molar ratio. The product is yellow and opaque with a pH in the range of 5 to 7. The formulation per milliliter is provided as the following:

Amphotericin B, USP	5 mg
DMPC	3.4 mg
DMPG	1.5 mg
Sodium Chloride, USP	9 mg
Water for Injection, USP, qs	1 mL

The product contains the following bolded note:

NOTE: Liposomal encapsulation or incorporation in a lipid complex can substantially affect a drug's functional properties relative to those of the unencapsulated or nonlipid-associated drug. In addition, different liposomal or lipid-complexed products with a common active ingredient may vary from one another in the chemical composition and physical form of the lipid component. Such differences may affect functional properties of these drug products (14).

AmBisome is amphotericin B liposome for injection. It is a sterile, nonpyrogenic lyophilized product for intravenous infusion; each vial contains 50 mg amphotericin B intercalated into a liposomal membrane consisting of approximately 213 mg of hydrogenated soy phosphatidylcholine, 52 mg of cholesterol, 84 mg of distearoyl phosphatidylglycerol, 0.64 mg alpha tocopherol, 900 mg sucrose, and 27 mg of disodium succinate hexahydrate as a buffer. When reconstituted with sterile water for injection, the pH of the solution is between 5.0 and 6.0. AmBisome is a true single bilayer liposomal drug delivery system. When the powder is reconstituted, multiple concentric bilayer membranes are formed; these are changed by microemulsification into single bilayer liposomes using a homogenizer. AmBisome contains liposomes that are less than 100 nm in diameter. Amphotericin B is a macrocyclic polyene antifungal antibiotic that is produced from a strain of *Streptomyces nodosus*.

Amphotec (Amphotericin B Cholesteryl Sulfate, Sequus Pharmaceuticals) is a sterile, pyrogen-free lyophilized powder for reconstitution and intravenous administration. It is a 1:1 molar ratio complex of amphotericin B and cholesteryl sulfate that upon reconstitution forms a colloidal dispersion of microscopic disk-shaped particles. Each 50-mg single-dose vial contains amphotericin B 50 mg, sodium cholesteryl sulfate 26.4 mg, tromethamine 5.64 mg, disodium edetate dihydrate 0.372 mg, lactose monohydrate 950 mg, and hydrochloric acid qs. The 100-mg single-dose vial contains amphotericin B 100 mg, sodium cholesteryl sulfate 52.8 mg, tromethamine 11.28 mg, disodium edetate dihydrate 0.744 mg, lactose monohydrate 1900 mg, and hydrochloric acid qs.

Amphotec is indicated for the treatment of invasive aspergillosis in patients when renal impairment or unacceptable toxicity precludes the use of amphotericin B deoxycholate in effective doses and in aspergillosis patients when prior amphotericin B deoxycholate therapy has failed.

The drug is reconstituted with sterile water for injection by rapidly adding the water to the vial; it is shaken gently by hand, rotating the vial until all the solids have dissolved. The fluid may be opalescent or clear. For infusion, it is further diluted in 5% dextrose injection. The product should not be reconstituted with any fluid other than sterile water for injection; do not reconstitute with dextrose or sodium chloride solutions. Also, for further dilution, it should not be admixed with sodium chloride or electrolytes. Solutions containing benzyl alcohol or any other bacteriostatic agent should not be used, as they may cause precipitation. An in-line filter should not be used, and the infusion admixture should not be mixed with other drugs. If infused using a Y-injection site or similar device, flush the line with 5% dextrose injection before and after infusion of Amphotec.

After reconstitution, the drug should be refrigerated and used within 24 hours; do not freeze. If further diluted with 5% dextrose injection, it should be refrigerated and used within 24 hours (15).

Daunorubicin citrate liposome injection (DaunoXome, NeXstar Pharmaceuticals) is an aqueous solution of daunorubicin citrate encapsulated with liposomes composed of distearoyl phosphatidylcholine and cholesterol (2:1 molar ratio), with a mean diameter of about 45 nm (range 35–65 nm). The weight ratio of lipid to drug is 18.7:1 (total lipid–daunorubicin base), equivalent to a 10:5:1 molar ratio of distearoyl phosphatidylcholine, cholesterol, and daunorubicin, respectively.

DaunoXome is formulated to maximize the selectivity of daunorubicin for solid tumors in situ. The liposomal formulation helps to protect the daunorubicin from chemical and enzymatic degradation, minimizes protein binding, and generally decreases uptake by normal tissues.

The product should be diluted 1:1 with 5% dextrose injection prior to administration. Each vial contains the equivalent of 50 mg daunorubicin base at a concentration of 2 mg/mL after preparation; it is recommended to be diluted to 1 mg/mL for administration. The only fluid recommended for preparation is 5% dextrose injection; it must not be mixed with a solution containing sodium chloride or benzyl alcohol or with any other solution. An in-line filter should not be used for the intravenous infusion of DaunoXome. The final product is a red translucent dispersion of liposomes that does scatter light but it should not be used if it appears opaque or has precipitate or foreign matter in it. It should be stored in a refrigerator (2–8°C; 36–46°F), do not freeze and protect from light (16).

Stealth Liposomes

Doxorubicin hydrochloride (Doxil) liposome injection consists of the drug encapsulated in Stealth liposomes for intravenous administration. Doxorubicin is a cytotoxic anthracycline antibiotic that is isolated from *Streptomyces peucetius* var. *caesius*. The product is available as a sterile translucent red liposomal dispersion containing in each 10-mL single-use glass vial 20 mg doxorubicin HCl at a pH of 6.5. The Stealth liposomes consist of 3.19 mg/mL of N-(carbonyl-methoxy polyethylene glycol 2000)-1,2-distearoyl-sn-glycero-3-phosphoethanolamine sodium salt, 9.58 mg/mL of fully hydrogenated soy phosphatidylcholine, and 3.19 mg/mL of cholesterol; also, each milliliter contains approximately 2 mg ammonium sulfate along with histidine as a buffer, sucrose for tonicity, and hydrochloric acid and/or sodium hydroxide for adjustment of pH. The doxorubicin is at least 90% encapsulated in the Stealth liposomes. These Stealth liposomes are protected from detection by the mononuclear phagocyte system by the coating with surface-bound methoxy polyethylene glycol; this is done to increase the blood circulation time. These liposomes have a half-life of approximately 55 hours in humans (17).

Pegylated Dosage Forms

Neulasta (pegfilgrastim) is a covalent conjugate of recombinant methionyl human granulocyte colony–stimulating factor (G-CSF) (Filgrastim) and monomethoxy polyethylene glycol (PEG). Filgrastim is a water-soluble 175-amino acid protein obtained from bacterial fermentation of a strain of *Escherichia coli*; it has a molecular weight of approximately 19 kD. Pegfilgrastim is produced by covalently bonding a 20-kD PEG molecule to the N-terminal methionyl residue of filgrastim, resulting in an average molecular weight of pegfilgrastim of approximately 39 kD. Neulasta is available in 0.6-mL prefilled syringes for subcutaneous injection. The syringe contains 6 mg of pegfilgrastim (based on protein weight), in a clear, colorless, sterile, preservative-free solution containing 0.35 mg acetate, 30 mg sorbitol, 0.02 mg polysorbate 20, and 0.02 mg sodium in water for injection; the pH of the injection is 4.0.

Pegasys (peginterferon alfa-2a), used in the treatment of hepatitis C virus, is a covalent conjugate of recombinant alfa-2a interferon (molecular weight approximately 20 kD) with a single branched bis-PEG chain of approximately 40 kD molecular weight. The PEG moiety is linked at a single site to the interferon alfa moiety via a stable amide bond to lysine; the final product has an approximate molecular weight of 60 kD.

Each vial of Pegasys contains approximately 1.2 mL of solution to deliver 1.0 mL of drug for subcutaneous administration. The 1.0-mL volume delivers 180 μg of drug product (expressed as the amount of interferon alfa-2a), 8 mg sodium chloride, 0.05 mg polysorbate 80, 10 mg benzyl alcohol, 2.62 mg sodium acetate trihydrate, and 0.05 mg acetic acid; the solution has a pH of 6.0 ± 0.01 and is colorless to light yellow.

Pegasys produces maximal serum concentrations at 72 to 96 hours after dosing that are sustained for up to 168 hours. In comparison to Roferon-A, the mean systemic clearance for Pegasys was 94 mL/hour, which is approximately one-hundredth of that for Roferon. The mean terminal half-life after subcutaneous dosing in patients with chronic hepatitis C was 80 hours (range 50 to 140 hours) compared to 5.1 hours (range 3.7 to 8.5 hours) for Roferon-A (18).

PEG-Intron (peginterferon alfa-2b Powder for Injection) is a covalent conjugate of recombinant alfa interferon with PEG; approximate molecular weight of the PEG portion is 12 kD, and the approximate molecular weight of the PEG-Intron molecule is 31 kD. The product is a white to off-white lyophilized powder supplied in 2-mL vials for subcutaneous use. Each vial contains 74, 118.4, 177.6, or 222 μg of PEG-Introl and 1.11 mg dibasic sodium phosphate anhydrous, 1.11 mg monobasic sodium phosphate dihydrate, 59.2 mg sucrose, and 0.074 mg polysorbate 80. After reconstitution with 0.7 mL of the supplied diluent, which is sterile water for injection, each vial contains PEG-Introl in strength of 100, 160, 240, or 300 μg/mL.

Compared to interferon alfa-2b, PEG-Intron has one-seventh the mean apparent clearance and a five-fold greater mean half-life, permitting a reduced dosing frequency. At effective therapeutic doses, PEG-Intron has approximately a 10-fold greater maximum concentration (C_{max}) and a 50-fold greater area under the curve than interferon alfa-2b (19).

Fusion Protein: Special Handling

Ontak

Ontak denileukin diftitox (Ontak) is included in this chapter because of its unusual nature and handling. Ontak is a fusion protein designed to direct the cytocidal action of diphtheria toxin to cells that express the interleukin (IL) 2 receptor. Ontak is a recombinant DNA–derived cytotoxic protein composed of the amino acid sequences for diphtheria toxin fragments A and B (Met_1-Thr_{387})-His followed by the sequences for IL-2 (Ala_1-Thr_{133}); it is produced in an *E. coli* expression system. Ontak has a molecular weight of 58 kD. The single-use vials (2 mL) contain 300 μg of recombinant denileukin diftitox in a sterile solution of 20 mM citric acid, 0.05 mM ethylenediaminetetraacetic acid (EDTA) and less than 1% polysorbate 20 in water for injection; the pH of the solution is between 6.9 and 7.2.

The drug is indicated in the treatment of patients with persistent or recurrent cutaneous T-cell lymphoma whose malignant cells express the CD25 component of the IL-2 receptor. It should be used only by physicians experienced in the use of antineoplastic therapy and management of patients with cancer. Use of this drug should be in patients managed in a facility equipped and staffed for cardiopulmonary resuscitation and where the patient can be closely monitored for an appropriate period based on their health status.

Ontak requires special handling as follows: (*a*) It must be brought to room temperature before preparing the dose. The vials may be thawed in the refrigerator for not more than 24 hours or at room temperature for 1 to 2 hours. (*b*) The solution in the vial may be mixed by gentle swirling: *do not vigorously shake Ontak solution.* (*c*) After thawing, a haze may be visible. This haze should clear when the solution is at room temperature. (*d*) Ontak solution must not be used unless the solution is clear, colorless, and without visible particulate matter. (*e*) *Ontak must not be refrozen.* A few administration items of interest: (*a*) Diluted Ontak solution should be prepared and held in plastic syringes or soft plastic intravenous bags. *Do not use a glass container* because adsorption to glass may occur in a dilute state. (*b*) The concentration of Ontak must be at least 15 µg/mL during all steps in the preparation of the solution for intravenous infusion. This is best accomplished by withdrawing the calculated dose from the vial or vials and injecting it into an empty infusion bag. Then, for each 1 mL of Ontak, no more than 9 mL of sterile saline without preservative should be added to the intravenous bag. (*c*) Ontak solution should not be physically mixed with any other drugs. (*d*) Do not administer Ontak solution through an in-line filter. (*e*) Prepared solutions of Ontak should be administered within 6 hours, using a syringe pump or intravenous infusion bag. (*f*) Unused portions of Ontak should be discarded immediately.

Prior to handling this drug, pharmacists, nurses, and physicians should carefully read and understand all of the precautions explained in the package labeling (20).

Implants

Implants are defined as sterile solid drug products made by compression, melting, or sintering. They generally consist of the drug and rate-controlling excipients.

Gliadel Wafer Implant

Polifeprosan 20 with carmustine implant (Gliadel Wafer), shown in Figures 20.7 to 20.9, is a sterile off-white to pale yellow wafer approximately 1.45 cm in diameter and 1 mm thick. Each wafer contains 192.3 mg of a biodegradable polyanhydride copolymer and 7.7 mg of

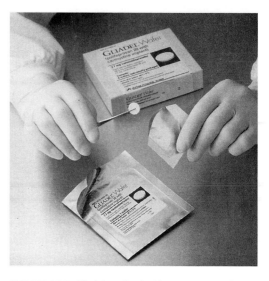

FIGURE 20.7 Gliadel wafer (polifeprosan 20 with carmustine implant) and packaging components. (Courtesy of Guilford Pharmaceuticals.)

carmustine. Polifeprosan 20 consists of poly[bis (p-carboxyphenoxy) propane: sebacic acid] in a 20:80 molar ratio and is used to control the local delivery of carmustine, which is distributed uniformly throughout the copolymer matrix.

Gliadel is designed to deliver the carmustine directly into the surgical cavity created when a brain tumor is resected, with numerous wafers being used depending upon the desired dose. When exposed to the aqueous environment in the resection cavity, the anhydride bonds in the copolymer are hydrolyzed, releasing the carmustine, carboxyphenoxypropane and sebacic acid. The active drug, carmustine, is released from the wafer and diffuses into the surrounding brain tissue, producing an antineoplastic effect by alkylating DNA and RNA.

In 3 weeks, more than 70% of the copolymer degrades, with carboxyphenoxypropane being eliminated by the kidney and sebacic acid being metabolized by the liver and expired as carbon dioxide.

Each wafer contains 7.7 mg of carmustine, and when eight wafers (the recommended dose) are used, a dose of 61.6 mg is delivered. The wafers are supplied in a single-dose treatment box containing eight individually pouched wafers. Each wafer is double-pouched in foil.

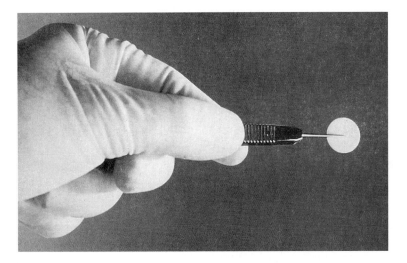

FIGURE 20.8 Gliadel wafer removed from sterile foil pouch in preparation for implantation. (Courtesy of Guilford Pharmaceuticals.)

The inner pouch is sterile; upon removing the outer foil pouch in an aseptic working environment, the inner pouch is treated as a sterile item. Gliadel wafers must be stored at or below −20°C (21).

Zoladex Implant

Goserelin acetate implant (Zoladex, Zeneca Pharmaceuticals) is a sterile, biodegradable product containing goserelin acetate, equivalent to 3.6 mg of drug, designed for subcutaneous injection with continuous release over 28 days. Goserelin acetate is dispersed in a matrix consisting of D,L-lactic and glycolic acids copolymer (13.3–14.3 mg/dose) containing less than 2.5% acetic acid and up to 12% goserelin-related substances. It is a sterile white to cream-colored cylinder 1 mm in diameter, preloaded in a special single-use syringe with a 16-gauge needle.

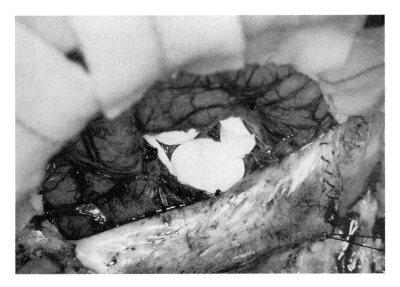

FIGURE 20.9 Gliadel wafer implanted in the brain. (Courtesy of Guilford Pharmaceuticals.)

The unit is packaged in a sealed light- and moisture-proof aluminum foil laminate pouch containing a desiccant capsule.

Zoladex is indicated for a number of disorders, including the palliative treatment of advanced carcinoma of the prostate, offering an alternative to orchiectomy and/or estrogen administration when the standard treatments are not indicated or are unacceptable to the patient. It is also used in the treatment of endometriosis and advanced breast cancer.

The product is administered subcutaneously into the upper abdominal wall using aseptic technique. It should be stored at room temperature and should not exceed 25°C.

Zoladex is also available as Zoladex 3-Month, containing the equivalent of 10.8 mg of goserelin. The base consists of a matrix of D,L-lactic and glycolic acids copolymer (12.82–14.76 mg/dose) containing less than 2% acetic acid and up to 10% goserelin-related substances and presented as a sterile white to cream-colored cylinder 1.5 mm in diameter, preloaded in a special single-use syringe with a 14-gauge needle and overwrap, as previously described. This preparation is designed for administration every 3 months (22).

Other Novel Delivery Systems

Definity is a vial of Perflutren Lipid Microspheres for preparing an injectable suspension. The vial contains components that upon activation yield perflutren lipid microspheres that are used as a diagnostic agent for contrast enhancement during echocardiographic procedures; it is administered intravenously. Prior to activation, the Definity vial contains 6.52 mg/mL octafluoropropane in the head space; each milliliter of the clear liquid contains 0.75 mg of a specific lipid blend, 103.5 mg of propylene glycol, 126.2 mg of glycerin, and 6.8 mg of sodium chloride in water for injection. The pH may be adjusted to 5.8 to 7.0 with either sodium hydroxide or hydrochloric acid. The perflutren vial must be activated prior to use with a mechanical shaking device (Vialmix). Upon activation, each milliliter of the milky white suspension contains a maximum of 1.2 $\times$ 10^{10} perflutren lipid microspheres and about 150 μL/mL of octafluoropropane. The microsphere particles have an average diameter of 1.2 to 3.3 μm (23).

Minocycline hydrochloride (Arestin) microspheres is a subgingival sustained-release product containing minocycline hydrochloride in a bioresorbable polymer, poly(glycolide-co-DL-lactide), or PGLA; it is for professional administration into periodontal pockets. Each unit dose cartridge delivers minocycline hydrochloride equivalent to 1 mg of minocycline free base (24).

Doxycycline hyclate (Atridox) 10% in the Atrigel delivery system is for controlled release in subgingival applications. It is composed of a two-syringe mixing system. Syringe A contains 450 mg of the Atrigel delivery system, which is a bioabsorbable, flowable polymeric formulation composed of 36.7% poly(DL-lactide) dissolved in 63.3% N-methyl-2-pyrrolidone. Syringe B contains doxycycline hyclate that is equivalent to 42.5 mg doxycycline. Once prepared, the product is a pale yellow to yellow viscous liquid with a concentration of 10% doxycycline hyclate in the gel. After professional application and upon contact with the crevicular fluid, the liquid product solidifies and allows for controlled release of drug over 7 days. Doxycycline is a broad-spectrum semisynthetic bacteriostatic tetracycline (25).

Cyanocobalamin (Nascobal Gel) for intranasal administration is used in the treatment of vitamin B_{12} deficiency, including pernicious anemia. It is self-administered as a nasal gel. Generally, 0.1 mL of the gel, containing 500 μg of cyanocobalamin, is administered intranasally once weekly. The cyanocobalamin is effectively absorbed through the nasal mucosa to produce therapeutic blood levels (26).

Autoinjection Systems

The EpiPen and EpiPen Jr. automatic injectors contain 2 mL of epinephrine injection for emergency intramuscular use. Each latex-free injector delivers 0.3 mg of Epinephrine Injection, USP, 1:1000 in a 0.3-mL volume. The remaining 1.7 mL (2.0–0.3 mL) remains in the injector after use and is not to be used. Each 0.3 mL of the solution contains 0.3 mg epinephrine, 1.8 mg sodium chloride, 0.5 mg sodium metabisulfite, hydrochloric acid to adjust the pH of the solution to 2.2 to 5.0 and water for injection (27).

Both EpiPen autoinjectors are designed as emergency supportive therapy of allergic reactions (anaphylaxis) and are not a replacement or substitute for immediate medical or hospital care. Epinephrine is a sympathomimetic amine that deteriorates rapidly on exposure to air or light, turning pink from oxidation to adrenochrome and brown from the formation of melanin. The EpiPen injectors should be checked immediately prior to use, and if there is any evidence of discoloration, they should be replaced. The activation cap on the units should not be removed until ready for use. The EpiPen injector should be stored in the provided tubes, since it is light sensitive, at room temperature; the units are not to be refrigerated.

Humulin N Pen contains NPH human insulin (rDNA origin) isophane suspension in a disposable insulin delivery device. It is packaged containing five 3-mL disposable insulin delivery devices containing NPH insulin 100 U/mL.

Safe-Needle Systems

With the implementation of the Needlestick Safety and Prevention Act, which requires the evaluation and implementation of "safer medical devices" as well as Occupational Safety and Health Administration (OSHA) requirements, new devices will be entering the market to enhance the safety of personnel responsible for injecting medications in patients.

Enoxaparin sodium injection (Lovenox) is now available in a prefilled syringe with an automatic safety device (28). The new device allows the use of normal injection technique; the needle shield is removed; the injection proceeds as usual; and the syringe/needle is removed from the injection site with the finger still on the plunger rod. Next, the syringe/needle is pointed away from you and others and the safety device is activated by firmly pushing on the plunger rod. The protective sleeve automatically covers the needle and an audible click is heard to confirm that the shield has been activated and covers the needle. The syringe/needle is then safely disposed of in the nearest sharps container.

REFERENCES

1. Physicians' Desk Reference, 57th ed. Montvale, NJ. Thomson PDR. 2003;1559–1566.
2. I Physicians' Desk Reference, 57th ed. Montvale, NJ. Thomson PDR. 2003;1136–1142.
3. Product Information. Livingston, NJ: Columbia Laboratories, 2003.
4. Product Literature. Palo Alto, CA: Alza, 2004.
5. Physicians' Desk Reference, 57th ed. Montvale, NJ. Thomson PDR. 2003;1433–1439.
6. Physicians' Desk Reference, 57th ed. Montvale, NJ. Thomson PDR. 2003;1529–1533.
7. Physicians' Desk Reference, 57th ed. Montvale, NJ. Thomson PDR. 2003;2275–2278.
8. Product Information. Research Triangle Park, NC: GlaxoWellcome, 2003.
9. Product Information. Palo Alto, CA: Alza, 1998.
10. Physicians' Desk Reference, 57th ed. Montvale, NJ. Thomson PDR. 2003;1347–1349.
11. Madan PL. Sustained-release drug delivery systems, part VI: Special devices. Pharm Manufact 1985;2:33–40.
12. Madan PL. Sustained-release drug delivery systems, part V: Parenteral products. Pharm Manufact 1985;2:51.
13. Physicians' Desk Reference, 57th ed. Montvale, NJ. Thomson PDR. 2003;1855–1857.
14. Physicians' Desk Reference, 57th ed. Montvale, NJ. Thomson PDR. 2003;1248–1250.
15. Physicians' Desk Reference, 57th ed. Montvale, NJ. Thomson PDR. 2003;1758–1761.
16. Physicians' Desk Reference, 57th ed. Montvale, NJ. Thomson PDR. 2003;1423–1425.
17. Physicians' Desk Reference, 57th ed. Montvale, NJ. Thomson PDR. 2003;2419–2423.
18. Physicians' Desk Reference, 57th ed. Montvale, NJ. Thomson PDR. 2003;583–585.
19. Product Information. Nutley, NJ: Hoffmann-LaRoche.
20. Physicians' Desk Reference, 57th ed. Montvale NJ. Thomson PDR. 2003;3059–3063.
21. Physicians' Desk Reference, 57th ed. Montvale, NJ. Thomson PDR. 2003;1826–1827.
22. Physicians' Desk Reference, 57th ed. Montvale, NJ. Thomson PDR. 2003;695–699.
23. Product Information. Plainsboro, NJ: Bristol MyersSquibb Medical Imaging, 2000.
24. Product Information. Warminster, PA: OraPharma, 2004.
25. Product Information. Newtown, PA: CollaGenex Pharmaceuticals, 2005.
26. Product Information. Hauppaugh, NY: Nastech Pharmaceutical, 2003.
27. Product Information. Indianapolis, IN: Eli Lilly, 2002.
28. Product Information. Bridgewater, NJ: Aventis Pharmaceuticals, 2003.

Definitions of Selected Drug Categories*

Abradant: an agent that removes an external layer, such as dental plaque. (Pumice)

Absorbent: a drug that takes up other chemicals into its substance, used to reduce the free availability of toxic chemicals. (Polycarbophil, gastrointestinal absorbent)

ACE Inhibitor: see Angiotensin Converting Enzyme Inhibitor.

Acidifier, Systemic: a drug that lowers internal body pH, useful in restoring normal pH in patients with systemic alkalosis. (Ammonium Chloride)

Acidifier, Urinary: a drug that lowers the pH of the renal filtrate and urine. (Sodium Dihydrogen Phosphate)

Adrenergic: a drug that activates organs innervated by the sympathetic nervous system; a sympathomimetic drug. (Epinephrine)

Adrenocorticosteroid, Anti-inflammatory: an adrenal cortex hormone that regulates organic metabolism and inhibits inflammatory response; a glucocorticoid. (Prednisolone)

Adrenocorticosteroid, Salt-regulating: an adrenal cortex hormone that regulates sodium/potassium balance in the body; a mineralcorticoid. (Desoxycorticosterone Acetate)

Adrenocorticotropic Hormone: a hormone that stimulates the adrenal cortex to produce glucocorticoids. (Corticotropin)

Adsorbent: a drug that binds other chemicals onto its surface, used to reduce the free availability of toxic chemicals. (Kaolin, gastrointestinal adsorbent)

Agonist: a drug that reacts with and activates physiological receptors and induces the associated biologic response. (Morphine, opioid receptor agonist; Isoproterenol, beta adrenergic receptor agonist)

Alcohol-Abuse Deterrent: a drug that alters physiology so that unpleasant symptoms follow ingestion of ethanol-containing products. (Disulfiram)

Alkalinizer, Systemic: a drug that raises internal

body pH, useful in restoring normal pH in patients with systemic acidosis. (Sodium Bicarbonate)

Alkylating Agent: an antineoplastic drug that attacks malignant cells by reacting covalently with their DNA. (Chlorambucil)

Alpha Receptor Agonist: a drug that activates sympathetic nervous system alpha receptors, e.g., to induce vasoconstriction. (Norepinephrine)

Alpha Receptor Antagonist: a drug that reacts asymptomatically with sympathetic nervous system alpha receptors and prevents their endogenous activation, e.g., to induce vasodilation. (Phentolamine)

Anabolic Steroid: an androgen analogue with relatively greater anabolic activity, used to treat catabolic disorders. (Methandrostenolone)

Analeptic: a central nervous system stimulant, sometimes used to simulate respiration during severe central nervous system depression. (Doxapram)

Analgesic: a drug that suppresses pain perception (nociception) without inducing unconsciousness. (Morphine Sulfate, opioid analgesic; Aspirin, nonopioid analgesic)

Androgen: a hormone that stimulates and maintains male reproductive function and sex characteristics. (Testosterone)

Anesthetic, General: a drug that eliminates pain perception by inducing unconsciousness. (Ether, inhalation anesthetic; Thiopental Sodium, intravenous anesthetic)

Anesthetic, Local: a drug that eliminates pain perception in a limited body area by local action on sensory nerves. (Procaine)

Anesthetic, Topical: a local anesthetic that is effective upon application to mucous membranes. (Tetracaine)

Angiotensin Converting Enzyme Inhibitor: a drug that inhibits biotransformation of angiotensin I into vasoconstricting angiotensin II, used to treat hypertension. (Captopril)

Anorexic: a drug that suppresses appetite, usually by elevating mood. (Phentermine)

Antacid: a drug that neutralizes excess gastric acid. (Aluminum Hydroxide Gel)

Antagonist: a drug that reacts asymptomatically with physiological receptors and prevents their

---

*Prepared by H. Douglas Johnson, Ph.D., Professor Emeritus of Pharmacology/Toxicology, College of Pharmacy, University of Georgia.

endogenous activation. (Naloxone, opioid receptor antagonist; Propranolol, beta adrenergic receptor antagonist)

Anthelmintic: a drug that eradicates intestinal worm infestations. (Thiabendazole)

Antiacne Agent: a drug that combats the lesions of acne vulgaris. (Tretinoin)

Antiadrenergic: a drug that inhibits response to sympathetic nerve impulses and adrenergic drugs; a sympatholytic drug. (Phentolamine, alpha adrenergic antagonist; Propranolol, beta adrenergic antagonist)

Antiamebic: a drugs that kills or inhibits protozoan parasites such as *Entamoeba histolytica*, causative agent of amebiasis. (Metronidazole, intestinal antiamebic; Chloroquine, extraintestinal antiamebic)

Antiandrogen: a drug that inhibits response to androgenic hormones.

Antianginal: a coronary vasodilator useful in preventing or treating attacks of angina pectoris. (Nitroglycerin)

Antiarrhythmic: a cardiac depressant useful in suppressing rhythm irregularities of the heart. (Procainamide)

Antiarthritic: a drug that reduces the joint inflammation of arthritis. (Prenisolone, glucocorticoid; Indomethacin, NSAID)

Antibacterial: a drug that kills or inhibits pathogenic bacteria. (Penicillin G, systemic antibacterial; Nitrofurantoin, urinary antibacterial; Bacitracin, topical antibacterial)

Anticholesterol Agent: a drug that lowers plasma cholesterol level. (Colestipol)

Anticholinergic: a drug that inhibits response to parasympathetic nerves impulses and cholinergic drugs; a parasympatholytic drug. (Atropine)

Anticholinesterase Antidote: a drug that reactivates cholinesterase enzyme after its inactivation by organophosphate poisons. (Pralidoxime)

Anticoagulant Antagonist: a drug that opposes overdosage of anticoagulant drugs. (Phytonadione, supplies vitamin K to oppose vitamin K–antagonist anticoagulants)

Anticoagulant, Systemic: a drug administered to slow clotting of circulating blood. (Warfarin)

Anticoagulant, for Storage of Whole Blood: a nontoxic agent added to collected blood to prevent clotting. (Anticoagulant Citrate Dextrose Solution)

Anticonvulsant: an antiepileptic drug administered prophylactically to prevent seizures, or a drug that arrests convulsions by inducing general central nervous system depression. (Phenytoin, antiepileptic prophylactic; Diazepam, central nervous system depressant anticonvulsant)

Antidepressant: a centrally acting drug that induces mood elevation, useful in treating mental depression. (Amitriptyline)

Antidiabetic: a drug that supplies insulin or stimulates secretion of insulin, useful in treating diabetes mellitus. (Insulin Injection, supplies insulin; Tolbutamide, stimulates insulin secretion)

Antidiarrheal: a drug that inhibits intestinal peristalsis, used to treat diarrhea. (Diphenoxylate)

Antidiuretic: a drug that promotes renal water reabsorption, thus reducing urine volume, used to treat neurogenic diabetes insipidus. (Desmopressin)

Antianemic: a drug used to treat anemia; see Hematopoietic, Hematinic.

Antibiotic: a drug originally of microbial origin used to kill or inhibit bacterial and other infections. (Penicillin, Tetracycline)

Antidote, General Purpose: a drug that reduces the effects of ingested poisons (or drug overdoses) by adsorbing toxic material. (Activated Charcoal)

Antidote, Specific: a drug that reduces the effects of a systemic poison (or drug overdose) by a mechanism that relates to the particular poison. (Dimercaprol, specific antidote for arsenic, mercury, and gold poisoning)

Antieczematic: a topical drug that aids in control of chronic exudative skin lesions. (Coal Tar)

Antiemetic: a drug that suppresses nausea and vomiting. (Prochlorperazine)

Antieneuretic: a drug that aids in control of bedwetting (enuresis). (Imipramine)

Antiepileptic: a drug that prevents epileptic seizures upon prophylactic administration. (Ethosuximide)

Antiestrogen: a drug that inhibits action of estrogenic hormones. (Tamoxifen)

Antifibrinolytic: a drug that promotes hemostasis by inhibiting clot dissolution (fibrinolysis). (Aminocaproic Acid)

Antifilarial: a drug that kills or inhibits pathogenic filarial worms. (Diethylcarbamazine)

Antiflatuent: a drug that reduces gastrointestinal gas. (Simethicone)

Antifungal, Systemic: a drug that kills or inhibits pathogenic fungi. (Griseofulvin)

Antifungal, Topical: a drug applied externally to kill or inhibit pathogenic fungi. (Tolnaftate)

Antiglaucoma Agent: a drug that lowers intraocular fluid pressure, used to treat glaucoma. (Methazolamide reduces fluid formation; Isofluorophate promotes fluid drainage)

Antigonadotropin: a drug that inhibits anterior pituitary secretion of gonadotropins, used to suppress ovarian malfunction. (Danazol)

Antigout Agent: a drug that reduces tissue deposits of uric acid in chronic gout or suppresses the intense inflammatory reaction of acute gout. (Allopurinol for chronic gout; Indomethacin for acute gout)

Antihemophilic: a drug that replaces blood clotting factors absent in the hereditary disease hemophilia. (Antihemophilic Factor)

Antiherpes Agent: a drug that inhibits replication of *Herpes simplex* virus, used to treat genital herpes. (Acyclovir)

Antihistaminic: a drug that antagonizes histamine action at H_1 histamine receptors, useful in suppressing the histamine-induced symptoms of allergy. (Chloropheniramine)

Antihyperlipidemic: a drug that lowers plasma cholesterol and lipid levels. (Clofibrate)

Antihypertensive: a drug that lowers arterial blood pressure, especially the elevated diastolic pressure of hypertension. (Guanethidine)

Antihypocalcemic: a drug that elevates plasma calcium level, useful in treating hypocalcemia. (Parathyroid Injection)

Antihypoglycemic: a drug that elevates plasma glucose level, useful in treating hypoglycemia. (Glucagon)

Anti-infective, Topical (or Local): a drug that kills or inhibits pathogenic microorganisms and is suitable for sterilizing skin and wounds. (Povidone Iodine Liquid Soap)

Anti-inflammatory: a drug that inhibits physiologic response to cell damage (inflammation). (Prednisolone, adrenocorticosteroid; Ibuprofen, nonsteroid)

Antileishmanial: a drug that kills or inhibits pathogenic protozoa of the genus *Leishmania*. (Hydroxystilbamidine Isethionate)

Antileprotic: a drug that kills or inhibits *Mycobacterium leprae*, causative agent of leprosy. (Dapsone)

Antimalarial: a drug that kills or inhibits protozoa of the genus *Plasmodium*, causative agents of malaria. (Chloroquine)

Antimanic: a drug that suppresses the excitement phase (mania) of bipolar disorder. (Lithium Carbonate)

Antimetabolite: a drug that attacks malignant cells or pathogenic cells by serving as a nonfunctional substitute for an essential metabolite. (Fluorouracil, antineoplastic antimetabolite)

Antimigraine Agent: a drug that reduces incidence or severity of migraine vascular headaches. (Methylsergide)

Anti–Motion Sickness Agent: a drug that suppresses motion-induced nausea, vomiting, and vertigo. (Dimenhydrinate)

Antimuscarinic: an anticholinergic drug that inhibits symptoms mediated by acetylcholine receptors of visceral organs (muscarinic receptors). (Atropine)

Antinauseant: a drug that suppresses nausea and vomiting; an antiemetic. (Ondansetron)

Antineoplastic: a drug that attacks malignant (neoplastic) cells in the body. (Chlorambucil, alkylating agent)

Antiparasitic: a drug that eradicates parasitic arthropods, helminths, protozoa, etc. (Lindane for scabies; Thiabendazole for intestinal worms; Metronidazole for amebic dysentery)

Antiparkinsonian (antidyskinetic): a drug that suppresses the neurologic disturbances and symptoms of parkinsonism. (Levodopa)

Antiperistaltic: a drug that inhibits intestinal motility; an antidiarrheal drug. (Diphenoxylate)

Antiplatelet Agent: a drug that inhibits aggregation of blood platelets, used to prevent heart attack. (Aspirin)

Antiprotozoal: a drug that kills or inhibits pathogenic protozoa. (Metronidazole)

Antipruritic: a drug that reduces itching (pruritus). (Trimeprazine, systemic antipruritic; Menthol, topical antipruritic)

Antipsoriatic: a drug that suppresses the lesions and symptoms of psoriasis. (Methotrexate, systemic antipsoriatic; Anthralin, topical antipsoriatic)

Antipsychotic: a drug that suppresses symptoms of psychoses of various diagnostic types. (Haloperidol)

Antipyretic: a drug that restores normal body temperature in the presence of fever. (Acetaminophen)

Antirachitic: a drug with vitamin D activity, useful in treating vitamin D deficiency and rickets. (Cholecalciferol)

Antirheumatic: an anti-inflammatory drug used to treat arthritis and rheumatoid disorders. (Indomethacin)

Antirickettsial: a drug that kills or inhibits pathogenic microorganisms of the genus *Rickettsia*. (Chloramphenicol)

Antischistosomal: a drug that kills or inhibits pathogenic flukes of the genus *Schistosoma*. (Oxaminiquine)

Antiscorbutic: a drug with vitamin C activity, useful in treating vitamin C deficiency and scurvy. (Ascorbic Acid)

Antiseborrheic: a drug that aids in the control of seborrheic dermatitis (dandruff). (Selenium Sulfide)

Antispasmodic: a drug that inhibits motility of visceral smooth muscles. (Atropine)

Antithyroid Agent: a drug that reduces thyroid hormone action, usually by inhibiting hormone synthesis. (Methimazole)

Antitreponemal: a drug that kills or inhibits *Treponema pallidum,* causative agent of syphilis. (Penicillin)

Antitrichomonal: a drug that kills or inhibits pathogenic protozoa of the genus *Trichomonas.* (Metronidazole)

Antitubercular: a drug that kills or inhibits *Mycobacterium tuberculosis,* causative agent of tuberculosis. (Isoniazid)

Antitussive: a drug that suppresses coughing. (Dextromethorphan)

Antiviral: a drug that kills or inhibits viral infections. (Idoxuridine, Ophthalmic Antiviral)

Antiviral, Prophylactic: a drug useful in preventing (rather than treating) viral infections. (Amantadine, prophylactic for influenza)

Antixerophthalmic: a drug with vitamin A activity, useful in treating vitamin A deficiency and xerophthalmia. (Vitamin A)

Anxiolytic: a drug that suppresses symptoms of anxiety. (Diazepam)

Astringent: a drug used topically to toughen and shrink tissues. (Aluminum Acetate Solution)

Astringent, Ophthalmic: a mild astringent suitable for use in the eye. (Zinc Sulfate)

Barbiturate: a sedative-hypnotic drug that contains the barbituric acid moiety in its chemical structure. (Phenobarbital)

Belladonna Alkaloid: a plant principle derived from *Atropa belladonna* and related species, with anticholinergic action. (Atropine)

Benzodiazepine: a sedative-anxiolytic-muscle relaxant drug that contains the benzodiazepine moiety in its chemical structure. (Diazepam)

Beta Receptor Agonist: a drug that activates sympathetic nervous system beta receptors, e.g., to induce bronchodilation. (Isoproterenol)

Beta Receptor Antagonist: a drug that reacts asymptomatically with sympathetic nervous system beta receptors and prevents their endogenous activation, e.g., to oppose sympathetic stimulation of the heart. (Propranolol)

Bone Metabolism Regulator: a drug that slows calcium turnover in bone, used to treat Paget's disease. (Etidronate)

Bronchodilator: a drug that expands bronchiolar airways, useful in treating asthma. (Isoproterenol, adrenergic bronchodilator; Oxytriphylline, smooth muscle relaxant bronchodilator)

Calcium Channel Blocker: an antianginal drug that acts by impairing function of transmembrane calcium channels of vascular smooth muscle cells. (Verapamil)

Carbonic Anhydrase Inhibitor: a drug that inhibits the enzyme carbonic anhydrase, the therapeutic effects of which are diuresis and reduced formation of intraocular fluid. (Acetazolamide)

Cardiac Depressant, Antiarrhythmic: a drug that depresses myocardial function, useful in treating cardiac arrhythmias. (Procainamide)

Cardiac Glycoside: a plant principle derived from *Digitalis purpurea* and related species, with cardiotonic action. (Digoxin)

Cardiotonic: a drug that increases myocardial contractile force, useful in treating congestive heart failure. (Digoxin)

Catecholamine Synthesis Inhibitor: a drug that inhibits biosynthesis of catecholamine neurotransmitters such as norepinephrine. (Metyrosine)

Cathartic: a drug that promotes defecation, usually considered stronger in action than a laxative. (Danthron)

Caustic: a topical drug that destroys tissue on contact, useful in removing skin lesions. (Toughened Silver Nitrate)

Centrally Acting Drug: a drug that produces its therapeutic effect by action on the central nervous system, usually designated by type of therapeutic action (sedative, hypnotic, anticonvulsant, etc.)

Cephalosporin: an antimicrobial drug that contains the cephalosporin moiety in its chemical structure. (Cefotaxime)

Chelating Agent: a complexing agent that binds metal ions into stable ring structures (chelates), useful in treating poisoning. (Edetate Calcium Disodium, chelating agent for lead)

Cholelitholytic: a drug that promotes dissolution of gallstones. (Ursodoxycholic acid)

Choleretic: a drug that increases bile secretion by the liver. (Dehydrocholic Acid)

Cholinergic: a drug that activates organs innervated by the parasympathetic nervous system; a parasympathomimetic drug. (Neostigmine, systemic cholinergic; Pilocarpine, ophthalmic cholinergic)

Chrysotherapeutic: a drug containing gold, used to treat rheumatoid arthritis. (Auranofin)

Coagulant: see Hemostatic, Systemic.

Contraceptive, Oral: an orally administered drug that prevents conception. Currently available oral contraceptives are for use by females. (Norethindrone Acetate and Ethinyl Estradiol Tablets)

Contraceptive, Topical: a spermicidal agent used topically in the vagina to prevent conception. (Nonoxynol-9)

Cycloplegic: an anticholinergic drug used topically in the eye to induce paralysis of accommodation (cycloplegia) and dilation of the pupil. (Cyclopentolate)

Decongestant, Nasal: an adrenergic drug used orally or topically to induce vasoconstriction in nasal passages. (Phenylephrine)

Demulcent: a bland viscous liquid, usually water-based, used to coat and soothe damaged or inflamed skin or mucous membranes. (Methylcellulose)

Dental Caries Prophylactic: a drug applied to the teeth to reduce the incidence of cavities. (Stannous Fluoride)

Dentin Desensitizer: a drug applied to the teeth to reduce the sensitivity of exposed subenamel dentin. (Zinc Chloride)

Depigmenting Agent: a drug that inhibits melanin production in the skin, used to induce general depigmentation in certain splotchy depigmented conditions (e.g., vitiligo). (Hydroquinone)

Detergent: an emulsifying agent used as a cleanser. (Hexachlorophene Liquid Soap, anti-infective detergent)

Diagnostic Aid: a drug used to determine the functional state of a body organ or to determine the presence of disease. (Peptavlon, gastric secretion indicator; Fluorescein Sodium, corneal trauma indicator)

Digestive Aid: a drug that promotes digestion, usually by supplementing a gastrointestinal enzyme. (Pancreatin)

Disinfectant: an agent that destroys microorganisms on contact and suitable for sterilizing inanimate objects. (Formaldehyde Solution)

Diuretic: a drug that promotes renal excretion of electrolytes and water, useful in treating generalized edema. (Furosemide, loop diuretic; Hydrochlorothiazide, thiazide diuretic; Triamterene, potassium-sparing diuretic)

Dopamine Receptor Agonist: a drug that activates dopamine receptors, e.g., to inhibit anterior pituitary secretion of prolactin. (Bromocriptine)

Emetic: a drug that induces vomiting, useful in expelling ingested but unabsorbed poisons. (Ipecac Syrup)

Emollient: a topical drug, especially an oil or fat, used to soften the skin and make it more pliable. (Cold Cream)

Ergot Alkaloid: a plant principle derived from the fungus *Claviceps purpura* grown on rye or other grains. (Ergonovine, uterine contractant; Ergotamine, migraine therapy)

Estrogen: a hormone that stimulates and maintains female reproductive organs and sex characteristics and functions in the uterine cycle. (Ethinyl Estradiol)

Expectorant: a drug that increases respiratory tract secretions, lowers their viscosity, and promotes removal. (Potassium Iodide)

Fecal Softener: a drug that promotes defecation by softening the feces. (Docusate)

Fertility Agent: a drug that promotes ovulation in women of low fertility or spermatogenesis in men of low fertility. (Clomiphene)

Fibrinolytic proteolytic: an enzyme drug used topically to hydrolyze exudates of infected and inflammatory lesions. (Fibrinolysin and Desoxyribonuclease, Bovine)

Galactokinetic: a drug used to initiate lactation after childbirth. (Oxytocin Nasal Spray)

Glucocorticoid: an adrenocortical hormone that regulates organic metabolism and inhibits inflammatory response. (Betamethasone)

Gonadotropin: a drug that supplies the gonad-stimulating actions of follicle-stimulating hormone (FSH) and/or luteinizing hormone (LH), used to promote fertility. (Menotropins contains FSH and LH, Human Chorionic Gonadotropin has LH-like activity)

Growth Hormone, Human: a drug that duplicates endogenous growth hormone, used in children to treat growth failure due to growth hormone lack. (Somatrem)

Heavy Metal Antagonist: a drug used as an antidote to poisoning with toxic metals such as arsenic and mercury. (Dimercaprol)

Hematopoietic: a vitamin that stimulates formation of blood cells, useful in treating vitamin-deficiency anemia. (Cyanocobalamin)

Hematinic: a drug that promotes hemoglobin formation by supplying iron. (Ferrous Sulfate)

Hemorheologic Agent: a drug that improves the flow properties of blood by reducing viscosity. (Pentoxyfylline)

Hemostatic, Local: a drug applied to a bleeding surface to promote clotting or to serve as a clot matrix. (Thrombin, clot promoter; Oxidized Cellulose, clot matrix)

Hemostatic, Systemic: a drug that stops bleeding by

inhibiting systemic fibrinolysis. (Aminocaproic Acid)

Histamine H₁ Receptor Antagonist: a drug used to combat the histamine-induced symptoms of allergy; an antihistamine (Chlorpheniramine)

Histamine H₂ Receptor Antagonist: a drug that inhibits histamine-mediated gastric acid secretion, used to treat peptic and duodenal ulcers. (Cimetidine)

Hormone: a drug that duplicates action of a physiologic cell regulator (hormone). (Insulin, Estradiol, Thyroxine)

Hydantoin: an antiepileptic drug that contains the hydantoin moiety in its chemical structure. (Phenytoin)

Hydrolytic, Injectible: an enzyme drug that promotes the diffusion of other injected drugs through connective tissues. (Hyaluronidase)

Hyperglycemic: a drug that elevates blood glucose level. (Glucagon)

Hypnotic: a central nervous system depressant used to induce sleep. (Flurazepam)

Hypotensive: see Antihypertensive.

Immunoglobulin: Antibody protein derived from blood serum, used to confer passive immunity to infectious disease. (See Immunizing Agent, Passive)

Immunizing Agent, Active: an antigen that induces antibody production against a pathogenic microorganism, used to provide permanent but delayed protection against infection. (Tetanus Toxoid)

Immunizing Agent, Passive: a drug containing antibodies against a pathogenic microorganism, used to provide immediate but temporary protection against infection. (Tetanus Immune Globulin, Rabies Immune Globulin)

Immunosuppressant: a drug that inhibits immune response to foreign materials, used to suppress rejection of tissue grafts. (Azathioprine)

Inotropic Agent: a drug that increases the contractile strength of heart muscle; a cardiotonic. (Digitoxin, Dopamine)

Ion Exchange Resin: a drug that in the gastrointestinal tract takes up ions present in a toxic amount with equivalent release of nontoxic ions. (Sodium Polystyrene Sulfonate, takes up potassium ions with release of sodium ions)

Irritant, Local: a drug that reacts weakly and nonspecifically with biologic tissue, used topically to induce a mild inflammatory response. (Camphor)

Keratolytic: a topical drug that toughens and protects skin. (Compound Benzoin Tincture)

Laxative: a drug that promotes defecation, usually considered milder in action than a cathartic. (Methylcellulose, bulk laxative; Mineral Oil, lubricant laxative; Sodium Phosphates Oral Solution, saline laxative)

Leprostatic: see Antileprotic.

Loop Diuretic: a diuretic with renal site of action in the thick ascending loop of Henle. (Furosemide)

MAO Inhibitor: see Monoamine Oxidase Inhibitor.

Metal Complexing Agent: a drug that binds metal ions, useful in treating metal poisoning. (Dimercaprol, complexing agent for arsenic, mercury, and gold)

Mineralocorticoid: an adrenocortical hormone that regulates sodium/potassium balance in the body. (Desoxycorticosterone Acetate)

Miotic: a cholinergic drug used topically in the eye to induce constriction of the pupil (miosis). (Pilocarpine)

Monoamine Oxidase Inhibitor: an antidepressant drug that inhibits the enzyme monoamine oxidase, thereby increasing catecholamine levels of neurons. (Isocarboxazid)

Monoclonal Antibody: a highly specific immunoglobulin produced by cell culture cloning. (Muromonab CD3, inactivates T lymphocytes that reject tissue grafts)

Mucolytic: a drug that hydrolyzes mucoproteins, useful in reducing the viscosity of pulmonary mucus. (Acetylcysteine)

Muscle Relaxant, Skeletal: a drug that inhibits contraction of voluntary muscles. (Dantrolene, Succinylcholine)

Muscle Relaxant, Smooth: a drug that inhibits contraction of visceral smooth muscles. (Aminophylline)

Mydriatic: an adrenergic drug used topically in the eye to induce dilation of the pupil (mydriasis). (Phenylephrine)

Narcotic: a drug that induces action by reacting with opioid receptors of the central nervous system, or a drug legally classified as a narcotic with regard to prescribing regulations.

Narcotic Antagonist: a drug that reacts with opioid receptors asymptomatically, used to terminate the action of narcotic drugs. (Naloxone)

Neuromuscular Blocking Agent: a drug that paralyzes skeletal muscles by preventing transmission of neural impulses to them. (Succinylcholine)

Nonsteroidal Anti-inflammatory Drug: an analgesic, anti-inflammatory drug that inhibits prostaglandin synthesis. (Indomethacin)

NSAID: see Nonsteroidal Anti-inflammatory Drug

Opioid: see Narcotic.

Opioid Antagonist: see Narcotic Antagonist.

Oxytoxic: a drug that stimulates uterine motility, used in obstetrics to initiate labor or to control postpartum hemorrhage. (Oxytocin)

Parasympatholytic: a drug that inhibits response to parasympathetic nerve impulses and to parasympathomimetic drugs; an anticholinergic drug. (Atropine)

Parasympathomimetic: a drug that activates organs innervated by the parasympathetic nervous system; a cholinergic drug. (Neostigmine)

Pediculicide: an insecticide suitable for eradicating louse infestations (pediculosis). (Lindane)

Penicillin Adjuvant: a drug that extends systemic duration of penicillin by inhibiting its renal excretion. (Probenecid)

Phenothiazine: an antipsychotic or antidepressant drug that contains the phenothiazine nucleus in its chemical structure. (Chloropromazine, antipsychotic; Imipramine, antidepressant)

Photosensitizer: a drug that increases cutaneous response to ultraviolet light, used with ultraviolet light to treat certain skin diseases (e.g., psoriasis). (Methoxsalen)

Pigmenting Agent: a drug that promotes melanin synthesis in the skin. (Trioxsalen, oral pigmenting agent; Methoxsalen, topical pigmenting agent)

Posterior Pituitary Hormone, Antidiuretic: a hormone that promotes renal reabsorption of water, useful in treating diabetes insipidus. (Vasopressin injection)

Potassium-sparing Diuretic: a diuretic that does not induce systemic potassium depletion as a side effect. (Triamterene)

Potentiator: an adjunctive drug that enhances the action of a primary drug, the total response being greater than the sum of the individual actions. (Hexafluorenium, potentiator for Succinylcholine)

Progestin: a progesterone-like hormone that stimulates the secretory phase of the uterine cycle. (Norethindrone)

Prostaglandin: a drug from the classes of cell-regulating hormones cyclized from arachidonic acid. (Alprostadil, maintains ductus arteriosus patency in newborn infants pending corrective surgery for congenital heart defects)

Prostaglandin Synthetase Inhibitor: a drug that inhibits prostaglandin synthesis and prostaglandin-induced symptoms such as inflammation; a nonsteroidal anti-inflammatory drug. (Ibuprofen)

Protectant: a topical drug that provides a physical barrier to the environment. (Zinc Gelatin, skin protectant; Methylcellulose, ophthalmic protectant)

Proteolytic, Injectable: an enzyme drug for injection into herniated lumbar intervertebral discs to reduce interdiscal pressure. (Chymopapain)

Prothrombogenic: a drug with vitamin K activity, useful in treating the hypoprothrombinemia of vitamin K deficiency or overdosage with a vitamin K antagonist. (Phytonadione)

Psychedelic: a drug (especially a street drug) that induces vivid sensory phenomena and hallucinations. (Mescaline)

Psychotherapeutic: a drug used to treat abnormal mental or emotional processes. (Chloropromazine, Haloperidol)

Rauwolfia Alkaloid: a plant principle derived from *Rauwolfia serpentina* and related species, with antihypertensive and antipsychotic actions. (Reserpine)

Radiographic Agent: see X-ray Contrast Medium.

Radiopharmaceutical: a drug containing a radioactive isotope, used for diagnostic or therapeutic purposes. (Iodinated Albumen with ^{125}I or ^{131}I)

Resin, Electrolyte Removing: see Ion Exchange Resin.

Rubefacient: a topical drug that induces mild skin irritation with erythema, used as a toughening agent. (Rubbing Alcohol)

Salt Substitute: a sodium-free alternative to sodium chloride used for flavoring foods. (Potassium Chloride)

Scabicide: an insecticide suitable for eradication of the itch mite *Sarcoptes scabiei* (scabies). (Lindane)

Sclerosing Agent: an irritant drug suitable for injection into varicose veins to induce their fibrosis and obliteration. (Morrhuate Sodium Injection)

Sedative: a central nervous system depressant used to induce mild relaxation. (Phenobarbital)

Specific: a drug specially adapted in its indicated use, usually because of a functional relationship between drug mechanism and disease pathophysiology.

Stimulant, Central: a drug that increases the functional state of the central nervous system, sometimes used in convulsive therapy of mental disorders. (Flurothyl)

Stimulant, Respiratory: a drug that selectively stimulates respiration, either by peripheral initiation of respiratory reflexes, or by selective central nervous system stimulation. (Carbon Dioxide, reflex respiratory stimulant; Ethamivan, central respiratory stimulant)

Sun Screening Agent: a skin protectant that absorbs light energy at wavelengths that cause sunburn. (ParaAminoBenzoic Acid, PABA)

Sulfonylurea: an oral antidiabetic drug that contains the sulfonylurea moiety in its chemical structure. (Tolazamide)

Suppressant: a drug that inhibits the progress of a disease but does not cure it.

Sympatholytic: a drug that inhibits response to sympathetic nerve impulses and to sympathomimetic drugs; an antiadrenergic drug. (Phentolamine, alpha sympatholytic; Propranolol, beta sympatholytic)

Sympathomimetic: a drug that activates organs innervated by the sympathetic nervous system; an adrenergic drug. (Epinephrine)

Systemically Acting Drug: a drug administered so as to reach systemic circulation, from which the drug diffuses into all tissues, including the site of the therapeutic action.

Thiazide Diuretic: a diuretic that contains the benzothiadiazide (thiazide) moiety in its chemical structure. (Hydrochlorothiazide)

Thrombolytic: an enzyme drug administered parenterally to solubilize blood clots. (Urokinase)

Thyroid Hormone: a hormone that maintains metabolic function and normal metabolic rate of tissues. (Levothyroxine)

Topically Acting Drug: a drug applied to the body surface for local therapeutic action.

Toxoid: a modified antigen from an infectious organism used as a vaccine. (Tetanus Toxoid)

Tranquilizer, Minor: an old term for an anxiolytic drug.

Tranquilizer: a drug (such as antipsychotic) used to suppress an acutely disturbed emotional state. (Trifluoperazine, antipsychotic)

Tricyclic Antidepressant: an antidepressant that contains the tricyclic phenothiazine nucleus in its chemical structure. (Imipramine)

Tuberculostatic: see Antitubercular.

Uricosuric: a drug that promotes renal excretion of uric acid, useful in treating chronic gout. (Probenecid)

Uterine Contractant: an obstetric drug used after placenta delivery to induce sustained uterine contraction to reduce bleeding. (Methylergonovine)

Uterine Contraction Inhibitor: a drug that inhibits uterine muscle contraction, used in preterm labor to prolong gestation. (Ritodrine)

Vaccine: an antigen-containing drug used to induce active immunity against an infectious disease. (Hepatitis B Vaccine, Rabies Vaccine)

Vasoconstrictor: a drug that narrows arterioles, usually to elevate blood pressure. See Vasopressor.

Vasodilator, Coronary: a drug that expands blood vessels in the heart and improves coronary blood flow, useful in treating angina pectoris; an antianginal drug. (Nitroglycerin)

Vasodilator, Peripheral: a drug that expands peripheral blood vessels and improves blood flow to the extremities of the body. (Minoxidil)

Vasopressor: an adrenergic drug administered to constrict arterioles and elevate arterial blood pressure. (Norepinephrine)

Vinca Alkaloid: a plant principle derived from *Vinca rosea* and related species, with antineoplastic action. (Vincristine)

Vitamin: an organic chemical essential in small amounts for normal metabolism, used therapeutically to supplement the vitamin content of foods.

Xanthine Alkaloid: a plant principle chemically related to xanthine, with central nervous system stimulant, smooth muscle relaxant, and diuretic actions. (Caffeine)

X-Ray Contrast Medium: a drug opaque to x-rays that assists visualization of an internal organ during radiographic examination. (Barium Sulfate, Iopanoic Acid)

Glossary of Pharmaceutical Terms

Active Ingredient: the ingredient or ingredients of a pharmaceutical product responsible for its pharmacologic activity (also medicament, drug substance, active pharmaceutical ingredient).

Aerosol: a dosage form that is packaged under pressure and contains therapeutically active ingredients that are released upon activation of an appropriate valve system.

Ampul: a final container that is all glass in which the open end, after filling with product, is sealed by heat (also ampoule, ampule, [French] carpule)

Aseptic: lacking disease-producing microorganisms; not the same as sterile.

Aseptic Processing: manufacturing dosage forms without terminal sterilization. The dosage form is sterile-filtered, then aseptically filled into the final package and aseptically sealed.

Bead: a solid dosage form in the shape of a small sphere. The dosage form generally contains multiple beads (also pellet).

Bolus: a large, long tablet intended for administration to animals.

Capsule: a solid dosage form in which the drug is enclosed within a hard or soft soluble container or shell.

Capsule, Delayed-release: a coated capsule or more commonly encapsulated granules that may be coated to resist releasing the drug in the stomach because the drug will irritate gastric mucosa or gastric fluid will inactivate the drug.

Capsule, Extended-release: a capsule that is formulated in such a manner as to make the contained medication available over an extended period following ingestion.

Capsule, Soft-shell: a solid dosage form in which one or more active ingredients, normally in solution or suspension or in the form of a paste, is filled into a one-piece shell.

Collodion: a liquid preparation composed of pyroxylin dissolved in a solvent mixture of alcohol and ether and applied externally.

Concentrate for Dip: a preparation containing one or more active ingredients usually in the form of a paste or solution; it is used to prepare a diluted suspension, emulsion, or solution of the active ingredient(s) for the prevention and treatment of ectoparasitic infestations of animals.

Cream: a semisolid dosage form containing one or more drug substances dissolved or dispersed in a suitable base.

Drops, Oral: a solution, emulsion, or suspension that is administered in small volumes, such as drops, by means of a suitable device.

Effervescent: a dosage form containing ingredients that rapidly release carbon dioxide when in contact with water.

Elixir: a clear, pleasantly flavored, sweetened hydroalcoholic liquid containing dissolved active ingredients intended for oral use.

Emulsion: a two-phase system in which one liquid is dispersed throughout another liquid in the form of small droplets.

Excipient: an inactive ingredient of a dosage form.

Extract: a concentrated preparation of vegetable or animal drug obtained by removal of the active constituents with suitable menstrua, by evaporation of all or nearly all of the solvent and by adjustment of the residual mass or powder to the prescribed standards.

Fluidextract: a liquid preparation of a vegetable drug containing alcohol as a solvent, preservative, or both and so made that unless otherwise specified in an individual monograph, each milliliter contains the therapeutic constituents of 1 g of the standard drug.

Foam: an emulsion packaged in a pressurized aerosol container that has a fluffy, semisolid consistency when dispensed.

Gel: a semisolid system consisting of either a suspension of small inorganic particles or large organic molecules interpenetrated by a liquid.

Granules: a preparation of dry aggregates of powder particles that may contain one or more active ingredients with or without other ingredients.

Implant: see pellet. a small sterile solid mass consisting of a highly purified drug with or without excipients made by compression or molding and put in place by injection or incision.

Infusion, Intramammary: a suspension of a drug in a suitable oil vehicle; intended for veterinary use only.

Inhalation: a solution or suspension of one or more drug substances administered by the nasal or oral respiratory route for local or systemic effect.

Injection: a preparation intended for parenteral administration or for constituting or diluting a parenteral article prior to administration.

Irrigation: a sterile solution intended to bathe or flush open wounds or body cavities.

Jelly: see gel.

Liniment: an alcoholic or oleaginous solution or emulsion applied by rubbing on the skin for treating pain and stiffness of underlying musculature.

Lotion: a fluid suspension or emulsion applied to the surface of the skin. See solution or suspension.

Lozenge: a solid preparation that is intended to dissolve or disintegrate slowly in the mouth.

Lyophilization: removal of water or other solvent from a frozen solution by sublimation caused by a combination of temperature and pressure differentials (also freeze drying).

Modified Release: a release pattern of the active ingredient from the dosage form that has been deliberately changed from that of the conventional form. Includes accelerated release, delayed release, extended release, pulsatile release, targeted release, and so on.

Molded Tablet: a tablet that has been formed by dampening the ingredients and pressing them into a mold, then removing and drying the resulting solid mass.

Mouthwash: an aqueous solution used to rinse the oral cavity.

Ointment: a semisolid preparation intended for external application to the skin or mucous membrane.

Ophthalmic Preparation: drug in dosage form intended to be applied to the eye.

Ophthalmic Ointment: a sterile ointment intended for application to the eye.

Ophthalmic Solution: a sterile solution, essentially free from foreign particles, suitably prepared and packaged for instillation into the eye.

Ophthalmic Suspension: a sterile liquid preparation containing solid particles dispersed in a liquid vehicle intended for application to the eye.

Ophthalmic Strip: a sterile single-use container or sterile impregnated paper strip containing the drug to be applied to the eye.

Orally Disintegrating: a solid oral dosage form that disintegrates rapidly in the mouth to facilitate release of the active ingredient.

Otic Solution: a solution intended for instillation in the outer ear.

Otic Suspension: a liquid preparation containing micronized particles intended for instillation in the outer ear.

Paste: a semisolid dosage form that contains one or more drug substances intended for topical application. It generally contains a high concentration of solids and has a stiff consistency.

Pellet: see bead. (Also a solid granule or regular shape prepared by compaction or by granulation.)

Pill: a solid spherical dosage form, usually prepared by a wet massing technique.

Plaster: a solid or semisolid mass supplied on a backing material and intended to provide prolonged contact with the skin.

Powder: an intimate mixture of dry, finely divided drug and/or chemicals that may be intended for internal (oral) or external (topical) use.

Premix: a mixture of one or more drug substances with a suitable vehicle.

Pulsatile Release: a release pattern of the active ingredient from the dosage form that is modified to release aliquots of the total dose at two or more time intervals.

Rinse: a solution used to cleanse by flushing.

Shampoo: a solution, emulsion, or suspension used to clean the hair and scalp.

Soap: the alkali salt(s) of one or more fatty acids.

Solution: a liquid preparation that contains one or more dissolved (molecularly dispersed) chemical substances in a suitable solvent or mixture of miscible solvents; may be oral, topical, otic, ophthalmic.

Spirit: an alcoholic or hydroalcoholic solution of volatile substances prepared usually by simple solution or by admixture of the ingredients.

Sterile: completely lacking living (viable) microbial life.

Sterility: an acceptably high level of probability that a product processed in an aseptic system does not contain viable microorganisms.

Stick: a slender, cylindrical dosage form of rigid consistency.

Suppository: a solid body adapted for introduction into the rectal, vaginal, or urethral orifice.

Suppository Tablet or Insert: a vaginal suppository prepared by compression of powdered materials into a suitable shape; can also be prepared by encapsulation in soft gelatin.

Suspension: a liquid preparation that consists of solid particles dispersed throughout a liquid phase in which the particles are not soluble; may be oral, topical, otic ophthalmic.

Syrup: a solution containing a high concentration of sucrose or other sugars. See solution.

System: a dosage form developed to allow for uniform release or targeting of drugs to the body.

System, Transdermal: a self-contained, discrete

dosage form that is designed to deliver drug(s) through the intact skin to the systemic circulation.

System, Ocular: a dosage form intended for placement in the lower conjunctival fornix, from which the drug diffuses through a membrane at a constant rate.

System, Intrauterine: a system that is intended for release of drug over a long period, such as a year.

Tablet: a solid dosage form containing medicinal substance(s) with or without diluents.

Tablet, Chewable: a tablet formulated so that it may be chewed, producing a pleasant-tasting residue that is easily swallowed and does not leave a bitter or unpleasant aftertaste.

Tablet, Delayed-release: a tablet with a coating that is intended to postpone release of the medication until the tablet has passed through the stomach.

Tablet, Extended-release: a tablet that is formulated so as to make the contained medication available over an extended period following ingestion.

Targeted Release: release of the active ingredient from a dosage form modified to preferentially deliver most of the drug to a specific region, organ, or tissue.

Terminal Sterilization: a process used to produce sterility in a final product contained in its final packaging system.

Tincture: an alcoholic or hydroalcoholic solution prepared from vegetable materials or from chemical substances.

Transdermal Delivery System, Electroporation: a transdermal delivery system enhanced by the application of short, high-voltage electric pulses to create aqueous pores in the lipid bilayer of skin and thereby facilitate drug diffusion.

Transdermal Delivery System, High Velocity Powder Particles: a transdermal drug delivery system using supersonic shock waves of helium gas to enhance drug diffusion through the skin.

Transdermal Delivery System, Iontophoresis: a transdermal drug delivery system enhanced by the use of applied electric current to facilitate drug diffusion through the skin.

Transdermal Delivery System, Phonophoresis: a transdermal drug delivery system enhanced by the application of low-frequency ultrasound to facilitate drug diffusion through the skin (also ultrasound, sonophoresis, ultrasonophoresis, ultraphonophoresis).

Transdermal Matrix Patch: a transdermal matrix system using a polymeric matrix containing drug intended for systemic delivery through the skin; generally the skin is the rate-controlling membrane for drug diffusion.

Transdermal Membrane Patch: a transdermal system containing a drug reservoir entrapped between backing and adhesive layers and a drug diffusion–controlling membrane; the reservoir is usually a semisolid dispersion or solution of the drug.

Troche: see lozenge.

Urethral: a dosage form intended for insertion into the urethra to provide a local effect of the active ingredient.

Validation: scientific study to prove that a process is doing what it is supposed to do and is under control.

Water, Aromatic: a clear, saturated aqueous solution (unless otherwise specified) of one or more volatile oils or other aromatic or volatile substances.

Systems and Techniques of Pharmaceutical Measurement

Appendix C

Knowledge and application of the systems of pharmaceutical measurement are essential to the practice of pharmacy. Whether applied to the compounding and dispensing of prescriptions in the community pharmacy, the filling of medication orders in the institutional pharmacy, or the large-scale industrial manufacture of pharmaceuticals, quantitative accuracy is essential in the preparation of safe and effective medications.

Pharmaceuticals prepared industrially undergo rigid in-process controls and final product assays to ensure conformance with the applicable standards for drug content. Prescriptions and medication orders filled extemporaneously in the community and institutional pharmacy usually lack the advantage of control by assay, and thus the pharmacist must be absolutely certain of the accuracy of all calculations and measurements employed. Calculations should be double-checked by the pharmacist and whenever possible by a colleague. The importance of accurate calculations and measurements cannot be overstated. For example, an error in the placement of a decimal point represents a *minimum* error of a factor of 10, and if it is applicable to the active ingredient, a critical drug underdosage or overdosage results.

The pharmacy student must have a working knowledge of the systems of pharmaceutical measurement, their application in pharmaceutical calculations, the factors used for conversion between the systems, and the proper techniques of weighing and measuring.

Systems of Pharmaceutical Measurement

Although pharmacy has moved toward the exclusive use of the metric system, two other systems of measurement, namely the *apothecary system* and the *avoirdupois system*, occasionally may be encountered. The metric system includes units or weight, volume and linear measure; the apothecary system includes units of weight and volume; and the avoirdupois system includes only units of weight. The metric system has replaced the apothecary system in virtually all pharmaceutical measurements and calculations, although some use remains, such as common reference to the dose of thyroid in *grains*, an apothecary system unit. The avoirdupois system is the *common* commercial system of weight used in the United States. It too is being replaced by the metric system, but at a much slower pace. The avoirdupois system is encountered by the pharmacist in the purchase of bulk chemicals and other items packaged and sold by the ounce or pound.

The Metric System

The metric system is the most widely used system in pharmacy. It is the system used in the *United States Pharmacopeia* (USP) and *National Formulary* (NF), by the federal Food and Drug Administration, in manufacturers' labeling of pharmaceutical products, and in most physicians' writing of prescriptions and medication orders.

In the metric system, the *gram* is the main unit of weight, the *liter* the main unit of volume, and the *meter* the main unit of length. Subunits and multiples of these basic units are indicated by the prefix notations and symbols shown in Table A.1.

In pharmacy, these are the most commonly used metric units:

Weight is expressed in terms of the kilogram (kg), gram (g), milligram (mg), or microgram (μg).

685

TABLE A.1 METRIC SYSTEM UNIT PREFIXES

MULTIPLICATION FACTOR	PREFIX	SYMBOL	TERM (USA)
1 000 000 000 000 000 000 $= 10^{18}$	exa	E	one quintillion
1 000 000 000 000 000 $= 10^{15}$	tera	T	one quadrillion
1 000 000 000 000 $= 10^{12}$	giga	G	one trillion
1 000 000 000 $= 10^{9}$	mega	M	one billion
1 000 000 $= 10^{6}$	kilo	k	one million
1 000 $= 10^{3}$	hecto	h	one thousand
100 $= 10^{2}$	deka	da	one hundred
10 $= 10$	peta	P	ten
0.1 $= 10^{-1}$	deci	d	one tenth
0.01 $= 10^{-2}$	centi	c	one hundredth
0.001 $= 10^{-3}$	milli	m	one thousandth
0.000 001 $= 10^{-6}$	micro	μ	one millionth
0.000 000 001 $= 10^{-9}$	nano	n	one billionth
0.000 000 000 001 $= 10^{-12}$	pico	p	one trillionth
0.000 000 000 000 001 $= 10^{-15}$	femto	f	one quadrillionth
0.000 000 000 000 000 001 $= 10^{-18}$	atto	a	one quintillionth

Adapted from American National Metric Council. *Metric Editorial Guide,* 4th ed. Washington: ANMC. The table is based on the International System of Units (SI, from the French, Le Système International d'Unites), as modified for use in the United States by the Secretary of Commerce.

Liquid measure is expressed in terms of the liter (L) or milliliter (mL).

Linear measure is expressed in terms of the meter (m), centimeter (cm), or millimeter (mm).

Area measure is expressed in terms of the square meter (m²) or square centimeter (cm²).

The metric weight scale in Figure A.1 is intended to depict the relationship between the units of weight in the metric system and to demonstrate an easy method of converting from one unit to another (1). In the example, 1.23 kg is to be converted to grams. On the scale, the gram position is three decimal places from the kilogram position. Thus, the decimal point is moved three places toward the right. In the other example, the conversion from milligrams to grams also requires movement of the decimal point three places, but this time to the left. The same method may be used to convert metric units of volume or length.

Table of Metric Weight

1 kg = 1000.000 g
1 hg = 100.000 g
1 Dg = 10.000 g
1 g = 1.000 g
1 dg = 0.100 g
1 cg = 0.010 g
1mg = 0.001 g
1 μg = 0.000001 g
1 ng = 0.0000000001 g
1 pg = 0.000000000001 g

hg, hectogram; Dg, dekagram; dg, decigram; cg, centigram; ng, nanogram; pg, picogram.

or

1 g = 0.001 kg
= 0.010 hg
= 0.100 Dg
= 10 dg
= 100 cg
= 1000 mg
= 1,000,000 μg
= 1,000,000,000 ng
= 1,000,000,000,000 pg

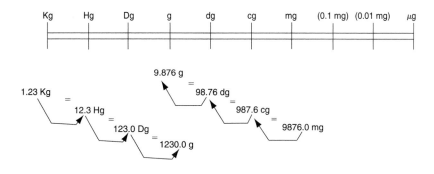

DECIMAL MOVEMENT

⊙→ TO CONVERT FROM LARGER TO SMALLER UNITS
←⊙ TO CONVERT FROM SMALLER TO LARGER UNITS

FIGURE A.1 Metric weight scale.

Table of Metric Volume

1 kL	=	1000.000 L
1 hL	=	100.000 L
1 DL	=	10.000 L
1 L	=	1.000 L
1 dL	=	0.100 L
1 cL	=	0.010 L
1 mL	=	0.001 L
1 μL	=	0.000001 L

kL, kiloliter; hL, hectoliter; DL, dekaliter; L, liter; dL, deciliter; cL, centiliter; mL, milliliter; μL, microliter.

or

1 L	=	0.0001 kL
	=	0.010 hL
	=	0.100 DL
	=	10 dL
	=	100 cL
	=	1000 mL
	=	1,000,000 μL

Table of Metric Length

1 km	=	1000.000 m
1 hm	=	100.000 m
1 Dm	=	10.000 m
1 m	=	1.000 m
1 dm	=	0.100 m
1 cm	=	0.010 m
1 mm	=	0.001 m
1 μm	=	0.000001 m
1 nm	=	0.000000001 m

km, kilometer; hm, hectometer; Dm, dekameter; m, meter; dm, decimeter; cm, centimeter; mm, millimeter; μm, micrometer; nm, nanometer.

or

1 m	=	0.001 km
	=	0.010 hm
	=	0.100 Dm
	=	10 dm
	=	100 cm
	=	1000 mm
	=	1,000,000 μm
	=	10,000,000,000 nm

The Apothecary System

The apothecary system provides for the measurement of both weight and volume. The tables of the system are presented below.

Table of Apothecaries' Fluid Measure

60 m	= 1 f℥[a]
8 f℥ (480 m)	= 1 f℥[a]
16 f℥	= 1 pt
2 pt (32 f℥)	= 1 qt
4 qt (8 pt)	= 1 gal

m, minim; f℥, fluidrachm; f℥, fluidounce; pt, pint; qt, quart; gal, gallon.

[a]When there is no doubt that the material referred to is a liquid, the *f* is usually omitted from this symbol. *Drachm* is also spelled *dram*.

Table of Apothecaries' Measure of Weight

20 gr	= 1 ℈
3 ℈ (60 gr)	= 1 ℨ
8 ℨ (480 gr)	= 1 ℥
12 ℥ (5760 gr)	= 1 lb

gr, grain; ℈, scruple; lb, pound.

The Avoirdupois System

The avoirdupois system is used in commerce to supply bulk chemicals and other items by weight, in ounces or pounds (e.g., epsom salts).

The grain is the same weight in the apothecary and avoirdupois systems. However, the ounce and the pound in the two systems differ in the number of grains per unit. The apothecary ounce contains 480 grains, whereas the avoirdupois ounce contains 437.5 grains. The apothecary pound contains 5760 grains, whereas the avoirdupois pound contains 7000 grains. Also, the symbols for the ounce and pound are different in the two systems.

Table of Avoirdupois Measure of Weight

437.5 gr	= 1 oz
16 oz (7000 gr)	= 1 lb

oz, avoirdupois ounce.

Intersystem Conversion

A pharmacist may convert the weight, volume, or dimensions of length from one system to another with conversion factors. Depending on the circumstances and requirements for accuracy, conversion factors of different exactness may be used. The following is a table of the factors commonly used in prescription practice. They are exact equivalents rounded off for practical application. Exact equivalents, used in the conversion of specific quantities in pharmaceutical formulas, may be found in the USP.

Useful Conversion Equivalents of Weight

1 g	= 15.432 gr
1 kg	= 2.2 lb (avoir)
1 gr	= 0.0648 g or 64.8 or 65 mg
1 ℥	= 31.1 g
1 oz (avoir)	= 28.35 g
1 lb (apoth)	= 373.2 g
1 lb (avoir)	= 453.6 or 454 g

Useful Conversion Equivalents of Volume

1 mL	= 16.23 ℳ
1 ℳ	= 0.06 mL
1 ʒ	= 3.69 mL
1 ℥	= 29.57 mL
1 pt	= 473 mL
1 gal (U.S.)	= 3785 mL
1 gal (British Imperial)	= 4546 mL

m, minim.

Conversion Equivalents of Length

1 inch	= 2.54 cm
1 meter	= 39.37 inches

Today there are very few occasions on which intersystem conversion is needed, owing to the almost exclusive use of the metric system in both product formulation and prescription compounding. However, when conversion is necessary or desired, it is a simple matter of selecting and applying the appropriate intersystem conversion factor.

For example, if one wishes to determine the number of milliliters in 8 f℥, the conversion factor that most directly relates milliliters and fluidounces is selected. That factor is 1 f℥ equals 29.57 mL; thus 8 f℥ equals 8 times 29.57 mL, or 236.56 mL.

Another example: how many 30-mL containers may be filled from 10 gal of a formulation? There is in 1 gal 3785 mL. Thus 10 gal equals 10 times 3785 mL, or 37,850 mL. By dividing this total number of milliliters by 30, the number of containers that may be filled is found to be 1,261.

Another example: how many 0.5-gr tablets may be prepared from 1 kg of a drug substance? Since 1 gr equals 64.8 mg, 0.5 gr equals 32.4 mg. Also, 1 kg equals 1000 g, or 1,000,000 mg. Since 32.4 is required for one tablet, 1,000,000 mg divided by 32.4 mg equals 30,864 tablets that may be prepared.

A final example: if a transdermal patch measures 30 mm square, what is this dimension in inches? The conversion factor, 1 inch equals 2.54 cm, may be expressed as 1 inch equals 25.4 mm. Thus, by dividing 30 mm by 25.4 mm/inch, one finds the patch is 1.18 inches square.

Quantitative Product Strength

The quantitative composition of certain pharmaceuticals, particularly liquids and semisolid dosage forms, often is expressed in terms of the *percentage strength* of the active and sometimes inactive ingredients. For some dilute solutions, the strength may be expressed in terms of its *ratio strength*. For most injections, many oral liquids, and some semisolid dosage forms, the quantity of active ingredient commonly is expressed as weight of drug per unit volume basis, such as milligrams of drug per milliliter of injection or oral liquid, or as weight of drug per unit weight of preparation, such as milligrams of drug per gram of ointment. The strength of solid dosage forms is given as the drug content (e.g., 5 mg) per dosage unit (e.g., tablets and capsules).

Percent, by definition, means parts per hundred. In pharmacy, percentage concentrations have specific meanings based on the physical character of the particular product or formulation. That is:

Percent weight in volume: Expressed % w/v, this defines grams of a constituent in 100 mL of a preparation (generally a liquid)

Percent volume in volume: Expressed % v/v, this defines milliliters of a constituent in 100 mL of a preparation (generally a liquid)

Percent weight in weight: Expressed % w/w, this defines grams of a constituent in 100 g of a preparation (generally a solid or semisolid, but also for liquid preparations prepared by weight)

Thus, a 5% w/v solution or suspension of a drug contains 5 g of the substance in each 100 mL of product; a 5% v/v preparation contains 5 mL of the substance in each 100 mL of product; and a 5% w/w preparation contains 5 g of the substance in each 100 g of product.

In the manufacture or compounding of pharmaceutical preparations, the pharmacist may calculate (*a*) the strength of an individual component in a product or (*b*) the amount of a component needed to achieve a desired percentage strength.

For example, what is the percentage strength, w/v, of a solution containing 15 g of drug in 500 mL? Since by definition percentage strength is in parts per hundred, just determine how many grams of drug are present in each 100 mL solution. Solving by proportion: 15 g/500 mL = (x) g/100 mL. The answer is 3 g, and thus the solution is 3 % w/v in strength.

Other examples: 3 mL of a liquid in 1 L of solution equals 0.3% v/v; 4 g of drug in 250 mL equals 1.6% w/v; and 8 g of drug in 40 g of product equals 20% w/w.

How many grams of drug are needed to prepare 400 mL of a 5% w/v preparation? In w/v problems, the specific gravity *of the preparation* is assumed to be the same as that of water (sp. gr. 1.0), so 1 mL is assumed to weigh 1 g. Therefore, in the problem example, the 400 mL is assumed to weigh 400 g, and 5% of 400 g = 20 g, the amount of drug needed.

A v/v problem example: How many mL of a liquid is needed to make 1 pt of a 0.1% v/v solution? There is in 1pt 473 mL, and 0.1% of that is 0.473 mL, the answer.

A w/w problem example: How many grams of zinc oxide powder should be used in preparing 120 g of a 20% w/w ointment? The answer is 20% of 120 g equals 24 g.

Ratio strength is sometimes used to express the strength of or to calculate the amount of a component needed to make a relatively dilute preparation. Compared to percentage strength designations, for example, a 0.1% w/v preparation (0.1 g/100 mL) is equivalent to 1 g/1000 mL, and may be expressed as a ratio strength of 1:1000 w/v. Ratio strength expressions use the w/v, v/v, and w/w designations in the same manner as percentage strength expressions. For example:

A 1:1000 w/v preparation of a solid constituent in a liquid preparation = 1 g of the solid constituent in 1000 mL of preparation.

A 1:1000 v/v preparation of a liquid constituent in a liquid preparation = 1 mL of constituent in 1000 mL of preparation.

A 1:1000 w/w/ preparation of a solid constituent in a solid or semisolid preparation = 1 g of constituent in 1000 g of preparation.

A ratio strength calculation: what is the ratio strength of 6000 mL of solution containing 3 g of drug? Whenever possible, it is preferable for ratio strengths to be expressed as 1:. In this example, if 3 g of drug is in 6000 mL of solution, 1 g of drug is contained in 2000 mL, and thus the ratio strength is 1:2000 w/v. Sometimes the answers do not come out as evenly; for example, what is the ratio strength of 0.3 mL of a liquid in 1 L of solution? In this instance, there is 0.3 mL in 1000 mL, equivalent to 3 mL in 10,000 mL, or a ratio strength of 3:10,000 v/v, or 1:3,333.3 v/v.

Another ratio strength calculation: In grams, how much drug is needed to make 5 L of a 1:400 w/v solution? By definition (of 1:400 w/v), 1 g of drug is needed for each 400 mL of solution. Since 5 L, or 5000 mL, of solution is to be prepared, the amount of drug required is found by solving 1 g/400 mL = (x) g/5000 mL, or 12.5 g.

Rather than being expressed in terms of percentage strength or ratio strength, the strength of some pharmaceutical preparations, particularly injections and sometimes oral liquids, is based on drug content per unit of volume, as milligrams per milliliter. Thus flexibility in dosing can be achieved by administering the volume of preparation that contains the desired dose.

Reducing and Enlarging Formulas

In the course of pharmaceutical manufacturing and in professional practice activities, it is often necessary to reduce or enlarge a pharmaceutical formulation to prepare the desired amount of product. A standard manufacturing formulation, or *master formula*, contains the quantitative amounts of each ingredient needed to prepare a specified quantity of product. When preparing other quantities, larger or smaller, the *quantitative relationship* of each component to the other in the formula must be maintained. For example, if there is 2 g of ingredient A and 10 mL of ingredient B (among other ingredients) in a formula for 1000 mL, one must use 0.2 g of ingredient A and 1 mL of ingredient B to make 100 mL, or one-tenth of the formula. If, on the other hand, a formula is to be enlarged—for example, from 1 L (1000 mL) of product to a gallon (3785 mL)—the amount of each ingredient required is 3.785 times that needed to prepare 1 L of product.

In these examples the quantity of product prepared is reduced or enlarged, but the quantitative relationship between each ingredient and the product strength remains unchanged.

Dosage Units

Drug dosage is selected by the prescriber based upon clinical considerations and the characteristics of the pharmacologic agent. Dosage forms (tablets, injections, transdermal patches) are used to administer the drug to the patient. Solid dosage forms, such as tablets and capsules, are generally prepared in various strengths to allow flexibility in dosing. The desired dose for a drug prepared in a liquid form may be provided by the volume administered. For example, if a liquid dosage form contains 5 mg of drug per milliliter and if a dose of 25 mg of drug is desired, 5 mL of the liquid may be administered. Commercially manufactured products are formulated to provide the drug in dosage forms and amounts convenient for administration. When the desired dosage or dosage form is commercially unavailable, the pharmacist may be called upon to compound the desired preparation.

Common Household Measure

Liquid and powder medications not packaged in unit dose systems are usually measured at home by the patient with common household measuring devices, such as the teaspoon or tablespoon. Although the household teaspoon may vary in volume capacity from approximately 3 to 8 mL, the American Standard Teaspoon has been established as having a volume of 4.93 ± 0.24 mL by the American National Standards Institute. For practical purposes, most pharmacy practitioners and pharmacy references use 5 mL as the capacity of the teaspoon. This is approximately equivalent to 1.33 f3, although physicians commonly use the drachm symbol to indicate a teaspoonful in their prescription directions to be transcribed

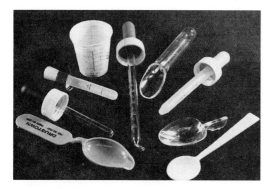

FIGURE A.2 Medicinal spoons of various shapes and capacities, calibrated medicine droppers, an oral medication tube, and a disposable medication cup.

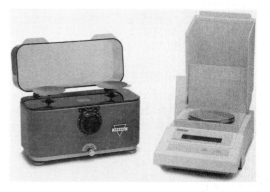

FIGURE A.3 Prescription balances: Torbal torsion balance (*left*) and Ohaus electronic balance. (Courtesy of Total Pharmacy Supply.)

by the pharmacist to the patient. The tablespoon is considered to have a capacity of 15 mL, equivalent to 3 teaspoonfuls or approximately 0.5 f℥.

Occasionally the pharmacist will provide a special medicinal spoon for the patient to use in measuring this medication. These spoons are available in half-teaspoon, teaspoon, and tablespoon capacities. Some manufacturers provide specially designed devices to be used by the patient in measuring medication. These include specially calibrated droppers, oral syringes, measuring wells or tubes, and calibrated bottle caps. In health care institutions, disposable measuring cups and unit dose containers are commonly employed in administering liquid medication. Examples of measuring devices are shown in Figure A.2.

Techniques of Pharmaceutical Measurement

Weighing and the Prescription Balance

In weighing materials, the selection of the instrument is based on the amount of material and the accuracy desired. In the large-scale manufacture of pharmaceuticals, large industrial *scales* of varying capacity and sensitivity are employed, and later, highly sensitive analytical balances are used in the quality control and analytical work.

In the hospital and community pharmacy, most weighing is done on either a *prescription balance* or an *electronic balance* (Fig. A.3). Prescription balances are termed *class III* (formerly class A) balances, which meet the prescribed standards of the National Institute of Standards and Technology. Every prescription department is required by law to have a prescription balance. The sensitivity of a balance is usually represented by the term *sensitivity requirement* (SR), the maximum change in load that will cause a specified change, one subdivision on the index plate, in the position of rest of the indicating element of the balance. The SR is determined in the following manner: (*a*) Level the balance. (*b*) Determine the rest point. (*c*) Place a 6-mg weight on one of the empty pans. (*d*) Look at the readout. The rest point should shift *not less than* one division on the index plate. The entire operation is repeated with a 10-g weight placed in the center of each balance pan. A class III balance has an SR of 6 mg with no load as well as with 10 g on each pan. This means that under these conditions, the addition of 6 mg of weight to one pan of the balance will disturb the equilibrium and move the balance pointer one division marking on the scale.

The USP directs that to avoid weighing errors of 5% or greater, which may be due to the limits of accuracy of the prescription balance, one must weigh a minimum of 120 mg of any material in each weighing (5% of 120 mg being the 6 mg SR, or error inherent with the balance). If a smaller weight of material is desired, it is directed that the pharmacist mix a larger calculated weight of the ingredient (120 mg or more), dilute it with a known weight of an inert dry diluent (as lactose), mix the two uniformly, and weigh an aliquot portion of the mixture (again 120 mg or more) calculated to contain the desired amount of agent. The class III balance with a capacity of 120 g should be used for all weighing required in prescription compounding.

The electronic balance is available in various sensitivities. The one most commonly used in prescription compounding has a readability of 0.001 mg; consequently, the least amount that can be weighed is 20 times that, or 20 mg. The electronic balance is much faster and easier to use than the prescription balance. The digital readout is easy to read and the balance is quite versatile and easy to clean, and it has a relatively small footprint.

Weights

Today, most pharmacies have a set of metric weights. Some commercial weight sets contain both the metric and apothecary systems. Prescription weights meet the National Bureau of Standards' specifications for analytical weights. Metric weights of 1 g and more and apothecaries' weights of 1 scruple and more are generally conical, with a narrow neck and head that allow them to be easily picked up with small forceps. Most of these weights are made of polished brass, and some are coated with nickel, chromium, or another material to resist corrosion. Fractional gram weights are made of aluminum and are generally square and flat with one raised end or corner for picking up with the forceps (Fig. A.4). Apothecaries' weights of 0.5 scruple are frequently coin-shaped brass, and those of 5 gr and less are usually bent aluminum wires, with each straight side representing 1 grain of weight. The half-grain weight is usually a smaller-gauge wire bent in half.

To prevent moisture and oils from the fingertips being deposited on the weights, all weights should be transferred with the forceps provided in each weight set.

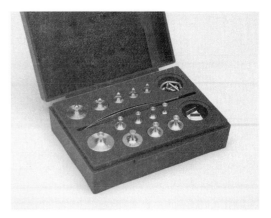

FIGURE A.4 Set of metric weights. (Courtesy of Mettler-Toledo, Inc.).

Care and Use of a Balance

First and foremost, the balance should be kept in a well-lighted location, placed on a firm, level counter approximately waist-high to the operator. The area should be as free from dust as is possible and in an area that is draft-free. There should be no corrosive vapors, high humidity, or vibration. When not in use, the balance should be clean and covered with the balance cover. Any agent spilled on the balance during use should be wiped off immediately with a soft brush or cloth. When not in use, the balance should always be kept with the weights off and the beam in the fixed or locked (arrested) position.

Before weighing an article, the balance must be made level. This is accomplished with the leveling screws on the bottom of the balance, according to the instructions accompanying the balance. The balance should be level both front to back and side to side, as indicated by the leveling bubble.

In using a prescription balance, neither the weights nor the substance to be weighed should be placed on the balance while the beam is free to oscillate. Before weighing, powder papers of equal size should be placed on both pans of the balance and the equilibrium of the balance tested by releasing the arresting knob. If the balance is off because of differences in the weight of the powder papers, additional weight may be added to the light pan by adding small tearings of powder papers. When balanced, the balance is placed in the arrested position and the desired weight added to the right-hand pan. Then an amount of substance considered to be approximately the desired weight is carefully placed on the left-hand pan with a spatula. The beam should then be slowly released by means of the locking device in the front of the balance. If the substance is in excess, the beam is fixed again and a small portion of the substance removed with the spatula. The process is continued until the two pans balance, as indicated by central position of the balance pointer. If the amount of weight on the balance is initially too little, the reverse process is undertaken. The powder paper used on the left-hand pan, intended to hold the substance to be weighed, is usually either folded diagonally or the edges turned up to contain the material being weighed.

In transferring material by spatula, the material may be lightly tapped from the spatula when the correct amount to be measured is approached. Usually this is done by holding the spatula with a small amount of material on it in the right hand and tapping the spatula with the forefinger. As material comes off the spatula, the left hand is working the balance-arresting mechanism, and the status of the weight is observed alternately with the tapping of the spatula. Most balances have a damping mechanism that slows down the oscillations and permits more rapid determinations of the balance or imbalance positions of the pans.

Once the material has been weighed, the balance beam is again put in the fixed position and the paper holding the weighed substance carefully removed. If more than a single weighing is to be performed, the paper is usually marked with the name of the substance it holds. After the final weighing, all weights are removed with the forceps and the balance cleaned, closed, and covered.

Most prescription balances contain built-in mechanisms whereby external weights are not required for weighing less than 1 g. Some balances use a rider, which may be shifted from the zero position toward the right side of the balance to add increments of weight marked on the scale in 10-mg units, up to 1 g. Another type of balance uses a central dial, calibrated in 10-mg units, to add weight up to 1 g. Both types of devices add the weight to the right-hand pan internally. In each case, the pharmacist may use a combination of the internal and external weights. For instance, if 1.2 g is to be weighed, the pharmacist can place a 1-g weight on the right hand pan and place the rider or adjust the dial to add 0.2 g. Care must always be exercised to bring the rider or dial to zero between weighings to maintain accuracy.

Most use of the prescription balance is weighing of powders or semisolid materials, such as ointments. However, liquids may also be weighed in tared (weighed) vessels of appropriate size. The pharmacist must always be certain to account for the weight of the vessel in calculating the amount of liquid weighed.

Materials should never be downweighed; that is, substances should never be placed on the pan with the balance in the unarrested position, forcing the pan to drop suddenly and forcefully. The sudden slamming down of the pan can do serious damage to the balance, affecting its sensitivity and accuracy.

The most common type of prescription balance is the torsion balance. It operates on the tension of taut wires, which when twisted by addition of weight, tend to twist back to the original position (Fig. A.3).

In using an electronic balance, first make sure the balance is clean and level. The balance should be calibrated daily. Many of these balances have internal calibration, and some use an external 200 g or 300 g weight. After calibration, a weighing boat or paper is placed on the balance pan and the Tare button is depressed to a reading of 0.000. Then, the required quantity of material is added to the weighing boat or paper; the dial constantly reads out the weight of material on the pan. Material can be easily removed or added to obtain the desired quantity.

Measuring Volume

The common instruments for pharmaceutical measurement are presented in Figure A.5. Two types of graduates, *conical* and *cylindrical*, are used in pharmacy. Cylindrical graduates are generally calibrated in metric units, whereas conical graduates may be graduated in both metric and apothecary or with a single scale of either of the systems. Graduates of both shapes are available in a wide variety of capacities, ranging from 5 to 1000 mL or more. Most graduates are made of a good-quality heat-treated glass, although graduates of polypropylene are also available. In measuring small volumes of liquids, less than 1.5 mL, the pharmacist should use a pipet as the one shown in Figure A.5. The bulky-looking device shown with the pipet is a pipet filler, used for drawing acids or other toxic solutions into the pipet without the mouth. The device, without being removed from the pipet, also allows for accurate delivery of the liquid.

In measuring volumes of liquids, the pharmacist should select the measuring device most appropriate to the volume of liquid to be measured and the desired degree of accuracy. With liquids, the more narrow the column of liquid, the more accurate is likely to be the measurement. Figure A.6 demonstrates this point. A reading error of the same dimension will produce a small-volume error with a pipet, a greater-volume error with a cylindrical graduate, and the largest error of volume with conical graduate. The greater the flare in the design

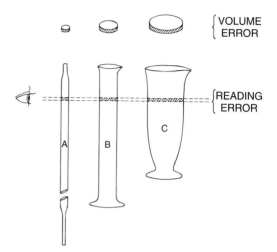

FIGURE A.6 The difference in the volume error occurring with the same reading error in measuring devices of different diameters.

of the conical graduate, the greater is the volume error.

In reading the level of liquid in a graduate, it is important to recognize the possibility of parallax error. Figure A.7 depicts this point. A liquid in a graduate tends to be drawn to the inner surface of the graduate and rises slightly against that surface and above its true meniscus. If one measures looking downward, it appears that the meniscus of the liquid is at this upper level, whereas it is slightly lower, at the actual level of the liquid the center of the graduate. Thus, measurements of liquids in graduates should be taken with the eyesight level with the liquid in the graduate.

If a pharmacist misreads a graduate, the *percentage of error* is affected by the volume of liquid. According to the USP, an acceptable 10-mL graduate cylinder with an internal diameter of 1.18 cm contains 0.109 mL of liquid in each millimeter of column. A reading error of 1 mm causes a percentage error of only 1.09% when 10 mL is being measured, 2.18% when 5 mL is being measured, 4.36% when 2.5 mL is being measured, and 7.26% when 1.5 mL is being measured. It is apparent that the greatest percentage error occurs when the smallest amount is being measured. Thus, the rule of thumb for measuring liquids in graduates is that a gradu-

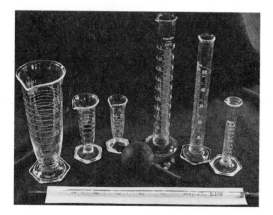

FIGURE A.5 Typical equipment for the pharmaceutical measurement of volume. Left, Conical graduates. Right, Cylindrical graduates. Front, a pipet for measurement of small volumes. Behind the pipet is a pipet filler, used instead of the mouth to draw acids and other dangerous liquids into the pipet.

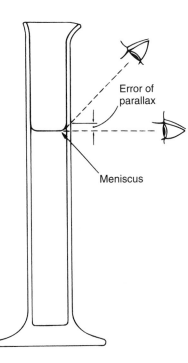

FIGURE A.7 Error in reading the meniscus of a liquid in a graduated cylinder when the reading is made from above the level of the liquid rather than at the same level.

Graduate Cylinder Size (mL)	Internal Diameter (cm)	Deviation in Actual Volume (mL)	Minimum Volume Measurable (mL)
5	0.98	0.075	3.00
10	1.18	0.109	4.36
25	1.95	0.296	11.84
50	2.24	0.394	15.76
100	2.58	0.522	20.88

For a 5% error, the minimum volumes measurable would be one-half of those stated. It is apparent that for accuracy, one should not use a graduate when the measurement would use only the bottom portion of the scale.

In using graduates, the pharmacist pours the liquid into the graduate slowly, observing the level. In measuring viscous liquids, adequate time must be allowed for the liquid to settle in the graduate, as some may run slowly down the inner sides of the graduate. It is best to attempt to pour such liquids toward the center of the graduate, avoiding contact with the sides. In emptying the graduate of its measured contents, adequate drain time should be allowed.

When pouring liquids from bottles, good pharmaceutical technique is to keep the label on the bottle facing up; this avoids the possibility of any errant liquid running down over the label as the bottle is righted after use. The bottle orifice should be wiped clean after each use.

ate should be used having a capacity *equal to or just exceeding* the volume to be measured.

According to Goldstein and Mattocks (2), based on a deviation of 1 mm from the mark and an allowable error of 2.5%, the smallest amounts that should be measured in cylindrical graduates having the stated internal diameters are as follows:

REFERENCES

1. Stoklosa MJ, Ansel HC. Pharmaceutical calculations, 10th ed. Baltimore: Williams & Wilkins, 1996.
2. Goldstein SW, Mattocks AM. How to measure accurately. J Am Pharm 1951;23:421.

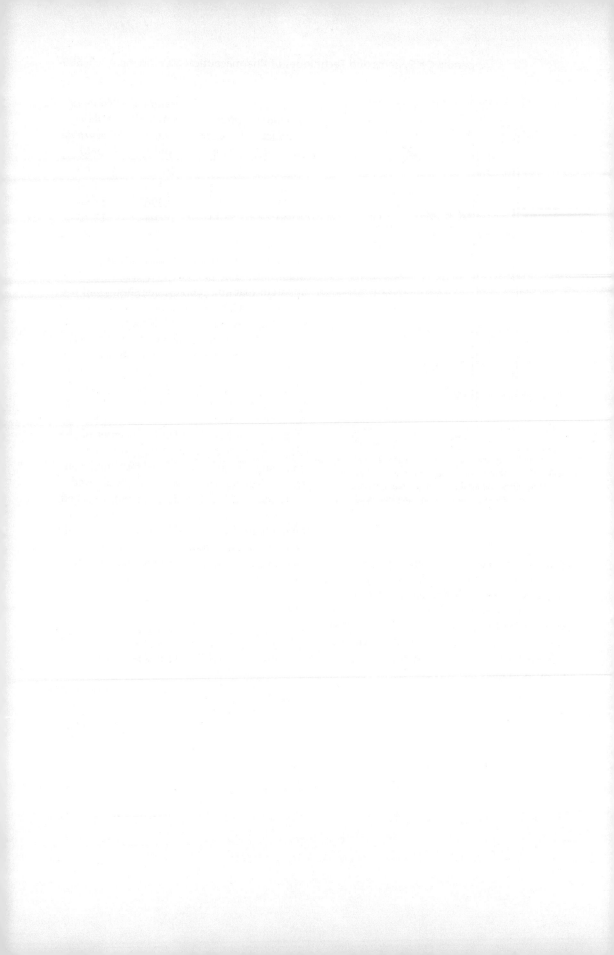

Index

Page numbers in *italics* denote figures; those followed by "t" denote tables; numbers followed by "c" indicate Physical Pharmacy Capsules.

A

Polyethylene terephthalate glycol, 84

Polymerase chain reaction, in biotechnology product preparation, 605–606

Polymerization, in drug degradation, 122

Polymethylmethacrylate contact lenses, 552

Polymorphism
  of crystals, 152
  in dosage form design, 100

Polymyxin B, in irrigation solutions, 501t

Polymyxin B sulfate, as preservative, 543

Polyoxy 40 stearate, as suppository base, 322

Polypropylene, in packaging, 84, 284

Polyvinyl alcohol
  as gelling agent, 421
  as thickening agent, 550

Polyvinyl chloride, in packaging, 84

Porosity
  of plastic, 85
  of powders, 191c

Portal circulation, bypass of, with rectal suppository route, 318–319

Positive controls, in clinical studies, 51

Positron emission tomography, 584–588
  advantages, 584
  principles, 584–585
  radiopharmaceuticals for, 586–588, 587t
  uses, 584–586

Positrons, 572

Posterior pituitary hormone, antidiuretic, 679

Postmarketing activities, for new drugs, 62

Potassium
  in enteral nutrition, 495–496
  in oral rehydration solutions, 351
  in parenteral therapy, 492

Potassium iodide
  saturated solution, 338–339
  stabilizers for, 121

Potassium permanganate, in pyrogen removal, 463

Potassium-sparing diuretics, 679

Potentiator, 679

Povidone, as gelling agent, 421

Povidone-iodine topical solution, 371

Powdered flavors, 133

Powders, 186–194
  angle of repose of, 190c
  blending of, 193–194, 194, 195
  blowers for, 196, 196
  bulkiness, 192c
  capsule filling with, 212–213, 212–215
  colorants for, 137
  definition, 186, 682
  degradation signs, 124
  density, 191c–192c
  flow properties, 190c
  granule preparation from, 198–199, 199
  medicated, 186, 194–198
    administration routes, 171
    aerosolized, 195, 195–196, 196
    bulk, 196
    divided, 196–198, 197

micronized
  for capsules, 210
  dissolution, 150
  for suspensions, 389
milled, for capsules, 210
papers for, 197, 197–198
particle size of, 187–188, 187t, 189c–191c
porosity, 191c
preparation, by comminution, 188, 192–193, 193c
reconstitution, for suspensions, 387, 403–404
for vaginal douches, 371–372
volume, 191c
wetting agents for, in suspensions, 396

Practice guidelines, radiopharmaceuticals, 590–596

"Practice Standards of the American Society of Health-System Pharmacists," 21–22

Precipitation, in parenteral nutrition mixtures, 491, 494

Preformulation studies, 42–43
  dissolution, 42
  membrane permeability, 106
  microscopic examination, 97
  particle size, 97–98, 100
  partition coefficient, 42, 106, 110c–111c
  pH, 100, 102c–105c
  phase rule, 97, 99c–100c
  physical description, 42–43, 96–97
  physical form, 42–43
  pKa (dissociation constant), 102c–103c, 106, 111
  polymorphism, 100
  solubility, 42, 100–103, 102c–105c
  stability, 42–43

Pregnancy
  drug responses in, 56, 57
  drug transfer in, 176
  influenza vaccines in, 530
  new drug testing in, 46
  vaccination in, 508, 532, 533
  varicella virus vaccines in, 531–532

Premix, definition, 682

Prescription
  label, 61, 88–89
  for radiopharmaceuticals, 593

Prescription balance, 691, 691–692, 693

Prescription Drug Marketing Act of 1987, 16

Preservatives, 125, 138–141, 140t
  antifungal, 127t
  antimicrobial, 127t
  compatibility, 139–140
  for contact lens solutions, 555
  container interactions with, 140
  for emulsions, 414
  general considerations, 139–140
  mode of action, 140, 140t
  for ointments, 281
  for ophthalmic preparations, 290, 542–543
  for parenterals, 457–458
  in pediatric patients, 398
  selection, 139
  for solutions, partitioning effect, 347
  with sterilization, 138